TABLE C *AUTOMATED LEUKOCYTE DIFFERENTIAL COUNTS, REFERENCE VALUES IN NORMAL MALE ADULTS**

Percentage	Coulter S+ STKR (80 Men) Mean	Central 95% Range	Technicon H1 (64 Men) Mean	Central 95% Range
Lymphocytes	36.1	22.3–49.9	31.3	18.3–44.2
Monocytes	4.1	0.7–7.5	5.5	2.6–8.5
Granulocytes	59.7	45.5–74.0	—	—
Neutrophils	—	—	58.8	45.5–73.1
Eosinophils	—	—	1.9	0.0–4.4
Basophils	—	—	0.7	0.2–1.2
LUC	—	—	1.8	0.0–4.9
Absolute Numbers				
Lymphocytes ($\times 10^9$/L)	2.4	1.2–3.5	2.06	0.9–3.22
Monocytes ($\times 10^9$/L)	0.3	0.0–0.5	0.37	0.12–0.62
Granulocytes ($\times 10^9$/L)	4.0	1.4–6.6	—	—
Neutrophils ($\times 10^9$/L)	—	—	4.01	1.31–6.71
Eosinophils ($\times 10^9$/L)	—	—	0.13	0.00–0.30
Basophils ($\times 10^9$/L)	—	—	0.05	0.01–0.09
LUC ($\times 10^9$/L)	—	—	0.12	0.00–0.31

* Data based on measurements from healthy, male medical students, age range 23–31 years, at an altitude of 4500 ft. LUC, large unstained cells.

(With permission: Lee, GR, Bithell, TC, Foerster, J., Athens, JW, Lukens, JN. Wintrobe's Clinical Hematology. 9th Edition. Philadelphia: Lea & Febiger, 1993.)

TABLE D *RED BLOOD CELL VALUES AT VARIOUS AGES: MEAN AND LOWER LIMIT OF NORMAL (-2 SD)**

Age	Hemoglobin (g/dl) Mean	-2 SD	Hematocrit (%) Mean	-2 SD	Red Cell Count (10^{12}/L) Mean	-2 SD	MCV (fl) Mean	-2 SD	MCH (pg) Mean	-2 SD	MCHC (g/dl) Mean	-2 SD
Birth (cord blood)	16.5	13.5	51	42	4.7	3.9	108	98	34	31	33	30
1 to 3 days (capillary)	18.5	14.5	56	45	5.3	4.0	108	95	34	31	33	29
1 week	17.5	13.5	54	42	5.1	3.9	107	88	34	28	33	28
2 weeks	16.5	12.5	51	39	4.9	3.6	105	86	34	28	33	28
1 month	14.0	10.0	43	31	4.2	3.0	104	85	34	28	33	29
2 months	11.5	9.0	35	28	3.8	2.7	96	77	30	26	33	29
3 to 6 months	11.5	9.5	35	29	3.8	3.1	91	74	30	25	33	30
0.5 to 2 years	12.0	10.5	36	33	4.5	3.7	78	70	27	23	33	30
2 to 6 years	12.5	11.5	37	34	4.6	3.9	81	75	27	24	34	31
6 to 12 years	13.5	11.5	40	35	4.6	4.0	86	77	29	25	34	31
12 to 18 years— female	14.0	12.0	41	36	4.6	4.1	90	78	30	25	34	31
male	14.5	13.0	43	37	4.9	4.5	88	78	30	25	34	31
18 to 49 years— female	14.0	12.0	41	36	4.6	4.0	90	80	30	26	34	31
male	15.5	13.5	47	41	5.2	4.5	90	80	30	26	34	31

* These data were compiled from several sources. Emphasis is on recent studies employing electronic counters and on the selection of populations that are likely to exclude individuals with iron deficiency. The mean $\pm$ 2 SD can be expected to include 95% of the observations in a normal population. MCV, mean corpuscular volume; MCH, mean corpuscular hemoglobin; MCHC, mean corpuscular hemoglobin concentration.

(From: Dallman P.R.: in *Pediatrics*, 16th Ed. ed A Rudolph. New York: Appleton-Century-Crofts, 1977; Lubin B.H.: Reference values in infancy and childhood. In *Hematology of Infancy and Childhood*, 3rd Ed, eds D. G. Nathan, F.A. Oski, Philadelphia: W.B. Saunders, 1987.)

(With permission: Lee, GR, Bithell, TC, Foerster, J., Athens, JW, Lukens, JN. Wintrobe's Clinical Hematology. 9th Edition. Philadelphia: Lea & Febiger, 1993.)

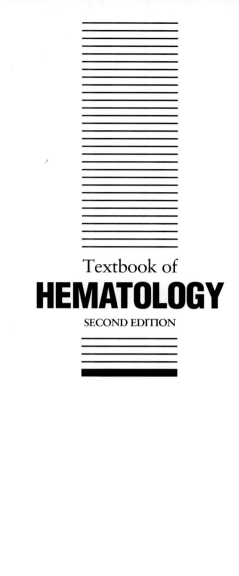

Textbook of
HEMATOLOGY
SECOND EDITION

Textbook of

HEMATOLOGY

SECOND EDITION

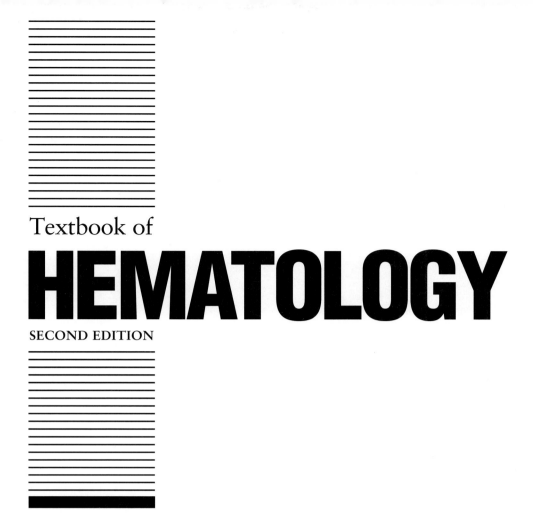

Shirlyn B. McKenzie, PhD, CLS

Professor and Chair
Department of Clinical Laboratory Sciences
School of Allied Health Sciences
The University of Texas Health Science Center at San Antonio
San Antonio, Texas

Williams & Wilkins

A WAVERLY COMPANY

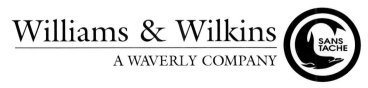

BALTIMORE • PHILADELPHIA • LONDON • PARIS • BANGKOK
BUENOS AIRES • HONG KONG • MUNICH • SYDNEY • TOKYO • WROCLAW   1996

Editor: Donna Balado
Managing Editor: Vicki Vaughn
Production Coordinator: Peter Carley
Book Project Editor: Robert D. Magee
Designer: Arlene Putterman
Typesetter: Maryland Composition
Printer: R. R. Donnelley
Color Separator: Maryland Composition
Binder: R. R. Donnelley

Library of Congress Cataloging-in-Publication Data

McKenzie, Shirlyn B.
    Texbook of hematology / Shirlyn B. McKenzie.—2nd ed.
        p.   cm.
    Includes bibliographical references and index.
    ISBN 0-683-18016-9
    1. Hematology.   I. Title.
    [DNLM: 1. Hematology.   2. Hematologic Diseases.   WH 100 M478t
1995]
    RB145.M39   1995
    616.1′5—dc20
DNLM/DLC
for Library of Congress   95-20705
                                                                 CIP

                                                                98   99
                                    2   3   4   5   6   7   8   9   10

To Gary,
the wind beneath my wings.

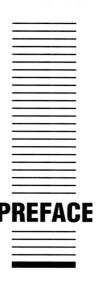

PREFACE

TEXTBOOK OF HEMATOLOGY, second edition, is a comprehensive text of hematology and hemostasis written for students in clinical laboratory science programs and for practicing laboratory professionals. Other health professional students and practitioners may also benefit from this book, including pathology residents, physician assistants and nurse pratitioners.

Because I believe that understanding hematologic/hemostatic diseases is dependent upon a thorough knowledge of normal processes, the book begins with normal hematopoiesis and progresses to hematopoietic disorders. Hemostasis adheres to a similar format with normal hemostatic functions discussed first, followed by hemostatic abnormalities. This text differs from hematology texts written by physicians in that it emphasizes the relationship between hematologic disease and diagnostic laboratory testing. Each chapter contains a discussion on the pathophysiologic aspects of the hematologic disease, a brief description of clinical findings and symptoms, and a discussion of laboratory findings associated with the disorder. Treatment is discussed in general terms to provide a complete picture of the disease and to alert the clinical laboratory professional to the expected hematologic changes when appropriate therapy is instituted.

● FEATURES OF THE SECOND EDITION

Although the primary goal of the second edition was to update the rapidly expanding information in hematology, I have also included several new chapters suggested by the book's users and contributors. It is a challenge to add this new material and still maintain a book with a realistic length suited to the readers' needs. This edition includes six new chapters. The three new chapters on body fluids, chromosome analysis, and molecular genetics are included to give a broader perspective of hematology and are somewhat unique to hematology textbooks for this audience. The three method chapters were added in response to numerous requests and suggestions from clinical laboratory science educators who used the first edition.

CHAPTER 20 ON CHROMOSOME ANALYSIS Malignant hematopoietic cells frequently have acquired chromosomal abnormalities. Some of these abnormalities are specific to a particular type or group of hematopoietic neoplasms. The detection of these abnormalities is often used for diagnosis, prognosis and patient follow-up after treatment. This chapter focuses on the practical uses of cytogenetic analysis in hematologic abnormalities and will acquaint the reader with basic terminology and techniques.

CHAPTER 21 ON MOLECULAR GENETICS Molecular genetics is the process of analyzing individual molecules of DNA to detect genetic defects. The growth in DNA technology has allowed its application in the clinical laboratory. This chapter discusses the technology in use and its application in the laboratory to uncover the genetic defects of certain hematologic diseases.

CHAPTER 22 ON BODY FLUIDS Hematology plays an important role in the morphologic evaluation of body fluids. Body fluid slides prepared by cytocentrifugation in the hematology laboratory are critical in the timely diagnosis of all types of malignancy as well as in detecting important benign disorders and infectious agents. This chapter is presented in an atlas format.

CHAPTERS 27, 28, LABORATORY METHODS These chapters discuss the tests performed in the hematology/coagulation laboratory. For each test, a brief description of the test procedure, its application, and potential sources of errors are given.

CHAPTER 29, AUTOMATION This chapter includes a description of the common hematology analyzers as well as semi-automated and automated coagulation instruments. Interpretation of histograms/cytograms derived from analysis of blood from patients with selected anemias and leukemias are illustrated and explained.

● Other Features of this Edition Include:

- An update and review of hematopoietic growth factors and an expanded section on bone marrow anatomy in Chapter 2. Several new diagrams and figures related to these topics are included.
- Chapter 4 on leukocytes is revised to include the new information gained in the rapidly evolving field of immunology.
- The chapters on acute leukemia, myelodysplastic syndromes, and lymphoproliferative disorders include the updated, ever expanding information on cellular markers and cytogenetics. In addition, the introductory chapter on leukemias includes a discussion of oncogenes and their role in the development of hematopoietic neoplasms.
- Disorders of hemostasis have been divided into two chapters—one on disorders of primary hemostasis (25) and one on disorders of secondary hemostasis and fibrinolysis (26). Chapter 26 on the disorders of secondary hemostasis includes the use of the International Normalized Ratio (INR) for patients on coumadin therapy and an expanded discussion of the conditions associated with thrombosis.
- Additional tables have been added to help students summarize and conceptualize important information.
- The number of color photographs of blood cells has been expanded to aid in the visualization of normal and abnormal cell morphology.
- All photographs are included within the chapters rather than on color plates to provide immediate reference to morphologic descriptions.
- More subheadings are added to help break lengthy material into more manageable text blocks.
- Case studies with questions found at the end of the chapters on abnormal hematopoiesis and hemostasis are used to emphasize salient points in the chapter. Instructors may want to ask additional questions related to these cases. The chapters on normal hematopoiesis and hemostasis are followed by multiple choice questions.
- Each chapter begins with a chapter outline and key terms and ends with a chapter summary. These were included as learning aids for the student.
- A glossary containing definitions to the italicized words in chapters will help students quickly determine the meaning of new terms.
- Reference values to the most commonly measured hematopoietic parameters are located on the front and back cover. Additional reference tables are included in the appendix. Critical limits are included when available.

● FEATURES RETAINED FROM THE FIRST EDITION

Features retained from the first edition are those that were considered unique strengths by users of the first edition. These include:

- Easy readability and logical flow of chapters

- Comprehensive, concise, well-organized format, including both normal and abnormal hematopoiesis and hemostasis, appropriate for either one or two levels of hematology coursework
- Explanation and correlation of laboratory tests to disease states
- Photographs at an appropriate magnification to emphasize detail without losing resolution

● ORGANIZATION OF THE SECOND EDITION

The first four chapters discuss normal hematopoiesis to give the student a thorough background in the physiology of the hematopoietic system and blood cells. The next eight chapters discuss anemias according to their functional classification with a merging of the morphologic classification. The next two chapters (13 and 14) cover the nonmalignant disorders affecting leukocytes. Chapters 15 through 19 address the malignant leukocyte disorders. This is followed by the new chapters on chromosome analysis (Chapter 20) and molecular genetics (Chapter 21). Body fluids (Chapter 22) completes discussion of hematology. Normal hemostasis is divided into two chapters, one on primary hemostasis (Chapter 23) and one on secondary hemostasis and fibrinolysis (Chapter 24). Disorders of primary hemostasis is covered in Chapter 25 and disorders of secondary hemostasis are covered in Chapter 26. The new procedure chapters (hematology, coagulation, automation) compose the last three chapters (27, 28, 29).

● COURSE SEQUENCING

This text is adaptable to variations in course offerings in clinical laboratory science programs. If there are two hematology courses, the first could include normal hematopoiesis, and introduction to anemia and non-neoplastic leukemia disorders. Some programs may also wish to include normal hemostasis and a few of the more common anemias, such as iron deficiency anemia and megaloblastic anemias. The second course could include the remaining anemias, malignant leukocyte disorders, cytogenetics, body fluids, and abnormal hemostasis. For programs with only one course, the topics could be presented in the order in which they appear. With the addition of laboratory procedures, the text may also be used in student laboratories or to help students prepare for student laboratories. For clinical laboratory technician (CLT) programs, the instructor should select appropriate topics and determine the depth of coverage.

Shirlyn B. McKenzie

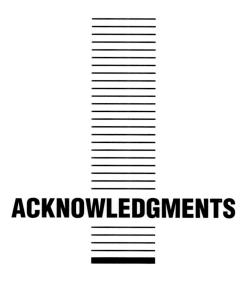

ACKNOWLEDGMENTS

I OWE a debt of gratitude to my contributors, Dr. Nan Clare, Kathryn Hansen, Dr. Margaret Gulley, Linda Larson, Cheryl Burns, and Judy Metz for adding their expertise to this book. A special thank you to Letitia Barnhart who prepared the glossary, a tedious, but important part of this new edition and to Cheryl Burns who provided many case studies and review questions. To Dr. William Ottinger for his in-depth review of the chapter on erythrocytes, to Dr. Linda Smith and Dr. Dennis Hohn for their review and suggestions on the hemolytic anemias, to David McGlasson for his review of the hemostasis chapters, to Jan Gaska for her library work, and to Denise Miller and Arthur Somoza for contributions to the art work, thank you. To Captain Ron Hickman for providing me with his collection of blood smears for photographs, I am grateful.

A special thank you to Donna Balado for her guidance, suggestions, support and patience during the preparation of this new edition. Thank you also to Bob Magee, project editor, for his helpful suggestions, understanding, attention to deadlines and reassurance throughout the production process and to Pete Carley, production coordinator.

To the many hematology instructors who have taken the time to send their comments and suggestions based on the first edition, thank you. It was my intention to incorporate as many of these suggestions as possible. Your help is greatly appreciated.

Finally, I want to recognize all those family members who helped me maintain my sense of reality throughout this consuming process. Thank you to Gary, Scott, Shawn, Belynda and Dora, for your support and understanding; to Lauren, who added the sunshine to my days spent at the desk; to my parents, George and Helen Olson, to Dorothy McKenzie Olson, Skipper and Sandy, Kathy and Dennis, Larry and Claudia, Gerald and Debbie, for your unconditional love and faith in me.

Shirlyn B. McKenzie

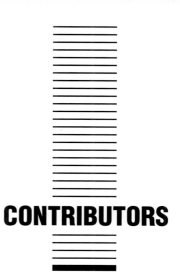

CONTRIBUTORS

Cheryl Burns, MS, CLS
University of Texas Health Science Center at San Antonio
Department of Clinical Laboratory Sciences
San Antonio, TX

C. Nan Clare, MD
University of Texas Health Science Center at San Antonio
Department of Pathology
San Antonio, TX

Margaret Gulley, MD
University of Texas Health Science Center at San Antonio
Department of Pathology
San Antonio, TX

Kathryn Hansen, MS, CLSp (CG)
University of Texas Health Science Center at San Antonio
Department of Pathology
San Antonio, TX

Linda Larson, MS, MT(ASCP)
University of North Dakota
Department of Pathology
Grand Forks, ND

Judy Metz, BS, MT(ASCP)
San Antonio, TX

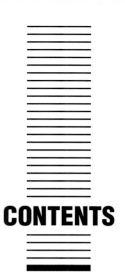

CONTENTS

Introduction

CHAPTER OUTLINE

KEY TERMS

hematology
hemostasis
diapedese
N:C ratio
ribosomes
endoplasmic reticulum
smooth endoplasmic
   reticulum
rough endoplasmic reticulum
Golgi apparatus
lysosomes
phagolysosomes
microfilaments
microtubules
nucleus
cytoplasm
nucleolus
mitochondria
euchromatin
heterochromatin
erythrocytes
leukocytes
platelets
thrombocytes

INTRODUCTION

Blood has been considered the essence of life for centuries. One of the Hippocratic writings from approximately 400 B.C. describes the body as being a composite of four humors: black bile, blood, phlegm, and yellow bile. Fahraeus, a 20th century Swedish physician, suggested that the theory of the four humors came from the observation of four distinct layers in clotted blood. In the process of clotting, blood separates into a dark-red, almost black, jelly-like clot, a thin layer of oxygenated red cells, a layer of white cells and platelets, and a layer of yellowish serum.[1] Health and disease were believed to occur as a result of an upset in the equilibrium of these humors. This may help explain why bloodletting to purge the body of its contaminated fluids was practiced from the time of Hippocrates until the 19th century.

The cellular composition of blood was not recognized until the invention of the microscope. With the help of a crude magnifying device that consisted of a biconvex lens, Leeuwenhoek (1632–1723) accurately described and measured the red blood cells (erythrocytes). The discovery of white blood cells (leukocytes) and platelets (thrombocytes) followed after microscope lenses were improved.

As a supplement to these categoric observations of blood cells, Karl Vierordt, in 1852, reported the first quantitative results of blood cell analysis.[2] His procedures for quantification were tedious and time-consuming. The blood was expelled from a calibrated capillary pipette onto a glass slide containing diluting fluid. All the cells in the blood mixture were counted with the aid of a micrometer in the eyepiece of the microscope. Students of hematology will appreciate the enormity of this task. After several years, attempts were made to correlate blood cell counts with various disease states.

Improved methods of blood examination in the 1920s and the growth of knowledge of blood physiology and blood-forming organs in the 1930s allowed anemias and other blood disorders to be studied on a rational basis. In some cases, the pathophysiology of hematopoietic disorders was realized only after the patient responded to experimental therapy. For example, clinical improvement of patients with certain macrocytic anemias was noted when liver, rich in vitamin B_{12}, was included in the patient's diet. From this observation came the discovery that vitamin B_{12} deficiency produces macrocytic anemia.

Contrary to early hematologists, modern hematologists recognize that alterations in the components of blood are the result of disease, not a primary cause of the disease. Under normal conditions, the production, release, and survival of blood cells are highly regulated to maintain a steady state of morphologically normal cells. Quantitative and qualitative hematologic abnormalities may result when an imbalance occurs among cell production in the bone marrow, release to the peripheral blood, and survival.[3]

NORMAL CHARACTERISTICS OF BLOOD

Composition of blood

Blood is composed of a liquid called plasma and cellular elements, including *leukocytes, platelets,* and *erythrocytes.* The normal adult has approximately six liters of this vital fluid, which composes 7% to 8% of total body weight. Plasma makes up approximately 55% of the blood volume, whereas 45% of the volume is composed of erythrocytes, and 1% of the volume is composed of leukocytes and thrombocytes. Variations in these blood elements are often the first sign of disease occurring in body tissue. Changes in diseased tissue often can be detected by laboratory tests that measure deviations from normal in blood constituents.

The principal component of plasma is water, which contains dissolved ions, proteins, carbohydrates, fats, hormones, vitamins, and enzymes. The principal ions necessary for normal cell function include calcium, sodium, potassium, chloride, magnesium, and hydrogen. The main protein constituent of plasma is albumin, which is the most important component in maintaining osmotic pressure. Albumin also acts as a carrier molecule, carrying compounds such as bilirubin and heme. Other blood proteins carry vitamins, minerals, and lipids. Immunoglobulins and complement are specialized blood proteins involved in immune defense. The coagulation proteins, responsible for maintaining normal *hemostasis,* circulate in the blood as inactive enzymes until they are needed for the coagulation process. An imbalance in these dissolved plasma constituents may indicate a disease in other body tissues.

Blood plasma also acts as a transport medium for cell nutrients and metabolites; for example, hormones manufactured in one tissue are transported by the blood to target tissue in other parts of the body. Bilirubin, the main catabolic residue of hemoglobin, is transported by albumin from the spleen to the liver for excretion. Blood urea nitrogen is carried to the kidney for filtration and excretion. Increased concentration of these normal catabolites may indicate either increased cellular metabolism or a defect in the organ responsible for their excretion. For example, in liver disease, the bilirubin level increases, indicating end organ disease. In hemolytic anemia, however, the bilirubin concentration may rise not because of liver disease, but because of the increased metabolism of hemoglobin.

When body cells die, they release their cellular constituents into surrounding tissue. Eventually some of these constituents reach the blood. Many of the constituents of body cells are specific for the cell's particular function; thus, an increased concentration of these constituents in the blood, especially enzymes, may indicate abnormal cell destruction in a specific organ.

Each of the three cellular constituents of blood has specific functions. Erythrocytes contain the vital protein hemoglobin, which is responsible for transport of oxygen and carbon dioxide between the lungs and body tissues. Leukocytes (of which there are five types) are responsible for defending the body against foreign antigens such as bacteria and viruses. Platelets are necessary for maintaining hemostasis. Blood cells circulate through blood vessels, which are distributed throughout every body tissue. Erythrocytes and platelets perform their functions without leaving the vessels, but leukocytes *diapedese* (pass through vessel walls) to tissues where they defend against invading foreign antigens. *Hematology* primarily is the study of these formed cellular blood elements.

Reference ranges for blood cell concentration

Physiologic differences in the concentration of cellular elements may occur according to race, age, sex, and geographic location; pathologic changes in specific blood cell concentrations may occur as the result of disease or injury. Whites have slightly higher leukocyte counts (0.5×10^9/L), higher hemoglobin levels (0.7 g/dL), higher hematocrit levels (0.017/L), and higher erythrocyte counts (0.05×10^{12}L/L) than blacks.[4] The greatest differences in reference ranges occur between newborns and adults. Generally, newborns have a higher erythrocyte concentration than any other age group. The erythrocytes also are larger than those of adults. After birth, erythrocytes decrease for the first 6 months of life, after which time they slowly increase. For children between the ages of 5 and 17, the hemoglobin level, hematocrit, mean corpuscular volume, mean corpuscular hemoglobin, and erythrocyte count increase with age.[4] The leukocyte concentration also is increased at birth but decreases after the first year of life. A common finding in young children is an absolute and relative lymphocytosis. After 12 years of age, males have higher hemoglobin, hematocrit, and erythrocyte levels than females. Tables A-D (inside cover) and Table E (endsheet) show hematologic reference ranges for various age groups.

Reference ranges of hematologic values must be determined in individual laboratories to account for the physiologic differences of groups of individuals within a specific geographic area. Reference values are determined by calculating the mean for a group of healthy individuals and reporting the reference range as the mean ± 2 standard deviations. This range represents the normal value for 95% of normal individuals. A value just below or just above this range is not necessarily abnormal; normal and abnormal overlap. Statistical probability indicates 5% of normal individuals will fall outside the ± 2 standard deviation range. The further a value falls from the reference range, however, the more likely the value is to be abnormal.

CELL MORPHOLOGY REVIEW

A basic understanding of cell morphology is essential to the study of hematology because many hematologic disorders are accompanied by abnormalities or changes in morphology of cellular or subcellular components as well as by changes in cell concentrations.

A cell is an intricate, complex structure consisting of a membrane-bound aqueous gel of proteins, carbohydrates, fats, inorganic materials, and nucleic acids. The nucleus, bound by a nuclear membrane, contains nucleic acids that control and direct the development, function, and division of the cell. The cytoplasm surrounds the nucleus and is bound by the cell membrane. The cytoplasm contains highly ordered organelles including: mitochondria, lysosomes, endoplasmic reticulum, Golgi apparatus, ribosomes, granules, microtubules, and microfilaments. Organelles are membrane-bound compartments with specific cellular functions (Fig. 1-1). The different kinds of organelles and the concentration of each is dependent on the function of the cell.

Cell membrane

The vital functions of the cell membrane provide selective permeability for the cell, thereby determining the interrelationships of the cell with its environment. The fluid mosaic membrane model was proposed by Singer and Nicholson in 1972.[5] The model proposes that the membrane is a bimolecular lipid complex with globular, structural, and enzymatic proteins integrated throughout the complex (Fig. 1-2). The phospholipid bilayer is arranged with the polar head groups of the lipids directed toward the outside and inside of the cell, and the long-chain hydrophobic hydrocarbons directed inward. The membrane lipids are mobile and can diffuse laterally throughout their own half of the bilayer or may flip-flop from one side of the bilayer to the other. Other lipids, in the form of cholesterol, lipoproteins, and lipopolysaccharides, also contribute to the basic framework of cell membranes. The lipid portion of the membrane accounts for the cell's high permeability to lipid-soluble substances.

The membrane proteins are the functional units of membranes providing selective permeability and structural stability. Proteins also are responsible for enzymatic catalysis and cell-to-cell recognition, as well as transport of specific substances. Membrane proteins may be divided into two groups, integral and peripheral, depending on their location and function. The integral proteins are considered to be interspersed throughout the lipid bilayer in a tightly embedded globular form. Some of the integral proteins may span the entire lipid bilayer, whereas others may only partially penetrate the membrane, with their hydrophobic end lying within the membrane and their hydrophilic portion protruding from the inner or outer membrane surface. Although proteins appear to be isolated from each other, they may move about in the plane of the membrane.

In addition to the integral proteins, there are peripheral proteins that are associated with one face of the bilayer membrane. Some peripheral proteins are noncovalently bound to integral proteins. Most are associated with the cytoplasmic side of the membrane.[6] These peripheral proteins on the cytoplasmic side of the membrane, such as spectrin and actin, form a lattice network to function as the cellular cytoskeleton and to hold many integral pro-

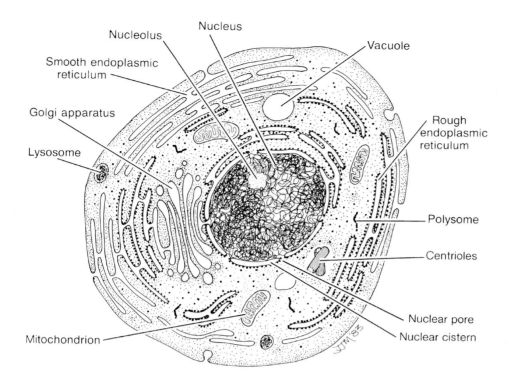

FIGURE 1-1. Drawing of a cell depicting the various organelles.

teins in a fixed position. The cytoskeleton imposes order on the membrane.

Carbohydrates, in branched or straight chains that are linked to membrane lipids (glycolipids) and proteins (glycoproteins), may extend from the outer surface of the membrane. The carbohydrates of the glycoproteins and glycolipids interact in the polar exterior environment of the cell to form a lattice network restricting the movement of the carbohydrates on the membrane. Functions of the carbohydrate moieties include specific binding, cell-to-cell recognition, and cell adhesion.

Many of the glycoproteins serve as receptors for extracellular molecules. Binding of an extracellular molecule to its specific protein receptor on the cell membrane may result in transduction of a signal to the cell's interior without passage of the extracellular molecule through the membrane. For example, when cell growth factors bind to their membrane receptors, the signal for the cell to proliferate or differentiate is transmitted from the membrane to the nucleus. This is accomplished by means of a change in the organization of the membrane receptors upon binding of the ligand. The receptor reorganization evokes latent tyrosine kinase activity in the cytoplasmic domain of the receptor. Binding of growth factor also may activate the cell through other biochemical pathways. Current research is focused on cellular receptors, their activation of

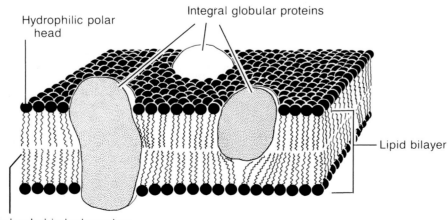

FIGURE 1-2. The fluid mosaic membrane model proposed by Singer and Nicholson.

biochemical cellular responses, and how they signal the nucleus.

Cytoplasm

Cytoplasm performs synthetic activities of the cell, including protein synthesis, growth, motility, and phagocytosis. The structural components, organelles, and other cellular inclusions lie within the cytoplasmic matrix. The hyaloplasm, a gel-like material, serves as a support and communication medium for the organelles. The composition of the cytoplasm depends on cellular function and maturity. The appearance of cytoplasm in fixed, stained cells is important in evaluating the morphology, classifying the cell, and determining the stage of differentiation. In blood cells stained with Romanowsky stains, the more immature or synthetically active the cell, the deeper blue the cytoplasm, as a result of the presence of ribonucleic acid (RNA), which has an affinity for the basophilic portion of the stain.

The volume of cytoplasm (C) in proportion to the nucleus (N), *N:C ratio*, varies depending on the type of cell and its maturity. Hematopoietic cells have a decreasing N:C ratio with increasing cell maturity. With the exception of megakaryocytes, the decreasing ratio occurs as a result of a decrease in nuclear size and an increase in cytoplasmic volume. The megakaryocyte increases in size as the cell matures; both the cytoplasm and the nucleus increase in size. The cytoplasm, however, increases proportionately more than the nucleus.

Ribosomes

The *ribosomes* are cellular "factories" that receive amino acid constituents, assemble them into polypeptide chains, and release the chains into the cytoplasm or the *endoplasmic reticulum* (ER), a network of communicating membranes. Ribosomes are composed of approximately half protein and half RNA. Single ribosomes become active in protein synthesis only after they are linked by messenger ribonucleic acid (mRNA) to form polyribosomes. Ribosomes may occur free in the cytoplasm or they may be associated with ER. Ribosomes that occur free in the cytoplasm are believed to synthesize protein needed to maintain cellular integrity; whereas, ribosomes that are associated with ER synthesize protein secreted by the cell. Cells rich in ribosomes, such as plasma cells, have a pronounced affinity for basic dyes.

Endoplasmic reticulum

Endoplasmic reticulum is composed of interconnecting, membrane-bound tubules and vesicles. These tubules may be continuous with the nuclear envelope and Golgi apparatus. Endoplasmic reticulum, considered morphologically, consists of two types, *smooth endoplasmic reticulum* (SER) and *rough endoplasmic reticulum* (RER). Although most ER appears to be RER, the amount of each type depends on the kind of cell and the state of its activity.

Cells that synthesize large amounts of secretory protein are rich in RER. Cells that synthesize protein that remains free in the cytoplasm, such as normoblasts, have little RER but many free ribosomes. Blood leukocytes, which synthesize membrane-bound protein products at certain phases in their life cycle, also may contain abundant RER.

Rough endoplasmic reticulum is studded with ribosomes on its outside surface. It may synthesize material for intracellular use, but most protein synthesized here is destined for secretion. The ribosomes on the surface of the RER synthesize protein and release it into the lumen of the RER. The protein may then be assembled into larger peptides. Subsequently, the peptides are channeled into the *Golgi apparatus*. In the Golgi, they are aggregated, condensed, and packaged within membranes.

Smooth ER, free of ribosomes, may be formed from RER and is often in continuity with RER. Smooth ER also may be contiguous with the Golgi complex. It is sometimes termed transitional ER because it may be contiguous with RER on one end and the Golgi complex on the other. From observations and experiments with cells rich in SER, several functions of this organelle have been postulated. Smooth ER may produce lipid, since SER is very abundant in liver cells synthesizing or storing fat. It also may be important in detoxification, because SER becomes more abundant in liver cells when barbiturates are ingested. During active stages of hormone synthesis, cells of the adrenals and testes are packed with SER. Thus, SER also may be involved in synthesis of certain hormones.

Golgi apparatus

The Golgi apparatus is composed of flattened sacs or cisternae, often curved and arranged in parallel arrays. The lumen of the cisternae are in continuity with each other through fenestrations (perforations) on their contiguous surfaces. The size of the Golgi apparatus depends on the cell type and function. Cells of the secretory type, such as the plasma cell, usually have large Golgi complexes. Promyelocytes and myelocytes, cells that are very active in granule formation, also have large Golgi complexes. The Golgi is usually adjacent to the nucleus and does not stain with Romanowsky stains or routine histologic stains. Its presence is indicated by a clear unstained area, usually adjacent to the nucleus.

Polypeptides, synthesized in RER, are channeled to the Golgi, where they are assembled into proteins, concentrated, packaged as membrane-bound organelles, and released into the cytoplasm. The Golgi membranes contain glucosyl, galactosyl transferases, and other enzymes necessary for the synthesis and coupling of carbohydrates with protein to form glycoproteins. The Golgi also synthesizes lipoprotein from the lipids produced in SER and the polypeptides produced in RER. The Golgi packages these proteins for release as membrane-bound granules.[6]

Lysosomes

Lysosomes are membrane-bound sacs that contain various hydrolytic enzymes. They vary greatly in size and morphology but may be identified cytochemically by specific reactions for acid phosphatase and other enzymes. The hydrolytic enzymes serve to degrade phagocytosed material or metabolites. Primary lysosomes move freely in the cytoplasm until they fuse with digestive vacuoles (phagosomes), whereupon they mix hydrolytic enzymes with the contents of the digestive vacuole, forming secondary lysosomes called phagolysosomes. Lysosomes also may be important in degradation of glycogen as well as in production and breakdown of hormones. For instance, inherited glycogen storage disease is characterized by an accumulation of glycogen in lysosomes. These lysosomes are deficient in the enzyme needed for glycogen breakdown.

Chediak-Higashi disease and chronic granulomatous disease are both characterized by increased incidence of infection, which is associated with lysosomal abnormalities. The lysosomal membranes in these disorders have appeared to be abnormally resistant to breakdown; thus, they cannot release their lysosomal contents, and, consequently, ingested bacteria are not killed by hydrolytic enzymes.

Mitochondria

Mitochondria function in numerous metabolic processes of the cell including oxidative phosphorylation, the main energy source of the cell. Glycolysis, an anaerobic reaction that occurs in the cytoplasm, produces a net gain of two adenosine triphosphate (ATP) molecules per mole of glucose, as the glucose is metabolized to pyruvic acid. Pyruvic acid enters the mitochondria, where it undergoes oxidative decarboxylation to an acetyl group. Here, acetyl is linked to coenzyme A (CoA), forming the active compound acetyl-CoA. The high energy acetyl-CoA then enters the Krebs cycle (tricarboxylic acid cycle), where it is oxidized to CO_2 and H_2O. Only one ATP is produced directly by one turn of the Krebs cycle. Most of the energy released from this cycle is trapped in the electron carriers, nicotinamide-adenine dinucleotide (NAD) and flavin adenine dinucleotide (FAD). The transfer of electrons from NAD and FAD to oxygen, through a series of electron transport carrier molecules, releases energy to synthesize additional ATP. The complete oxidation of 1 mole of glucose yields 38 ATP. This oxidative phosphorylation is also called cell respiration.

The mitochondrion consists of the following two membranes: an outer, smooth membrane and inner membrane with numerous foldings called mitochondrial cristae. These cristae greatly increase the surface area of the inner membrane, which increases the respiratory activity of the cell. The inner chamber beneath the inner membrane is the mitochondrial matrix. The compartment between the inner and outer membrane is the intermembrane space or intracristal space. Enzymes for the Krebs cycle are located in the mitochondrial matrix. The enzyme system and electron carriers of oxidative phosphorylation are contained within the inner membrane of the mitochondria.

Mitochondria do not stain with Romanowsky stains; therefore, they appear as clear areas within the cytoplasm.

The number, size, shape, and structural organization of the mitochondria are related to the physiologic state of the cell. All blood cells contain mitochondria except mature erythrocytes. Thus, in erythrocytes, the cellular supply of ATP is limited to that gained from anaerobic glycolysis, two ATP per mole of glucose.

Microfilaments

Microfilaments vary in size and number, depending on cell type and activity. The filaments are most highly developed in muscle cells. Two classes of filaments, one approximately 70 Å in diameter, composed of actin, and one about 150 Å in diameter, composed of myosin, are organized in parallel bundles. The mechanical–chemical interaction of these filaments causes contraction of the cell. Cells that are not specialized for contraction have thinner, less conspicuous filaments. These filaments are important for motility of the cell as well as for a supportive cytoskeletal network.

Microtubules

Microtubules are hollow cylinders 200 Å to 270 Å in diameter with electron dense walls 50 Å to 75 Å thick. Although randomly scattered and few in number in most cells, microtubules may develop transiently during alterations in cell shapes. Their presence and positioning during development of spermatozoa into elongated cells suggest that microtubules may be important in creating cell shape by contributing to the cellular cytoskeleton. During mitotic cellular division, microtubules increase in numbers to form the spindle apparatus. They attach to chromosomes and may be responsible for chromosome movement.

Nucleus

The *nucleus* contains the genetic material, deoxyribonucleic acid (DNA), responsible for the regulation of all cellular functions. The abundant nuclear material, chromatin, consists of DNA and structural proteins. Two kinds of chromatin are visible with light microscopy, *euchromatin* and *heterochromatin*. Euchromatin is a lighter staining chromatin believed to consist of unwound or loosely twisted chromatin. Heterochromatin appears deeply stained in lumps or granules because of tightly twisted or folded chromatin strands. The ratio of euchromatin to heterochromatin is dependent on the activity of the cell. Euchromatin is dispersed metabolically active chromatin; whereas heterochromatin is inactive. Usually the younger, more active blood cells have fine threadlike euchromatin, rather than deep staining heterochromatin. Most active cells contain from one to four pale blue-staining *nucleoli* (nucleolus—singular) within the nucleus. The nucleolus consists of RNA and other protein. The nucleolus of very young blood cells is easily seen with brightfield microscopy on thin stained smears. Evidence suggests that the nucleolus is important in ribonucleoprotein synthesis.

The nuclear contents are surrounded by a double membrane, the nuclear envelope. The inner membrane in some cell types is lined with fine filaments, fibrous lamina, which may lend mechanical support to the envelope. The outer membrane of the envelope, on the cytoplasmic side, may be studded with ribosomes and is often continuous with ER. The gap between the two membranes (500 Å) is called the perinuclear cistern. Throughout the nuclear envelope, at points where the inner and outer membranes are continuous with one another, there are nuclear pores approximately 500 Å in diameter. The pores act as semipermeable membranes excluding some substances entirely and others only partially. Thus, there is a means of communication between the nucleus and *cytoplasm*.

● SUMMARY

Blood is composed of plasma and cells. There are three general types of blood cells: erythrocytes, leukocytes, and thrombocytes or platelets. The cells compose approximately 45% to 50% of the volume of blood. Hematology is the study of blood, particularly of the cells.

The blood cells circulate within the vessels, maintaining a rather constant concentration. Reference ranges vary depending on sex, age, geographic location, and, to a lesser extent, race. Changes in concentration may occur as a result of disease or tissue injury.

The cell is an intricate, complex structure bound by a membrane. The membrane is a phospholipid bilayer with integral proteins throughout. This membrane has receptors that bind extracellular molecules and transmit messages to the cell's nucleus. Within the cell are the cytoplasm with numerous organelles and the nucleus. The cellular organelles include ribosomes, which assemble amino acids into protein chains; endoplasmic reticulum, which synthesizes and transports protein to the Golgi apparatus; the Golgi apparatus, which assembles proteins into organelles; lysosomes, which contain hydrolytic enzymes; and mitochondria, which function in oxidative phosphorylation as well as other metabolic processes. Microfilaments and microtubules vary in number depending on cell type and/or activity. Microfilaments function in cell contraction, whereas microtubules are probably important in maintaining cell shape. The nucleus contains the genetic material, DNA, which regulates all cell functions.

Many hematologic disorders are accompanied by abnormalities in these cellular and subcellular components.

● REVIEW QUESTIONS

1. In which group of individuals would you expect to find the highest reference ranges for hemoglobin, hematocrit, and erythrocyte count?
   a. newborns
   b. males older than 12 years of age
   c. females older than 17 years of age
   d. children between 1 and 5 years of age

2. These cells are important in the transport of oxygen and carbon dioxide between the lungs and body tissues:
   a. platelets
   b. leukocytes
   c. thrombocytes
   d. erythrocytes

3. Forty-five percent of the volume of blood is composed of:
   a. plasma
   b. erythrocytes
   c. leukocytes
   d. platelets

4. Alterations in the concentration of blood cells generally are the result of:
   a. bone marrow abnormalities
   b. an inadequate diet
   c. disease
   d. dehydration

5. Leukocytes are necessary for:
   a. defense against foreign antigens
   b. hemostasis
   c. oxygen transport
   d. excretion of cellular metabolites

6. Selective cellular permeability and structural stability is provided by:
   a. membrane lipids
   b. membrane proteins
   c. ribosomes
   d. the nucleus

7. Rough endoplasmic reticulum is important in:
   a. synthesizing lipid
   b. synthesizing hormones
   c. synthesizing and assembling proteins
   d. phagocytosis

8. Abnormalities of these organelles is associated with an increased incidence of infection:
   a. Golgi apparatus
   b. mitochondria
   c. ribosomes
   d. lysosomes

REFERENCES

1. Wintrobe, M.M.: Blood, Pure and Eloquent. New York, McGraw-Hill, 1980.
2. Vierordt, K.: Zahlungen der Blutkorperchen des Menschen. Arch. Physiol. Heilk., 11:327, 1852.
3. Miale, J.B.: Laboratory Medicine: Hematology, 6th Ed. St. Louis, Mosby, 1982.
4. Bao, W, Dalferes, E.R., Srinivasan, B.R., Webber, L.S., and Berenson, G.S.: Normative distribution of complete blood count from early childhood through adolescence: The Bogulusa Heart Study. Prev. Med. 22:825, 1993.
5. Singer, S.J., and Nicholson, G.L.: The fluid mosaic model of the structure of cell membranes. Science 175:720, 1972.
6. Morrow, J.S.: Plasma membrane dynamics and organization. In: Hematology: Basic Principles and Procedures. Edited by R. Hoffman, E.J. Benz, S.J. Shattil, B. Furie, H.J. Cohen. New York: Churchill-Livingstone. 1995.

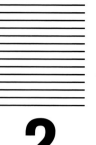

Structure and function of hematopoietic organs and development of blood cells

2

CHAPTER OUTLINE

KEY TERMS

hematopoiesis
erythropoiesis
primitive erythropoiesis
megaloblastic
Gower hemoglobin
Portland hemoglobin
medullary hematopoiesis
extramedullary hematopoiesis
myelopoiesis
megakaryopoiesis
hematopoietic system
*mononuclear phagocyte
  system*
culling
pitting
splenectomy
erythroblastic island
*myeloid to erythroid ratio
  (M:E)*
hyperplastic
hyperplasia
hypoplastic
aplasia
pluripotential stem cell
*hematopoietic inductive
  microenvironment*
unilineage
hematopoietic growth factors
apoptosis
cytokines

INTRODUCTION

Hematopoiesis (hemat = blood; poiesis = formation) is the term used to describe the formation and development of blood cells. Cellular differentiation, proliferation, and maturation of blood cells take place in the hematopoietic tissue, which consists primarily of bone marrow. Only mature cells are released into the peripheral blood. The link between the bone marrow and blood cell production was not established until it was recognized that blood formation was a continuous process. Before 1850, it was believed that blood cells formed in the fetus were viable until death of the host and that there was no need for a continuous source of new elements.

DEVELOPMENT OF HEMATOPOIESIS

Hematopoiesis begins as early as the nineteenth day after fertilization in the yolk sac of the human embryo. At about the third month of embryonic life, the fetal liver becomes the chief site of blood cell production, and the yolk sac discontinues its role in hematopoiesis. At this time, hematopoiesis also begins to a lesser degree in the spleen, kidney, thymus, and lymph nodes. Lymph nodes continue as an important site of lymphopoiesis throughout life, but blood cell production in the liver, spleen, kidney, and thymus discontinues or decreases as the bone marrow becomes active in hematopoiesis. Bone marrow becomes the primary site of hematopoiesis in the third trimester of gestation. It continues as the primary source of blood production after birth and throughout adult life (Fig. 2-1).

Although leukocytic and platelet precursors may be present in the yolk sac, most hematopoietic activity at this site is confined to *erythropoiesis* (erythrocyte formation). Cell production at this time is called *primitive erythropoiesis* because the embryonic erythroblasts and hemoglobin are not typical of that seen in later developing erythroblasts. The embryonic erythroblasts in the yolk sac arise from clusters of cells in the mesenchyme called "blood islands." Embryonic erythroblasts have a *megaloblastic* appearance with coarse clumped chromatin. Megaloblastic is the term used to describe abnormal erythrocyte progenitor cells in which nuclear maturation lags behind cytoplasmic maturation, and the cells are abnormally large. The megaloblastic appearance of embryonic erythroblasts, however, is not the result of abnormal hematopoiesis. The hemoglobin in these cells consists of the embryonic varieties, *Gower 1, Gower 2,* and *Portland*. Leukocyte and platelet formation *(myelopoiesis and megakaryopoiesis)* begin in the fetal liver, but production of these cells is not considered significant until the onset of hematopoiesis in the bone marrow.

Hematopoiesis in the bone marrow is called *medullary hematopoiesis. Extramedullary hematopoiesis* denotes blood cell production in hematopoietic tissue other than bone marrow (extraskeletal), which does not usually occur in adults. After birth, in certain hematologic disorders such as sickle cell anemia, thalassemia and leukemia, extramedullary hematopoiesis may occur in the liver and spleen. Organomegaly frequently accompanies significant hematopoietic activity at these sites.

HEMATOPOIETIC TISSUE

The *hematopoietic system* includes tissues and organs involved in the proliferation, maturation, and destruction of blood cells. These organs and tissues include the mononuclear phagocyte sytem, spleen, lymph nodes, thymus, bone marrow, and liver.

Mononuclear phagocyte system

The *mononuclear phagocyte system* is a collection of monocytes and macrophages, found both intravascularly and extravascularly, whose primary functions are phagocytic and immunologic. In the past, the term reticuloendothelial system (RES) was used to encompass monocytes and macrophages as well as vascular endothelial cells, reticular cells, dendritic cells, and lymph germinal center cells. The term, mononuclear phagocyte system, is more specific and includes (1) circulating blood monocytes; (2) fixed macrophages of the bone marrow, liver (Kupffer cells), spleen, lymph nodes; and (3) free macrophages in the spleen, lymph nodes, lungs, serous cavities, and other tissues. The cells of this system are responsible for engulfing particulate matter and denatured protein and for removing effete or damaged cells. The macrophages and monocytes also exhibit an immune function that includes the processing of antigen for presentation to lymphocytes, and the secretion of mitogens for enhancement of lymphocyte activation and transformation. These cells also secrete growth factors that stimulate the proliferation and differentiation of hematopoietic cells.

Spleen

The spleen is located in the upper left quadrant, beneath the diaphragm, and to the left of the stomach. This organ's

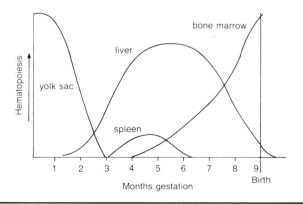

FIGURE 2-1. Location of hematopoiesis during fetal development. At birth, most blood cell production is limited to the marrow.

functions were considered a mystery in the earliest days of medicine. Attempts to solve this mystery resulted in suggestions that the spleen might have such functions as controlling one's emotions, supporting a healthy liver, or maintaining body symmetry. After several emergency *splenectomies* (singular, splenectomy; removal of the spleen) were performed without causing permanent harm to the patients, it was recognized that the spleen was not essential to life. The removal of the spleen also has led to clarification of splenic function as a discriminatory filter. Splenic functions will be better understood after a brief description of the splenic architecture and blood flow.

SPLENIC ARCHITECTURE
The spleen, enclosed by a capsule of connective tissue, contains the largest collection of lymphocytes and mononuclear phagocytes in the body (Fig. 2-2). These cells, together with a reticular meshwork, are concentrated in different areas of the spleen, contributing to the formation of the following three types of pulp (tissue within the capsule): white pulp, red pulp, and the marginal zone. The indented, medial aspect of the organ (hilus) is where the blood vessels, lymphatic vessels, and nerves penetrate to the pulp. The connective tissue extending into the organ from the capsule (trabeculae) divides the pulp into communicating compartments.

The white pulp (primarily lymphocytes), a visible grayish white zone, is composed of lymphatic nodules and the periarterial lymphatic sheath. Within the nodules, there are germinal centers consisting of a mixture of B lymphocytes, reticulum cells, and phagocytic macrophages. The periarterial lymphatic sheath surrounds arteries as they enter the spleen. This sheath is packed with T-lymphocytes and macrophages. The white pulp is where the immune response is initiated. In some cases of heightened immunologic activity, the white pulp may increase to occupy half the volume of the spleen (it normally composes 20% or less). White pulp is surrounded by a marginal zone, a reticular meshwork containing blood vessels, free cells, and narrow interstices. This zone lies at the junction of the white pulp and red pulp. The red pulp contains the sinuses and cords. The sinuses are dilated vascular spaces for ve-

nous blood. The red color of the red pulp is caused by the presence of blood in the sinuses. The cords are composed of masses of reticular tissue and macrophages, which lie between the sinuses.

SPLENIC BLOOD FLOW
The spleen is richly supplied with blood. It receives 5% of the total cardiac output, a blood volume of 300 mL/minute. Blood enters the spleen through the splenic artery, which branches into many vessels in the trabeculae. Vessel branches may terminate in the white pulp, red pulp, or marginal zone. Blood entering the spleen may follow either the rapid transit pathway (closed circulation) or the slow transit pathway (open circulation). The rapid transit pathway is a relatively unobstructed blood flow route whereby blood enters the sinuses in red pulp from arteries and passes directly to the venous collecting system. In contrast, blood entering the slow transit pathway moves sluggishly through a circuitous route of macrophage-lined cords before it gains access to the sinuses. Plasma in the cords freely enters the sinuses, but erythrocytes meet resistance at the sinus wall as they squeeze through the tiny openings in the sinus walls. This skimming of the plasma from blood in the cords to the sinuses sharply increases the concentration of erythrocytes in the cords. Sluggish blood flow and continued erythrocyte metabolic activity in cords results in a splenic environment that is hypoxic, acidic, and hypoglycemic. Hypoxia and hypoglycemia occur as erythrocytes continue to use the limited oxygen and glucose. Metabolic byproducts create the acidic environment. Normal erythrocytes can tolerate this brief assault from the splenic environment emerging undamaged.

SPLENIC FUNCTIONS
Blood that empties into the white pulp and marginal zone takes the slow transit pathway. The slow transit pathway is very important to splenic function, which includes culling, pitting, immune defense, and storage.

The discriminatory filtering and destruction of senescent or damaged erythrocytes by the spleen is termed *culling*. Cells entering the spleen through the slow transit pathway become concentrated in the hypoglycemic, hy-

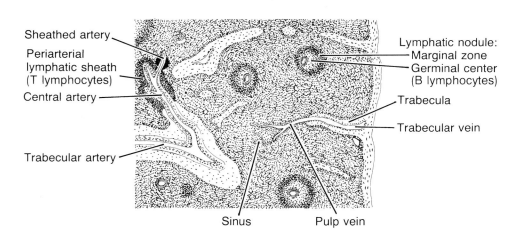

Sheathed artery
Periarterial lymphatic sheath (T lymphocytes)
Central artery
Trabecular artery
Lymphatic nodule:
Marginal zone
Germinal center (B lymphocytes)
Trabecula
Trabecular vein
Sinus
Pulp vein

FIGURE 2-2. Schematic drawing of splenic tissue.

poxic cords, a hazardous environment for aged or damaged erythrocytes. The activity of the adenosine triphosphate (ATP) fueled cation pump of erythrocytes is increased in cells with damaged membranes. Thus, these cells require extra energy in the form of ATP (produced through glycolysis) to maintain osmotic equilibrium. Because of the low glucose concentration and slow circulation in the splenic cords, the supply of glucose in damaged or senile erythrocytes is rapidly diminished. This decreases the availability of ATP and contributes to the demise of these cells. Slow passage through a macrophage-rich route allows the phagocytic cells to remove these old or damaged erythrocytes before or during their squeeze through the 3-μm pores to cords and sinuses. Normal erythrocytes withstand this adverse environment and eventually re-enter the circulation.

Pitting refers to the spleen's ability to "pluck out" inclusions from intact erythrocytes without destroying them. The pinched off cell membrane can reseal itself, but the cell cannot synthesize lipids and proteins for new membrane due to its lack of cellular organelles. Therefore, extensive pitting causes a reduced surface area-to-volume ratio, resulting in the formation of spherocytes. Inclusions removed from erythrocytes in this manner include Howell-Jolly bodies, Pappenheimer bodies, and Heinz bodies. Blood cells with antibodies attached to membrane bound antigens also are susceptible to pitting by macrophages. The macrophage removes the antigen–antibody complex and the attached membrane. The presence of spherocytes on a blood film is evidence that the erythrocyte has undergone membrane assault in the spleen.

The spleen is an important line of immune defense in blood-borne infections because of its rich supply of lymphocytes and phagocytic cells, as well as its unique circulation. Blood-borne antigens are forced into close contact with phagocytes and lymphocytes, which allows for recognition of the antigens' foreignness and leads to antigen phagocytosis and antibody formation.

The immunologic function of the spleen is probably less important in the well-developed immune system of the adult than in the less-developed immune system of the child. Young children who undergo *splenectomy* may develop overwhelming, often fatal, infections with pneumococcus or *Haemophilus influenzae*. This also may be a rare complication of splenectomy in adults.

Sequestering approximately one third of the platelet mass, the spleen acts as a reservoir for platelets. Massive splenomegaly may result in a pooling of 80% to 90% of the platelets, producing peripheral blood thrombocytopenia. Conditions associated with an enlargement of the spleen also are frequently accompanied by leukopenia and anemia, the result of splenic pooling and sequestration of leukocytes and erythrocytes. Removal of the spleen results in a transient thrombocytosis, with a return to normal in approximately 10 days.

Although the spleen is not essential to life, splenectomy does produce characteristic erythrocyte abnormalities easily noted on blood smears by experienced laboratory scientists. After splenectomy, the erythrocytes contain granular inclusions such as Howell-Jolly bodies, Pappenheimer

bodies, and occasionally Heinz bodies (only observed with supravital stains or unstained wet preparations). Abnormal shapes, such as acanthocytes and target cells, also may be seen. Target cells, cells with an excess membrane to volume ratio, have several mechanisms of formation. In patients who have undergone splenectomy, these cells are probably formed as a result of excess lipid on the membrane since the spleen normally grooms the excess lipid from reticulocytes (young erythrocytes) in their maturation process.

Erythrocyte lifespan is not increased after splenectomy. The culling function of the spleen is assumed by other organs, primarily the liver. Even when a spleen is present, the liver, because of its larger blood flow, is responsible for removing most of the particulate matter of the blood. The liver, however, is not as effective as the spleen in filtering abnormal erythrocytes. This is probably because of the rapid flow of blood past hepatic macrophages.

HYPERSPLENISM

In a number of conditions, the spleen may become enlarged and, through exaggeration of its normal activities of filtering and phagocytosing, cause anemia, leukopenia, thrombocytopenia, or combinations of cytopenias. The plasma volume also may increase exacerbating the cytopenias through a dilutional effect. Although exceptions exist, a diagnosis of hypersplenism is made when four conditions are met (Table 2-1): (1) the presence of anemia, leukopenia or thrombocytopenia in the peripheral blood; (2) the existence of a cellular or hyperplastic bone marrow corresponding to the peripheral blood cytopenias; (3) the occurrence of splenomegaly; and (4) the correction of cytopenias after splenectomy.

Hypersplenism has been categorized into two types: primary and secondary. The primary type occurs when no underlying disease can be identified. In primary hypersplenism, the spleen functions abnormally, causing disease. The most common cause of primary hypersplenism is congestive splenomegaly associated with cirrhosis of the liver and portal hypertension. A number of other vascular abnormalities also may cause or contribute to the condition, such as thrombosis of the splenic or portal veins. Leukopenia is the most consistent peripheral blood finding, but anemia and thrombocytopenia also may occur.

Secondary hypersplenism occurs in cases where an underlying disorder causes the splenic abnormalities. The causes of secondary hypersplenism are many and varied. Inflammatory and infectious diseases are believed to cause splenomegaly by an increase in the defensive functions of

TABLE 2-1 *FOUR CONDITIONS NECESSARY FOR A DIAGNOSIS OF HYPERSPLENISM*

1. anemia, leukopenia or thrombocytopenia
2. cellular or hyperplastic bone marrow corresponding to peripheral blood cytopenias
3. splenomegaly
4. correction of cytopenias after splenectomy

the spleen. For example, an increase in the clearing of particulate matter may lead to an increase in the number of macrophages; whereas, an increase in antibody production may cause hyperplasia of lymphoid cells. Disorders in which the macrophages accumulate large quantities of undigestible substances are characterized by splenomegaly; some of these disorders, such as Gaucher's disease, will be discussed in a later chapter. Neoplasms or benign tumors, in which the abnormal cells occupy much of the splenic volume, may cause splenomegaly. The tumor cells, however, may incapacitate the spleen. In these cases, the peripheral blood will show evidence of hyposplenism. Several blood disorders may cause splenomegaly that occurs secondary to compensatory (or workload) hypertrophy of this organ. In these disorders, the blood cells are intrinsically abnormal or coated with antibody, and they are removed from circulation in large numbers (e.g., hereditary spherocytosis, idiopathic thrombocytopenic purpura). An outstanding feature of myelofibrosis, a disorder in which the bone marrow is progressively replaced with fibrous tissue, is splenomegaly. In these cases, the spleen contains foci of extramedullary blood formation.

The effects of hypersplenism may be relieved by splenectomy. However, this procedure is not always advisable, especially when the spleen is performing a constructive role, such as antibody production or filtration of protozoa or bacteria. Splenectomy appears to be most beneficial in patients with hereditary or acquired hemolytic disorders and in idiopathic thrombocytopenic purpura. The blood cells are still abnormal after splenectomy, but the site of their destruction is removed. Consequently, the cells have a more normal lifespan.

●
Lymph nodes

The lymphatic system is composed of lymph nodes and lymphatic vessels, which drain into the left and right lymphatic duct. The vessels originate in connective tissue spaces. They carry lymph in one direction toward the lymphatic ducts near the neck where lymph enters the blood. Lymph is formed from blood fluid that escapes into connective tissue. The bean-shaped lymph nodes occur in groups or chains along the larger lymphatic capillaries. Nodes are composed of lymphocytes, macrophages, and a reticular meshwork surrounded by a capsule. Lymph nodes act as filters, removing foreign particles from lymph by phagocytic cells. Thus, they are extremely important in immune defense. As antigens pass through the nodes, they contact and stimulate immunocompetent lymphocytes to proliferate and differentiate into effector cells (cells that participate in the immune response).

Lymph nodes contain an inner area called the medulla and an outer area called the cortex (Fig. 2-3). Fibrous trabeculae extend inward from the capsule to form irregular communicating compartments within the parenchyma. The medulla, which surrounds the efferent lymphatics, consists of cords of plasma cells that lie between sinusoids. The cortex contains clumps of cells called follicles surrounded by T-lymphocytes and macrophages. The central portions of follicles, known as geminal centers, contain B-lymphocytes and vary in structure in relation to their state of activity. A stimulated node may have germinal centers filled with proliferating lymphocytes, whereas a resting node contains follicles with small normal appearing lymphs and macrophages.

●
Thymus

The thymus is a lymphopoietic organ located in the upper part of the anterior mediastinum. The thymus is a well-developed organ at birth and continues to increase in size until puberty. After puberty, however, it begins to atrophy, until, in old age it appears barely recognizable. It is a bilobular organ demarcated into a cortex and medulla. The cortex is densely packed with small lymphocytes and a few macrophages. The central medulla is less cellular, containing lymphocytes mixed with medullary epithelial cells and macrophages.

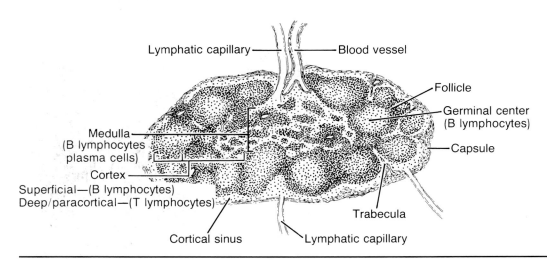

FIGURE 2-3. Schematic drawing of a lymph node. Notice the location of T and B lymphocyte populations.

The primary purpose of the thymus is to serve as a compartment for maturation of T-lymphocytes. The thymic hormone, thymosin, is important in the maturation of virgin lymphocytes into immunocompetent T-lymphocytes. Thymosin extracts and thymic grafts have been shown to restore immunologic function in animals that have undergone thymectomy. The thymus is responsible for supplying the T-lymphocyte–dependent areas of lymph nodes, spleen, and other peripheral lymphoid tissue with immunocompetent T-lymphocytes.

● Bone marrow

Blood-forming tissue located between the trabeculae of spongy bone is known as bone marrow. This major hematopoietic organ is a rich, cellular, highly vascularized, loose connective tissue that has a volume of 30 to 50 mL/kg body weight. The marrow is composed of two major compartments: the hematopoietic compartment and the vascular compartment. The hematopoietic compartment, also known as the hematopoietic cords, is the site of formation and maturation of blood cells (Fig. 2-4). This compartment includes both hematopoietic cells (functional element) and stromal cells (supporting tissue). Hematopoietic cells are only transient residents of the marrow, and, when they mature, they move toward a sinus. These mature cells traverse the endothelial cell lining of the sinus and eventually gain access to the peripheral blood through the vascular compartment. The vascular compartment of bone marrow is composed of the nutrient artery, central longitudinal vein, arterioles, and sinuses.

HEMATOPOIETIC MARROW ARCHITECTURE

There is a pattern to the arrangement of hematopoietic cells within the marrow cavity. Erythroblasts constitute between 25% and 30% of the marrow cells and are produced near the sinuses. A common finding among these developing cells is the *erythroblastic island*. The island is a composite of a single macrophage surrounded by erythroblasts in varying states of maturation. The macrophage cytoplasm extends out to surround the erythroblasts. Dur-

ing this close association, it is suspected that the developing erythrocytes acquire iron from the macrophages. The least mature cells are closest to the center of the island, and the more mature cells are at the periphery.

Granulocytes are produced in nests, close to the trabeculae and arterioles. These nests are not quite as apparent morphologically as erythroblastic islands. Developing granulocytes are associated with a distinct reticular cell. At the metamyelocyte stage they begin moving toward the sinus.

Lymphocytes are produced in lymph nodules, which are randomly dispersed throughout the marrow. Lymphoid stem cells may leave the bone marrow and travel to the thymus, where they mature to T-lymphocytes. Some lymphocytes remain in the bone marrow, where they mature into B-lymphocytes.

Megakaryocytes lie adjacent to the endothelium of sinusoidal walls and discharge platelets directly into the lumen of the sinus. Cytoplasmic processes of the megakaryocyte penetrate the sinus wall and form long proplatelet processes. Pieces of these proplatelets pinch off to form platelets (Fig. 2-5).

When bone marrow is aspirated or biopsied for examination, the specimens may contain at least two other types of cells normally associated with bone: osteoblasts and osteoclasts. These cells are dislodged during puncturing of the bone by the needle in collection of the marrow specimen. Osteoblasts are large cells (up to 30 μm in diameter) that resemble plasma cells except that the perinuclear halo (Golgi apparatus) is detached from the nuclear membrane and, in Romanowsky-stained specimens, appears as an unstained area away from the nucleus. In addition, the cytoplasm of osteoblasts is less basophilic, and the nucleus has a finer chromatin pattern than plasma cells. They are normally found in groups. These cells synthesize matrix and can be seen in the marrow of children and in the marrow of individuals with metabolic bone diseases. The cells are alkaline phosphatase positive. Osteoclasts are even larger than osteoblasts and may reach up to 100 μm in diameter. The cells are granular and may have either acidophilic or basophilic cytoplasm. They resemble mega-

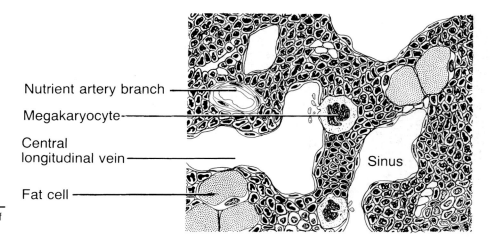

Nutrient artery branch

Megakaryocyte

Central longitudinal vein

Fat cell

Sinus

FIGURE 2-4. Schematic drawing of a section of bone marrow.

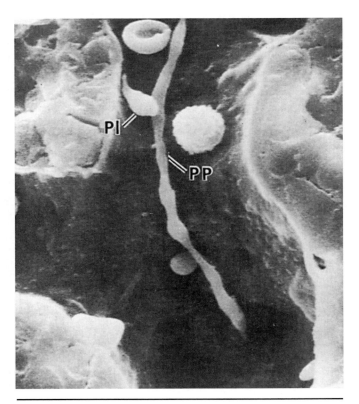

FIGURE 2-5. Scanning electron micrograph of the luminal face of the myeloid sinus wall with an intraluminal segment of a proplatelet process (pp) showing periodic constriction along its length. PL: platelet displaying tear-drop shape. (With permission from: DeBruyn PPH: Structural substrates of bone marrow function. Semin Hematol, 18: 179, 1981.)

karyocytes except that the nuclei are usually discrete and often contain nucleoli.

Mast cells (tissue basophils) are not normally found in the bone marrow but may be present in certain conditions including aplastic anemia, chronic blood loss, anaphylaxis, and tumors of the lymphoid tissue involving bone marrow. The cells are large (20 to 25 μm) with numerous, coarse granules that stain deeply basophilic. The nucleus is round, not bilobed like the basophil.

RED AND YELLOW HEMATOPOIETIC MARROW

The bone marrow is composed of hematopoietically active red marrow and hematopoietically inactive fatty yellow marrow. Hematopoietic red marrow lies adjacent to the endosteum. It contains both myeloid and erythroid precursors with a normal *myeloid to erythroid ratio (M:E)* of 1.5:1 to 4:1. The fatty yellow marrow occupies the central cavity, surrounds the blood vessels, and is composed of adipocytes.

Bone marrow hematopoietic cellularity is measured in relative terms of percentage of hematopoietic red marrow to total bone marrow cellularity (red plus yellow marrow). In adults, approximately half of the marrow is red and the other half is yellow. Thus, normal cellularity is 50%. For the first 4 years of life, nearly all the marrow cavities are composed of red hematopoietic marrow. After 4 years

of age, the red marrow in shafts of long bones is gradually replaced by yellow fatty tissue. By the age of 25 years, hematopoiesis is limited to the marrow of the skull, ribs, sternum, scapulae, clavicles, vertebrae, pelvis, upper half of the sacrum, and proximal ends of the long bones. Cellularity in these areas may decrease after age 70. Little information is available on the effect of aging on human bone marrow function. At the present time, animal and human data indicate that marrow stem cells do not wear out.[2] Most evidence supports the theory that decreased cellularity accompanying aging is due to decreased hematopoietic growth factor responsiveness.

Bone forms a rigid compartment for the marrow. Thus, any change in volume of the hematopoietic elements, which occurs in many anemias and leukemias, must be compensated for by a change in the space-occupying adipocytes (yellow marrow). Normal red marrow can respond to stimuli and increase its activity several times the normal rate. As a result, the red marrow becomes *hyperplastic* and replaces portions of the fatty yellow marrow. *Hyperplasia* accompanies conditions with increased or ineffective hematopoiesis. The degree of hyperplasia is related to the severity and duration of the pathologic state. Acute blood loss may cause erythropoietic tissue to temporarily replace fatty tissue, whereas severe chronic anemia may cause erythropoiesis to be so intense that it not only replaces fatty marrow but it also causes osteoporosis, coarse trabeculation of the bone, and cortical thinning. In malignant diseases that invade or originate in the bone marrow such as leukemia, proliferating abnormal cells may replace both normal hematopoietic tissue and fat.

In contrast, the hematopoietic tissue may become inactive or *hypoplastic*. Fat cells then increase, providing a cushion for the marrow. Environmental factors such as chemicals and toxins may suppress hematopoiesis, whereas other types of hematopoietic suppression may be genetically determined. Myeloproliferative disease, which begins as a hypercellular disease, frequently terminates in a state of *aplasia* in which hematopoietic tissue is replaced by fibrous tissue.

STROMA

The bone marrow stroma forms a favorable microenvironment for sustained proliferation of hematopoietic cells. It forms a meshwork of long, highly anastomosing branches that provides a three-dimensional scaffolding for hematopoietic cells. The stroma is composed of two major cell types: macrophages and the reticular cells. The stromal cells produce an extracellular matrix of collagen, glycoproteins, proteoglycans, and other proteins.[1]

Macrophages There are two subpopulations of macrophages, the perisinal and the central macrophages. The perisinal macrophages are located in the vicinity of the marrow sinuses and function as a part of the blood–marrow barrier. They phagocytose the extruded nuclei of mature erythrocytes as they move into the lumen of the sinus from the hematopoietic marrow and phagocytose abnormal cells as they migrate to the sinus. Processes of these cells also can penetrate the endothelium of the sinus and remove senescent cells in the sinus. The central macrophages serve as the center of the erythroblastic islands discussed above. It is believed that these cells supply the developing erythroblasts with iron. Macrophages stain acid phosphatase positive.

Reticular cells The reticular cells are groups of cells that form a reticulum or syncytium. These cells are associated with reticular fibers, which they produce and which form a three-dimensional supporting network that holds the vascular sinuses and hematopoietic elements. The fibers can be visualized with light microscopy and after silver staining. The reticular cells are alkaline phosphatase positive.

MARROW CIRCULATION

The vascular supply of bone marrow is served by a nutrient artery and a central longitudinal vein, which traverse the bone through the bone foramina and span the marrow cavity (Fig. 2-6). The nutrient artery branches and coils around the central longitudinal vein. Arterioles radiate outward from the nutrient artery to endosteum (membrane that lines the marrow cavity of bone). Another source of arterial blood for the marrow is the periosteal capillaries (the periosteum is the membrane that covers the surface of bone). These periosteal capillaries and the capillary branches of the nutrient artery form a juncture with the venous sinuses as the capillaries reenter the marrow. The sinuses, lined by single endothelial cells, gather into wider collecting sinuses, which open into the central longitudinal vein. The central longitudinal vein continues through the length of the marrow and exits through the foramina where the nutrient artery entered. The central vein is then known as the comitant vein.

BLOOD CELL EGRESS FROM THE MARROW TO THE BLOOD

The mechanism by which the mature hematopoietic cell navigates its passage from the hematopoietic cords past the sinus wall barrier into the sinus (thus gaining access to the blood) is still unknown. Special properties of the maturing hematopoietic cell as well as the sinus wall have been suggested as central features in the cell's interaction with the sinus wall. The adventitial cell, a reticular cell, creates a discontinuous layer on the abluminal side (marrow side) of the sinus wall while endothelial cells line the luminal side (inside of sinus) of the sinus in a continuous layer. The adventitial cell extends its long cytoplasmic processes deep into the marrow cords forming a part of the reticular meshwork that supports hematopoietic cells. Studies have revealed that as blood cell traffic across the sinus increases, the adventitial cells contract, creating a less continuous layer over the abluminal sinus wall. In areas where the adventitial layer contracts creating spaces between adventitial cells, it also retracts from the sinus endothelium, creating a subcompartment between the adventitial layer and the sinus endothelial layer where mature cells accumulate. This allows the mature hematopoietic cells access to more interaction sites on the abluminal side of the sinus endothelial surface.

The passage of hematopoietic cells across the endothelium into the lumen of the sinus is transendothelial. The blood cell presses against the abluminal membrane of the sinus endothelial cell, forcing it into contact with the luminal surface of the cell. The two membranes fuse. Then, under pressure from the passing cell, the membrane separates, creating a pore through which the hematopoietic cell enters the lumen of the sinus. These pores are only 2 to 3 μm in diameter.

Because of the small size of the endothelial cell pores, blood cells must have the ability to deform so that they can squeeze through the sinusoidal lining. Progressive increases in deformability and motility have been noted as granulocytic cells mature from the myeloblast to the segmented granulocyte. This facilitates the movement of cells into the sinus lumen. Other factors contributing to the orderly release of cells from the bone marrow may include humoral and neural influences.

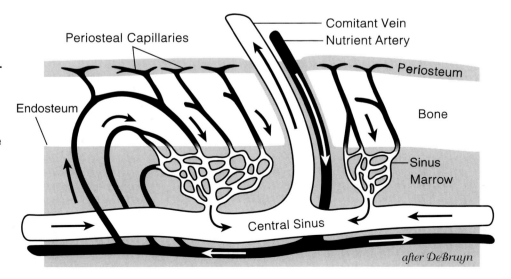

FIGURE 2-6. Diagram of the microcirculation of bone marrow. The major arterial supply to the marrow is from periosteal capillaries and from capillary branches of the nutrient artery, which have traversed the bony enclosure of the marrow through the bone foramina. These capillaries join with the venous sinuses as they reenter the marrow. The sinuses gather into wider collecting sinuses which then open into the central longitudinal vein (central sinus). (Adapted from: DeBruyn PPH: Structural substrates of bone marrow function. Semin Hematol, 18: 179, 1981.)

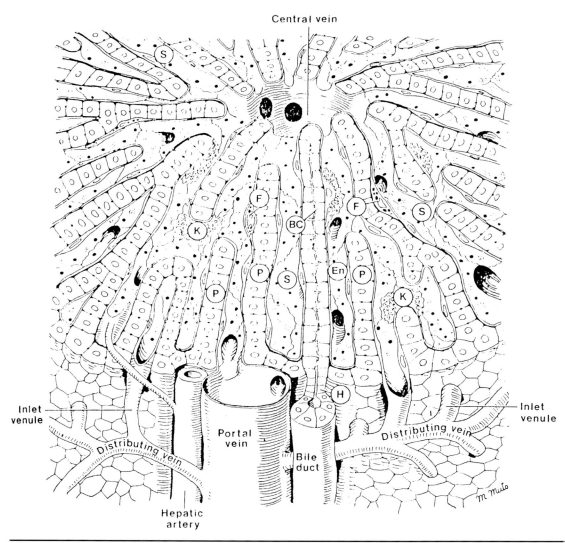

FIGURE 2-7. Three-dimensional aspect of the normal liver. In the upper center, the central vein; in the lower center, the portal vein. BC, bile canaliculi; P, liver plates; H. Hering canal; K, Kupffer cells; S, sinusoid; F, fat-storing cell; En, sinusoid endothelial cell. (Courtesy of: Junqueira, L.C., Carneiro, J.: Basic Histology, 4th Ed. Los Altos, Lange Medical Publishers, 1983.)

● Liver

The liver is the largest organ in the body, weighing approximately 3 pounds in the adult. It is located beneath the diaphragm in the upper abdomen. Its circulatory system is unique in that it has a dual blood supply provided by the hepatic artery and the portal vein. Blood from the portal vein comes from the alimentary canal, the pancreas, and the spleen. This rich supply of blood is mainly responsible for the red to red-brown color of the organ.

The liver consists of a large number of functional units called the hepatic lobules. In cross-section, the lobules appear hexagonal-shaped (Fig. 2-7). Each lobule consists of a central vein (branch of the hepatic vein) surrounded by irregular interconnecting plates of hepatic cells (hepatocytes) that radiate outward like spokes of a wheel from the hub. Sinusoids separate these plates of hepatocytes.

Small channel-like spaces between adjacent hepatocytes form the bile canaliculi. These tubes collect bile and convey it to the hepatic ducts. At the periphery of the lobules lie the portal areas (usually 3 to 6 per lobule). Each portal area consists of three tiny tubes, a venule (a branch of the portal vein), an arteriole(a branch of the hepatic artery), and a bile duct. Lymphatic vessels also may be present.

Branches of the portal vein and hepatic artery both drain into sinusoids. These channels then empty into the central vein. The sinusoids are separated from hepatocytes by a space, Disse's space. The lumen of sinusoids are lined by two types of cells, epithelial cells and Kupffer cells. Small intercellular spaces between the epithelial cells make the lining discontinuous and allow plasma direct access to the hepatocytes. The lining does, however, hold back erythrocytes. The second type of cell in the sinusoidal lining, the Kupffer cell, is usually stellate in shape due to protruding cytoplasmic processes and is attached to epithelial cells. The processes may extend into or across the sinusoidal lumen. These cells have morphologic features of typical macrophages and are actively phagocytic. Although the liver is not as discriminate a filter as the spleen, the Kupffer cells endocytose large quantities of matter present in the blood, including fibrinogen derivatives, fibrin degradation products, activated coagulation proteins, damaged platelets, damaged leukocytes, and aged or damaged erythrocytes. The spleen is more efficient in removing slightly damaged erythrocytes and in pitting inclusions in erythrocytes because of the relatively static environment of blood cells in the spleen's macrophage lined cords. A third type of cell may be present in the liver sinusoidal lining on the side that faces the perisinusoidal space, the lipocyte, a cell that accumulates lipids. The function of this cell is obscure.

In addition to its filtering function for blood cells, the liver detoxifies various drugs and substances by oxidation, methylation, and conjugation. Bilirubin, one of the metabolic products of hemoglobin catabolism, is conjugated by the liver enzyme, glucuronyl transferase, and excreted in the bile. Bile aids in the emulsification and absorption of fats in the digestive canal. Other functions of the liver include the metabolism of proteins, fats, and carbohydrates and the storage of iron and vitamins A, B, and D.

In the fetus, the liver is the main site of hematopoiesis from the third month of gestation until shortly before birth. This hematopoietic function is retained after birth. When the bone marrow loses its capacity to make blood cells due to invasion by malignant cells or fibrous tissue, hematopoiesis may, to some extent, resume in the liver.

● DERIVATION OF BLOOD CELLS

Mature blood cells have a limited lifespan and, with the exception of lymphocytes, are incapable of self-renewal. Replacement of effete peripheral hematopoietic cells is the function of more primitive cells in the bone marrow called stem cells. Stem cells are characterized by their ability to differentiate into distinct cell lines with specialized functions, and their ability to regenerate themselves to maintain the stem cell compartment.

● History of the stem cell concept

The monophyletic theory of blood cell development proposes a common precursor cell, the *pluripotential stem cell*, which, under the influence of humoral factors, may give rise to each of the principle blood cell lines. The pluripotential cell is capable of self-renewal, proliferation, and differentiation into all hematopoietic cell lines.

Clinical and experimental evidence strongly supports the monophyletic theory. Based on this evidence, hematopoietic cells may be divided into three cellular compartments dependent on maturity. In order of increasing maturity, these compartments are (1) primitive multipotential cells capable of self-renewal and differentiation into all blood cell lines, (2) committed progenitor cells destined

to proliferate and develop into distinct cell lines, and (3) mature cells with specialized functions that have lost the capability to proliferate.

In 1961, Till and McCulloch[3] demonstrated the potential of single stem cells to repopulate the spleen of heavily irradiated mice with all blood cell lines. Mice were lethally irradiated to completely destroy all hematopoietic cells. These mice were then intravenously transfused with normal marrow cells from donor mice. In the early stages of recovery, the spleens and marrow of these transfused animals showed macroscopic nodules of proliferating hematopoietic cells. Although in the first 7 to 8 days the nodules each contained only one cell line (erythrocytic, myelocytic, or megakaryocytic), nodules present at 14 days showed mixed cell populations. The cell that formed the colony was termed the colony-forming unit spleen (CFU-S). It has been suggested that perhaps the nodules appearing at 7 days were formed from more mature unipotent committed stem cells, whereas the 14-day nodules were derived from a more primitive multipotential stem cell.[4] It also is interesting to note that the nodules appeared in specific areas of the spleen according to their predominant cell line. The erythrocytic nodules were present on the spleen surface, the megakaryocytic nodules grew beneath the capsule, and the myelocytic nodules grew within the spleen. This preference for certain areas of the spleen may be caused by the influence of the local environment, called the *hematopoietic inductive microenvironment* (HIM), on the hematopoietic stem cell. Studies of the bone marrow stromal influence on hematopoiesis, in mice and hamsters, have suggested that normal stroma is essential for supporting normal hematopoiesis.[5,6]

Further experiments provided direct evidence for the existence of pluripotential stem cells. Donor marrow cells from mice were irradiated severely enough to cause chromosomal aberrations and then injected into lethally irradiated recipients. Different hematopoietic cell types with the same unique abnormal karyotype were found in splenic nodules.[7] In addition, cell suspensions from these nodules could be injected into other irradiated mice to form new splenic nodules with similar chromosomal abnormalities. These studies indicate that a single marrow cell exists that is not only capable of differentiating into different hematopoietic cell types but also is capable of self-renewal.

● Questions surrounding the lymphocytic stem cell

Questions have been raised as to whether the lymphocytes orginate from the same stem cell as other hematopoietic cell lines. Chromosomal marker research suggests that the lymphocyte and other hematopoietic cells have in common a primitive stem cell that gives rise to both myeloid and lymphoid progenitors (Fig. 2-8). For example, a single G6PD isoenzyme has been found in all hematopoietic cells including T- and B-lymphocytes in a patient with sideroblastic anemia (a stem cell disorder) and G6PD mosaicism.[8] Females inherit two X chromosomes, one from each parent. However, only one of the two X chromosomes in each cell is active. The process of X inactivation

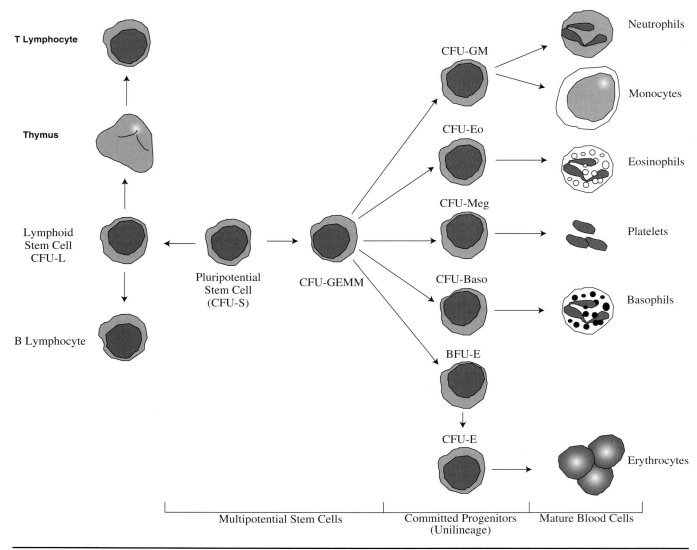

FIGURE 2-8. The differentiation of blood cells from a pluripotential stem cell. The pluripotential stem cell and the colony forming unit-granulocyte, erythrocyte, macrophage, megakaryocyte (CFU-GEMM) have the potential to differentiate into one of several cell lines and are therefore termed multipotential stem cells. The committed progenitors, colony-forming unit-granulocyte, macrophage (CFU-GM), colony-forming unit-eosinophil (CFU-EO), colony-forming unit-megakaryocyte (CFU-Meg), colony-forming unit-basophil (CFU-Baso), burst-forming unit-erythroid (BFU-E), and colony-forming unit-erythroid (CFU-E), differentiate into only one cell line (unilineage) except for CFU-GM which is bipotential. The BFU-E is more immature than the CFU-E. The mature blood cells are those found in the peripheral blood. The lymphoid stem cell (CFU-L) may differentiate into either T- or B-lymphocytes.

of one of the two X chromosomes in embryogenesis is random. G6PD is an enzyme whose genetic mode of transmission is on the X chromosome; thus, in females, who are heterozygous for two different G6PD isoenzymes (one inherited from the mother and the other from the father), two populations of hematopoietic cells exist. One population contains the maternal isoenzyme, and one population contains the paternal isoenzyme. All cells derived from the same stem cell, however, have the same G6PD isoenzyme. Thus, a single isoenzyme, found in all hematopoietic cells in heterozygous patients with hematopoietic stem cell disorders, indicates the hematopoietic cell population, including lymphocytes, probably originated from a single abnormal pluripotential stem cell.

Further evidence for a common hematopoietic stem cell

for all blood cells is provided from studies on patients with chronic myelogeneous leukemia (CML). The malignant cells in this disorder have been found to carry an abnormal chromosome, the Philadelphia chromosome. Early studies found this abnormal karyotype in erythrocyte precursors, granulocytes, and megakaryocytes but absent in lymphocytes. These data suggested that lymphocytes were derived from a stem cell distinctly different from the stem cell for other hematopoietic cells. Contrary to these earlier studies, more recent studies have demonstrated that the abnormal Philadelphia chromosome can be found in B-lymphocytes as well as other blood cell lines in some patients with CML. Patients with CML frequently enter a myeloblastic crisis in which masses of malignant myeloblasts fill the bone marrow and enter the peripheral blood. Results of cell marker studies and cytochemical stains have shown that a small portion of blastic crises in CML are caused by proliferation of malignant lymphoblasts rather than myeloblasts. This suggests that the malignant cell in CML is probably a primitive stem cell that is capable of differentiating into myeloblasts or lymphoblasts. Disease-associated karyotypes are not definite proof of clonality of cells. However, these findings, together with studies of G6PD isoenzymes, indicate the lymphocytic cell line may be derived from a primitive multipotential stem cell that is capable of differentiating into lymphocytes as well as other blood cells.

Cell cycle

The cell cycle, the period between two mitotic events, has four phases: postmitotic rest (G1), DNA synthesis (S), premitotic (G2), and mitotic (M) (Fig. 2-9). After mitosis, the cells may re-enter the cell cycle or enter a dormant, nondividing phase (G0). Some G0 cells can re-enter the cell cycle while others are terminally differentiated and do not divide again. The entry of quiescent G0 cells into the S phase requires initiation by two environmental signals or growth stimuli. For example, the activation of T-lymphocytes requires PHA and IL-2 and the activation of B-lymphocytes requires binding of surface immunoglobulin plus B-cell growth factor. These stimuli activate genes and gene products that control the initiation of cellular DNA synthesis.

Stem cell renewal and differentiation

The stem cell pool comprises approximately 1 to 2×10^6 cells. Despite this low number, these cells are responsible for the generation of more than 10^{11} cells per day on a continual basis. Surprisingly, only a small number of stem cells are dividing at one time (less than 5%). Most are in the quiescent phase, the G_0 state. To maintain the stem cell pool while continually producing cells to replace senescent differentiated blood cells, stem cells must be capable of balanced self-renewal and differentiation. This might occur in one of two ways[9] (Fig. 2-10). First, a stem cell may divide into two daughter cells, one of which is committed to differentiate while the other remains in the stem cell pool. Alternatively, for every stem cell that produces two daughter cells, both of which differentiate, an-

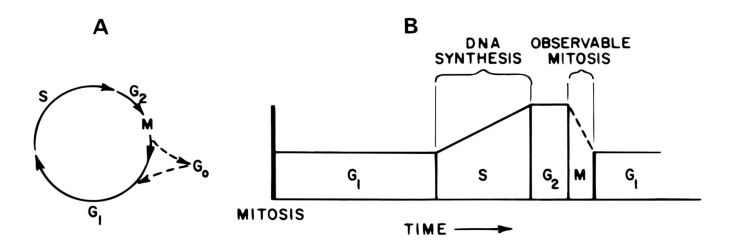

A

B

DNA SYNTHESIS   OBSERVABLE MITOSIS

MITOSIS   TIME ⟶

G_1 — NUCLEUS CONTAINS DIPLOID DNA

S — PERIOD OF DNA REPLICATION

G_2 — NUCLEUS CONTAINS TETRAPLOID DNA

M — PERIOD OF MITOSIS

G_0 — RESTING STATE. HAS POTENTIAL FOR DIVISION

GENERATION TIME — TIME FROM ONE MITOSIS TO THE NEXT

FIGURE 2-9. The four phases of the cell generative cycle. (With permission from: Wintrobe's Hematology, Philadelphia: Lea & Febiger, 1993.)

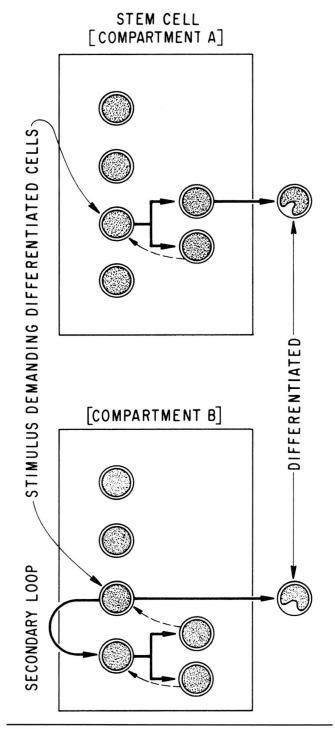

STEM CELL
[COMPARTMENT A]

STIMULUS DEMANDING DIFFERENTIATED CELLS

[COMPARTMENT B]

SECONDARY LOOP

DIFFERENTIATED

FIGURE 2-10. Models of stem cell replication. It has been suggested that division in stem cell compartments may be asymmetric (A) or symmetric (B). Compartment size is maintained in (A) by stimuli that demand differentiated cells and trigger cellular division. In this model, one daughter cell matures and the other remains a stem cell. In (B), the stimuli that demand differentiated cells deplete the stem cell compartment by inducing cellular differentiation of the stem cell but a secondary loop recognizes compartment depletion and induces stem cell division to maintain the compartment size. (With permission from: Wintrobe's Hematology, Philadelphia: Lea & Febiger, 1993.)

other stem cell divides to produce two daughter stem cells that remain in the stem cell pool. Either of these processes would maintain the stem cell pool at a constant size while producing progeny that differentiate and replace senescent cells. The daughter cells of stem cells retain the ability to generate cells of all hematopoietic lineages. With additional divisions, however, the progeny of daughter cells become progressively restricted to differentiate into fewer and fewer lineages until eventually they become restricted to a single cell line *(unilineage)*. These unilineage cells, referred to as committed progenitors, give rise to identifiable hematopoietic precursor cells such as erythroblasts and myeloblasts (Fig. 2-8).

Hematopoietic stem cell model

In vitro methods for growing human hematopoietic stem cells in soft agar culture have provided further evidence for the hierarchical model of hematopoiesis (Fig. 2-11). The pluripotential stem cell gives rise to multipotential stem cells, which then differentiate into committed stem cells. These committed stem cells then develop into mature, nonproliferating cells. With the exception of the pluripotential stem cell, the nomenclature for the progenitor cells is based on the mature progeny that they produce in culture systems. "Pluripotential" is the descriptive term used to identify the parent hematopoietic stem cell that gives rise to all other progenitor stem cells. Till and McCulloch[3] termed this cell the CFU-S. This cell also has been referred to as the totipotential stem cell.

The myeloid stem cell, called the colony-forming unit-granulocyte, erythrocyte, monocyte, megakaryocyte (CFU-GEMM), and the lymphoid stem cell, called the colony-forming unit-lymphocyte (CFU-L), are derived from the pluripotential stem cell. These two progenitor cells have a limited capacity for self-renewal but can still differentiate into several cell lines. Therefore, these progenitor cells are called multipotential stem cells. Eventually, under the control of specific hematopoietic growth factors (described in the next section), the multipotential cells become committed to one cell line and are then appropriately termed unilineage or committed progenitor cells. Each of these committed progenitor cells is named for the cell line to which it is committed (e.g., CFU-Meg for megakaryocytic cell line, CFU-E for erythroid cell line, CFU-M for monocytic cell line, and CFU-G for granulocytic cell line). Each committed progenitor cell differentiates into morphologically identifiable blood cells: platelets, erythrocytes, monocytes, and granulocytes.

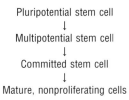

Pluripotential stem cell
↓
Multipotential stem cell
↓
Committed stem cell
↓
Mature, nonproliferating cells

FIGURE 2-11 *Hierarchical Hematopoietic Model*

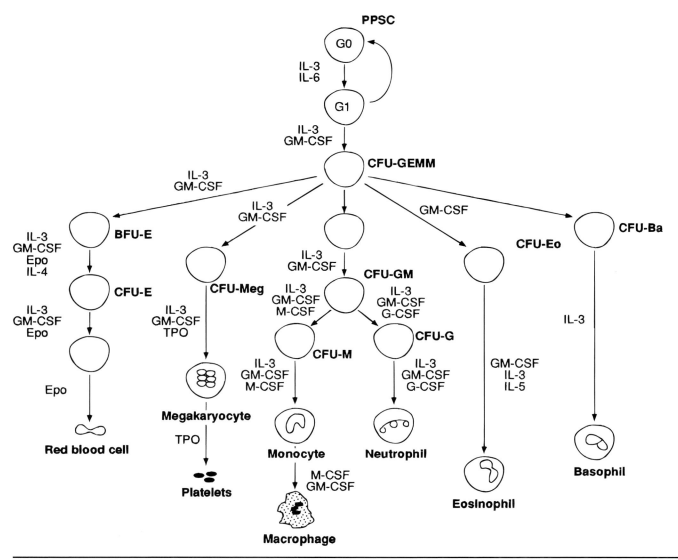

FIGURE 2-12. The pluripotential stem cell (PPSC) gives rise to erythrocytes, platelets, monocytes, macrophages, and granulocytes. This cell also can differentiate into lymphoid cells. Under specific stimulation from growth factors, IL-3, IL-6, and GM-CSF, the PPSC differentiates to the colony-forming unit-granulocyte, erythoid, macrophage, megakaryocyte (CFU-GEMM). The CFU-GEMM then randomly differentiates into granulocytes, erythrocytes, monocytes, and megakaryocytes under the influence of specific growth factors, erythropoietin (Epo), thrombopoietin (TPO), granulocyte-monocyte colony-stimulating factor (GM-CSF), granulocyte colony-stimulating factor (G-CSF), macrophage colony-stimulating factor (M-CSF). Interleukin-5 (IL-5) appears to be the specific factor needed for differentiation into eosinophils. (Adapted from Smith and Yee, Pharmacotherapy 12 (2, Pt. 2), 11s, 1992.)

MYELOID STEM CELL (CFU-GEMM)

The multipotential progenitor cell committed to differentiate into granulocytes, monocytes, platelets, and erythrocytes is termed the CFU-GEMM. Under the influence of specific growth factors, this cell can differentiate to form one of the specific hematopoietic cell lines.[10] (Fig. 2-12).

Erythropoiesis In the erythroid culture system, progenitor cells give rise to two distinct types of erythroid colonies in the presence of the erythroid growth factor, erythropoietin (EPO). A primitive progenitor cell, burst-forming unit-erythroid (BFU-E), derived from CFU-GEMM, is rela-tively insensitive to erythropoietin and forms large colonies after 14 days in the form of bursts. Another type of colony grows to a maximal size in 7 to 8 days, matures, and degenerates. The erythropoietin-sensitive progenitor of this colony is termed colony-forming unit-erythroid (CFU-E). The CFU-E, a descendant of BFU-E, gives rise to the first recognizable erythrocyte precursor, the pronor-moblast. These progenitor cells are induced to proliferate and differentiate by several growth factors acting synergis-tically with erythropoietin, including granulocyte-macro-phage colony-stimulating factor (GM-CSF), interleukin-3 (IL-3), interleukin-4 (IL-4).

$$\text{CFU-GEMM} \xrightarrow{\substack{\text{IL-3} \\ \text{GM-CSF}}} \text{BFU-E} \xrightarrow{\substack{\text{IL-4, EPO} \\ \text{IL-3, GM-CSF}}}$$

$$\text{CFU-E} \xrightarrow{\text{EPO}} \text{Pronormoblast}$$

At each step in differentiation, the cells take on more specific characteristics of erythrocytes. At the CFU-E stage, the cells develop the Rh antigens and erythropoietin receptors.

Granulopoiesis and monopoiesis Granulocytes and monocytes are derived from a common bipotential stem cell, colony-forming unit-granulocyte, monocyte (CFU-GM) that is derived from the CFU-GEMM. Specific growth factors for granulocytes and monocytes, acting synergistically with GM-CSF or IL-3, appear to determine which path of differentiation the CFU-GM takes. Monocyte colony-stimulating factor (M-CSF) will induce monocyte differentiation, while granulocyte colony-stimulating factor (G-CSF) induces neutrophil granulocyte differentiation.

$$\text{CFU-GEMM} \xrightarrow{\text{IL-3, GM-CSF}} \text{CFU-GM} \xrightarrow{\substack{\text{IL-3, CM-CSF} \\ \text{G-CSF}}}$$

$$\text{CFU-G} \rightarrow \text{Granulocytes}$$

$$\text{CFU-GEMM} \xrightarrow{\text{IL-3, GM-CSF}} \text{CFU-GM} \xrightarrow{\substack{\text{IL-3, GM-CSF} \\ \text{M-CSF}}}$$

$$\text{CFU-M} \rightarrow \text{Monocytes/macrophages}$$

Eosinophils are derived directly from the CFU-GEMM under the influence of the growth factors GM-CSF, IL-3, and IL-5.

$$\text{CFU-GEMM} \rightarrow \text{CFU-Eo} \xrightarrow{\substack{\text{IL-3, GM-CSF} \\ \text{IL-5}}} \text{Eosinophils}$$

Basophils also are derived directly from the CFU-GEMM under the influence of IL-3.

$$\text{CFU-GEMM} \rightarrow \text{CFU-Ba} \xrightarrow{\text{IL-3}} \text{Basophils}$$

Thrombopoiesis Platelets (thrombocytes) are derived from CFU-GEMM. CFU-Meg is induced to proliferate and differentiate into megakaryocytes by the growth factors IL-3 and GM-CSF, while megakaryocytes are stimulated to increase in size and to produce platelets by a substance termed thrombopoietin (TPO).

$$\text{CFU-GEMM} \xrightarrow{\text{IL-3, GM-CSF}} \text{CFU-Meg} \xrightarrow{\substack{\text{IL-3, GM-CSF} \\ \text{TPO}}}$$

$$\text{Megakaryocyte} \xrightarrow{\text{TPO}} \text{Platelets}$$

LYMPHOID STEM CELL

The lymphoid stem cell is derived from the pluripotential stem cell and gives rise to T- and B-lymphocytes. Lymphocytes mature at multiple sites, including the bone marrow, thymus, lymph nodes, and spleen. Multiple growth factors

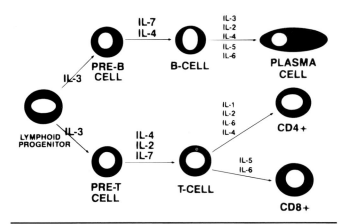

FIGURE 2-13. Growth factors influencing lymphopoiesis. Some of the factors involved in regulating growth and differentiation of lymphoid cells are sufficient to induce growth and/or differentiation while others act synergistically. (IL-interleukin; CD4-helper T-lymphocyte; CD8-suppressor T-lymphocyte) (With permission from: Hoffman R, Benz EJ, Shattil SJ, Furie B, Cohen HJ [eds]: Hematology: Basic principles and procedures. New York: Churchill Livingstone, 1991.)

play a role in T- and B-lymphocyte growth and development, most of which act synergistically (Fig. 2-13).

● Growth factors and the control of hematopoiesis

The regulation of hematopoietic stem cell differentiation and expansion is critical because this determines the concentration of various cell lines in the marrow and eventually in the peripheral blood. Hematopoietic progenitor cell survival, self-renewal, proliferation, and differentiation is governed by specific glycoproteins called *hematopoietic growth factors*. It appears that growth factors play an important role in regulating blood cell production through suppression of *apoptosis*, often referred to as programmed cell death.[11,12]

Growth factors belong to a group of soluble mediators called *cytokines*. Cytokines aid in communication between cells. They are produced by a number of different cells and have an effect on cells in the local environment. Each growth factor has multiple functions, creating a complex cell-to-cell communication system. Bagby and Segal have simplified this functional complexity of growth factors into eight general rules (Table 2-2). Of special note is that many of these factors act synergistically with other growth factors. Some do not act on hematopoietic cells directly but rather stimulate other cells to produce specific growth factors. These growth factors and their specific activities are listed in Table 2-3.

CHARACTERISTICS OF GROWTH FACTORS

Growth factors can be divided into two nomenclature groups: colony-stimulating factors (CSFs) and interleukins (ILs). The CSFs include: Stem cell factor (SCF; c-Kit ligand), GM-CSF, G-CSF, M-CSF, EPO, and TPO. Interleukins are named in order of discovery (e.g., IL-1,

TABLE 2-2 *GENERAL RULES OF HEMATOPOIETIC GROWTH FACTORS AND INTERLEUKIN BIOLOGY*

1. Each hematopoietic growth factor or interleukin exhibits mutiple biologic activities.
2. Growth factors and interleukins that induce proliferation of hematopoietic precursor cells often enhance the functional activity of the terminally differentiated progeny of those precursor cells.
3. Factors that stimulate hematopoiesis can do so directly or indirectly.
4. Most of the hematopoietic growth factors and cytokines function synergistically with others.
5. The hematopoietic regulatory cytokine network is organized hierarchically.
6. The network exhibits many signal amplification circuits.
7. The genes encoding these proteins share important functional and structural similarities.
8. Structural or regulatory abnormalities of hematopoietic growth factor or growth factor gene expression may result in abnormalities of hematopoiesis.

(With permission from: Hoffman R, et al (Ed): Hematology: Basic principles and procedures. New York: Churchill Livingston, 1991.)

IL-2, and so forth). The growth factors promote growth and maturation of hematopoietic progenitors and moderate the functional activity of mature cells. They may act on the same cells that produce them. Growth factors are secreted by a number of different cells, including monocytes, macrophages, activated T-lymphocytes, fibroblasts, and endothelial cells (Fig. 2-14).

The growth factors interact with their target by means of unique transmembrane cell receptors. The number of receptors on a cell's surface is small, and only a low level of receptors need to bind the factor for the factor to have an effect on the cell. Once the factor binds, a signal is transmitted from the surface to the cell's nucleus. Several mechanisms of signal transduction have been described, including activation of tyrosine kinase activity and conformation change of a GTP-binding protein.[13,14] In the case of the latter, GTP-protein activates phosphatidyl-inositol-biphosphate phosphodiesterase (PPDE). The PPDE breaks down a lipid membrane and releases two messengers: diacylglycerol and inositol triphosphate. This results in an increase in intracellular calcium ions and activation of protein kinase C. The result is an increase in protein synthesis,

TABLE 2-3 *HEMATOPOIETIC GROWTH FACTORS AND SOME OF THEIR CHARACTERISTICS*

Factor*	Cells Stimulated	Production Sources	Chromosomal Location
M-CSF (CSF-1)	Monocytes	Endothelial cells, monocytes, fibroblasts	5q33.1
GM-CSF	All granulocytes, megakaryocytes, erythrocytes, stem cells, leukemic blasts	T cells, endothelial cells, fibroblasts	5q23-31
G-CSF	Granulocytes, macrophages, endothelial cells, fibroblasts, leukemic blasts	Endothelial cells, placenta, monocytes	17q11-22
IL-1	Stimulates expression of growth factors by other cells. Mediates inflammation	Monocytes, macrophages, endothelial cells	2q
IL-2	T- and B-lymphocytes	T-lymphocytes	4q
IL-3	Granulocytes, erythroid cells, multipotential progenitors, leukemic blasts	T cells	5q23-31
IL-4	B, T cells	T cells	5q31
IL-5	B cells, CFU-Eo	T cells	5q31
IL-6	B, T cells, CFU-GEMM, CFU-GM, BFU-E, macrophages, neural cells, hepatocytes	Fibroblasts, leukocytes, epithelial cells	7p15
IL-7	B cells	Leukocytes	8q12-13
IL-8	T cells, neutrophils	Leukocytes	4
IL-9	BFU-E, CFU-GEMM	Lymphocytes	5q31
IL-11	B, T cells, CFU-GEMM, CFU-GM, macrophages, BFU-E, CFU-E, megakaryocytes, leukemic blasts	Macrophages	NI
Erythropoietin	CFU-E, BFU-E	Kidney, liver	7q11-22
c-kit ligand ("stem cell factor," SCF; steel factor)	Primitive progenitors	NI	NI

* CSF, colony-stimulating factor; GM, granulocyte-macrophage; IL, interleukin; CFU, colony-forming unit; BFU, burst-forming unit; GEMM, granulocytes, erythroid cells, macrophages, megakaryocytes; NI, not identified.

(Adapted from Lee GR: Wintrobe's Clinical Hematology, 9th Ed. Philadelphia, Lea & Febiger, 1993.)

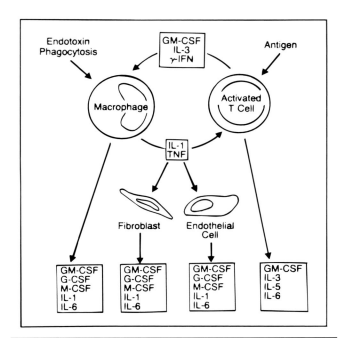

FIGURE 2-14. Cellular sources of colony-stimulating growth factors and interleukins and regulators of their production. IL-3: interleukin-3; TNF: tumor necrosis factor; IL-1: interleukin-1; IL-5: interleukin-5; IL-6: interleukin-6; γ-interferon: gamma-interferon; GM-CSF: granulocyte-monocyte colony stimulating factor; G-CSF: granulocyte colony stimulating factor; M-CSF: macrophage colony stimulating factor. (With permission from: Groopman JE, Molina JM, and Scadden DT: Hematopoietic growth factors. N Engl J Med, 321 (21): 1449, 1989.)

cell proliferation, differentiation, or activation. The exact mechanism of how the signal is transmitted to the nucleus is unknown.

Growth factors and their receptors also have been shown to be involved in malignant transformation of cells. Proto-oncogenes code for proteins involved in cell proliferation or differentiation, including growth factors and their receptors. Proto-oncogenes can be transformed to oncogenes by a process called oncogene activation. Oncogenes are genes whose abnormal expression or product leads to malignant transformation. Activation of the proto-oncogenes that code for growth factors and their receptors may lead to enhanced and uncontrolled cell growth. This will be discussed further in Chapter 17.

Most of the growth factors are glycoproteins with a molecular weight in the range of 14,000 to 90,000 Daltons. They are effective in picomolar concentration and often are not detectable in the circulating blood. They tend to function in the microenvironment of the bone marrow.[15] Stromal cells in the bone marrow microenvironment serve to support stem cell renewal, proliferation, and differentiation by secreting specific hematopoietic growth factors as well as by providing physical support and points of adhesion. In vitro experiments reveal that without stromal cells, stem cells in culture will differentiate and die, even in the presence of growth factors. Culture systems with stromal cells, however, support hematopoiesis for

weeks to months. Thus, it appears that stromal cells as well as growth factors play a vital part in hematopoietic cell differentiation and proliferation. It also has been shown that stromal cells secrete factors that are chemotactic for hematopoietic stem cells, thus guiding these cells toward stromal cells.[16]

A model has been proposed for the regulation of hematopoietic progenitor cells in the bone marrow[17] (Fig. 2-15). According to this model, hematopoietic progenitor cells attach to the stroma of the bone marrow by specific receptors and are influenced by growth factors produced locally by the stromal cells (endogenous growth factor) as well as by growth factors that adhere to the matrix molecules of the marrow that are produced by cells in other locations (exogenous growth factor).

MULTILINEAGE GROWTH FACTORS

Several growth factors influence the activity of a wide spectrum of progenitor cells and are called multilineage growth factors. These include IL-3, GM-CSF, IL-1, IL-6, IL-11, and SCF. Although these factors can initiate proliferation in several cell lines, other factors, working synergistically, are necessary for the production of mature cells in these lineages.[18]

Interleukin-3 This growth factor influences the activities of cells from the pluripotential stem cell to the mature progeny of the myeloid cell line. It acts synergistically with lineage-specific growth factors (EPO, TPO, M-CSF, G-CSF) to induce cells committed to a specific lineage.

Granulocyte-macrophage colony-stimulating factor The release of this factor is regulated by IL-1 and IL-2. It acts at various points in the development of the myeloid cell line but in a narrower spectrum than IL-3. It is the chief promoter of granulocyte and monocyte differentiation. However, it must work with other growth factors for inducing this specific cell lineage maturation.

This growth factor also affects the function of mature cells. It decreases neutrophil chemotaxis, increases neutrophil margination and adhesion to the endothelium, enhances phagocytosis, oxidation, and degranulation at the site of inflammation.[15] It also stimulates production of IL-1 (thus, enhancing its own production) and tumor necrosis factor by monocytes, increases cytotoxicity of macrophages and eosinophils, and stimulates basophils to release histamine.

Interleukin-1 This interleukin has numerous endocrine, metabolic, and hematologic effects. Two forms are recognized: α-IL-1 and β-IL-1. The synthesis of each is directed by separate genes, but they bind to the same receptor binding sites. Their effect on hematopoiesis is not direct but rather indirect: IL-1 stimulates other cells to increase synthesis of growth factors. The broad effect of this interleukin is in large part due to its ability to stimulate the expression of other growth factors by bone marrow stromal cells including IL-6, GM-CSF, and G-CSF.

Interleukin-6 This interleukin has diverse activity at many points in hematopoietic differentiation. It rarely acts alone

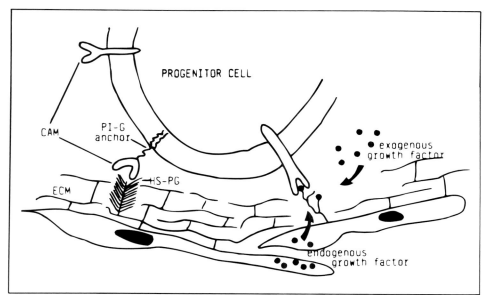

FIGURE 2-15. A model for regulation of hematopoietic progenitor cells in the microenvironment of the bone marrow. The hematopoietic progenitor cell attaches to bone marrow stromal cells via specific receptors and ligands. The progenitor cells are then influenced by both endogenous and exogenous growth factors. (CAM: cell adhesion molecule; HS-PG: heparin sulfate proteoglycan; ECM: extracellular matrix; PI-G: phosphatidylinositol-glycan). (With permission from: Gordon MY, Ford AM and Greaves MF: Cell interactions and gene expression in early hematopoiesis. Int J Cell Cloning, 8:11-25, Suppl 1; 1990).

but rather synergistically with IL-3 to stimulate the growth of CFU-GEMM, BFU-E, and CFU-Meg. It also can work with IL-4 and G-CSF or M-CSF and appears to be important for megakaryocyte development.

Interleukin-11   Research indicates that IL-11 may promote CFU-GM, CFU-GEMM, and BFU-E. Interleukin-11 (IL-11), in synergy with IL-3 and IL-4, shortens the G_0 phase of early myeloid progenitor cells and, in synergy with IL-3, increases the number, size and ploidy of megakaryocyte colonies. Evidence indicates it may increase the number of circulating neutrophils. This cytokine also stimulates the development of IgG producing B-lymphocytes in a T-lymphocyte dependent process. IL-11 inhibits adipogenesis and may play a role in mediating the conversion of active red marrow to yellow marrow.

Stem cell factor (SCF)[19–21]   This growth factor exists in both membrane-bound and soluble forms.[22] The SCF receptor is c-kit, encoded by a proto-oncogene on chromosome 4. Alone, SCF has little biologic activity in vitro, but it synergizes with a variety of growth factors to stimulate colony formation in the early stages of hematopoiesis. It has little effect on lineage committment.

LINEAGE-SPECIFIC GROWTH FACTORS

The remainder of the growth factors have a narrower spectrum of influence and work synergistically with the multilineage growth factors to induce maturation along a specific cell line. These include G-CSF, M-CSF, EPO, TPO, and the remaining interleukins.

Granulocyte colony-stimulating factor   The primary function of this growth factor is to induce the differentiation of GM-CFU to G-CFU. It acts synergistically with GM-CSF or IL-3. Recently, it has been suggested that G-CSF can act synergistically with IL-3 to induce differentiation

and maturation of other cell lineages including the megakaryocytic cell line.[23] It also influences the function of mature cells. It increases migration, phagocytosis, and oxidative metabolism of neutrophils and enhances antibody-dependent cytotoxicity.[15]

Erythropoietin   This growth factor is a hormone since it is not produced close to the site of its action but rather is produced by the kidney and must travel to the bone marrow to influence erythrocyte production. Its release is regulated by the oxygen needs of the body. It may have its earliest influence on the BFU-E but is most influential on the CFU-E and later progeny. The reticulocyte and more mature erythrocytes do not have receptors for EPO and thus are not influenced by this growth factor.

Monocyte colony-stimulating factor   This was the first growth factor described, thus its alternate name, CSF-1. Its function is to stimulate CFU-GM to differentiate into monocytes and macrophages. The cell receptor for this factor is encoded by the proto-oncogene, c-*fms*. It has been suggested that specific alterations in this proto-oncogene may lead to altered expression or function of the receptor, which, in turn, may lead to leukemic cell transformation.[24] This factor also has an effect on the function of monocytes. It stimulates monocytes to produce G-CSF, tumor necrosis factor, IL-1, and interferons. It also increases tumoricidal activity and antibody-dependent cytotoxicity.

Thrombopoietin   This growth factor stimulates the maturation of megakaryocytes and influences the production of platelets. The gene encoding this factor has not yet been cloned.

Interleukin-2   This interleukin stimulates the proliferation and activation of T and B lymphocytes and NK cells. It also has an inhibitory effect on granulocyte, monocyte, and erythroid cell lines.

Interleukin-4　This interleukin stimulates the proliferation and activation of B-lymphocytes, helper T-lymphocytes, cytotoxic T-lymphocytes, mast cells, and fibroblasts. It promotes the switching of immunoglobulin synthesis by B lymphocytes from IgM to IgG and IgE. It interacts with IL-2 to suppress B-lymphocyte proliferation and to upregulate T-lymphocytes. It promotes growth of BFU-E or CFU-E in the presence of EPO and of CFU-GM in the presence of G-CSF and GM-CSF.

Interleukin-5　This interleukin acts on both lymphoid and myeloid cells. Together with GM-CSF it promotes the proliferation and differentiation of eosinophils. It also stimulates the development of B-lymphocytes and activates cytotoxic T-lymphocytes.

Interleukin-7, interleukin-8, interleukin-9　These interleukins have only recently been described. IL-7 stimulates the growth of lymphocytes and probably megakaryocytes. IL-8 is chemotactic for neutrophils, and IL-9 influences megakaryocyte and erythroid colony formation.[15]

CLINICAL USE OF HEMATOPOIETIC GROWTH FACTORS

The cloning and characterization of genes encoding the hematopoietic growth factors have allowed scientists to produce the factors in large quantity using recombinant DNA technology. This has opened the door for using growth factors in therapeutic regimens for hematopoietic disorders. Growth factor therapy shows promise in a variety of hematopoietic disorders.

Stimulation of erythropoiesis in renal disease　Therapy with recombinant human erythropoietin (r-HuEPO) has been used in patients with end-stage renal disease. Nearly all dialysis patients respond by reaching target hematocrit levels within 8 to 12 weeks.[25]

Recovery from treatment-induced myelosuppression　G-CSF and GM-CSF have been used to accelerate bone marrow recovery after intense chemo- or radiotherapy. This treatment may reduce the mortality and morbidity associated with infectious complications due to myelosuppression in these patients.

Therapy of myelodysplastic syndromes　Growth factors are being used to overcome cytopenias and enhance cellular function. If effective, infectious morbidity may be reduced.[26]

Enhanced killing of malignant cells　The growth factors may induce malignant cells into the S phase so that the cells are more sensitive to killing by cycle-specific agents.

Priming of bone marrow for donation　Growth factors may be used to prime the bone marrow of donors for marrow transplantation.

Stimulation of malignant cells to differentiate　Growth factors may be useful in decreasing leukemic cell self-renewal by inducing the cells to differentiate.[23]

Enhancement of the acute phase reaction　Since several factors enhance the acute phase reaction, they may be useful in helping to fight infections.

Enhancement of the immune system　Some factors, especially the interleukins, may stimulate the immune response in the immunosuppressed and also enhance immunosurveillance for cancer cells.

Stimulation of marrow cells in bone marrow transplantation[27]　Growth factors may speed neutrophil recovery in patients who undergo autologous or allogeneic bone marrow transplantation, thus reducing morbidity associated with neutropenia. Erythropoietin also is being studied as treatment in these patients.

Treatment in bone marrow failure[28]　IL-3 has been used in treatment of bone marrow failure, and G-CSF has shown success in treating congenital agranulocytosis.

Utilization of growth factors in combination　Combining growth factors is just beginning to be evaluated. When preceded by therapy with IL-3, GM-CSF produces a dramatic increase in progenitor cells in the peripheral blood.[29] Thus, peripheral blood could be used for harvesting progenitor cells to be used in rescuing patients after high-dose intensified chemotherapy.

It appears that clinical use of hematopoietic growth factors may allow physicians to manipulate and regulate the entire hematopoietic system.[30]

● SUMMARY

The hematopoietic system includes the tissues and organs involved in the proliferation, maturation, and destruction of blood cells. These tissues and organs include the mononuclear phagocyte system, spleen, lymph nodes, thymus, bone marrow, and liver. The bone marrow is the primary site of blood cell production after birth. The marrow is composed of about 50% hematopoietically active red marrow and 50% hematopoietically inactive yellow marrow. The red marrow has a normal ratio of myeloid to erythroid precursors of 1.5:1 to 4:1. Red marrow can increase its activity and replace some of the yellow marrow when needed. The spleen is important in culling erythrocytes and pitting erythrocyte inclusions. The liver also removes damaged or aged erythrocytes, leukocytes, and platelets but is not as discriminatory a filter as the spleen.

Blood cells are derived from pluripotential stem cells in the bone marrow. Under the influence of specific hematopoietic growth factors, this cell may proliferate and differentiate into all hematopoietic cell lines. The stem cells are capable of self-renewal. Hematopoietic progenitor cells are stimulated to proliferate and differentiate by hematopoietic growth factors. The growth factors include colony-stimulating factors and interleukins. They interact with their target cell by means of unique transmembrane cell receptors. Upon attachment of the growth factor to its receptor, a signal is sent across the cell membrane to the cytoplasm and eventually the nucleus. These factors tend to function in the microenvironment of the marrow. Stromal cells in the marrow also play a vital role in cell differentiaion and proliferation.

REVIEW QUESTIONS

1. In a patient with chronic blood loss and increased erythropoietin stimulation, the bone marrow will probably show:
   a. increased M:E ratio
   b. erythrocyte hyperplasia
   c. erythrocyte hypoplasia
   d. increased yellow marrow

2. A growth factor that influences differentiation of the CFU-GM into granulocytes is:
   a. M-CSF
   b. IL-1
   c. SCF
   d. G-CSF

3. The central cell in the erythroblastic island is the:
   a. macrophage
   b. erythroblast
   c. megakaryocyte
   d. Kupffer cell

4. A M:E ratio of 1:2 in the bone marrow is:
   a. normal for adults
   b. decreased
   c. increased
   d. normal for infants

5. With extensive pitting of erythrocyte inclusions by the spleen, one would expect to find which of the following on a peripheral blood smear?
   a. target cells
   b. erythrocyte fragments
   c. spherocytes
   d. macrocytes

6. In hypersplenism one would expect to find:
   a. thrombocytosis
   b. bone marrow hypoplasia
   c. bone marrow hyperplasia
   d. leukocytosis

7. The following cell is most sensitive to erythropoietin stimulation:
   a. reticulocyte
   b. CFU-GEMM
   c. BFU-E
   d. CFU-E

8. All hematopoietic cells are derived from the CFU-GEMM except:
   a. lymphocytes
   b. platelets
   c. erythrocytes
   d. granulocytes

9. This organ is important in maturation of T-lymphocytes:
   a. lymph nodes
   b. liver
   c. spleen
   d. thymus

10. Bone marrow stroma is composed of these two major cell types:
    a. macrophages and adipocytes
    b. macrophages and reticular cells
    c. reticular cells and adipocytes
    d. myeloid and erythroid precursors

REFERENCES

1. Montiel, M.: Bone Marrow. In Clinical hematology and fundamentals of hemostasis. Edited by D. Harmening. Philadelphia, FA Davis, Co., 1992.
2. Baldwin, J.G.: Hematopoietic function in the elderly. Arch Intern Med 148: 2544, 1988.
3. Till, J.E., McCulloch, E.A.: A direct measurement of the radiation sensitivity of normal mouse bone marrow cells. Radiat Res 14:213, 1961.
4. Magli, M.C., Iscove, N.N., Odartchenko, N.: Transient nature of early haemopoietic spleen colonies. Nature 295:527, 1982.
5. McCulloch, E.A., et al: The cellular basis of the genetically determined hematopoietic defect in anemic mice of genotype SI/SId. Blood 26:399,1965.
6. Eastment, E. Ruscetti, F.W.: Generation of erythropoiesis in long-term bone marrow suspension cultures. J Supramolec Struct Cell Biochem(Suppl):lll, 1981.
7. Becker, A.J., McCulloch, E.A., Till, J.E.: Cytological demonstration of the clonal nature of spleen colonies derived from transplanted mouse marrow cells. Nature 197:452, 1963.
8. Prchal, J.T., et al: A common progenitor for human myeloid and lymphoidcells. Nature 274:590, 1978.
9. Emerson, S.F.: The stem cell model of hematopoiesis. In Hematology: Basic principles and procedures. Edited by R. Hoffman, E.J. Benz, S.J. Shattil, B. Furie, H.J. Cohen. New York, Churchill Livingstone, 1995.
10. Calabretta, B. and Baserga, R.: Control of cell growth and differentiation. In Hematology: Basic principles and procedures. Edited by R. Hoffman, E.J. Benz, S.J. Shattil, B. Furie, H.J. Cohen. New York, Churchill Livingstone, 1995.
11. Williams, GT, Smith CA, Spooncer E, Dexter TM, Taylor DR: Hematopoietic colony stimulating factors promote cell survival by suppressing apoptosis. Nature 343:76, 1990.
12. Koichiro, M and Krantz, SB: Apoptosis of human erythroid colony-forming cells is decreased by stem cell factor and insulin-like growth factor as well as erythropoietin. J Cell Phys 156:264, 1993.
13. Mertelsmann R.: Hematopoietic cytokines: From biology and pathophysiology to clinical application. Leukemia 7 Suppl 2:5168-77, 1993
14. Urhovac, R., Kusec R, Jaksic B.: Myeloid hemapoietic growth factors. Int J Clin Pharm Ther Tox 31(5):241, 1993.
15. Smith, S.P. and Yee, G.C.: Hematopoiesis. Pharmacotherapy 12 (2 Pt. 2): 11s, 1992.
16. Cherry, B, et al. Production of hematopoietic stem cell-chemotactic factor by bone marrow stromal cells. Blood 83(4):964, 1994.
17. Gordon, M.Y., Ford, A.M., and Greaves, M.F.: Cell interactions and gene expression in early hematopoiesis. Int J Cell Clon 8:11, Suppl 1, 1990.
18. Morstyn, G. and Burgess, A.W.: Hemopoietic growth factors: A review. Cancer Res 48: 5624, 1988.

19. Morstyn, G., et al. Stem cell factor is a potent synergistic factor in hematopoiesis. Oncology 51:205, 1994.

20. Galli, MC, Giardina, PV, Migliaccio AR, Migliaccio, G.: The biology of stem cell factor, a new hematopoietic growth factor involved in stem cell regulation. Int J Clin Lab Res 23:70, 1993.

21. McNiece, IK, Zsebo, KM: The role of stem cell factor in the hematopoietic system. Cancer Invest 11(6):724, 1993.

22. Langley, KE, et al. Soluble stem cell factor in human serum. Blood 81(3):656, 1993.

23. Gabrilove, J.L.: Introduction and overview of hematopoietic growth factors. Sem Hemat 26 (2, Suppl 2), 1, 1989.

24. Sherr, C.J.: Regulation of mononuclear phagocyte proliferation by colony-stimulating factor-1. Inter J Cell Clon 8 (Suppl 1): 46, 1989.

25. Adamson, J.W.: The promise of recombinant human erythropoietin. Sem Hematol 26 (2, Suppl 2): 5, 1989.

26. Arcenas, AG and Vadhan-R.: Hematopoietic growth factor therapy of myelodysplastic syndromes. Leukemia and Lymphoma suppl 2 (2):65, 1993.

27. Nemunaitis, J.: Use of hematopoietic growth factors in marrow transplantation. Curr Opin Oncol 6(2):139, 1994.

28. Castro-Malaspina, H: Aplastic anemia: Current concepts on pathogenesis and therapy. Mouv Rev Fr Hematol 35:183, 1993.

29. Kanz, L., Brugger, W., Brass, K., and Mertelsmann, R.: Combination of cytokines: current status and future prospects. Br J Haematol 79 (Suppl 1): 96, 1991.

30. Appelbaum, F.R.: The clinical use of hematopoietic growth factors. Sem Hematol 26 (3, Suppl. 3): 7, 1989.

The erythrocyte

3

KEY TERMS

normoblast
erythroblast
reticulocyte
pronormoblast
basophilic normoblast
polychromatophilic
 normoblast
orthochromatic normoblast
pyknotic
polychromatophilic
 erythrocyte
siderocytes
culled
integral proteins
peripheral proteins
glycolysis
hexose monophosphate
 shunt (HMP)
methemoglobin reductase
 pathway
Rapoport-Leubering shunt
Embden-Meyerhoff pathway
anemia
erythrocytosis
erythroprotein
heme
oxygen affinity
Bohr effect

INTRODUCTION

The erythrocyte (red blood cell) was one of the first microscopic elements recognized and described after the discovery of the microscope. For centuries, these corpuscles were considered inert particles with no function. In 1817, Francois Magendie diluted blood with water, found no microscopic corpuscles, and erroneously surmised that the erythrocytes seen by others probably were air bubbles.[1] We now know that erythrocytes suspended in water will burst, which explains Magendie's negative findings. Magendie eventually recognized his mistake and later provided a morphologic description of the erythrocyte. It was not until 1865, however, when Hoppe-Seyler discovered the oxygen-carrying capacity of the red pigment (hemoglobin) within the corpuscles, that the function of these "globules" began to be understood. Today, we recognize the erythrocyte as being one of the most highly specialized cells in the body.

MATURATION

Erythropoiesis is normally an orderly process through which the peripheral concentration of erythrocytes is maintained in a steady state. Hormonal stimulation of the committed erythroid stem cells (BFU and CFU-E) results in proliferation, differentiation, and maturation of precursor cells in the bone marrow. Nucleated erythrocyte precursors in the bone marrow are collectively called *normoblasts* or *erythroblasts*. The anuclear erythrocyte, a terminally differentiated cell, leaves the marrow and gains entry to the peripheral blood. Young erythrocytes with residual RNA are more accurately referred to as reticulocytes.

Bone marrow normoblast maturation occurs in an orderly and well-defined sequence. The process involves a gradual decrease in cell size, together with condensation and eventual expulsion of the nucleus. As the normoblast matures, there is a gradual increase in hemoglobin production. Although the stages of erythrocyte maturation are usually described in step-like fashion, the actual maturation is a gradual process. Some cells on a bone marrow smear may not conform to all of the particular criteria of a certain stage, and a judgment must be made. The more experience an individual has in examining blood and bone marrow specimens, the easier it becomes to make these judgments. The stages in order from most immature to mature cell are: pronormoblast (rubriblast), basophilic normoblast (prorubricyte), polychromatophilic normoblast (rubricyte), orthochromatic normoblast (metarubricyte), reticulocyte, and erythrocyte (Table 3-1).

The normoblasts generally spend from 5 to 7 days in the proliferating and maturing compartment of the bone marrow. After maturation in the bone marrow, the reticulocyte is released into the marrow sinuses and gains access to the peripheral blood. The released reticulocyte continues its maturation in the peripheral blood for another day. The mature circulating erythrocyte has a lifespan of 100 to 120 days. This lengthy lifespan accounts for the relatively small amount of erythroid marrow in comparison to the large circulating erythrocyte mass. A description of each stage in maturation as it appears on Wright's stained smears follows.

Pronormoblast

The *pronormoblast* (Fig. 3-1), the earliest recognizable erythrocyte precursor, is a unipotent cell originating from the pluripotent stem cell. It is committed to the erythrocytic lineage. Each pronormoblast produces between 8 and 32 mature erythrocytes. The pronormoblast is a large round cell with a diameter of 12 to 20 μm and a high nuclear:cytoplasmic ratio (N:C). The large bluish-purple staining nucleus takes up most of the cell volume and is surrounded by a small to moderate amount of deeply basophilic cytoplasm. The round homogeneous staining nucleus contains a fine linear network of chromatin often referred to as "lacy" chromatin. Although the chromatin pattern of the pronormoblast is fine, it appears coarser than that of any of the white cell blasts. One or more lighter staining nucleoli are readily visible. Frequently, the Golgi apparatus appears as a large unstained area adjacent to the nucleus. The unstained area surrounding the nucleus, the perinuclear halo, represents the mitochondria. Hemoglobin synthesis may be occurring at this stage, but, because of the large number of basophilic ribosomes, its visible presence is obscured. Upon specific stimulation,

TABLE 3-1 CHARACTERISTICS OF THE DEVELOPMENTAL STAGES OF THE ERYTHROCYTE AS SEEN ON ROMANOWSKY STAINED SMEARS

Cell	Cytoplasm	Nucleus
Pronormoblast	moderate amount; deep blue	large; fine chromatin pattern; nucleoli present
Basophilic normoblast	more than in pronormoblast; deep blue	coarsening of chromatin; nucleoli absent or indistinct
Polychromatophilic normoblast	abundant; grey-blue	chromatin irregular and clumped
Orthochromatic normoblast	pink to orange-pink; may have bluish tinge	chromatin heavily condensed
Reticulocyte	pink with bluish-tinge (polychromatophilic)	absent
Erythrocyte	pink to orange-pink	absent

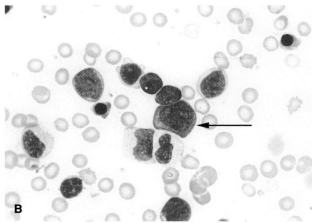

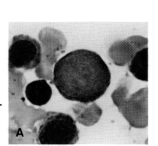

FIGURE 3-1. A, Pronormoblast (bone marrow, 250×, Wright-Giemsa stain). B, Pronormoblast (250×, Wright-Giemsa stain).

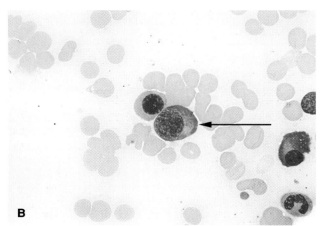

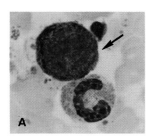

FIGURE 3-2. A, Basophilic normoblast (bone marrow, 250×, Wright-Giemsa stain). B, late basophilic normoblast (bone marrow, 250×, Wright-Giemsa stain).

the pronormoblast divides and matures to the basophilic normoblast.

Basophilic normoblast

The *basophilic normoblast* (Fig. 3-2) is smaller than the pronormoblast, ranging in size from 10 to 16 μm. The N:C ratio is decreased. The more abundant cytoplasm is deeply basophilic and is often more pronounced than in the pronormoblast. Varying amounts of hemoglobin may tinge the cytoplasm shades of pink. The nucleus shows a coarsening of the chromatin pattern and an absence of nucleoli. Occasionally, an indistinct nucleolus may be seen. A few small masses of clumped chromatin may be seen along the rim of the nuclear membrane.

Polychromatophilic normoblast

The *polychromatophilic normoblast* (Fig. 3-3) is reduced in size to 10 to 12 μm. The N:C ratio also is decreased. Nuclear chromatin is irregular and coarsely clumped. The most characteristic change of the cell at this stage is the presence of abundant grey-blue cytoplasm. The staining

properties of the cytoplasm are due to the synthesis of large amounts of hemoglobin (acidophilic) and decreasing numbers of ribosomes (basophilic). Thus, the cell derives its descriptive name, polychromatophilic, from the appearance of the cytoplasm. This is the last stage capable of mitosis.

Orthochromatic normoblast

The *orthochromatic normoblast* (Fig. 3-4) is between 8 and 10 μm in diameter. The nucleus, which occupies approximately one fourth of the cell volume, contains heavily condensed chromatin. Late stages are accompanied by

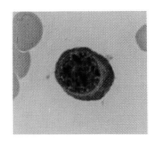

FIGURE 3-3. Polychromatophilic normoblast (bone marrow, 250×, Wright-Giemsa stain).

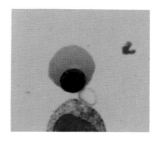

FIGURE 3-4. Orthochromatophilic normoblast (bone marrow, 250×, Wright-Giemsa stain).

a structureless *(pyknotic)*, fragmented nucleus, often eccentrically placed or partially extruded. The cytoplasm is predominantly pink or orange-pink with only a tinge of blue. These cells cannot synthesize DNA and thus, cannot divide.

Reticulocyte

The *reticulocyte* (Fig. 3-5) is a young erythrocyte without a nucleus but with residual RNA and mitochondria in the cytoplasm. The residual RNA gives the young cell a bluish tinge with Wright's stain. The cell is appropriately described as a *polychromatophilic erythrocyte*. After 2 to 2½ days in the bone marrow, the reticulocyte is released into the vascular sinuses of the marrow. Here it gains access to the peripheral blood. Reticulocyte maturation continues in the peripheral blood for another day.

Reticulocytes are slightly larger (8 to 10 μm) than mature erythrocytes and compose about 1% of circulating erythrocytes (50×10^9/L). These cells may be identified in vitro by reaction with supravital stains, new methylene blue, or brilliant cresyl blue, which cause precipitation of the RNA. In this method, the reticulocytes are identified by the presence of punctate purplish-blue inclusions.

Approximately 65% of the cell's hemoglobin is made during the normoblast stages. The remaining 35% of cellular hemoglobin is made during the reticulocyte stage. Normally, reticulocytes contain small amounts of iron that are dispersed throughout the cytoplasm in the form of hemosiderin or ferritin. These iron-containing cells are called *siderocytes* and may be identified with Perls' Prussian blue stain for iron. The spleen is responsible for removal of these excess granules, and the normal mature erythrocyte is devoid of granular inclusions.

Erythrocyte

The erythrocyte is a biconcave disc approximately 7 to 7.5 μm in diameter and 80 to 100 fL in volume. It stains pink to orange because of the large amount of the intracellular acidophilic protein, hemoglobin. The cell has lost its residual RNA and mitochondria as well as some important enzymes; therefore, it is incapable of synthesizing new protein or lipid. The normal erythrocyte lifespan is 100 to 120 days.

ERYTHROCYTE MEMBRANE

Membrane function

A normal intact membrane is absolutely essential for normal erythrocyte function and survival. Inherited or acquired abnormalities in membrane structure or composition may lead to severe anemia.

Around the beginning of the 20th century, investigations began that established the complexity of the erythrocyte membrane. Hedin performed experiments that demonstrated the osmotic properties and selective permeability of the erythrocyte.[2] He found that erythrocyte volume increased in hypotonic solutions and in solutions such as urea or glycerol. Solutions of sodium chloride or sucrose, however, caused shrinking of the cell. Antigenic properties of the membrane were recognized several years later by Landsteiner. He discovered that human sera caused clumping of the erythrocytes in different individuals. He originally divided these individuals into three groups, A, B, and C, according to their erythrocyte agglutination patterns with human sera.[3] Today, we use the terminology group A, B, and O to identify blood types on these agglutination patterns. Hundreds of other erythrocyte antigens have been identified in the last 80 years. Most have been discovered since 1940.

Studies of blood circulation have determined that the 7 μm erythrocyte must be a flexible (deformable) corpuscle to squeeze through the tiny 3 μm fenestrations of the capillaries of the spleen. The cell's deformability is not only a property of the erythrocyte membrane but also of the fluidity of the cell's content, mainly hemoglobin. Reversible deformability of the membrane occurs when the cell changes geometric shape but the surface area remains constant. Any decrease in deformability of membrane or fluidity of content results in decreased erythrocyte deformability. Consequently, the cell becomes trapped in the splenic cords and is destroyed by macrophages. Decreased deformability also leads to fragmentation of the cell under the normal stress of circulation. The erythrocyte could be compared with a plastic sandwich bag partially filled with

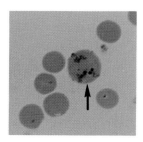

FIGURE 3-5. Reticulocyte (new methylene blue stain, 850×, peripheral blood).

TABLE 3-2 *ERYTHROCYTE MEMBRANE COMPOSITION*

I. Lipids
   A. Unesterified cholesterol
   B. Phospholipids
      cephalin
      lecithin
      sphingomyelelin
      phosphatidylserine
   C. Glycolipids
II. Proteins
   A. Integral proteins
      glycophorins A, B, C
      band 3
   B. Peripheral proteins
      spectrin
      actin
      ankyrin (band 2.1)
      band 4.2
      band 4.1
      adducin
      band 4.9 (dematin)
      tropomyosin

water. The deformability of the plastic and the fluidity of the contents make it easy to distort the bag into various shapes. If the plastic is replaced with glass or if the fluid content is made rigid by freezing, the bag will lose its deformability and break under forces that tend to distort it.

Membrane composition

The erythrocyte membrane is a biphospholipid protein complex composed of 52% protein, 40% lipid, and 8% carbohydrate (Table 3-2).[4] This chemical structure and composition control the membrane functions of transport and flexibility and determine the membrane's antigenic properties. Any defect in structure or alteration in chemical composition may alter any or all functions and lead to premature death of the cell. Mature erythrocytes lack the cellular organelles (nucleus and mitochondria) and enzymes necessary to synthesize new lipid and protein; thus, extensive damage to the membrane cannot be repaired, and the damaged cell will be selected (*culled*) and removed from the circulation by the spleen.

LIPID COMPOSITION

Approximately 95% of the lipid content of the membrane consists of equal amounts of unesterified cholesterol and phospholipids. The remaining lipids are free fatty acids and glycolipids. Cholesterol affects the surface area of the cell and is responsible for the passive cation permeability of the membrane. It appears that membrane cholesterol exists in free equilibrium with plasma cholesterol. Thus, it is not surprising that increases in free plasma cholesterol, such as occurs in lecithin-cholesterol acyl transferase (LCAT) deficiency, result in accumulation of cholesterol on erythrocyte membranes. These cholesterol-loaded erythrocytes appear distorted with the formation of target cells and spicules. Studies on the effects of cholesterol in model membranes indicate that an increase in the cholesterol to phospholipid ratio increases the microviscosity and the degree of order of the membrane. Reticulocytes normally contain more membrane cholesterol than older erythrocytes. This excess cholesterol is removed from the reticulocytes during maturation by the spleen. Patients who have undergone splenectomy usually have increased numbers of target cells on a blood smear because of the abnormal accumulation of cholesterol on the membrane.

Although minor traces of other phospholipids, such as lysolecithin, are present, there are four main types of phospholipids—phosphatidylethanolamine (cephalin), phosphatidylcholine (lecithin), sphingomyelin, and phosphatidylserine—found in the erythrocyte membrane. Exchange between phospholipids of the membrane and plasma may occur, especially with lecithin. There is a direct correlation between the fatty acid content of the diet and the plasma. Therefore, the fatty acid content of the diet may have an effect on the fatty acid composition of phospholipids in the erythrocyte membrane.

The phospholipid molecules are arranged with polar heads directed to the inside and outside of the cell and the hydrophobic tails directed to the interior of the bilayer. Considerable evidence exists that the mobility of phospholipids within the membrane contribute to membrane fluidity. Intramolecular movement of the hydrophobic tails is accompanied by lateral movement of molecules through the lipid layer. It is interesting to note that lipid associated with membrane penetrating proteins (integral proteins) appears to diffuse as a unit with the proteins. The function of these lipid-associated proteins is intimately involved with the lipid. Membrane enzymes associated with lipid require the presence of the lipid for full enzymatic activity.

A small portion of membrane lipids are glycolipids in the form of glycosphingolipid. The two groups of glycosphingolipid, cerebrosides and gangliosides, are sugar derivatives of ceramides. Glycolipids are responsible for some antigenic properties of the membrane.

PROTEIN COMPOSITION

Erythrocyte membrane proteins are of two types: integral proteins and peripheral proteins (Fig. 3-6). Integral proteins are firmly entrenched in the lipid bilayer, whereas peripheral proteins are outside the lipid framework on the cytoplasmic side of the membrane but attached to the membrane lipids or integral proteins by ionic and hydrogen bonds. Both types of membrane protein are synthesized during cell development. The proteins are usually identified by a number according to their separation by polyacrylamide gel electrophoresis in sodium dodecyl sulfate (Fig. 3-7).

Integral proteins consist of two types: glycophorins and band 3 protein.

Glycophorins The three major glycophorins, glycophorins A, B, and C, are made up of three domains, the cyto-

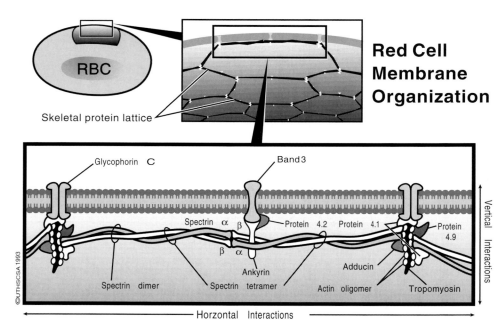

Red Cell Membrane Organization

FIGURE 3-6. A model of the organization of the erythrocyte membrane showing the peripheral and integral proteins and lipids. Spectrin is the predominant protein of the skeletal protein lattice. Spectrin dimers join head-to-head to form spectrin tetramers. At the tail end, spectrin tetramers come together at the junctional complex. This complex is composed of actin oligomer and stabilized by tropmyosin, which sits in the groove of the actin filaments. Band 4.9 protein (dematin) binds to actin and bundles actin filaments. Spectrin is attached to actin by protein 4.1, which also attaches the skeletal lattice to the lipid membrane via its interaction with glycophorin C. Adducin binds to two spectrin heterodimers. Ankyrin links the skeletal protein network to the inner side of the lipid bilayer via band 3. Protein 4.2 interacts with ankyrin and band 3.

plasmic domain, the hydrophobic domain, which spans the bilayer, and the extracellular domain on the exterior surface of the membrane.[4] The extracellular domain is glycosylated. Glycophorin A carries the MN antigens, glycophorin B carries the Ss antigens, and glycophorin C carries the Gerbich antigen. Glycophorin C also plays a role in attaching the skeletal protein network on the cytoplasmic side to the bilipid layer through its interaction with protein 4.1. The carboxyl (COOH) group of sialic acid, which is attached to the membrane glycophorins, imparts a strong negative charge to the exterior of the cell. This charge is important in reducing erythrocyte interaction.

Band 3 protein Band 3 is important in attaching the skeletal protein network to the lipid bilayer and will be discussed below.

Peripheral membrane proteins are organized into a two-dimensional lattice network directly laminating the inner side of the membrane lipid bilayer. The horizontal interactions of this lattice are parallel to the plane of the membrane and serve as a skeletal support for the membrane lipid layer. The vertical interactions are perpendicular to the plane of the membrane and serve to attach the lattice network to the lipid layer of the membrane. The skeletal proteins give membranes their viscoelastic properties and contribute to cell shape, deformability, and membrane stability. It is not unusual to find that defects in this erythrocyte cytoskeleton are associated with abnormal cell shape, abnormal stability, and hemolytic anemia.

The peripheral proteins include spectrin, actin, ankyrin (band 2.1), band 4.2, band 4.1, adducin, band 4.9 (dematin), and tropomyosin.

Spectrin, actin, band 4.1, adducin, band 4.9, and tropomyosin provide the structural framework for the lipid bilayer, while ankyrin interacts with band 4.2 and band 3 to attach the structural skeleton to the lipid layer of the membrane.

The skeletal protein lattice consists of highly ordered hexagons (sometimes hepatagons and pentagons) (Fig. 3-6). Spectrin is the predominant structural protein of the lattice that forms the arms of the hexagon. Spectrin is a long dimeric protein composed of two chains, α (band 1) and β (band 2), that are intertwined. These dimeric chains associate head-to-head to form tetramers. The tail regions

BAND #	PROTEIN	~ MOLECULAR WEIGHT	~#/CELL
1	SPECTRIN (α chain)	240,000	200,000
2	SPECTRIN (β chain)	220,000	200,000
2.1	ANKYRIN	215,000	100,000
3	PROTEIN 3	~90,000	1,200,000
4.1	PROTEIN 4.1	80,000	200,000
4.9	PROTEIN 4.9	48,000	100,000
5	ACTIN	42,000	500,000
6	G3PD	36,000	
7	TROPOMYOSIN	29,000	
	GLOBIN	17,000	

FIGURE 3-7. Polyacrylamide gel electrophoresis in sodium dodecyl sulfate of the major red cell membrane proteins. Proteins are identified according to the band number as separated by this process. (With permission from: Platt, O.S.: Inherited disorders of red cell membrane proteins. In: Genetically Abnormal Red Cells. Volume II, Edited by R.O. Nagel. Boca Raton, CRC Press, 1988.)

of the spectrin tetramers come together in hexagons at the junctional complexes. The junctional complexes are composed of short actin oligomers associated with other proteins. The interaction between actin and spectrin is not completely understood, but the association of these two proteins requires band 4.1 protein. Adducin promotes the binding of spectrin to actin but presumably competes with band 4.1 protein for a binding site. Tropomyosin is believed to sit in the groove of the actin oligomers, increasing actin stability. Band 4.9 protein appears to interact with actin, but little is known about its function.[6]

This skeletal lattice is attached to the membrane by several associations. Ankyrin serves to link the skeletal protein network to the inner side of the lipid bilayer. It binds near the center of the spectrin tetramers (a short distance from the head-to-head association site) to band 3 protein, an integral membrane protein. There is one ankyrin molecule for each spectrin tetramer. Band 4.2 protein interacts with ankyrin and band 3. Band 3 protein supports an oligosaccharide on the outside surface of the membrane that can express the I and i blood group antigen. On the cytoplasmic side of the membrane, band 3 binds hemoglobin and glycolytic enzymes in addition to ankyrin.[6] Band 3 protein is the anion transporter, exchanging HCO_3^- or Cl^- across the membrane. At the distal end of the spectrin tetramer, spectrin is bound to the membrane via band 4.1 protein and glycophorin C.

The skeletal proteins are not static but rather are in a continuous disassociation-association equilibrium with each other and with attachment sites. This occurs in response to various physical and chemical stimuli that affect the erythrocytes' journey while moving throughout the body.

Another membrane component that deserves mention because of its effect on the membrane is calcium. Most intracellular calcium (80%) is found in association with the erythrocyte membrane. Calcium is maintained at an extremely low intracellular concentration by the activity of an adenosine triphosphate (ATP)-fueled pump. Conditions that allow accumulation of this cation in the erythrocyte result in irreversible echinocyte formation and reduced deformability. The abnormal erythrocyte shape is assumed to be produced by calcium-induced irreversible cross-linking and alteration of the cytoskeletal proteins.

● ERYTHROCYTE METABOLISM

Before the 1930's, it was noted that *glycolysis* occurred in blood after it left the body, but contradictory data existed as to the reason for this process. Subsequently, researchers with meticulous sterile techniques proved that glycolysis does not occur in plasma but instead occurs within individual blood cells. Previous studies had used plasma contaminated with bacteria, which explained the observed glycolysis in plasma in these studies. Today, it is recognized that although glycolysis occurs in all blood cells, erythrocytes, because of their large numbers, are responsible for most glucose metabolism.

Studies by Gustav Embden and Otto Meyerhof con-

TABLE 3-3 *IMPORTANT METABOLIC PATHWAYS IN THE ERYTHROCYTE*

Metabolic Pathway	Function
Embden-Meyerhof pathway	Provides ATP for regulation of intracellular cation concentration (Na, K, Ca, Mg) via cation pumps
Hexose-monophosphate shunt	Provides NADPH and glutathione to reduce cellular oxidants
Rapoport-Leubering	Forms 2,3-BPG which facilitates oxygen release to the tissues
Methemoglobin reductase	Protects hemoglobin from oxidation via NADH and methemoglobin reductase

cerning glycolysis resulted in the step-by-step description of anaerobic glucose breakdown to lactate. The pathway they proposed served as an outline for later studies, which also revealed the details of intermediate steps such as production of 2,3-bisphosphoglycerate (2,3-BPG) also known as 2,3-DPG. The descriptive process of glycolysis led to the understanding of the metabolic processes of the erythrocyte. Much of the elucidation of these processes and their importance to the erythrocyte is the result of investigations of anemic patients. For example, in some individuals given primaquine, a prophylatic drug for malaria, severe hemolytic anemia with the presence of Heinz bodies developed. Studies revealed that glutathione was grossly deficient in these individuals after the drug was administered. The defect was identified as glucose-6-phosphate dehydrogenase (G6PD) deficiency, an enzyme in the hexose monophosphate (HMP) shunt that is responsible for the recycling of glutathione and, thus, the reduction of oxidants.

The metabolism of the erythrocyte is limited because of the absence of a nucleus, mitochondria, and other subcellular organelles. Although the binding, transport, and release of O_2 and CO_2 is a passive process not requiring energy, a variety of energy-dependent metabolic processes occur that are essential to cell viability. The most important metabolic pathways in the mature erythrocyte require glucose as a substrate. These pathways include (1) *Embden-Meyerhof pathway*, (2) *hexose-monophosphate shunt*, (3) *methemoglobin reductase pathway*, and (4) *Rapoport-Luebering shunt*. These pathways contribute energy for maintaining (1) high intracellular K^+, low intracellular Na^+, and very low intracellular Ca^{++} (cation pump); (2) hemoglobin in reduced form; (3) high levels of reduced glutathione; (4) membrane integrity and deformability (Table 3-3).

● Embden-Meyerhoff pathway

The erythrocyte obtains its energy in the form of ATP from glucose breakdown in the Embden-Meyerhoff pathway (Fig. 3-8). Approximately 90% to 95% of the cell's glucose consumption is used by this pathway. Normal erythrocytes have no glycogen deposits. They depend en-

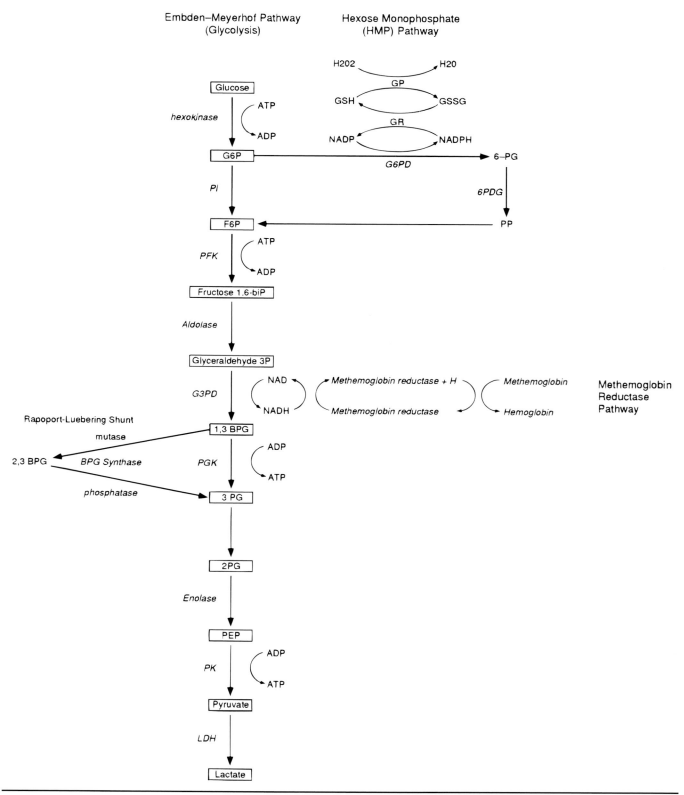

FIGURE 3-8. The erythrocyte metabolic pathways. The Embden-Meyerhof Pathway is the major source of energy for the erythrocyte through production of ATP. The hexose-monophosphate pathway is important for reducing oxidants by coupling oxidative metabolism with pyridine nucleotide (NADP) and glutathione (GSSG) reduction. The methemoglobin reductase pathway supports methemoglobin reduction. The Rapoport-Luebering shunt produces 2,3 BPG, (also known as 2,3 DPG) which alters oxygen affinity. (BPG—bisphosphoglycerate).

TABLE 3-4 *CONCENTRATION OF CATIONS IN THE RBC VS PLASMA*

Cation	RBC (mmoles/L)	Plasma (mmoles/L)
Sodium	5.4–7.0	135–145
Potassium	98–106	3.6–5.0
Calcium	0.0059–0.019	21–26.5
Magnesium	3.06	0.65–1.05

tirely on environmental glucose for glycolysis. Glucose enters the cell by facilitated diffusion, an energy-free process. The glucose is metabolized to lactate, producing a net gain of two moles of ATP per mole of glucose.

Adequate amounts of ATP are necessary to maintain erythrocyte shape, flexibility, and membrane integrity through regulation of intracellular cation concentration. The cations, Na^+, K^+, Ca^{++}, and Mg^{++}, are maintained in the erythrocyte at levels much different than in plasma (Table 3-4). Sodium and Ca^{++} are more concentrated in the plasma while K^+ and Mg^{++} are more concentrated within the cell. Normally, erythrocyte osmotic equilibrium is maintained both by the selective permeability of the membrane and by the cation pumps located in the cell membrane. The Na^+, K^+ pump hydrolyzes one mole of ATP in the expulsion of $3Na^+$ and the uptake of $2K^+$. Calcium is maintained in low concentration by the action of a similar but separate cation pump that also uses ATP for fuel. Excess Ca^{++} leakage into the cell or failure of the pump causes rigid shrunken cells with protrusions (echinocytes). Calcium also plays a role in maintaining low membrane permeability to Na^+ and K^+. An increase in intracellular calcium is associated with excess K^+ leakage from the cell. Magnesium is another major intracellular cation. This divalent cation reacts with ATP to form the substrate complex, Mg-ATP, for Ca^{++}, Mg^{++}-ATPase (calcium cation pump). Although Mg^{++} itself is necessary for active extrusion of Ca^{++} from the cell through this complex formation, Mg^{++} is not moved out of the cell in the process.

Enormous amounts of ATP are needed to maintain normal levels of these intracellular cations against their concentration gradients. Increased osmotic fragility is noted in cells with abnormally permeable membranes and/or decreased production of ATP. Upon the exhaustion of glucose, the fuel for the cation pumps is no longer available. Thus, cells cannot maintain normal intracellular cation concentrations, which leads to cell death.

● **Hexose monophosphate shunt**

Five percent of cellular glucose enters the oxidative HMP shunt, an ancillary system for producing reducing substances (Fig. 3-8). This pathway produces reduced nicotinamide adenine dinucleotidephosphate (NADPH) and glutathione.

Reduced glutathione (GSH) protects the cell from per-

manent oxidant injury. Oxidants within the cell will oxidize hemoglobin sulfhydryl (-SH) groups unless the oxidants are reduced by GSH. This reduction process oxidizes glutathione (GSSG), which in turn is reduced back to GSH by adequate levels of NADPH. The erythrocyte normally maintains a large ratio of NADPH to $NADP^+$. Failure to maintain reducing power through adequate levels of GSH or NADPH leads to oxidation of hemoglobin -SH groups, followed by denaturation and precipitation of hemoglobin in the form of Heinz bodies. Heinz bodies attach to the cell membrane and are removed from the cell with a portion of the membrane by macrophages in the spleen. If large portions of the membrane are damaged in this manner, the whole cell may be removed. Reduced glutathione also is responsible for maintaining reduced -SH groups at the membrane level. Decreases in GSH lead to oxidant injury of membrane -SH groups, resulting in leaky cell membranes. Cellular depletion of ATP may then occur because of increased consumption of energy by the cation pump.

● **Methemoglobin reductase pathway**

The methemoglobin reductase pathway, an offshoot of the Embden-Meyerhof pathway, is essential to maintain heme iron in the reduced state, Fe^{++} (Fig. 3-8). Hemoglobin with iron in the ferric state, Fe^{+++}, is known as methemoglobin. This form of hemoglobin cannot combine with oxygen. Methemoglobin reductase together with NADH produced by the Embden-Meyerhof pathway protect the heme iron from oxidation. In the absence of this system, the 2% of methemoglobin formed daily will eventually build up to 20% to 40%, severely limiting the oxygen-carrying capacity of the blood. Challenges by oxidant drugs can interfere with methemoglobin reductase and cause even higher levels of methemoglobin. This results in cyanosis.

● **Rapoport-Leubering shunt**

The Rapoport-Leubering shunt is a part of the Embden-Meyerhof pathway (Fig. 3-8). This pathway bypasses the formation of 3-phosphoglycerate and ATP from 1,3-diphosphoglycerate (1,3 DPG). Instead, 1,3 DPG forms 2,3 diphosphoglycerate catalyzed by a mutase and DPG synthase. Thus, the erthrocyte sacrifices one of its two ATP producing steps to form 2,3-DPG. DPG is present in the erythrocyte in a concentration of one mole BPG/mole hemoglobin and binds strongly to deoxyhemoglobin, holding the hemoglobin in the deoxygenated state and facilitating oxygen release. Increases in BPG concentration facilitate the release of oxygen to the tissues by causing a decrease in hemoglobin affinity for oxygen. Thus, the erythrocyte has a built-in mechanism for regulation of oxygen delivery to the tissues.

● **ERYTHROCYTE KINETICS**

In the middle of the 19th century, Dr. Jourdanet, a French physician practicing in the highlands of Mexico, noted that patients with altitude sickness exhibited symptoms similar to those of patients with anemia at sea level.[1] Patients with altitude sickness, however, had no decrease in red corpuscles, as was typical of anemic patients at sea level. He also noted that his surgical patients in the highlands had more than the normal number of red corpuscles and that their blood flowed more slowly than normal. He believed that the increased number of red corpuscles in an individual at high altitude compensated for the reduced atmospheric pressure of oxygen. It was not until 1890, however, that the increase in erythrocytes was accepted as an acquired adjustment to high altitude. The adjustment was noted by Viault, when he observed an increase in his own erythrocytes after an ascent to 15,000 feet.

Over the following decades, it was discovered that the stimulation of erythropoiesis in the bone marrow in response to decreased oxygen pressure was the result of a hormone, erythropoietin. Erythropoietin is released into the peripheral blood by renal tissue sensitive to hypoxia. It is now recognized that through this hormonal control, erythrocyte mass is closely regulated and is normally maintained in a steady state within narrow limits.

● Erythrocyte concentration

The normal erythrocyte concentration varies with sex, age, and geographic location. A high erythrocyte count (5.2×10^{12}/L) and hemoglobin concentration (19 g/dL) at birth are followed by a gradual decrease, which continues until approximately the second or third month of extrauterine life. At this time, erythrocyte and hemoglobin values reach a nadir of 3.5×10^{12}/L and 10 to 11 g/dL, respectively.

This erythrocyte decrease in infancy is sometimes called the "physiologic anemia" of the newborn. The most likely cause for physiologic anemia of the newborn is a cessation of bone marrow erythropoiesis after birth due to an extremely low concentration of erythropoietin. Erythropoietin levels are high in the fetus because of the relatively hypoxic environment in vivo and the high oxygen affinity of hemoglobin F (fetal hemoglobin). After birth, however, when the lungs replace the placenta as a means of providing oxygen, the arterial blood oxygen saturation rises from 45% to 95%. Erythropoietin cannot be detected in the plasma from about the first week of extrauterine life until the second or third month. Reticulocytes reflect the differences in bone marrow activity at this time. At birth and for the next few days, the reticulocyte count is high (mean, 3.2%). Within 1 week, the count drops to 0.5% and remains low until about the second month. A very gradual rise in hemoglobin and erythrocyte concentration continues from the second month after birth until adult levels are reached at about 17 years of age.[8] Males have a higher erythrocyte concentration than females, but this difference does not become apparent until adolescence (approximately 12 years of age). Older individuals (older than 70 years of age) have erythrocyte concentrations within the reference range.[9,10]

Individuals living at high altitudes have higher mean erythrocyte concentrations than those living at sea level.

Decreases in the partial pressure of atmospheric oxygen at high altitudes results in a physiologic increase in erythrocytes. This is in an attempt by the body to provide adequate tissue oxygenation.

DECREASED ERYTHROCYTE MASS

A decrease in the erythrocyte mass and consequently in hemoglobin concentration results in tissue hypoxia. This causes the prevalent hematologic disorder called *anemia*. This decrease in erythrocytes in proportion to plasma produces decreased blood viscosity, which may, at least partially, compensate for the anemia by increasing the rate of blood flow to hypoxic tissues. Anemia, although not a diagnosis in itself, is an important clinical sign of many different pathologies (iron deficiency, hemolysis, malignancy, and so forth). If the underlying pathology is successfully treated, erythrocyte concentration returns to normal.

INCREASED ERYTHROCYTE MASS

Increased erythrocyte mass, *erythrocytosis,* is seen much less frequently than decreased erythrocyte mass. Many of the clinical signs of erythrocytosis are related to the accompanying increase in blood viscosity. Erythrocytosis may be either relative or absolute. Relative increases are produced by a decrease in plasma volume with a normal erythrocyte mass such as occurs in dehydration. Recently, it has been shown that mental stress and orthostatic exercise are associated with a relative increase in erthrocyte concentration.[11] Absolute eythrocytosis is due to an actual increase in erythrocyte mass. This condition may be found in disorders that prevent adequate tissue oxygenation, such as high oxygen-affinity hemoglobins and pulmonary disorders. Rarely, erythrocytosis is caused by a primary defect associated with unregulated proliferation of committed erythroid stem cells.

● Erythropoietin

Erythropoietin (EPO) is a thermostable, nondialyzable, glycoprotein renal hormone, with a molecular weight (MW) of approximately 34,000 Daltons. It stimulates erythropoiesis in the bone marrow.[12] Erythropoietin is secreted by the kidney in response to cellular hypoxia. The hypoxic signal is detected by oxygen sensors located in the kidneys. This feedback control of erythropoiesis is the mechanism by which the body maintains optimal erythrocyte mass for tissue oxygenation. Erythropoietin has been defined in biologic terms to have an activity of 7000 units (U) per mg protein.[1] Normal plasma contains between 3 and 8 mU of EPO per milliliter of plasma. Erythropoietin also may be found in the urine at concentrations proportional to those found in the plasma, normally approximately 1 to 4 mU/mL.

In anemia, the actual titer of EPO is related to both hemoglobin concentration and the pathophysiology of the anemia. For example, patients with pure erythrocyte aplasia show EPO titers 4 times greater than patients with iron deficiency anemia and 10 times greater than those with megaloblastic anemia, even though hemoglobin concentration in all three types of anemia may be similar. Serum EPO levels are significant because they reflect not only EPO production but also its disappearance from the blood or utilization by the bone marrow. Between 3 and 8 mU/mL EPO can maintain normal steady-state erythropoiesis, whereas it takes between 2000 and 5000 mU/mL EPO to increase erythropoiesis to 10 times normal, which is necessary in severe bleeding or hemolytic anemia. The reason for this steep increase in EPO is unknown.

Patients with renal disease and those who have undergone nephrectomy usually are anemic but continue to make erythrocytes and produce limited amounts of EPO in response to hypoxia. These findings suggest that an extrarenal source of erythropoietin exists, most probably the liver; however, studies of anemic rats have demonstrated that the ability of the extrarenal tissue in rats to produce EPO is limited to about 20% of the total EPO concentration. In addition, the adult liver appears to require a more severe hypoxic stimulus for EPO production than the kidney. The role of the liver in EPO production is probably associated with its role in EPO production during the fetal and neonatal periods. In sheep, the switch from liver to kidney production of EPO is initiated in untero but is not complete until after birth.[13] This is probably a genetically predetermined event.[14]

The most important action of EPO is stimulation of committed stem cells, BFU-E and CFU-E, to proliferate and differentiate. Erythropoietin receptors on the cell membrane increase as the BFU-E matures to the CFU-E. These receptors decrease as pronormoblasts mature and are absent on the reticulocyte. The activity of the more immature BFU-E also is influenced by other growth factors, IL-3 and GM-CSF. The CFU-E, however, appear to be primarily controlled by EPO.

Other effects of EPO include decreasing cell maturation time, increasing rate of hemoglobin synthesis, and stimulating early release of bone marrow reticulocytes (stress or shift reticulocytes).

The normal bone marrow can increase erythropoiesis 5- to 10-fold in response to the appropriate EPO stimulation, if sufficient iron is available. In hemolytic anemia, there is a readily available supply of iron recycled from erythrocytes destroyed in vivo, which results in a sustained increase in erythropoiesis. The rate of erythropoiesis in blood loss anemia, where iron is lost from the body, however, is dependent on pre-existing iron stores. This rate of erythropoiesis usually does not exceed 2.5 times normal, unless large parenteral or oral doses of iron are administered.

Initially, increased erythropoietic activity is noted as a hypercellular bone marrow. The space, normally occupied by fat, is gradually taken over by hematopoietic cells. Large sustained increases in erythropoiesis, as is seen in chronic hemolytic anemias, may be accompanied by expansion of the marrow cavities. Expansion of the marrow cavity at the expense of cortical bone may cause bone deformities in children and pathologic fractures in adults. Hematopoiesis outside the bone marrow, extramedullary hematopoiesis, also may occur in chronic anemias. This type of hematopoiesis occurs primarily in the spleen and liver and may result in hepatosplenomegaly.

In addition to oxygen, other factors may have an influence on erythropoietin production and erythropoietic activity. It is well documented that testosterone stimulates erythropoiesis, which partially explains the difference in hemoglobin concentrations according to sex and age. Research has shown, however, that testosterone is unable to stimulate erythropoiesis in nephrectomized mice. It is probable that testosterone stimulates EPO production by the kidney rather than by directly stimulating the bone marrow unipotent stem cell.

Hormones from the pituitary, thyroid, and adrenal glands also effect erythropoiesis. Anemic patients with hypopituitarism, hypothyroidism, and adrenocortical insufficiency show an increase in erythrocyte concentration when the appropriate deficient hormone is administered. The reduction of EPO in hypothyroidism is probably the result of the reduced demand for cellular oxygen by metabolically inactive or hypoactive tissue.

Hypothalmus stimulation may cause an increase in release of EPO from the kidney, which could explain the association of polycythemia and cerebellar tumors. A number of other tumors have been reported to cause an inappropriate increase in erythropoietin production.

●
HEMOGLOBIN

The function of erythrocytes is to transport oxygen from the lungs to the tissue and carbon dioxide from tissue to lungs. Hemoglobin is the highly specialized intracellular erythrocyte protein responsible for performing this gaseous transport. Each gram of hemoglobin can carry 1.34 mL of oxygen.

Hemoglobin occupies approximately 33% of the volume of the erythrocyte and accounts for 90% of the cell's dry weight. Each cell contains between 27 and 32 pg of hemoglobin. In anemic states, the cell may contain less hemoglobin, thereby decreasing the oxygen-carrying capacity of the blood. The erythrocyte's membrane and its metabolic pathways are responsible for protecting and maintaining the hemoglobin molecule in its functional state. Abnormalities in the membrane that alter its permeability or alterations of the cell's enzyme systems may cause changes in the structure and/or function of the hemoglobin molecule and affect the capacity of this protein to deliver oxygen.

Although hemoglobin is synthesized as early as the pronormoblast stage, most hemoglobin synthesized during the nucleated red cell phase occurs in the polychromatophilic stage. Altogether, 65% of the cell's hemoglobin is made before the extrusion of the nucleus. The lack of a nucleus prevents the reticulocyte from programming the cell to make new RNA for protein synthesis, but residual RNA and mitochondria in the reticulocyte enable the cell to make the remaining 35% of the cell's hemoglobin. The mature erythrocyte contains no nucleus or mitochondria and is unable to program or synthesize new protein.

Hemoglobin concentration in the body is the result of

a fine balance between production and destruction of erythrocytes. The normal hemoglobin concentration in an adult male is approximately 15 g/dL, with a total blood volume of approximately 5000 mL. Therefore, the total body mass of hemoglobin is approximately 750 g.

$$15 \text{ g/dL} \times 5000 \text{ mL} \times 1 \text{ dL/100 mL} = 750 \text{ g}$$

Since the normal erythrocyte lifespan is 120 days, 1/120 of the total amount of hemoglobin must be synthesized each day to maintain a steady-state concentration. This amounts to approximately 6.25 g of new hemoglobin per day.

$$\frac{750 \text{ g}}{120 \text{ days}} = 6.25 \text{ g/day}$$

If each erythrocyte carries 30 pg of hemoglobin, 2×10^{11} new erythrocytes must be produced each day.

$$\frac{6.25 \text{ g/day}}{30 \text{ pg/cell}} \times 10^{12} \text{ pg/g} = 2 \times 10^{11} \text{ cells/day}$$

This figure amounts to a turnover of approximately 4% of the total erythrocyte population per day. The normal reticulocyte count is 0.8% to 2.5% for males and 0.8% to 4.0% for females.

● Structure

A molecule of hemoglobin contains four subunits (tetramer), each subunit containing a heme that is nestled in a hydrophobic crevice of a protein chain, globin (Fig. 3-9).

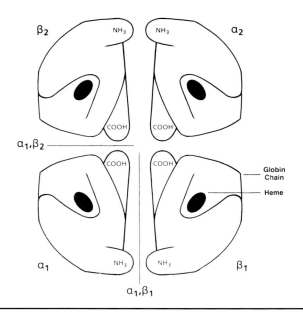

FIGURE 3-9. Hemoglobin is a molecule composed of four subunits. Each subunit has a globin chain with a heme nestled in a hydrophobic crevice. There are four different types of globin chains, α, β, δ, and γ, that occur in pairs. The globin chains present determine the type of hemoglobin. Depicted here is a hemoglobin A consisting of 2β and 2α chains. The contacts between the unlike chains α1 and β1 and α1 and β2 are important in maintaining the stability of the molecule. There is little contact between like chains α1 α2 and β1 β2.

Heme is a tetrapyrrole ring with a ferrous iron located in the center of the ring. This iron is complexed (coordination complex) with the F8 histidine of the associated globin chain. There are two identical pairs of globin chains in the hemoglobin tetramer. Each chain is wound up into 8 spiral or helical segments and attached by short, nonhelical segments. The helical segments are lettered A to H, starting at the amino end. The folding of the chains place the heme near the exterior of the molecule, where it is readily accessible to oxygen. Each heme can carry one molecule of oxygen; thus, each hemoglobin molecule can carry four molecules of oxygen.

Different types of hemoglobin are formed, dependent on the composition of the associated globin chain tetrads. The composition of these globin chains is responsible for the different functional and physical properties of hemoglobin. In normal adults, there are four types of globin chains produced: α, β, δ, and γ. A pair of α-chains combines with a pair of β, δ, or γ chains to form one of three types of hemoglobin: hemoglobin A, hemoglobin A_2, and hemoglobin F, respectively. The arrangement of each globin chain is similar. The α-chain has 141 amino acids while β-, δ-, and γ-chains have 146 amino acids. Hemoglobin A is the major adult hemoglobin, usually constituting 97% of the total hemoglobin. Hemoglobin A_2 and hemoglobin F are minor hemoglobins.

The four globin chains are held together by noncovalent bonds in a tetrahedral array, giving the hemoglobin molecule a nearly spherical shape. Although there is little contact between pairs of like chains (α, α and β, β), there is close contact between unlike chains (α and β). These close contacts between $\alpha_1\beta_1$ or $\alpha_2\beta_2$ allow little movement between the subunits. These α and β contacts are important in maintaining stability of the molecule. However, some conformational change of the hemoglobin molecule must occur to facilitate oxygen uptake and release under physiologic conditions. The $\alpha_1\beta_2$ and $\alpha_2\beta_1$ contacts are less firm and allow conformational change of the molecule as it goes from the oxygenated to the deoxygenated form. In the deoxygenated form, the distance between the β-chains increases by 7Å. Complete loss of the $\alpha_1\beta_2$ contact causes the dissociation of hemoglobin into dimers, $\alpha_1\beta_1$ or $\alpha_2\beta_2$.

HEME SYNTHESIS

Porphyrins are metabolically active only when chelated. *Heme* is an iron-chelated porphyrin ring that always functions as a prosthetic group of a protein. The porphyrin ring is composed of a flat tetrapyrrole ring with iron (Fe^{++}) inserted into the center. The iron is held in place by a coordination complex. Porphyrin ring synthesis starts in the mitochondria, continues in the cytoplasm, and then re-enters the mitochondria to incorporate iron. The final step in hemoglobin synthesis occurs in the cytoplasm; heme leaves the mitochondria to combine with the globin chains in the cytoplasm.

Heme synthesis begins with the condensation of glycine and succinyl coenzyme A (CoA) to form δ-aminolevulinic

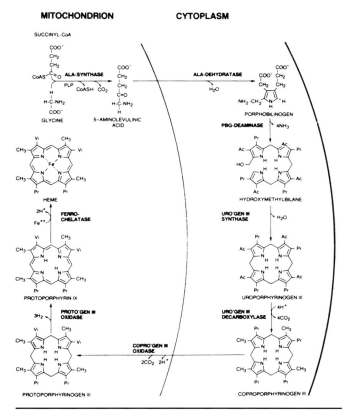

FIGURE 3-10. The synthesis of heme begins in the mitochondria with the condensation of glycine and succinlyl CoA. The product, Δ-aminolevulinate, leaves the mitochondria to form the pyrrole ring, porphobilinogen. The combination of four pyrroles to form a linear tetrapyrrole, the cyclizing of the linear form to uroporphyrinogen and the decarboxylation of the side chains to form coproporhyrinogen occurs in the cytoplasm. The final reactions, the formation of protoporphyrin IX and insertion of iron into the ring, occur in the mitochondria. (With permission from: Tietz NW: Fundamentals of Clinical Chemistry. Philadelphia: W. B. Saunders, 1987.)

of coproporphyrinogen III. Inside the mitochondria, the enzyme coproporphyrinogen-oxidative decarboxylase catalyzes the unsaturation of the porphyrin ring and conversion of propionate side chains to vinyl groups, forming protoporphyrinogen IX. Protoporphyrinogen is oxidized to protoporphyrin IX by protoporphyrinogen oxidase. The final step in the mitochondria is the chelation of iron with the protoporphyrin ring catalyzed by ferrochelatase.

GLOBIN SYNTHESIS

The synthesis of globin peptide chains occurs on polyribosomes in the cytoplasm. The type of chain synthesized is under genetic control. Most cells produce α- and β-chains for the formation of HbA, the major adult hemoglobin. Heme is inserted into the hydrophobic pocket near the surface of each globin chain (Fig. 3-11). An α and β globin chain combine to form the $\alpha\beta$ dimer. Two $\alpha\beta$ dimers combine to form the stable $\alpha_2\beta_2$ globin tetramer.

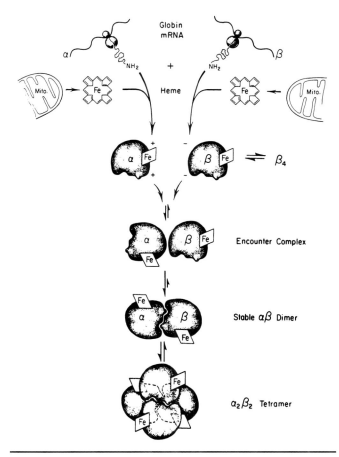

FIGURE 3-11. Assembly of hemoglobin. The α and β globin polypeptides are translated on their respective mRNAs. On binding of heme, the protein folds into its native three-dimensional structure. The binding of α and β hemoglobin subunits to each other is facilitated by electrostatic attraction. An unstable intermediate encounter complex can rearrange to form the stable $\alpha\beta$ dimer. Two dimers combine to form the functional $\alpha2\beta2$ tetramer. (With permission: Bunn HF: Subunit assembly of hemoglobin: An important determinant of hematologic phenotype. Blood, 69:1, 1987.)

acid (Δ-ALA) (Fig. 3-10). This reaction occurs in the mitochondria in the presence of pyridoxal phosphate, CoA, ferrous iron, and Δ-ALA synthetase. This reaction is an important control site in the synthesis of heme. The Δ-ALA leaves the mitochondria, and, in the cytoplasm, two linear Δ-ALA condense and cyclize to form the pyrrole, porphobilinogen. This dehydration reaction is catalyzed by the cytoplasmic enzyme, ALA dehydratase. This important intermediate, porphobilinogen, is the primary building block for formation of all natural tetrapyrroles, including not only heme but also cobalamins. In the next reaction, four porphobilinogen molecules condense to form a linear tetrapyrrole (hydroxymethylbilane), which subsequently cyclize to form uroporphyrinogen III. The cyclization reaction requires both uroporphyrinogen-I synthetase (porphobilinogendeaminase) and uroporphyrinogen-III cosynthetase. In the absence of cosynthetase, only the symmetric type I isomer, which has no physiologic role, is formed. Decarboxylation of the side chains of uroporphyrinogen, catalyzed by the cytoplasmic enzyme uroporphyrinogen decarboxylase results in the formation

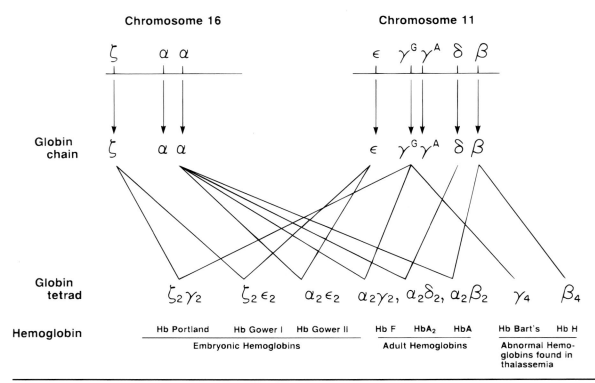

FIGURE 3-12. The genes for the globin chains are located on chromosome 11 and 16. The ζ chain appears to be the embryonic equivalent of the α chain, both of which are located on chromosome 16. Note the α gene is duplicated. The other globin genes are located on chromosome 11. The chains combine in two pairs to form the embryonic, fetal, and adult hemoglobins. One or more of the α genes are missing in an inherited condition called α thalassemia. Due to the shortage of α chains, the β and γ chains may form a tetrad of identical chains, β4 or γ4. These are hemoglobins with abnormal function.

● Ontogeny of hemoglobin

TYPES OF HEMOGLOBIN

Intrauterine erythropoiesis is associated with the production of embryonic hemoglobins, Gower I, Gower II, and Portland, in the first trimester of gestation. These embryonic hemoglobins are made from the combination of embryonic globin chains, $\zeta(\zeta)$ and $\epsilon(\epsilon)$ in pairs, or embryonic chains in combination with α (γ) and τ (τ) chains (Fig. 3-12). These primitive hemoglobins are detectable during hematopoiesis in the yolk sac and are not usually detectable after 8 weeks gestation because the production of embryonic chains ceases at this time.

Hemoglobin F (HbF) ($\alpha_2\gamma_2$) is the predominate hemoglobin formed during liver and bone marrow erythropoiesis in the fetus. HbF composes 90% to 95% of the total hemoglobin production in the fetus until 34 to 36 weeks of gestation. In adults, hemoglobin A (HbA), which consists of two α chains and two β chains ($\alpha_2\beta_2$), is the major hemoglobin. Although HbA is found as early as 9 weeks gestation, β-chain synthesis does not exceed that of γ-chain synthesis until after birth. Thus, the normal full-term infant has from 50% to 85% HbF. After birth, the percentage of HbA increases with the age of the infant until normal adult levels are reached by the end of the first year of life. HbF production constitutes less than 2% of the total hemoglobin of adults.

Most, if not all HbF in adults is restricted to a few erythrocytes sometimes referred to as F cells (less than 8% erythrocytes). From 13% to 25% of the hemoglobin in these F cells is HbF. The switch from HbF to HbA after birth is incomplete and, in part, reversible. For example, patients with hemoglobinopathies or anemia may have increased levels of HbF, often proportionate to the decrease in HbA. In bone marrow recovering from suppression, HbF levels often rise. This is due to small increases in HbF production within F cells in addition to an increase in the number of erythroblasts producing HbF.

HbA$_2$ appears late in fetal life, composes less than 1% of the total hemoglobin at birth, and reaches normal adult values after 1 year (1.8% to 3.5%).

CONTROL OF GLOBIN CHAIN SYNTHESIS

Globin chain synthesis is directed by eight genetic loci per haploid genome (Fig. 3-12). The genes controlling ζ-chain synthesis and the two genes controlling α-chain synthesis are located on chromosome 16. The ζ-chain, the fetal equivalent of the α-chain, is synthesized very early in embryonic development. After 8 weeks, ζ-chain synthesis is replaced by α-chain synthesis. All other globin genes are arranged in linear fashion in order of activation on chromosome 11. The ϵ-gene is located at one end of chromosome 11 and as it switches off, two γ-genes are activated. One γ-gene directs the production of a γ-chain with glycine at 136 position, γ^G, while the other directs the production of a γ-chain with alanine at 136 position, γ^A. The γ^G synthesis predominates before birth (3 : 1) but γ^G and γ^A synthesis are equal (1 : 1) in adults. The next two genes on chromosome 11, δ and β, are switched on to a small degree when the γ genes are activated, but they are not fully activated until γ-chain synthesis is switched off at about 35 weeks of gestation. The δ-chain differs from the β chain by only 10 of 146 amino acids, but the rate of synthesis of the δ-chain is only 1/40 that of the β-chain.

The mechanism governing the switch from γ chain synthesis to β chain synthesis after birth is not understood. Several hypotheses have been proposed to explain the switch: (1) stem cell clones exist with different globin chain biosynthetic capabilities; (2) the hematopoietic environment or a modulating factor may be responsible for programming cells to express specific globin chains; (3) chain production may be programmed according to the ontogenetic stage of the erythroid precursors.

It is unlikely that HbF is dependent on the clonal nature of erythroblasts. Studies of patients with clonal disorders such as polycythemia vera and chronic myelogenous leukemia show distribution of F cell frequency similar to that of the normal population. If HbF production were limited to particular clones, one would expect that when these clones became neoplastic, there would be a rise in HbF.

It also is unlikely that the environment of the developing stem cell determines the production of either γ or β chains since both HbA and HbF are synthesized in fetal liver, spleen, and bone marrow.

Studies have suggested that the synthesis of different globin chains occurs in sequence dependent on developmental stage. In vitro cultures of BFU-E from fetal liver, umbilical cord blood (neonatal), and adult blood show HbF production from these three sources to be, in decreasing concentration, fetal, neonatal, and adult. Moreover, the switch from fetal to adult hemoglobin synthesis is closely related to gestational age in humans. Premature infants switch over to adult hemoglobin synthesis later after birth than full-term infants. Likewise, postmature infants produce more hemoglobin A from birth. In one study, a 2-year-old boy with refractory acute leukemia was transplanted with liver cells from twin fetuses at an 18-week gestational age.[15,16] Within 2 weeks, regeneration of hematopoietic cells in the marrow occured. At 3 weeks after transplant, the bone marrow and peripheral blood cells were analyzed for globin chain synthesis. Typical fetal patterns of globin chain synthesis were revealed: the ratio of γ to γ plus β chains = 0.87 to 0.98. These findings suggest that the perinatal switch from Hgb F to Hgb A synthesis is probably time-controlled by a developmental clock. The clone of stem cells is gradually reprogrammed during the perinatal period, leading to a switching from γ-chain production to β-chain production.

● Regulation of hemoglobin synthesis

The key rate-limiting step in heme synthesis appears to be the initial reaction of glycine and succinyl-CoA to form Δ-ALA. Heme regulates this reaction by suppression of the synthesis and inhibition of the activity of Δ-ALA synthase. Studies of porphyrias, disorders characterized by the accumulation of heme precursors, show that heme suppression of Δ-ALA synthase synthesis is the major control mechanism for heme synthesis. Conversely, increased utilization or demand for heme will induce an increase in synthesis of Δ-ALA synthase. Any metabolic change that affects heme formation or degradation has the potential to affect heme biosynthesis.

Small amounts of free protoporphyrin and coproporphyrin are present in both normoblasts and erythrocytes. This free porphyrin may represent incomplete hemoglobin synthesis or residual products occurring after completion of hemoglobin synthesis. However, in pathologic conditions associated with inhibition or stimulation of heme biosynthesis, the concentration of free porphyrins increases. Normal free erythrocyte protoporphyrin (FEP, now referred to as zinc protoporphyrin, ZPP) concentration is 16 to 67 μg/dL of erythrocytes. Free coproporphyrin levels are lower, 0.7 to 2.3 μg/dL. Reference ranges for porphyrins and porphyrin precursors in the urine, feces, and erythrocytes are located in Table J in the Appendix.

Iron uptake by the developing erythrocyte is not finely regulated, and a block in heme synthesis, as occurs in lead poisoning, may lead to increased amounts of mitochondrial and/or cytoplasmic deposits of iron. Conversely, heme has been shown to inhibit the release of iron from transferrin, a feedback mechanism limiting the iron supply to the developing normoblast. Approximately 80% to 90% of the iron taken into the normoblast is converted into heme within an hour. The remainder is converted to ferritin or hemosiderin. In the absence of adequate amounts of iron, the erythrocyte continues to synthesize porphyrin, which accumulates in cells as zinc protoporphyrin.

The rate of globin synthesis is governed primarily by the rate at which the DNA code is transcribed to mRNA but is also modified by processing of mRNA, by the translational events of mRNA, and by the stability of globin mRNA. The α and β chains normally are synthesized in equal amounts.

The regulation of heme and globin synthesis are highly interrelated. If globin synthesis decreases, such as occurs in thalassemia, then porphyrin synthesis also decreases. If heme synthesis decreases, as in iron deficiency, then globin synthesis decreases.

● Function

The function of hemoglobin is transport and exchange of respiratory gases. The ease with which hemoglobin binds and releases oxygen is known as *oxygen affinity*. Increased oxygen affinity means the hemoglobin does not readily give up its oxygen, whereas decreased oxygen affinity means the hemoglobin releases its oxygen more readily. Hemoglobin-oxygen affinity is physiologically responsive and adjustable. Varying environmental conditions or physiologic demand for oxygen results in changes in erythrocyte parameters, which directly effect the oxygen affin-

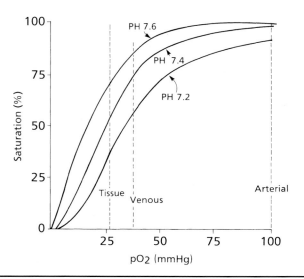

FIGURE 3-13. The oxygen affinity of hemoglobin is depicted by the oxygen dissociation curve (ODC). At a pH of 7.4 and an oxygen tension (PO2) of 26 mmHg hemoglobin is 50% saturated. If the pH increases to 7.6, the suture is shifted left, indicating increased oxygen affinity. Conversely, if the pH drops to 7.2, the curve is shifted right, indicating decreased oxygen affinity.

ity. In particular, pO_2, pH (H+), pCO_2, 2,3-DPG, and temperature effect oxygen affinity. Rapidly metabolizing tissue produces CO_2 and acid (H+) as well as heat. These factors decrease oxygen affinity and promote the release of oxygen from hemoglobin to the tissue. However, in the alveolar capillaries of the lungs, the high pO_2 and low pCO_2 drives off CO_2 and reduces H+, promoting the uptake of oxygen by hemoglobin (increasing oxygen affinity). Thus, pO_2, CO_2, and H+ facilitate the transport and exchange of respiratory gases.

Hemoglobin affinity for oxygen determines the proportion of oxygen released to the tissues or loaded onto the cell at a given oxygen pressure (pO_2). This may be graphically represented by the hemoglobin-oxygen dissociation graph (Fig. 3-13). If hemoglobin-oxygen saturation is plotted versus the partial pressure of oxygen (pO_2), a sigmoid-shaped curve results. Oxygen affinity of hemoglobin is usually expressed as the pO_2 at which 50% of the hemoglobin is saturated with oxygen (P_{50}). The P_{50} in humans is normally about 26 mmHg. When the curve is shifted to the right, oxygen affinity is decreased, which means more oxygen is released to the tissues at a higher oxygen tension. When the curve is shifted to the left, oxygen affinity is increased, and less oxygen is released to the tissues at a given oxygen tension.

The explanation for the sigmoid shape of the oxygen dissociation curve (ODC) is that hemoglobin is an allosteric protein. This refers to the way the binding of oxygen by a hemoglobin molecule depends on the interaction of the four heme groups, sometimes referred to as heme–heme interaction. The interaction of the heme groups is the result of movements within the molecule or tetramer triggered by the uptake of a single molecule of oxygen by one heme group. (Hemoglobin with oxygen is called oxyhemoglobin; hemoglobin without oxygen is called deoxyhemoglobin.) In the deoxy form, heme iron is 0.4 to 0.6 Å out of the plane of the porphyrin ring, displacing or moving the F8 histidine of the globin chain. Upon uptake of oxygen by one heme subunit, this iron moves into the plane of the porphyrin pulling the histidine with it. This movement causes other conformational changes within the subunit that lead to destabilization of the interactions between α and β globin chain subunits, consequently altering the deoxyhemoglobin structure. This alteration of the quaternary structure of deoxyhemoglobin triggered by the uptake of oxygen by one heme group facilitates the binding of oxygen by the other three heme units. Fewer subunit crosslinks need to be broken to bind each subsequent oxygen molecule. This cooperative binding of oxygen makes hemoglobin a very efficient oxygen transporter.

The sigmoid shape of the ODC results in the release of large quantities of oxygen from hemoglobin during small physiologic changes in pO_2. Note that the steepest part of the curve occurs at oxygen tensions found in tissues. This is physiologically of great importance for it allows the transfer of oxygen from the lungs to the tissues with only small changes in oxygen tension. The pO_2 in the arteries is about 95 to 100 mmHg. In the veins, the pO_2 drops to about 40 mmHg. The ODC shows that the oxygen saturation of hemoglobin drops from 100% in the arteries to 75% in the veins. This indicates hemoglobin gives up about 25% of its oxygen to the tissues (5 mL of O_2 per 100 mL blood).

The ODC can be altered, not only by pO_2, but also by the action of pCO_2, pH, and temperature. A decrease in pH enhances the release of oxygen from hemoglobin (decreases oxygen affinity), shifting the curve to the right. An increase in CO_2 and temperature also decrease the oxygen affinity of hemoglobin. The effects of pH on hemoglobin–oxygen affinity is known as the *Bohr effect*. The Bohr effect, an example of the acid-base equilibrium of hemoglobin, is one of the most important buffer systems of the body. A molecule of hemoglobin can accept a H^+ when it releases a molecule of oxygen (Fig. 3-14). Deoxyhemoglobin accepts and holds on to the H^+ better than oxyhemoglobin. In the tissues, the H^+ concentration is higher because of the presence of lactic acid and CO_2. When blood reaches tissue, the affinity of hemoglobin for oxygen is decreased by the H^+, thereby permitting the more efficient unloading of oxygen at these sites.

$$HHb + O_2 \longrightarrow Hb (O_2) + H^+$$
(T conformational state)   (R conformational state)

Thus, proton binding facilitates O_2 release and minimizes changes in the hydrogen ion concentration of the blood when tissue metabolism is releasing CO_2 and lactic acid. If there is a simultaneous decrease in the tissue pO_2, as occurs in heavy exercise, up to 75% of the hemoglobin oxygen can be released as the erythrocytes pass through the capillaries.

Carbon dioxide is carried to the lungs by three separate mechanisms: dissolved CO_2, bicarbonate, and bound to

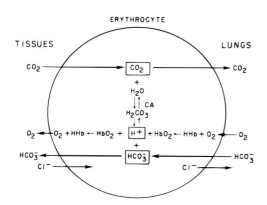

FIGURE 3-14. Interrelations of oxygen and carbon dioxide transport in the erythrocyte. Arrows to the left indicate direction of reactions taking place in the tissues; those to the right in the lungs. In the tissue, CO_2 diffuses into the erythrocyte and in the presence of carbonic anhydrase (CA), reacts with water to form bicarbonic acid. The bicarbonic acid dissociates into bicarbonate (HCO_3-) and a proton (H+). The HCO_3- is exchanged for chloride (Cl-) in the plasms (chloride shift). The proton is accepted by oxyhemoglobin (HbO_2) which, through the Bohr effect, facilitates the dissociation of oxygen. These reactions are reversed in the lungs because of the low pCO_2 and high pO_2. (From: Lee GR: Wintrobe's Clinical Hematology. Philadelphia, Lea & Febiger, 1993).

the N-terminus groups of hemoglobin (carbamino hemoglobin). Most of the carbon dioxide (70%) transported by the blood is in the form of bicarbonate, which is produced when carbon dioxide diffuses from the plasma into the erythrocyte. In the presence of the erythrocyte enzyme, carbonic anhydrase (CA), CO_2 reacts with water to form bicarbonic acid:

$$H_2O + CO_2 \xrightarrow{CA} H_2CO_3$$

Hydrogen ion and bicarbonate are liberated from carbonic acid and the H+ accepted by deoxyhemoglobin. (Fig. 3-14)

$$H_2CO_3 \longrightarrow H+ + HCO_3-$$

Hemoglobin histidine residues buffer approximately 50% of the H+ generated from bicarbonate production. Plasma proteins and phosphate buffer about 10% of the H+. The remaining 40% of the H+ is absorbed by the Bohr effect (see above). The free bicarbonate diffuses out of the erythrocyte into the plasma in exchange for plasma Cl- that diffuses into the cell, a phenomenon called the chloride shift. The bicarbonate is carried to the lungs by the plasma, where the pCO_2 is low. Here the bicarbonate is rapidly converted back into CO_2 and H_2O and expired.

Approximately 13% to 15% of the total CO_2 exchanged by the erythrocyte in respiration is through carbamino hemoglobin. Deoxyhemoglobin directly binds 0.4 moles of CO_2 per mole hemoglobin. Carbon dioxide reacts with uncharged N-terminal amino groups of the four globin chains to form carbamino hemoglobin. The remaining CO_2 is dissolved in the plasma and carried to the lungs.

A byproduct of the glycolytic pathway, 2,3-DPG, oc-

curs in the erythrocyte at almost equimolar quantities with hemoglobin. Its function is to modulate the oxygen affinity of hemoglobin. In the absence of DPG, the P_{50} of hemoglobin is 10 mmHg. Thus, hemoglobin affinity for oxygen in the absence of DPG is very high, and little oxygen would be released to the tissues. In the presence of physiologic concentrations of DPG, the P_{50} of hemoglobin is approximately 26 mmHg. Therefore, DPG decreases the oxygen affinity of hemoglobin by a factor of 2.6. Very little oxygen would be unloaded in the tissues where the pO_2 is about 26 mmHg, in the absence of DPG.

DPG binds preferentially to deoxyhemoglobin in a 1:1 ratio. The binding site for DPG is a cavity between the β globin chain subunits. DPG stabilizes the quaternary structure of deoxyhemoglobin by binding to the positive charges on both β chains, thereby crosslinking the chains. This stabilized deoxyhemoglobin form is known as the T (tense) structure. At high PO_2, such as that found in normal lungs, the oxygen saturates the hemoglobin. This changes the quartenary conformation, and DPG is released. The fully oxygenated form of hemoglobin is known as the R (relaxed) structure.

Several physiologic mechanisms of oxygen delivery can be explained by this hemoglobin–DPG interaction. When a person goes from sea level to high altitudes, the body adapts to the decreased atmospheric pressure of oxygen by releasing more oxygen to the tissues. This adaptation is mediated by increases of DPG in the erythrocyte, usually noted within 36 hours of ascent. (Erythrocyte mass also increases as a part of the adaptive mechanism to decreased pO_2.)

Fetal hemoglobin, HbF, has a high oxygen affinity compared with adult hemoglobin, HbA, facilitating the transfer of oxygen in utero from the maternal to the fetal circulation. Fetal blood's higher oxygen affinity is due in part to the fact that hemoglobin F binds DPG less stongly than hemoglobin A. The concentration of erythrocyte DPG is similar in adult and fetal cells, but because hemoglobin F does not bind DPG, fetal erythrocytes have a higher oxygen affinity than adult cells.

Blood stored at 4°C in acid-citrate dextrose loses 2,3-DPG rapidly in the first week of storage. A great deal of blood storage research has concentrated on maintenance of DPG without a concomitant fall in erythrocyte ATP. It is the decrease in DPG and ATP that limits the shelf life of stored blood. In most patients, transfused blood with low DPG levels does not constitute a problem. Normal levels of intracellular DPG are achieved within 8 to 24 hours after infusion. However, when large amounts of blood are transfused or in exchange transfusions, tissue hypoxia may occur due to the proportionally high quantity of transfused blood with low quantities of intracellular 2,3-DPG.

Acquired abnormal hemoglobins

The acquired abnormal hemoglobins are hemoglobins that have been altered post-translationally to produce molecules with comprimised oxygen transport, thereby causing hypoxia and/or cyanosis. The degree of hypoxia is related to the decrease in normal hemoglobin, while the degree of cyanosis is related to the concentration of the abnormal hemoglobin.

METHEMOGLOBIN

Methemoglobin is hemoglobin with iron in the ferric state (Fe^{+++}), which is incapable of reversibly combining with oxygen. Its very high oxygen affinity makes it useless as a respiratory pigment.[17] Normally, 2% methemoglobin is formed every day. At this concentration, the abnormal pigment is not harmful as the reduction in oxygen carrying capacity of the blood is insignificant. The accumulation of higher concentrations is held in control by several reducing systems: NADH methemoglobin reductase I, ascorbic acid, GSH, NADH methemoglobin reductase II, and NADPH methemoglobin reductase. Of these reducing systems, the most important, accounting for more than 60% of the reduction of methemoglobin, is NADH methemoglobin reductase I.

Methemoglobin formation may be the result of exposure to environmental toxicants. Increased levels of methemoglobin are formed when an individual is exposed to certain oxidizing chemicals or drugs. If the offending agent is removed, methemoglobinemia disappears within 24 to 48 hours.

Infants are more susceptible to methemoglobin production because HbF is more readily converted to methemoglobin and also because infants' erythrocytes are deficient in the reducing enzymes. Foods, drugs, or water high in nitrites may cause methemoglobinemia in this segment of the population.

Cyanosis develops when methemoglobin levels exceed 10% while hypoxia is produced at levels exceeding 60%. Methemoglobin may be reduced by medical treatment with methylene blue or ascorbic acid, which speeds up reduction by NADPH-reducing enzymes. In some cases of severe methemoglobinemia, exchange transfusions are helpful.

Methemoglobinemia also may result from congenital defects in the reducing systems mentioned above or from the presence of an abnormal hemoglobin. The most severe methemoglobinemia is caused by a deficiency or abnormality of the enzyme NADH methemoglobin reductase I. In this condition, cyanosis is observed from birth, and methemoglobin levels reach 10% to 20%. The oxygen affinity of normal hemoglobin is increased in these children, resulting in increased erythropoiesis and subsequently higher than normal hemoglobin levels. The hereditary structural hemoglobin variant, HbM, also results in methemoglobinemia. HbM is produced by amino acid substitutions in the globin chains near the heme pocket that stabilize the iron in the oxidized, Fe^{+++} state. Methemoglobinemia caused by these hereditary defects cannot be reduced by treatment with methylene blue or ascorbic acid.

Laboratory diagnosis of methemoglobinemia involves demonstration of a maximum absorbance band at a wavelength of 630 nm at pH 7.0 to 7.4. If cyanide is added to the hemolysate, the band disappears, and the change in absorbance is directly proportional to the concentration of methemoglobin. Differentiation of acquired from hereditary types of methemoglobin requires assay of NADH-methemoglobin reductase and hemoglobin electrophoresis. Enzyme activity is only reduced in hereditary NADH-methemoglobin reductase deficiency and hemoglobin electrophoresis is only abnormal in HbM disease. The acquired types of methemoglobinemia show normal enzyme activity and a normal electrophoresis pattern (Table 3-5).

TABLE 3-5 *LABORATORY DIFFERENTIATION OF METHEMOGLOBINEMIA*

Methemoglobinemia Resulting From	Methemoglobin Level	Enzyme Activity	Hemoglobin Electrophoresis
Hereditary enzyme deficiency	Increased	Decreased	Normal
Toxic substance exposure	Increased	Normal	Normal
Hemoglobin M disease	Increased	Normal	Abnormal

(From: Harmening DM: Clinical Hematology and Fundamentals of Hemostasis. Philadelphia, FA Davis, 1992.)

SULFHEMOGLOBIN

Sulfhemoglobin is a stable compound formed when sulfur combines with the heme of hemoglobin. The green sulfhemoglobin compound is so stable that the erythrocyte carries it until the cell disappears from circulation. Sulfhemoglobin cannot carry oxygen and cannot be reduced by ascorbic acid or methylene blue. However, sulfhemoglobin can combine with carbon monoxide to form carboxysulfhemoglobin. Normal levels of sulfhemoglobin do not exceed 2.2%. Cyanosis is produced at levels exceeding 3% to 4%. Sulfhemoglobinemia accompanies methemoglobinemia, which usually precedes it. Sulfhemoglobin is formed after exposure of blood to trinitroluene or acetanilid, phenacetin, and sulfonamides. It also is found to be elevated in severe constipation and in bacteremia with *Clostridium welchii*. Diagnosis of sulfhemoglobinemia is made spectrophotometrically by demonstrating an absorption band at 620 nm. This is the only abnormal hemoglobin pigment not measured by the cyanmethemoglobin method for determining hemoglobin concentration.

CARBOXYHEMOGLOBIN

Carboxyhemoglobin is formed when hemoglobin is exposed to carbon monoxide. Hemoglobin affinity for carbon monoxide is more than 200 times greater than its affinity for oxygen. Carboxyhemoglobin is incapable of transporting oxygen. High levels of carboxyhemoglobin impart a cherry-red color to the blood and skin. However, high levels of carboxyhemoglobin, together with high levels of deoxyhemoglobin, may give blood a purple-pink color.

Normally, blood carries small amounts of carboxyhemoglobin formed from the carbon monoxide produced during heme catabolism. The normal level of carboxyhemoglobin varies depending on individuals' smoking habits and their environment. City dwellers have higher levels than country dwellers due to the carbon monoxide produced from automobiles. For nonsmokers, the range is from a low of 0.1% in the country to 6.9% in large cities. For smokers, the range is from a low of 0.26% in the country to a high of 11.9% in large cities. As is the case with methemoglobinemia, carboxyhemoglobin has an impact on oxygen delivery because it destroys the molecule's cooperativity. Acute carboxyhemoglobinemia causes irreversible tissue damage and death from anoxia. Chronic carboxyhemoglobinemia is accompanied by increased oxygen affinity and polycythemia.

Carboxyhemoglobin is commonly measured in whole blood by the method of Tietz and Fiereck.[18] Blood hemolysate is treated with sodium hydrosulfite (dithionite), which reduces the oxyhemoglobin and methemoglobin to deoxyhemoglobin. This leaves only deoxyhemoglobin and carboxyhemoglobin in the specimen. These two hemoglobins have similar absorbances at 555 nm, but carboxyhemoglobin has a greater absorbance at 541 nm. Absorbance is measured at both wavelengths, and the ratio of A541 to A555 shows a linear relation to the amount of carboxyhemoglobin[19] (Fig. 3-15).

Glycosylated hemoglobin

Glycosylated hemoglobin, Hgb A_1, is a minor component of normal adult hemoglobin and is composed of subgroups. The most important subgroup is Hgb A_{1C},

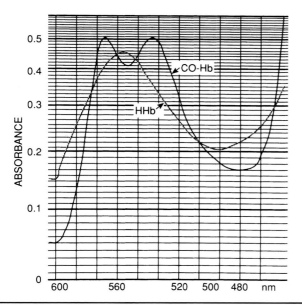

FIGURE 3-15. Absorbance spectra of carboxyhemoglobin (CO-Hb) and reduced hemoglobin (HHb). In the CO-Hb method of Tietz and Fiereck, measurements are taken at 555 nm, where the two species have similar absorbances, and at 541 nm, where CO-Hb has a greater absorbance. (With permission from: Anderson SC, Cockayne S: Clinical Chemistry: Concepts and Applications. Philadelphia: W. B. Saunders, 1992.)

which has glucose irreversibly attached to the β chains. Hgb A_{1C} is produced throughout the life of the erythrocyte, its synthesis dependent on the time averaged concentration of blood glucose. If young cells are exposed to extremely high concentrations of glucose (e.g., 400 mg/dL) for several hours, the concentration of Hb A_{1C} increases both with concentration and time of exposure. For this reason, older erythrocytes contain more Hgb A_{1C} than younger erythrocytes. Measurement of Hgb A_{1C} is routinely used as an indicator of control of blood glucose levels in diabetics because it represents a time-averaged blood glucose level. Glycosylated hemoglobin reflects the mean glucose values during the preceding 4 to 8 weeks.

Average levels of Hgb A_{1C} are 7.5% in diabetics and 3.5% in healthy individuals. Hgb A_{1C} may be measured by elution from affinity columns, immunoassay, gel electrofocusing, high-performance liquid chromatography, and electrophoresis.

ERYTHROCYTE DESTRUCTION

Erythrocyte destruction is normally the result of senescence, since replacement of cellular constituents by synthesis is practically nonexistent in the mature erythrocyte. Erythrocyte aging is characterized by a decline in cellular enzyme systems, especially of those in the glycolytic pathway, which in turn leads to decreased ATP production and a loss of adequate reducing systems. Consequently, the cell loses the ability to maintain its shape, its deformability, and its membrane integrity. About 90% of aged erythrocyte destruction is extravascular, taking place in the histiocytic cells of the spleen, liver, and bone marrow. The remaining 10% is catabolized intravascularly, whereby the erythrocyte releases hemoglobin directly into the bloodstream.

Extravascular

Most extravascular destruction of erythrocytes takes place in the macrophages (histiocytes) of the spleen. Aged erythrocytes have more rigid, leaky membranes, and move slowly and with difficulty through the small apertures of the macrophage-lined cords of the spleen. In addition, the glucose supply in the spleen is low, limiting the energy-producing process of glycolysis within the erythrocyte. Aged erythrocytes usually have increased permeability to cations, and the cells very quickly deplete the cellular level of ATP as attempts are made to maintain osmotic equilibrium by pumping these excess cations out of the cell. Thus, the splenic environment is well suited for culling aged erythrocytes.

Within the macrophage, the hemoglobin molecule is broken down into iron, heme, and globin (Fig. 3-16). The essential elements, iron and globin, are conserved and reused for new hemoglobin or other protein synthesis. Heme iron may be stored as ferritin or hemosiderin within the macrophage, but most is released to the transport protein, transferrin. If released to transferrin, the iron is deliv-

EXTRAVASCULAR HEMOGLOBIN DEGRADATION

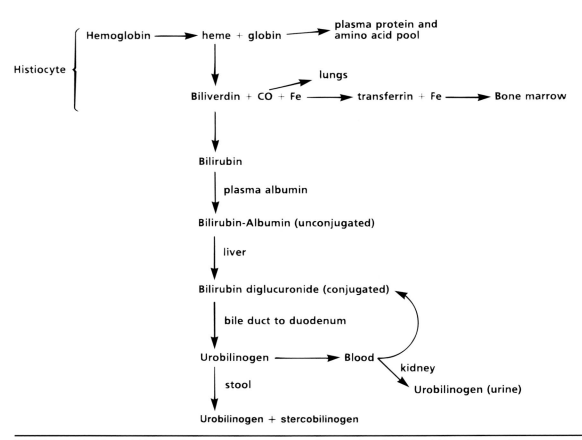

FIGURE 3-16. Most hemoglobin degradation occurs within the macrophages of the spleen. The globin and iron portions are conserved and reused. Heme is reduced to bilirubin, eventually degraded to urobilinogen, and excreted in the feces. Thus, indirect indicators of erythrocyte or erythrocyte destruction include the blood bilirubin level and urobilinogen concentration in the feces.

ered to developing normoblasts in the bone marrow. This endogenous iron exchange is responsible for about 80% of the iron passing through the transferrin pool. Thus, iron from the normal erythrocyte aging process is conserved and reused. The globin portion of the hemoglobin molecule is broken down and recycled into the amino acid pool.

Heme is further catabolized and excreted in the feces. The α-methane bridge of the porphyrin ring is cleaved, producing a mole of carbon monoxide and biliverdin. Carbon monoxide is released to the bloodstream, where it is carried by erythrocytes as carboxyhemoglobin to the lungs and expired. The remaining portion of the porphyrin ring, biliverdin, is rapidly reduced within the cell to bilirubin. Bilirubin, released from the macrophage, is complexed with plasma albumin and carried to the liver. Upon uptake by the liver, bilirubin is conjugated to bilirubin glucuronide by the enzyme, bilirubin UDP-glucuronyl-transferase, present in the ER of the liver. Once conjugated, bilirubin becomes polar and lipid insoluble. Bilirubin glucuronide is excreted into the bile and reaches the intestinal tract where it is converted into urobilinogen by

intestinal bacterial flora. Most urobilinogen is excreted in the feces, where it is quickly oxidized to urobilin or stercobilin. A small amount of urobilinogen is reabsorbed from the intestine, enters the portal circulation, and is again excreted into the gut by the liver. Some of the reabsorbed urobilinogen is filtered by the kidney and appears in the urine.

● Intravascular

The small amount of hemoglobin released into the peripheral bloodstream through intravascular erythrocyte breakdown undergoes dissociation into α-β dimers (Fig. 3-17). These dimers are quickly bound to the plasma glycoprotein, *haptoglobin* (Hp), in a 1:1 ratio. Haptoglobin is an α_2-globulin present in plasma at a concentration of 50 to 200 mg/dL. The HpHb complex prevents the filtering of the hemoglobin dimers by the kidney by virtue of the complex size. The haptoglobin carries hemoglobin dimers to the liver, where hemoglobin is processed within the hepatocyte in a manner similar to that of hemoglobin in extravascular destruction.

INTRAVASCULAR HEMOGLOBIN DEGRADATION

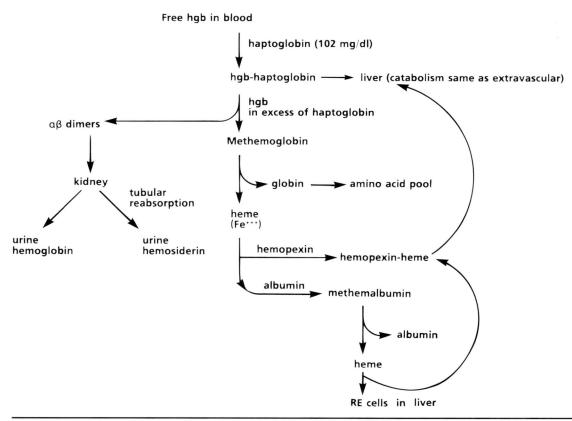

FIGURE 3-17. When the erythrocyte is destroyed within the vascular system, hemoglobin is released directly into the blood. Normally, the free hemoglobin quickly complexes with haptoglobin, and the complex is degraded in the liver. In severe hemolytic states, haptoglobin may become depleted, and free hemoglobin dimers are filtered by the kidney. During haptoglobin depletion, in addition to filtering by the kidney, some hemoglobin is quickly oxidized to methemoglobin and bound to either hemopexin or albumin for eventual degradation in the liver.

The HpHb complex is cleared very rapidly from the bloodstream, with a T1/2 disappearance rate between 10 and 30 minutes. The haptoglobin concentration may be depleted very rapidly in acute hemolytic states because the liver fails to synthesize haptoglobin in compensatory levels. Haptoglobin however is an acute phase reactant, and increased concentrations may be found in inflammatory, infectious, or neoplastic conditions. Therefore, patients with hemolytic anemia accompanied by an underlying infectious or inflammatory process may have normal haptoglobin levels. When haptoglobin is depleted, as in severe hemolysis, free $\alpha\beta$ dimers may be filtered by the kidney and reabsorbed by the proximal tubular cells at a maximum rate of 1.4 mg/minute. Dimers passing through the kidney in excess of the reabsorption capabilities of the tubular cells will appear in the urine as free hemoglobin. Dimers reabsorbed by the tubular cells are catabolized to bilirubin and iron, both of which eventually enter the plasma pool. However, some iron remains in the tubular cell and is complexed to storage proteins forming ferritin and hemosiderin. Eventually, the iron-loaded tubular cells

are sloughed off and excreted in the urine. The iron inclusions can be visualized with the Prussian blue stain. Thus, the presence of iron in the urine (hemosidinuria) is a sign of recent increased intravascular hemolysis.

In the absence of haptoglobin, hemoglobin not excreted by the kidney is either cleared directly by hepatic uptake or may be oxidized to methemoglobin. Heme dissociates from methemoglobin and avidly binds to a β-globulin glycoprotein, hemopexin. Hemopexin is synthesized in the liver and combines with heme in a 1:1 ratio. The hemopexin–heme complex is cleared from the plasma slowly with a T1/2 disappearance of 7 to 8 hours. When hemopexin becomes depleted, the dissociated oxidized heme combines with plasma albumin in a 1:1 ratio to form methalbumin. Methalbumin clearance by the liver also is very slow. In fact, methalbumin may only be a temporary combining form for heme until more hemopexin or haptoglobin becomes available. Heme is probably transferred from methalbumin to hemopexin for clearance by the liver as it becomes available. When present in large quantity, methalbumin and hemopexin–heme complexes impart a brownish color to the plasma. Schumm's test is designed to detect these abnormal compounds spectrophotometrically.

SUMMARY

Erythrocytes are derived from the unipotent committed stem cells BFU-E and CFU-E. Erythropoietin, a growth hormone produced in renal tissues, stimulates erythropoiesis and is responsible for maintaining a steady-state erythrocyte mass. Morphologic developmental stages of the erythroid cell include (in order of increasing maturity) the pronormoblast, basophilic normoblast, polychromatophilic normoblast, orthochromatic normoblast, reticulocyte, and the erythrocyte. As the cell matures, hemoglobin production increases, changing the color of the cytoplasm on Wright-stained blood smears from deep blue to grey to pinkish red. The nucleus gradually becomes pkynotic and is extruded from the cell at the orthochromatic stage.

The erythrocyte membrane is a bilipid-protein complex that is important in maintaining cellular deformability and selective permeability. As the cell ages, it becomes rigid, leaky, and is culled in the spleen. The normal erythrocyte lifespan is 100 to 120 days.

The erythrocyte derives its energy and reducing power from glycolysis and ancillary pathways. The Embden-Meyerhoff pathway provides ATP to help the cell maintain erythrocyte shape, flexibility, and membrane integrity through regulation of intracellular cation permeability. The hexose-monophosphate shunt provides reducing power to protect the cell from permanent oxidant injury. The methemoglobin reductase pathway helps protect heme from oxidation. The Rapoport-Leubering shunt facilitates oxygen delivery to the tissue.

The erythrocyte concentration varies with sex, age, and geographic location. Higher concentrations are found in males and newborns and at high altitudes. Decreases below the reference range result in a condition called anemia. This condition causes tissue hypoxia. Increased erythrocyte concentration (erythrocytosis) is less common.

Hemoglobin, the intracellular protein in erythrocytes, is a tetramer with four protein chains and a tetrapyrrole ring (heme) nestled in the hydrophobic crevice of each protein chain. Each hemoglobin molecule is capable of combining with four molecules of oxygen. The ease with which hemoglobin binds and releases oxygen is known as oxygen affinity. Hemoglobin-oxygen affinity is physiologically adjustable. In particular, pO_2, pH, pCO_2, 2,3-DPG, and temperature affect oxygen affinity.

Different types of hemoglobin exist dependent on the combination of globin chain pairs. Most adult hemoglobin is hemoglobin A, which is composed of two α and two β globin chains. At birth, most hemoglobin is hemoglobin F (two α and two γ chains).

Destruction of aged erythrocytes occurs in the macrophages of the spleen and liver. The essential elements, globin and iron, are conserved and reused. The heme portion of the molecule is catabolized to bilirubin and excreted via the intestinal tract. Intravascular erythrocyte breakdown releases hemoglobin directly into the blood. Here, the molecule dissociates into α and β dimers, which bind to the carrier protein, haptoglobin. Haptoglobin carries the dimers to the liver where they are further catabolized to bilirubin and excreted.

REVIEW QUESTIONS

1. The earliest recognizable erythroid precursor on a Wright-stained smear of the bone marrow is:
   a. Pronormoblast
   b. Basophilic normoblast
   c. CFU-E
   d. BFU-E

2. A physician ordered a reticulocyte count on an anemic patient. The reticulocyte count was 9% and the erythrocyte count was 3.5×10^{12}/L. These results suggest that:
   a. there is an increase in intravascular hemolysis
   b. there is an increase in extravascular hemolysis
   c. the bone marrow is producing erythrocytes at an increased rate
   d. the bone marrow is not producing erythrocytes at an increased rate

3. Erythrocytes that contain a marked decrease in spectrin would most likely cause:
   a. an increase in membrane permeability
   b. methemoglobinemia
   c. an absence of the MN antigens
   d. decreased erythrocyte membrane stability

4. This metabolic pathway facilitates oxygen release from hemoglobin to the tissues:
   a. Embden-Meyerhoff
   b. Hexose-monophosphate shunt
   c. Rapoport-Leubering
   d. Methemoglobin reductase

5. The reference range for erythrocyte concentration is lowest in:
   a. newborns
   b. adolescent males
   c. adults older than 70 years of age
   d. 2-month-old infant

6. Relative erythrocytosis may be found:
   a. in pulmonary disorders
   b. at high altitudes
   c. with high oxygen affinity hemoglobins
   d. in dehydration

7. This renal hormone simulates erythropoiesis in the bone marrow:
   a. IL-1
   b. erythropoietin
   c. granulopoietin
   d. thrombopoietin

8. These pairs of chains make up the majority of hemoglobin found in normal adults:

a. $\alpha_2 \beta_2$
b. $\alpha_2 \gamma_2$
c. $\alpha_2 \delta_2$
d. $\zeta_2 \tau_2$

9. A shift to the right in the ODC occurs when there is a(n):
   a. increase in O_2
   b. increase in CO_2
   c. increase in pH
   d. decrease in CO_2

10. The sigmoid shape of the ODC is due to:
    a. the cooperative binding of O_2 by hemoglobin
    b. the Bohr effect
    c. the presence of glycosylated hemoglobin
    d. erythropoietin

11. Haptoglobin may become depleted in:
    a. inflammatory conditions
    b. acute hemolytic anemia
    c. infectious diseases
    d. kidney disease

12. This form of hemoglobin has iron in the ferric state:
    a. sulfhemoglobin
    b. carboxyhemoglobin
    c. methemoglobin
    d. deoxyhemoglobin

REFERENCES ●

1. Wintrobe, M.M.: Blood, Pure and Eloquent. New York: McGraw-Hill, 1980.
2. Hedin, S.G.: Uber die Permeabilitaet der Blutkorperchen. Pflugers Arch 68:229, 1897.
3. Landsteiner, K.: Uber Agglutinationserscheinungen normalen menschlichen Blutes. Wien Klin Wochenschr 14:1132, 1901.
4. Mohandas, N.: The red cell membrane. In: Hematology Basic Principles and Practice. Edited by R. Hoffman, E.J. Benz Jr., S.F. Shattil, B. Furie, H.J. Cohen. New York: Churchill Livingstone, 1995.
5. Palek, J., Lambert, S.: Genetics of the red cell membrane skeleton. Semin Hematol 27: 290, 1990.
6. Platt, O.S.: Inherited disorders of red cell membrane proteins. In: Genetically Abnormal Red Cells. Edited by R.L. Nagel. Boca Raton, Florida: CRC Press, 1988.
7. Viault, F.: Sur l'augmentation considerable du nombre des globules ranges dans le sang chez les habitants des haute plateaux de l'amerique du sud. CR Acad Sci (Paris) 119:917, 1890.
8. Bao, W., et. al: Normative distribution of complete blood count from early childhood through adolescence: The Bogalusa Heart Study. Prev Med 22:825, 1993.
9. Cavalieri, T.A., Chopra, A., Bryman, PN: When outside the norm is normal: interpreting lab data in the aged. Geriat 47:66, 1992.
10. Kosower, N.S.: Altered properties of erythrocytes in the aged. Am J Hematol 42:241, 1993.
11. Muldoon, M.F., Bachen, E.A., Manuch, S.B.: Acute cholesterol responses to mental stress and change in posture. Arch Intern Med 152:775–780, 1992.
12. Wang, F.F., Kung, C.K., Goldwasser, E.: Some chemical properties of human erythropoietin. Endocrinology 116:2286, 1985.
13. Zanjani, E.D., Ascensao, J.L., McGlave, P.B., Banisadre, M., Ash, R.C.: Studies on the liver to kidney switch of erythropoietin production. J Clin Invest 67:1183, 1981.
14. Zanjani, E.D., Ascensao, J.L.: Erythropoietin. Transfusion 29:46, 1989.
15. Peschle, C., et al.: Regulation of Hb synthesis in ontogenesis and erythropoietic differentiation: In vitro studies on fetal liver, cord blood, normal adult blood or marrow, and blood from HPFH patients. In: Hemoglobins in Development and Differentiation. Edited by G. Stamatoyannopoulos, A.W. Nienhuis. New York: Alan R. Liss, 1980.
16. Papayannopoulou, T.H., et al.: Fetal to adult hematopoietic cell transplantation in humans: insights into hemoglobin switching. Blood 67:99, 1986.
17. Rodgers, G.P., Schechter, A.N.: Molecular pathology of the hemoglobin molecule. In: Hematology Basic Principles and Practice. Edited by R. Hoffman, E.J. Benz Jr., S.F. Shattil, B. Furie, H.J. Cohen. New York: Churchill Livingstone, 1995.
18. Tietz, N.W., Fiereck, E.A.: The spectrophotometric measurement of carboxyhemoglobin. Ann Clin Lab Sci 3:36, 1973.
19. Anderson, S.C., Cockayne, S.: Clinical Chemistry. Concepts and Applications. Philadelphia: W. B. Saunders, 1993.

The Leukocyte

4

KEY TERMS

non-specific granules
azurophilic granules
myeloblast
promyelocyte
myelocyte
primary granules
specific granules
secondary granules
metamyelocyte
band (stab)
polymorphonuclear neutrophil
leukocytosis
leukopenia
granulocytopenia
neutropenia
agranulocytosis
granulocytosis
neutrophilia
marginal pool
circulating pool
diapedesing
mitotic pool
post-mitotic pool
opsonins
phagosome
phagolysosome
pyrogen
monoblast
monocyte
promonocyte
eosinophil
basophil
erythrophagocytosis
immune response
antigen-dependent
  lymphopoiesis
antigen-independent
  lymphopoiesis
lymphoblast
prolymphocyte
lymphocyte
immunocompetent
reactive lymphocyte
stimulated lymphocyte
activated lymphocyte
transformed lymphocyte
atypical lymphocyte
leukocytoid lymphocyte
virocyte
immunoblast
Downey cells
effector lymphocytes
plasma cells
plasmacytoid lymphocyte
flame cells
Mott cells
Russell bodies
Dutcher bodies

immunoglobulin
hypogammaglobulinemia
polyclonal gammopathies
monoclonal gammopathies
immune response
cell mediated immunity
humoral immunity

INTRODUCTION

The colorless, less plentiful white corpuscles of the blood, leukocytes, were overlooked until the advent of improved microscopic lenses. William Hewson first observed leukocytes in the blood in the 18th century. He believed that these nucleated cells came from the nucleated cells in the lymph and that they eventually emerged from the spleen as red cells.[1] In the 19th century, the interest in leukocytes intensified with studies on inflammation and microbial infection.

EARLY DISCOVERIES OF LEUKOCYTE FUNCTION

The association of pus in areas of inflammation with the leukocytes of blood was suggested by William Addison in 1843.[1] He recognized a similarity in the nucleated cells found in the exudates (pus cells) of pimples and boils to those of nucleated cells in the peripheral blood. Previously, it had been determined that the microvasculature of the body was closed; thus, the idea of a hemic source of pus cells (which were found outside the microvasculature) was considered unlikely. Several years later, Augustus Waller observed the migration of leukocytes between adjacent epithelial cells in the walls of capillaries in a hyperextended, fixed frog's tongue. Julius Cohnheim confirmed this observation in 1867. Cohnheim found that vitally stained blood corpuscles of implanted corneal tissue in frogs could later be found in the frog's subcutaneous lymph sac.[2] This provided evidence that blood cells could leave the vasculature and enter the tissue. Subsequently, the defensive nature of inflammation and pus formation was suggested by Metchnikov when he observed the presence of nucleated blood cells surrounding a thorn introduced beneath the skin of a larval starfish.[3] Up to this time, the prevailing opinion of pathologists was that leukocytes were exploited by micro-organisms as sites of microbial proliferation and dissemination to tissues.

These observations by early hematologists have helped establish the function of blood leukocytes as a defense system of the body against foreign invaders and noninfectious challenges (tissue necrosis). We now know that the vascular system is only a temporary residence for leukocytes. The main function of the vasculature is to transport and distribute leukocytes to every body tissue. In response to chemotactic stimuli, blood leukocytes randomly adhere to the luminal surface of the vascular endothelium and exit to the tissue to carry on their function.

The era of morphologic hematology began in 1877 with Paul Ehrlich's discovery of a triacid stain.[4] The stain, used in conjunction with improved compound microscopes, allowed differentiation of leukocytes on fixed blood smears according to nuclear and cytoplasmic characteristics. Ehrlich's categories of leukocytes were of a descriptive nature: acidophil, basophil, neutrophil, lymphocytes, large mononuclears (large lymphocytes), and large mononuclears with indented nuclei (monocytes). The acidophil (acid loving) had an affinity for the acid part of

the stain, giving the cytoplasmic granules an orange-pink color. The basophil (base loving) had an affinity for the basic part of the stain, yielding bluish-black cytoplasmic granules. The neutrophil took up both acid and basic portions of the stain, giving the cell a pinkish-blue cytoplasm. All these granular cells had segmented nuclei. The nongranular, mononuclear cells included monocytes and lymphocytes. Monocytes were the largest cells and contained a single large nucleus often in a horseshoe shape. The terminology today for blood leukocytes is similar to Ehrlich's classification: *eosinophils, basophils, neutrophils, lymphocytes,* and *monocytes.*

Many of Ehrlich's observations and Metchnikov's experiments provided the groundwork for understanding the leukocytes as defenders against infection. Ehrlich recognized that variations in numbers of leukocytes accompanied specific pathologic conditions, such as eosinophilia in asthma, parasitic infection, and dermatitis, as well as neutrophilia in bacterial infections.

It is now recognized that defensive function includes two separate but interrelated events: phagocytosis and the subsequent development of the immune response. Granulocytes and monocytes are responsible for phagocytosis, while monocytes and lymphocytes interact to produce an effective immune response.

LEUKOCYTE CONCENTRATIONS IN THE PERIPHERAL BLOOD

Leukocytes develop from primitive pluripotential stem cells in the bone marrow. Upon specific hematopoietic growth hormone stimulation, the stem cell proliferates and differentiates into the various types of leukocytes: granulocytes (which include neutrophils, eosinophils, and basophils), monocytes, and lymphocytes. Upon maturation, these cells may be released into the peripheral blood or may remain in the bone marrow storage pool until needed.

The total peripheral blood leukocyte count is high at birth, 9 to 30×10^9/L. A few immature granulocytic cells (myelocytes, metamyelocytes) may be seen in the first few days of life; however, immature leukocytes are not present in the peripheral blood after this age except in disease. In a week, the leukocyte count drops to between 5 to 21×10^9/L. A gradual decline occurs until the age of 8 years, at which time the leukocyte concentration averages 8×10^9/L. The Bogalusa Heart Study found that in children between the ages of 5 and 17, females had, on the average, leukocyte counts 0.5×10^9/L higher than males.[5] Adult values average from 3.5 to 11.0×10^9/L, with slightly lower concentrations in blacks. There are conflicting reports on the reference range for older adults. Some hematologists do not believe the reference range for older adults is different from that of other adults, while others believe the range is somewhat lower (3 to 9×10^9/L). It is, however, generally accepted that the lymphocyte count is lower in older adults; this decrease is due primarily to a decrease in T-lymphocytes. Decreased leukocyte counts in the elderly may be due to drugs or sepsis.[6]

●
Calculation of the absolute cell count

An increase or decrease in the total number of leukocytes may be caused by an altered concentration of all leukocyte types or, more commonly, is limited to an alteration in one specific type of leukocyte. For this reason, an abnormal total leukocyte count should be followed by a leukocyte differential count. A leukocyte differential count enumerates each leukocyte type among a total of 100 leukocytes. The differential results are reported in the percentage of each type counted. To accurately interpret whether an increase or decrease in cell types exists, however, it is necessary to calculate the absolute concentration using the results of the total leukocyte count and the differential (relative concentration) in the following manner:

relative differential count
$$\text{(\%)} \times \underset{\text{(WBC/L)}}{\text{total leukocyte count}} = \underset{\text{(cells/L)}}{\text{absolute count}}$$

The usefulness of this calculation is emphasized in the following example. Two different blood specimens both had a relative lymphocyte concentration of 60%. One had a total leukocyte count of 3×10^9/L and the other a total leukocyte count of 9×10^9/L. The relative lymphocyte concentration on both specimens appears elevated (normal is 20% to 40%); however, calculation of the absolute concentration (normally 1.5 to 4.0×10^9/L) shows that only one specimen has an absolute increase in lymphocytes; the other is normal:

$$0.6 \times 3 \times 10^9/L = 1.8 \times 10^9/L \text{ (normal)}$$
$$0.6 \times 9 \times 10^9/L = 5.4 \times 10^9/L \text{ (increased)}$$

NEUTROPHILS

The neutrophil is the most numerous leukocyte in the adult peripheral blood, 54% to 62% (2 to 7×10^9/L). At birth, neutrophil concentration is about 60%; this level drops to 30% by 4 to 6 months of age. After 4 years of life, the concentration of neutrophils gradually increases until adult values are reached at 6 years of age. Most peripheral blood neutrophils are mature segmented forms; however, a few nonsegmented forms (bands) may be seen in normal specimens. Most variations in the total leukocyte count are due to an increase or decrease in neutrophils.

EOSINOPHILS

Eosinophil concentrations are maintained at 1% to 3% (0 to 0.45×10^9/L) throughout life. It is possible that no eosinophils may be seen on a 100-cell differential; however, careful scanning of the entire smear should reveal an occasional eosinophil.

BASOPHILS

Basophils are the least plentiful cells in the peripheral blood, 0% to 1% (0 to 0.2×10^9/L). It is common not to find basophils on a 100-cell differential; the finding of an absolute basophilia, however, is very important since it frequently indicates the presence of a hematologic malignancy.

MONOCYTES

Monocytes usually compose from 4% to 10% (0.2 to 0.8 $\times 10^9$/L) of leukocytes. Occasionally, reactive lymphocytes may resemble monocytes. This gives even the experienced clinical laboratory scientist difficulty in the differentiation of the two cells.

LYMPHOCYTES

The lymphocyte concentration varies with the age of the individual. About 30% of the leukocytes at birth are lymphocytes. This increases to 60% at about 4 to 6 months and remains at this level until 4 years of age. Then a gradual decline occurs until a level of 34% at 21 years is reached. The concentration in adults ranges from 20% to 40% (1.5 to 4.0×10^9/L). After age 65, lymphocytes decrease in both sexes.

●
NEUTROPHILS

●
Neutrophil maturation

The neutrophil orginates from the CFU-GEMM stem cell. This stem cell is induced to differentiate into the CFU-GM cell by the growth factors GM-CSF and IL-3. GM-CSF, IL-3, and G-CSF selectively promote the proliferation, differentiation, and maturation of neutrophils from the CFU-GM.

The neutrophil undergoes six morphologically identifiable stages in the process of maturation from the unipotential stem cell to the functional segmented neutrophil: (1) myeloblast, (2) promyelocyte (progranulocyte), (3) myelocyte, (4) metamyelocyte, (5) band or unsegmented granulocyte, and (6) segmented granulocyte or polymorphonuclear neutrophil (PMN).

During this maturation process, there is an obvious progressive change in the nucleus. The nucleoli disappear, the chromatin condenses, and the once round mass indents and eventually segments. These nuclear changes are accompanied by distinct cytoplasmic changes. The scanty, agranular, basophilic cytoplasm of the earliest stage is gradually replaced by a voluminous, pink-staining granular cytoplasm in the mature differentiated stage (Fig. 4-1) (Table 4-1).

MYELOBLAST

The *myeloblast* (Fig. 4-2) is the earliest recognizable neutrophil precursor. The myeloblast ranges in size from 14 to 20 μm in diameter and has a high nuclear to cytoplasmic (N:C) ratio. The nucleus is usually round or oval and contains delicate, lacy, evenly stained chromatin. There are from three to five large highly developed nucleoli. There is no condensation of chromatin on the smooth nuclear membrane. The small to moderate amount of cytoplasm is agranular, staining deep blue at

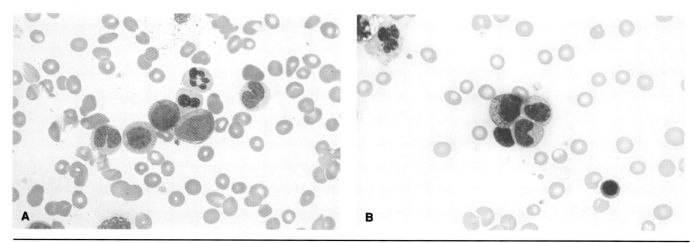

FIGURE 4-1. A, Compare the chromatin pattern of the nucleus and the cytoplasmic changes in the various stages of neutrophil development shown in this illustration. Left to right: band neutrophil, myelocyte, promyelocyte, myeloblast, band neutrophil. Segmented neutrophils are above the blast (BM). **B,** Compare the nuclear and cytoplasmic features at the various stages of neutrophil development shown in this picture. The three nucleated cells in the center are (clockwise beginning at 2 o'clock): myelocyte, metamyelocyte, promyelocyte. Bottom right side is a nucleated erythrocyte. At about 7 o'clock a bare nucleus lies between the metamyelocyte and promyelocyte. (Bone marrow 250×, Wright-Giemsa stain.)

the periphery and lighter blue toward the nucleus. These cells may stain positive for peroxidase, even though granules are not evident. When positive, peroxidase helps differentiate myeloblasts from lymphoblasts. A distinct unstained area adjacent to the nucleus representing the Golgi apparatus may be seen.

PROMYELOCYTE

The *promyelocyte* (Fig. 4-3) is recognized by the presence of large, blue-black *primary granules*, also called *nonspecific* or *azurophilic granules*. The primary granules have

a phospholipid membrane that stains with the lipophilic stain, Sudan black B. The granules contain a number of enzymes and other substances. The granules can be shown, by cytochemical techniques, to contain a number of enzymes and other substances: acid phosphatase, myeloperoxidase, acid hydrolases, lysozyme, sulfated mucopolysaccharides, and other basic proteins. The promyelocyte size varies from 15 to 21 μm depending on the stage of the mitotic cycle of the cell. A promyelocyte appears larger than the myeloblast. The basophilic cytoplasm is similar to that of the blast. The nucleus is still quite large.

TABLE 4-1   *CHARACTERISTICS OF CELLS IN THE MATURATION STAGES OF THE NEUTROPHIL*

Cell Stage	Size (μm)	Granules	Cytoplasm	Nucleus	N:C Ratio
Myeloblast	14–20	Absent	Deep blue	Round or oval; delicate, lacy chromatin; 3–5 nucleoli	High
Promyelocyte	15–21	Large, blue-black, azurophilic (non-specific)	Deep blue	Round or oval; chromatin lacy but more condensed than blast; nucleoli present	High but less than myeloblast
Myelocyte	16–24	Small pinkish-red specific granules; some azurophilic granules present	Light pink but may have patches of blue	Round; chromatin more condensed than in promyelocyte; nucleoli usually absent	Decreased from progranulocyte
Metamyelocyte	12–18	Predominance of small pinkish-red specific granules; few azurophilic granules present	Pink	Chromatin condensed; stains dark purple; kidney-bean shape	Decreased
Band (nonsegmented)	9–15	Abundant small, pinkish-red; specific granules	Pink	Chromatin is pyknotic at ends of horseshoe shaped nucleus. Stains dark purple	Decreased
Polymorphonuclear (segmented)	9–15	As in band	Pink	Nucleus is segmented into 2–4 lobes; chromatin condensed; stains dark purple	Decreased

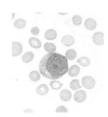

FIGURE 4-2. Myeloblast (arrow) (Bone marrow 250×, Wright-Giemsa stain).

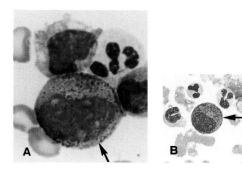

FIGURE 4-3. A, Promyelocyte (Bone marrow 250×, Wright-Giemsa stain); **B**, Promyelocyte (Bone marrow 250×, Wright-Giemsa stain).

The chromatin structure, although coarser than that of the blast, is still open and rather lacy, staining light purple-blue. Several nucleoli are visible at this stage.

MYELOCYTE

The *myelocyte* (Fig. 4-4), 16 to 24 μm in diameter, is the stage at which the *specific* or *secondary* granules appear. These neutrophilic granules are small, sand-like granules, with a pink-red to pink-violet tint. The secondary granules, like the primary granules, are surrounded by a phospholipid membrane that stains with Sudan black B. Large primary azurophilic granules may still be apparent, but their synthesis has ceased. Their concentration likewise decreases with mitotic divisions. The secondary granules contain alkaline phosphatase and lysozyme but not acid phosphatase or peroxidase. Several other enzymes, such as amino peptidase, collagenase, and basic proteins have

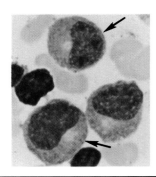

FIGURE 4-5. Metamyelocyte (Bone marrow 250×, Wright-Giemsa stain).

been identified in the secondary granules.[7] The cytoplasm becomes acidophilic, staining a light pink color. The nucleus is reduced in size; the nuclear chromatin appears more condensed and more darkly stained than that in the progranulocyte. Nucleoli may be seen in the early myelocyte but are usually absent. The nucleus is round or oval and frequently eccentric. Later stages of the myelocyte may show a flattening of one side of the nucleus. A clear light area is visible next to the nucleus, which represents the Golgi apparatus. The N:C ratio is decreased. This is the last stage capable of mitotic division.

METAMYELOCYTE

Metamyelocytes (juvenile) (Fig. 4-5) are slightly smaller, 12 to 18 μm in diameter, than myelocytes, but their most apparent differentiating characteristic is nuclear indentation. The indentation gives the nucleus a kidney bean shape. The nuclear chromatin is condensed, ill-defined, and stains dark purple. Nucleoli are not visible. The cytoplasm is pink with a predominance of secondary granules.

BAND GRANULOCYTE

The metamyelocyte becomes a *band* (stab) (Fig. 4-6) when the indentation of the nucleus is more than half the diameter of the hypothetical round nucleus. This indentation gives the nucleus a horseshoe shape appearance. The chromatin shows degenerative changes with pyknosis at either end of the nucleus. The cell is slightly smaller in diameter, 9 to 15 μm, than the metamyelocyte. The cytoplasm appears pinkish as in the previous stage. This is the first stage that may normally be found in the peripheral blood.

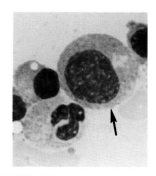

FIGURE 4-4. Myelocyte (Bone marrow 250×, Wright-Giemsa stain).

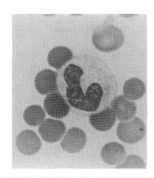

FIGURE 4-6. Band neutrophil (PB, 250×, Wright-Giemsa stain).

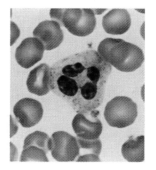

FIGURE 4-7. Segmented neutrophil (PB, 250×, Wright-Giemsa stain).

Depending on the criteria for differentiating bands from more mature neutrophils, the normal concentration of bands in peripheral blood varies from 1% to 10%.[8]

POLYMORPHONUCLEAR NEUTROPHIL

Although similar in size to the band form, the *polymorphonuclear neutrophil (PMN)* (Fig. 4-7) is recognized, as its name implies, by a segmented nucleus with two or more lobes connected by a thin nuclear filament. The chromatin is condensed and stains a deep purple-black. Most neutrophils have from two to four nuclear lobes. More than five lobes is abnormal, and the cell is classified as a hypersegmented PMN. The lobes are often touching or superimposed on one another, which sometimes makes it difficult to differentiate the cell as a band or as a PMN. If there is a doubt as to whether the cell is a band or PMN, it should be called a PMN. Another difficulty in classifying the segmented stage is the determination of whether the connecting isthmus between lobes is a filament or a band. It is generally accepted that if the connecting filament is wide enough to discern a chromatin pattern, then the cell is classified as a band (Fig. 4-8). If there is no visible chromatin pattern in the connecting isthmus, it is a filament and the cell is classified as a segmented PMN.

Only one active X chromosome is needed for a normal functioning cell. In females with two X chromosomes, one

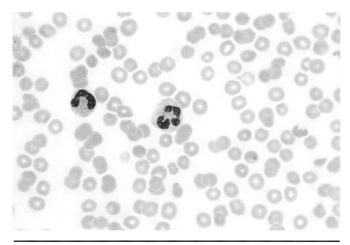

FIGURE 4-8. Left to right: band neutrophil and segmented neutrophil (peripheral blood, 250×, Wright-Giemsa stain).

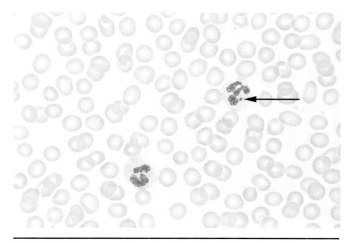

FIGURE 4-9. The segmented neutrophil on the left has a Barr body extending from the nucleus. See text for explanation (peripheral blood, 250×, Wright-Giemsa stain).

is randomly inactivated in each cell of the female embryo and remains inactive in all daughter cells (Lyons hypothesis). This inactive X chromosome remains unextended and appears as a sex chromatin body. This body in neutrophils assumes a drumstick shape, becomes exteriorized, and appears as an appendage of the nucleus. These appendages, called Barr bodies, may be identified in 1% to 5% of the circulating PMNs of females (Fig. 4-9).

The cytoplasm of the mature PMN contains many secondary granules and stains a pink color. Primary granules may be present but because of their scarcity and loss of staining quality, may not be readily identified.

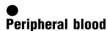

Peripheral blood

NEUTROPHIL KINETICS

Neutrophils constitute the majority of circulating leukocytes. The absolute number varies between 2.0 and 7.0 × 10^9/L. Diurnal variations commonly occur with higher levels in the afternoon and lower levels in the morning. This variation within the normal range may be associated with the individual's activity level.

Alterations in the concentration of peripheral blood is often the first sign of an underlying pathology (Table 4-2). A normal leukocyte count does not rule out the presence of disease, but *leukocytosis* (an increase in leukocytes) or *leukopenia* (a decrease in leukocytes) are important clues to disease processes and deserve further investigation. This investigation should include a leukocyte differential count to identify the concentration of different types of leukocytes. *Granulocytopenia* defines a decrease in all types of granulocytes (i.e., eosinophils, basophils, and neutrophils). *Neutropenia* is a more specific term denoting a decrease in only neutrophils. Neutropenia exists if the absolute neutrophil count falls below 2.0 × 10^9/L. When the neutrophil count falls below 0.5 × 10^9/L, the condition is called *agranulocytosis* and the patient is at high risk of

TABLE 4-2 *TERMS ASSOCIATED WITH ABNORMAL CONCENTRATIONS OF LEUKOCYTES*

TERMS ASSOCIATED WITH INCREASES OF CELLS	TYPE(S) OF CELLS AFFECTED
Leukocytosis	General increase in total leukocyte concentration
Granulocytosis	Neutrophils, eosinophils, and/or basophils
Neutrophilia	Neutrophils
Eosinophilia	Eosinophils
Basophilia	Basophils
Monocytosis	Monocytes
Lymphocytosis	Lymphocytes

TERMS ASSOCIATED WITH DECREASES OF CELLS	
Leukopenia	General decrease in total leukocyte concentration
Granulocytopenia	Neutrophils, eosinophils and/or basophils
Agranulocytosis	Neutrophils
Neutropenia	Neutrophils
Monocytopenia	Monocytes
Lymphocytopenia	Lymphocytes

developing an infection if not isolated from the normal environment. *Granulocytosis* is a term used to denote an increase in all granulocytes. *Neutrophilia* is a more specific term indicating an increase in neutrophils only. Neutrophilia occurs when the absolute number of neutrophils exceeds 7×10^9/L. This condition is most often a result of the body's reactive response to bacterial infection, metabolic intoxication, drug intoxication, or tissue necrosis.

Not all blood neutrophils are circulating freely at the same time. About half the total blood neutrophil concentration is temporarily marginated along the vessel walls *(marginal pool)*, while the other half is circulating *(circulating pool)*. Thus, if all marginated neutrophils were to circulate freely, the total neutrophil count would double. The two pools, because they are in equilibrium, rapidly and freely exchange neutrophils. Certain physiologic events may decrease the marginal pool, temporarily increasing the circulating pool. Most neutrophils disappear into the tissues from the marginal pool in response to antigenic stimulation. The average neutrophil circulates approximately 10 hours in the blood before diapedesing to the tissues, although a few die of senescence. *Diapedesing* refers to the outward movement of circulating neutrophils through intact blood vessel walls to the tissues (transendothelial migration).

BONE MARROW

Neutrophils in the bone marrow can be divided into two pools (Fig. 4-10): (1) the *mitotic pool* and (2) the *postmitotic pool.*

The mitotic pool, also called the proliferating pool, includes cells capable of DNA synthesis: myeloblasts, promyelocytes, and myelocytes. Cells spend about 3 to 6 days in this proliferating pool, undergoing 4 or 5 cell divisions. Three of these divisions occur in the myelocyte stage, but the number of divisions is probably not constant.[7] The myelocyte pool is approximately four times the size of the promyelocyte pool.

The postmitotic pool, also known as the maturation storage pool, includes metamyelocytes, bands, and segmented neutrophils. Cells spend about 5 to 7 days in this compartment before they are released to the peripheral blood. The storage pool contains 15 to 20 times as many cells as are circulating in the peripheral blood. When needed, segmented neutrophils and bands can be released from the storage pool to the peripheral blood, increasing the total leukocyte count almost immediately.

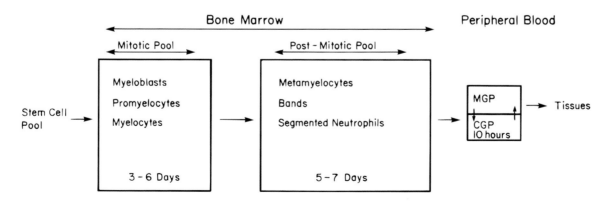

Approximate ratios of cells according to maturation

1 : 3 : 12 : 16 : 12 : 7

FIGURE 4-10. Neutrophils are produced from stem cells in the bone marrow and spend about 1 to 2 weeks in this maturation compartment. Most neutrophils are released to the peripheral blood as segmented forms. When the demand for these cells is increased, more immature forms may be released. Half the neutrophils in the peripheral blood are in the marginating pool; the other half are in the circulating pool. Neutrophils spend about 10 hours in the blood before marginating and exiting randomly to tissue. (Adapted from Boggs, D.R., Winkelstein, A.: White Cell Manual. 4th Ed. Philadelphia: F. A. Davis Co., 1983.)

BONE MARROW RELEASE OF NEUTROPHILS

The normal marrow transit times for neutrophil precursors may be decreased under conditions of stress (e.g., severe infection). Transit time could be decreased as a result of several mechanisms: (1) acceleration of maturation, (2) skipped cellular divisions, and (3) early release of cells from the marrow.

Normally, input of neutrophils from the bone marrow to the blood equals output of the neutrophils from the blood to the tissues, maintaining a relatively steady state concentration in the peripheral blood. However, when the demand for neutrophils is increased such as in infectious states, the neutrophil concentration in the peripheral blood can increase almost immediately as neutrophils from the bone marrow storage pool are released. Depending on the strength and duration of the stimulus, the bone marrow stem cells also may be induced to proliferate and differentiate to form additional neutrophils.

The mechanism that regulates the production and release of neutrophils is not completely understood but it most likely includes a feedback loop between the circulating neutrophils and the bone marrow. The growth factors, including GM-CSF, interleukin-1 (IL-1) (leukocyte pyrogen), and tumor necrosis factor (TNF), have been shown to induce neutrophilia when infused into rats and monkeys.[9,10] The anaphylatoxin, C5a, also has been shown to induce neutrophilia in rabbits when it is given intravenously in microgram quantities.[11] Although IL-1 and TNF may play a role in increasing the neutrophil concentration in response to pathologic conditions in humans, GM-CSF is probably the primary humoral feedback substance in the normal steady-state. This factor also activates the functional activity of neutrophils. The most potent producers of GM-CSF are T-lymphocytes.

Interleukin-1 is produced by almost all cells, and there is evidence that it regulates most processes of inflammation. IL-1 stimulates the production of GM-CSF and G-CSF and stimulates its own production. This may partially explain the leukocytosis that accompanies inflammatory processes. IL-1 also upregulates the receptors for colony-stimulating factors (CSF) on hematopoietic stem cells, thus stimulating hematopoiesis.

The vascular endothelial cell that forms the inner lining of blood vessels also generates cytokines that govern activation and recruitment of leukocytes. Thus, endothelial cells may be important in recruiting neutrophils to the earliest phases of inflammation and injury.

The release mechanism of the bone marrow storage pool is selective in normal, steady-state kinetics, releasing only segmented neutrophils and a few band neutrophils. The mechanisms controlling this regulated release are not fully understood. The release is partially regulated by the small pore size in the vascular endothelium of bone marrow sinusoids, and by the ability of the mature segmented neutrophil to deform enough to squeeze through the narrow opening. Immature cells are less deformable and cannot penetrate the small pores; however, when an increased demand for neutrophils exists, a greater proportion of less mature neutrophils are released into the peripheral blood.

Generally, the elderly appear more susceptible to infection. Studies suggest that aging has no effect on the basal level of neutrophil counts or bone marrow neutrophil reserves. There may, however, be a significant reduction in the ability to mobilize bone marrow neutrophil reserves into the peripheral blood.[12] Newborns also have an increased susceptibility to infections. Premature infants are even more vulnerable than full-term infants. The most likely factors responsible for this inadequate defense against invading pathogens in newborns are a diminished neutrophil storage pool and an impaired ability of the neutrophil to migrate to the site of infection.[13]

● Neutrophil function

Neutrophils leave the vasculature and migrate to areas of tissue damage or infection. This is accomplished by adhesion of the neutrophils to the endothelial cells of the blood vessel wall and subsequent migration of the adhered neutrophils into the tissue. Once in the tissue, the neurophil phagocytoses and kills invading organisms and interacts in other physiologic processes.

ADHERENCE

Leukocyte migration to the tissue is regulated by mechanisms of leukocyte-endothelial cell (EC) recognition. It is proposed that this recognition requires three sequential events: (1) primary adhesion of leukocytes and ECs (reversible), (2) activation of the leukocyte by chemoattractant or cell contact mediated signals that trigger expression of secondary leukocyte adhesion receptors (activation-dependent receptors), and (3) strong, sustained attachment of the leukocyte to the endothelial cell (activation-dependent binding)[14] (Table 4-3).

Within minutes of tissue injury, neutrophils interact with the walls of venules in a loose fashion, rolling along the affected area. This slows the transit of neutrophils through the area. The rolling neutrophils may then be activated by stimulating factors, known as chemoattractants. Activation causes the neutrophil to express activation-dependent adhesion receptors, resulting in rapid arrest of the rolling motion and firm adhesion to the EC. Adhesion molecules and their receptors present on the leukocytes and EC act to tether the cells together or induce activation-dependent adhesion events.

Based on molecular structure, there are three families of adhesion receptors mediating interaction of the leukocyte with the immune system and endothelium: β_2-integrins, selectins, and the immunoglobulin superfamily. These adhesion receptors and their ligands (counter-receptors) are critical for every step of cell recruitment to sites of tissue injury, including margination along vessel walls, diapedesis, and chemotaxis. Each adhesion receptor is a transmembrane protein with three domains: extracellular, transmembrane, and intracellular. The binding of a ligand to the extracellular domain sends a signal across the membrane to the interior of the cell. The transduction of this signal to the cell's interior is probably mediated by phosphorylation of a "G" protein (guanine nucleotide-binding protein) located within the receptor's intracellular do-

TABLE 4-3 *ADHESION MOLECULES IMPORTANT IN LEUKOCYTE-ENDOTHELIAL CELL INTERACTIONS*

Molecules	CD Designation	Expressed by	Counter-Receptor (Ligand)
I. β_2-integrins			
LFA-1	CD11a-CD18	Activated leukocytes	ICAM-1 ICAM-2 (both on EC)
MAC-1	CD11b-CD18	Activated leukocytes	ICAM-1 on EC Others?
gp150/95	CD11c-CD18	Activated leukocytes	ICAM-1 on EC Others?
II. Selectins			
L-selectin	CD62L	Leukocytes	E-selectin?
E-selectin	CD62E	Activated ECs	Unknown receptor on neutrophils, monocytes memory T-lymphocytes
P-selectin	CD62P	Activated ECs and platelets	Unknown receptor on neutrophils & monocytes
III. Immunoglobulin Supergene Family			
ICAM-1	CD54	EC	LFA-1 (CD11a-CD18) MAC-1 (CD11b-CD18) on activated leukocytes
ICAM-2	CD102	EC	LFA-1 (CD11a-CD18) on activated leukocytes
LFA-2	CD2	T-lymphocytes	LFA-3 (CD-58) on EC
LFA-3	CD58	EC	CD2 on T-lymphocytes
VCAM-1	CD106	EC	VLA-4 (CD49d) on monocytes, lymphocytes, eosinophils, basophils
T cell receptor	CD3	T lymphocytes	Antigen
CD4	CD4	T_H lymphocytes	MHC Class II
CD8	CD8	T_S lymphocytes	MHC Class I
MHC Class II	—	B-lymphocytes Activated T-lymphocytes Monocytes	CD4 on T_H lymphocytes
MHC Class I	—	Nucleated cells	CD8 on T_S lymphocytes

main. The phosphorylated protein may acquire enzyme activity, thus creating breakdown products that function as secondary messengers to the cell's interior apparatus. These secondary messengers have been shown to affect calcium flux, NADPH oxidase activity, cytoskeleton assembly, and phagocytosis.

Integrins Integrin receptors interact with a variety of ligands, including matrix glycoproteins, complement, and other cells. The receptors' intracellular domains react with the cell's cytoskeleton, thus providing a transmembrane link between the extracellular ligand and the cytoskeleton. The integrin receptors are necessary for normal leukocyte motility and transendothelial migration.

There are at least three β_2-integrins present in the leukocyte plasma membranes: LFA-1 (CD 11a-CD18), Mac-1 (CD11b-CD18), and gp 150/95 (CD11c-CD18).[15] These are activation dependent receptors that are maximally expressed on activated cells. Each of the three integrin activation receptors has an α-subunit (CD11a, CD11b, CD11c) noncovalently linked to a common β-subunit (CD-18). LFA-1 receptor is involved in cell-to-cell interactions and is crucial in the adhesion of all leukocytic cells.[16] The endothelial cell counter-receptors for LFA-1 are intracellular adhesion molecules 1 and 2 (ICAM-1 and ICAM-2).

The gp 150/95 and Mac-1 counter-receptor on endothelial cells is ICAM-1 and possibly other unidentified counter-receptors. Mac-1 is also known as the C3 recep-

tor. Mac-1 binds complement (C3bi), which serves as a pathway for activated neutrophils to trigger phagocytosis and the respiratory burst.

Selectins There are three members of the selectin family of membrane glycoproteins: L-selectin, E-selectin, and P-selectin. L-selectin is present at high levels on circulating resting neutrophils, on lymphocytes, and monocytes. It mediates the rolling of the unactivated neutrophil on cytokine activated ECs. The EC counter-receptor for L-selectin may be E-selectin (ELAM-1). This suggests that L-selectin plays a role in leukocyte extravasation at sites of injury.

Both E-selectin and P-selectin are present on activated ECs. E-selectin promotes the adhesion of neutrophils, monocytes, and a subset of memory T-lymphocytes to the EC, thus, helping regulate migration of these cells into tissue areas of inflammation. E-selectin is transiently synthesized by ECs 2 to 8 hours after stimulation by tumor necrosis factor-alpha (TNF-α), IL-1, or lipopolysaccharide (LPS). P-selectin, located in EC secretory granules, is rapidly translocated to the cell membrane after stimulation with histamine or complement 5b-9 complex, peroxides, or thrombin. Its membrane expression is transient, paralleling neutrophil and monocyte adhesion to activated ECs at sites of tissue injury. The counter-receptors for E-selectin and P-selectin have not been characterized at the molecular level.[17]

Immunoglobulin supergene family This family of adhesion receptors shares an immunoglobulin domain of 90 to 100 amino acids sandwiched between two sheets of antiparallel β-strands usually linked by a disulfide bond (Table 4-3). Members of this family of adhesion receptors include ICAM-1, ICAM-2, VCAM-1, LFA-2, LFA-3, TCR, CD4, CD8, MHC class II, and MHC class I.

The LFA-2 receptor found on T-lymphocytes may be activated by binding LFA-3 on the EC. The LFA-2 receptor may subsequently synergize with signals generated by the T-cell receptor (TCR) and enhance the T-lymphocyte immune response.

ICAM-1, located on EC, reacts with the integrins LFA-1 and Mac-1 on leukocytes. Its expression is induced by inflammatory cytokines such as TNF and IL-1. ICAM-2 on EC binds only to LFA-1 on leukocytes and does not appear to be induced by inflammatory mediators. Both ICAM-1 and ICAM-2 mediate cellular responses during the inflammatory response.

VCAM-1 also is expressed on EC in response to inflammatory cytokines. It reacts with VLA-4 on monocytes, lymphocytes, eosinophils, and basophils. It serves to recruit these cells to areas of inflammation.

The T-cell receptor, C4 and C8 (antigen-specific receptors found on T-lymphocytes), and MHC Class II and MHC Class I molecules are important in T-lymphocyte activation and regulate their interaction with other cells in the immune response. These receptors and molecules will be discussed later in this chapter.

MIGRATION

After adherence to the endothelial cell, the neutrophils use pseudopods to squeeze through endothelial cells. Migration beneath the endothelium occurs until the neutrophil passes the basement membrane and periendothelial cells.[18] Migration is enhanced when the EC is activated by IL-1 and/or TNF. The β_2-integrins on leukocytes appear to be important in mediating transendothelial migration.

Neutrophil movement is directed by the binding of chemoattractant molecules and extracellular matrix proteins to specific leukocyte receptors. Chemoattractants include C5a, leukotriene-B$_4$ (LTB$_4$), platelet-activating factor (PAF), crystal-induced chemotactic factor (CCF), N-Formyl-Met-Leu-Phe (f-MLF), and IL-8.[14] It has been demonstrated that when these chemotactic factors are infused into rabbits, an initial neutropenia is followed by a rapid increase in circulating neutrophils and leukocytosis.[19] Other chemoattractants include: C3a; secretions from mast cells, lymphocytes, macrophages and other neutrophils; proteins from the activated coagulation cascade, including the kinin activation pathway; and products from bacteria and viruses. Most leukocyte receptors for extracellular matrix proteins such as fibronectin, collagen, and laminin, belong to the β_1-integrin family.

PHAGOCYTOSIS

Once in the area of inflammation, the neutrophil must recognize the particle as foreign before attachment occurs and phagocytosis begins. Some micro-organisms or particles may be recognized without surface modification, whereas others must be *opsonized* (coated with antibody and/or complement) to make them more palatable to the neutrophil. Two *opsonins* are well-defined, IgG and complement component C3b. The antibody binds to the micro-organism/particle by means of its Fab region, while the Fc region of the antibody attaches to the Fc receptor on the neutrophil membrane. Thus, the antibody forms a connecting link between the micro-organism/particle and the neutrophil. The neutrophil also has receptors for activated complement. (Some bacteria with polysaccharide capsules avoid recognition, thus reducing the effectiveness of phagocytosis.) Following recognition and attachment, the particle is surrounded by extended pseudopods of the neutrophil (Fig. 4-11). As the pseudopods touch, they fuse and pinch off, forming a *phagosome* that is bound by the cytoplasmic membrane turned inside out. A plasma membrane-bound oxidase is activated during ingestion. This oxidase causes enzymatic reduction of oxygen, resulting in the formation of microbactericidal metabolites.

Next, primary and specific granules fuse with the digestive vacuole and dispel their contents into the lumen of the vacuole, forming the *phagolysosome*. This fusion and release is known as degranulation. Some enzymes of the granules may play a role in the killing of the micro-organism, but the direct effect of the granular contents is digestion of the already killed organism. The segregation of the digestive enzymes and oxygen metabolites within the phagolysosome protects the cell from self-injury as it attacks microbes. Following digestion of the phagocytosed material by contents of the granules, the material is exocytosed. Most neutrophils die in the inflammatory exudate and are phagocytosed by macrophages.

In addition to their primary functions of phagocytosis and killing of micro-organisms, neutrophils interact in other physiologic processes. Neutrophils stimulate coagulation by releasing a substance that triggers prekallikrein to become kallikrein. Kallikrein activates the first contact factor of coagulation, thus initiating the extrinsic coagulation pathway. Kallikrein also converts kininogen to kinin. Kinins are responsible for vascular dilation and increased vessel permeability. Kinins, chemotactic for neutrophils, attract them to sites of inflammation. Neutrophils initially activate kinin production, but as the cells accumulate, they break down kinins. Neutrophils also contain *pyrogen*, a substance that acts on the hypothalmus to produce fever. This endogenous pyrogen is now known as IL-1.

Neutrophil metabolism

Neutrophils derive most of their energy from anaerobic glycolysis. The hexose-monophosphate (HMP) shunt, which provides reducing power through production of NADPH, also is active in these cells, especially during the process of phagocytosis. Little energy is derived from the tricarboxylic acid cycle because of the scarcity of mitochondria. The neutrophil has both oxygen-dependent and oxygen-independent mechanisms for killing phagocytosed bacteria (Table 4-4). The oxygen-dependent mechanisms are the most important, although those not requiring oxygen may be important in killing certain types of micro-organisms under specific conditions.

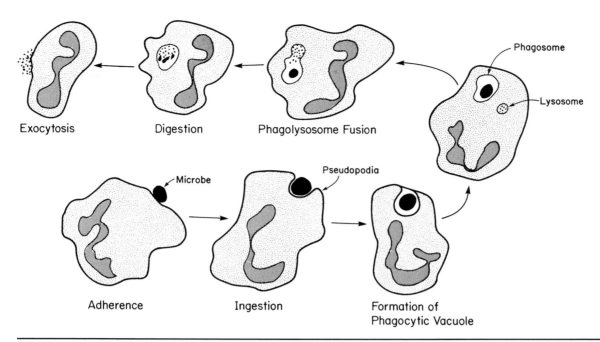

FIGURE 4-11. Phagocytosis begins with recognition and attachment of the microbe to the neutrophil. The microbe is then internalized forming a phagocytic vacuole. Next, the lysosome fuses with the vacuole, forming a phagolysosome, and releases its contents into the vacuole to help kill and digest the microbe. This is followed by extrusion of the vacuole contents from the neutrophil (exocytosis). (Courtesy Denise Miller.)

Phagocytosis is accompanied by an energy-dependent respiratory burst that generates oxidizing compounds through the HMP shunt. These oxidizing compounds produced from partial oxygen reduction are important agents in killing ingested organisms. Activation of a membrane-bound oxidase that uses NADPH as an electron donor (it may also use NADH) produces superoxide (O_2-) from oxygen. Hydrogen peroxide (H_2O_2) is generated from superoxide either spontaneously or catalyzed by superoxide dismutase:

$$2O_2 + 2NADPH \rightarrow 2O_2^- + 2NADP^+ + 2H^+$$
$$\rightarrow H_2O_2 + O_2 + 2NADP^+$$

The increased $NADP^+$ produced from this reaction activates the HMP shunt.

TABLE 4-4 *NEUTROPHIL ANTIMICROBIAL SYSTEMS*

1. Oxygen-dependent
   A. Myeloperoxidase-independent
      —Hydrogen peroxide (H_2O_2)
      —Superoxide anion (O_2^-)
      —Hydroxyl radicals (OH^-)
      —Singlet oxygen ($^1O_2$)
   B. Myeloperoxidase-dependent
      (forms oxidized halogens)

2. Oxygen-independent
   —Acid pH of phagosome
   —Lysozyme (primary granules)
   —Lactoferrin (secondary granules)
   —Cationic proteins (primary granules)

Hydrogen peroxide is the important bactericidal compound of oxygen metabolism in neutrophils. However, its killing effect is potentiated by the formation of OCl^-, a highly reactive oxidizing radical that is a potent antimicrobial. The reaction requires myeloperoxidase, an enzyme localized in the primary granules of neutrophils.

$$H_2O_2 + Cl^- \xrightarrow{\text{myeloperoxidase}} OCl^- + H_2O$$

Defects in the production of H_2O_2 may cause severe and fatal infections. However, myeloperoxidase deficiency does not usually result in an increased incidence of bacterial infection unless there are other concomitant host defects. Myeloperoxidase deficiency is partially compensated for by an increase in activity of myeloperoxidase-independent systems.

Some micro-organisms can produce H_2O_2, contributing to the microbicidal activity of neutrophils. The H_2O_2 formed may be toxic to the organism that formed it or to other microbial species. This H_2O_2 of microbial origin is particularly important when the leukocytic generation of H_2O_2 is defective, as in chronic granulomatous disease.

The ability of the neutrophil to produce superoxide and reoxidize the product to oxygen can be measured in the laboratory by the redox dye, nitroblue tetrazolium. The dye is reduced to a blue formazan during the normal oxygen metabolism that occurs with ingestion. If oxygen is not metabolized, the dye is not reduced and remains yellow.

The HMP shunt is also stimulated by the process of glutathione (GSH) detoxification of H_2O_2 catalyzed by the enzyme glutathione peroxidase. In this process, gluta-thione is oxidized (GSSG). In turn, GSSG is reduced back to GSH by NADPH (from the HMP shunt) catalyzed by the enzyme glutathione reductase. There is a concomitant increase in $NADP^+$, stimulating the HMP shunt.

$$2GSH + H_2O_2 \xrightarrow[\text{peroxidase}]{\text{glutathione}} GSSG + 2H_2O$$

$$GSSG + 2NADPH \xrightarrow[\text{reductase}]{\text{glutathione}} 2GSH + 2NADP^+$$

Some of the bactericidal oxygen-independent factors of neutrophils include the acid pH of the phagosome and the presence of lysozyme from primary granules, which is capable of hydrolyzing bacterial cell wall components. Lactoferrin from secondary granules inhibits bacterial growth (bacteriostatic) by binding iron, an essential microbial nutrient. Cationic proteins from neutrophil primary granules are released in the phagosome, coat the bacteria, and kill them.

All micro-organisms are not killed by the same mechanism; consequently, specific defects in the neutrophil metabolism may result in infection by certain types of micro-organisms but not by other types. Some virulent organisms may overcome the neutrophil defense system. These surviving organisms may then multiply and kill the neutrophil. The organisms are freed in the process, and the neutrophil releases its enzymes into the tissue. This causes tissue damage and inflammation.

Studies of granulocyte metabolism have identified a variety of metabolic pathways in addition to glycolysis. Some of these pathways are more active at the myeloblast stage and decrease or disappear with maturity of the cell:

1. Granulocytes are able to synthesize pyrimidines de novo. The activity of the enzymes involved is highest in myeloblasts and decreases with cellular maturity.
2. Granulocytes cannot perform the early steps of purine synthesis, but they are capable of synthesizing purines from small precursors.
3. DNA synthesis is most active in the immature cells. DNA polymerase activity decreases with maturity of the granulocytes.
4. RNA synthesis is directed by DNA in both mature and immature cells. It is apparent, however, that only certain regions of the chromosome corresponding to euchromatin are transcribed. Myeloblasts have the highest rate of RNA activity. RNA synthesis also increases after particle ingestion.
5. Myeloblasts incorporate amino acids into protein at a high rate. This activity decreases in circulating granulocytes.
6. Granulocytes are capable of synthesizing lipids and using them as an energy source. Lipid turnover and biosynthesis is increased in phagocytosis due to loss of cytoplasmic membrane in formation of the phagosome.
7. The synthesis of arachidonic acid is stimulated when neutrophils are exposed to chemotactic factors. Arachidonic acid is the precursor substance of prostaglandin and thromboxane, potent modulators of the inflammatory response, and platelet aggregation.

EOSINOPHILS

The eosinophil originates from the multipotential or multilineage cell, CFU-GEMM. The CFU-GEMM is induced to differentiate into CFU-Eo by the action of the growth factors, GM-CSF and IL-3, and IL-5. Only IL-5 has lineage specificity for eosinophils and is the major cytokine required for eosinophil production.

The eosinophil undergoes a morphologic maturation similar to the neutrophil. It is not possible to morphologically differentiate eosinophilic precursors from neutrophilic precursors with the light microscope until the myelocyte stage, when the typical acidophilic crystalloid granules of the eosinophil appear. Granule formation begins in the promyelocyte, with small coreless granules. The myelocyte eosinophil contains large, eosin-staining, crystalloid granules. Maturation from the myelocyte to the metamyelocyte, band, and segmented stages is similar to that described for neutrophils with gradual nuclear indentation and segmentation. There is no appreciable change in the cytoplasm in these latter stages of development. The reddish-orange spherical granules are uniform in size and evenly distributed throughout the cell. Because of the low percentage of eosinophils in the bone marrow, no useful purpose is served by differentiating the eosinophil into its maturational stages (e.g., eosinophilic myelocyte) when the count is normal. Bone marrow maturation and storage time is about 9 days.

The mature eosinophil (Fig. 4-12) is from 12 to 17 μm in diameter. The nucleus usually has no more than two or three lobes, and the cytoplasm is completely filled with granules. The granules are bound by a phospholipid membrane and have a central crystalloid core surrounded by a matrix. These granules contain four major proteins: major basic protein (MBP), eosinophil cationic protein (ECP), eosinophil peroxidase (EPO), and eosinophil-derived neurotoxin (EDN), also known as protein x (EPX)[20] (Table 4-5). The MBP is located in the crystalloid core, while the other three proteins are found in the granule matrix. Granules also contain the enzymes acid phosphatase, glycuronidase, cathepsins, aryl-sulphatase, histaminase, collagenase, and catalase.

Eosinophil concentration and kinetics

Eosinophils have a concentration in peripheral blood of less than 0.45×10^9/L (1% to 3%), with a mean of 0.35

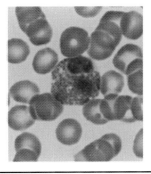

FIGURE 4-12. Eosinophil (PB, 250×, Wright-Giemsa stain).

TABLE 4-5 *MAJOR PROTEINS OF EOSINOPHIL GRANULES*

1. Major Basic Protein (MBP)
   —cytotoxic for protozoans and helminth parasites
   —stimulates release of histamine from mast cells and basophils

2. Eosinophil Cationic Protein (ECP)
   —capable of killing mammalian and non-mammalian cells
   —stimulates release of histamine from mast cells and basophils
   —inhibition of T-lymphocyte proliferation
   —preactivates plasminogen
   —enhances mucus production in the bronchi
   —stimulation of glycosaminoglycan production by fibroblasts

3. Eosinophil-Derived Neurotoxin (EDN) (also known as eosinophil Protein X)
   —ability to provoke cerebral and cerebellar dysfunction in animals
   —inhibitor of T-cell responses

4. Eosinophil peroxidase (EPO)
   —combines with H_2O_2 and halide ions to produce a potent bactericidal and helminthicidal action
   —cytotoxic for tumor and host cells
   —stimulates histamine release and degranulation of most cells
   —diminishes roles of other inflammatory cells by inactivating leukotrienes.

$\times~10^9$/L. The cell shows a diurnal variation of highest concentrations in the morning and lowest concentrations in the afternoon. During the first 3 months of life, the eosinophil count may be three times as high as in the adult.

Very little is known about the kinetics of eosinophils. Most of the body's eosinophil population is below the epithelial layer in tissues that are exposed to the external environment such as the nasal passages, skin, and urinary tract. These cells spend very little time in the peripheral blood (1 to 8 hours) before migrating to the tissues where they may live for several weeks. Tissue eosinophils may re-enter the circulation and bone marrow.

Eosinophil function

Eosinophils have multiple biologic functions and contribute to a variety of immune defense mechanisms. Their production and function are influenced by the cellular arm of the immune system.[20] Eosinophils are associated with allergic reactions, parasitic infections, and chronic inflammation. Their major defensive role is host defense against helminth parasites via a complex interaction of the eosinophils, immune system, and parasite. They also are capable of phagocytosing bacteria.

The eosinophils are proinflammatory cells that are capable of either protecting or damaging the host, depending on the situation.[20] Eosinophils respond to and have membrane receptors for the same chemotaxins as neutrophils: IgG and complement. The cell membrane also possesses receptors for IgE and histamine. The density of these receptors increase when the cell is activated. Especially chemotactic for eosinophils are products released from basophils and mast cells, lymphokines from sensitized lymphocytes, and antigen/antibody reactions of allergy. The cytokines IL-3, IL-5, and GM-CSF promote the adherance of eosinophils and induce chemoattractant-induced adhesion.[21] Transendothelial migration is 10-fold greater in the presence of these cytokines.

Eosinophils have a β_2-integrin–independent mechanism for recruitment into the tissues. This was first suggested when eosinophils and mononuclear leukocytes but not neutrophils were found at sites of infection in children with congenital β_2-integrin deficiency. Eosinophil recruitment appears to be modulated by the eosinophil adhesion receptor, very late activation antigen-4 (VLA-4) and its ligand on EC, VCAM-1. VCAM-1 has been shown to be expressed on EC when the vascular endothelium is activated with IL-1, TNF, or IL-4. Changes in eosinophil adhesion molecule expression occur during eosinophil migration. This implies that dynamic changes in cell adhesion molecules are involved in cell recruitment to areas of inflammation.

The eosinophil liberates substances that can neutralize mast cell and basophil products, thereby modulating the allergic response. Evidence suggests a direct correlation between the degree of eosinophilia and severity of inflammatory diseases such as asthma. In these conditions, the cytotoxic potential of eosinophils is turned against the host's own tissue.

● BASOPHILS

Basophils (Fig. 4-13), the smallest of the granulocytes (10 to 14 μm), originate from the multilineage stem cell CFU-GEMM in the bone marrow. The CFU-GEMM is induced to differentiate to the CFU-Ba by both GM-CSF and IL-3. Basophil colonies develop from the CFU-Ba under the influence of IL-3.

Basophils undergo a maturation process similar to that described for the neutrophil. The first recognizable stage is the promyelocyte, although this stage is very difficult to differentiate from the promyelocyte of the neutrophil or eosinophil. The basophilic promyelocyte is smaller (12 μm) with a higher N:C ratio than the promyelocyte of neutrophils or eosinophils. As with the eosinophils, the various stages of the maturing basophil are characterized by gradual indentation and segmentation of the nucleus.

The basophilic myelocyte, metamyelocyte, band, and segmented forms are easily discernible from other granulocytes because of the presence of large (0.2 to 1 μm) purple-black granules unevenly distributed throughout the cytoplasm. The granules were originally believed to be basophilic (hence came the name basophil). It is now well established that the "basophilic" granules are actu-

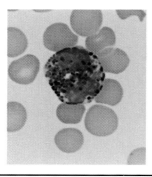

FIGURE 4-13. Basophil (peripheral blood, 250×, Wright-Giemsa stain).

ally metachromatic. The granules contain histamine and heparin. The granules have been called "suicide bags" because the release of large numbers of these granules in anaphylactic shock may cause death of the host. Their solubility in water causes the cellular granules to appear scanty on stained smears. Frequently, only a few deeply stained granules overlie the nucleus while the remaining granules have a washed-out appearance. The nucleus is usually bilobular in the mature basophil, but its actual conformation is often obscured by the overlying granules. The cytoplasm may appear rose- or lavender-colored or may not stain at all. Because there are so few of these blood cells in bone marrow and peripheral blood, there is no advantage in classifying the basophil into maturation categories.

The relation between basophils and tissue mast cells continues to be investigated. The origin of mast cells is not certain, but these cells may share a common hematopoietic stem cell with the basophil. It is difficult to differentiate the mast cell and basophil precursors in the bone marrow, although there are some differences (Table 4-6). The basophil has a segmented nucleus, whereas the mast cell has a single round nucleus and many more granules than the basophil. In fact, the mast cell granules almost obscure identification of the nucleus. The enzyme content and ultrastructure of the granules are additional properties that help distinguish the two cells. Mast cell granules contain acid phosphatase, protease, and alkaline phosphatase. Basophil granules do not contain these enzymes, but they are positive for peroxidase. Both cells are cytochemically positive with the periodic acid–Schiff (PAS) reaction, but the positivity in basophils is more intense

TABLE 4-6 *COMPARISON OF THE CHARACTERISTICS OF BASOPHILS AND MAST CELLS*

Characteristics	Basophils	Mast Cells
Origin	Hematopoietic Stem Cell	Hematopoietic Stem Cell
Site Maturation	Bone Marrow	Connective or Mucosal Tissue
Proliferative Potential	no	yes
Life Span	days	weeks to months
Size	small	large
Nucleus	segmented	round
Granules	few, small (peroxidase positive)	many, large (acid phosphatase, alkaline phosphatase positive)
Key Cytokine Regulating Development	IL-3	Stem cell factor (SCF)
Surface Receptors:		
IL-3	present	absent
c-kit (receptor for SCF)	absent	present
IgE receptor	present	present

than that of mast cells. Mast cells, which are long-lived and have proliferative potential, are found in bone marrow and tissue but not in peripheral blood. Basophils are endstage cells incapable of proliferation and spend only hours in the blood. Basophils are present in bone marrow, peripheral blood, and tissue.

Mast cells and basophils express different surface antigens. Mast cells have an antigen profile similar to that of macrophages, whereas basophils have a profile similar to that of other granulocytes.[22]

Basophil concentration

Basophils constitute less than $0.2 \times 10^9/L$ (0% to 1%) of the total leukocytes. Although they are scarce, it is not difficult to identify them on a blood smear. Even when the granules are washed out, the few deep-staining granules remaining are certain identification markers of this cell.

Basophil function

The basophil and mast cell function as mediators of inflammatory responses, especially those of hypersensitivity. These cells have membrane receptors for IgE. When IgE attaches to the receptor, the cell is activated and degranulation is initiated. Degranulation releases enzymes that are vasoactive, bronchoconstrictive, and chemotactic (especially for eosinophils). This release of mediators initiates the classic clinical signs of immediate hypersensitivity. These cells can synthesize more granules after degranulation occurs. Basophils and mast cells express CD40L, the ligand for CD40, an antigen on B-lymphocytes. The interaction of B-lymphocyte CD40 and basophil CD 40L in conjunction with IL-4 can induce IgE synthesis by B-lymphocytes.[23] Thus, basophils may play an important role in inducing and maintaining allergic reactions.

In addition to IgE, other mediators may activate basophils and mast cells, including complement fragments C3a, C4a, and C5a; histamine-releasing factors secreted by platelets and mononuclear peripheral blood cells; drugs.[24]

Recruitment of basophils into sites of inflammation in the tissues is mediated by adhesion molecules present on both eosinophils and basophils. Some of these molecules are not present on neutrophils (i.e., VLA-4). This may help explain the preferential recruitment of eosinophils and basophils into extravascular inflammatory sites associated with hypersensitivity and allergic responses.

MONOCYTES

The monocyte is produced in the bone marrow from a bipotential stem cell (CFU-GM) that is capable of maturing into either monocytes or granulocytes. The differentiation and growth of CFU-GM into monocytes in culture is dependent on the action of GM-CSF, IL-3, and M-CSF. It is believed that these growth factors also are the regulators of in vivo monocytopoiesis. Monocytes and macrophages can be stimulated by T-lymphocytes and endotoxin to liberate M-CSF. This may be one mechanism for the monocytosis associated with some infections. The M-CSF also activates the secretory and phagocytic activity of monocytes and macrophages.

Neoplastic clonal proliferation of neutrophils, such as occurs in CML, frequently shows proliferation of monocytes as well as neutrophils, and acute myelomonocytic leukemia involves unregulated proliferation of both monoblasts and myeloblasts. The bipotential stem cell, CFU-GM, is most likely the neoplastic cell in these disorders.

● Monocyte maturation

The monocyte precursors in the bone marrow are the monoblast and promonocyte. These cells are found in abundance only in leukemic processes of the monocyte system. The monoblast of the marrow cannot be morphologically distinguished from the myeloblast by light microscopy unless there is marked proliferation of the monocytic series, as occurs in monocytic leukemia. It is not known whether the leukemic process of maturation simulates normal monocytopoiesis. Cytochemical stains frequently are used to help differentiate myeloblasts and monoblasts.

The promonocyte is usually the first stage to develop morphologic characteristics that allow it to be differentiated as a monocyte precursor by light microscopy. The identification of early monocyte precursors is aided by observing folds or indentations in the nucleus and by their association with mature monocytes.

MONOBLAST

The *monoblast* (Fig. 4-14) has abundant agranular blue-grey cytoplasm. The nucleus is most often ovoid or round but may be folded or indented. The light blue-purple nuclear chromatin is finely dispersed (lacy), and several nucleoli are easily identified. Differentiation of the monoblast from the myeloblast may be possible with special cytochemical stains. The monoblast has nonspecific esterase activity demonstrated by reaction with the substrates α-naphthyl butyrate or naphthol AS-D acetate (NASDA). The NASDA activity is inhibited by sodium fluoride. The myeloblast has both specific esterase activity (demonstrated by reaction with the substrate naphthol AS-D chloroacetate) and nonspecific esterase activity, but the nonspecific esterases are not inhibited by sodium fluoride.

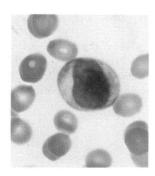

FIGURE 4-15. Promonocyte (peripheral blood, 250×, Wright-Giemsa stain).

PROMONOCYTE

The *promonocyte* (Fig. 4-15) is an intermediate form between the monoblast and monocyte. The cell is large, 12 to 20 μm in diameter, with abundant blue-grey cytoplasm. Fine azurophilic granules may be present. The nucleus is most often irregular and deeply indented with a fine chromatin network. Chromatin filaments are coarser than the monoblast. Nucleoli may be present. Cytochemical stains for nonspecific esterase, peroxidase, acid phosphatase, and arylsulfatase are positive.

MATURE MONOCYTE

The mature monocyte (Fig. 4-16) has variable morphologic characteristics dependent on its activity. The cell adheres to glass and spreads or sends out numerous psuedopods resulting in a wide variation of size and shape on blood smears. The cells range in size from 12 to 20 μm with an average of 18 μm, making them the largest cells in peripheral blood. The blue-grey cytoplasm is evenly dispersed with fine dust-like membrane-bound granules, which give the cell cytoplasm the appearance of "ground-glass." Electron-microscopic cytochemistry reveals two types of granules. One type contains peroxidase, acid phosphatase, and arylsulfatase, suggesting that these granules are similar to the lysosomes (azurophilic granules) of neutrophils. Less is known about the content of the other type of granule, but, unlike the specific granules of neutrophils, it does not contain alkaline phosphatase. The lipid membrane of the granules stain with Sudan black B.

The nucleus is irregular, frequently horseshoe- or bean-shaped, and possesses numerous folds, giving the appearance of brain-like convolutions. Sometimes nucleoli may

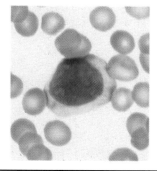

FIGURE 4-14. Monoblast (peripheral blood, 250×, Wright-Giemsa stain).

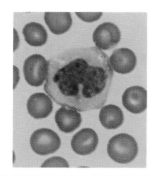

FIGURE 4-16. Monocyte (peripheral blood, 250×, Wright-Giemsa stain).

be seen. The chromatin is loose and linear, forming a lacy pattern in comparison to the clumped dense chromatin of mature lymphocytes or granulocytes. Monocytes, however, are sometimes difficult to distinguish from large lymphocytes, especially in reactive states when there are many reactive lymphocytes.

MACROPHAGE

The monocyte eventually leaves the blood and enters the tissues, where it matures into a macrophage. The transition from monocyte to macrophage is characterized by progressive cellular enlargement. The nucleus becomes round, nucleoli appear, and the cytoplasm appears blue. As it matures, the macrophage loses peroxidase, but reveals increases in endoplasmic reticulum (ER), lysosomes, and mitochondria. Also, granules are noted in the maturing macrophage. These cells can live for months in the tissues. Macrophages do not normally re-enter the blood, but, in areas of inflammation, some may gain access to the lymph, eventually entering the blood.

Macrophages, collectively known as histiocytes, develop different cytochemical and morphologic characteristics that depend on the site of maturation and habitation in tissue. These cells are given more specific names, dependent on their location in the body. For example, macrophages in the liver are known as Kupffer cells, those in the lung as alveolar macrophages, those in the skin as Langerhans cells, and those in the brain as microglial cells.

Macrophages may proliferate in the tissue, especially in areas of inflammation, thereby increasing the number of cells at these sites. Occasionally, two or more macrophages fuse to produce giant multinucleated cells. This occurs in granulomatous lesions, where many macrophages are tightly packed together. Fusion also occurs when particulate matter is too large for one cell to ingest or when two cells simultaneously ingest a particle.

Monocyte kinetics

The promonocytes undergo two or three divisions before maturing into monocytes. Bone marrow transit time is about 60 hours. In contrast to the large neutrophil storage pool, there is no reserve pool of monocytes in the bone marrow, most are released within a day after their derivation from promonocytes.[18] Monocytes diapedese into the tissues in a random manner after an average transit time in the vascular space of 12 to 14 hours.

The total vascular monocyte pool consists of a marginal and a circulating pool. The marginating pool is about three times the size of the circulating pool. Monocytes in the circulating peripheral blood number about 0.2 to 0.8 $\times$ 10^9/L in the normal adult or about 4% to 10% of the total leukocytes. Children have a slightly higher concentration. Absolute monocytosis prevails in the first 2 weeks of life, with a mean of 1×10^9/L.

Monocyte metabolism and function

It has been known since the experiments of Metchnikov that monocytes and macrophages function as phagocytes.

In addition to their phagocytic function, these cells secrete a variety of substances that affect the function of other cells, especially that of lymphocytes. Lymphocytes, in turn, secrete soluble products, lymphokines, that modulate monocytic functions.

Monocytes (and macrophages) ingest and kill micro-organisms. They are especially important in inhibiting the growth of intracellular micro-organisms. This inhibition requires cellular activation (enhancement of function) of monocytes by soluble products of T-lymphocytes. The killing by activated monocytes is nonspecific (i.e., the secretions from Listeria-sensitized T-cells will activate a killing mechanism in monocytes not only to Listeria but to other micro-organisms). Activation also may occur as the result of the actions of other substances on monocytes such as endotoxins and naturally occurring opsonins. Activation results in the production of many large granules, enhanced phagocytosis, and an increase in the HMP shunt.

Monocytes/macrophages have some ability to bind directly to micro-organisms, but binding is enhanced if the micro-organism has been opsonized by complement or immunoglobin (Fig. 4-17). Macrophages possess receptors for the Fc component of IgG and for the complement component C3b. Following attachment, the opsonized organism is ingested in a manner similar to that for neutrophils (Fig. 4-11). Primary lysosomes fuse with the phagosome, releasing hydrolytic enzymes and other microbicidal substances. The most powerful microbicidal substances of monocytes and macrophages are products of oxygen metabolism: superoxide (O_2^-), singlet oxygen ($^1O_2$), hydroxyl radical (OH^-), and hydrogen peroxide (H_2O_2).

Activated macrophages attach to tumor cells and kill them by a direct cytolytic effect. If the tumor cell has immunoglobulin attached, the macrophage Fc receptor attaches to the Fc portion of the immunoglobulin and exerts a lytic effect on the tumor cell.

Macrophages are important as scavengers, phagocytosing cellular debris, effete cells, and other particulate matter. Monocytes in the blood ingest activated clotting factors, thus limiting the coagulation process. They also ingest denatured protein and antigen–antibody complexes. Macrophages lining the blood vessels remove toxic substances from the blood, preventing their escape into tissues. The macrophages of the spleen are important in removing aged erythrocytes from the blood; they conserve the iron of hemoglobin by either storing it for future use or by releasing it to transferrin for use by developing normoblasts in the bone marrow. The splenic macrophages, by virtue of their Fc receptor, also remove cells sensitized with antibody. In autoimmune hemolytic anemias or in autoimmune thrombocytopenia, the spleen is sometimes removed to prevent premature destruction of these antibody-coated cells and the resulting cytopenias.

In some pathologic conditions, for unknown reasons, erythrocytes are randomly phagocytosed and destroyed by monocytes and macrophages in the blood and bone marrow (erythrophagocytosis) (Fig. 4-18). *Erythrophagocytosis* is readily identified when the ingested erythrocytes still contain hemoglobin. At times, erythrocyte digestion

**Phagocyte - Microorganism Binding
in the Presence of Opsonins**

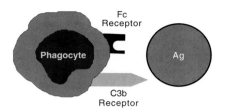

Phagocyte binding of microorganism
without antibody or complement.

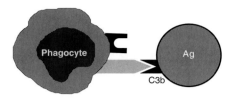

Phagocyte binding of microorganism is
enhanced when complement (opsonin) is
attached.

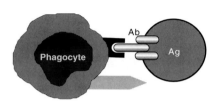

Phagocyte binding of microorganism is
enhanced when antibody (opsonin) is
attached.

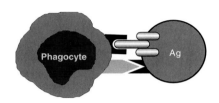

Phagocyte binding of microorganism
when both complement and antibody are
attached is stronger than if either
opsonin were present alone.

FIGURE 4-17. Phagocyte micro-organism
binding in the presence of opsonins.
(Courtesy of Denise Miller.)

can be inferred by the finding of ghost spheres within the macrophage.

The monocyte–macrophage system plays a major role in initiating and regulating the immune response. Macrophages phagocytize and degrade both soluble and particulate substances that are foreign to the host. Through unknown mechanisms, they spare critical portions of these antigens known as antigenic determinant sites or epitopes. These antigenic determinants on the macrophage membrane are presented to antigen-dependent T-lymphocytes.

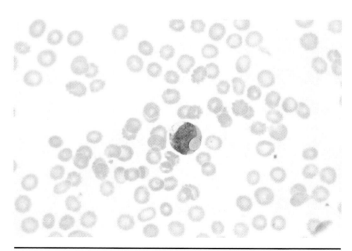

FIGURE 4-18. Erythrophagocytosis by a monocyte (PB; 250×; Wright-Giemsa stain).

Thus, monocytes/macrophages are known as antigen-presenting cells (APC). In addition to antigen presentation, the APC provides cell surface molecules known as major histocompatibility complex (MHC) antigens and a secretory product, IL-1. Antigen-specific T-lymphocyte proliferation requires antigen presentation in context with cell surface MHC antigens, and stimulation with soluable mediators such as IL-1 or IL-2. T-lymphocytes will only respond to foreign antigens when the antigens are displayed on APCs that have the same MHC phenotype as the lymphocyte itself.[25]

Macrophages stimulate the proliferation and differentiation of lymphocytes through secretion of cytokines. They secrete IL-1, which stimulates T-lymphocytes to secrete interleukin-2 (IL-2). IL-2 is a growth factor that stimulates the proliferation of other T-lymphocytes. In addition, IL-2 acts in synergy with interferon (IFN) to activate macrophages.[26] Prostaglandins are arachidonic metabolites that, when released from macrophages, inhibit the functions of activated lymphocytes. Activated lymphocytes, in turn, secrete lymphokines that regulate the function of macrophages. For these interdependent reactions to occur between the macrophage and lymphocyte, the two cell populations must express compatible MHC antigens.

Macrophages release a variety of substances that are involved in host defense or that may affect the function of other cells in addition to IL-1. Other secretory products that are involved in host defense include lysozymes, complement components, and IFN (an antiviral compound).

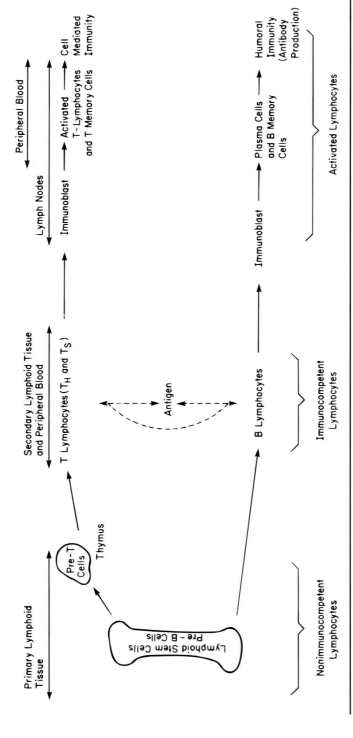

FIGURE 4-19. Lymphocytes originate from the lymphoid stem cell (derived from the pluripotential stem cell) in the bone marrow. Lymphocytes that mature in the thymus become T-lymphocytes and those that mature in the bone marrow become B-lymphocytes. Three morphologic stages can be identified in this development to T and B cells: lymphoblast, prolymphocyte, and lymphocyte. Upon encounter with antigen, these immunocompetent T and B lymphocytes undergo blast transformation, usually in the lymph nodes, to form effector lymphocytes. The B-lymphocytes eventually emerge as plasma cells. Effector T-lymphocytes, however, are morphologically indistinguishable from the original T-lymphocytes. The recognizable morphologic stages of blast transformation include activated lymphocytes, immunoblasts, plasmacytoid lymphocytes (B cells), and plasma cells (B cells). Marker studies of these cells indicate that some morphologic stages may represent several stages of immunologic maturation.

Secreted substances that modulate other cells include: hematopoietic growth factors (G-CSF, M-CSF, GM-CSF), factors that stimulate the growth of new capillaries, factors that stimulate and suppress the activity of lymphocytes, chemotactic substances for neutrophils, and a substance that stimulates the hepatocyte to secrete fibrinogen. Activated macrophages also release, after death, enzymes such as collagenase, elastase, and neutral proteinase that hydrolyze tissue components.

● LYMPHOCYTES

For many years after its discovery, the lymphocyte was considered an insignificant component of blood and lymph. Since 1960, major advances in immunology have targeted the lymphocyte as directing the activities of all other cells in the *immune response*. The lymphocyte's primary function is to react with antigen and, together with monocytes, modulate the immune response.

● Maturation

As already discussed, the lymphoid cell line arises from the pluripotential stem cell found in the bone marrow. The pluripotential stem cell gives rise to two committed stem cells: the lymphoid stem cell and the hematopoietic stem cell. The lymphoid stem cell differentiates and matures, under the inductive influence of selective microenvironments, into two types of morphologically identical but immunologically and functionally diverse lymphocytes, T-lymphocytes and B-lymphocytes.

Lymphopoiesis can be divided into two different phases: *antigen-independent lymphopoiesis* and *antigen-dependent lymphopoiesis* (Fig. 4-19). Antigen-independent lymphopoiesis takes place within the primary lymphoid tissue (bone marrow, thymus, fetal liver, yolk sac). This type of lymphopoiesis begins with the committed lymphoid stem cell and results in the formation of immunocompetent T-lymphocytes and B-lymphocytes (nicknamed "virgin" lymphocytes because they have not yet reacted with antigen). Antigen-dependent lymphopoiesis occurs in the secondary lymphoid tissue (adult bone marrow, spleen, lymph nodes, gut-associated lymphoid tissue), and it begins with antigenic stimulation of the immunocompetent T- and B-lymphocytes. This type of lymphopoiesis results in the formation of effector T- and B-lymphocytes that mediate the immune response through the production of lymphokines by T-lymphocytes and antibodies by B-lymphocytes.

The morphologic criteria that are used to identify the stages of antigen-independent lymphopoiesis do not give precise information to distinguish between T- and B-lymphocyte categories. It does, however give information on the degree of maturation and activity of these cells. Morphologic assessment of lymphocyte populations is sufficient in most cases. When there is a need to differentiate the T or B specificity of these cells (as in malignant proliferations), monoclonal antibodies are most commonly used.

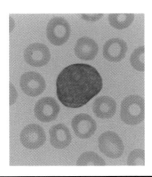

FIGURE 4-20. Lymphoblast (PB, 250×, Wright-Giemsa stain).

ANTIGEN-INDEPENDENT LYMPHOPOIESIS

Three stages of bone marrow morphologic maturation are recognized: lymphoblast, prolymphocyte, and lymphocyte.

Lymphoblast   The *lymphoblast* (Fig. 4-20) is about 10 to 18 μm in diameter with a high N:C ratio. The nuclear chromatin is lacy and fine, but it appears more smudged or heavy than that of myeloblasts. One or two well-defined pale blue nucleoli are visible. The nuclear membrane is dense, and a perinuclear clear zone can be seen. The agranular cytoplasm is more scanty than in other white cell blasts and stains deep blue. There are subtle differences, but lymphoblasts are usually morphologically indistinguishable from myeloblasts. Cytochemical stains are needed to identify their lymphoid origin. Unlike myeloblasts, the lymphoblasts have no peroxidase, lipid, or esterase but contain acid phosphatase; sometimes deposits of glycogen are present. Both T- and B-lymphoblasts contain a DNA polymerase, terminal deoxynucleotidyl-transferase (TdT). It is believed that this enzyme is a specific marker for immature lymphoid cells that are in an intermediate developmental stage between the stem cell and differentiated T- and B-lymphocytes. Special stains may sometimes be used to help differentiate T- and B-lymphoblasts. Lymphoblasts of T-lymphocyte potential contain alpha-naphthyl acid esterase, whereas B-lymphoblasts may contain small amounts of immunoglobulin or the μ heavy chain immunoglobulin. The immunoglobulin can be detected using immunofluorescent techniques.

Prolymphocyte   The *prolymphocyte* (Fig. 4-21) is very difficult to distinguish in normal bone marrow specimens.

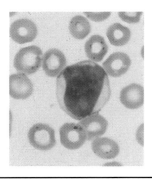

FIGURE 4-21. Prolymphocyte (PB, 250×, Wright-Giemsa stain).

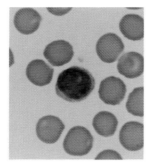

FIGURE 4-22. Lymphocyte (PB, 250×, Wright-Giemsa stain).

The prolymphocyte is slightly smaller than the lymphoblast with a lower N : C ratio. The nuclear chromatin is clumped but more finely dispersed than that of the lymphocyte. Nucleoli are usually present. The cytoplasm is light blue and agranular.

Lymphocyte The mature lymphocyte (Fig. 4-22) has extreme size variability, which is primarily dependent on the amount of cytoplasm present. These mature cells are generally classified as large and small lymphocytes, but the classification is somewhat arbitrary because intermediate forms always are present. There is no advantage in separating the lymphocytes into these two morphologic types. The lymphocyte count should reflect the total of the large and small forms.

Small lymphocytes range in size from 7 to 10 μm and make up the majority of all lymphocytes. In these cells, the nucleus is about the size of an erythrocyte and occupies about 90% of the cell area. The chromatin is deeply condensed and lumpy, staining a deep, dark purple color. Nucleoli, although always present, are only occasionally visible with the light microscope as small, light areas within the nucleus. The nucleus is surrounded by a small amount of sky-blue cytoplasm. A few azurophilic granules and vacuoles may be present. Lymphocytes are motile and may present a peculiar "hand mirror" shape on stained blood smears. These cells have the nucleus in the rounded anterior portion trailed by an elongated section of cytoplasm known as the uropod. Small lymphocytes include a diversity of functional subsets including resting, immunocompetent T- and B-lymphocytes, differentiated T-effector, and T- and B-memory lymphocytes.

Large lymphocytes are heterogeneous and range in size from 11 to 16 μm in diameter. The nucleus may be slightly larger than in the small lymphocyte, but the difference in cell size is mainly attributable to a larger amount of cytoplasm. The cytoplasm may be lighter blue with peripheral basophilia, or it may be darker than the cytoplasm of small lymphocytes. Azurophilic granules may be prominent. These granules differ from those of the myelocytic cells in that they are peroxidase-negative. The nuclear chromatin appears similar to that of the small lymphocyte, and the nucleus may be slightly indented. These large cells, like the small lymphocytes, probably represent a diversity of functional subsets.

ANTIGEN-DEPENDENT LYMPHOPOIESIS (BLAST TRANSFORMATION)

During development into *immunocompetent* T- and B-lymphocytes, the cells acquire specific receptors for antigen, which commit them to an antigen specificity. Contact and binding of this specific antigen to receptors on immunocompetent lymphocytes begins a complex sequence of cellular events known as blast transformation (blastogenesis). The end result is a clonal amplification of cells responsible for the overt expression of immunity to the specific antigen. The series of events, usually occurring within the lymph node, include cell enlargement, an increase in DNA synthesis, enlargement of the nucleolus, an increase in the rough endoplasmic reticulum, and mitosis. These transformed cells, called immunoblasts, apparently have the option of differentiating into memory cells or effector cells that are capable of mediating the immune response.

Reactive lymphocyte One form of an antigen-stimulated lymphocyte is the *reactive lymphocyte* (Fig. 4-23). Although this cell's place in the blast transformation process is not certain, it may be a precursor to the immunoblast. The reactive lymphocyte exhibits a variety of morphologic features and is usually bizarrely shaped. The cell is larger than resting (unstimulated) lymphocytes with an increase in diffuse or localized basophilia of the cytoplasm. Frequently, the basophilia is intense near the periphery of the cytoplasmic membrane. Azurophilic granules may be increased in number, and vacuoles are sometimes present. The cytoplasmic membrane is easily indented by surrounding erythrocytes, which give the cell a scallop shape. The nucleus may be round but is more frequently elongated, stretched, or irregular. The chromatin becomes more dispersed, staining lighter than the chromatin of a resting lymphocyte. Nucleoli may be seen when the chromatin pattern is fine and dispersed.

The reactive lymphocyte is also referred to as *stimulated, transformed, atypical, activated,* and *leukocytoid.* A few reactive lymphocytes may be seen in the blood of healthy individuals, but they are found in increased concentrations in viral infections. For this reason, the reactive lymphocyte also has been called a *virocyte.*

Immunoblast The *immunoblast* (Fig. 4-24) is the next stage in blast transformation. The cell is characterized by prominent nucleoli and a fine nuclear chromatin pattern (but coarser than that of other leukocyte blasts). The large

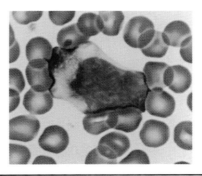

FIGURE 4-23. Reactive lymphocyte (PB, 250×, Wright-Giemsa stain).

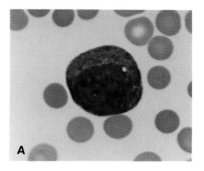

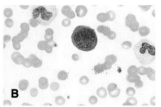

A

B

FIGURE 4-24. A, Immunoblast (PB, peripheral blood, 250×, Wright-Giemsa stain); **B**, Immunoblast (PB, peripheral blood, 250×, Wright-Giemsa stain).

nucleus is usually central and stains a purple-blue color. The abundant cytoplasm stains an intense blue color due to the high density of polyribosomes. The cell is large, ranging in size from 12 to 25 μm.

Reactive lymphocytes and immunoblasts may be either T- or B-lymphocytes. Final definition requires cell marker studies. In the past, reactive lymphocytes and immunoblasts were referred to as *Downey cells,* and were classified as Types I, II, or III, depending on various morphologic criteria. This classification is obsolete as the various types of Downey cells are actually morphologic variations accompanying the process of blast transformation.

The immunoblast proliferates increasing the pool of cells programmed to respond to the initial antigen. These programmed daughter cells *(effector lymphocytes)* mature into cells that mediate the efferent arm of the immune response. The daughter cells of the B-immunoblasts, which mediate humoral immunity, are plasmacytoid lymphocytes (Fig. 4-25) and plasma cells Fig. 4-26). The plasmacytoid lymphocyte (lymphocytoid plasma cell) is believed to be an immediate precursor of the plasma cell. It gains its descriptive name from its morphologic similarity to the lymphocyte but has marked cytoplasmic basophilia similar to that of plasma cells. The plasma cell has an eccentric nucleus with clumped chromatin; abundant, deeply basophilic cytoplasm; and a prominent paranuclear unstained area (Golgi complex). These cells will be discussed in more detail in the section on B-lymphocytes.

In contrast to the progeny of the B-immunoblast, the daughter cells produced from the T-immunoblast, T-effector lymphocytes, are morphologically indistinguishable from the original unsensitized lymphocytes.

A number of the T- and B-immunoblast daughter cells alternatively form T- and B-memory cells. Memory cells are morphologically similar to the resting lymphocytes. They retain the memory of the stimulating antigen and are capable of eliciting a secondary immune response when challenged again by the same antigen.

The reactive lymphocyte is commonly found in the blood during viral infection; however, the immunoblast, plasmacytoid lymphocyte, and plasma cell are usually only found in lymph nodes and other secondary lymphoid tissue. During intense stimulation of the immune system, however, these transformed cells may be found in the peripheral blood due to recirculation.

T-lymphocytes

A portion of the bone marrow lymphoid precursor cells migrate to the thymus where they proliferate and differentiate to acquire cellular characteristics of T-lymphocytes. Lymphopoiesis, at this stage, is independent of antigen stimulation.

T-LYMPHOCYTE DEVELOPMENT

It is believed that the hormone, thymosin, synthesized and secreted by epithelial cells in the thymus, has an influence on T-lymphocyte maturation. Intrathymic death for potential T-lymphocytes is high, about 95%; consequently, only a small portion leave the thymus as immunocompetent T-lymphocytes.

T-lymphocytes diversify late in thymic maturation into either T-helper (T_H) or T-cytotoxic/suppressor (T_C/T_S) lymphocytes (Fig. 4-27).

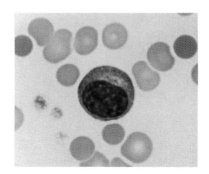

FIGURE 4-25. Plasmacytoid lymph (proplasmocyte). (PB, 250×, Wright-Giemsa stain).

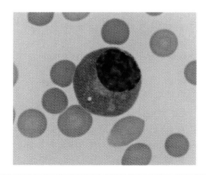

FIGURE 4-26. Plasma cell (PB, 250×, Wright-Giemsa stain).

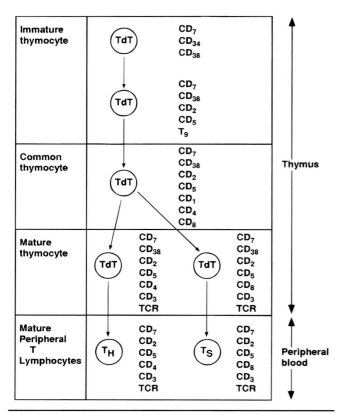

FIGURE 4-27. Immunologic maturation of the T-lymphocyte from the committed lymphocyte stem cell to the peripheral blood T-helper and T-suppressor lymphocytes. Monoclonal antibodies have identified at least three intrathymic stages of maturation before the cells are released to the peripheral blood as mature T-lymphocytes. Differentiation into either helper or suppressor lymphocytes occurs at the last intrathymic stage of maturation. (CD = cluster of differentiation antigens; TCR = T-cell receptor; T9 = a CD number has not yet been assigned to this antigen.)

These subsets are phenotypically and functionally distinct but morphologically indistinguishable from each other. The immunocompetent T-lymphocytes enter the circulation and subsequently populate the paracortical areas of the lymph nodes and the periarteriolar region of white pulp in the spleen. About 60% to 80% of peripheral blood lymphocytes are T-lymphocytes. The helper-to-suppressor cell ratio in the circulation is 2:1.

The thymus functions primarily during fetal life and the first few years after birth; thus, the T-lymphoid system is fully developed at birth. Surgical removal of the thymus after birth does not severely impair immunologic defense; however, lack of thymic development in the fetus (Di George symdrome) results in the absence of T-lymphocytes and severe impairment of the cellular immune response. T-lymphocytes confer protection against antigens that have the ability to avoid contact with antibody by residing and replicating within the cells of the host; thus, serious infection with intracellular parasites, bacteria, fungi, and viruses may occur if T-lymphocytes are deficient.

The phenotypic features of lymphocytes that allow them to be identified as T-lymphocyte or B-lymphocyte include enzymes, surface receptors, and other membrane antigens. This differentiation is possible throughout antigen-independent and antigen-dependent lymphopoiesis. T-lymphocytes contain a variety of enzymes including nonspecific esterases, β-glucuronidase, N-acetyl-β-glucosaminidase, and a dot-like pattern of acid phosphatase positivity. TdT is present in immature thymocytes in the thymus but is absent from mature peripheral blood T-lymphocytes.

MEMBRANE MARKERS

Lymphocyte subpopulations were first identified by virtue of their unique surface receptors. Surface receptors have a binding affinity for certain ligands. Binding of sheep red blood cells (SRBC) by T-lymphocytes via the "E" receptor has been the most useful marker for identifying these cells. The "E" receptor, now known as the lymphocyte function antigen-3 receptor (LFA-3) (CD2) on the T-lymphocyte binds SRBC and forms a rosette. The lymphocyte is in the center of the rosette and the SRBCs form the petals (Fig. 4-28). The receptor is present primarily on mature thymocytes and peripheral blood T-lymphocytes. T-lymphocytes also possess receptors for the Fc portion of IgM and IgG (CD16). It was originally believed that the different Fc receptors identified distinct subpopulations of T-lymphocytes. It is now known that T-lymphocytes can change the specificity of their Fc receptor upon antigenic stimulation.

An extensive panel of monoclonal antibodies has been developed to recognize developmental surface antigens on T-lymphocytes. The monoclonals developed by Coulter Corporation (Hialeah, FL) were designated by the letter "T" followed by a number from 1 to 11 (i.e., T1, T2, and so forth). A second panel was developed by Becton-Dickenson (Mountain View, CA), which used the letters "Leu" followed by numbers. A third panel, developed by

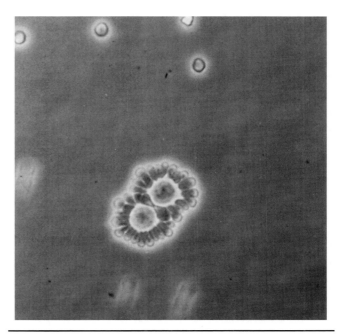

FIGURE 4-28. Sheep erythrocytes bind to T-lymphocyte, forming a rosette. (From Wintrobe's Clinical Hematology, 1993.)

Ortho-Diagnostics, used the letters "OKT" followed by numbers. If a cell reacted with a particular monoclonal antibody, the cell was said to be positive. Thus, one laboratory may label a particular cell population T1-positive, while another labels it Leu1-positive, even though both recognize the same antigen. In an effort to avoid confusion from these numerous terms identifying monoclonal antibodies to the same antigens, the World Health Organization has suggested that the abbreviation CD for "cluster of differentiation" followed by numbers be used to identify specific cell differentiation antigens. In this system, a cell is positive for a particular CD antigen if it reacts with a specific antibody, eliminating the confusing multiple trade names associated with monoclonal antibodies. For instance, a cell reacting with the monoclonal antibodies T1 or Leu1 are CD5 positive. Dako Corporation (Carpinteria, CA) uses the CD terminology to identify its monoclonal antibodies, thus avoiding the use of two different terminology systems. Other cells such as B-lymphocytes, monocytes, and granulocytes also possess surface antigens that can be identified by monoclonal antibodies. Some antigens are lineage-specific while others are shared with a variety of cells. Selected CD antigens and their corresponding monoclonal antibodies are listed in the Appendix (Table M).

It is possible to define distinct stages of intrathymic differentiation of T-lymphocytes using monoclonal probes to identify the presence of CD antigens on the cell surface. Some antigenic determinants appear in a very early developmental stage of the cell and disappear with maturity; other unique determinants appear on more mature cells. Using these probes, it was found that developing T-lymphocytes may be divided into three discrete intrathymic stages (Fig. 4-27): immature thymocyte, common thymocyte, and the mature thymocyte.

Early immature cortical thymocytes express nuclear TdT, CD34 and CD38, CD2, CD5, CD7, and T9 (no CD number yet assigned). As the cell matures to the common thymocyte, it loses T9 and CD34 and acquires CD1, CD4, and CD8. In the last stage, the mature thymocyte stage, the cell loses CD1 and expresses the new antigen, CD3. At this stage, thymocytes retain either CD4 or CD8 but not both. The CD4 lymphocytes are helper lymphocytes while those with CD8 are suppressor lymphocytes. CD4 and CD8 are members of the immunoglobulin supergene family of adhesion molecules. Mature peripheral T-lymphocytes lose CD38, but this antigen can be re-expressed when the cell is activated.[27] The CD25 antigen is associated with the IL-2 receptor and is present on activated T-lymphocytes.

About 60% to 80% of peripheral blood T-lymphocytes are helper cells. They are also the predominant T-lymphocytes of the lymph nodes. Suppressor cells make up only 35% of peripheral blood T-lymphocytes but are the predominant T-lymphocyte found in the bone marrow. The normal T_4/T_8 ratio in circulating blood is 2:1. The balance between T_4 and T_8 must be maintained for normal activity of the immune system. This ratio may be depressed in viral infections, immune deficiency states, and acquired immune deficiency syndrome (AIDS). The ratio may be increased in other disorders such as acute graft-versus-host disease, scleroderma, and multiple sclerosis.

THE T-LYMPHOCYTE ANTIGEN RECEPTOR

The T-lymphocyte has an antigen receptor on its surface that is responsible for initiating the cellular immune response. The receptor, T-cell receptor (TCR), is a heterodimer of two peptide chains linked by a disulphide bond near the membrane (Fig. 4-29). This receptor is a member of the immunoglobulin supergene family of adhesion molecules. There are two groups of TCR defined by the nature of the heterodimer chains, TCR1 (gamma and delta chains) and TCR2 (alpha and beta chains). Most T-lymphocytes express the TCR1 protein. The organization of the TCR chains is similar to that of the immunoglobulin chains. Each TCR chain is composed of a variable region that binds antigen and a constant region that anchors the TCR to the cell membrane. The variable (V), gene is made from three DNA segments, variable (V), diversity (D), and joining (J) in the beta and delta genes but only two segments, V and J, in the alpha and gamma genes. A complete V gene is translocated to a constant (C) gene to form the TCR chain. Before synthesis, there is a rearrangement of the genes coding for this receptor. Rearrangement and recombination of the V, D, and J segments and subsequent joining with a C gene provide a diversity of TCR chains. This diversity allows the T-lymphocyte to recognize many different antigens.

The TCR is expressed in a molecular complex with three other polypeptide chains on the cell membrane. The three chains are not covalently linked, but each chain is a transmembrane peptide. These three chains comprise the CD3 subunit. It is believed that the CD3 complex mediates extracellular to intracellular signal transduction when antigen in the context of MHC molecules binds to the TCR. Since antigenic stimulation of T-lymphocytes is MHC-restricted, T-lymphocytes will only respond to foreign antigens that are displayed on APCs that have the same MHC phenotype. The different subsets of T-lymphocytes recognize different classes of MHC molecules. Suppressor T-lymphocytes recognize Class I MHC molecules by a specific receptor related to the CD8 antigen. Helper T-lymphocytes recognize Class II MHC molecules recognized by another specific receptor related to the CD4 antigen.

● B-lymphocytes

Potential B-lymphocytes, produced from the committed lymphoid stem cell, mature in the bone marrow. This maturation is independent of antigen stimulation. The immunocompetent, mature B-lymphocytes then enter the blood and migrate to the germinal centers (follicles) and medullary cords of lymph nodes, to the germinal centers of the spleen, and to the other secondary lymphoid tissue. Antigenic stimulation causes the B-lymphocyte to undergo proliferation and differentiation into immunoglobulin (antibody)-secreting plasma cells in the germinal centers of the secondary lymphoid tissues. The immunoglobulin recognizes and binds to foreign antigen. B-lymphocytes compose 15% to 30% of peripheral blood lymphocytes.

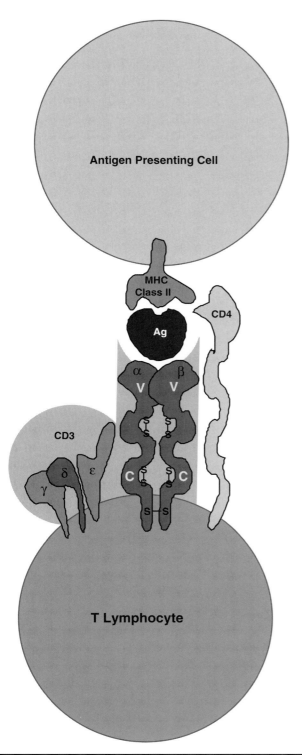

FIGURE 4-29. The T-lymphocyte has an antigen receptor on its surface (TCR) that is composed of two peptide chains linked by a disulfide bond. This receptor is expressed in a complex with CD3. This TCR is probably in close proximity to an MHC restricted receptor (CD4 or CD8) that recognizes the appropriate MHC molecule on antigen presenting cells (APCs). The helper T-lymphocyte receptor (CD4), shown here, recognizes Class II MHC molecules while the suppressor T-lymphocytes receptor (CD8) recognizes Class I MHC molecules.

B-lymphocytes possess certain phenotypic features, distinct from those of T-lymphocytes, which allow these cells to be identified. The enzyme TdT may be found on very young B cells but is not present on subsequent stages. The esterase and acid phosphatase stains are either negative or appear positive in a scattered granular pattern.

B-LYMPHOCYTE DEVELOPMENT
The pre-B lymphocyte, not stimulated by antigen, synthesizes the heavy chain of IgM, the μ chain. At this stage, this chain remains in the cytoplasm and is not combined with the light chain of IgM to form a complete immunoglobulin molecule. The next stage of development, the early B-lymphocyte, is characterized by the disappearance of the cytoplasmic μ heavy chains, and the subsequent appearance of the surface membrane IgM that contains the normal immunoglobulin structure of two light and two heavy chains. This IgM is different from the IgM secreted and found in the blood in that it has several additional amino acids on its heavy chains that serve as an anchor to the membrane. Membrane IgD can be identified after the appearance of IgM. B-lymphocytes are not capable of reacting with antigen until they develop both IgM and IgD on their surface. A dramatic decrease in membrane IgD is noted after cell stimulation.[29] Two more immunoglobulin classes, IgG and IgA, may develop on the cell surface later in ontogeny. Most mature B-lymphocytes possess only one class of immunoglobulin on their membrane, although a small percentage may express IgG and IgA together with IgM and IgD. Surface-bound immunoglobulin serves as a receptor for a particular antigen.

When stimulated by antigen, mature B-lymphocytes undergo proliferation and transformation into plasma cells. This is the antigen-dependent phase of lymphopoiesis for B-lymphocytes. These cells are committed to secreting large amounts of specific, single-class immunoglobulin. Plasma cells are rich in cytoplasmic immunoglobulin but contain little or no surface immunoglobulin. These cells produce only one of the five classes of immunoglobulin. Plasma cells are the fully-activated form of B-lymphocyte maturation whose primary function is formation and secretion of immunoglobulin that recognizes a particular antigen.

MEMBRANE MARKERS
In addition to immunoglobulin, other membrane markers are present at various stages in B-lymphocyte development. Early B-lymphocytes develop complement receptors for the complement components C3b (immune adherence) and C3d, which remain with the cell through the plasma cell stage. An Fc receptor for the Fc component of IgG is also present on early and mature B-lymphocytes.

B-lymphocytes may be identified in vitro by virtue of these complement receptors and surface membrane immunoglobulin. Erythrocytes from mice rosette with B-lymphocytes as do sheep erythrocytes that are coated with antibody and complement (EAC). EAC attaches to B-lymphocytes by means of the B-lymphocyte complement receptors. Another technique for B-lymphocyte identification involves demonstration of surface membrane im-

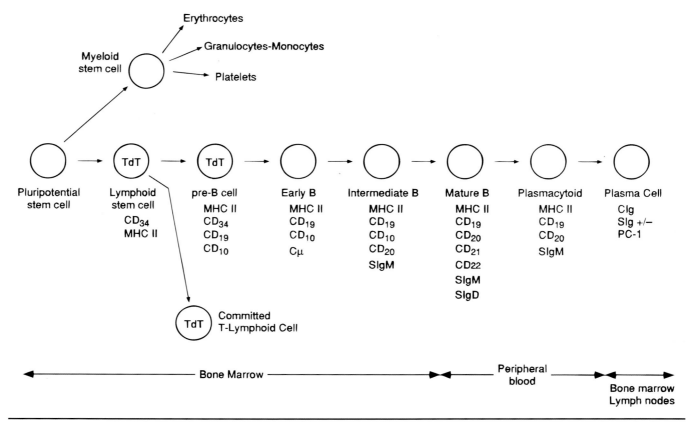

FIGURE 4-30. Immunologic maturation of the B-lymphocyte from the pluripotential stem cell to the plasma cell. Each stage of maturation can be defined by specific antigens (CD) that appear sequentially on the developing cell. Stem cells, pre-B lymphocytes, early B-lymphocytes, and intermediate B-lymphocytes are normally found in the bone marrow. The mature B-lymphocyte is found in the peripheral blood. When stimulated by antigen the B-lymphocytes undergo maturation to plasma cells, in the lymph nodes or bone marrow. ($C\mu$ = cytoplasmic μ chains; SIg = surface membrane immunoglobulin; CIg = cytoplasmic immunoglobulin; MHC II = class II HLA antigens; CD = cluster of differentiation antigens.)

munoglobulin by fluorescein conjugated antisera to the different classes of immunoglobulins.

In most cases, identification of B-lymphocytes is now done using flow cytometry and a panel of antibodies to surface antigens. Monoclonal antibodies have defined specific B-lymphocyte antigens that correspond to the stage of differentiation of the cell (Fig. 4-30).[30] Some antigens span most of the stages of B-lymphocyte differentiation while others are expressed at limited stages in differentiation. These monoclonal probes have been used to divide B-lymphocytes into three general developmental levels: pre–B-lymphocyte, intermediate B-lymphocyte, and secretory B-lymphocyte. Each level may contain several stages of immunologic maturation. This immunologic maturation of B-lymphocytes can be roughly correlated to the morphologic maturation. The pre–B-lymphocyte level corresponds to the bone marrow lymphoblast and prolymphocyte stages. The intermediate B-lymphocyte level corresponds to the more mature peripheral blood B lymphocyte, whereas the secretory B-lymphocyte level corresponds to the activated B-lymphocyte and plasma cell.

Some surface antigens appear on the B-lymphocyte before immunoglobulin can be detected. These include MHC molecules, CD34, CD19, and CD10. CD34 is a hematopoietic stem cell antigen and may be present on a variety of stem cells already committed to a particular lineage. The CD19 antigen is the earliest B-lymphocyte specific antigen and is retained until the latest stages of cell activation. Thus, it defines most cells of B-lymphocyte lineage. This is followed by the appearance of CD10. The CD10 antigen, common acute lymphoblastic leukemia antigen (CALLA), was originally believed to be a specific marker of leukemia cells in acute lymphoblastic leukemia. It is now known that CALLA is present on a small percentage (less than 3%) of normal bone marrow cells. The CALLA antigen is found only on pre-B and early B-lymphocytes; the antigen disappears with cell maturity. Heavy chains of IgM can be found in the cytoplasm of early B-lymphocytes. The acquisition of CD20 and surface membrane IgM (SIgM) mark the next stage of the intermediate B-lymphocyte. The loss of CD10 and acquisition of CD21 and CD22 identify the mature stage. The CD21 antigen is associated with the C3d receptor. Surface membrane-bound IgD also appears at the mature stage. The PC-1 antigen is the most limited membrane antigen, present only on the terminally differentiated B lymphocytes, the plasma cells.

Additional B-lymphocyte antigens are consistently

being identified; therefore, this antigenic description should not be considered complete and final.

PLASMA CELLS

Stimulated B-lymphocytes, cells that have encountered antigen to which they have been programmed to respond, undergo transformation from reactive lymphocytes to immunoblasts, to plasmacytoid lymphocytes, and finally to plasma cells in the lymph nodes. *Plasma cells,* the progeny of B-immunoblasts, represent the fully-activated mature B-lymphocyte. The intermediate stage in this transformation, the *plasmacytoid lymphocyte* (also called lymphocytoid plasma cell, intermediate form, Turk cell) may be identified. The plasmacytoid lymphocyte ranges in size from 15 to 20 μm. The nuclear chromatin is less clumped (more immature) than that of a plasma cell, and there may be a single visible nucleolus. The nucleus is central or slightly eccentric, and the cytoplasm is deeply basophilic. The plasmacytoid lymphocyte has the CD19 and CD20 antigens of lymphocytes and the PC-1 antigen of the plasma cell. In addition, the cell has some cytoplasmic immunoglobulin as well as surface membrane immunoglobulin. This cell is occasionally seen in the peripheral blood of patients with viral infection.

Plasma cells are round or slightly oval with a diameter from 9 to 20 μm. The rough endoplasmic reticulum is well developed, and the cytoplasm expands because of the production of large amounts of immunoglobulin. With an increase in cytoplasmic immunoglobulin, the secretory capacity of the cell is increased. Surface membrane immunoglobulin is usually absent. The nucleus is off to one side and contains block-like radial masses of chromatin often referred to as the cartwheel or wheel spoke arrangement. Nucleoli are not present. The paranuclear Golgi complex is obvious and surrounded by deeply basophilic cytoplasm. The cytoplasm stains red with pyronine (pyroninophilic) because of the high RNA content. Azurophilic granules may be present as well as rod-like crystal inclusions. The plasma cell has lost the CD19 and CD20 antigens but retains the PC-1 antigen. Plasma cells are not normally present in the peripheral blood or lymph and constitute less than 4% of the cells in the bone marrow. Most plasma cells are found in the medullary cords of lymph nodes, although intense stimulation of the immune system may cause them to be found in the peripheral blood. Plasma cells may be noted in the blood in rubeola, infectious mononucleosis, toxoplasmosis, syphilis, tuberculosis, and multiple myeloma.

Morphologic variations of plasma cells include *flame cells* and *Mott cells* (Fig. 4-31). Flame cells are named for their reddish-purple cytoplasm. The red tinge is caused by a glycoprotein produced in the RER, and the purple tinge is caused by the presence of ribosomes. These cells contain more immunoglobulin than normal plasma cells. At one time, flame cells were believed to be associated with IgA multiple myeloma. It is now recognized that these cells can be seen in a variety of pathologies and occasionally may be found in normal bone marrow.

Mott cells, also called grape cells, are plasma cells filled with globules. These globules most often contain immuno-

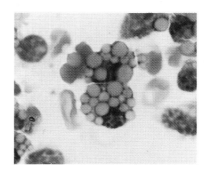

FIGURE 4-31. Mott cells (grape cells); (BM, 250×, Wright-Giemsa stain).

globulin (Russell bodies). *Russell bodies* normally stain blue-violet or pink, but, in the staining process, the globulin may dissolve and the cell then appears to be filled with colorless vacuoles. The globules form as a result of accumulation of material in the RER, SER, and the Golgi complex caused by obstruction of secretion. This pathologic plasma cell is associated with chronic plasmocyte hyperplasia, parasitic infection, and malignant tumors.

Intranuclear membrane bound inclusion bodies, *Dutcher bodies,* have been described in plasma cells from patients with dysproteinemias. These inclusions stain with PAS, indicating that they contain glycogen or glycoprotein. Dutcher bodies are most often found in neoplastic plasma cells.

● Immunoglobulin

Immunoglobulin (antibody) is a unique molecule produced by B-lymphocytes and plasma cells and consists of two pairs of polypeptide chains: two heavy and two light chains linked together by disulfide bonds (Fig. 4-32). The number and arrangement of these bonds are specific for the various immunoglobulin classes. There are five types of heavy chains, μ, γ, δ, α, and ϵ, but within a given immunoglobulin molecule the two heavy chains are identical. The two heavy chains determine the class of the antibody, of which there are five: IgM, IgG, IgA, IgE, and IgD. The two classes of light chains are kappa and lambda, of which there are many subclasses. As with the heavy chains, the two light chains within an immunoglobulin molecule are identical. Either kappa or lambda chains may be found in association with any of the various heavy chains.

Each heavy and light immunoglobulin chain consists of a variable region and a constant region. The constant region is the same for all antibodies of the same class, but the variable region is different in each immunoglobulin. The constant region mediates effector functions such as cell lysis by complement. Together, the variable regions of the light and heavy chains determine the antibody combining site. Rearrangement of gene segments of the heavy chain variable regions and of the gene segments of the light chain variable regions allow a diverse repertoire of immunoglobulin specificity for foreign antigens.

Internal homologies, called homologous regions, exist within the immunoglobulin molecule. Each homologous region folds into a compact domain containing between

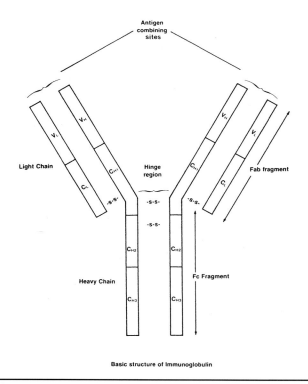

Basic structure of Immunoglobulin

FIGURE 4-32. Schematic drawing of an IgG molecule. The four peptide chains are indicated by the double lines and the disulfide bonds between the chains are indicated by -s-s-. The variable domains are indicated by V and the constant regions by C. The variable regions have variable amino acid sequencing depending on the antibody specificity while the constant regions have a constant sequence among immunoglobulins of the same class. The two heavy chains (H) determine the class of immunoglobulin, in this case for IgG. The two light chains may be either kappa or lambda.

110 and 120 amino acid residues; each domain serves a distinctive molecular function such as complement fixation or antigen-combining site. Light chains have two domains, whereas heavy chains have four or five domains. Each of the classes and subclasses of immunoglobulin has distinct physical and biologic properties (Table 4-7).

The immunoglobulin molecule may be divided into three separate portions by enzymatic digestion with papain: (1) two Fab fragments, the antibody-combining frag-

ments; and (2) one Fc fragment, the crystalizable fragment. The two Fab portions are composed of the variable regions of heavy and light chains. These two fragments contain the two antibody-combining sites. The Fc portion contains the constant regions of the heavy chains and is responsible for complement binding, skin fixation, and placental transport, as well as binding the immunoglobulin to cellular Fc receptors.

IMMUNOGLOBULIN GENE REARRANGEMENT

During B-lymphocyte development, there is a rearrangement of the gene segments coding for immunoglobulin (Fig. 4-33). This is one of first features that allows the cell

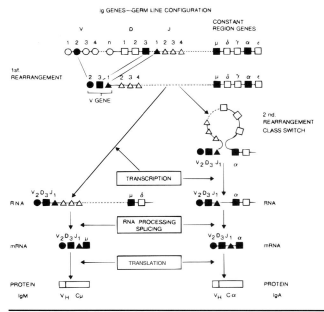

FIGURE 4-33. Immunoglobulin gene rearrangement of the heavy chain genes. As the B-lymphocyte differentiates, the germ-line configeration (top line) of DNA segments from the V, D, and J regions rearrange to produce the variable (V) region of the chain. Transcription of this variable gene with the first in line constant region gene (μ gene) gives rise to an RNA transcript. The intervening section of the chromosome is spliced giving rise to the mature mRNA. This is translated to the complete μ-heavy chain of Ig. (Adapted from Lee, G.R., et al: Wintrobe's Clinical Hematology, 1993).

TABLE 4-7 *SOME BIOLOGIC AND PHYSICAL PROPERTIES OF HUMAN IMMUNOGLOBULINS*

Class	Sedimentation Coefficient	Heavy Chain	Molecular Weight (Daltons)	Number of Subclasses	Mean Serum Concentration (g/L)	Complement Fixation	Crosses Placenta
IgG	7s	$\gamma1, \gamma2, \gamma3, \gamma4$	150,000	4	11	+	+
IgM	19s	μ	950,000	2	1.5	+	−
IgA	7s, 9s, 11s	$\alpha1, \alpha2,$	160,000 (monomer) 320,000 (dimer)	2	2.4	−	−
IgD	7s	δ	185,000	1	0.03	−	−
IgE	8s	ϵ	190,000	1	<0.005	−	−

to be recognized as a B-lymphocyte. Heavy chain gene rearrangement occurs in the B-lymphocyte progenitor cells, and light chain gene rearrangement occurs at the pre–B-lymphocyte stage.[26]

The gene segment rearrangement process involves random selection of coding sequences from menus of three serially arranged DNA segments and recombination to form a unique coding sequence and antibody specificity. The three gene segments that encode antibody specificity of the immunoglobulin heavy chains make up the complete variable (V) region gene and include: variable (VH), diversity (DH), and joining (JH) segments. Rearrangement and recombination of the VH, DH, and JH variable region gene segments and subsequent joining with the μ constant region gene, allow the B-lymphocyte to produce a variety of specific immunoglobulins of the IgM class that can react with foreign antigens. Further recombination of specific VH/DH/JH complexes with different constant region genes ([gamma], [delta], [alpha], [epsilon]) allow the B-lymphocyte to switch from production of IgM to another immunoglobulin class (IgG, IgD, IgA, IgE) without losing antibody specificity.

The kappa and lambda light chains also may rearrange gene segments to provide additional immunoglobulin diversity. Light chain-variable gene segments include the variable and joining regions, but there is no diversity region.[28]

IMMUNOGLOBIN G

Immunoglobulin G represents about 80% of the total serum immunoglobulin and is composed of four subclasses, IgG1, IgG2, IgG3, and IgG4. The subclasses of IgG may be identified by antigenic and structural differences in the heavy chain. Some antigens provoke an antibody response of all IgG subclasses; others elicit an antibody response within one subclass. IgG1 and IgG3 are capable of activating complement by the classic pathway. IgG2 is minimally active in complement activation, and IgG4 activates complement only by the alternate pathway. All IgG subclasses can bind to the Fc receptor on neutrophils, but only IgG1 and IgG3 can bind to monocyte Fc receptors. IgG is capable of crossing the maternal-fetal membranes. It is also the major immunoglobulin found in extravascular spaces, where it diffuses to neutralize toxin and to opsonize bacteria for phagocytosis. IgG is the major antibody produced during the secondary immune response. Optimum reactivity with antigen in vitro occurs at 37° C.

IMMUNOGLOBULIN M

Immunoglobulin M is composed of five subunits linked by disulfide bonds that make it the largest of the five antibody classes. The J chain, a nonimmunoglobulin, is bound to the IgM pentamer by disulfide bonds and aids in maintaining the tertiary structure of the molecule. IgM antibodies are the first antibodies formed in the immune response and the heavy chain, μ, is the first immunoglobulin chain produced in the maturation of B lymphocytes. These immunoglobulins avidly fix complement and have optimum

reactivity with antigen in vitro at temperatures below 37° C.

IMMUNOGLOBULIN A

Immunoglobulin A represents only 5% to 15% of serum immunoglobulins but is the predominant immunoglobulin in external secretions such as tears and saliva. It is believed that IgA protects the body against invasion by bacteria and viruses that enter the body through mucous membrane routes. Secretory IgA (sIgA) consists of an IgA dimer attached to a secretory component by disulfide bonds. The secretory component is synthesized by epithelial cells and is linked to IgA before it is secreted externally. The J chain also is found in polymer forms of IgA. The role of serum IgA is unknown. Its origin is probably from a clone of plasma cells different from the plasma cells producing sIgA as suggested by studies showing that radiolabeled serum IgA does not appear in external secretions.

IMMUNOGLOBULIN D

Immunoglobulin D is a minor component of serum but is often found with IgM on the surface of B-lymphocytes. The role of IgD in the immune response is unknown; however, IgD antibodies have been found in 40% of patients with lupus erythematosus and in 20% of patients with rheumatoid arthritis. This immunoglobulin does not fix complement.

IMMUNOGLOBULIN E

Immunoglobulin E, also known as "reagin," is responsible for the immune response of allergies. Basophils contain surface receptors for the Fc region of IgE. Attachment of the antigen–antibody complex to the basophil by this receptor triggers the release of histamine. Histamine is the most important mediator of immediate hypersensitivity reactions.

IMMUNOGLOBULIN PRODUCTION

Antibody production by a clone of plasma cells is limited to one class of heavy chain and one class of light chain. Plasma cells normally have large amounts of cytoplasmic immunoglobulin, but usually have no surface immunoglobulin. Stimulated B-lymphocytes may contain small amounts of cytoplasmic immunoglobulin of any one of the five classes of immunoglobulin; the same immunoglobulin class is present on the membrane.

The rate-limiting step in antibody production is the synthesis of heavy chain. A balance between production of heavy and light chains assures that there is no excess of one or the other. Neoplastic diseases of plasma cells, however, upset this balance; excesses of light chains or heavy chains may then be found in both serum and urine.

Alterations in immunoglobulin production may be classified as hypogammaglobulinemia, polyclonal gammopathy, and monoclonal gammopathy. These conditions are most commonly detected by serum protein electrophoresis, as each class of immunoglobulin has a specific electrical charge that permits migration in an electrical field. *Hypogammaglobulinemia* is characterized by a decrease in the total concentration of immunoglobulins. Decreases of this type, which are mostly of a hereditary nature, will be discussed in Chapter 14. *Polyclonal gammopathies* result in an increase in immunoglobulin of more than one class. This benign alteration is frequently seen in viral or bacterial infections. *Monoclonal gammopathies* are characterized by an increase in one specific class of immunoglobulin with identical heavy and light chains. This type of alteration is usually the result of unregulated proliferation (neoplastic) of one clone of plasma cell. This pathologic condition will be discussed in Chapter 19.

● T-lymphocyte and B-lymphocyte function

The T-lymphocyte, B-lymphocyte, and macrophage interact in a series of events that allows the body to attack and eliminate foreign antigens. This series of events is known collectively as the *immune response* (IR). The T-lymphocytes are responsible for part of the IR known as *cell-mediated immunity* (CMI). CMI requires interaction among histocompatible macrophages, T-lymphocytes, and antigen. It is independent of antibody production by B-lymphocytes. There are at least three important functional subsets of T-lymphocytes involved in the IR: helper T-lymphocytes (TH), suppressor T-lymphocytes (Ts), and cytotoxic T-lymphocytes (Tc). When these cells become activated in the IR, they proliferate and produce lymphokines.

Lymphokines are cytokines released primarily from T-lymphocytes that influence the function of other lymphocytes, macrophages, and other body cells (Table 4-8).

TABLE 4-8 *SOME SOLUBLE MEDIATORS RELEASED FROM T-LYMPHOCYTES AND THEIR EFFECT ON OTHER CELLS*

Lymphokine	Action
Macrophage chemotactic factor (MCF)	Attracts and accumulates macrophages
Macrophage inhibition factor (MIF)	Prevents migration of macrophages from site of inflammation
Macrophage activating factor (MAF)	Stimulates macrophages to kill intracellular organisms
γ-Interferon	Inhibits intracellular viral multiplication
Leukocyte inhibition factor (LIF)	Immobilizes neutrophils
Lymphocytotoxin	Kills nonlymphocytic cells
Transfer factor	Stimulates pre-committed T-lymphocytes mediating delayed hypersensitivity
IL-2	Induces proliferation and activation of other lymphocytes
IL-4	Stimulates proliferation of B-lymphocytes
IL-5	Stimulates proliferation/differentiation of B-lymphocytes
IL-6	Stimulates proliferation/differentiation of B-lymphocytes

TABLE 4-9 *MAJOR HISTOCOMPATIBILITY COMPLEX ANTIGENS*

Class I	Class II	Class III
HLA-A	HLA-D (Ia)	Complement components
HLA-B	HLA-DP	
HLA-C	HLA-DQ	
	HLA-DR	

B-lymphocytes also can secrete lymphokines. Under the influence of lymphokines, monocytes can produce monocyte-derived cytokines. Many lymphokines work in synergy.

The B-lymphocytes are responsible for the part of the IR known as *humoral immunity* (i.e., the production of antibodies). To accomplish effective humoral immunity, the peripheral B-lymphocyte must be activated and it must differentiate to a plasma cell.

The ability of the body to mount an IR against a particular foreign antigen is controlled by IR genes located in the major histocompatibility complex (MHC) on chromosome 6. These genes code for histocompatible antigens found on the surface of essentially all nucleated cells. The term used to describe the MHC gene cluster in humans is the human leukocyte antigen (HLA) region (Table 4-9). The HLA genes are located in specific regions within the complex known as HLA-A, HLA-B, HLA-C, HLA-D, and HLA-DR. The regions are classified according to their structure and specific role in the IR. HLA-A, HLA-B, and HLA-C genes code for Class I cell surface recognition proteins (on essentially all nucleated cells). These proteins are needed by Tc to distinguish self from nonself. HLA-D genes code for Class II antigens on the B-lymphocyte, monocyte, macrophage, and activated T-lymphocytes. The Class II antigens also are known as Ia antigens. These antigens determine the ability of immune cells to cooperate and interact in the IR. The D region is arranged into at least three subregions, DP, DQ, and DR. The Class III genes code for components of the complement system.[31]

T-LYMPHOCYTE FUNCTION

The IR generally begins with antigen recognition by macrophages followed by phagocytosis and degradation of the antigen. In this process, certain critical immunologic determinants of the antigen are preserved and presented to T_H-lymphocytes in the context of MHC II molecules (Fig. 4-34). The T_H-lymphocytes bind to the antigen on the surface of the macrophage by means of the TCR. The activated macrophage elaborates a monokine, IL-1. The binding of antigen/MHC II, plus the effect of IL-1, stimulates a sequence of biochemical and morphologic events in the T_H-lymphocyte that results in proliferation and differentiation of specifically sensitized T-lymphocytes. The sensitized (activated) T_H-lymphocyte secretes IL-2 as well as other lymphokines. These lymphokines affect other macrophages and lymphocytes. The activated T_H lymphocytes develop IL-2 receptors on their surface through

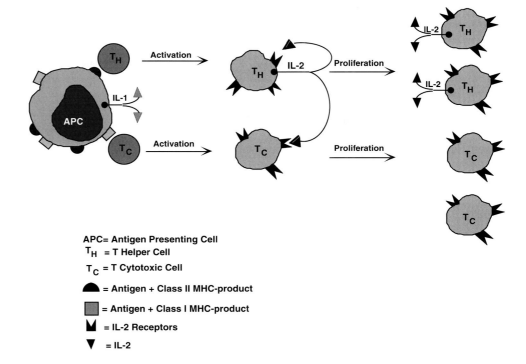

FIGURE 4-34. Activation and proliferation of T-lymphocytes requires two signals. The signals for the T$_H$-lymphocyte (CD4+) are the binding of processed antigen and the MHCII molecules on the APC via the TCR and CD4 receptor and the binding of IL-1 secreted by APC. The activated T$_H$-lymphocyte is stimulated to secrete IL-2. The first signal for Tc-lymphocyte (CD8+) activation is the binding of processed antigen in complex with MHCI molecules on the APC. IL-2 provides the second signal for Tc-lymphocyte activation and proliferation. IL-2 also stimulates activated T$_H$-lymphocytes to proliferate. (Adapted from: Zucker-Franklin D, Greaves MF, Grossi CE, Marmont AM: Atlas of Blood Cells. Philadelphia, Lea & Febiger, 1988.

APC= Antigen Presenting Cell
T$_H$ = T Helper Cell
T$_C$ = T Cytotoxic Cell
= Antigen + Class II MHC-product
= Antigen + Class I MHC-product
= IL-2 Receptors
= IL-2

which the cell binds IL-2, stimulating the cell to proliferate.

There are two populations of T$_H$-lymphocytes that differ in their helper function but cannot be distinguished by cell markers, T1 and T2. The T1 lymphocytes require physical contact between the B-lymphocyte and T-lymphocyte through the TCR of the T$_H$-lymphocyte and the antigen/MHCII molecule complex on the B-lymphocyte to stimulate the B-lymphocyte. The T2 population does not require physical contact with B-lymphocytes but mediates B-lymphocyte function through release of soluble mediators. This soluble mediator mechanism is not MHC restricted.

The T$_S$-lymphocytes also possess receptors for IL-2, and the binding of this lymphokine stimulates the activity of these cells. The T$_S$-lymphocytes, identified by the CD8 antigen, serve to suppress the immune response. They may suppress other T-lymphocytes or stop B-lymphocytes from producing antibodies.

Within the population of T-lymphocytes are the cytotoxic lymphocytes (T$_C$), also known as T-effector cells. Normally, in the healthy individual, there are few T$_C$-lymphocytes. The T$_C$-lymphocytes function in antigen-specific, MHC Class I-restricted cytolysis. The binding of antigen and Class I molecules of the macrophage plus the binding of IL-2 to specific receptors on the T$_C$-lymphocyte stimulates the cell to proliferate. The T$_C$-lymphocyte recognizes and destroys virus-modified autologous cells. This cell also is believed to be responsible for the graft-versus-host response, which occurs in individuals with allogeneic transplants. In graft-versus-host disease (GVHD), the immunosuppressed recipient receiving the graft is unable to mount an immune response against the grafted tissue. The

grafted tissue, however, contains T$_C$-lymphocytes capable of mounting an attack on host antigens.

In addition to the production of activated T-lymphocytes that directly participate in CMI, each type of activated T-lymphocyte can produce memory cells. These memory cells retain the memory of the stimulating antigen; when the same antigen is re-encountered, they elicit a more rapid and effective immunologic response.

B-LYMPHOCYTE FUNCTION
The functional activity of the B-lymphocyte includes the synthesis and secretion of antibodies. The surface immunoglobulin on the B-lymphocyte serves as the receptor for the processed antigen, which is bound to both the macrophage and the T$_H$-lymphocyte. In addition to binding the antigen presented by the macrophage, the B-lymphocyte MHC II molecules bind to the T$_H$-lymphocyte MHCII receptors. This three-cell complex, T$_H$-lymphocyte, macrophage, B-lymphocyte, initiates B-lymphocyte immunoblast formation. The immunoblast transforms to an antibody-secreting plasma cell. In addition to forming plasma cells, activated B-lymphocytes may form memory B-lymphocytes. T$_H$-lymphocytes may mediate activation of B-lymphocytes through secretion of lymphokines which does not require physical contact between the two cells. The activated T$_H$-lymphocyte secretes B-cell (lymphocyte) growth factors (BCGF) and differentiation factors (IL-2, IL-4, IL-5, and IL-6) that stimulate the B-lymphocyte to proliferate.

Polymeric antigens of identical repeating units may stimulate B-lymphocytes directly without the aid of T$_H$-lymphocytes. Unlike T$_H$-lymphocytes, B-lymphocytes do not need to recognize MHC to recognize antigen but can bind free antigen or antigen complexed with APC.[26] These antigens are known as T-independent antigens. More complex antigens, however, require T_H-lymphocyte participation and are known as T-dependent antigens.

It is evident that the activation of the IR, successful elimination of the antigen, and subsequent suppression of the IR require the interaction of histocompatible macrophages, T-lymphocytes, and B-lymphocytes. Derangements in this complex system may impair the normal immune response. Recurrent infection or the inability to deal with mico-organisms reflects immunodeficiency. Alterations also may occur that prevent lymphocytes from differentiating self-antigens from foreign-antigens. The clinical consequences of this upset are autoimmune disorders.

● Null cells

T- and B-lymphocytes account for all but approximately 10% of peripheral blood lymphocytes. A third population of lymphoid cells, which does not express either T- or B-lymphocyte markers, is the null cell. Not all null cells are, however, lymphocytes. The lymphoid null cell has a receptor for the Fc fragment of IgG. There are three subsets of null lymphoid cells: large granular lymphocytes (LGLs), natural killer (NK) cells, and killer (K) cells. There is evidence to believe that the natural killer cells and killer cells are specific types of large granular lymphocytes.

LARGE GRANULAR LYMPHOCYTES
These null cells are large with a high cytoplasmic to nuclear ratio, pale blue cytoplasm, and azurophilic granules. They do not adhere to surfaces or phagocytose. Some of these cells possess the CD2, CD3, or CD8 T-lymphocyte markers as well as monocyte antigens. The Fc receptor for IgG (CD16), however, is the most characteristic marker. The LGL cells mediate two cytolytic activities: natural killing and antibody-dependent cellular cytotoxicity (ADCC).

NATURAL KILLER CELLS
Natural killing is the function of this unsensitized NK null cell. Because these cells resemble LGLs, the term NK cell and LGL are often used interchangeably. However, cells other than LGL have NK activity. The term natural killer is a functional description while LGL is a morphologic description. Some NK cells have the CD2 marker but lack the mature T-lymphocyte marker, CD3, while other NK cells have a mature T-lymphocyte phenotype with CD2, CD3, and a functional TCR. A third group of NK cells has no T-lymphocyte markers. It is unclear as to whether the diversity of NK cells represent cells from a single lineage with a diversity of receptors or several distinct lineages. The diversity also may be related to the state of cellular activation. Unlike the Tc-lymphocytes, no previous sensitization is necessary for the lytic activity of NK cells, and cytolysis is not MHC-restricted. The lymphoid cell attaches to viral infected cells or tumor cells and spontaneously lyses the target cell. Interferon appears to increase the activity of NK cells.

KILLER CELLS
The K cells are the lymphoid element responsible for ADCC. There is increasing evidence that these cells may actually be an activated form of NK cells. Thus, they are sometimes referred to as lymphokine activated killer (LAK) cells. These cells possess complement receptors as well as Fc receptors but do not carry sIg. K cells may attach to IgG-coated tumor cells by means of their receptor for Fc, and they may exert a lytic effect on the target cell without any prior sensitization. The activity of K cells may be important in killing tumor cells or virally infected cells. The K cells also have been implicated as the effector cell of some autoimmune disorders. Any self cell coated with IgG may be a target for the action of K cells. For this reason, the action of K cells has been termed, antibody-dependent cellular cytotoxicity.

● Adhesion molecules of the immune response

Adhesion receptors are important in the congregation of lymphoid cells at sites of infection[32] (Table 4-10). The TCR recognizes antigen bound to monocytes/macrophages. The leukocyte function-related antigens, LFA-1 (on activated leukocytes), and LFA-3 (on EC) are important in the antigen-independent adhesion of activated T-lymphocytes, localizing these cells in sites of antigen accumulation. LFA-1 on T-lymphocytes is required for the lymphocyte's interaction with other cells, most likely by promoting adherance. The ligand for LFA-1 is the intracellular adhesion molecule on EC, ICAM-1, which modulates inflammatory responses by up-regulation or down-regulation of expression. Inflammatory mediators such as lipopolysaccharide, IL-1, and TNF cause strong expression of ICAM-1 in tissues, thus increasing adherance of lymphocytes and monocytes with LFA-1 in areas of inflammation. LFA-3 antigen is expressed on endothelial cells and is the ligand for CD2 on T-lymphocytes. Reaction of CD2 with its ligand generates an activation signal in the T-lymphocyte.

The B_1-integrin subfamily of very late activation (VLA) molecules appear on lymphocytes several weeks after antigen stimulation. They also are expressed on other leukocytes. The six VLA molecules, VLA-1 through VLA-6, are recognized as CD49a through CD49f, respectively. VLA-4 binds to VCAM-1 receptor on EC, a member of the superimmunoglobulin family. VLA-4 and VLA-6 also are present on eosinophils and basophils but not neutrophils. The VCAM-1 receptor is induced by inflammatory mediators on the endothelium. Other B_1-integrin molecules bind to extracellular matrix components such as collagen and are expressed on many nonhematopoietic cells and other leukocytes.

● Lymphocyte metabolism and kinetics

Lymphocytes contain all the enzymes of the glycolytic and tricarboxylic acid cycle. Glucose enters the cell through facilitated diffusion and is catabolized to produce ATP through oxidative phosphorylation. The ATP is used for

TABLE 4-10 *ADHESION MOLECULES INVOLVED IN THE INTERACTION OF LYMPHOCYTES WITH OTHER CELLS IN THE IMMUNE RESPONSE. (EC = ENDOTHELIAL CELL; CD = CLUSTER OF DIFFERENTIATION; LFA = LEUKOCYTE FUNCTION-RELATED ANTIGEN; VLA = VERY LATE ACTIVATION)*

Adhesion Molecule	CD Designation	Expressed by	Counter-ligand	Function
LFA-1	CD11a-CD18	Activated leukocytes	ICAM-1, ICAM-2 on endothelial cells	Mediates interaction of lymphocytes with other cells possibly by promoting adherence to target cells in site of antigen.
CD2	CD2	T-lymphocytes Monocytes	LFA-3 (CD58) on EC	Promotes adherence of the monocytes and T-lymphocytes to EC and mediates activation of T-lymphocytes.
CD4	CD4	T_H-lymphocytes	Class II Molecules	Enhances adhesion of T_H-lymphocytes to other cells and mediates activation of T_H-lymphocytes.
CD8	CD8	T_S-lymphocytes	Class I Molecules	Enhances adhesion and activation of T_S-lymphocytes; promotes avidity of cytotoxic T-lymphocytes and target cell.
VLA1, VLA2, VLA3, VLA4, VLA5, VLA6	CD49a, CD49b, CD49c, CD49d, CD49e, CD49f	Lymphocytes (VLA-1 also on eosinophils and basophils)	For VLA4 ligand is VCAM-1 on EC	Increase adhesion of cells in area of inflammation.

recirculation and locomotion, as well as replacement of lipids, replacement of proteins, and maintenance of ionic equilibrium. The HMP shunt provides only a fraction of the needed energy, but it is important for purine and pyrimidine synthesis and for providing the reducing energy by production of NADPH.

Lymphocytes have a peripheral blood concentration in adults from 1.5 to 4.0 × 10⁹/L (20% to 40% of blood leukocytes). The normal lymphocyte count in the first 10 years of life ranges from 1.5 to 11.0 × 10⁹/L, depending on the age of the child. At birth, the mean lymphocyte count is 5.5 × 10⁹/L (30%). This value rises to a mean value of 7 × 10⁹/L (60%) in the next 6 months. A gradual decrease in lymphocytes is noted from 4 years of age until normal adult values are reached in the second decade.[33]

Although many immune functions are well conserved throughout life, some investigators believe that there is a derangement of some immune responses in the elderly, which contributes to increased risk of morbidity and mortality in this group. In the healthy elderly, there is a decrease in absolute numbers of lymphocytes. This is due to a decrease in both T_H- and T_S-lymphocytes. There is an increase, however, in activated T-lymphocytes, NK cells, and T-lymphocytes that mediate non-MHC restricted cytotoxicity.[33]

Although lymphocytes are the second most numerous intravascular leukocyte in adults, peripheral blood lymphocytes comprise only 5% of the total body lymphocyte concentration. Ninety-five percent of the lymphocytes are located in extravascular tissue of the lymph nodes and spleen. There is a continuous movement of lymphocytes between the intravascular and extravascular compartments. Lymphocytes from lymph nodes enter the lymph and gain entry to the blood as the lymph drains into the right lymphatic duct and the thoracic duct. When blood lymphocytes are stimulated by an antigen, they migrate to specific areas of lymphoid tissue where they undergo proliferation and transformation into effector cells. These cells also can pass directly through the cytoplasm of post-capillary or high endothelial venule cells (emperipolesis) as they recirculate between intravascular or extravascular compartments. Because of this unique recirculation, proliferation, and transformation, it is difficult to determine the lifespan of lymphocytes. The cells leave and re-enter the blood many times. It is generally agreed that most lymphocytes (80%) in the peripheral blood are long-lived, with a lifespan from a few months to 20 years. These long-lived lymphocytes include both T- and B-lymphocytes, but the majority are T-lymphocytes. These cells spend most of their lifespan in a prolonged, intermitotic, G_o phase. The remaining 20% of the lymphocytes live from a few hours to 5 days. These short-lived lymphocytes include both T- and B-lymphocytes, but most are B-lymphocytes.

SUMMARY

Leukocytes include five morphologically and functionally distinct types of nucleated blood cells: neutrophils, eosinophils, basophils, monocytes, and lymphocytes. The leukocytes develop from the pluripotential stem cell in the bone marrow. Under the influence of hematopoietic growth factors, the stem cell matures into terminally differentiated cells. These cells circulate only a matter of hours in the peripheral blood before diapedesing to the tissues.

The leukocytes serve as the defenders of the body against foreign invaders and noninfectious challenges. This is accomplished by the cells' participation in phagocytosis and the immune response. They are attracted to sites of inflammation, infection, or tissue injury by chemoattractants. They leave the circulation using special adhesion molecules and their ligands located on the leukocytes and endothelial cells of the vessel walls. Neutrophils and monocytes are active in phagocytosis while eosinophils function in defending the body against parasites. Eosinophils also are involved in allergic reactions and chronic inflammation. Basophils are involved in allergic reactions releasing histamine and heparin when activated via the binding of IgE to membrane Fc receptors.

There are two types of lymphocytes—T and B. Lymphocytes have an antigen-independent and antigen-dependent maturation process. In the antigen-independent maturation process, B-lymphocytes mature in the bone marrow, while T-lymphocytes mature in the thymus. There are at least two different types of T-lymphocytes: helper T-lymphocytes (T_H) and suppressor T-lymphocytes (T_S). The lymphoblast from the bone marrow matures and acquires cellular characteristics of a T- or B-lymphocyte. In the antigen-dependent maturation process, these mature, immunocompetent T- and B-lymphocytes undergo a series of cellular events in response to encounters with antigen. This is known as blast transformation. The end result is a clonal amplification of lymphocytes, responsible for immunity to the specific antigen that stimulated transformation. Reactive lymphocytes are the most common form of antigen-stimulated lymphocyte found in the peripheral blood.

T- and B-lymphocytes have separate but related functions in the immune response. Monocytes/macrophages phagocytose antigens, preserving critical immunologic determinants that are presented to the T_H-lymphocytes. The T_H-lymphocytes bind to the antigen and the MHC molecules on the surface of the macrophage by means of the TCR. Cytokines released by the macrophage and T_H-lymphocyte activate the lymphocyte. T_S-lymphocytes also are activated by the released cytokines and serve to suppress the immune response. The functional activity of the B-lymphocyte includes the synthesis and secretion of antibodies. Surface immunoglobulin serves as the B-lymphocyte receptor for the processed antigen that is bound to the macrophage and T_H-lymphocyte. The B-lymphocyte also binds to the MHC receptors on the T_H-lymphocyte. As a result of this interaction, the B-lymphocyte transforms to an antibody-secreting plasma cell.

Monocytes function as phagocytes and secrete a variety of cytokines that affect the function of other cells, especially that of lymphocytes. As described above, monocytes play a major role in initiating and regulating the immune response. These cells also are referred to as APC.

The concentration of leukocytes in the peripheral blood is at a steady state. The total leukocyte count is normally between 3.5 and 11×10^9/L. An increase in the number of leukocytes (leukocytosis) serves as an indicator of infection or inflammation. This increase may be caused by an increased concentration of all cell types or, more commonly, of only one particular type. Neutrophils are the most plentiful leukocytes (54% to 62%) in the adult and tend to increase in bacterial infections or inflammation. Lymphocytes are the next most plentiful cell (20% to 40%). Reactive forms of the lymphocyte may be seen in the presence of viral infections. Monocytes usually compose from 4% to 10% of leukocytes. Basophils and eosin-

ophils are the least plentiful cells, composing only 0% to 1% and 1% to 3%, respectively. Infants generally have higher total leukocyte counts and higher lymphocyte counts than adults, while older adults generally have a decrease in the absolute number of lymphocytes.

● REVIEW QUESTIONS

1. A leukocyte count and differential in a 40-year-old white man was 5.4×10^9/L. There were 20% neutrophils, 58% lymphocytes, 20% monocytes, and 2% eosinophils. This respresents:
   a. absolute lymphocytosis
   b. relative neutrophilia
   c. absolute neutropenia
   d. leukopenia

2. Which of the following is a cause of neutrophilia:
   a. viral infection
   b. acute bacterial infection
   c. allergic reactions
   d. myeloperoxidase deficiency.

3. B-lymphocytes can be distinguished from T-lymphocytes by:
   a. morphology on Romanowsky-stained smears
   b. size of the cell
   c. monoclonal antibodies to surface antigens
   d. presence of granules

4. The plasma cell develops from the:
   a. basophil
   b. T-lymphocyte
   c. B-lymphocyte
   d. monocyte

5. In the neutrophil series of leukocyte development, the earliest stage to normally appear in the peripheral blood is the:
   a. myeloblast
   b. promyelocyte
   c. myelocyte
   d. band

6. The primary function of neutrophils is:
   a. a mediator of hypersensitivity
   b. control of parasitic infections
   c. initiation of the immune response
   d. phagocytic defense against microorganisms

7. The primary hematopoietic growth factor responsible for inducing neutrophil differentiation and maturation from the CFU-GEMM is:
   a. IL-3
   b. G-CSF
   c. GM-CSF
   d. M-CSF

8. Leukocyte migration to the tissue is regulated by leukocyte-endothelial cell recognition, which requires:
   a. interaction of adhesion molecules and their receptors

b. activation of membrane oxidase

c. leukocyte degranulation

d. opsonins

9. Immunoglobulin diversity is provided by:

a. activation of specific immunoglobulin genes in the B-lymphocyte for each antigen encountered

b. selective translation of portions of immunoglobulin mRNA in the B-lymphocyte

c. Rearrangement and recombination of gene coding sequences for immunoglobulin in the B-lymphocyte

d. Rearrangement and recombination of the TCR genes in the T-lymphocyte

10. This is the first heavy immunoglobulin chain produced in the maturing B-lymphocyte:

a. α

b. β

c. μ

d. γ

● REFERENCES

1. Wintrobe, M.M.: Blood, Pure and Eloquent. New York: McGraw-Hill, 1980.
2. Cohnhein, J.F.: Uber entzuendung und Eiterung. Arch Pathol Anat Physiol Klin Med, 40:179, 1867.
3. Metchnikov, I.: Uber die Beziehung der Phagocyten zu Milzbrandbacillen. Arch Pathol Anat, 97:502, 1884.
4. Ehrlich, P.: Beitrag zur Kenntnis der Anilinfarbungen und ihrer Verwendung in der mikroskopischen Technik. Arch Mikr Anat, 13:263, 1877.
5. Bao, W., et al.: Normative distribution of complete blood count from early childhood through adolescence: The Bogalusa Heart Study. Prev Med, 22:825, 1993.
6. Cavalieri, T.A., Chopra, A., Bryman, P.N.: When outside the norm is normal: interpreting lab data in the aged. Geriatr, 47:66, 1992.
7. Wintrobe, M.M., et al.: Clinical Hematology. 9th Ed. Philadelphia: Lea and Febiger, 1993.
8. Novak, R.W.: The beleaguered band count. Clin Lab Med, 13:895, 1993.
9. Ulich, T.R., et al.: Kinetics and mechanisms of recombinant human interleukin 1 and tumor necrosis factor-induced changes in circulating numbers of neutrophils and lymphocytes. J Immuno, 139:3406, 1987.
10. Clark, S.C., Kamen, R.: The human hematopoietic colony-stimulating factors. Science, 236:1229, 1987.
11. Kajita, T., Hugli, T.E.: C5a-induced neutrophilia. Am J Pathol, 137:467, 1990.
12. Chatta, G.S., et al.: Aging and Marrow neutrophil reserves. J Am Geriatr Soc, 42:77, 1994.
13. Etzioni, A.: Neutrophil function in the newborn—a review. Isr J Med Sci, 30:328, 1994.
14. Butcher, E.C.: Leukocyte-endothelial cell recognition: Three (or more) steps to specificity and diversity. Cell, 67:1033, 1991.
15. Arnaout, M.A.: Structure and function of the leukocyte adhesion molecules CD11/CD18. Blood, 75:1037, 1990.
16. Alvarez, V., et al.: Differentially regulated cell surface expression of leukocyte adhesion receptors on neutrophils. Kidney Intern, 40:899, 1991.
17. Zimmerman, G.A., Prescott, S.M., McIntyre, T.M.: Endothelial cell interactions with granulocytes: tethering and signaling molecules. Immunol Today, 13:93, 1992.
18. Athens, J.W.: Granulocytes—neutrophils. In: Wintrobe's Clinical Hematology. Edited by G.R. Lee, T.C. Bithell, J. Foerster, J.W. Athens, J.N. Lukens. Philadelphia: Lea and Febiger, 1993.
19. Jagels, M.A., Hugli, T.E.: Neutrophil chemotactic factors promote leukocytosis. J Immunol, 148:1119, 1992.
20. Jones, D.G.: The eosinophil. J Comp Path, 108:317, 1993.
21. Bochner, B.S., Schleimer, R.P.: The role of adhesion molecules in human eosinophil and basophil recruitment. J Allergy Clin Immunol, 94:427, 1994.
22. Kiatmura, Y., Kasugai, T., Arizono, N., Matsuda, H.: Development of mast cells and basophils: Processes and regulation mechanisms. Am J Med Sci, 306:185, 1993.
23. Gauchat, J-F., et al.: Induction of human IgE synthesis in B-cells by mast cells and basophils. Nature, 365:340, 1993.
24. Gotze, O.: The potential role of basophilic leukocytes and mast cells. Nephrol Dial Transplant, 9[suppl 2]:57, 1994.
25. Cronenberger, J.H., Jennette, J.C.: Immunology: Basic concepts, diseases, and laboratory methods. Norwalk, Connecticut: Appleton and Lange, 1988.
26. Roitt, I., Brostoff, J., Male, D.: Immunology. St. Louis: C. V. Mosby, 1989.
27. Deegan, M.J.: Membrane antigen analysis in the diagnosis of lymphoid leukemias and lymphomas. Arch Pathol Lab Med, 113:606, 1989.
28. Gill, J.I., Gulley, M.L.: Immunoglobulin and T-cell receptor gene rearrangement. Hem Onc Clinics North Amer, 8:751, 1994.
29. Yuan, D.: Regulation of gene expression during B cell differentiation. In: B-Lymphocyte Differentiation. Edited by J. C. Cambier. Boca Raton, Florida: CRC Press Inc., 1986.
30. Anderson, K.C., et al.: Expression of human B cell-associated antigens on leukemias and lymphomas: A model of human B cell diferentiation. Blood, 63:1424, 1984.
31. Cronenberger, H.: Nonimmune and immune defenses: A review. J Med Tech, 2:701, 1985.
32. Springer, T.A.: Adhesion receptors of the immune response. Nature, 346:425, 1990.
33. Samsoni, P., et al.: Lymphocyte subsets and natural killer cell activity in healthy old people and centenarians. Blood, 82:2767, 1993.

General aspects and classifications of anemia

5

INTRODUCTION

Anemia, a decrease in erythrocyte mass, is one of the most common problems encountered in clinical medicine. However, anemia is not a disease but rather the expression of an underlying disorder or disease; it is an important clinical marker of a disorder that may be basic or complex. Therefore, once the diagnosis of anemia is made, the physician must determine its exact cause. Treating anemia without identifying its cause may not only be ineffective, but could lead to more serious problems. For example, if a patient experiencing iron deficiency anemia due to chronic blood loss were given iron or a blood transfusion, the hemoglobin level may temporarily rise; however, if the cause of the iron deficiency is not isolated and treated, serious complications of the primary disease may develop, and the anemia would probably return after cessation of treatment. Thus, it is necessary to understand the pathogenesis of an anemia to institute correct treatment.[1]

Anemia is functionally defined as a decrease in the competence of blood to carry oxygen to tissues, thereby causing tissue hypoxia. In clinical medicine, it refers to a decrease in the normal concentration of hemoglobin or erythrocytes.

NORMAL ERTHROCYTE KINETICS

To understand how anemia develops, it is necessary to understand normal erythrocyte kinetics. Total erythrocyte mass (M) in the steady state is equal to the number of new erythrocytes produced per day (P) times the erythrocyte life span (S) (100 to 120 days):

$$\begin{array}{ccccc} M & = & P & \times & S \\ \text{Mass} & & \text{Production} & & \text{Survival} \end{array}$$

Thus, the average 70-kg man with 2 liters of erythrocytes must produce 20 mL of new erythrocytes each day to replace the 20 mL normally lost due to cell senescence.[2]

$$\frac{2000 \text{ mL (M)}}{100 \text{ days (S)}} = 20 \text{ mL/day (P)}$$

From this formula, it can be seen that if the survival time of the erythrocyte is decreased by half, the bone marrow must double production to maintain the mass at 2000 mL.

$$\frac{2000 \text{ mL (M)}}{50 \text{ days (S)}} = 40 \text{ mL/day (P)}$$

New erythrocytes are released from the bone marrow as reticulocytes. Thus, increased production of erythrocytes is reflected by an increase in the absolute reticulocyte count in the peripheral blood. The bone marrow can compensate for decreased survival in this manner, if the iron supply is adequate, until production is increased to a level 5 to 10 times normal, which is the maximal functional capacity of the marrow. Thus, if all necessary raw products for cell synthesis are readily available, erythrocyte lifespan may decrease to about 18 days before marrow

compensation is inadequate and anemia develops. If, however, bone marrow production of erythrocytes does not increase when the erythrocyte survival is decreased, the erythrocyte mass cannot be maintained and anemia develops. There is no mechanism for increasing erythrocyte lifespan to help accommodate an inadequate bone marrow response.

Thus, anemia may develop if (1) erythrocyte loss or destruction exceeds the maximal capacity of bone marrow erthrocyte production or (2) the bone marrow erythrocyte production is impaired.

INTERPRETATION OF ABNORMAL HEMOGLOBIN CONCENTRATIONS

Diagnosis of anemia is usually made after discovery of a decreased hemoglobin concentration. Hemoglobin is the carrier protein of oxygen; thus, it is expected that a decrease in its concentration is accompanied by a decrease in oxygen delivery to tissues. Although this is usually true, there are at least three reasons why care should be exercised in interpreting abnormal hemoglobin values.

First, it is important to distinguish between relative and absolute hemoglobin concentration. Relative hemoglobin concentration (grams of hemoglobin per deciliter of blood) signifies the mass of hemoglobin in relation to the volume of plasma. This is the way hemoglobin is normally measured in the laboratory. Absolute hemoglobin concentration is the actual total hemoglobin mass independent of plasma volume.

There are a few instances when an abnormal relative hemoglobin concentration does not necessarily signify anemia. In *hypervolemia*, the total blood volume increases. This is primarily caused by a plasma volume increase while the erythrocyte mass remains stable. In this case, the relative hemoglobin concentration, reported in gm/dL, will appear falsely decreased because of the increase in plasma volume. Also, a normal relative hemoglobin concentration does not necessarily reflect a normal absolute total hemoglobin mass. For instance, in the hypovolemia accompanying acute hemorrhage, erythrocyte mass and plasma are both decreased proportionately, thereby maintaining a normal relative hemoglobin concentration. Within a few hours after hemorrhage has ceased, the blood volume adjusts upward with an increase in plasma volume, which thereby dilutes the remaining erythrocytes. Consequently, hemoglobin concentration decreases. Thus, the hemoglobin concentration may appear normal for a period of time after hemorrhage, even though the absolute hemoglobin mass is decreased.

A second reason for using care in interpreting hemoglobin values is that at high altitudes, where partial pressure of atmospheric oxygen is lower, there is a physiologic increase in hemoglobin mass to assure adequate oxygen delivery to the tissues. The hemoglobin reference range at high altitudes is higher than the reference range at lower altitudes. Therefore, signs of anemia at high altitudes may occur at higher hemoglobin levels than at sea level. Diagnosis of anemia requires an upward adjustment of hemoglobin and hematocrit values dependent on the altitude.[3] Cigarette smoking has a similar effect on hemoglobin. The hemoglobin reference range for cigarette smokers is higher than in nonsmokers.

Finally, a third reason that hemoglobin concentration should be interpreted with care is that, in individuals with rare hemoglobin structural variants, function of the hemoglobin molecule may be altered. Structurally abnormal hemoglobins may not carry and release oxygen as efficiently as normal hemoglobin. For example, hemoglobins that have a high oxygen affinity may not release adequate oxygen to the tissues. With high-affinity hemoglobins, bone marrow compensates for the hypoxia by producing more erythrocytes in response to increased erythropoietin. This results in erythrocytosis and increased hemoglobin concentration (both absolute and relative). In this case, hemoglobin levels in the reference range may not represent enough hemoglobin for adequate oxygen delivery to tissues.

CAUSES OF TISSUE HYPOXIA NOT RELATED TO THE HEMATOPOIETIC SYSTEM

There are several mechanisms by which tissue hypoxia may be produced independent of a defect in the hematopoietic system. As discussed, hypoxia may result from a decrease in the partial pressure of oxygen as occurs at high altitudes. Likewise, decreased capillary exchange of oxygen in the lungs, as occurs in emphysema, may produce hypoxia. In both of these cases, hypoxia is not due to a defect in the hematopoietic system. In fact, the bone marrow responds to these types of hypoxia by increasing the erythrocyte mass, thereby producing erythrocytosis. If, however, the hypoxia is due to a defect in the erythrocytic oxygen transport system, as is the case in structurally abnormal hemoglobins, or decreased erythrocyte mass, as in anemia, the hematopoietic system is involved.

In most cases, the clinical findings are integrated with the laboratory findings by the physician to correctly diagnose the illness. The examples mentioned serve to emphasize the fact that the physician, when making a diagnosis of anemia, cannot depend solely on laboratory results but also must consider a pathophysiologic approach.

ADAPTATIONS TO ANEMIA

Signs and symptoms of anemia range from slight fatigue or barely noticeable physiologic changes to life-threatening reactions depending on the rate of onset, the severity of blood loss, and the ability of the body to adapt (Table 5-1). With rapid loss of blood as occurs in acute hemor-

TABLE 5-1 *FACTORS AFFECTING THE PRESENCE OF SYMPTOMS IN ANEMIA*

1. Rate of onset of blood loss
2. Severity of blood loss
3. Ability of the body to adapt to decreases in hemoglobin concentration

TABLE 5-2 *ADAPTATIONS TO ANEMIA*

I. Increase in Oxygenated Blood Flow
   —increase in cardiac rate
   —increase in cardiac output
   —increase in circulation rate
   —preferential increase in blood flow to vital organs

II. Increase in Oxygen Utilization by Tissues
   —increase in 2,3-BPG in erythrocytes
   —decreased oxygen affinity of hemoglobin in tissues due to Bohr effect

rhage, clinical manifestations are related to hypovolemia and vary with the amount of blood lost. A normal person may lose up to 1000 mL or 20% of total blood volume, and not exhibit clinical signs of the loss at rest; but with mild exercise, tachycardia is common.[4] Severe blood loss of 1500 to 2000 mL or 30% to 40% of total blood volume leads to circulatory collapse and shock. Death is imminent if the acute loss reaches 50% of total blood volume (2500 ml).

Slow-developing anemias may show an equally severe drop in hemoglobin, as is seen in acute blood loss, but the threat of shock or death is not usually present. The reason for this apparent discrepancy is that the body, in slow-developing anemias, has several adaptive mechanisms that allow organs to function at hemoglobin levels of up to 50% less than normal. The adaptive mechanisms are of two types: an increase in the oxygenated blood flow to the tissues and an increase in oxygen utilization by the tissues (Table 5-2).

Increase in oxygenated blood flow

Oxygenated blood flow to the tissues may be increased by increasing the cardiac rate, the cardiac output, and the circulation rate. Oxygen uptake by hemoglobin in the alveoli of the lungs is increased by deepening the amount of inspiration and increasing the respiration rate. In anemia, decreased blood viscosity due to the decrease in erythrocytes and decreased peripheral resistance help to increase the circulation rate, delivering oxygen to tissues at an increased rate. Blood flow to the vital organs, the heart and brain, may preferentially increase; while flow to tissues with low oxygen requirements and normally high blood supply, such as skin and the kidneys, is decreased. Experiments using anemic rats with a 50% decrease in hematocrit showed a 115% increase in blood flow to the heart and an 85% increase to the brain.[5]

Increase in oxygen utilization by tissue

An important compensatory mechanism at the cellular level, which allows the tissue to extract more oxygen from the hemoglobin, involves an increase in 2,3-DPG (2,3-diphosphoglycerate; also referred to as 2,3-BPG or 2,3-bisphosphoglycerate) within the erythrocytes. An increase in erythrocyte 2,3-DPG is accompanied by a shift to the right in the oxygen dissociation curve, permitting the tissues to extract more oxygen from the blood even though the PO_2

remains constant. It is not clear exactly how anemia stimulates this increase in cellular 2,3-DPG. Another adaptive mechanism at the cellular level involves the Bohr effect. The scarcity of oxygen causes anaerobic glycolysis by muscles and other tissue to produce a build-up of lactic acid. This tissue acidosis decreases hemoglobin's affinity for oxygen in the capillaries, thus releasing more oxygen to the tissues. At oxygen tensions in the lung, this small change in oxygen affinity does not appear to affect the uptake of oxygen by hemoglobin.

These same adaptive mechanisms that occur with anemia are apparent in healthy individuals during vigorous exercise. With exercise, the heart may increase the flow of blood to tissues 5 to 10 times normal, and the amount of oxygen released to the tissue may double.

Even with these physiologic adaptations, anemic patients respond differently to similar changes in hemoglobin levels. The extent of the physiologic adaptations are influenced by:

1. severity of the anemia;
2. competency of the cardiovascular and respiratory systems;
3. oxygen requirement of the individual (physical and metabolic activity);
4. duration of the anemia;
5. the disease or condition that caused the anemia;
6. the presence and severity of coexisting disease.

● DIAGNOSIS OF ANEMIA

The diagnosis of anemia and determination of its cause is made through a combination of information received from the patient history, the physical examination, and the laboratory investigation (Table 5-3).

● History

The patient's history, including symptoms, may reveal some important clues as to the cause of the anemia. Information solicited by the physician should include dietary habits, medication taken, possible exposure to chemicals or toxins, and description and duration of the symptoms. The most common complaint is fatigue. Muscle weakness and fatigue develop when there is not enough oxygen available to burn fuel for production of energy. Severe drops in hemoglobin may lead to a variety of additional symptoms. When oxygen to the brain is decreased, headache, vertigo, and syncope may occur. Dyspnea and palpitations from exertion, or occasionally while at rest, are not uncommon complaints. The patient should be questioned as to any overt signs of blood loss, such as hematuria, hematemesis, and bloody or black stools. Family history may help define the rarer hereditary types of hematologic disorders. Sickle cell anemia and thalassemia are frequently manifest to some degree in several members of the immediate family.

TABLE 5-3 *DIAGNOSIS OF ANEMIA AND DETERMINATION OF ITS CAUSE REQUIRES INFORMATION OBTAINED FROM THE PATIENT HISTORY, PHYSICAL EXAMINATION AND LABORATORY DATA*

I. Patient history
  Dietary habits
  Medications
  Exposure to chemicals and toxins
  Symptoms and their duration:
  a. Fatigue
  b. Muscle weakness
  c. Headache
  d. Vertigo
  e. Syncope
  f. Dyspnea
  g. Palpitations
  Previous record of abnormal blood examination
  Family history of abnormal blood examination

II. Signs of anemia obtained by physical examination
  a. Splenomegaly
  b. Hepatomegaly
  c. Skin pallor
  d. Pale conjunctiva
  e. Hypotension
  f. Jaundice
  g. Koilonychia
  h. Bone deformities in congenital anemias
  i. Smooth tongue
  j. Neurological dysfunction

III. Laboratory investigation
  a. Erythrocyte count
  b. Hematocrit
  c. Hemoglobin
  d. Erythrocyte indices: MCV, MCH, MCHC
  e. Reticulocyte count and reticulocyte production index
  f. Blood smear examination
  g. Leukocyte and platelet quantitative and qualitative examination
  h. Bone marrow examination (depending upon results of other laboratory tests and patient clinical data)
  i. Tests to measure erythrocyte destruction depending upon other information available: serum bilirubin, urine hemosiderin, haptoglobin, methalbumin, lactate dehydrogenase (LDH)

● Physical examination

Physical examination of the patient helps the physician detect the adverse effects of a long-standing anemia (Table 5-3). Organomegaly of the spleen and liver are of primary importance in establishing the extent of involvement of the hematopoietic system in production and destruction of erythrocytes. Massive splenomegaly is characteristic of some hereditary chronic anemias. The spleen also may become enlarged in some autoimmune hemolytic anemias when the spleen is the primary site of destruction of antibody-sensitized erythrocytes. Heart abnormalities may occur as a result of the increased cardiac workload associated with the physiologic adaptations to anemia. Usually cardiac problems occur only with chronic or severe anemias. Changes in epithelial tissue from oxygen deprivation will be noted in some patients. Skin pallor is easily noted in most white patients, but because of variability in natural skin tone, pale conjunctiva is a more reliable indicator of anemia. The presence of bruises, ecchymoses, and petechiae indicate that the platelets may be involved in the disorder that is producing the anemia. Anemia also may occur secondary to a defect in hemostasis.[1] Hypotension may accompany significant decreases in blood volume.

In addition to the general physical findings associated with anemia, specific clinical signs that are associated with a particular type of anemia may occur. These include jaundice in hemolytic anemias, koilonychia in iron deficiency, bone deformities and extramedullary hematopoietic tissue masses in the hereditary hemoglobinopathies, a smooth tongue in megaloblastic anemia, and neurologic dysfunction in pernicious anemia.

In addition to determining the extent of anemic manifestations, physical examination helps to establish the underlying disease process causing the anemia. Some disorders associated with anemia include chronic diseases such as rheumatoid arthritis, as well as malignancies, gastrointestinal lesions, kidney disease, parasitic infection, and liver dysfunction.

●
Laboratory investigation

After the physical examination and patient history, the physician will order laboratory tests if he suspects the patient has anemia. Initially, routine tests are performed to determine if anemia is present and to evaluate erythrocyte production and destruction/loss (Table 5-4). These tests include determination of hemoglobin and hematocrit, enumeration of erythrocytes and reticulocytes, examination of a blood smear, calculation of erythrocyte indices, and measurement of the bilirubin concentration. In addition, the urine and stool may be examined for the presence of blood. These routine tests are followed by a protocol of specific diagnostic tests that help establish the pathophysiology of the anemia. These specific tests will be discussed in the appropriate chapters on anemia.

ERYTHROCYTE COUNT, HEMATOCRIT AND HEMOGLOBIN

Determination of the erythrocyte count, hematocrit, and hemoglobin are routine laboratory tests used to screen for the presence of anemia. These parameters may be mea-

TABLE 5-4 *ROUTINE LABORATORY TESTS USED TO ESTABLISH THE PRESENCE OF ANEMIA AND TO EVALUATE ERYTHROCYTE DESTRUCTION/LOSS*

Hemoglobin

Hematocrit

Erythrocyte count

Reticulocyte count

Blood smear examination

Erythrocyte indices

Bilirubin

Urine and stool analysis for blood

TABLE 5-5 *HEMOGLOBIN (Hb) AND HEMATOCRIT (Hct) CUTOFFS FOR A DIAGNOSIS OF ANEMIA IN CHILDREN, NONPREGNANT FEMALES AND MALES*

Age (yrs)/Sex	Hb (g/dL)	Hct (%)
Both sexes		
1–1.9	11.0	33.0
2–4.9	11.2	34.0
5–7.9	11.4	34.5
8–11.9	11.6	35.0
Female		
12–14.9	11.8	35.5
15–17.9	12.0	36.0
≥18	12.0	36.0
Male		
12–14.9	12.3	37.0
15–17.9	12.6	38.0
≥18	13.6	41.0

* Based on fifth percentile values from the Second National Health and Nutrition Examination Survey after excluding persons with a higher likelihood of iron deficiency.

(From: Center for Disease Control. Morbidity and Mortality Weekly Report, 38 (22), June 8, 1989.)

sured on automated instruments or by manual methods. A decrease below two standard deviations from the reference range for the age and sex of the individual should be followed by other laboratory tests to help establish criteria for diagnosis. The Centers for Disease Control and Prevention (CDC)-recommended cutoff values for a diagnosis of anemia according to age and sex are provided in Table 5-5. Upward adjustment for these cutoff values should be used for individuals living at high altitudes and for those who smoke. These CDC-recommended adjustments are included in Tables 5-6 and 5-7. Hemoglobin and hematocrit values also vary in pregnancy, with a gradual decrease in the first two trimesters and a rise during the third trimester (Table 5-8).

TABLE 5-6 *ALTITUDE ADJUSTMENTS FOR HEMOGLOBIN (Hb) AND HEMATOCRIT (Hct) CUTOFFS FOR A DIAGNOSIS OF ANEMIA*

Altitude (ft)	Hb (g/dL)	Hct (%)
<3000	0.0	0.0
3000–3999	+ 0.2	+ 0.5
4000–4999	+ 0.3	+ 1.0
5000–5999	+ 0.5	+ 1.5
6000–6999	+ 0.7	+ 2.0
7000–7999	+ 1.0	+ 3.0
8000–8999	+ 1.3	+ 4.0
9000–9999	+ 1.6	+ 5.0
>10,000	+ 2.0	+ 6.0

(From: Center for Disease Control. Morbidity and Mortality Weekly Report, 38 (22), June 8, 1989.)

TABLE 5-7 *ADJUSTMENTS FOR HEMOGLOBIN (Hb) AND HEMATOCRIT (Hct) IN SMOKERS*

Characteristic	Hb (gm/dL)	Hct (%)
Nonsmoker	0.0	0.0
Smoker (all)	+ 0.3	+ 1.0
½–1 pack/day	+ 0.3	+ 1.0
1–2 packs/day	+ 0.5	+ 1.5
>2 packs/day	+ 0.7	+ 2.0

(From: Center for Disease Control. Morbidity and Mortality Weekly Report, 38 (22), June 8, 1989.)

Erythrocyte cell count The erythrocytes compose about 45% of the blood volume. As discussed in Chapter 3, the highest normal erythrocyte counts are seen at birth. The neonatal erythrocyte population is macrocytic and contains between 2% and 6% reticulocytes (young erythrocytes released from the bone marrow within the last 24 hours). In addition, from 3 to 10 nucleated erythrocytes per 100 leukocytes may be observed in the peripheral blood during the first week of life. A gradual decrease in erythrocytes occurs for the 2 months after birth. This decline is followed by a gradual increase until normal adult values are reached at about 14 years of age. A difference in erythrocyte values between sexes is noted at puberty, females having lower values than males. This may partly be explained by the theory that the male hormone, testosterone, stimulates erythropoiesis. The erythrocyte count changes very little in normal older adults and increases slightly after menopause.[6] Normal reference ranges for elderly ambulatory clinic patients are given in Table 5-9. At high altitudes, a compensatory physiologic increase in erythrocytes proportional to the decrease in arterial oxygen saturation of hemoglobin is noted. Heavy smokers also may compensate for a decrease in oxygen saturation by increasing the number of erythrocytes.

Hematocrit The volume of packed erythrocytes after centrifugation in relation to the volume of whole blood expressed in liter/liter (sometimes in percentage) is known as the *hematocrit* (or PCV: packed cell volume). The hematocrit in percent is about three times the hemoglobin

TABLE 5-8 *HEMOGLOBIN CUTOFFS FOR A DIAGNOSIS OF ANEMIA IN PREGNANCY BY MONTH AND TRIMESTER**

Gestation (wks)	12	16	20	24	28	32	36	40
Trimester	1†	2	2†	2	3	3†	3	term
Mean Hb (g/dL)	12.2	11.8	11.6	11.6	11.8	12.1	12.5	12.9
5th percentile Hb values (g/dL)	11.0	10.6	10.5	10.5	10.7	11.0	11.4	11.9
§Equivalent 5th percentile Hct values (%)	33.0	32.0	32.0	32.0	32.0	33.0	34.0	36.0

* Based on pooled data from four European surveys of healthy women taking iron supplements.

† Hb values adopted for the trimester-specific cutoffs.

§ Hematocrit.

(From: Center for Disease Control. Morbidity and Mortality Weekly Report, 38 (22), June 8, 1989.)

TABLE 5-9 *COMPARISON OF RED BLOOD CELL MEASUREMENTS OF ELDERLY (OVER 65 YEARS) AND ELDERLY NONANEMIC WITH A GENERAL POPULATION OF INDIVIDUALS*

	Red Cell Count (10¹²/L)	Hemoglobin (gm/dL)	Hematocrit (%)	MCV (fL)	MCH (pg)	MCHC (gm/dL)
Males						
All ages	5.40 ± 0.78	16.00 ± 1.96	47.00 ± 4.90	87.00 ± 4.90	29.00 ± 1.96	34.00 ± 1.96
Elderly (106)	4.68 ± 1.01	14.09 ± 3.43	42.18 ± 9.50	88.97 ± 16.88	30.32 ± 6.19	33.54 ± 2.98
Elderly nonanemic (98)	4.72 ± 0.96	14.34 ± 2.84	42.82 ± 8.17	90.49 ± 14.44	30.54 ± 4.90	33.64 ± 2.53
Females						
All ages	4.80 ± 0.59	14.00 ± 1.96	42.00 ± 4.90	87.00 ± 4.90	29.00 ± 1.96	34.00 ± 1.98
Elderly (186)	4.45 ± 1.12	13.37 ± 3.08	40.12 ± 8.92	90.26 ± 15.44	30.30 ± 5.14	33.42 ± 2.49
Elderly nonanemic (177)	4.49 ± 1.03	13.54 ± 2.71	40.59 ± 8.01	90.28 ± 13.72	30.35 ± 4.51	33.48 ± 2.43

MCV, MCH, MCHC = mean corpuscular volume, hemoglobin, hemoglobin concentration.

(From: Freedman, M.L. Iron deficiency in the elderly. Hosp. Pract. [Off]. 21(3A): 115–122, 127, 130, 1986.)

concentration (e.g., hemoglobin 12 gm/dL $\times$ 3 = 36% hematocrit). A small amount of plasma (1% to 4%) is trapped in the packed cell layer during centrifugation, leading to a false-positive error (but insignificant) in the hematocrit. When the hematocrit is calculated from the erythrocyte count and erythrocyte volume (erythrocyte count $\times$ erythrocyte volume = hematocrit) on electronic cell counters, this error is absent.

Certain clinical situations can falsely elevate the hematocrit. Swelling of the erythrocyte occurs in hyperglycemia and hypernatremia, raising the erythrocyte volume (MCV) and, therefore, the hematocrit. On electronic cell counters that use isotonic saline as a diluent, this osmotic effect can be overcome by allowing the cells to equilibrate in the saline solution before counting. In cases of extreme leukocytosis, the hematocrit may be affected. This error can be minimized when reading a centrifuged hematocrit by taking care not to include the leukocyte layer in the calculations. When using electronic cell counters, the blood should be diluted before analyzing to minimize errors of leukocytosis. The results are then multiplied by the reciprocal of the dilution used.

The hematocrit differs according to age, sex, and geographic location similar to that described for erythrocytes. The highest normal value, 0.61 L/L, is seen in newborns, followed by a gradual decrease, and reaching a nadir at 2 months of age. The hematocrit then increases until normal adult values (about 0.45 L/L) are reached at 14 years of age. Females have lower values than males.

Care should be taken when interpreting the hematocrit since it is calculated in a relative term, as discussed earlier for hemoglobin, rather than an actual mass. For example, either an absolute decrease in erythrocytes or an absolute increase in plasma volume may give a low hematocrit value. An absolute decrease in plasma volume with normal erythrocyte mass may give an elevated hematocrit value. When large volumes of blood are lost rapidly as in hemorrhage, immediate hematocrit values may appear normal because both erythrocytes and plasma are being lost in the same proportion. In time, the body will attempt to replace blood volume with tissue fluid, which will produce a dilutional effect on remaining erythrocytes and a decrease in hematocrit.

Hemoglobin Hemoglobin concentration is an indirect measurement of the oxygen-carrying capacity of blood. For this protein to be measured, the erythrocytes are lysed, releasing their contents. The free hemoglobin is then reacted with potassium cyanide and potassium ferricyanide to form the stable pigment, cyanmethemoglobin. The optical density of the solution measured spectrophotometrically is directly proportional to the hemoglobin concentration.

As would be expected, hemoglobin values vary according to age and sex, similar to the variations noted in erythrocyte and hematocrit values. The highest normal value at birth, 19 g/dL, declines after the first week of extrauterine life. The decline occurs as an adjustment to improved oxygenation of the blood after birth as the lungs replace the placenta as the site of oxygen exchange.[1] After a low

of 10 to 11 g/dL at 2 months, the concentration gradually rises until adult values are reached at 14 years. Values are similar in boys and girls until about age 9, when the hemoglobin concentration rises faster in boys. Adult females have lower concentrations than males, and blacks have concentrations that average 0.5 g/dL lower than whites. Pregnant women have a lower hemoglobin level, probably due to placental hormones and/or variations in the extracellular fluid volume.

There is a diurnal variation in hemoglobin, hematocrit, and erythrocyte values. The highest values occur in the morning and the lowest in the evening. Cigarette smoking causes an increase in hemoglobin concentration that is probably mediated by exposure to carbon monoxide. As compensation for decreased oxygen-carrying capacity, smokers maintain higher levels of hemoglobin than nonsmokers. Furthermore, there is a direct dose-response relationship between the amount smoked and the hemoglobin level (Table 5-7).[7]

Variations also are reported to occur as a result of blood drawing techniques. Hemoglobin values are about 0.7 g/dL higher if the patient's blood is obtained while the individual is in an upright rather than supine position. Prolonged vasoconstriction by the tourniquet may cause hemoconcentration of the sample and elevate the hemoglobin.

ERYTHROCYTE INDICES

The erythrocyte indices are extremely helpful in classifying the erythrocytes as to their size and hemoglobin content. Hemoglobin, hematocrit, and erythrocyte count are used to calculate the three indices: *mean corpuscular volume* (MCV), *mean corpuscular hemoglobin concentration* (MCHC), and *mean corpuscular hemoglobin* (MCH). The indices give the clinical laboratory scientist a clue as to what the erythrocytes should look like on the stained blood film. Since abnormal erythrocyte morphology is characteristic of distinct types of anemia, the indices are useful for initial classification of anemic states.

Mean cell volume The MCV indicates the average volume of individual erythrocytes in femtoliters (fL). It may be measured directly on some automated cell counters; for instance, on the Coulter counters, as blood cells pass singly through an orifice through which an electric current is flowing, the cell produces a voltage pulse, the magnitude of which is proportional to the cell volume. The MCV, however, also may be calculated from the hematocrit and erythrocyte count.

$$\text{MCV (fL)} = \frac{\text{hematocrit (L/L)}}{\text{erythrocyte count } (\times 10^2/\text{L})}$$

Example: A patient has a hematocrit of 0.45 L/L and an erythrocyte count of 5×10^{12}/L.

$$\text{MCV (fL)} = \frac{0.45\text{L/L}}{5 \times 10^{12}/\text{L}} = 90 \times 10^{-15} \text{ L or 90 fL}$$

The MCV is used to classify cells as normocytic, microcytic, or macrocytic. Normocytic cells have an MCV between 80 and 100 fL. Cells less than 80 fL are microcytic, whereas cells greater than 100 fL are macrocytic. Abnormalities in the MCV are clues to disease processes of the hematopoietic system; they are useful in preliminary assessment of anemia pathophysiology.

This index usually correlates with the appearance of cells on stained blood smears (i.e., cells with an increased MCV appear larger [macrocytes] and cells with a decreased MCV [microcytes] appear smaller) (Table 5-10). It must, however, be remembered that MCV is a measurement of volume, whereas estimation of the size of flattened cells on a blood smear is a measurement of cell diameter. Cell diameter and cell volume are not the same. Spherocytes usually have a normal or only slightly decreased volume (MCV), but on a stained smear they are unable to flatten as much as normal erythrocytes because of a decreased surface area and increased rigidity. Spherocytes, therefore, appear to have a smaller diameter than normal cells. Conversely, target cells may appear larger due to an increased diameter, but the MCV is usually normal.

Mean corpuscular hemoglobin concentration The MCHC is the average concentration of hemoglobin in grams in a deciliter of erythrocytes (g/L in SI units). (This parameter has commonly been expressed in the past as a percentage.) The MCHC is calculated from the hemoglobin and hematocrit as follows:

$$\text{MCHC (g/dL)} = \frac{\text{Hemoglobin (gm/dL)}}{\text{Hematocrit (L/L)}}$$

Example: A patient has a hemoglobin concentration of 15 g/dL and a hematocrit of 0.45 L/L.

$$\text{MCHC (g/dL)} = \frac{15 \text{ g/dL}}{0.45 \text{ L/L}} = 33$$

This index indicates whether the general cell population is normochromic, hypochromic, or hyperchromic (Table 5-11). The reference range for MCHC is 32 to 36 g/dL. An MCHC below 32 g/dL indicates hypochromic cells, whereas an MCHC between 32 and 36 g/dL indi-

TABLE 5-10 *RED BLOOD CELL ANISOCYTOSIS CORRELATION WITH COULTER S PARAMETER MCV*

Smear Evaluation	MCV Coulter S
Marked microcytosis	↓65
Moderate microcytosis	66–75
Slight microcytosis	
Male	76–79
Female	76–80
Normal	
Male	80–94
Female	81–100
Slight macrocytosis	
Male	95–108
Female	101–108
Moderate macrocytosis	109–120
Marked macrocytosis	↑120

(From O'Connor BH: A color atlas and instruction manual of peripheral blood cell. morphology. (Baltimore, Williams & Wilkins, 1984.)

TABLE 5-11 *RED BLOOD CELL HYPOCHROMIA CORRELATION WITH COULTER S PARAMETER MCHC*

Smear Evaluation	MCHC Coulter S
Normochromia	31.5–36
Hypochromia	
Slight	30.0–31.5
Moderate	29.0–30.5
Marked	↓29

Note: Recheck any MCHC over 36% for hemolysis, cold agglutinins, or insufficient blood in relation to EDTA.

(From O'Connor BH: A color atlas and instruction manual of peripheral blood cell. morphology. (Baltimore, Williams & Wilkins, 1984.)

cates normochromic cells. The term hyperchromic should be used sparingly. The only erythrocyte that is hyperchromic, with an MCHC greater than 36 g/dL, is the spherocyte. Spherocytes have a decreased surface-to-volume ratio because of a loss of membrane but have not lost an appreciable amount of their hemoglobin.

Mean corpuscular hemoglobin The MCH is a measurement of the average weight of hemoglobin in individual erythrocytes. The MCH may be calculated as follows:

$$\text{MCH (pg)} = \frac{\text{hemoglobin (g/dL)} \times 10}{\text{erythrocyte count} (\times 10^{12}/\text{L})}$$

Example: A patient has a hemoglobin concentration of 15 g/dL and an erythrocyte count of $5 \times 10^{12}/\text{L}$

$$\text{MCH (pg)} = \frac{15 \text{ g/dL}}{5 \times 10^{12}/\text{L}} = 30 \text{ pg}$$

The reference range of MCH for normocytic cells is 26 to 34 pg.

When evaluating cells for hemoglobin content using MCH, it is important to take into consideration the size of the cells (MCV). The MCH should always correlate with the MCV and MCHC. Smaller cells normally contain less hemoglobin, and larger cells normally contain more hemoglobin. In some anemias, a decrease or increase in cell size (MCV) is associated with a proportional decrease or increase in the amount of hemoglobin within the cell (MCH), resulting in a normochromic cell (normal MCHC). In other anemias, however, the decrease in the amount of hemoglobin within the cell (MCH) is substantially more than the decrease in cell size and the cell appears hypochromic (decreased MCHC). It is important to understand this concept because microcytic cells with an MCH less than 26 pg are not necessarily hypochromic and macrocytes with an MCH greater than 34 pg are not usually hyperchromic. The MCH does not take into account the size of a cell; thus, it should not be interpreted without taking into consideration the MCV. More information is available from the MCHC.

Falsely elevated MCHC, MCH and MCV, as determined on automated cell counters, may occur if the patient's erythrocytes are agglutinated by cold autoagglutinins. On Coulter counters, the clumps of erythrocytes pass through the orifice of the counter together, and the instrument sizes the clumps as individual cells. The MCV, conse-

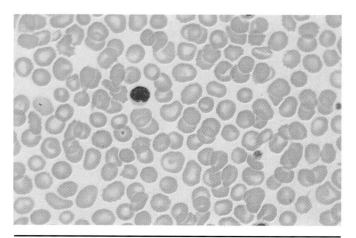

FIGURE 5-1. Peripheral blood from a newborn; note the macrocytic erythrocytes. (250× original magnification; Wright-Giemsa stain.)

quently, appears grossly elevated, and the erythrocyte count erroneously low. As a result, the calculated hematocrit also is erroneously low. The hemoglobin determination is unaffected because erythrocytes are lysed for determination of this parameter. This leads to a false elevation of the MCHC (normal hemoglobin/falsely low hematocrit) and of the MCH (normal hemoglobin/falsely low erythrocyte count).

Developmental changes in erythrocyte indices The MCV is increased to a mean of 108 fL at birth but decreases to a mean of 77 fL between the ages of 6 months and 2 years (Fig. 5-1).[1] It increases to a mean of 80 fL by 5 years of age but does not reach the adult mean of 90 fL until about 18 years of age. The MCH changes in parallel to the MCV throughout infancy and childhood. The MCHC, however, remains constant within the adult range. Between the ages of 12 and 17 years, males have a higher MCHC and lower MCH and MCV than females.[8]

Red cell distribution width (RDW) Since the MCV represents an average of erythrocyte volume, it is less reliable in describing the erythrocyte population when there is considerable variation in erythrocyte size (*anisocytosis*).[9] The RDW is a calculated index provided by some hematology analyzers to help identify anisocytosis. The *RDW* is the coefficient of variation of erythrocyte volume distribution. It is calculated as follows:

$$\frac{\text{standard deviation} \times 100}{\text{mean MCV}} = \text{RDW}$$

The normal RDW is between 11.5% and 13.5%. All abnormalities found to this time are on the high side, indicating an increase in the heterogeneity of erythrocyte size. A low RDW would mean a more uniform erythrocyte population. It would be difficult to understand a decreased RDW, since little or no variability in size is considered normal.

Caution must be used in interpreting the RDW since it is a reflection of the ratio of the standard deviation of cell size and the mean MCV. An increased standard deviation (heterogeneous cell population) with a high MCV may give a normal RDW. Conversely, a normal standard deviation (homogeneous cell population) with a low MCV may give an increased RDW. Examination of the erythrocyte histogram and stained blood smear will give the scientist clues as to the accuracy of the RDW in these cases. When the standard deviation increases, indicating a true variability in cell size, the base of the erythrocyte histogram with cell size on the x-axis will be broader than usual.

RETICULOCYTE COUNT

Immature, anuclear erythrocytes containing organelles and an extensive ribosomal system for hemoglobin synthesis are known as *reticulocytes*.

Reticulocytes usually spend 2 to 3 days in the bone marrow and an additional day in the peripheral blood before becoming mature erythrocytes. The peripheral blood reticulocyte count indicates the degree of effective bone marrow activity and is one of the most useful and cost-effective laboratory tests in classifying the pathophysiology of anemia. Reticulocytes may sometimes be identified as polychromatophilic erythrocytes on Romanowsky-stained smears (Fig. 5-2). The *polychromatophilia* is due to the presence of basophilic ribosomes (RNA). Definitive identification of these cells is made by staining blood with a supravital stain such as new methylene blue. This stain causes residual RNA to aggregate into a reticulum and precipitate as deep bluish-purple inclusions (Fig. 5-3). The number of reticulocytes is determined by identifying the number of reticulocytes in 1000 erythrocytes. The reticulocyte count is usually reported as a percentage, but also may be reported in absolute numbers, the number of reticulocytes per liter of blood.

The percentage of reticulocytes in whole blood is 0.8% to 4.0% or about 18 to 50 × 10⁹/L in a healthy individual. In the healthy aged, there appears to be a decrease in the

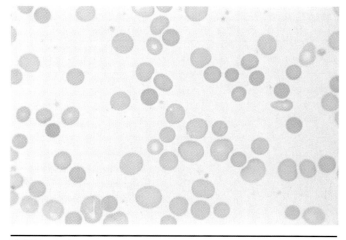

FIGURE 5-2. The large erythrocytes with a bluish tinge are polychromatophilic erythrocytes. They are larger than the more mature erythrocytes. (Peripheral blood; 250× original magnification; Wright-Giemsa stain.)

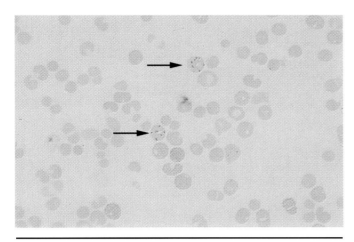

FIGURE 5-3. The erythrocytes with the particulate inclusions are reticulocytes. The inclusions represent reticulum that stains with the supravital stain brilliant cresyl blue. (Peripheral blood, 250× original magnification.)

lifespan of the erythrocyte.[10] This is compensated for by an active bone marrow so that the hemoglobin and hematocrit remain in the reference range of other adults. There is, however, a slight reticulocytosis, reflecting the increased production of erythrocytes.

Corrected reticulocyte count In anemia, a more accurate index of erythropoietic activity is needed than the relative reticulocyte count. When reported as a percentage, it does not indicate the relation between the peripheral blood erythrocyte mass and the number of reticulocytes being produced. Since increased bone marrow production of erythrocytes is the expected response to anemia, a reticulocyte count in the reference range of 0.5% to 1.5% is never normal for an anemic individual. For instance, in a healthy male with a 5×10^{12}/L erythrocyte count and 1% reticulocyte count, the absolute number of reticulocytes released is 50×10^9/L.

$$(0.01) \times (5 \times 10^{12}/L) = 50 \times 10^9/L$$

In an anemic male with a 2.0×10^{12}/L erythrocyte count, 19% hematocrit, and 1% reticulocyte, the absolute number of new cells released is 20×10^9/L, hardly enough to stabilize even the anemic erythrocyte mass.

$$(0.01) \times (2.0 \times 10^9/L) = 20 \times 10^9/L$$

In the anemic individual, the relative reticulocyte count appears normal (1%), but he is actually making 30×10^9/L less erythrocytes than the normal male with the same relative reticulocyte count.

The corrected reticulocyte count overcomes this dilutional problem and is useful in evaluating the bone marrow response in anemia. The correction makes adjustments proportional to the severity of the anemia.[11] The formula for corrected reticulocyte count uses the patient's hematocrit in comparison to a normal hematocrit (0.45 L/L).

$$\frac{\text{Patient's hematocrit}}{0.45 \text{ L/L}} \times \text{reticulocyte count}$$

In the anemic male mentioned above, the corrected reticulocyte count would be:

$$\frac{0.19 \text{ L/L} \times 1\%}{0.45 \text{ L/L}} = 0.4\%$$

Reticulocyte production index An additional reticulocyte correction is needed if large polychromatophilic macrocytes are seen on the blood smear. With increasing erythropoietin stimulation, the bone marrow releases reticulocytes before their normal 2- to 3-day marrow maturation period. These immature reticulocytes appear as large polychromatophilic erythrocytes (shift or stress reticulocytes) on the blood smear. This means the additional bone marrow maturation time is added to peripheral blood maturation time, and it takes longer than the normal 1 day for the peripheral blood reticulocyte to lose its reticulum and become a mature erythrocyte. The more severe the anemia, the earlier the reticulocyte is released. In a stimulated marrow, hematocrit levels of 0.35 L/L, 0.25 L/L, and 0.15 L/L are associated with early reticulocyte release and a prolongation of the reticulocyte maturation in peripheral blood to approximately 1.5, 2.0, and 2.5 days, respectively (Fig. 5-4). To correct for the prolongation of maturation of these circulating shift reticulocytes, the following formula is used:

$$\frac{\text{Patient's hematocrit}}{0.45 \text{ L/L}} \times \frac{\text{reticulocyte}}{\text{count}} \times \frac{1}{\substack{\text{maturation time of} \\ \text{shift reticulocytes} \\ \text{based on hematocrit}}}$$

This correction is known as the *reticulocyte production index* (RPI).

The RPI is a good indicator of the adequacy of the bone marrow response in anemia. Generally speaking, an RPI greater than 2 indicates an appropriate bone marrow response, whereas an RPI less than 2 indicates an inadequate compensatory bone marrow response (hypoproliferation) or an ineffective bone marrow response. When used in this way, the reticulocyte count provides a direction for the course of investigation concerning anemia pathophysiology. For example, an anemic male with an erythrocyte count of 2.0×10^{12}/L, hematocrit of 18%, and polychromatophilic macrocytes on the blood smear has a reticulocyte count of 3%, increased in terms of the uncorrected, relative reticulocyte count. The absolute reticulocyte concentration also is slightly above normal:

$$(0.03) \times (2.0 \times 10^{12}/L) = 60 \times 10^9/L$$

Calculation of the RPI, however, indicates his marrow is not adequately responding to the anemia.

$$\frac{0.18}{0.45} \times 3 \times \frac{1}{2.5} = 0.5$$

Based on this calculation, his anemia appears to be associated with an impaired erythropoietic mechanism. Impaired erythropoiesis may be due to an insufficient pro-

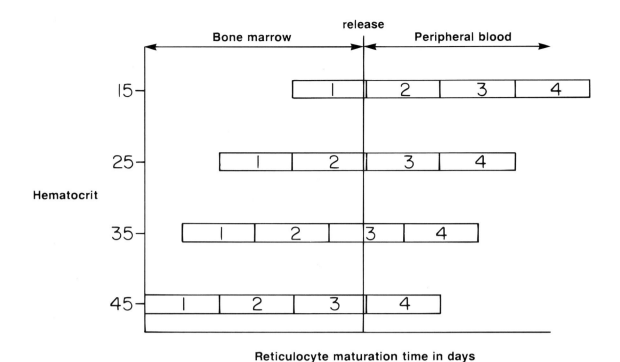

Reticulocyte maturation time in days

FIGURE 5-4. The correlation of hematocrit (given here as a percentage) with the reticulocyte maturation time. As anemia worsens, the reticulocyte is released earlier from the bone marrow and spends a longer time maturing in the peripheral blood.

duction of erythrocytes (hypoproliferative defect) or production of defective erythrocytes that are destroyed in the marrow (ineffective erythropoiesis). Other diagnostic tests and bone marrow examination would help differentiate between these two defects.

BLOOD SMEAR EXAMINATION

The erythrocyte is sometimes called a discocyte because of its biconcave shape. On a Romanowsky-stained blood smear, the erythrocyte appears as a $7\,\mu$m disc with a central area of pallor that is surrounded by a rim of pink-staining hemoglobin. The area of pallor is caused by the closeness occurring between the two concave portions of the membrane when the cell becomes flattened on a glass slide. Normally, the area of pallor occupies about one third the diameter of the cell. The area of pallor is not seen in erythrocytes suspended in saline or plasma and viewed with the light microscope.

This normal morphology of the erythrocyte may be altered by various pathologic conditions intrinsic or extrinsic to the cell. Careful examination of a stained blood smear will reveal these morphologic aberrations. *Poikilocytosis* is the general term used to describe a nonspecific variation in the shape of erythrocytes (Fig. 5-5). *Anisocytosis* denotes a nonspecific variation in the size of the cells. Some variation in size is normal because of the variation in age of the erythrocytes, younger cells being larger and older cells smaller. Some shapes and sizes, however, are particularly characteristic of serious underlying hematologic disorders or malignancy. These include nucleated erythrocytes (except in newborns), schistocytes, teardrop erythrocyte shape, spherocytes, and marked

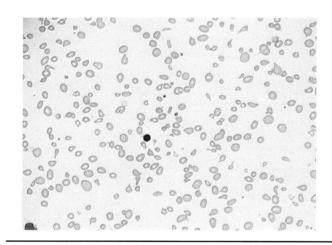

FIGURE 5-5. Erythrocytes with marked anisocytosis and poikilocytosis (PB; 100X original magnification; Wright stain). (Adapted from: Hillman RS & Finch CA: Red cell manual. 6th Ed. Philadelphia, FA Davis, 1992.)

erythrocyte shape abnormalities in normocytic anemia without evidence of hemolysis.[12] It is important to keep in mind that some abnormal morphology can be artifactual because of poorly made or improperly stained smears. If artifactual morphology is suspected, the erythrocytes should be examined in a wet preparation. If the abnormal morphology is present in this preparation, the possibility of artifacts can be eliminated.

Poikilocytes Poikilocytosis (Table 5-12) is usually reported as slight, moderate, or marked, depending on the

TABLE 5-12 *ABNORMALITIES IN THE SHAPE OF ERYTHROCYTES*

Terminology	Synonyms	Description	Associated Disease States
Poikilocytosis	—	Increased variation in the shape of red cells	See disease states associated with specific poikilocytes on this table
Echinocyte (sea urchin)	Burr cell; crenated cell	Spiculated red cells with short equally spaced projections over the entire surface	Liver disease; uremia; pyruvate kinase deficiency; peptic ulcers; cancer of stomach; heparin therapy
Acanthocyte (spike)	Spur cell	Red cells with spicules of varying length irregularly distributed over the surface	Abetalipoproteinemia; alcoholic liver disease; disorders of lipid metabolism; post splenectomy; fat malabsorption; retinitis pigmentosa
Elliptocyte (oval)	Ovalocyte; pencil cell; cigar cell	Oval to elongated ellipsoid cell with central area of pallor and hemoglobin at both ends	Hereditary elliptocytosis; iron deficiency anemia; thalassemia; anemia associated with leukemia
Drepanocytes (sickle)	Sickle cells	Red cells containing polymerized HbS showing various shapes: sickle shaped, crescent or boat shaped	Sickle cell disorders
Dacryocyte (tear)	Tear drop; tennis racquet cell	Round cell with a single elongated or pointed extremity; usually microcytic and/or hypochromic	Myelophthisic anemias; thalassemias
Codocyte (bell)	Target cell; Mexican hat cell	Thin bell-shaped cells with an increased surface to volume ratio; on stained blood smears they assume the appearance of a target with a bull's eye in the center, surrounded by an achromic zone and outer ring of hemoglobin; osmotic fragility is decreased	Hemoglobinopathies; thalassemias; obstructive liver disease; iron deficiency anemia; splenectomy; renal disease; LCAT deficiency
Schistocytes (cut)	Schizocyte; fragmented cell	Fragments of red cells; variety of shapes including triangles, comma shaped; microcytic	Microangiopathic hemolytic anemias; heart-valve hemolysis; DIC; severe burns; uremia
Keratocytes (horn)	Helmet cells; horn-shaped cells	Red cells with one or several notches with projections that look like horns on either end	Microangiopathic hemolytic anemias; heart-valve hemolysis; Heinz body hemolytic anemia; glomerulonephritis; cavernous hemangiomas
Spherocyte	—	Spherocytic red cells with dense hemoglobin content (hyperchromatic); lack an area of central pallor osmotic fragility is increased	Hereditary spherocytosis; immune hemolytic anemias; severe burns; ABO incompatibility; Heinz-body anemias
Stomatocytes (mouth)	Mouth cell; cup form; mushroom cap	Uniconcave red cells with the shape of a very thick cup; on stained blood smears cells have an oval or slit-like area of central pallor	Hereditary stomatocytosis; spherocytosis; alcoholic cirrhosis; anemia associated with Rh null disease; lead intoxication; neoplasms
Leptocytes (thin)	Thin cell	Thin, flat cell with hemoglobin at periphery; usually cup shaped, MCV is decreased but diameter of cell is normal	Thalassemia; iron deficiency anemia; hemoglobinopathies; liver disease
Knizocytes	—	Red cells with more than two concavities; on stained blood smears there is a dark stick of hemoglobin in center with a pale area on either end	Conditions in which spherocytes are found
Xerocytes		Dense, irregularly contracted cells; hemoglobin may be concentrated at periphery of the cell	Familial xerocytosis

number of abnormal forms seen. In most laboratories, this measurement is subjective, with no criteria for each degree of abnormality. It has been suggested that to standardize this measurement, the scientist should count the number of each type of poikilocyte in 10 different fields; divide by 10 to derive an average per field; and report as slight, moderate, or marked according to preset criteria (Table 5-13).[13] In this procedure, total poikilocytosis is a sum of the mean per field for each individual shape. For example, if a smear has the following mean values per field: ovalocytes, 6; stomatocytes, 4; and target cells, 3; total poikilocytosis (13) is moderate.

Figure 5-6A illustrates normal erythrocytes and 5-6B illustrates poikilocytes. Following is a description of spe-cific types of poikilocytes, their physiologic significance and disorders with which they are associated.

ECHINOCYTES *Echinocytes,* also called burr cells (Fig. 5-7A), are usually smaller than normal erythrocytes with regular, spine-like projections on their surface. The characteristic appearance is not related to tonicity of the medium in which the cells are suspended. The shape change is instead believed to be the result of an increase in the area of the outer leaflet of lipid bilayer compared with the inner layer. Echinocyte formation is reversible (i.e., the cell can revert to a discocyte). Echinocytes may eventually assume the shape of a spherocyte, presumably because of grooming

TABLE 5-13 *MEAN RANGES FOR POIKILOCYTOSIS OF RED BLOOD CELLS/10 FIELDS*

Abnormal Shape	Normal	Slight	Moderate	Marked
Spherocyte	0	1–5	6–15	↑15
Acanthocyte	0	1–5	6–15	↑15
Sickle cell	0	1–5	6–15	↑15
Rouleaux forms	0	1–5	6–15	↑15
Envelope forms	0–1	2–5	6–15	↑15
Tear drop forms	0–1	2–5	6–15	↑15
Bizarre forms	0–1	2–5	6–15	↑15
Tailed rbc forms	0–1	2–5	6–15	↑15
Target cells	0–1	2–5	6–15	↑15
Schistocytes	0–1	2–5	6–15	↑15
Ovalocytes	0–1	2–5	6–15	↑15
Elliptocytes	0–1	2–5	6–15	↑15
Burr cells	0–1	2–5	6–15	↑15
Stomatocytes	0–1	2–5	6–15	↑15
Blister cells	0–1	2–5	6–15	↑15

(From: O'Connor BH: A color atlas and instruction manual of peripheral blood cell morphology. Baltimore, Williams & Wilkins, 1994.)

(removal) of the membrane spines by the spleen; in this circumstance, the cell cannot revert to a normal shape.

Normal discocytes may be transformed into echinocytes under certain in vitro conditions. Echinocytes are a common artifact in stained blood smears because of the glass effect of the slide. The glass releases certain basic substances, raising the pH of the medium surrounding the cell, and inducing echinocyte formation. Plasma provides a buffering effect on the cells, and for this reason blood films made from whole blood may show only certain areas of echinocyte transformation. To determine the in vivo or in vitro nature of echinocytes, it may be necessary to enclose a drop of blood between two plastic coverslips (wet preparation) and observe the unstained individual erythrocytes. If there are no echinocytes in the wet preparation, but they were noted on the stained blood smears, the cell abnormality occurred as an in vitro event.

Echinocytes have been reported to occur in vivo in a variety of conditions including liver disease, pyruvate kinase deficiency, uremia, peptic ulcers, and cancer of the stomach, as well as in newborns with liver disease and in patients receiving heparin therapy. Echinocytes appear within several days in blood stored at 4° C. Consequently, blood from patients receiving transfusions may show the presence of echinocytes if blood is taken from the patient immediately after transfusion; however, a few minutes after transfusion, the buffering action of patient's plasma causes the transfused echinocyte to assume a normal discoid shape.

STOMATOCYTES *Stomatocytes* (Fig. 5-7B), in wet preparations, appear as small cup-shaped uniconcave discs. After staining, these cells exhibit a slit-like (mouth-like) area of pallor. Normal discocytes may be transformed under certain conditions to stomatocytes and, eventually, to spherostomatocytes. The stomatocyte shape is reversible, but the spherostomatocyte is not. Cationic drugs and low pH cause a gradual loss of biconcavity, leading to the stomatocyte and eventually formation of a sphere. Stomatocytosis is the opposite of echinocytosis; the shape change in stomatocytosis is believed to be the result of an increase in the area of the inner bilayer of the lipid leaflet membrane.

Since the abnormal shape can be artifactual on stained blood smears, care should be taken in identifying stomatocytes. Stomatocytes in vivo are characteristic of a rare autosomal-dominant hemolytic anemia called hereditary stomatocytosis. Stomatocytes also are associated with spherocytosis, alcoholic cirrhosis, lead intoxication, Rh

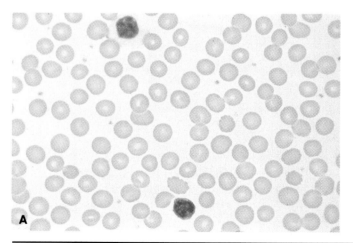

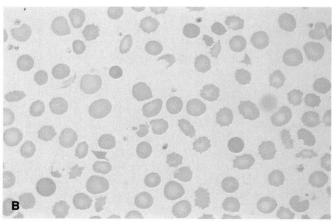

FIGURE 5-6. A, Normocytic, normochromic erythrocytes. Compare the size of the cells to the nucleus of the lymphocytes. (250× original magnification; Wright-Giemsa stain) **B,** Poikilocytosis with acanthocytes, helmet cell, elliptocytes, echinocytes, schistocytes, and spherocytes. There is also anisocytosis with microcytes and macrocytes. At least two of the macrocytes are polychromatophilic indicating that they are reticulocytes. (250× original magnification; Wright-Giemsa stain.)

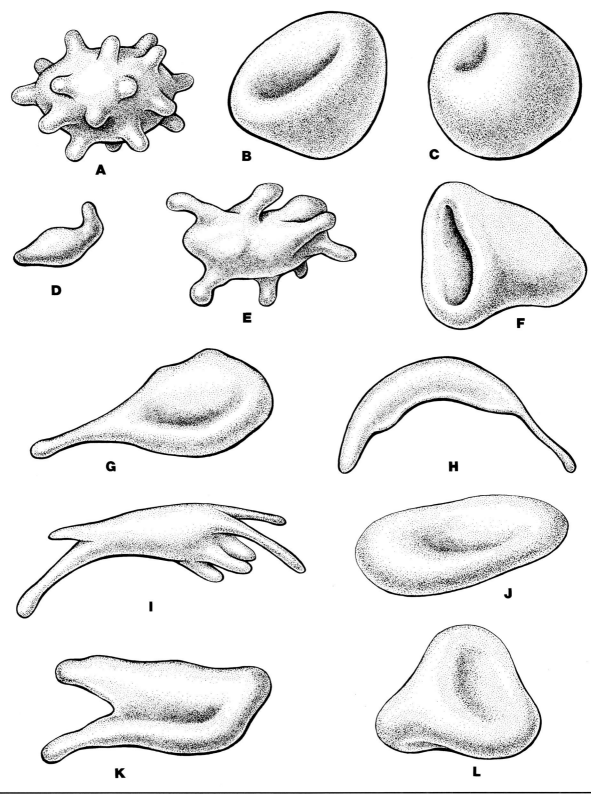

FIGURE 5-7. Drawings of various poikilocytes. **A.** Echinocyte **B.** Stomatocyte **C.** Spherocyte **D.** Schistocyte **E.** Acanthocyte **F.** Codocyte (target cell) **G.** Dacryocyte (tear drop) **H.** Drepanocyte (sickle cell) **I.** Drepanocyte (holly leaf) **J.** Elliptocyte **K.** Keratocyte (helmet cell) **L.** Knizocyte

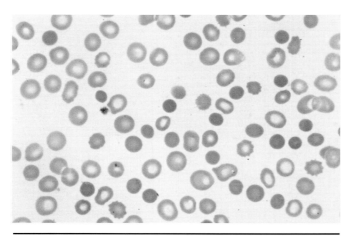

FIGURE 5-8. Spherocytes. Note the densely staining, small, spherocytic cells. These cells lack the central area of pallor. (PB; 250× original magnification.)

null disease, neoplasms, and in conditions that alter the sodium permeability of the erythrocyte membrane.

SPHEROCYTES Spherocytes (Fig. 5-7C) are erythrocytes that have lost their biconcavity resulting from a decreased surface-to-volume ratio. On stained blood smears, the spherocyte appears as a densely stained sphere lacking a central area of pallor (Fig. 5-8). Although the cell appears microcytic on stained blood smears, the volume is usually normal because of the increased cell thickness. The spherocyte is the only erythrocyte that may be classified as hyperchromic because of the increased MCHC. Spherocytes have increased osmotic fragility, with hemolysis beginning in NaCl concentrations of about 0.6% and complete at about 0.4%. Autohemolysis (in vitro suspension of patients' cells and serum) is increased. Spherocytes, which are less deformable than discocytes, have a decreased lifespan and are removed in the spleen. Spherocytes are present in hereditary spherocytosis, immune hemolytic anemias, Heinz-body anemias, and in severe burns.

SCHISTOCYTES Schistocytes (Fig. 5-7D) are erythrocyte fragments caused by mechanical damage to the cell. They appear in a variety of shapes: triangular, comma-shaped, helmet-shaped, in addition to other forms. Since schistocytes are fragments of erythrocytes, they are usually microcytic. They maintain normal deformability, but their survival in the blood stream is reduced. The fragments may assume a spherical shape and hemolyze or they may be removed in the spleen.

Schistocytes may be found whenever blood vessel pathology is present. Erythrocyte fragmentation is particularly associated with intravascular fibrin formation. Erythrocytes become hung up on fibrin strands in the vessels (termed "the clothesline effect"). The force of blood flow may release the distressed cell intact, or the cell may be fragmented by the fibrin strand, producing schistocytes. This mechanism of erythrocyte damage predominates in disseminated intravascular coagulation (DIC), microangiopathic hemolytic anemias, and thrombotic thrombocytopenic pupura (TTP). Schistocytes also may be seen in valvular lesions, uremia, and March hemoglobinuria. Spheroschistocytes, seen in severe burn victims, are the result of heat damage to spectrin protein in the membrane cytoskeleton.

ACANTHOCYTES Acanthocytes, or spur cells (Fig. 5-7E), are small spherical cells with irregular thorn-like projections. Often the projections will have small bulb-like tips. These cells have membranes with altered lipid content. Acanthocytes have a normal lifespan with a normal to slightly decreased osmotic fragility. Acanthocytes may be seen in liver disease, abetalipropoteinemia (congenital acanthocytosis), fat malabsorption, disorders of lipid metabolism, and retinitis pigmentosa.

LEPTOCYTES Leptocytes are thin, flat, cells with normal or greater than normal diameter. Although the diameter of the cell is normal or increased, the MCV is usually decreased. The cells have an increased surface-to-volume ratio either as a result of decreased hemoglobin content or increased surface area. The leptocyte is usually cup-shaped, like stomatocytes, but the cup has little depth. Target cells may be formed from leptocytes when the depth of the cup increases. Leptocytes are seen in liver disease and in anemias characterized by hypochromic erythrocytes such as iron deficiency anemia and thalassemia.

CODOCYTES Codocytes (Fig. 5-7F), also called Mexican hat cells or target cells, are thin, bell-shaped cells with an increased surface-to-volume ratio. On stained blood smears, the cells have the appearance of a target with a bull's eye in the center (Fig. 5-9). The bull's eye is surrounded by an achromic zone and a thin, outer ring of pink-staining hemoglobin. The typical appearance of these cells is only discernible in the area of the slide where the cells are well separated. Erythrocyte shape cannot be evaluated in the extreme outer feather edge, where all cells are flattened.

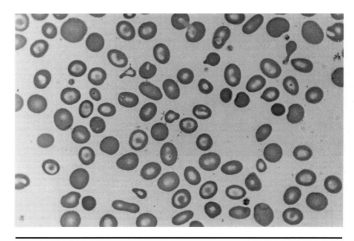

FIGURE 5-9. This blood film shows a variety of poikilocytes. There are codocytes (target cells), elliptocytes, teardrop forms, and spherocytes. There also is anisocytosis with some small erythrocytes and larger forms. (250× original magnification; Wright-Giemsa stain.)

Target cells may appear as artifacts when smears are made in a high humidity environment or when a wet smear is blown dry rather than fan dried. Target cells have decreased osmotic fragility due to the increased surface-to-volume ratio of the cell.

Target cells may be seen in disorders in which there is an increase in membrane lipids such as liver disease, hereditary deficiency of lecithin-cholesterol acyl transferase (LCAT), after splenectomy, and in renal disease. Increased surface-to-volume ratio also may occur as a result of diminution of corpuscular hemoglobin as in iron deficiency anemia and thalassemia. Target cells may occur in some hemoglobinopathies, especially hemoglobin S and hemoglobin C disease.

DACRYOCYTES *Dacryocytes*, also called teardrops (Figs. 5-7G and 5-9), are erythrocytes that are elongated at one end, forming a teardrop or pear-shaped cell. Some teardrops may form after erythrocytes with cellular inclusions have transversed the spleen. Erythrocytes with inclusions are more rigid in the area of the inclusion, and this portion of the cell has more difficulty passing through the splenic filter than the rest of the cell. As a result, the cell is stretched into an abnormal shape. The teardrop cannot return to its original shape because the cell has either been stretched beyond the limits of deformability of the membrane or the cell has been in the abnormal shape for too long a time. This is most likely the mechanism of formation of teardrops observed in thalassemia when Heinz bodies are present. Teardrops also are observed in myelofibrosis with myeloid metaplasia and metastatic cancer to the bone marrow. The mechanism of formation of dacryocytes in these pathologic states is unknown.

DREPANOCYTES *Drepanocytes*, also called sickle cells (Fig. 5-7H), are elongated, crescent-shaped erythrocytes with pointed ends. Some forms have more rounded ends with a flat rather than concave side. These modified forms of sickle shape may be capable of reversing to the normal discocyte. Sickle cell formation may be observed in wet preparations or in stained blood smears from patients with sickle cell anemia. The hemoglobin within the cell is abnormal and polymerizes into rods at decreased oxygen tension or decreased pH. The cell first transforms into a holly-leaf shape (Fig. 5-7I). Then, as the hemoglobin polymerization continues, it transforms into a sickle-shaped cell. Some holly-leaf forms may be observed on stained blood smears in addition to the typical sickle shape. The sickle cell has decreased osmotic fragility but increased mechanical fragility. Even in anemic individuals, the irregular shape of the cell decreases the erythrocyte sedimentation rate by inhibiting rouleaux formation.

ELLIPTOCYTES *Elliptocytes*, also called pencil cells and cigar cells (Figs. 5-7J and 5-9), vary from elongated oval shapes (ovalocytes) to elongated rod-like cells. They have a central area of biconcavity with hemoglobin concentrated at both ends. Elliptocytes are formed after the erythrocyte matures and leaves the bone marrow because reticulocytes in patients with elliptocytosis are normal in shape. The

mechanism of formation is not known. The osmotic fragility of elliptocytes is normal except in hemolytic hereditary elliptocytosis when osmotic fragility is increased. Autohemolysis, at 48 hours, is increased but is corrected by the addition of both glucose and ATP, suggesting that elliptocytes have abnormal membrane permeability. Rouleaux formation is normal. Elliptocytes are the predominant shape of erythrocytes in hereditary elliptocytosis. These abnormal shapes also may occur in iron deficiency, thalassemia, and anemia associated with leukemia. Megaloblastic anemia is associated with abnormally large oval erythrocytes called *macroovalocytes*.

KERATOCYTES *Keratocytes*, also called *helmet cells* (Fig. 5-7K), are cells with a concavity on one side and two horn-like protrusions on either end. They are produced by impalement on a fibrin strand. The two halves of the erythrocyte hang over the strand as saddlebags, the membranes of the touching sides fuse, producing a vacuole-like inclusion on one side. This cell with an eccentric vacuole is called a "blister cell." The vacuole bursts, leaving a notch with two spicules on the ends. It also has been suggested that these cells may result from repeated collisions in abnormalities of the circulation. Keratocytes are seen in disseminated intravascular coagulation (DIC), microangiopathic hemolytic anemia, glomerulonephritis, cavernous hemangiomas, and hemolytic anemia resulting from mechanical trauma.

KNIZOCYTES *Knizocytes* (Fig. 5-7L) are cells with more than two concavities. The appearance of this cell on stained blood smears may vary depending on how the cell comes to rest on the flat surface; however, most knizocytes have a dark-staining stick in the center with a pale area on either side surrounded by a rim of pink staining hemoglobin. The mechanism of formation is unknown. Knizocytes are associated with spherocytosis.

Anisocytes Anisocytosis, variation in cell size, may be detected by examining the blood smear and/or by reviewing the MCV and RDW. Normal erythrocytes have a diameter of about 7 to 8 μm and a cell volume of 80 to 100 fL. If the majority of cells are larger than normal, the cells are macrocytic; if smaller than normal, they are microcytic (Table 5-14). If there is a significant variation in size with microcytic, normocytic, and macrocytic cells present, the MCV may be normal because it is an average of cell size. In this case, the RDW is helpful. An RDW more than 14.5 suggests that the erythrocytes are heterogeneous in size, which makes the MCV less reliable.[9] Microscopic examination of the cells is especially helpful when the RDW is elevated. To evaluate erythrocyte size microscopically, the cells are compared with the nucleus of a normal small lymphocyte. Normocytic erythrocytes are about the same size as the lymphocyte nucleus. Figure 5-10 shows erythrocytes with a marked degree of anisocytosis.

MACROCYTES *Macrocytes* are larger than normal erythrocytes having a diameter greater than 8.0 μm and a mean corpuscular volume more than 100 fL. The cell usually

TABLE 5-14 *ABNORMALITIES IN ERYTHROCYTE SIZE*

Terminology	Description	Associated Disease States
Anisocytosis	Increased variation in the range of red cell sizes	See disease states associated with microcytes and macrocytes below
Microcytosis	Red cells with a reduced volume (<80 fL)	Iron deficiency anemia; thalassemia; sideroblastic anemia
Macrocytosis	Red cells with an increased volume (>100 fL)	Megaloblastic anemias; hemolytic anemia; recovery from acute hemorrhage; liver disease; asplenia; aplastic anemia; myelodysplasia; endocrinopathies

contains an adequate amount of hemoglobin, resulting in a normal MCHC. Macrocytes are associated with liver disease, asplenia, aplastic anemia, endocrinopathies, and myelodysplasia. They also are associated with impaired DNA synthesis such as occurs in cobalamin (vitamin B12), or folate deficiency. Young erythrocytes are normally larger than mature erythrocytes, but, within a day of entering the blood stream, are groomed by the spleen to normal size.

MICROCYTES *Microcytes* are erythrocytes with a diameter less than 7.0 μm and a mean corpuscular volume less than 80 fL. The cell is usually hypochromic (Fig. 5-11) but may be normochromic. Microcytes in the shape of spheres (microspherocytes) are usually hyperchromic. Microcytes are usually associated with defective hemoglobin formation such as occurs in iron deficiency, sideroblastic anemia, and thalassemia.

Variation in hemoglobin (color) Normal erythrocytes have an MCH of approximately 30 pg. On stained smears, the erythrocyte has a central area of pallor approximately one third the diameter of the cell. In certain conditions, the cells may contain less hemoglobin than normal. The only erythrocyte that contains more hemoglobin than normal in relation to its volume is the spherocyte. Spherocytes lack a central area of pallor and stain uniformly dense.

HYPOCHROMIC CELLS *Hypochromic* cells are poorly hemoglobinized erythrocytes with an exaggerated area of pallor (more than one third the diameter of the cell) on Romanowsky-stained blood smears. Hypochromic cells, although occasionally normocytic, are usually microcytic (Fig. 5-11). The result of decreased or impaired hemoglobin synthesis, hypochromic cells are associated with iron deficiency, sideroblastic anemia, thalassemia, and anemia of chronic disease.

POLYCHROMATOPHILIC ERYTHROCYTES *Polychromatophilic erythrocytes* (reticulocytes) are usually larger than normal cells with a bluish tinge on Romanowsky-stained blood smears. The bluish tinge is caused by the presence of residual RNA in the cytoplasm. Large numbers of these cells are associated with decreased erythrocyte survival or hemorrhage and an erythroid hyperplastic marrow (Table 5-15).

Erythrocyte inclusions The erythrocyte inclusions are described here as they appear on Romanowsky-stained blood smears unless otherwise stated.

BASOPHILIC STIPPLING Erythrocytes with *basophilic stippling* (Figs. 5-12 and 5-13A) are cells with bluish-black granular inclusions distributed throughout the entire volume of the cell. The granules may vary in size and distribution from

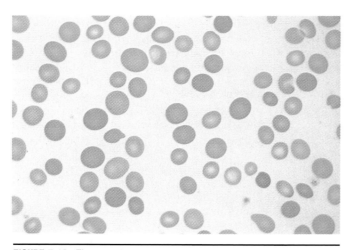

FIGURE 5-10. These erythrocytes show marked anisocytosis. (MCV-104 fL; RDW-30.2). (PB; 250× original magnification; Wright-Giemsa stain).

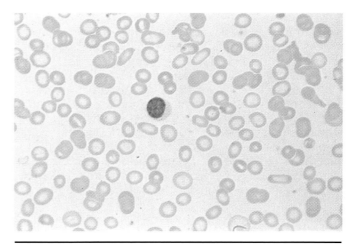

FIGURE 5-11. Microcytic, hypochromic erythrocytes. Compare the size of the erythrocytes with the nucleus of the lymphocyte. Normocytic cells are about the same size as the nucleus. There is only a thin rim of hemoglobin around the periphery of the cells indicating they are hypochromic. (PB, 250× original magnification; Wright-Giemsa stain)

TABLE 5-15 *VARIATIONS IN ERYTHROCYTE COLOR*

Terminology	Description	Associated Disease States
Hypochromia	Decreased concentration of hemoglobin in the red cell; red cells have an increased area of central pallor (>⅓ diameter of cell)	Iron deficiency anemia; thalassemia; other anemias associated with a defect in hemoglobin production
Polychromasia	Young red cells containing residual RNA; stain a pinkish-gray to pinkish-blue color on Wright's stained blood smears; usually appear slightly larger than mature red cells	Hemolytic anemias; newborns; recovery from acute hemorrhage

small and diffuse to coarse and punctate. The granules, which are composed of aggregated ribosomes, are sometimes associated with mitochondria and siderosomes. It is believed that basophilic stippling is not present in living cells; instead, stippling is probably produced during preparation of the blood smear or during the staining process. Electron microscopy has not shown an intracellular structure similar to basophilic stippling.[11] Cells dried slowly or stained rapidly may demonstrate fine, diffuse stippling as an artifact. Pathologic basophilic stippling is more coarse and punctate and is seen in lead poisoning, thalassemia, and other disorders of hemoglobin synthesis.

HOWELL-JOLLY BODIES *Howell-Jolly bodies* (Fig. 5-13B) are dark purple or violet spherical granules in the erythrocyte. These inclusions are nuclear (DNA) fragments usually occurring singly in cells, rarely more than two per cell. Howell-Jolly bodies are associated with nuclear maturation abnormalities such as megaloblastic anemia. They also are seen in some hemolytic anemias, in severe anemia, and after splenectomy or in functional asplenia.

CABOT RINGS *Cabot rings* are reddish-violet erythrocytic inclusions usually occurring in the formation of a figure eight or oval ring (Fig. 5-14). Cabot rings are believed to be remnents of spindle fibers, which form during mitosis. They occur in severe anemias and in dyserythropoiesis.

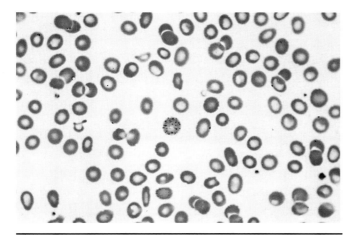

FIGURE 5-12. Basophilic stippling in mature erythrocytes. These inclusions are composed of aggregated ribosomes. (Peripheral blood, Wright-Giemsa stain, 250×.)

HEINZ BODIES *Heinz bodies* do not stain with Romanowsky stains but can be visualized with supravital stains or with phase microscopy in the living cell. They appear as 2- to 3-μm round masses lying just under or attached to the cell membrane. Heinz bodies are composed of aggregated, denatured hemoglobin. They are associated with enzymopathies, toxins or drugs that affect hemoglobin, unstable hemoglobin disorders, and after splenectomy.

SIDEROBLASTS *Sideroblasts* are nucleated erythrocytes that contain stainable iron granules; whereas siderocytes are nonnucleated erythrocytes containing iron granules (Fig. 5-13C). Sideroblasts and siderocytes may be identified with Perls Prussian blue iron stain, which stains ferritin aggregates a blue color. Finely dispersed ferritin cannot be visualized by this technique. It is hypothesized that when ferritin is not used rapidly by the erythrocyte, it aggregates and forms hemosiderin. Thus, hemosiderin represents an abundant supply of iron to the normoblast or an abnormality in iron use by the cell. About 50% to 70% of all erythroblasts in the marrow contain iron, which can be visualized with Perl's Prussian blue stain. This number decreases in some pathologic states and may be markedly increased in others. Reticulocytes and erythrocytes in the peripheral blood do not normally contain ferritin aggregates.

PAPPENHEIMER BODIES *Pappenheimer bodies* are secondary lysosomes, variable in their composition of iron and protein, or mitochondria with iron micelles (Fig. 5-15). This type of iron granule appears as small irregular basophilic deposits in erythrocytes and normoblasts and stains in both Romanowsky and Prussian blue stains. Romanowsky stains visualize Pappenheimer bodies by staining the protein matrix of the granule; whereas Prussian blue stain is responsible for staining the iron portion of the granule. They occur only in pathologic states.[11] Pappenheimer bodies are seen in sideroblastic anemia and thalassemias (Table 5-16).

Variation in erythrocyte distribution on stained smears On a well-made blood smear, the erythrocytes are evenly distributed and well separated on the feather edge of the smear. Stacking or aggregating of cells is associated with certain pathologic states (Table 5-17).

ROULEAU (PL. ROULEAUX) *Rouleau* is an alignment of erythrocytes one on top of another, resembling a stack of coins (Fig. 5-16). This phenomenon occurs normally when blood is collected and allowed to stand in tubes. It also can be seen

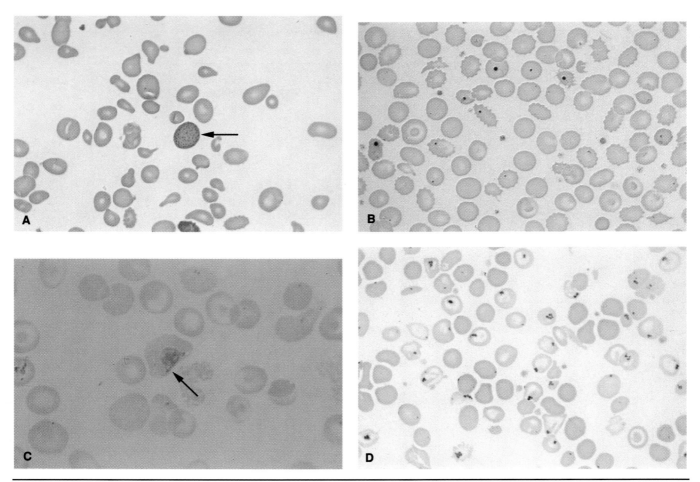

FIGURE 5-13. A, Erythrocyte with basophilic stippling, (PB; 250 × original magnification; Wright-Giemsa stain). This cell is also polychromatophilic. It is somewhat unusual to find this combination within a single cell. **B,** Howell-Jolly bodies in erythrocytes. These bodies are the single round purple inclusions. (Peripheral blood; 250×.) **C,** The erythroblast in the center contains cytoplasmic iron granules. This cell is referred to as a sideroblast. These granules do not stain with Romanowsky stains. (Bone marrow, Perl's Prussian stain, 250×.) **D,** These erythrocytes contain iron granules called Pappenheimer bodies. These bodies will stain with both Romanowsky and Perl's Prussian blue stains. (Peripheral blood, Wright-Giemsa stain, 250×.)

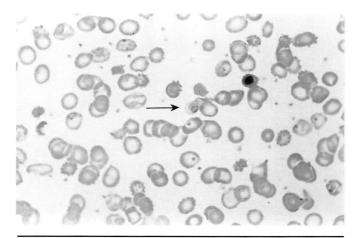

FIGURE 5-14. Cabot's ring. The arrow is pointing to a cell with a Cabot ring. This is from a case of dyserythropoiesis. (PB; 250× original magnification)

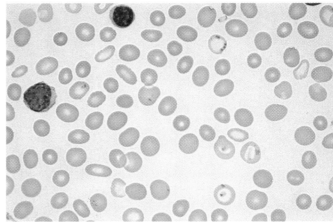

FIGURE 5-15. Pappenheimer bodies. These bodies are not as numerous as the ones in Fig 5-13D above but they are more typical morphologically. (PB; 250× original magnification; Wright-Giemsa stain.)

TABLE 5-16 *ABNORMAL ERYTHROCYTE INCLUSIONS*

Terminology	Description	Associated Disease States
Howell-Jolly bodies	Small, round bodies composed of DNA usually located eccentrically in the red cell; usually occurs singly, rarely more than 2 per cell; stains dark purple with Wright's stain	Post splenectomy; megaloblastic anemias; some hemolytic anemias; functional asplenia; severe anemia
Basophilic stippling	Round or irregularly shaped granules of variable number and size distributed throughout the red cell; composed of aggregates of ribosomes (RNA); stain bluish-black with Wright's stain	Lead poisoning; anemias associated with abnormal hemoglobin synthesis; thalassemia
Cabot rings	Appear as a figure-eight, ring or incomplete ring; thought to be composed of the microtubules of the mitotic spindle; stain reddish-violet with Wright's stain	Severe anemias; dyserythropoiesis
Pappenheimer bodies	Iron containing bodies usually found at the periphery of the cell; visible with Prussian blue stain, and with Wright's stain	Sideroblastic anemia; thalassemia; other severe anemias
Heinz bodies	Bodies composed of denatured or precipitated hemoglobin; not visible on Wright's stained blood smears; with supravital stain appear as purple shaped bodies of varying size, usually close to the cell membrane; can also be observed with phase microscopy on wet preparations	G-6-PD deficiency; unstable hemoglobin disorders; oxidizing drugs or toxins; post splenectomy
Reticulofilamentous substance	Artifactual aggregation of ribosomes; not visible on Wright's stained smears; supravital stain must be used (new methylene blue), appears as deep blue reticular network	Normal reticulocytes

TABLE 5-17 *ABNORMALITIES IN ERYTHROCYTE ARRANGEMENT*

Terminology	Description	Associated Disease States
Rouleaux	Red blood cells arranged in rolls or stacks; usually associated with abnormal or increased plasma proteins; red blood cells can be dispersed by mixing cells with saline	Multiple myeloma and other gammopathies
Agglutination	Irregular clumps of red blood cells from antigen-antibody reaction	Cold agglutinins; autoimmune hemolytic anemias

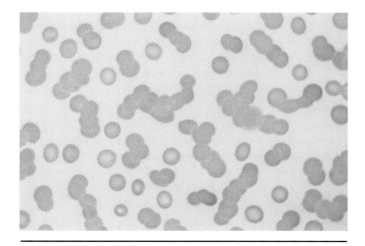

FIGURE 5-16. Rouleaux. The erythrocytes are stacked on one another like a stack of coins. This blood smear is from a patient with multiple myeloma, a malignant plasma cell disorder. The background of the slide has a bluish hue due to the large amount of protein in the plasma. (250× original magnification; Wright-Giemsa stain.)

in the thick portion of blood smears. In certain pathologic states that are accompanied by an increase in fibrinogen or globulins, rouleaux become marked and are readily seen in the feather edge of blood smears. When the erythrocyte assumes abnormal shapes, such as sickled forms, the occurrence of rouleaux is inhibited. The formation of rouleaux also is inhibited when erythrocytes are suspended in saline.

AGGLUTINATION In the presence of IgM antibodies (cold agglutinins) directed against erythrocyte antigens, erythrocytes may *agglutinate*, forming irregular clusters of varying sizes (Fig. 5-17). These clusters are readily differentiated from rouleaux by their irregular conformations (grape-like clusters). On automated cell counters, a blood count with a grossly elevated MCV and low erythrocyte count but a normal hemoglobin is suggestive of the presence of cold-reacting erythrocyte agglutinins. The effect of cold agglutinins is overcome by keeping the blood specimen at 37° C. When performing blood counts, the diluting fluid also must be kept at 37° C.

LEUKOCYTE AND PLATELET ABNORMALITIES

Some nutritional deficiencies, stem cell disorders, and bone marrow abnormalities affect the production, func-

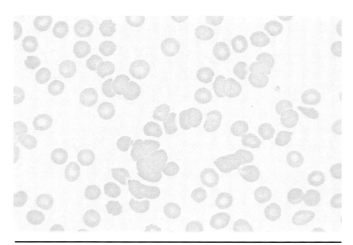

FIGURE 5-17. This blood smear is from a patient with cold agglutinin disease. Notice the clumping of the erythrocytes. (PB; 250× original magnification; Wright-Giemsa stain.)

tion, and/or morphology of all hematopoietic cells; thus, evaluation of the quantity and morphology of platelets and granulocytes may supply additional important data as to the cause of anemia.

BONE MARROW EXAMINATION

Bone marrow examination is important in helping the physician arrive at a definitive diagnosis in anemic patients when other laboratory tests are not conclusive. It also is important in diagnosis and management of therapy for hematopoietic system disorders, especially in malignancy. Bone marrow examination also is of diagnostic utility in any unexplained excess or deficiency of peripheral blood cells, in splenomegaly, fever of unknown origin, in the workup of dysproteinemia or lysosomal storage disease, and in human immunodeficiency virus infection.[14] The marrow is the central location for production of all blood cells. Therefore, much information pertaining to production and maturation of cells can be obtained from a bone marrow aspiration and biopsy. Marrow aspirates provide a good specimen for morphologic evaluation of fat cells, endothelial cells, and hematologic cells, while biopsy specimens are preferred for evaluation of cellularity and marrow achitecture.[15]

Contraindications of bone marrow aspiration or biopsy include hereditary bleeding disorders such as hemophilia. Thrombocytopenia is not considered a contraindication and bone marrow examination is in fact useful in identifying the cause of this disorder.

Obtaining the specimen The bone marrow aspiration/biopsy is performed by a physician. Bone marrow is obtained by needle aspiration and/or biopsy from the posterior iliac crest or sternum in adults and from the tibia or anterior iliac crest in infants. The iliac crest is a safer site to obtain a biopsy specimen than the sternum because there is little risk of soft tissue or organ damage in this area. Furthermore, if the procedure is performed at the iliac crest, it usually causes less apprehension in the patient, to whom this site is not visible. The site for aspira-

tion is identified by palpation before preparing the site for puncture. After cleansing and sterilizing the area, a local anesthetic is injected. A large bore needle is then inserted through the skin and into the bone. When no resistance to the needle is felt, it has reached the marrow. After removal of the stylet, a glass syringe is attached to the needle and the marrow is aspirated. If biopsy material is needed, a biopsy needle cuts away a core of marrow with a twisting action (a Jamshidi needle is most popular). Biopsy specimens are placed directly into fixative solution until processed as a histologic specimen.

Preparation of the specimen The procedure for preparing marrow aspirates for examination is not standardized. Many methods are used, including stained smears, squash preparations (made by placing the specimen between two slides and pulling the slides apart in opposite directions), sections of clotted marrow, buffy coat preparations, and particle concentration smears.[16] Regardless of the method used, it is important that aspirate material contain particulate matter for examination and exhibit a minimum of cellular disruption for accurate differential counts.

The most frequently used bone marrow preparation technique is described here.[17] The laboratory scientist assists the physician at the patient's bedside. After aspirating the sample, the physician hands the syringe to the laboratory scientist. A portion of aspirate from the syringe is immediately transferred to a Petri dish. If a good sample was obtained, spicules and glossy particles of fat should be visible. Direct smears are made by placing a particle and a small amount of blood from the aspirate onto a slide and distributing it with a spreader slide, similar to making a peripheral blood smear. If a small amount of 22.4% polymerized bovine albumin is added to the specimen before making direct smears, cellular disruption is minimal.[15] The remaining clotted blood in the dish is placed into a fixative so that the stained sections of the clot can be used for cytologic study. A third portion of the aspirate is placed into a tube containing the anticoagulant, EDTA. After adequate mixing, a sample of this anticoagulated marrow is placed onto a watch glass. The fluid portion around the particles is removed, placed in a Wintrobe tube, and centrifuged. The centrifuged specimen will have four layers: fat and perivascular layer (1% to 3%); plasma; nucleated myeloid and erythroid cells (5% to 8%), also called the buffy coat layer; and erythrocytes. The volume (in percentages) of each layer is recorded. There are no reference ranges for plasma and erythrocyte layers, as this depends on the amount of dilution of the bone marrow with sinusoidal blood. Buffy coat (concentrate) smears are made from the nucleated cell layer. The marrow particles remaining on the watch glass after the fluid is removed are placed on a slide and gently crushed with another slide or coverslip. A smear is made by pulling the slides in opposite directions parallel to their surfaces (particle smears). Usually the direct smears, the buffy coat smear and the particle smears are stained with Wright's stain.

Microscopic examination of the bone marrow specimen The stained aspirate preparation should be examined under low power magnification (100×) to evaluate overall cellularity and determine the number of megakaryocytes, plasma cells, osteoclasts, osteoblasts, and mast cells. Megakaryocytes are easily identified because of their large size and multinuclearity. Abnormal cellular elements such as tumor cells, lipid-packed macrophages, lymphoma cells, and granulomas also can be detected under low power.[4]

Aspirates are valuable for quantifying hematopoietic precursors and for visualizing details of cellular structure. Under high power (1000×), the orderly process of cellular maturation is evaluated. The proliferation and maturation processes of hematopoietic cells normally result in a quantitative pyramid of cells with blasts at the top and the most mature cells at the bottom (Table F, see Endsheet). A bone marrow differential derived from counting 300 to 500 nucleated hematopoietic cells will reveal possible abnormalities in the pyramid.

The determination of the myeloid to erythroid (M:E) ratio helps define the sizes of the two major cellular components of the marrow (myeloid and erythroid).[16] The ratio is determined by calculating the ratio of the number of granulocytes and their precursors to the number of nucleated erythroid precursors (monocytes and lymphocytes are not included in the M:E ratio). The normal ratio is between 1.5 to 1 and 3.5 to 1, reflecting the predominance of myeloid elements. If one of the two cell systems (myeloid or erythroid) is considered normal, inferences can be made from an abnormality in this ratio. For example, if the erythroid series appears normal in both concentration and morphology, an increased ratio signifies an increase in myeloid production.

Next, the details of nuclear and cytoplasmic development should be examined. Morphologic variations may denote specific abnormalities (e.g., megaloblastic anemia, myelodysplasia).

If bone marrow fragments or spicules are present, cellularity may be evaluated by determining the cell to fat ratio. Cellularity, however, is best determined in biopsied material. It is important for the examiner to know the age of the patient because marrow cellularity (and the resulting differential count) varies greatly among different age groups. A normal adult has about a 1:1 ratio of fat to hematopoietic tissue (indicating a 50% cellularity). A young child has the highest cellularity with about 65% hematopoietic tissue whereas, in the elderly, hematopoietic tissue decreases to about 30%.

Evaluation of iron stores A stain for iron (Prussian blue) is routinely performed on both histologic sections and film preparations of marrow so iron stores may be assessed. The presence of hemosiderin (iron deposits) in macrophages signifies a normal supply of iron, but its distribution in the normoblast may signify abnormalities in its utilization by the cell. Normal iron distribution in the developing normoblast is random or diffuse. Iron deposits concentrated in mitochondria that surround the nucleus (ringed sideroblast) are an important diagnostic feature of an anemia with improper utilization of iron.

Bone marrow biopsy Although needle aspiration is good for preparation of films used in evaluating cellular structure, it disrupts normal marrow structure. Occasionally, aspiration results in a "dry tap" due to fibrosis, aplasia, malignancy, granuloma, or packed cellular marrow. Infrequently, dry taps are due to faulty technique. Another problem with aspirates is that aspirate film preparations often are diluted with peripheral blood, making estimation of hematopoietic cellularity difficult and erroneous. A bone marrow biopsy overcomes these problems. Bone marrow biopsy provides a core of material for evaluation of architecture of the marrow. The core of biopsied marrow is placed on a piece of gauze to absorb excess blood. Several touch preparations are then made by gently touching the core to a slide several times along the slide's surface. Next, the biopsied specimen is placed in a fixative, decalcified, embedded in paraffin or plastic and sectioned in the histology laboratory. These treatments cause the morphology of individual cells to be less distinct than they are in aspirates: however, tumor cells, fibrosis, aplasia, hypoplasia, and hyperplasia are readily discernible by this technique. *Hyperplasia*, an increase in hematopoietic cells, is seen in conditions with a defect in cell survival, in ineffective erythropoiesis, and in neoplasms of the hematopoietic system. *Hypoplasia* is a decrease in hematopoietic cells accompanied by an increase in fat and/or fibrous tissue. Hypoplasia is seen in stem cell disorders, bone marrow tumors, and fibrosis. Stains routinely used on bone marrow aspirate and biopsy sections are noted in Table 5-18.

Ancillary studies Immunohistochemical and immunocytochemical studies using monoclonal antibodies can be done on bone marrow tissue sections embedded in paraffin or on imprints or smears. These studies assist in the identification of cell types and subtypes, by recognition of specific cell antigens.

Flow cytometry may be used to define the ploidy (DNA content) of cells or to provide a cell marker profile. Heparinized bone marrow aspirate material at room temperature is the specimen of choice for flow analysis. When aspirates cannot be obtained due to marrow pathology,

TABLE 5-18 *STAINS OF BONE MARROW ASPIRATES AND BIOPSY SECTION PREPARATIONS*

Stains of Bone Marrow Aspirate and Biopsy Section Preparation

Section Preparations
Hematoxylin & Eosin (H & E)
Prussian blue (iron stain)
Silver stain (reticulin stain)
Immunohistochemical stains

Aspirate Preparations
Wright's stain
Periodic acid-Schiff PAS, (for glycogen or glycoprotein)
Trichrome stain (assess fibrosis and visualize protein globules, Russell bodies)
Fungal and acid-fast bacilli, AFB, (for organisms)
Congo red (for amyloid)
Mucicarmine (for mucin produced by metastatic adenocarcinoma)
Acid or alkaline phosphatase
Immunocytochemical stains

collagenase digestion of the trephine biopsy specimen provides cell suspensions that can be used for immunophenotyping by flow cytometry.[18]

Cytogenetic studies may be performed when malignancy is suspected or diagnosed. These studies may demonstrate chromosomal changes that are characteristic of certain malignant disorders or may be used to help identify disease remission or progression.

Molecular studies may be used to identify DNA alterations not detectable by cytogenetic studies. This includes rearrangement of T- and B-lymphocyte receptor genes and the bcr/abl translocation in Philadelphia chromosome-negative chronic myelocytic leukemia (CML).

TESTS FOR ERYTHROCYTE DESTRUCTION

Tests of erythrocyte destruction are important in evaluating erythrocyte survival. If the hemoglobin concentration is stable over at least several days in an anemic patient, then the measurements of erythrocyte production including marrow cellularity and RPI are indirect measurements of erythrocyte destruction. Serum unconjugated bilirubin is primarily derived from hemoglobin catabolism; its concentration in the absence of hepatobiliary disease may yield further information concerning erythrokinetics. Increased unconjugated bilirubin is indicative of increased hemoglobin catabolism, either intravascular or extravascular. Conversely, chronic and acute blood loss and hypoproliferative anemias result in decreased serum bilirubin since the number of erythrocytes catabolized is decreased. Cytoplasmic maturation abnormalities in the erythrocyte also may be accompanied by decreased serum bilirubin, even though there is an increase in erythrocyte destruction. This is because when insufficient hemoglobin is being synthesized (hypochromic cells), less hemoglobin is being catabolized. Thus, the bilirubin level should always be interpreted together with the degree of anemia. For example, a bilirubin within the normal range should be considered elevated in a patient with a 5 g/dL hemoglobin concentration.

Other laboratory tests are used to evaluate erythrocyte turnover or blood loss. Hemosiderin in urine, decreased haptoglobin, and increased methalbumin are associated with increased intravascular hemolysis. Certain biochemical constituents that are concentrated in blood cells are indicators of the degree of cellular turnover; thus, in anemias associated with ineffective erythropoiesis or hemolysis, these products will be increased in the blood. The most commonly measured constituents of this type include uric acid, the main end product of purine metabolism, and lactate dehydrogenase (LDH), an enzyme that is present in the cell cytoplasm.

The choice of laboratory tests for diagnoses of anemia should depend on the tests' degrees of specificity and sensitivity. A highly sensitive test is one that will likely be positive when the anemia is present. A highly specific test is one that will likely be negative when the anemia is not present. Highly sensitive tests are good for screening for anemia, and highly specific tests are good for confirming the presence of the anemia. Table 5-19 shows a variety of tests used in diagnosing anemia together with their rates of sensitivity and specificity.

CLASSIFICATION OF ANEMIA

The purpose of the classification of anemias is to enable the physician to identify the associated erythrokinetic lesion by using laboratory test results in addition to other clinical data. The classification also is useful to laboratory scientists when correlating various test results for accuracy and when making suggestions for additional follow-up tests.

Although specific diagnosis is the ultimate goal of any anemia classification system, it must be kept in mind that

TABLE 5-19 *OPERATING CHARACTERISTICS OF DISCRIMINATING TESTS USED IN DIAGNOSING ANEMIA*

Test	*Sensitivity (%)*	*Specificity (%)*	*Disease*
RDW > 15	87–100	66	Iron deficiency anemia
Ferritin < 12	65–97	99	Iron deficiency anemia
Transferrin saturation < 16	95	70–95	Iron deficiency anemia
Reticulocyte count	62–90	99(> 10%)	Hemolysis
Coombs' test	90	?95	Autoimmune hemolytic anemia
MCHC > 36	?100	100*	Hereditary spherocytosis
Splenomegaly	100	?	Hereditary spherocytosis
MCV > 105	11	95	Vitamin B_{12} or folic acid deficiency
MCV < 100	100	?40–50	Iron deficiency anemia
MCV < 80	100	?	Thalassemia
Hemosiderin (urine)	100	?	Paroxysmal nocturnal hemoglobinuria

MCHC, mean corpuscular hemoglobin concentration; MCV, mean corpuscular volume; RDW, red cell distribution width.

* Provided that artifacts are excluded.

(From: Djulbegović B., Hadley T., Pašić R.: A new algorithm for diagnosis of anemia. Postgrad. Med. 85(5): 119–130, 1989.)

anemia frequently develops from more than one mechanism, complicating correlation and interpretation of laboratory test results. In addition, complicating factors may alter the typical findings of a specific anemia. For example, pre-existing iron deficiency may inhibit the reticulocytosis that normally accompanies acute blood loss or mask the macrocytic features of folic acid deficiency. In these cases, laboratory test results may depend on which mechanism predominates.

Anemias may be classified by either morphology or pathophysiology (function).

Morphologic classification

Anemias may be initially classified morphologically according to the average size and hemoglobin concentration of the erythrocytes as indicated by the erythrocyte indices. This morphologic classification is helpful because MCV, MCH and MCHC are known at the time anemia is diagnosed, and certain causes of anemia characteristically produce a specific size of erythrocytes (large, small, or normal) and a specific hemoglobin content (normal or abnormal). The general categories of a morphologic classification include macrocytic-normochromic, normocytic-normochromic, and microcytic-hypochromic.

It must again be stressed that, although an anemia may initially seem to belong in one of these categories, the morphologic expression may be the result of a combination of factors. For example, a combined deficiency of iron and folate may result in a normal MCV even though iron deficiency is normally microcytic and folate deficiency is normally macrocytic. These complicated cases usually can be detected by examining the blood smear for specifics of erythrocyte morphology.

A morphologic assessment of anemia, however, is not sufficient; determining the pathophysiology of anemia through additional laboratory tests yields even more meaningful information. In addition, patient history and physical examination are essential to differential diagnosis within given classifications.

Functional classification

Considering that the normal bone marrow compensatory response to decreased peripheral blood hemoglobin levels is an increase in erythrocyte production, persistent anemia may be expected as the result of three pathophysiologic mechanisms: (1) a proliferation defect; (2) a maturation defect; or (3) a survival defect (increased destruction). These are considered to be the three functional classifications of anemia. Functional classification uses the RPI and/or serum iron studies to categorize an anemia. Proliferation and maturation defects usually have an RPI less than 2 while survival defects are characterized by an RPI greater than 2. Serum iron studies are most helpful in identifying the pathophysiology of anemias resulting from maturational defects accompanied by microcytic cells since the RPI is variable in these cases.

Although some anemias may be the result of several mechanisms, one mechanism is usually dominant. The initial step in approaching an anemic patient is the identification of this dominant mechanism. If the functional and morphologic classifications of anemia are combined, the result is a classification using the RPI, iron studies, and morphology of the erythrocyte (Fig. 5-18). If an anemia does not fit into any of these categories, the anemia is probably multifactorial.

PROLIFERATIVE DEFECTS

These defects are characterized by decreased proliferation, maturation, and release rates of erythrocytes in response to anemia. The most characteristic laboratory findings of proliferation defects are normocytic-normochromic erythrocytes and an RPI less than 2, signifying a marrow output of reticulocytes inappropriate to the degree of anemia. Serum bilirubin levels are normal or decreased because of the decrease in cell production. The bone marrow is hypocellular with normal or increased iron stores. Decreased proliferation may be caused by inappropriate erythropoietin production. This tropic basis is responsible for the anemias associated with malignancies, chronic renal disease, and certain endocrinopathies.

Conversely, erythropoietic stimulating mechanisms may be normal, but the bone marrow may fail to respond to the stimulus appropriately. This occurs when the bone marrow is infiltrated with fibrous, neoplastic or granulomatous tissue, or when the marrow is damaged by chemicals, drugs, or radiation. It is possible to differentiate these causes of hypoproliferation by observing if either all three cell lines are affected or only the erythrocytes are involved. If the proliferation defect is due to inappropriate erythropoietin production, decreased proliferation is limited to the erythrocytic cell line. In contrast, marrow damage or infiltration is characterized by hypoplasia of normal hematopoietic cells in the bone marrow, producing *pancytopenia* in the peripheral blood. In addition, marrow infiltration is accompanied by poikilocytosis and a leukoerythroblastic reaction in the peripheral blood presumably caused by damage of the normal sinusoidal barrier.

Most proliferative defects also are associated with decreased erythrocyte lifespan; however, survival is only moderately decreased and could easily be compensated for by a normal marrow or a normal stimulus. Rarely is hypoproliferation caused by an abnormality in the hematopoietic stem cells.

MATURATION DEFECTS

These defects disrupt the orderly process of either nuclear or cytoplasmic development producing qualitatively abnormal cells. The erythrocytes are macrocytic in nuclear defects and microcytic in cytoplasmic defects. Despite the abnormal maturation process, the marrow increases production of erythrocytes, resulting in bone marrow erythroid hyperplasia. Through unknown mechanisms, the marrow recognizes the cells as being intrinsically abnormal and destroys most of them before they can be released to the peripheral blood (ineffective erythropoiesis). Since many of the abnormal erythrocytes are not released to the peripheral blood, the RPI is usually less than 2. Poikilo-

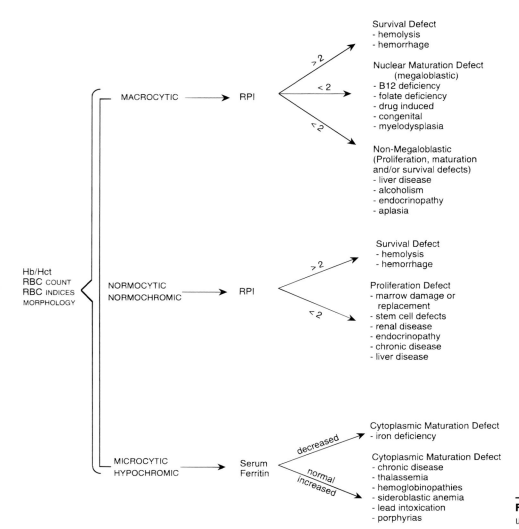

FIGURE 5-18. Classification of anemias using erythrocyte indices and iron studies.

cytes, indicative of abnormal erythropoiesis, are frequently present in direct proportion to the severity of the anemia.

Cytoplasmic maturation defects are caused by abnormal hemoglobin production. Therefore, the defect is limited to the erythroid cell line. Hemoglobin production may be impaired because of one or more of the following: limited iron supply; defective iron utilization; decreased globin synthesis; and defective porphyrin synthesis. Most erythrocytes of cytoplasmic maturation defects are microcytic and hypochromic with a variable degree of poikilocytosis. These anemias are best differentiated using the result of iron studies.

Since all developing hematopoietic cells have nuclei, nuclear maturation defects affect all hematopoietic cell lines and probably other body cells as well. As a result, the peripheral blood reflects not only anemia but also pancytopenia with characteristic morphologic changes apparent in all cell lines. The distinctive morphologic changes in cell lines are collectively termed *megaloblastic*.

The cytologic clues of megaloblastosis in the erythroid cell line include (1) large erythroblasts with large nuclei

and loose chromatin; (2) nuclear/cytoplasmic asynchrony with hemoglobin production progressing normally but nuclear maturation lagging; and (3) macrocytic erythrocytes with a normal hemoglobin concentration. Granulocytes also exhibit distinct morphologic changes such as large size and nuclear hypersegmentation. Platelets show marked variation in size.

SURVIVAL DEFECTS

These defects are the result of premature loss of circulating erythrocytes either by hemorrhage or hemolysis. In this type of defect, bone marrow proliferation increases, and maturation is orderly. This is the only functional defect in which the RPI is typically greater than 2. The blood film reflects this increased erythropoietic activity by the presence of polychromatophilic macrocytes ("shift" reticulocytes).

In contrast to poikilocytes that are formed in the bone marrow as a result of dyserythropoiesis typical of proliferation and maturation defects, poikilocytes (schistocytes and spherocytes) of a survival defect are formed after the cell leaves the marrow. The schistocyte is the result of mechanical trauma to the cell such as shearing by fibrin strands or damage by passage through abnormal capillaries. Spherocytes indicate extravascular erythrocyte membrane damage. Generally, the erythrocyte population is normocytic and normochromic. It is possible, however, that macrocytosis may prevail, depending on the degree of reticulocytosis, or that microcytosis may predominate, depending on the number of schistocytes or microspherocytes.

Other indications of decreased erythrocyte survival may include increased serum bilirubin, decreased haptoglobin, increased methalbumin, hemosiderinuria, hemoglobinuria, hemoglobinemia, increased exhaled CO, and increased urine or fecal urobilinogen.

A knowledge of the functional and morphologic classification of anemias is necessary to design a cost-effective laboratory testing approach that aids in specific diagnosis. Only appropriate tests that help identify the cause of anemia should be performed in the laboratory work-up. Figure 5-19 shows general schemas of laboratory testing that are useful in diagnosing anemias. It should be remembered that the patient's clinical history and physical examination are always performed by the physician before beginning a laboratory work-up. The information gained in these areas may eliminate the need for some tests and/or suggest additional tests. These schemas will gain more meaning as the student reads the following chapters on each group of anemias.

Classification using the red cell distribution width

It has been suggested that the classification of anemias use the terms heterogeneous (increased RDW) and homogeneous (decreased RDW) in conjunction with the descriptive morphologic terms microcytic, normocytic, and macro-

cytic (e.g., homogeneous macrocytic, heterogeneous macrocytic[22]) (Table 5-20).

A study of anemic individuals provided the following information regarding the relation between categories of anemia and RDW.[19]

1. Hypoproliferative anemias have a normal RDW regardless of the MCV.
2. Maturational defect anemias have an increased RDW regardless of the MCV or the degree of anemia. The RDW is increased in these individuals before anemia develops or before abnormal cells can be identified on the smear.
3. The RDW is normal after acute hemorrhage if iron supplies are adequate.
4. Uncompensated hemolytic anemias have a high RDW while compensated hemolytic states have a normal RDW.

SUMMARY

Anemia is a decrease in the competence of blood to carry oxygen to the tissues due to a decrease in the concentration of hemoglobin. Diagnosis of anemia is made through a combination of information from the patient history, physical examination, and laboratory investigation. Initially, routine laboratory tests are performed to determine the presence of anemia and to evaluate erythrocyte production and destruction. These tests include hemoglobin, hematocrit, erythrocyte count, reticulocyte count, blood smear examination, erythrocyte indices, and serum bilirubin. More specific tests may be performed based on the results of these routine tests.

The erythrocyte indices may be used to determine the size and hemoglobin content of erythrocytes. Because some anemias are characterized by specific erythrocyte morphology, the indices are helpful in intially classifying the anemia.

The reticulocyte count is routinely reported in relative terms: the number of reticulocytes per erythrocytes in percent. More information is available by calculation of the absolute count, corrected reticulocyte count (corrected for degree of anemia), and reticulocyte production index (corrected for degree of anemia and for early release of reticulocytes from the bone marrow). Generally, in an anemic patient, the reticulocyte count should be increased if the bone marrow is responding by increasing production of cells.

Examination of the blood film is helpful in assessing anisocytosis and poikilocytosis. Anisocytosis is a variation in erythrocyte size. It also is calculated and expressed as the red cell distribution width (RDW) on some automated cell counters. Macrocytes are erythrocytes with a volume greater than 100 fL while microcytes have a cell volume less than 80 fL. It is not uncommon to find a variety of cell sizes in some anemias. Poikilocytosis is a variation in cell shape. Specific shapes give clues to the cause of anemia. For example, drepanocytes are typically found in sickle cell anemia, while dacryocytes are observed in myelofibrosis with myeloid metaplasia.

TABLE 5-20   *CLASSIFICATION OF ANEMIAS BY MCV AND RDW*

	Normal RDW	Increased RDW
Normocytic	Acute hemorrhage Splenic pooling Chronic disease Chronic leukemia Chronic liver disease	Immune hemolytic anemia Early iron, B$_{12}$ or folate deficiency Sideroblastic anemia Myelofibrosis
Microcytic	Heterozygous thalassemia Chronic disease	Iron deficiency Homozygous thalassemia HgB S/B^{thal} HgB H disease Hemolytic anemia with schistocytes
Macrocytic	Myelodysplastic syndromes Aplastic anemia	Immune hemolytic anemia with marked reticulocytosis B$_{12}$ or folate deficiency CLL with high lymph count

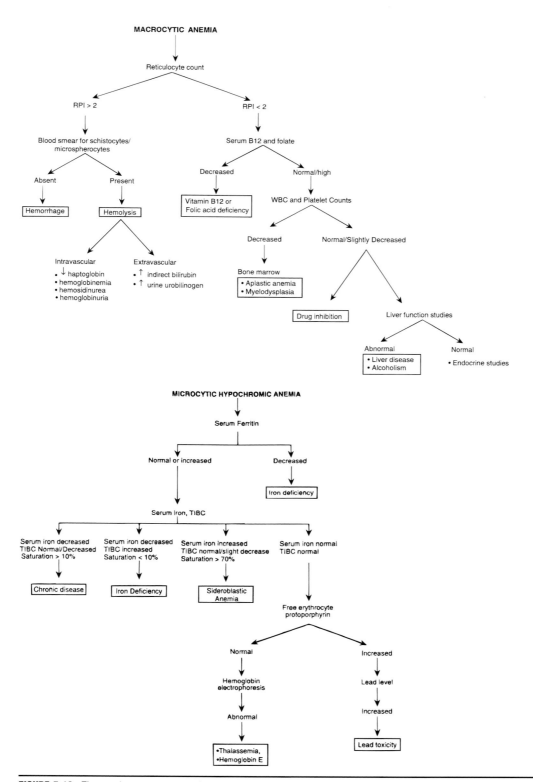

FIGURE 5-19. These schema are a general guide to the laboratory work-up of anemia. The red cell indices and the appearance of the cells on a stained blood smear will give the first important clue to morphologic classification. The results of the next tests in the schema, the RPI and iron studies, will give clues to the pathophysiologic mechanisms involved. Note that most causes of anemia can be determined without performing a bone marrow examination. This procedure is usually reserved for those anemias that appear to be caused by a stem cell defect, marrow damage, or marrow replacement.

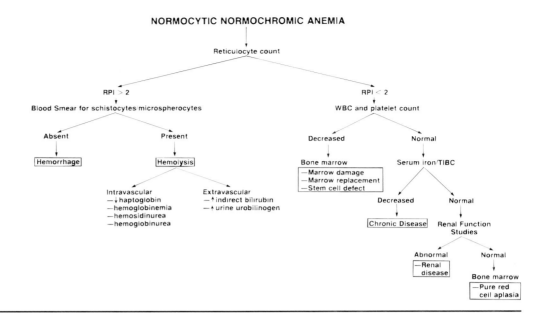

FIGURE 5-19. *(continued)*

Erythrocyte inclusions, when present, also are helpful in determining the cause of anemia. Pappenheimer bodies indicate faulty iron metabolism, and Howell-Jolly bodies are found in megaloblastic anemia, after splenectomy, and in some hemolytic anemias.

Bone marrow examination is indicated if laboratory tests give inconclusive results. Bone marrow is examined for cellularity, cellular structure, M:E ratio, and iron stores. Bone marrow aspirates are best for examining details of cellular structure, while biopsy material is superior for evaluating marrow structure and for identifying the presence of tumor cells.

Anemias are generally classified by a functional or morphologic scheme or by a combination of the two. The morphologic classification includes three general categories based on erythrocyte indices: normocytic-normochromic, macrocytic-normochromic, and microcytic-hypochromic. The functional classification uses the reticulocyte production index (RPI) and serum iron studies to classify the anemias according to pathophysiology: proliferation defect, maturation defect, and survival defect. These classifications help the scientist and physician design a cost-effective approach to reach a specific diagnosis.

REVIEW QUESTIONS

A patient has the following results: erythrocyte count, 2.5 $\times 10^{12}$/L; hemoglobin, 5.3 g/dL; hematocrit, 0.17 L/L; reticulocyte count, 1%. Use this information to answer the questions below.

1. Calculate the absolute reticulocyte count and the RPI, and choose the correct answer:
   a. Absolute count, 25 $\times 10^9$/L; RPI, 0.15
   b. Absolute count, 250 $\times 10^9$/L; RPI, 0.15
   c. Absolute count, 170 $\times 10^9$/L; RPI, 0.38
   d. Absolute count, 100 $\times 10^9$/L; RPI, 1.5

2. What are the erythrocyte indices in the above patient?

	MCV	MCH	MCHC
a.	47	28	31
b.	80	21	41
c.	68	21	31
d.	80	28	41

3. How would you classify the above cell population morphologically?
   a. normocytic, normochromic
   b. macrocytic, normochromic
   c. microcytic, normochromic
   d. microcytic, hypochromic

4. If the above cell population was homogeneous (absence of anisocytosis), what may the RDW show?
   a. false increase
   b. false decrease
   c. normal range
   d. true increase

5. Given the schema shown in Figure 5-19, what laboratory test is probably the most important to follow up on the cause of this anemia?
   a. reticulocyte count
   b. serum iron
   c. WBC and platelet count
   d. serum ferritin

6. Why may the serum bilirubin results be misleading as an indicator of erythrocyte destruction in this patient?
   a. The cells are not being destroyed at an increased rate and the liver is not excreting the bilirubin due to liver failure.

b. The cells are being produced in the bone marrow and released as fast as they are being destroyed so the bilirubin will be normal.

c. The cells may be destroyed at an increased rate but the hypochromic cells do not release much hemoglobin and hence, less bilirubin is formed.

d. The cells are not destroyed as fast in anemic individuals as in normal individuals and the bilirubin will be falsely decreased.

7. A peripheral blood smear that has a mixture of macrocytes, microcytes and normal erythrocytes present can best be described by which term?
   a. poikilocytosis
   b. polychromatophilia
   c. megaloblastosis
   d. anisocytosis

8. Which of the following erythrocyte inclusions cannot be stained and visualized with Romanowsky stains?
   a. Pappenheimer bodies
   b. Howell-Jolly bodies
   c. Heinz bodies
   d. Basophilic stippling

9. Which of the following laboratory tests is most specific for vitamins B12 or folic acid deficiency?
   a. low ferritin
   b. high RDW
   c. Coomb's test
   d. MCV >105

10. In an anemia caused by hemorrhage or hemolysis what would you expect to find in your laboratory investigation?
   a. presence of polychromatophilic macrocytes on the peripheral blood smear
   b. A hypoplastic bone marrow
   c. Megaloblastosis in the bone marrow and pancytopenia in the peripheral blood
   d. An RPI less than 2

REFERENCES

1. Wintrobe, M.M., Lukens, J.N., Lee, G.R.: The approach to the patient with anemia. In Wintrobe's Clinical Hematology. Edited by G.R. Lee, T.C. Bithell, J. Foerster, J.W. Athens, J.N. Lukens. Philadelphia: Lea & Febiger, 1993.
2. Crosby, W.H.: Reticulocyte counts. Arch. Intern. Med., 141:1747, 1981.
3. Center for Disease Control. CDC criteria for anemia in children and childbearing-aged women. MMWR, 38:400, 1989.
4. Williams, W.J., Beutler, E., Erslev, A.J., Lichtman, M.A.: Hematology. 4th Ed. New York: McGraw-Hill, 1990.
5. Woodson, R.D., Auebach, S.: Effect of increased oxygen affinity and anemia on cardiac output and its distribution. J. Appl. Physiol., 53:1299, 1982.
6. Scott, R.B.: Common blood disorders: A primary care approach. Geriatrics, 48:72, 1993.
7. Nordenberg, D., Yip, R., Binkin, N.J.: The effect of cigarette smoking on hemoglobin levels and anemia screening. JAMA, 264:1556, 1990.
8. Weihang, B., Dalferes, E.R., Srinivasan, A.R., Webber, L.S., Berensen, G.S.: Normative distribution of complete blood count from early childhood through adolescence: The Bogalusa Heart Study. Prev. Med. 22:825, 1993.
9. Brown, R.G.: Determining the cause of anemia. Postgrad. Med., 89:161, 1991.
10. Kosower, N.S.: Altered properties of erythrocytes in the aged. Am. J. Hematol;. 42:241, 1993.
11. Friedman, E.W.: Reticulocyte counts: How to use them, what they mean. Diagn. Med., 7(6):29, 1984.
12. Christensen, D.J.: Diagnosis of anemia. Postgrad. Med., 73:293, 1983.
13. O'Connor, B.H.: A Color Atlas and Instruction Manual of Peripheral Blood Cell Morphology. Baltimore, Williams & Wilkins, 1984.
14. Hyun, BH, Stevenson A.J., Hanau, C.A.: Fundamentals of bone marrow examination. Hem. Onc. Clin. North Am. 8(4):651, 1994.
15. Paulsen, K.: Bone marrow sampling and processing. Clin. Lab. Sci., 6:159, 1993.
16. Trubowitz, S., Davis, S. (eds.): The Human Bone Marrow: Anatomy, Physiology and Pathophysiology. Vol. II. Boca Raton: CRC Press, 1982.
17. Brown, B.A.: Hematology: Principles and Procedures. 6th Ed. Philadelphia: Lea & Febiger, 1993.
18. Maung, Z.T., Bown, N.P., Hamilton, P.J.: Collagenase digestion of bone marrow trephine biopsy specimens: an important adjunct to hematological diagnosis when marrow aspiration fails. J. Clin. Pathol. 46(6):576, 1993.
19. Bessman, J.D., Gilmer, P.R., Gardner, F.H.: Improved classification of anemias by MCV and RDW. Am. J. Clin. Pathol., 80:332, 1983.

Anemia of defective heme synthesis

6

KEY TERMS

Sideropenic
Sideroachrestic
Transferrin
Ferritin
Apoferritin
Hemosiderin
Ropheocytosis
Chlorosis
Pica
Hemosiderosis
Refractory Anemia with
  Ringed Sideroblasts
  (RARS)
Plumbism

TABLE 6-1 *CAUSES OF DEFECTIVE HEMOGLOBIN PRODUCTION THAT MAY RESULT IN A MICROCYTIC HYPOCHROMIC ANEMIA*

1. Defects in heme synthesis
   a) faulty iron metabolism
      —Iron deficiency
      —Defective iron utilization
   b) defective porphyrin metabolism
2. Defects in globin synthesis (thalassemias): deletion or mutation affecting globin genes

INTRODUCTION

Defective hemoglobin production may be due to disturbances in either heme or globin synthesis (Table 6-1). The result of this cytoplasmic maturation defect is microcytic, hypochromic anemia. Defective heme synthesis may be caused by faulty iron metabolism (lack of iron, defective iron utilization) or defective porphyrin metabolism (Fig. 6-1). Defective globin synthesis is caused by a deletion or defect of globin genes. These globin deletions and defects are the result of a hereditary condition known as thalassemia. Thalassemias will be discussed in Chapter 7.

The anemias discussed in this chapter are those defects in heme synthesis caused by faulty iron metabolism: *sideropenic* anemia and *sideroachrestic* anemia. Sideropenic anemia is characterized by a deficiency of iron for heme

synthesis due to limited dietary intake of iron, malabsorption of iron, or increased iron loss. Sideropenic anemia is referred to as iron deficiency anemia. Sideroachrestic anemias are characterized by adequate or excess stores of iron but there is a block in the insertion of iron into the protoporphyrin ring to form heme. This block may be the result of an acquired or inherited defect in porphyrin synthesis (sideroblastic anemia) or by defective reuse of iron from the macrophage (anemia of chronic disease).

For convenience, the erythropoietic porphyrias, congenital defects in porphyrin metabolism, also are included in this chapter. Except for erythropoietic porphyria type, the porphyrias, generally are not characterized by the presence of anemia.

IRON METABOLISM

Iron is required by every cell in the body. It has vital roles in oxidative metabolism, cellular growth and proliferation, and oxygen transport and storage.[1] To serve in these functions, iron must be bound to protein compounds. Iron in inorganic compounds or in ionized forms is potentially dangerous. If the amount of iron in the body exceeds the capacity for safe transport and storage in the protein bound form, iron toxicity may develop, causing damage to cells. Conversely, if too little iron is available, the synthesis of physiologically active iron compounds is limited, and critical metabolic processes are inhibited.

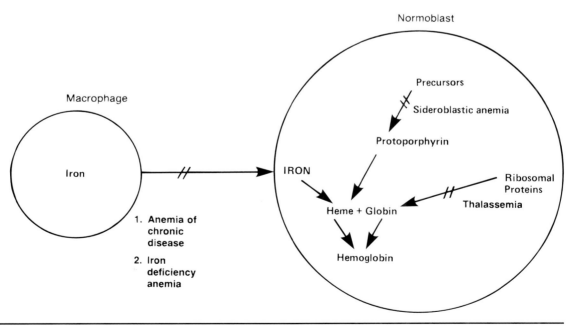

FIGURE 6-1. Sites of defective synthesis of hemoglobin resulting in microcytic, hypochromic anemia. In anemia of chronic disease, a block in release of iron from the macrophage prevents use of iron for hemoglobin synthesis by the developing normoblast. In iron deficiency anemia, an absence of iron in the macrophage means there is a lack of iron delivered to the developing normoblast. In sideroblastic anemia a block in porphyrin synthesis causes iron to build up in the mitochondria of the normoblast. Thalassemia is characterized by defective synthesis of globin chains, but heme synthesis is normal. (// = block or defect at this point of the hemoglobin synthesis pathway.)

Distribution

Iron-containing compounds in the body are one of two types: (1) compounds that serve in metabolic or enzymatic functions; and (2) compounds that serve as storage forms for iron.[1,2] The first category of compounds includes hemoglobin, myoglobin, cytochromes, and other proteins that serve in the transport and utilization of oxygen. These compounds account for 25 to 55 mg iron/kg body weight, 90% to 95% of which is in hemoglobin. The second type of compounds include ferritin and hemosiderin. These storage compounds account for 5 to 25 mg of iron/kg body weight. Thus, the total iron concentration in the body is approximately 2 to 4 gm (Table 6-2).

Hemoglobin constitutes the major fraction of body iron, with a concentration of 1 gm iron/kg of erythrocytes or 0.5 mg iron/mL blood. After iron is incorporated into hemoglobin, it remains there until the erythrocyte is removed from circulation and the hemoglobin is degraded in the macrophages of the spleen and liver. Approximately 85% of the iron derived from hemoglobin catabolism is promptly recycled to the plasma, where it is bound to the transport protein, *transferrin,* and delivered to the erythroid marrow for heme synthesis. This iron recycling provides most of the marrow's daily requirement for erythropoiesis.

Ferritin, the major storage form of iron, is predominately found in the bone marrow, spleen, and liver. Ferritin is composed of ferric hydroxide miscelles surrounded by a protein shell and is 17% to 33% iron by weight. The protein shell without the ferric hydroxide miscelles is called *apoferritin.* Ferritin is a water-soluble form of iron that cannot be visualized by microscopy and does not stain with iron stains. Its synthesis is directly proportional to the total amount of iron stores. It functions in recycling iron for hematopoiesis and is a readily available form of iron.

Hemosiderin is a water-insoluble, heterogeneous iron-protein aggregate containing up to 50% of its weight in iron. It is readily visualized in unstained tissue specimens as irregular, golden brown granules, and it stains blue with Prussian blue iron stain. It is a long-term storage form of iron that is not readily mobilized. Hemosiderin appears to be derived from ferritin.

The ratio of ferritin to hemosiderin varies with the total body iron concentration. At lower iron concentrations, the ferritin form predominates, whereas at higher concentrations the majority of storage iron exists as hemosiderin.

Absorption

The amount of iron absorbed is dependent on: (1) the condition of mucosal cells in the GI tract; (2) intraluminal factors; (3) dietary iron intake; (4) tissue iron stores; and (5) hematopoietic activity of bone marrow (Table 6-3).

The major regulation of body iron equilibrium is accomplished through absorption in the mucosal cells of the duodenum. Absorption decreases progressively as iron passes further down the gastrointestinal (GI) tract. Dietary iron must be exposed to the intestinal absorptive surface at sufficient intervals to permit adequate absorption by mucosal cells; thus, increased motility of nutrients through the gastrointestinal tract or decreased absorptive surface area may result in decreased iron absorption.

Absorption depends not only on the amount of iron present in the diet but also on the form of iron ingested and the food mixture eaten. Thus, the quantity of iron absorbed cannot be predicted from the amount of iron ingested. Dietary iron exists in two forms: non-heme iron present in vegetables and whole grains, and heme iron present primarily in red meats in the form of hemoglobin. The ferric complexes of non-heme iron are not easily absorbed. During digestion, ferric complexes are broken down, iron is reduced to the ferrous form, and bound to high molecular weight chelators. Chelators, including gastric HCl, dietary lactic acid, and ascorbic acid, help stabilize iron in the soluble, more easily absorbed ferrous form. Certain sugars, amino acids, and amines also aid in absorption by preventing the precipitation and polymerization of iron complexes. In contrast, other agents found in the diet such as carbonates, oxalates, phosphates, phytates, and tannates combine with iron to form insoluble complexes that cannot be absorbed. Thus, although non-

TABLE 6-2 *APPROXIMATE COMPOSITION AND DISTRIBUTION OF THE IRON-CONTAINING COMPOUNDS IN ADULTS*

Compound	Total Amount (g)	Iron Content Male (g)	Iron Content Female (g)	Percent of Total Iron
Heme compounds:				
Hemoglobin	800	2.4	1.7	65–80
Myoglobin (muscle hemoglobin)	40	0.14	0.12	3.5
Heme enzymes and cytochromes	5.8	0.01	0.01	0.5
Nonheme compounds:				
Transferrin	7.5	0.003	0.003	0.1
Iron-sulfur proteins	—	—	—	—
Ferritin	3.0	0.7–1.5	0.7–1.5	—
Hemosiderin	—	—	—	—
Total storage iron	—	1.0–1.5	1.2–1.5	30
Total Iron		4.0	2.0	100

TABLE 6-3 *FACTORS AFFECTING IRON ABSORPTION IN THE GI TRACT*

1. Condition of mucosal cells in the GI tract
2. Intraluminal factors: parasites, toxins, intestinal motility
3. Dietary iron intake: amount and forms ingested
4. Tissue iron stores: amount of storage iron is inversely related to the amount absorbed
5. Hematopoietic activity of bone marrow: rate of activity is directly related to the amount absorbed

heme iron represents the majority of dietary iron, only 2% of this form is actually absorbed in the duodenum.

Heme iron is more readily absorbed than non-heme iron. The presence of other agents in the intestinal lumen, such as phosphates and ascorbic acid, do not affect the absorption of this form of iron. Heme is split from the globin portion of hemoglobin in the lumen of the intestine. Heme is then assimilated directly by the mucosal cells. Once inside the mucosal cell, iron is believed to be released from heme by heme oxygenase. The iron then appears to enter the same iron pool as non-heme iron.

There appears to be a predetermined setpoint of iron stores, which results in a negative correlation between the amount of iron absorbed and iron stores.[2] The efficiency of intestinal absorption of iron increases in response to accelerated erythropoietic activity and depletion of body iron stores. For instance, bleeding, hypoxia, or hemolysis results in accelerated erythrocyte production and enhanced iron absorption. Increased iron uptake in hemolytic anemias that result from extravascular hemolysis may lead to an excess of iron in various organs because the body does not actually lose the iron released from erythrocytes hemolyzed in vivo. Rather, the iron is recycled to the marrow for erythropoiesis or it enters the storage iron pool. Conversely, diminished erythropoiesis, such as occurs in starvation, decreases the absorption of iron.

Iron deficiency anemia due to a lack of dietary iron is usually treated with daily oral doses of ferrous salts. The efficiency of absorption of this therapeutic iron is greatest during initial treatment, when body stores are depleted. Increased absorption occurs up to 6 months after hemoglobin values return to normal or until iron stores are replenished. Absorption of dietary iron also is increased from 10% to 20% in early stages of developing iron deficiency.

● Transport

TRANSFERRIN

Once in the mucosal cell, iron may combine with apoferritin to form ferritin, or it may cross into the plasma and bind in the ferric form to the carrier protein, transferrin (Fig. 6-2). Transferrin is a true plasma transport protein that mediates iron exchange between tissues. It is not lost in delivering iron to the cells but returns to the plasma and is reused.

Transferrin, a B_1-globulin, is a single polypeptide chain with a molecular mass of 79,570 Daltons and a half-life of about 8 days. It is synthesized in the liver. It is composed of two homologous lobes, each of which is further divided into two dissimilar domains. Each lobe contains a single iron-binding site located in a cleft between the two do-

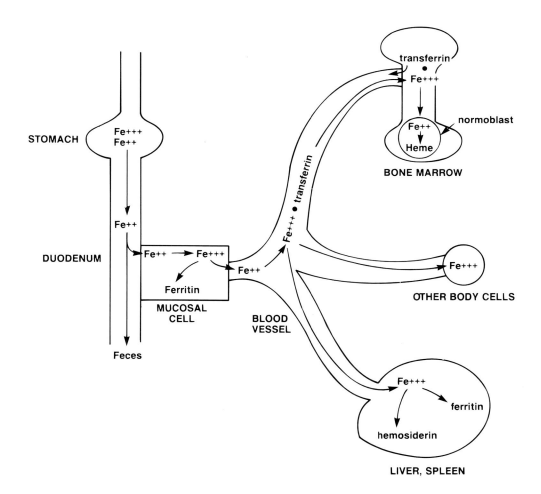

FIGURE 6-2. The transport of iron absorbed from food complexes.

mains. The binding of a ferric iron to either site is random. If only one transferrin lobe binds an iron molecule, it is termed monoferric transferrin, whereas if both sites are occupied it is diferric transferrin.

Each gram of transferrin can bind 1.25 μg of iron. Enough transferrin is present in plasma to bind 253 to 435 μg of iron per deciliter of plasma. This is referred to as the total iron binding capacity (TIBC). Serum iron concentration is about 70 to 201 μg/dL and almost all (95%) of this iron is complexed with transferrin; thus, transferrin is about one third saturated with iron (serum iron/TIBC $\times$ 100 = % saturation of transferrin). The reserve iron-binding capacity of transferrin is referred to as the serum unsaturated iron binding capacity (UIBC).

Laboratory screening to determine iron status includes measurement of serum iron and frequently calculation of percent saturation of transferrin. Transferrin may be measured directly and the transferrin saturation calculated as: serum iron/transferrin $\times$ 2/100.[3] Transferrin also may be functionally measured as the maximum amount of iron able to be bound in the serum (TIBC). An excess of ammonium ferric citrate is added to serum to saturate the transferrin iron binding sites. The unbound iron is removed and the iron content of the serum is determined. This is the TIBC. The measured serum iron and TIBC are usually used to calculate the percent saturation: serum Fe/TIBC $\times$ 100 = % saturation.

As a general rule, changes in the quantity of total body storage iron are accompanied by fluctuations in the serum iron and transferrin (TIBC). As storage iron increases, serum iron increases, TIBC decreases and transferrin saturation increases; conversely, if storage iron is decreased or absent, serum iron decreases, TIBC increases and transferrin saturation decreases (Fig. 6-3). A transferrin saturation below 15% is an indicator of iron deficiency, while saturation over 55% is diagnostic for iron overload or hemochromatosis.

Transferrin appears to be equally distributed between the plasma and extravascular space. Through circulation in the interstitial space, it exchanges iron with all cells of the body. The majority of transferrin-bound iron is delivered to the developing bone marrow normoblasts, where the iron is released for use in heme synthesis. Iron in excess of requirements for hemoglobin synthesis is deposited in tissue for storage. Some transferrin-bound iron is derived from iron absorbed by mucosal cells; however, most of the iron bound to this protein is derived from the monocyte–macrophage system. The major flow of iron in the body is therefore unidirectional, passing from transferrin to erythroid marrow; then to erythrocytes; and finally to macrophages when the senescent erythrocyte is removed and degraded by liver, bone marrow, and splenic macrophages. Released iron from hemoglobin catabolism in the monocyte–macrophage system enters the plasma and is again bound to transferrin for transfer to the marrow (Fig. 6-4). In patients with congenital deficiencies of transferrin, iron accumulates in the liver and spleen, but little iron is present in the developing normoblasts. These findings emphasize the importance of transferrin to iron transport.

TRANSFERRIN RECEPTOR

Transferrin releases iron at specific receptor sites on the developing cell, referred to as the transferrin receptor. Transferrin receptors are expressed on virtually all cells, but the number per cell is a function of cellular iron re-

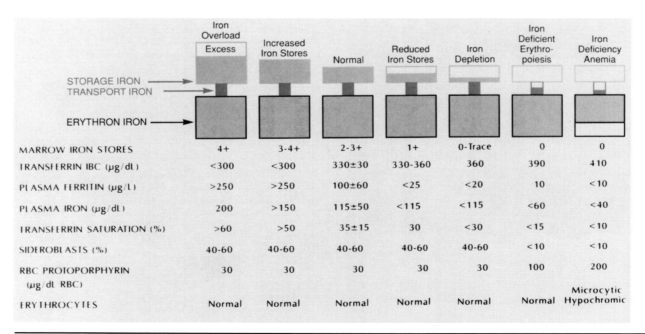

	Iron Overload Excess	Increased Iron Stores	Normal	Reduced Iron Stores	Iron Depletion	Iron Deficient Erythro- poiesis	Iron Deficiency Anemia
MARROW IRON STORES	4+	3-4+	2-3+	1+	0-Trace	0	0
TRANSFERRIN IBC (µg/dL)	<300	<300	330±30	330-360	360	390	410
PLASMA FERRITIN (µg/L)	>250	>250	100±60	<25	<20	10	<10
PLASMA IRON (µg/dL)	200	>150	115±50	<115	<115	<60	<40
TRANSFERRIN SATURATION (%)	>60	>50	35±15	30	<30	<15	<10
SIDEROBLASTS (%)	40-60	40-60	40-60	40-60	40-60	<10	<10
RBC PROTOPORPHYRIN (µg/dl RBC)	30	30	30	30	30	100	200
ERYTHROCYTES	Normal	Normal	Normal	Normal	Normal	Normal	Microcytic Hypochromic

FIGURE 6-3. The distribution and stores of iron as body iron content changes from increased iron content to decreased iron content. The boxes show how storage iron, transport iron and erythron (erythrocyte) iron changes with a continuum of changes in iron stores. Note that the erythrocytes do not exhibit morphologic changes until iron stores are depleted. (With permission from: Herbert, V. Anemias. In Paige, O.M. (ed). Clinical Nutrition. Philadelphia: Mosby, 1988.)

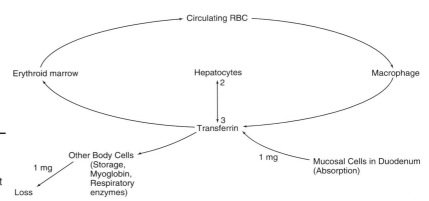

FIGURE 6-4. The daily iron cycle. Most iron is recycled from the erythrocytes to the bone marrow. Only a small amount of iron is lost from the body through loss of iron containing cells. To maintain iron balance, a similar amount of iron is absorbed from the duodenum.

quirements. The synthesis of the receptor is controlled via an iron-dependent negative feedback in cells.[4] Those cells with high iron requirements have high numbers of transferrin receptors. Cells with high iron requirements include erythroid precursors, the cells of the placenta, and cells of the liver.

The transferrin receptor is a transmembrane glycoprotein dimer with two identical subunits, each of which can bind a molecule of transferrin. Thus, if each subunit of the receptor binds a diferric transferrin molecule, the receptor carries four atoms of iron. The affinity of the transferrin receptor for diferric transferrin is greatest at a physiologic pH of 7.4. At a lower pH of 5, there is no difference in affinity of the receptor for apotransferrin or diferric transferrin. When transferrin has a normal saturation of iron (about 33%) and the rate of erythropoiesis is normal, most of the iron delivered to the normoblasts is in the diferric form. At about 19% transferrin saturation, equal amounts of monoferric and diferric transferrin are bound to the receptor, and at lower saturations most receptor-bound iron is in the monoferric form.[1]

Iron enters the cell in an energy- and temperature-dependent process called *ropheocytosis*. After binding of transferrin to the receptor, the transferrin-receptor complex rapidly clusters with other transferrin-receptor complexes on the cell membrane and the membrane invaginates, forming a pit with the complex inside (Fig. 6-5). The invagination seals over to form an internal endosome. In the interior of the cell, the endosome fuses with an acidic vesicle, placing the complex in an environment with a pH below 5.5. At this stage, iron is released from transferrin and made available for cellular use. The acidified environment in the endosome decreases the affinity between iron and transferrin while it increases the affinity of transferrin for the transferrin receptor. The endosome is transported back to the surface of the cell, where the neutral pH of the plasma causes a decrease in the affinity of transferrin for the receptor. Consequently, the transferrin is released to the plasma, making both it and the receptor available for recycling.

● Storage

The largest non-heme iron stores in the body are hemosiderin and ferritin. Storage iron provides a readily available iron supply in the event of increased iron loss through bleeding. Depletion of these storage compounds reflect an excess iron loss over that which is absorbed. The direction of iron flow in the hepatocytes, the main iron storage depot, depends on the plasma iron concentration. With iron depletion, plasma iron falls, and the hepatocyte releases more of its storage iron to transferrin. Conversely, an increase in plasma iron results in an increase of iron delivered to the hepatocyte for storage.

Apoferritin is a spherical protein shell consisting of 24 subunits that surround a ferric oxyhydroxide crystalline core. Each apoferritin molecule can store up to 4500 iron atoms within its shell. When the apoferritin carries iron in its core, it is known as ferritin. Ferritin acts as the primary storage compound for the body's iron needs and can readily release its store of iron if plasma iron levels decrease. It is also an important antioxidant that protects cells against ferrous iron-catalyzed oxidative damage.

Isoferritins exist that are composed of two primary subunits, heart (H) and liver (L) in different proportions. Isoferritins in the erythrocytes are rich in the H subunit while isoferritins in the liver are rich in the L subunits.

Ferritin is primarily an intracellular protein, but small amounts enter the blood through active secretion or cell lysis. Serum ferritin derived from liver and spleen is rich in the L subunit. The amount of circulating ferritin parallels the concentration of storage iron in the body. Therefore, laboratory tests for serum ferritin are a reliable index of iron stores; 1 ng/mL of serum ferritin indicates about 8 mg of storage iron. Serum ferritin does not exhibit diurnal variations associated with serum iron levels. Decreased serum ferritin levels may be the first indication of developing iron deficiency anemia. Ferritin levels become abnormal before the exhaustion of mobilizable iron stores, whereas abnormalities in the TIBC and serum iron may become detectable only when iron stores are depleted. Generally, ferritin levels less than 12 μg/L indicate depletion of iron stores while levels greater than 1000 μg/L indicate iron overload.[5] Care should be used in interpreting serum ferritin levels, however, since nonspecific increases may be seen in malignancy, chronic infections, and liver disease, as well as in chronic inflammatory disorders, even though storage iron is normal or decreased. Thus, concomitant iron deficiency can be masked in these conditions if other tests of iron status are not considered. Table

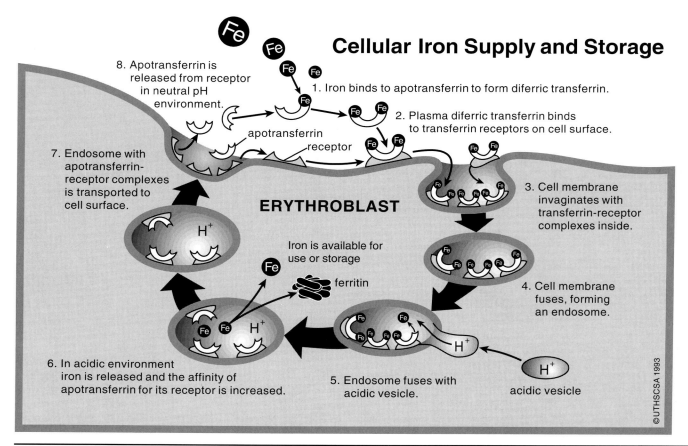

Cellular Iron Supply and Storage

8. Apotransferrin is released from receptor in neutral pH environment.

1. Iron binds to apotransferrin to form diferric transferrin.

apotransferrin receptor

2. Plasma diferric transferrin binds to transferrin receptors on cell surface.

7. Endosome with apotransferrin-receptor complexes is transported to cell surface.

ERYTHROBLAST

3. Cell membrane invaginates with transferrin-receptor complexes inside.

Iron is available for use or storage

ferritin

4. Cell membrane fuses, forming an endosome.

6. In acidic environment iron is released and the affinity of apotransferrin for its receptor is increased.

5. Endosome fuses with acidic vesicle.

acidic vesicle

©UTHSCSA 1993

FIGURE 6-5. Iron binds to apotransferrin in the plasma forming mono or diferric transferrin. Transferrin binds to transferrin receptors on the cell surface. The transferrin-receptor complex enters the cell where the iron is released. The apotransferrin-receptor complex is transported to the cell surface where the apotransferrin is released to the plasma for reutilization. (Adapted from: Hoffman, R., Benz, E.J., Shattil, S.J., Furie, B., Cohen, H.J. (eds): Hematology: Basic Principles and Procedures. New York: Churchill Livingstone, 1991.)

6-4 shows the variations in tissue iron in various disease states.

In addition to serum ferritin, estimation of storage iron may be made on bone marrow tissue sections. Sideroblasts are normoblasts that contain iron granules. These granules can be stained with Prussian blue stain. All developing normoblasts and reticulocytes contain dispersed ferritin molecules necessary for heme synthesis, but only 30% to 60% contain iron aggregates (hemosiderin) large enough to be visualized with the light microscope. Hemosiderin appears as yellow to brown refractile pigment on unstained specimens. On Prussian blue-stained specimens, the iron appears as blue intracellular particles. Stores may be graded from 0 to 4+ or as markedly reduced, normal, or increased. Bone marrow macrophages also contain ferritin and hemosiderin if body iron stores are normal. Normally, mature erythrocytes do not contain iron aggregates because any excess iron in the cell after hemoglobin synthesis is complete is removed by splenic macrophages.

● Ferrokinetics

Quantitative measurement of internal iron exchange (ferrokinetics) is useful in understanding the pathophysiology of certain erythropoietic disorders. Ferrokinetic studies monitor the movement of radioactively labeled iron (^{59}Fe) from the plasma to the bone marrow and into circulating erythrocytes. Plasma iron is labeled by intravenous injection of a tracer amount of radioiron. The labeled iron binds to transferrin for transport. Its clearance from the plasma can be followed by counting the radioactivity that remains in the plasma at intervals. The rate at which iron leaves the plasma is called the plasma iron transport rate (PIT). The PIT is a good indicator of total erythropoiesis (effective and ineffective) and correlates well with the erythroid cellularity of bone marrow. Tissue need is the primary determinant of PIT. The PIT may be expressed as a total daily rate (mg/day) or as a rate per volume of blood (Table 6-5).

Normal turnover is about 0.6 to 0.8 mg/dL/day; thus, for a blood volume of 5 liters, the normal iron turnover is approximately 30 mg/day. If total plasma iron is 3 to 4 mg, then complete turnover occurs every 2½ to 3 hours.

The amount of iron used for effective hemoglobin synthesis also can be measured by determining the amount of labeled iron incorporated into circulating erythrocytes over time. This is termed the erythrocyte iron turnover rate (EIT). Normally, approximately 80% of the labeled

TABLE 6-4 *EFFECTS OF DISEASE ON TISSUE IRON*

Disease	Iron/Total Iron-Binding Capacity	Ferritin	Bone Marrow Iron
Iron deficiency anemia	Low	Low	Absent
Anemia of chronic disease	Normal or low	Normal or high	Abundant
Anemia of chronic renal disease	Normal or high	Normal or high	Abundant
Anemia of chronic liver disease	High	High	Abundant
Anemia of hypothyroidism	Normal	Normal	Normal
Sideroblastic anemias	High	High	Abundant with ringed sideroblasts
Hypoplastic and aplastic anemias	High	High	Abundant
Polycythemia vera	Low	Low	Low or absent
Hemolytic anemia	Normal	Normal	Normal
Megaloblastic anemia	High	High	Abundant
Thalassemia minor	Normal	Normal	Normal

(From: Freedman, M.L.: Iron deficiency in the elderly. Hosp. Prac., 21(3A):115, 1986.)

iron (0.56 mg/day/dL) can be accounted for in circulating erythrocytes within 21 days. The EIT is a good measure of effective erythropoiesis and correlates with the reticulocyte production index.

The discrepancy that exists between the rate at which iron leaves the plasma (PIT = 0.7 mg/day/dL) and the rate at which it moves from marrow to circulating erythrocytes (EIT = 0.56 mg/day/dL) suggests that the red cell utilization (RCU) of iron is less than 100%. Studies to interpret these results conclude that plasma iron is in equilibrium with one or more functional compartments, possibly the bone marrow and liver. Some of the labeled iron may enter this tissue. In addition, 5% to 10% of bone marrow iron is involved in ineffective erythropoiesis, causing a loss of the labeled iron by intramedullary destruction of abnormal erythrocytes. Ferrokinetic studies also are of practical value in locating sites of medullary and extramedullary erythropoiesis by counting surface radioactivity over the liver, spleen, and sacrum.

● Requirements

NORMAL IRON REQUIREMENTS

Normally, humans maintain a relatively constant body concentration of iron throughout life. This is accomplished by remaining in a positive iron balance during growing years and establishing equilibrium between loss and absorption in adult life. Human ability to excrete iron

TABLE 6-5 *BASIC FERROKINETIC MEASUREMENTS*

Measurement	Calculation	Average Normal Value
$t\frac{1}{2}$*	Graphically, from semilogarithmic plot of plasma radioactivity disappearance	86 minutes
PIT	$\dfrac{0.693}{t\frac{1}{2}} \times$ plasma Fe (mg/ml) $\times$ plasma vol (ml) $\times$ 1440 min/day -or- $\dfrac{\text{plasma Fe } (\mu g/dl) \times 100 - VPRC}{t\frac{1}{2} \times 100}$	26 mg/day -or- 0.7 mg/day/dl blood
RCU	$\dfrac{\text{day 14 radioactivity/ml blood} \times 100}{\text{0 time radioactivity/ml blood}}$ -or- $\dfrac{\text{day 14 radioactivity/ml RBC} \times \text{red cell mass (ml)} \times 100}{\text{total injected radioactivity}}$	80%
EIT	PIT $\times$ RCU	21 mg/day -or- 0.56 mg/day/dl blood
MTT	Graphically, from a semilogarithmic plot, the time at which 100 − RCU = 50%	3.5 days

* Abbreviations: $t\frac{1}{2}$, plasma Fe half-disappearance time; PIT, plasma iron transport rate; RCU, red blood utilization; EIT, erythrocyte iron turnover rate; MTT, marrow transit time; VPRC, volume of packed red cells. (From: Lee, G.R., Bithell, T.C., Foerster, J., Athens, J.W., Lukens, J.N.: Wintrobe's Clinical Hematology. Philadelphia: Lea & Febiger, 1993.)

to achieve this balance is extremely limited. As mentioned previously, major control of iron repletion is achieved by regulation of absorption to fit body needs. Although a normal diet contains about 15 mg of iron per day, only 5% to 10% is absorbed in the gastrointestinal tract. When the body's need for iron increases, there is a limited capacity to absorb more iron. If consistent alterations in iron balance occur, either iron deficiency or iron overload (*hemosiderosis*) can occur. Increased or decreased amounts of iron may cause a variety of clinical abnormalities.

Body iron is conserved by reutilization so that daily absorption and loss are small. Total body iron lost through body secretions of urine, sweat, bile, and desquamation of cells lining the gastrointestinal tract amounts to about 1 mg/day. Normal erythrocyte aging results in destruction of 20 to 25 mL of erythrocytes/day (10 to 12 mg iron) in splenic and hepatic macrophages, but most of this hemoglobin iron is transported by transferrin from the monocyte–macrophage system to the bone marrow, where it is reused by developing normoblasts. The total daily requirement is thus about 1 mg, enough to replace the iron lost through sweat, urine, bile, and desquamation.

FACTORS THAT INCREASE IRON REQUIREMENTS
Normal physiologic factors affecting daily requirements for iron include menstruation, pregnancy, and growth. In a female with a 14 g/dL hemoglobin concentration, normal monthly menstrual blood loss amounts to 41 to 46 mL or 20 to 23 mg iron loss. Thus, the average daily iron loss in menstruating females is twice that of their male counterparts. To maintain total body iron balance, menstruating females must absorb about 2 mg of iron daily.

The daily iron requirement during pregnancy is about 3.4 mg; if spread out at a daily average over the three trimesters, it would be about 1000 mg per pregnancy. The fetus accumulates 250 mg of this iron from maternal stores via the placenta; added to this is the iron requirement for increased maternal blood volume and iron loss at delivery due to bleeding. A single pregnancy without supplemental iron could exhaust iron stores.

In infancy, rapid growth of body size and hemoglobin mass require more iron in proportion to food intake than at any other time of life. During the first 6 months of life, an infant synthesizes 50 g of new hemoglobin. In addition, iron is needed for tissue growth. At birth, normal iron stores of 30 mg are adequate to see the infant through the first 4 to 5 months of life but may be quickly depleted in an infant on an iron deficient, milk-only diet. Milk is a poor source of iron and will not satisfy the needs of a developing infant. Even less iron is absorbed from cow's milk than mother's milk because the higher calcium concentration in cow's milk inhibits absorption. Premature infants are at an even higher risk of rapid iron depletion because much of the placental transfer of iron occurs in the last trimester of pregnancy and they have a faster rate of postnatal growth than full-term infants.[6] It is recommended that full-term infants begin iron supplements no later than 4 months of age and that low birth-weight infants begin no later than 2 months of age.[6] Iron requirements also are high in childhood and adolescence, especially in menstruating females.

Chronic blood loss increases the need for iron since about 0.5 mg is lost per milliliter of blood lost. Iron stores may be used if enough iron is not absorbed to make up for the loss.

● IRON DEFICIENCY ANEMIA

Iron deficiency is the most common nutritional deficiency in the world. It is prevalent in countries where grain is the mainstay of the diet or meat is scarce. Unfortunately, these also are countries where hookworm infestation is endemic. The combination of decreased availability of dietary iron and chronic blood loss from parasitic infection puts these individuals in double jeopardy of development of iron deficiency anemia. Malnutrition is associated with not only decreased iron intake but also decreased intake of other essential nutrients including folate. Thus, causes of anemia associated with malnutrition may be multifactorial.

● Historical aspects

In America, between 1870 and 1920, *chlorosis,* a term used to describe the condition of iron deficiency, was so common in young women it was believed that every female had some form of the disease during puberty. The term chlorosis was coined because of the greenish tinge of the skin in these patients; however, often the greenish hue was not apparent but pallor was pronounced. Other classic clinical signs and symptoms of anemia were present, including shortness of breath on exertion, lethargy, and heart palpitations. These chlorotic girls were found to have decreased numbers of red corpuscles and an increase in the proportion of serum to cells. Some of the chlorotic girls also were noted to have perverted appetites, craving substances such as chalk, cinders, charcoal, and bugs. As therapy for these patients, doctors prescribed iron salts, even though the exact nature of the disease had not been identified.

Some physicians linked chlorosis to dietary habits, while others implicated menstruation as a possible cause of the disease because chlorosis affected girls in puberty but not boys. It has been proposed that the prevalence of chlorosis during this time was not only due to poor dietary habits but also was related to the cultural and social values of the times.[7] It was fashionable to be a chlorotic girl, as they were considered the most attractive and fertile females. To compound the problem, eating red meat was linked to sexual immorality among young women; hence, the refusal of meat was considered a social virtue.

Although iron deficiency in the United States is still the most common nutritional deficiency, it is not nearly as prevalent as it was at the turn of the century. In the United States today, young children and females of child-bearing age are more likely to acquire iron deficiency anemia from an iron deficient diet than the rest of the population. Iron deficiency in males is almost always due to blood loss.

● Pathophysiology

Iron deficiency may occur due to blood loss, increased demands for iron, malabsorption, or poor diet. In malabsorption or with an iron deficient diet, iron stores may become depleted over a period of years. With blood loss or an increase in the demand for iron (e.g., infancy), iron depletion may occur more rapidly, sometimes over a period of months.

CAUSES OF IRON DEFICIENCY

In most developed countries, inadequate dietary intake of iron is rarely the cause of anemia (except in infancy, pregnancy, and adolescence). Diet and socioeconomic status, however, are factors in the development of iron deficiency in children. Infants who are fed iron-fortified formula or breast milk have reduced prevalence of iron deficiency anemia. Children from low-income families have an increased prevalence.

The average adult male in the United States ingests many times more iron than is required; it would take an adult male about 8 years to develop iron deficiency anemia if he absorbed no iron during those years. Therefore, iron deficiency in this segment of the population is almost always due to chronic blood loss from the gastrointestinal or genitourinary tracts. Gastrointestinal lesions leading to blood loss include peptic ulcers, hiatus hernia, malignancies, alcoholic gastritis, excessive salicylate ingestion, hookworm infestation, and hemorrhoids. Genitourinary tract blood loss occurs less frequently; it may result from lesions within the genitourinary system.

Less often, blood loss is the result of intravascular hemolysis. If haptoglobin (a plasma hemoglobin-binding protein) becomes depleted, the free circulating hemoglobin is filtered by the kidneys and appears in the urine (hemoglobinuria). This results in a loss of iron, the amount of which is proportional to the amount of hemoglobin in the urine. Some of the hemoglobin is reabsorbed by the renal tubules, resulting in the deposition of iron in renal tubular cells and eventual sloughing of these cells in the urine. Such is the case with paroxysmal nocturnal hemoglobinuria or malfunctioning prosthetic heart valves. This loss of iron-loaded tubular cells amplifies iron loss in conditions associated with intravascular hemolysis.

Malabsorption is an uncommon cause of iron deficiency except in malabsorption syndromes (such as sprue), after gastrectomy, in atrophic gastritis, and in achlorhydria. Gastrectomy results in impaired iron absorption due to the absence of gastric juice, which helps to solubilize and reduce dietary iron into the more easily absorbed ferrous form. In addition, with the loss of the reservoir function of the stomach, nutrients may transit rapidly through the duodenum, allowing little time for iron absorption. Iron deficiency anemia is frequently accompanied by atrophic gastritis and achlorhydria, but it is unknown whether achlorhydria and gastritis are causes of iron malabsorption or the iron deficiency is a cause of atrophic gastritis and hence achlorhydria. In these patients, therapy with oral iron may be ineffective due to poor iron absorption.[8]

STAGES OF IRON DEFICIENCY

Iron deficiency, defined as a diminished total body iron content, develops in sequential stages over a period of negative iron balance. These stages include: (1) iron depletion, (2) iron deficient erythropoiesis, and (3) iron deficiency anemia. Thus, iron deficiency may range in severity from reduced iron stores with no functional effect to severe anemia with deficiencies of tissue iron-containing enzymes.[5]

Laboratory evaluation of iron status is helpful in defining these three stages (Table 6-6). During the iron depletion stage, iron stores are exhausted as indicated by a de-

TABLE 6-6 *IRON VALUES IN THE DEVELOPMENT OF IRON DEFICIENCY ANEMIA*

		Tissue Iron Stores	Hemoglobin (g/dl)	Serum Iron (μg/dl)	TIBC (μg/dl)	Saturation (%)	Serum Ferritin (μg/L)	Daily Iron Absorption (%)	RBC Morphology
Stage 1 Iron Depletion		↓	N	N	N or sl↑	N	↓	10–15%	N
Stage 2 Iron Deficient Erythropoiesis		↓	N	↓	↑	↓	↓	10–20%	N
Stage 3 Iron Deficiency Anemia		↓	↓	↓	↑	↓	↓	10–20%	Hypochromic, Microcytic
Normal	♂	2+	13–18	65–185	240–440	30	30–340	5–10%	Normochromic, Normocytic
	♀	2+	12–16	65–185	240–440	30	20–148	5–10%	Normochromic, Normocytic

N = Normal
↓ = Decreased
↑ = Increased
TIBC = Total iron binding capacity

crease in serum ferritin. Values less than 12 μg/L indicate depletion of iron stores. The iron stores are apparently mobilized to supply the iron for erythropoiesis. Iron absorption in the gut is usually increased at this stage in an attempt to compensate for the negative iron flow. Anemia and/or erythrocyte morphologic changes are not present. Although the traditional erythrocyte parameters (hemoglobin, hematocrit, erythrocyte count) are normal, the red cell distribution width (RDW) is frequently elevated and may be the first indication of a developing iron deficiency in the nonanemic patient. The elevated RDW indicates the need for evaluating the iron status of the patient. In hospitalized patients, the RDW is not as specific and the ferritin not as sensitive in detecting iron deficiency.[9] Hospitalized patients have a high incidence of other diseases that may affect these parameters. For instance, liver disease is associated with an increase in the RDW, whereas infection, inflammation, and chronic diseases may cause a falsely elevated serum ferritin even in the presence of iron deficiency.

In the second stage of iron deficiency, iron stores have been depleted. Serum iron and serum ferritin are decreased, and the TIBC is increased. This results in a decrease in the percent saturation of transferrin. With continued negative iron flow, the iron available for erythropoiesis is limited primarily to the amount of iron recycled. In addition to the abnormal results of iron studies, the iron deficient erythropoiesis stage is reflected by the absence of bone marrow sideroblasts and an increase in erythrocyte protoporphyrin, often referred to as free erythrocyte protoporphyrin (FEP). It is now believed that most of the erythrocyte protoporphyrin (EP) formed in the absence of iron complexes with zinc forming zinc protoporphyrin (ZPP). Thus, the protoporphyrin is not actually "free." Prior to the discovery of ZPP, acid extraction procedures were used to assay erythrocyte protoporphyrins. The acid extraction caused the loss of zinc and the formation of free protoporphyrin. Hematofluorometers can now be used to measure ZPP directly. The measurement of ZPP is a sensitive index of this second stage of iron deficiency characterized by increased EP. Anemia and hypochromia are still not detectable, but the erythrocytes may become slightly microcytic. It is believed that microcytosis precedes hypochromia.

The evaluation of EP is useful when attempting to identify the cause of microcytic hypochromic anemia. The concentration of EP is affected by heme synthesis, the iron supply, and the rate of erythropoiesis. In iron deficient erythropoiesis, the erythrocyte continues to make porphyrin, even in the absence of sufficient iron to insert into the protoporphyrin ring to form heme. As a result, the protoporphyrin accumulates in the cell, remaining there for the entire erythrocyte lifespan. Erythrocytes with excess EP fluoresce with ultraviolet (UV) light. The EP also is increased in the anemia of chronic disease, lead poisoning, erythropoietic protoporphyria, some sideroblastic anemias, and conditions with markedly increased levels of erythropoiesis (e.g., sickle cell anemia). Although EP may be increased in some thalassemia patients, the increase is only moderate (mean value, 85 μg/dL erythrocytes) com-

pared with iron deficiency (mean value, 284 μg/dL erythrocytes).[10] The normal reference range is 16 to 67 μg/dL.

A long-standing negative iron flow eventually leads to the last stage of iron deficiency—iron deficiency anemia. Blood loss may significantly shorten the time for this stage to develop. All laboratory tests for iron status (serum ferritin, TIBC, serum iron, percent saturation) become markedly abnormal, and the EP is elevated even more than in the previous stage. The most significant finding is the classic microcytic hypochromic anemia.

It is apparent then, that when iron-deficient microcytic hypochromic anemia is present, the situation represents the advanced stage of severely deficient total body iron.

Clinical features

The onset of iron deficiency anemia is insidious, usually occurring over a period of months to years. Early stages of iron deficiency usually show no clinical manifestations, but with complete depletion of iron stores, anemia develops and clinical symptoms appear. Symptoms such as weakness and lethargy are considered to be related to hypoxia due to the decrease in hemoglobin. A variety of other abnormalities may occur due to an absence of tissue iron in iron-containing enzymes. These include koilonychia (concavity of nails), glossitis, pharyngeal webs, muscle dysfunction, impaired thermogenesis, and gastritis.

A curious manifestation of iron deficiency is the *pica* syndrome. Pica is a perversion of appetite that leads to bizarre eating practices. The most common dysphagias described in patients with iron deficiency include ice-eating (phagophagia), dirt (clay)-eating (geophagia), and starch-eating (amylophagia). Clay acts as an ion exchange resin and can interfere with iron absorption. Starch does not interfere directly with iron absorption, but is a poor source of iron and when ingested in large quantities may exacerbate the iron deficiency. In one study of 55 patients with iron deficiency anemia, 58% had pica and of these 88% had phagophagia.[11] Among some cultural groups, pica is a practiced custom that may lead to the development of iron deficiency; thus, among some populations, pica may be a cause rather than a manifestation of iron deficiency.

Symptoms reported to occur in iron deficient children include: irritability, loss of memory, and difficulties in learning. Deficiencies of the immune system have been attributed to iron-related impairment of host defense mechanisms, including decreased blastogenic response of lymphocytes to antigenic stimulation.

In the absence of iron in the gut, other metals are absorbed in increased amounts. This can be significant when a person is exposed to toxic metals such as lead, cadmium, and plutonium.

Laboratory findings

Laboratory tests are essential to an accurate diagnoses of iron deficiency.

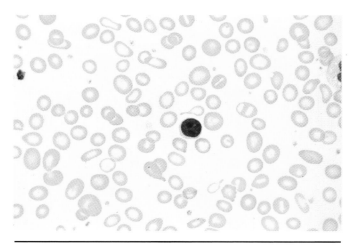

FIGURE 6-6. Microcytic, hypochromic anemia of iron deficiency. (PB; 250× original magnification; Wright-Giemsa stain.)

PERIPHERAL BLOOD

The blood picture in well-developed iron deficiency is microcytic (MCV, 55 to 74 fL), hypochromic (MCHC, 22 to 31 g/dL; MCH, 14 to 26 pg) (Fig. 6-6). Because iron deficiency develops in stages, any gradation between the well-developed microcytic hypochromic iron deficient picture and normal may occur. When the anemia is mild, the morphologic aspects of the erythrocyte are little affected. With progressive severity, the characteristic features of a cytoplasmic maturation defect appear. Microcytosis and anisocytosis, characterized by an increased RDW, are usually the first morphologic signs to develop even before anemia develops. The ZPP is markedly elevated. The erythrocyte count and hematocrit are not good indicators of the degree of anemia since they are often not proportionate to the severe decrease in hemoglobin (mean, 84 g/L). This typical blood picture may be masked if the patient has a concurrent folate deficiency. In these cases, microcytosis may only become apparent after folic acid replacement therapy.[12]

The blood film demonstrates progressively abnormal poikilocytosis. The most frequent poikilocytes are target cells and elliptocytes. Nucleated erythrocytes may be seen if hemorrhage has occurred. Both the relative and absolute number of reticulocytes may be normal or even slightly increased, but the reticulocyte count is decreased in relation to the severity of the anemia, with an RPI less than 2.

The leukocyte count is usually normal but may be increased due to chronic marrow stimulation in long-standing cases or after hemorrhage. With concomitant hookworm infestation, eosinophilia may be present.

Platelets may be normal, increased, or decreased. Thrombocytopenia may occur in patients with severe or long-standing anemia, especially if accompanied by folate deficiency. Thrombocytosis frequently accompanies iron deficiency. It has been proposed that thrombocytosis is related to iron deficiency caused by chronic blood loss. Numeric changes seen in platelets are corrected with treatment that replenishes iron stores.

ERYTHROCYTE PROTOPORPHYRIN STUDIES

When insufficient iron is available to developing normoblasts, erythrocyte protoporphyrin (EP) accumulates in the cell and can be detected as ZPP. Since ZPP persists throughout the lifespan of the cell, a measure of ZPP provides a retrospective indicator of iron availability at the time of cell maturation. The ZPP measurement correlates with plasma ferritin concentration but is more cost-effective.

The level of ZPP may be used as a screening test to differentiate iron deficiency and thalassemia which are the two most common causes of microcytic hypochromic anemia. ZPP is usually not elevated in thalassemia. An increase in ZPP has been reported in some thalassemia patients, but the increase is moderate when compared with that found in iron deficiency.[10] When laboratory analysis reveals a high ZPP combined with a high RDW, iron deficiency is strongly suggested.[10] The RDW is normal or only slightly elevated in thalassemia trait.

In patients with lead poisoning, the ZPP cannot be used to distinguish iron deficiency and thalassemia because lead inhibits ferrochelatase, the enzyme needed to incorporate iron into the protoporphyrin ring.[13] Consequently, the free erythrocyte protoporphyrin complexes with zinc. Hence, ZPP is increased in lead poisoning whether or not iron is available.

The ZPP assay shows higher sensitivity in detecting iron deficiency in elderly patients with chronic inflammation than either TIBC or serum ferritin since both may be falsely increased in this condition.[14]

ZPP may be tested by a quantitative method or a qualitative screening method. Both tests are based on the fluorescent properties of ZPP. The hematofluorometer is a simple instrument dedicated to measurement of ZPP. The results are reported as a molar ratio, mmol ZPP/mol heme.

IRON STUDIES

The serum iron is decreased, usually less than 30 μg/dL, the TIBC is increased and transferrin saturation is decreased to less than 15%. Serum iron concentration has a diurnal variation with highest levels in the morning so sampling time is an important consideration. It has been suggested that since the diagnostic sensitivity of TIBC is inferior to the ferritin assay in the diagnosis of iron deficiency, the TIBC should no longer be used for this purpose.[15] Serum ferritin levels, which correlate closely with storage iron levels, are decreased in all stages of iron deficiency and may be the first indication of a developing iron deficiency. Once serum ferritin levels fall below 12 μg/L, the levels may no longer correlate with storage iron because stores are exhausted. Serum ferritin, however, is an acute phase reactant and may appear normal or even increased in concomitant inflammatory conditions. Serum ferritin is an important test to differentiate iron deficiency anemia from other microcytic hypochromic anemias. Levels are normal in the anemia of chronic disease unless complicated by iron deficiency, and increased in sideroblastic anemia and thalassemia.

It has been suggested that for detecting concomitant iron deficiency and anemia of chronic disease, the lower limit of serum ferritin to detect the iron deficiency should be raised from 12 to 50 μg/L.[16] In one study of patients with rheumatoid arthritis, it was found that in patients whose ferritin levels were less than 70 μg/L, iron deficiency was always present.[17] If iron status in patients with chronic disease or inflammation is evaluated using a combination of serum ferritin (using the lower normal limit of 50 μg/L) and MCV (using the lower normal limit of 80 fL), the specificity and predictive value of the combined tests are 100% but the sensitivity is only 79%.[16] If TIBC (using the lower normal limit of 50 μmoL/L) is added to the above protocol, the reliability of estimating iron status is very good. It has been suggested that the combination of serum ferritin, MCV, and TIBC testing may eliminate the need for costly, inconvenient, and sometimes painful bone marrow examination to assess iron stores in patients with inflammation or chronic disease.[16] It also has been suggested that the threshold level of serum ferritin for a diagnosis of iron deficiency in the aged subject be raised since serum ferritin levels rise with age.[18]

SERUM TRANSFERRIN RECEPTOR ASSAYS

Small concentrations of transferrin receptor can be identified in serum by sensitive immunoassay techniques. This receptor in serum is a truncated form of the intact protein found on the cell membrane. Serum transferrin receptor assays using the enzyme-linked immmunosorbent assay technique with monoclonal antibodies has proved useful in detecting and differentiating iron deficiency anemia and anemia of chronic disease. Patients with iron deficiency have a mean serum transferrin receptor level (13.91 ± 4.63 mg/l) more than two times that of mean receptor levels in healthy individuals (5.36 ± 0.82 mg/L). Conversely, patients with chronic disease have mean levels almost identical to those of healthy individuals. The serum transferrin receptor level also is in the normal range in patients with acute infection and acute hepatitis.[19]

In iron deficiency anemia, there is a significant negative correlation between hemoglobin and serum transferrin receptor level[19] (Table 6-7). Receptor levels also parallel the reticulocyte count, suggesting that the receptor level may reflect the turnover of transferrin receptors as cells mature.[20] Thus, the serum transferrin receptor level may provide an index of erythrocyte production in the marrow.

BONE MARROW

The bone marrow shows mild to moderate erythroid hyperplasia with a decreased myeloid to erythroid (M:E) ratio. Total cellularity often is moderately increased. This increase in marrow erythropoietic activity without a corresponding increase in peripheral blood reticulocytes suggests an ineffective erthropoietic component. With appropriate iron therapy, the erythroid hyperplasia initially increases and then returns to normal. A common finding (not exclusive to iron deficiency anemia) is the presence of poorly hemoglobinized normoblasts with scanty ragged (irregular) cytoplasm. This change is most evident at the polychromatophilic stage. Erythroid nuclear abnormalities are sometimes present and may resemble the changes found in dyserythropoietic anemia. These changes include budding, karyorrhexis, nuclear fragmentation, and multinuclearity. Stains for iron reveal an absence of hemosiderin in the macrophages, an invariable characteristic of iron deficiency. Sideroblasts are markedly reduced or absent.

Evaluation of iron stores using serum iron studies and/or serum transferrin receptor assays eliminate the need for bone marrow examination in almost all cases.

● Therapy

Once the cause of the anemia has been established, the principles of treatment are to treat the underlying disorder (e.g., bleeding ulcer), administer iron, and observe the response. The anemia is usually corrected by the oral administration of ferrous sulfate. Intolerance of iron preparations caused by gastrointestinal upsets may complicate iron therapy, but this usually can be avoided by giving the iron supplements with food or by administering smaller

TABLE 6-7 *COMPARISON OF IRON STATUS PARAMETERS BETWEEN GROUPS OF PATIENTS WITH VARIOUS DISEASES*

Patient Group	Hemoglobin (gm/L)*	MCV (fl)*	Serum Iron (μg/dl)*	TIBC (μg/dl)*	Saturation (%)*	Ferritin (μg/L)†	Transferrin Receptor (mg/L)*
Normal controls (n = 17)	143 ± 12	93 ± 3	75 ± 28	377 ± 67	20 ± 8	43 (23–80)	5.36 ± 0.82
Iron-deficiency anemia (n = 17)	95 ± 12	74 ± 8	21 ± 15	428 ± 76	5 ± 4	7 (4–12)	13.91 ± 4.63
Acute infection (n = 15)	139 ± 12	88 ± 5	32 ± 23	302 ± 120	14 ± 15	252 (103–613)	5.11 ± 1.42
Anemia of chronic disease (n = 41)	102 ± 12	84 ± 7	35 ± 25	257 ± 87	14 ± 11	220 (86–559)	5.65 ± 1.91
Acute hepatitis (n = 5)	144 ± 8	94 ± 4	121 ± 72	400 ± 70	33 ± 24	2438 (1071–5552)	4.80 ± 1.19
Chronic liver disease with anemia (n = 10)	111 ± 13	97 ± 9	52 ± 32	193 ± 80	28 ± 19	280 (116–677)	5.98 ± 2.06

* Data expressed as mean ± S.D.
† Data expressed as geometric mean ± S.D.
RCMI = red cell mean index
MCV = mean cell volume
TIBC = total iron binding capacity
(From: Ferguson BJ, et al.: Serum transferrin receptor distinguishes the anemia of chronic disease from iron deficiency anemia. *Journal of Laboratory and Clinical Medicine* 119: 385, 1992)

doses. However, iron absorption may decrease as much as 50% when taken with food. Parenteral iron therapy, which is more dangerous and expensive than oral iron therapy, may, on rare occasion, be indicated for unusual circumstances.

Iron deficient patients treated with iron experience a return of strength, appetite, and a feeling of well-being within 3 to 5 days, whereas the anemia is not alleviated for weeks. The dysphagias also are corrected before the anemia is relieved.

Reticulocyte response to iron therapy begins at about the third day after the start of therapy, peaks at about the eighth to tenth day (4% to 10% reticulocytes), and declines thereafter. If therapy is successful, the hemoglobin should rise until levels within normal limits are established, usually within 6 to 10 weeks. To restore iron stores, extended therapy with small amounts of iron salts may be required (usually 6 months) after the hemoglobin has returned to normal.

● ANEMIAS CAUSED BY ABNORMAL IRON METABOLISM

Anemias caused by abnormal iron metabolism are the result of either a block in the incorporation of iron into the protoporphyrin ring to form heme or defective iron reutilization (usually the result of a slow release of iron from macrophages). Although absorbed at normal rates in these anemias, iron is used at less than normal rates for erythropoiesis. This results in a lack of iron for hemoglobin synthesis and a blood picture similar to that of iron deficiency anemia. In contrast to iron deficiency, however, the positive iron balance in these anemias may lead to an increase in iron stores, predominantly in the spleen, liver, and bone marrow. Serum ferritin levels above 250 μg/L in the male or above 200 μg/L in the female indicate increased iron stores.

The anemias discussed in this section include sideroblastic anemia and the anemia of chronic disease. Lead poisoning also is included because of its pathophysiologic relation to these anemias through a block in heme synthesis.

● Sideroblastic anemias

Sideroblastic anemia (SA) is the result of diverse clinical and biochemical manifestations that reflect multiple underlying pathogenic mechanisms. However, all types are characterized by: (1) an increase in total body iron, (2) the presence of ringed sideroblasts in the bone marrow, and (3) hypochromic anemia (Table 6-8).

TABLE 6-8 *CHARACTERISTICS OF SIDEROBLASTIC ANEMIAS*

1. Increase in total body iron
2. Ringed sideroblasts in BM
3. Hypochromic anemia

TABLE 6-9 *CLASSIFICATION OF SIDEROBLASTIC ANEMIA*

I. Hereditary
  A. Sex-linked
  B. Autosomal recessive

II. Acquired
  A. Idiopathic refractory sideroblastic anemia (IRSA) or refractory anemia with ringed sideroblasts (RARS)
  B. Secondary to drugs, toxins, lead
  C. Secondary associated with malignancy

CLASSIFICATION

The classification of sideroblastic anemia is arbitrary at best, and one may find many different schemes of classification. The classification given in Table 6-9 is one of the most descriptive. There are two major groups, those that are inherited and those that are acquired. Most patients with the hereditary form of sideroblastic anemia are males, which suggests that it is a sex-linked recessive trait. Although some carrier females show morphologically abnormal erythrocytes, only the affected males demonstrate the typical findings of sideroblastic anemia. In rare instances, both sexes are equally affected, implying that there may be another hereditary form that is transmitted in an autosomal recessive manner. In these hereditary forms, anemia may become apparent in infancy but most commonly appears in young adulthood. Rarely, symptoms may not occur until age 60.

The acquired forms of sideroblastic anemia are more common than the hereditary forms. The acquired forms are classified according to whether the basis of the anemia is unknown (idiopathic type) or is secondary to an underlying disease or toxin (secondary type). The idiopathic form, *refractory anemia with ringed sideroblasts* (RARS), may affect either sex in adult life. RARS is included in a group of stem cell disorders called myelodysplastic syndromes. These syndromes have similar hematologic findings and a tendency to terminate in acute leukemia. The acquired secondary sideroblastic anemias are associated with malignancy, drugs, or other toxic substances. In the secondary types, once the underlying disorder is effectively treated or the toxin removed, the anemia abates.

PATHOPHYSIOLOGY

Studies of patients with sideroblastic anemia have shown disturbances of the enzymes regulating heme synthesis. Ringed sideroblasts are a specific finding for these heme enzyme abnormalities. Ringed sideroblasts are formed from an accumulation of nonferritin iron in the mitochondria which circle the normoblast nucleus. The mitochondria eventually rupture as they become laden with iron. When stained with Prussian blue, the iron appears as blue punctate deposits circling all or part of the nucleus. Normally, iron within the normoblasts is deposited diffusely throughout the cytoplasm.

Hereditary sideroblastic anemia Defective heme synthesis appears to be involved in the pathogenesis of the hereditary form of sideroblastic anemia. The most well-documented heme enzyme abnormality in the hereditary sex-linked form of sideroblastic anemia is decreased erythropoietic Δ-ALA-synthase. The formation of Δ-ALA from glycine and succinyl CoA in the presence of pyridoxal phosphate and Δ-ALA-synthase is the rate-limiting step in heme synthesis. Recently, two different forms of Δ-ALA synthase have been identified, the nonerythroid or hepatic form and the erythroid form.[21,22] The nonerythroid form is coded for by a gene expressed in all tissues and has been assigned to the chromosomal region 3p21. The erythroid form is coded for by a gene that has been assigned to the Xp21-q21 chromosomal region (female sex chromosome). In some cases, there is a clinical response to pharmacologic doses of pyridoxine. Thus, in these cases, it is possible that a mutation in the sex-linked gene for Δ-ALA synthase produces an enzyme with decreased affinity for pyridoxine. It also is possible that an abnormal Δ-ALA-synthase with increased sensitivity to a mitochondrial protease is produced.

Acquired sideroblastic anemia

REFRACTORY ANEMIA WITH RINGED SIDEROBLASTS In patients with the acquired idiopathic form of sideroblastic anemia, RARS, studies have documented multiple mitochondrial enzymatic defects in addition to decreased Δ-ALA synthase activity. It has been suggested that the primary defect may be an abnormality of mitochondrial iron metabolism. In the majority of SA, iron uptake by the developing erythroblast is normal; however, increased sequestration of stromal iron may occur even before full establishment of heme synthesis. This could have an adverse effect on heme synthesis by inhibiting the activity of mitochrondrial enzymes.

Approximately 10% of RARS terminate in acute leukemia (most commonly myeloid or erythroid) or other malignancy. This may occur within a few months of the diagnosis of RARS or may occur up to 7 years later. As mentioned previously, this form of sideroblastic anemia is now considered to be the result of a stem cell disorder. It is discussed in more detail in the chapter on myelodysplastic syndromes (Chapter 16).

SECONDARY TO DRUGS OR TOXINS Acquired sideroblastic anemia, secondary to drugs/toxins, is the result of the drugs' or toxins' interference with the activity of heme enzymes. The most common drugs associated with this type of anemia are chemotherapeutic drugs, antituberculosis drugs, chloramphenicols, alcohol, and lead. Lead poisoning may cause a sideroblastic-like anemia.

LEAD POISONING Lead poisoning *(plumbism)* has been recognized for centuries. In children, it generally results from ingestion of flaked lead-based paint from painted articles. In adults, it is primarily the result of inhalation of lead or lead compounds from industrial processes. Lead serves no physiologic purpose. Clinically, lead toxicity is associated with hyperactivity, low IQ, concentration disorders, hearing loss, and impaired growth and development.

Thirty-three states in the United States require labora-

tories and physicians to report elevated blood lead levels to the state health department. Twenty-three of these states also report elevated blood lead levels to the Center for Disease Control (CDC). In 1994, there were 12,137 reports of adults with elevated blood lead levels of which 5,619 were new cases (not reported the previous year).[23] The proportion of new cases in the lower reporting levels decreased but increased in the $> 60\mu g/dL$ category. In the first quarter of 1995, the number of reports of elevated blood lead levels increased by 10% over the same reporting period in 1994. The number of reports at the 25 to $39\mu g/dL$ level increased but reports at all higher levels decreased.

Although lead poisoning consistently shortens the erythrocyte lifespan, the anemia accompanying plumbism is not primarily the result of hemolysis but rather the result of a marked abnormality in heme synthesis. Once ingested, lead passes through the blood to the bone marrow, where it accumulates in the mitochondria of normoblasts and inhibits cellular enzymes involved in heme synthesis. The heme enzymes most sensitive to lead inhibition are Δ-aminolevulinic acid dehydrase (Δ-ALA-D) and ferrocheletase (heme synthase). The effect of lead on ferrochelatase is competitive inhibition with iron. Other enzymes may be affected at higher lead concentrations. Thus, the synthesis of heme is primarily disturbed at the conversion of Δ-ALA to porphobilinogen (Δ-ALA-D), and at the incorporation of iron into protoporphyrin to form heme (ferrochelatase). As a result, there is an increase in urine excretion of Δ-ALA. The erythrocyte protoporphyrin also is strikingly increased, causing the cells to fluoresce with UV light. Urine coproporphyrin also is excessively increased. Iron accumulates in the cell.

Studies have revealed that microcytic, hypochromic anemia is not characteristic of elevated lead levels in children[24] (Table 6-10). Evidence suggests that if a microcytic anemia is present, it is most likely due to complications of iron deficiency or to the presence of alpha-thalassemia trait.[13,24,25] In one study, it was found that 33% of black children with lead poisoning and microcytosis had alpha-

TABLE 6-10 *HEMATOLOGIC VALUES FROM CHILDREN WITH NORMAL IRON LEVELS BUT INCREASED BLOOD LEAD LEVELS*

	Blood Lead Levels ($\mu g/dL$)		
	<29 (n = 53)	30–50 (n = 40)	>51 (n = 16)
Hb (g/L)	123	123	123
Hct (L/L)	0.36	0.36	0.37
MCV (fL)	79.5	78.5	74.6
MCHC (%)	34.0	34.0	33.4
Reticulocyte Count (%)	1.4	1.6	2.0

(From: Carraccio, C.L., Bergman, G.E. and Daley, B.P. Combined iron deficiency and lead poisoning in children. Effect on REP levels. *Clinical Pediatrics* 26, 644, 1987.)

TABLE 6-11 *1991 CDC GUIDELINES FOR EVALUATING AND TREATING CHILDHOOD LEAD POISONING*

Blood Lead Level	Decision
<10 μg/dL	Not considered to indicate lead poisoning
10–14 μg/dL	Increased monitoring suggested. If high lead poisoning prevalence in child's community, intervene with community-wide lead poisoning prevention.
15–19 μg/dL	Evaluate child and environment for sources of lead exposure if levels persist. Parents should receive education on lead poisoning prevention and nutrition. Retest more frequently.
20–44 μg/dL	Full medical evaluation is indicated. Remove sources of lead from child's environment. Drug treatment may be necessary.
45–69 μg/dL	Treat with chelators. Remove child to a lead-free environment until sources of lead exposure have been eliminated.
>70 μg/dL	Medical emergency; immediate therapy indicated.

thalassemia trait.[14] Coexistent iron deficiency and lead poisoning put children at a higher risk of developing even more serious lead poisoning because these children not only absorb larger portions of lead in iron deficient states, but the competitive inhibition of ferrochelatase by lead is even greater in the absence of iron. Thus, it is critical to make a diagnosis of iron deficiency when it coexists with lead poisoning.

In 1991, the Centers for Disease Control and Prevention (CDC) set a new acceptable blood lead level at 10 μg/dL or less, down from the 30 μg/dL level set in the mid-1970s. They also recommended five decision levels for evaluation and treatment depending on the lead level (Table 6-11). Although screening for lead by the ZPP measurement has been used in the past, it is no longer recommended as an appropriate screening tool since ZPP is unaffected until lead levels reach approximately 20 μg/dL,[25,26] and it is now apparant that lead levels less than 20 μg/dL can impair neuropsychologic development. ZPP may be useful as a screening tool in children with very high lead levels, but screening should generally be done by direct lead measurements.

Erythrocyte protoporphyrin cannot be used to differentiate iron deficiency and thalassemia in the presence of lead poisoning because of an increase in erythrocyte protoporphyrin caused by lead in thalassemia. Other tests, including iron studies to detect iron deficiency, hemoglobin electrophoresis and tests for hemoglobin H inclusions to detect thalassemias, may be indicated. If thalassemia is suspected, testing of parents may be helpful. The RDW also may be helpful. An RDW of less than 17 suggests thalassemia, while an RDW greater than 17 suggests iron deficiency.

ALCOHOLISM Sideroblastic anemia is a common finding in chronic alcohol intoxication, occurring in up to 31% of hospitalized alcoholics. Studies show that sideroblastic anemia is particularly common among alcoholics with a poor diet. This type of SA is associated with a concomitant decrease in folic acid and megaloblastosis. When the patient refrains from ethanol ingestion for 1 week, the ringed sideroblasts disappear. The alcohol is believed to inhibit the synthesis of pyridoxal phosphate and exacerbate the effect of folate deficiency. Alcoholics with a poor diet also may have an inadequate intake of pyridoxal phosphate. Alcohol is directly toxic to mitochondria.

SECONDARY TO MALIGNANCY Ringed sideroblasts may be found in diseases other than sideroblastic anemia. For example, ringed sideroblasts often are associated with hematologic malignancies (e.g., leukemia, malignant histiocytosis, multiple myeloma, lymphoma). Some investigators believe that the presence of ringed sideroblasts in these orders suggests that the malignancy may be the result of an abnormal clone of pluripotential stem cells that affects the erythrocyte as well as other cell lines. Occasionally, ringed sideroblasts appear in the bone marrow after treatment of malignant disease (e.g., multiple myeloma, Hodgkin's disease). This is a very poor prognostic sign, as these cases almost always terminate in acute leukemia.

CLINICAL FEATURES

In patients with acquired sideroblastic anemias secondary to drugs or malignancy, the manifestations of the underlying disorder are dominant. Patients with hereditary sideroblastic anemia or RARS, however, generally show primary signs and symptoms of anemia. In hereditary sideroblastic anemias, most patients also show signs associated with iron overload, including hepatomegaly, splenomegaly, and diabetes. In the latter stages of the disease, cardiac function may be affected.

LABORATORY FINDINGS

Peripheral blood The anemia is usually moderate to severe. A dimorphic picture of normochromic and hypochromic cells is characteristically seen in inherited and acquired forms of sideroblastic anemia (Fig. 6-7). Dual populations of macrocytes and microcytes also may be found. Mild macrocytosis is found in a significant minority of patients and is especially prevalent in RARS and in the sideroblastic anemia associated with alcoholism; a few hyochromic cells, however, are almost always found. If a dimorphic erythrocyte population is present, the MCV, MCH, and MCHC may be normal because these parameters are an average of all erythrocytes, thus emphasizing the need for careful examination of the blood smear. The RDW and erythrocyte histogram/cytogram are useful in detecting these dual populations. The RDW is increased and the histogram shows two peaks, representing the dual population. Poikilocytosis and target cells may be present. Erythrocytes may contain Pappenheimer bodies (iron deposits) (Fig. 6-8). When Pappenheimer bodies are present, reticulocyte counts must be performed carefully because both RNA and these iron-containing Pappenheimer bodies take up supravital stains. Basophilic stippling may be

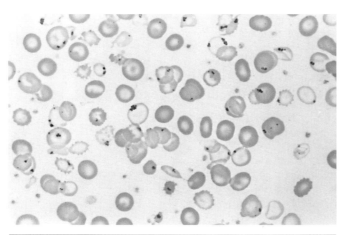

FIGURE 6-7. A blood film from a patient with sideroblastic anemia. Two populations of erythrocytes are present: hypochromic and normochromic. This is the dimorphic blood picture typical of sideroblastic anemia. Note also the numerous inclusions (Pappenheimer bodies). (PB; 250× original magnification; Wright-Giemsa stain.)

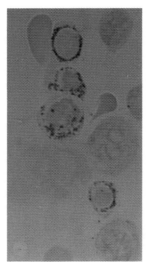

FIGURE 6-9. Ringed sideroblasts (Perl's Prussian blue stain; BM; 250× original magnification).

seen in any of the sideroblastic anemias. However, coarse, punctate, basophilic stippling resulting from aggregated ribosomes and degenerating mitochrondria is a particularly characteristic feature of lead poisoning. The erythrocyte protoporphyrin level in erythrocytes is typically increased. Rarely, nucleated erythrocytes may be present. Even though the bone marrow is usually hyperplastic, the reticulocyte production index is less than 2, indicating the anemia has an ineffective erythropoietic component. Leukocyte and platelet counts are usually normal but may be decreased. Thrombocytosis is found in about a third of patients. The serum bilirubin may be slightly increased (usually less than 2.0 mg/dL).

Iron studies Iron studies show increased serum iron, normal or decreased TIBC with increased saturation levels (sometimes reaching 100%), and increased serum ferritin. Plasma iron turnover is increased with defective iron utilization. These iron kinetic studies suggest an ineffective erythropoietic component.

Bone marrow Bone marrow changes include erythroid hyperplasia often accompanied by various degrees of megaloblastosis. The megaloblastosis is sometimes responsive to folate, which indicates the presence of a complicating folate deficiency. Normoblasts appear poorly hemoglobinized, with scanty, frayed cytoplasm. Macrophages contain increased amounts of storage iron. Ringed sideroblasts (Fig. 6-9) constitute over 40% of the normoblasts. The ringed sideroblasts must be present for the diagnosis of sideroblastic anemia; however, as mentioned previously, it is important to recognize that other disease entities may have ringed sideroblasts present without involving a diagnosis of sideroblastic anemia. These entities include megaloblastic anemia, primary bone marrow disorders, and malignancies. Chemotherapy also may be accompanied by the presence of ringed sideroblasts.

THERAPY

Pyridoxine therapy is generally tried on patients with the hereditary form of sideroblastic anemia; less than half experience a return to normal hemoglobin levels with this form of therapy. Folic acid also is administered to those with megaloblastic features. Sometimes the risk of hemochromatosis is lessened by removal of excess body iron (usually by phlebotomy). Some patients live for many years tolerating their anemia well, while others die because of complications of iron overload, infections, or bone marrow failure.

Idiopathic sideroblastic anemia (RARS) is refractory to all therapy and requires blood transfusion to maintain an adequate hemoglobin level. With each blood transfusion, however, about 250 mg of iron is given to a patient already overloaded with iron. New techniques to increase iron mobilization and excretion with the chelator, desferrioxamine, may prove useful in these patients. Pyridoxine (large nonphysiologic doses) and folic acid therapy may rarely

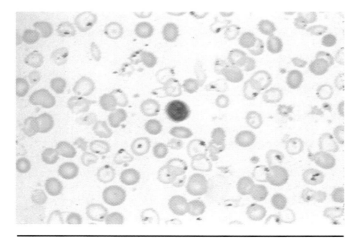

FIGURE 6-8. Sideroblastic anemia, note numerous Pappenheimer bodies and dual cell population—hypochromic and normochromic. (PB; 250× original magnification; Wright-Giemsa stain.)

elicit a hematologic response. Most often, the disease is marked by progressive debility and death from secondary causes (infection, secondary hemochromatosis) or by development of acute leukemia.

Secondary sideroblastic anemia resulting from a disease, toxin, or drug may be corrected by successful treatment of the disease or by elimination of the toxin/drug.

● Anemia of chronic disease

The anemia of chronic disease (ACD) is usually defined as the anemia that occurs in patients with chronic infections (including acquired immune deficiency syndrome), inflammatory disorders, or neoplastic disorders not due to bleeding, hemolysis, or marrow involvement and characterized by hypoferremia but normal iron stores (Table 6-12).[27] Other diseases found to be associated with ACD include congestive heart failure, thrombophlebitis, deep leg vein thrombosis, and ischemic heart disease.[28] The anemia appears to be a specific entity and does not relate to any nutritional deficiency. Anemias associated with renal, endocrine, or hepatic insufficiency are usually excluded from ACD.

Anemia of chronic disease is the most common anemia among hospitalized patients. In one study of patients admitted to an acute geriatric ward, 24% were found to be anemic and 35% of these patients had ACD.[29] Anemia is present in up to 50% of patients with malignant solid tumors and is the most common hematologic abnormality in cancer patients. Often anemia is the clue that leads to a diagnosis of cancer. The most common anemia in these patients is ACD. There is a rough correlation between the degree of anemia and the extent of underlying disease.[30]

PATHOPHYSIOLOGY
Several faulty mechanisms of heme synthesis may be attributed to this anemia. First, it is hypothesized that the anemia occurs as the result of cytokine inhibition of erythropoietin (EPO) production and EPO action on stem cells.[31] These cytokines are produced as a result of the immune response and/or inflammatory process. In general, the EPO levels in patients with anemia of chronic disease are lower than in anemic patients with similar hemoglobin levels but absence of chronic disease.[32,33] This finding suggests a blunted EPO response to anemia in ACD. Two cytokines, IL-1 and tumor necrosis factor (TNF), that play a significant role in inflammation and the immune response are increased in many patients with ACD. These cytokines may contribute to the development of ACD by inhibiting EPO production and marrow erythropoiesis.[27] Pharmacologic doses of EPO overcome this inhibitory effect and correct the anemia in some patients with ACD.[27] Second, there appears to be a block in the release of iron from macrophages for recycling resulting in a diminished iron flow to the bone marrow normoblasts. It is possible that the cytokines affect the release of iron from the macrophage as well as inhibiting erythropoiesis. Third, the erythrocyte survival time is shortened as a result of extracorpuscular factors. The reason for the decreased erythrocyte lifespan is unknown, but several mechanisms have been suggested, including nonspecific macrophage activation, hemolytic factors elaborated by tumors, vascular factors, and the presence of bacterial toxins capable of hemolyzing erythrocytes. Of these three mechanisms, inhibited EPO production with impaired erythropoiesis is probably the most important.

CLINICAL FINDINGS
The signs and symptoms of the anemia of chronic disease are usually those associated with the underlying disorder. Rarely severe, the degree of the anemia correlates with the activity of the underlying disease.

LABORATORY FINDINGS

Peripheral blood A mild anemia with a hemoglobin of not less than 90 g/L and hematocrit of not less than 0.27 L/L is characteristic. Erythrocytes are usually normocytic, normochromic but may present as normocytic, hypochromic or, in long-standing cases, microcytic, hypochromic. In contrast to iron deficiency anemia, in anemia of chronic disease hypochromia of erythrocytes precedes the microcytosis. The reticulocyte production index is less than 2. The leukocyte count and platelet count are normal, unless changed due to the primary disease state.

Iron studies Iron studies show decreased plasma iron (10 to 70 μg/dL), decreased TIBC (100 to 300 μg/dL), low transferrin saturation (10% to 25%), and normal or in-

TABLE 6-12 *CONDITIONS ASSOCIATED WITH THE ANEMIA OF CHRONIC DISORDERS*

Chronic infections
   Pulmonary infections: abscesses, emphysema, tuberculosis, pneumonia
   Subacute bacterial endocarditis
   Pelvic inflammatory disease
   Osteomyelitis
   Chronic urinary tract infections
   Chronic fungal disease
   Meningitis

Chronic, noninfectious inflammations
   Rheumatoid arthritis
   Rheumatic fever
   Systemic lupus erythematosus
   Severe trauma
   Thermal injury
   Adjuvant disease in rats
   Sterile abscesses

Malignant diseases
   Carcinoma
   Hodgkin's disease
   Lymphosarcoma
   Leukemia
   Multiple myeloma

Miscellaneous
   Alcoholic liver disease
   Congestive heart failure
   Thrombophlebitis
   Ischemic heart disease

"Idiopathic"

(From: Lee, E.R., Bithell, T.C., Foerster, J., Athens, J.W., Lukens, J.N.: Wintrobe's clinical hematology. Philadelphia: Lea & Febiger, 1993.)

TABLE 6-13 *DIFFERENTIAL DIAGNOSIS OF ANEMIAS CAUSED BY DEFECTIVE HEMOGLOBIN SYNTHESIS*

	Serum Iron	TIBC	% Saturation	Serum Ferritin	ZPP	Bone Marrow Macrophage Iron	Bone Marrow Sideroblasts	Hemoglobin Electrophoresis
Iron Deficiency Anemia	↓	↑	↓	↓	↑	↓	↓	N
Sideroblastic Anemia	↑	N or ↓	↑	↑	N or ↑	↑	↑ ringed forms	N
Anemia of Chronic Disease	↓	N or ↓	↓	N or ↑	N or ↑	N or ↑	↓	N
Thalassemia Trait	N	N	N	↑	N	N or ↑	N or ↑	↑A_2 N or ↑F

TIBC = Total iron binding capacity; ZPP = zinc protoporphyrin; ↓ = decreased; ↑ = increased; N = Normal

creased serum ferritin. Serum ferritin may be helpful in distinguishing this anemia from iron deficiency anemia. Although serum iron and percent saturation are low in both anemias, serum ferritin, which reflects body iron stores, is normal or increased in chronic disease and low in iron deficiency (Table 6-13).

It is important to keep in mind that ferritin is an acute phase reactant and is very often increased in infectious and inflammatory conditions. Therefore in ACD, serum ferritin may be normal even if concurrent iron deficiency exists. If serum ferritin falls in the range of 20 to 100 μg/L in anemia of chronic disease, another means of assessing iron should be considered such as serum transferrin receptor assay or bone marrow examination.[34] Serum transferrin receptor is high in iron deficiency but normal in uncomplicated anemia of chronic disease.

Erythrocyte protoporphyrin Since ACD is partially due to iron deficient erythropoiesis, the ZPP levels are markedly increased.[35,36]

Bone marrow The bone marrow usually shows an increased M:E ratio because of a decrease in erythrocyte precursors. The proportion of younger normoblasts is increased. Poor hemoglobin production is apparent, especially in the polychromatophilic normoblasts. The proportion of sideroblasts decreases to less than 30%; however, the macrophages appear to have increased amounts of hemosiderin. This finding helps to distinguish the anemia of chronic disease from iron deficiency anemia. In iron deficiency, there is an absence of macrophage iron as well as an absence of sideroblasts.

THERAPY

The anemia is alleviated by successful treatment of the underlying disease. The anemia is usually mild and nonprogressive; thus, transfusion is rarely warranted, except in older patients with vascular disease and circulatory insufficiency.

Hemochromatosis

Iron overload is said to exist when total body iron is in excess of 4 g. Hemochromatosis is a term used to describe the clinical disorder that results in parenchymal tissue damage from iron overload. Hemochromatosis may occur when there is an inappropriate increase in the intestinal absorption of iron (primary idiopathic hemochromatosis, hepatic cirrhosis) or with chronic transfusion therapy (in each blood transfusion, the patient receives about 250 mg of iron). The danger of hemochromatosis lies in the fact that excess iron deposits are stored not only in macrophages but also in hepatocytes, cardiac cells, endocrine cells, and other parenchymal tissue. These excess iron deposits interfere with the normal function of these cells or may even cause cell death. This situation has potential fatal consequences, especially in relation to cardiac tissue.

In hemochromatosis, the serum ferritin and serum iron levels are elevated but the TIBC is normal or low. The saturation of transferrin is high, sometimes approaching 100%. Biopsy of liver and bone marrow reveal massive iron deposits. Anemia is not usually present unless there are complicating conditions.

Treatment of hemochromatosis includes the infusion of iron chelators (e.g., desferrioxamine) to help bind iron and excrete it in the urine. Only a very small amount of iron is released from the storage pool and is available for complex formation at one time; thus, continuous infusion of the chelator removes this iron over a long period of time. Chelator therapy is the primary form of treatment for transfusion induced hemochromatosis. For idoipathic hemochromatosis, phlebotomy is usually the treatment. Each unit of blood removed eliminates about 250 mg of iron. It is suggested that following initial venesection therapy to deplete iron stores, iron status be monitored annually by serum ferritin levels.[37]

PORPHYRIAS

Porphyrins are synthesized in most tissue, but the liver and bone marrow are the major sites of synthesis. Porphyrins are required for heme synthesis and for enzymes that function in oxidation-reduction reactions and electron transport.

The porphyrias are a group of inherited disorders characterized by a block in porphyrin synthesis. Abnormal porphyrin metabolism is due to a defect in one or more enzymes in the pathway of heme synthesis. As a result of these enzyme deficiencies, porphyrins accumulate in tissues and large amounts are excreted in the urine and/or feces. These excess porphyrin deposits cause most of the symptoms and clinical findings associated with porphyria.

TABLE 6-14 *CLASSIFICATION AND CHARACTERISTICS OF THE PORPHYRIAS*

| Porphyria | Mode of Inheritance | Probable Enzymatic Defect | Metabolites in Excess | | | Tissue Source |
			Urine	Feces	Erythroid Cells	
Erythropoietic Porphyria	Autosomal recessive	Uroporphyrinogen III cosynthetase	Uroporphyrin I Coproporphyrin I	Coproporphyrin I Uroporphyrin I	Uroporphyrin I Coproporhyrin I	Erythropoietic
Erythropoietic Protoporphyria	Autosomal dominant	Ferrocheletase	Normal	Protoporphyrin	Protoporphyrin	Erythropoietic and occasionally hepatic
Acute Intermittent Porphyria	Autosomal dominant	Uroporphyrinogen I synthetase	δ-ALA, Porphobilinogen	Normal	Normal	Hepatic
Hereditary Coproporphyria	Autosomal dominant	Coproporphyrinogen oxidase	Coproporphyrin III	Coproporphyrin III	Normal	Hepatic
Variegate Porphyria	Autosomal dominant	Protoporphyrinogen oxidase	Porphobilinogen, δ-ALA	Protoporphyrin Coproporphyrin	Normal	Hepatic
Porphyria Cutanea Tarda	Autosomal dominant	Uroporphyrinogen decarboxylase	Uroporphyrin I Uroporphyrin III	Protoporphyrin (normal to slight) Coproporphyrin (normal to slight)	Normal	Hepatic

The most common findings include photosensitivity, abdominal pain, and neuropathy (motor dysfunction, sensory loss, and mental disturbances). There is, however, adequate production of heme for hemoglobin synthesis.

The porphyrias, although rare, have received wide recognition and stimulated interest because the disease affected the royal families of England and Scotland, especially those descended from Mary, Queen of Scots. Historians have described George III as suffering from a mental and physical disorder believed to have been porphyria, which affected his ability to rule. Princess Charlotte, the granddaughter of George III and heir to the throne, died in childbirth; her death was attributed to an acute porphyria attack at the time of delivery.[38]

Two forms of porphyria, erythropoietic and hepatic, are expressed depending on the primary site of defective porphyrin metabolism, the bone marrow or the liver (Table 6-14). Only the erythropoietic porphyrias affect the erythrocytes. Therefore, these porphyrias will be discussed here.

●
Pathophysiology

The erythropoietic prophyrias result from an abnormality of the enzymes in the heme biosynthetic pathway within the normoblasts of the bone marrow. At least two types exist: erythropoietic porphyria (EP) and erythropoietic protoporphyria (EPP). These two types are classified according to the particular enzyme defect and to the excessive porphyrin intermediaries produced. Although EP is associated with hemolytic anemia, anemia in EPP is rare.

Porphyrins are functionless products produced by the irreversible oxidation of series I and series III porphyrinogens. Porphyrinogens of the III series are the precursors of heme, whereas, the series I porphyrinogens are func-

tionless, dead end compounds. Normally, in heme synthesis, most porphyrinogens are readily converted to heme and very small amounts of the porphyrins are formed. If, for some reason, excessive amounts of porphyrinogen are produced, the oxidized porphyrin compounds also increase. Porphyrins are resonating compounds; thus, erythrocytes that contain these substances can be shown to fluoresce with UV light.

ERYTHROPOIETIC PORPHYRIA (GUNTHER'S DISEASE)

Erythropoietic porphyria (EP), also referred to as congenital erythropoietic porphyria (CEP), is characterized by the presence of excessive amounts of series I porphyrins: uroporphyrin I (Uro I) and coproporphyrin I (Copro I). There is no known physiologic function for the series I isomers. They cannot be used in heme synthesis. In normal heme synthesis, both isomers I and III are formed but in a 1:10,000 ratio. In erythropoietic porphyria, the large amount of series I porphyrins suggests there is a defect in uroporphyrinogen III cosynthetase channeling the porphobilinogen into the functionless Uro I isomer (Fig. 6-10). On the other hand, enough Uro III is produced to generate adequate amounts of heme. This suggests that a deficiency of cosynthetase may not be the only enzyme abnormality. Another possibility for the excessive amounts of Uro I isomer is hyperactivity of the uroporphyrin I synthetase. The support for either of these hypotheses requires purification, characterization, and accurate measurement of these enzymes.

The excess porphyrins are deposited in body tissues and excreted in urine and feces. Their presence can be verified by intense fluorescence with ultraviolet light (400 to 410 nm). The cause of the hemolytic anemia that accompanies EP is unknown, but it is believed to be closely associated with the excessive porphyrin deposits within erythrocytes. This is supported by the finding that normal erythrocytes

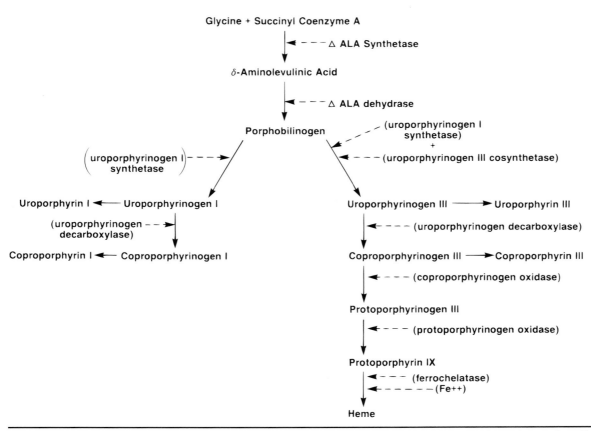

FIGURE 6-10. The formation of heme from glycine and succinyl-coenzyme A involves the production of porphyrinogen intermediates. Normally, only very small amounts of the series I isomers are formed. However, in the hereditary condition erythropoietic porphyria, there is an abnormality in this pathway and large amounts of the funtionless series I isomers are formed. These isomers are oxidized to porphyrin and accumulate in the tissues. Another form of porphyria, erythropoietic protoporphyria is characterized by excessive production of protoporphyrin.

infused into EP patients have a normal lifespan. The erythrocytes in EP may be subject to photohemolysis as they pass through the dermal capillaries that are exposed to UV light. The erythrocytes show increased photohemolysis in vitro but it is uncertain as to whether this is also an in vivo phenomenon.

ERYTHROPOIETIC PROTOPORPHYRIA
Erythropoietic protoporphyria (EPP) is characterized by an overproduction of protoporphyrin, the immediate precursor of heme. This suggests a defect in ferrochelatase (Fig. 6-10). The activity of this enzyme has been measured in bone marrow, reticulocytes, peripheral blood, and the liver from EPP patients, and its activity is consistently decreased. Adequate amounts of heme are produced, however, and no anemia is present. Excess protoporphyrin can be found in the blood and feces but, due to its insolubility in water, protoporphyrin is not present in the urine. This porphyria is believed to be of both erythropoietic and hepatic origin.

● Clinical features
Erythropoietic porphyria is a rare autosomal recessive disease with less than 100 cases reported. EPP is inherited as

an autosomal dominant trait but recessive inheritance is possible.[39] About 300 cases of EPP have been reported, but the actual rate of occurrence is probably masked due to the subtlety of the clinical signs and the absence of colored porphyrins in the urine.

The first signs of EP occur in infancy. The urine is colored pink to reddish brown, depending on the amount of uroporphyrin excreted. This is usually first noted as a pink stain on the infant's diaper. The excess porphyrins in the skin create an extreme photosensitivity to sunlight. Vesicular or bullous eruptions appear on bared areas shortly after exposure. The lesions heal slowly and may become infected. Repeated eruptions and skin injury cause scarring and may lead to severe mutilation of the face, ears, and hands. The excess porphyrin stains the teeth a dirty brown. In UV light, the teeth fluorese bright red. Hypertrichosis affects the entire body but is especially present in exposed areas. The hair may be blonde and downy or coarse and dark. Splenomegaly is a consistent finding and is usually progressive with the disease. A mild to severe hemolytic anemia is present with erythrocyte lifespan decreased to as little as 18 days. Patients with EP never exhibit the abdominal pain or neurologic and psychotic signs associated with hepatic porphyrias.

Clinical signs of EPP are more subtle, and its course is relatively mild in comparison to EP. Photosensitivity is not severe and scarring is usually absent. Sunlight exposure leads to erythema and urticaria. Protoporphyrin accumulates in the erythrocytes, which causes them to fluoresce intensely, but there is no hemolytic anemia. Occasionally hepatic damage occurs.

Laboratory findings

ERYTHROPOIETIC PORPHYRIA

The peripheral blood in EP exhibits a mild to severe normocytic anemia with anisocytosis and poikilocytosis. The blood smear reveals significant polychromatophilia and nucleated erythrocytes. Reticulocytes are increased. The erythrocytes fluoresce with UV light.

The bone marrow in EP shows erythroid hyperplasia. A large portion of the normoblasts demonstrate intense fluorescence with UV light. The fluorescence is localized principally in the nuclei. The fact that not all normoblasts fluoresce suggests that two populations of erythrocytes exist of which one is normal.

There is an increase in plasma iron turnover with a decrease in iron utilization. This suggests the anemia may be partly caused by an ineffective erythropoietic component. Serum iron and storage iron are usually normal.

Haptoglobin is absent and unconjugated bilirubin, urinary, and fecal urobilinogen are increased.

Large amounts of uroporphyrin I and coproporphyrin I are excreted in the urine and feces. These isomers also are found in the plasma and in erythrocytes. Series III isomers of these porphyrins also are increased.

ERYTHROPOIETIC PROTOPORPHYRIA

The blood and bone marrow in EPP usually reveal no abnormalities on routine examination; however, with UV light, the cytoplasm of normoblasts fluoresce intensely. The erythrocytes, plasma, and feces contain large amounts of protoporphyrin. The protoporphyrins are not found in the urine. The protoporphyrin in erythrocytes is free (FEP), not bound to zinc as in iron deficiency anemia and lead poisoning.[40] The FEP is higher than in other disorders associated with an increase in erythrocyte protoporphyrin levels. It would be expected that this block in heme synthesis occurring in the reaction just before insertion of iron into the porphyrin ring would cause an accumulation of iron within the normoblasts. The fact that this iron build-up does not occur cannot be explained.

Prognosis and therapy

Individuals with EP do not usually survive beyond the fifth decade of life. Attempts to decrease the excess porphyrins have been unsuccessful, but the quality of life for EP patients has improved by minimizing the scarring and mutilation with effective dermatologic treatment. Avoidance of exposure to sunlight is critical. Splenectomy has sometimes resulted in a decrease of porphyrin production and helped ameliorate the hemolytic anemia. Evidence for long-term success with splenectomy, however, is questionable. Blood transfusion in conjunction with administra-

tion of chelators to reduce iron overload suppresses erythropoiesis and decreases or eliminates symptoms. Treatment of EPP is aimed at protecting the skin from sunlight and minimizing the toxic effects of protoporphyrin on the liver. In most patients with EPP, high doses of β-carotene improve tolerance to sunlight. Blood transfusions and hematin may be used to suppress erythropoiesis. Splenectomy may be helpful if hemolysis and splenomegaly are prominent. Cholestyramine may promote excretion of liver protoporphyrin.[41]

SUMMARY

Hemoglobin synthesis requires adequate production of heme and globin. Inadequate amounts of either may result in microcytic, hypochromic anemia. Defects in heme synthesis may be due to faulty iron or porphyrin metabolism. Defects in globin synthesis are due to genetic defects that affect production of the globin chains. These globin defects are known as thalassemias. The anemias with a faulty iron metabolic component include iron deficiency, ACD, and SA. Iron deficiency anemia is due to inadequate amounts of iron for heme synthesis. This iron deficiency usually occurs due to blood loss or a nutritional deficiency of iron. ACD has several pathophysiologic mechanisms: decreased erythropoiesis, block in reutilization of macrophage iron, and a decreased erythrocyte survival. The erythrocytes are normocytic normochromic but in some cases are microcytic hypochromic. SA is due to defective porphyrin synthesis and a block in the insertion of iron into the poryphyrin ring to form heme. The erythrocyte population in SA characteristically contains cells that are normochromic as well as cells that are hypochromic (dual population). There are ringed sideroblasts in the bone marrow.

Iron studies are helpful in differentiating these disorders. Serum transferrin is increased and saturation decreased if total body iron is decreased, whereas if storage iron is normal or increased, the serum transferrin is normal or decreased with normal or increased saturation. Serum ferritin is a reliable indicator of iron stores except in the presence of inflammation or infection when it is falsely increased. The serum transferrin receptor assay is useful in differentiating iron deficiency and ACD. Levels are increased in iron deficiency and normal in ACD.

Hemochromatosis is a disorder characterized by total body iron excess. This may be due to chronic transfusion or inappropriate increase in intestinal absorption. Serum iron studies reflect the excessive iron overload with increased serum ferritin and a very high saturation of transferrin.

The porphyrias are a heterogeneous group of hereditary disorders that are due to a block in porphyrin synthesis. The defect is in a critical enzyme in the porphyrin metabolic pathway. Only two porphyrias have a erythropoietic component, EP and EPP. Excess porphyrins are deposited in body tissues and excreted in feces and/or urine. Erythrocytes have very high levels of free erythrocyte protoporphyrin. In EP, the erythrocytes have decreased survival but in EPP, survival appears normal.

REVIEW QUESTIONS

An 83-year-old man was admitted to a local hospital with recurrent urinary tract bleeding and an infection associated with prostatitis.

Admission Laboratory Data:
RBC: 4.15×10^{12}/L
Hb: 81 gm/L
Hct: 0.26 L/L
PLT: 174×10^9/L
WBC: 2.8×10^9/L

Differential:
Segmented Neutrophils: 71%
Band Neutrophils: 9%
Lymphocytes: 18%
Monocytes: 2%

RBC morphology: Red cells show mild hypochromasia with marked microcytosis. Marked poikilocytosis is present with 3+ target cells, 2+ elliptocytes, 1+ echinocytes, 1+ schistocytes, and rare spherocytes.

Laboratory Data for Anemia Work-up:
Reticulocyte count: 2.6%
Serum Iron: 18 μg/dL
Total iron-binding capacity (TIBC): 425 μg/dL
Transferrin saturation: 4.2%

1. Which anemia of defective heme synthesis does this case probably represent?
   a. sideroblastic anemia
   b. anemia of chronic disease
   c. iron deficiency anemia
   d. erythropoietic porphyria

2. Which laboratory result is most useful in distinguishing iron deficiency anemia from anemia of chronic disease?
   a. serum iron
   b. MCV
   c. hemoglobin
   d. transferrin receptor

3. If a serum ferritin and zinc protoporphyrin (ZPP) were performed on the patient described in question 1, which set of results would you expect?
   a. serum ferritin decreased; ZPP increased
   b. serum ferritin normal; ZPP decreased
   c. serum ferritin increased; ZPP increased
   d. serum ferritin decreased; ZPP decreased

4. What is the most common cause of iron deficiency?
   a. poor diet
   b. chronic blood loss
   c. malabsorption
   d. increased iron requirement

5. What is the iron transport protein?
   a. ferritin
   b. transferrin
   c. hemosiderin
   d. albumin

6. If a serum transferrin receptor assay were performed on an iron deficient individual, what would you expect the results to be?
   a. increased
   b. decreased
   c. normal

7. If a child with lead poisoning also had a significant microcytic, hypochromic anemia, what complicating pathology (pathologies) should be considered?
   a. iron deficiency
   b. thalassemia
   c. iron deficiency and thalassemia
   d. sideroblastic anemia

8. Screening for lead by the ZPP measurement is not an appropriate screening tool for elevated blood lead levels in children because:
   a. the ZPP is not affected until blood lead levels reach 20 μg/dL
   b. lead poisoning does not cause elevation of ZPP in children
   c. the procedure is more expensive and difficult to perform than direct lead measurements
   d. changes in the hemoglobin concentration and erythrocyte indices are more accurate indicators of lead poisoning

9. Which of the following statements is true concerning sideroblastic anemia?
   a. the hereditary form occurs most frequently in females
   b. there are ringed sideroblasts in the bone marrow
   c. there is a deficiency of iron delivered to the developing normoblasts
   d. it almost always terminates in acute leukemia

10. Which of the following set of results is most characteristic of ACD?
    a. plasma iron decreased, TIBC increased, transferrin saturation increased, ferritin decreased
    b. plasma iron increased, TIBC decreased, transferrin saturation increased, ferritin decreased
    c. plasma iron decreased, TIBC increased, transferrin saturation decreased, ferritin increased
    d. plasma iron decreased, TIBC decreased, transferrin saturation decreased, ferritin normal or increased

REFERENCES

1. Brittenham, G.M.: Disorders of iron metabolism: Iron deficiency and overload. In Hematology: Basic Principles and Practice. Edited by R. Hoffman, E.J. Benz Jr., S.J. Shattil, B. Furie, H.J. Cohen. New York: Churchill Livingstone, 1995.
2. Gaven, M.W., McCarthy, D.M., Garry, P.J.: Evidence that iron stores regulate iron absorption—a setpoint theory. Am. J. Clin. Nutr., 59:1376, 1994.
3. Beilby, J., et al.: Transferrin index: an alternative method for calculating the iron saturation of transferrin. Clin. Chem., 38:2078, 1992.
4. Testa, U., Pelosi, E., Peschle, C.: The transferrin receptor. Crit. Rev. Oncol., 4(3):241, 1993.

5. Fairweather-Tait, S.: Iron. Int. J. Vitam. Nutr. Res., 63(4):296, 1993.
6. Oski, F.A.: Iron deficiency in infancy and childhood. N. Engl. J. Med., 329(3):190, 1993.
7. Brumberg, J.J.: Chlorotic girls, 1870–1920: a historical perspective on female adolescence. Child. Dev., 53:1468, 1982.
8. Ovaert, C., Backy, A.: Iron deficiency is not always simple. Arch. Fr. Pediatr., 50:697, 1993.
9. Thompson, W.G., Meola, T., Lipkin, M.Jr., Freedman, M.L.: Red cell distribution width, mean corpuscular volume, and transferrin saturation in the diagnosis of iron deficiency. Arch. Intern. Med., 148:2128, 1988.
10. Junca, J., Flores, A., Roy, C., Alberti, R., Milla, F.: Red cell distribution width, free erythrocyte protoporphyrin, and England-Fraser index in the differential diagnosis of microcytosis due to iron deficiency or beta-thalassemia trait. A study of 200 cases of microcytic anemia. Hematol. Pathol., 5:33, 1991.
11. Rector, W.G. Jr.: Pica: Its frequency and significance in patients with iron-deficiency anemia due to chronic gastrointestinal blood loss. J. Gen. Intern. Med., 4:512, 1989.
12. Carmel, R., Weiner, J.M., Johnson, C.S.: Iron deficiency occurs frequently in patients with pernicious anemia. JAMA, 257:1081, 1987.
13. Bhambhani, K., Aronow, R.: Lead poisoning and thalassemia trait or iron deficiency. The value of the red blood cell distribution width. Am. J. Dis. Child., 144:1231, 1990.
14. Lowenstein, W., et al.: Free erythrocyte protoporphyrin assay in the diagnosis of iron deficiency in the anemic aged subject. A prospective study of 103 anemic patients Ann. Med. Intern., 142:13, 1991.
15. Withold, W., et al.: Efficacy of transferrin determination in human sera in the diagnosis of iron deficiency. Eur. J. Clin. Chem. Clin. Biochem., 32:19, 1994.
16. Vreugdenhil, G., Baltus, C.A., van Eijk, H.G., Swaak, A.J.: Anaemia of chronic disease: Diagnostic significance of erythrocyte and serological parameters in iron deficient rheumatoid arthritis patients. Br. J. Rheumatol., 29:105, 1990.
17. Coenen, J.L., et al.: Measurements of serum ferritin used to predict concentrations of iron in bone marrow in anemia of chronic disease. Clin. Chem., 37:560, 1991.
18. Sahay, R., Scott, B.B.: Iron deficiency anemia—how far to investigate? Gut, 34:1427, 1993.
19. Ferguson, B.J., et al.: Serum transferrin receptor distinguishes the anemia of chronic disease from iron deficiency anemia. J. Lab. Clin. Med., 119:385, 1992.
20. Kohgo, Y., et al.: Serum transferrin receptor as a new index of erythropoiesis. Blood, 70:1955, 1987.
21. Cox, T.C., et al.: Erythroid 5-aminolevulinate synthase is located on the X-chromosome. Am. J. Hum. Genet., 46:107, 1990.
22. Sutherland, G.R,. et al.: 5-aminolevulinate synthase is at 3p21 and thus not the primary defect in x-linked sideroblastic anemia. Am. J. Hum. Genet., 43:331, 1988.
23. MMWR, 44:515,1995.
24. Carraccio, C.L., Bergman, G.E., Daley, B.P.: Combined iron deficiency and lead poisoning in children. Effect on FEP levels. Clin. Pediatr., 26:644, 1987.
25. Clark, M., Royal, J., Seeler, R.: Interaction of iron deficiency and lead and the hematologic findings in children with severe lead poisoning. Pediatr., 81:247, 1988.
26. Rainey, P.M.: Lead—a heavy burden for small children. Clin. Chem. News., 18(6):37, 1992.
27. Means, R.T. Jr., Krantz, S.B.: Progress in understanding the pathogenesis of the anemia of chronic disease. Blood, 80:1639, 1992.
28. Cash, J.M., Sears, D.A.: The anemia of chronic disease: spectrum of associated diseases in a series of unselected hospitalized patients. Am. J Med., 87:638, 1989.
29. Joosten, E., et al.: Prevalence and causes of anaemia in a geriatric hospitalized population. Gerontol., 38:111, 1992.
30. Dutcher, J.P.: Hematologic abnormalities in patients with nonhematologic malignancies. Hem. Onc. Clin. North. Am., 1:281, 1987.
31. Krantz, S.B.: Pathogenesis and treatment of the anemia of chronic disease. Am. J. Med. Sci., 307:353, 1994.
32. Miller, C.B., et al.: Decreased erythropoietin response in patients with the anemia of cancer. N. Engl. J. Med., 322:1689, 1990.
33. Baer, A.N., Dessypris, E.N., Goldwasser, E., Krantz, S.B.: Blunted erythropoietin response to anemia in rheumatoid arthritis. Br. J. Haematol., 66:559, 1987.
34. Ferguson, B.J., et al.: Serum transferrin receptor distinguishes the anemia of chronic disease from iron deficiency anemia. J. Lab. Clin. Med., 19:385, 1992.
35. Hastka, J., et al.: Zinc protoporphyrin in anemia of chronic disorders. Blood, 81:1200, 1993.
36. Garrett, S., Worwood, M.: Zinc protoporphyrin and iron-deficient erythropoiesis. Acta. Haematol., 91:21, 1994.
37. Adams, P.C., Kertesz, A.E., Valberg, L.S.: Rate of iron reaccumulation following iron depletion in hereditary hemochromatosis. Implications for venesection therapy. J. Clin. Gastroenterol., 16(3):207, 1993.
38. Miale, J.B.: Laboratory Medicine: Hematology. 6th Ed., St. Louis: CV Mosby Co., 1982.
39. Mascaro, J.M.: Porphyrias in children. Pediatr. Dermatol., 9:371, 1992.
40. Paslin, D.A.: The porphyrias. Int. J. Dermatol., 312:527, 1992.
41. Desnick, R.J., Anderson, K.E.: Heme biosynthesis and its disorders: The porphyrias and sideroblastic anemias. In: Hematology: Basic Principles and Practice. Edited by R. Hoffman, E.J. Benz Jr., S.J. Shattil, B. Furie, H.J. Cohen. New York: Churchill Livingstone, 1995.

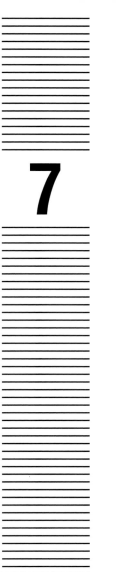

Anemias caused by abnormalities in globin biosynthesis

7

CHAPTER OUTLINE

KEY TERMS

hemoglobinopathies
thalassemias
congenital Heinz body
  hemolytic anemias
vaso-occlusive crises
autosplenectomy

INTRODUCTION

Clinical diseases that result from a genetically determined abnormality of the structure or synthesis of the hemoglobin molecule are called *hemoglobinopathies*. The abnormality is associated with the globin chains; the heme portion of the molecule is normal. The globin abnormality may be either a qualitative defect in the globin chain (structural abnormality) or a quantitative defect in globin synthesis.

Qualitatively abnormal hemoglobin molecules are the result of genetic mutations involving amino acid deletions or substitutions in the globin protein chain. These mutations cause structural variation in one of the globin chain classes (structural hemoglobin variants). The nomenclature of these disorders is discussed in a later section. The most common clinical disorder of this type of mutation is sickle cell anemia.

The quantitative globin disorders are the result of various genetic defects that cause reduced synthesis of structurally normal globin chains. The quantitative disorders are known collectively as the *thalassemias*.

As a result of the globin chain defects, hemoglobinopathies are frequently, but not always, associated with a chronic hemolytic anemia. Clinical expression of the hemoglobinopathy varies depending on the class of globin chain involved (α, β, δ, or γ), the severity of hemolysis, and the compensatory production of other normal globin chains.[1] Some of the hemoglobinopathies produce no clinical signs or symptoms of disease and are identified only through population studies specifically designed to reveal "silent" carriers. As discovery of silent carriers increases, the incidence of these genetic disorders is proving to be much higher than originally thought. This is especially true for the thalassemias. About 100,000 to 200,000 individuals are born each year with a severe form of thalassemia. It is believed that hemoglobinopathies are the most common lethal hereditary diseases in humans.[2,3]

Hemoglobinopathies are found worldwide but occur most commonly in African blacks and ethnic groups from the Mediterranean basin and southeast Asia. The geographic locations where the quantitative and qualitative hemoglobin disorders are found frequently overlap; thus, it is not uncommon for individuals to have a structural hemoglobin variant together with a form of thalassemia. This may partly explain the wide variety of clinical findings associated with hemoglobinopathies.

The first part of this chapter discusses the structural hemoglobin variants, and the second part discusses the thalassemias.

STRUCTURAL HEMOGLOBIN VARIANTS

Identification of hemoglobin variants

The largest group of hemoglobinopathies results from an inherited structural change in one of the globin chains; however, synthesis of the abnormal chain is usually not impaired. Any of the globin chain classes, α, β, δ, or γ, may be affected.

The most common structural hemoglobinopathy, sickle cell anemia, was recorded by James Herrick of Chicago in 1910.[4] Herrick described the typical crescent-shaped sickled erythrocytes in a young black student from the West Indies. After this initial report, additional cases of the disease were described, and the clinical pattern of sickle cell anemia was established. The pathophysiologic aspects of the disease, however, remained a mystery until Linus Pauling in 1949 discovered the altered electrophoretic mobility of the hemoglobin in patients with sickle cell disease.[5] The altered electrical charge of the molecule was ascribed to a molecular abnormality of the globin chain. More than 300 abnormal hemoglobins have since been discovered.

Most structural hemoglobin variants result from a single amino acid substitution or deletion in the non-α polypeptide globin chain. Substitutions and deletions, however, do not necessarily alter the physical (solubility and stability) or functional properties of the hemoglobin molecule. Only when the mutation affects these properties does clinical disease result. In fact, the majority of the structural variants result in no clinical or hematologic abnormality and have only been discovered by population studies or through family studies. Certain substitutions at critical interaction sites, however, may alter the structure of the hemoglobin molecule in such a way as to profoundly affect its function, solubility, or stability. These phenotypic variants produce both clinical and hematologic abnormalities of varying severity, depending on the nature and site of the mutation.

HEMOGLOBIN ELECTROPHORESIS

Hemoglobin carries an electrical charge resulting from the presence of carboxyl (COOH) and protonated (H+) nitrogen groups. The type and strength of the charge depends on both the amino acid sequence of the hemoglobin molecule and the pH of the surrounding medium. Many amino acid substitutions alter this electrophoretic charge of the molecule, enabling detection of a structural hemoglobin variant by hemoglobin electrophoresis. It is important to understand, however, that different substitutions may cause identical changes in the net charge of the molecule; thus, two different mutant hemoglobins may have identical electrophoretic mobility.

In hemoglobin electrophoresis, a red blood cell lysate is applied to one end of a cellulose acetate strip, which has been soaked with buffer at a desired pH. A current applied to the strip allows the different hemoglobin molecules with characteristic electrical charges to migrate along the strip at different rates. After a specified period of time, the strip is removed and stained. The amount of hemoglobin in each band is then quantitated by scanning densitometry. Routine hemoglobin electrophoresis is performed on cellulose acetate strips at pH 8.5. Those hemoglobins that migrate faster than HbA are "fast" hemoglobins; those that migrate between the point of origin and HbA are "slow" hemoglobins. The electrophoretic pattern for the more common structural hemoglobin variants are shown in Figure 7-1.

Electrophoresis also may be done on citrate agar at pH

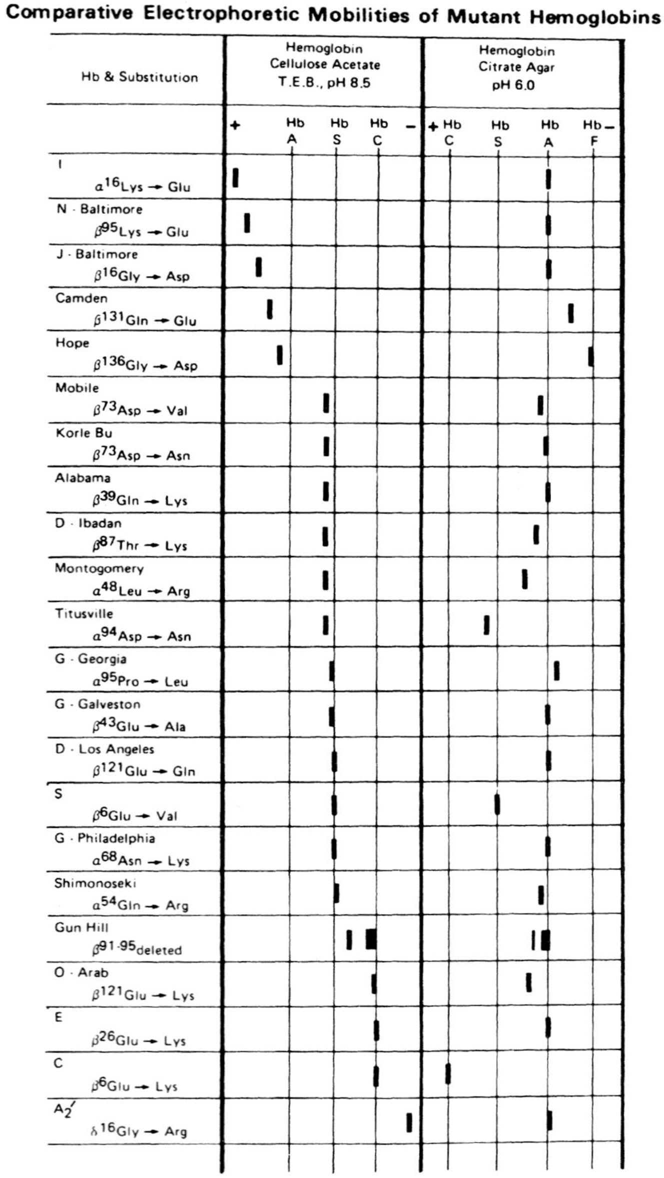

Comparative Electrophoretic Mobilities of Mutant Hemoglobins

Hb & Substitution	Hemoglobin Cellulose Acetate T.E.B., pH 8.5				Hemoglobin Citrate Agar pH 6.0				
	+	Hb A	Hb S	Hb C	− / +	Hb C	Hb S	Hb A	Hb F
I — α^{16} Lys → Glu									
N · Baltimore — β^{95} Lys → Glu									
J · Baltimore — β^{16} Gly → Asp									
Camden — β^{131} Gln → Glu									
Hope — β^{136} Gly → Asp									
Mobile — β^{73} Asp → Val									
Korle Bu — β^{73} Asp → Asn									
Alabama — β^{39} Gln → Lys									
D · Ibadan — β^{87} Thr → Lys									
Montgomery — α^{48} Leu → Arg									
Titusville — α^{94} Asp → Asn									
G · Georgia — α^{95} Pro → Leu									
G · Galveston — β^{43} Glu → Ala									
D · Los Angeles — β^{121} Glu → Gln									
S — β^{6} Glu → Val									
G · Philadelphia — α^{68} Asn → Lys									
Shimonoseki — α^{54} Gln → Arg									
Gun Hill — $\beta^{91\text{-}95}$ deleted									
O · Arab — β^{121} Glu → Lys									
E — β^{26} Glu → Lys									
C — β^{6} Glu → Lys									
A_2' — δ^{16} Gly → Arg									

FIGURE 7-1. Electrophoretic pattern of common structural hemoglobin variants. Electrophoresis is usually performed on cellulose acetate at a pH of 8.4. Further testing on citrate agar at pH 6.2 allows separation of those hemoglobins that have similar patterns at pH 8.4. (From Schneider RG et al: Abnormal hemoglobins in a quarter million people. Blood 48:629, 1976).

6.0. This allows separation of hemoglobins that migrate together on cellulose acetate. In particular, on cellulose acetate at pH 8.5, HbD and HbG will migrate with HbS, whereas HbE and HbO will migrate with HbC. These variants can, however, be separated by electrophoresis on citrate agar at pH 6.0.

HbF QUANTITATION

Most clinically symptomatic hemoglobinopathies involve abnormalities of the β-globin chain, resulting in a decrease or absence of HbA ($\alpha_2\beta_2$) and a compensatory increase in HbF ($\alpha_2\gamma_2$) and/or HbA$_2$ ($\alpha_2\delta_2$). Typically, an elevation in HbF and/or HbA$_2$ is the clue to the presence of a hemoglobinopathy. HbF is quantitated by the alkali denaturation test. Its distribution among the erythrocyte population, however, is evaluated by the acid elution test. These tests are based on the fact that HbF is more resistant to alkali and acid treatment than other hemoglobins. Hemoglobin F is frequently elevated in other hematologic disorders as well as in hemoglobinopathies.

Alkali denaturation HbF concentrations greater than 10% can be measured accurately by electrophoresis and densitometry. Smaller, but significant increases in HbF, can be measured more accurately by alkali denaturation. In the alkali denaturation test, a known volume of washed erythrocytes are lysed and 1.2N NaOH is added to the hemolysate. HbF resists denaturation in this medium, whereas HbA is denatured. The denatured HbA is then precipitated from solution by ammonium sulfate leaving HbF in the filtrate. The filtrate is measured spectrophotometrically. The amount of HbF is expressed as a percentage of the total hemoglobin, which is measured by the standard cyanomethemoglobin method.

$$\frac{\text{HbF by alkali denaturation}}{\text{Total Hb by cyanmethemoglobin}} \times 100 = \%\ \text{HbF}$$

Acid elution The acid elution test (Betke-Kleihauer test) is helpful in determining the distribution of HbF among erythrocytes on a blood smear. All hemoglobins except HbF are eluted from the erythrocyte by citric acid–phosphate buffer at pH 3.3. After elution, the slide is stained and examined. Those erythrocytes that contained HbA appear as ghosts with a visible cell membrane but a lack of stainable hemoglobin; those erythrocytes containing HbF stain darkly. This test is important in distinguishing hereditary persistence of fetal hemoglobin (HPFH) from other hemoglobinopathies with a characteristic increase in HbF concentration. In HPFH, the HbF is evenly distributed among erythrocytes, whereas in other hematologic disorders with high levels of HbF, the HbF is restricted to a few erythrocytes (heterogeneous distribution).

HbA$_2$ QUANTITATION

HbA$_2$ estimation is useful in diagnosis of β-thalassemia trait. In this disorder, the HbA$_2$ may be elevated up to 7% of the total hemoglobin. HbA$_2$ can be separated from other hemoglobins by electrophoresis on cellulose acetate, but its quantitation is most reliable when the A$_2$ band is eluted from the cellulose acetate and measured spectrophotometrically. Column chromatography also gives accurate and reproducible results.

OTHER TESTS

Other tests for abnormal hemoglobins are based on altered physical properties of the structural variants. These include solubility tests, heat precipitation tests, and tests for Heinz bodies. Descriptions of these tests are included in the following discussion of specific structural variants.

TECHNIQUES FOR DETECTING SPECIFIC MUTATIONS AT THE MOLECULAR LEVEL

Techniques are now available to identify the specific molecular defect of hemoglobin disorders.[6] These techniques are discussed in Chapter 22. The polymerase chain reaction (PCR) has been incorporated into all diagnostic procedures for identifying point mutations because it enhances sensitivity and reduces the amount of DNA required and time for analysis. Southern blotting is the technique used to detect deletions and has been used extensively to characterize the α-thalassemias. Methods to detect deletions using the PCR technique are being developed.

Prenatal diagnosis may be carried out in the first trimester of pregnancy using DNA from chorionic villi. In the highly heterogenous β-thalassemias, DNA analysis is first done on the parents to detect the mutations. Once identified, the same mutations are searched for in the chorionic villi. In hemoglobinopathies caused by a single mutation, such as sickle cell anemia, only the DNA of fetal origin needs to be studied.

● Nomenclature

The first abnormal hemoglobin discovered was called HbS (S for sickle) because it was associated with crescent-shaped erythrocytes. Subsequently, other hemoglobin variants were discovered, and they were given successive letters of the alphabet according to electrophoretic mobility beginning with the letter C. The letter A was already used to describe the normal adult hemoglobin, HbA. The letter B was not used to avoid confusion with the ABO blood group system. The letter F had been designated to describe fetal hemoglobin, HbF. The letter M was given to those hemoglobins that tended to form methemoglobin.

As more and more variants were discovered, it was recognized that the alphabetical system was not sufficient, and another nomenclature system was needed. It also became apparent that some variants with the same letter designation (same electrophoretic mobility) had different structural variations. Thus, subsequent hemoglobins were given common names according to the geographic area in which they were discovered (e.g., Hb Ft. Worth). If the hemoglobin had the electrophoretic mobility of a previous lettered hemoglobin, that letter is used in addition to the geographic area (e.g., HbG Honolulu).

An international committee has attempted to create a semblance of order out of the confusion surrounding hemoglobin nomenclature. They recommend that all variants be given a scientific designation as well as a common name. The scientific designation includes the following: (1) the mutated chain, (2) the amino acid position affected, (3) the helical position of mutation, and (4) the amino acid substitution. For example, HbS would be designated as β6 (A3) Glu → Val. The mutation is in the β-chain affecting the amino acid in the sixth position of the chain located in the A3 helix position. The amino acid valine is substituted for glutamic acid. Hemoglobins with amino acid deletions include the word "missing" after the amino acid and helix designation (e.g., β56–59 [D7–E3] miss-

ing). The advantage of the helical designation is that amino acid substitutions in the same helix may lead to similar functional and structural alterations of the hemoglobin molecule, allowing a better understanding of the clinical manifestations of each.[7]

Not all globin chain defects cause symptoms of disease and, thus, many go undetected. Only those that cause symptoms are likely to be brought to the attention of a physician. The majority of abnormal hemoglobins discovered have been those that affect the β-chain. One possible explanation for this greater frequency is that the β-chain is a constituent of the major adult hemoglobin, HbA. Thus, an alteration of this chain produces a quantity of abnormal hemoglobin that is sufficient to produce symptoms of disease.

Although the α-chain is also a constituent of HbA, fewer hemoglobin variants have been linked to an abnormality in this chain. This could be explained by the fact that four α-genes exist, two on each homologous chromosome. This means from one to four genes may be mutated producing varying amounts of the abnormal hemoglobin from 25% to 100%. It is unlikely, however, that all four genes would be affected; thus, hemoglobins with α-chain defects usually constitute a smaller proportion of the total hemoglobin than those with β-chain defects. Symptoms of disease in α-chain defects, if present, may be mild and frequently go unnoticed. Those substitutions affecting the δ- or γ-chains are not clinically significant because these chains are constituents of the minor adult hemoglobins, HbA$_2$ and HbF. They are not likely to produce symptoms and therefore are not easily detected.

If an individual is homozygous for the gene coding for a structural globin mutant of the β-chain, no HbA is produced, and the term "disease" or anemia is used to describe the specific disorder (i.e., sickle cell anemia). If, however, one of the genes coding for the β-chain is normal, and the other β-gene codes for a structural variant, both HbA and the abnormal hemoglobin are produced, and the term "trait" is used to describe the heterozygous disorder (i.e., sickle cell trait). The abnormal hemoglobin usually accounts for less than 50% of the total hemoglobin in the "trait" form, whereas, in the homozygous state of "disease," the abnormal hemoglobin constitutes more than 50% of the total hemoglobin. This lower concentration of abnormal hemoglobin in the heterozygous state probably occurs because the α-chains have a stronger attraction to bind with normal β-chains than with the abnormal β-chains. If the variant hemoglobin constitutes greater than 50% of the total hemoglobin and the patient is known, through family studies, to be heterozygous for the mutant gene, then the patient has probably inherited two different abnormal hemoglobin genes (doubly heterozygous). The possibility that the patient has inherited a form of thalassemia with the hemoglobin variant also should be considered.

● Pathophysiology

The structural hemoglobin variants cause symptoms if the amino acid substitution occurs at a critical site of the mole-

TABLE 7-1 *CHANGES IN THE HEMOGLOBIN MOLECULE CAUSED BY GENETIC MUTATION IN GLOBIN CHAINS*

Change	Example
1. Decreased solubility	Hb S; Hb C
2. Decreased stability	Congenital Heinz body hemolytic anemias
3. Altered oxygen affinity	Hb M; Hb Chesapeake

cule. Most mutations cause clinical signs of disease because the mutation affects the solubility, function (oxygen-affinity) and/or stability of the hemoglobin molecule (Table 7-1).

ALTERED SOLUBILITY

If a nonpolar amino acid is substituted for a polar residue near the surface of the chain, the solubility of the hemoglobin molecule may be affected. Hemoglobin S is an example of this type of substitution. In the deoxygenated state, the hemoglobin S molecule polymerizes into insoluble, rigid aggregates. The majority of surface substitutions, however, do not affect the tertiary structure, heme function, or subunit interactions and are therefore innocuous.

ALTERED FUNCTION

Polar amino acid substitutions for nonpolar residues near the hydrophobic crevice of the globin chain that contains the heme (heme pocket) may affect the oxygen affinity of hemoglobin by stabilizing heme iron in the ferric state. The normal nonpolar heme pocket helps maintain heme iron in the reduced ferrous state. Most structural variants affecting the heme pocket are caused by a substitution of tyrosine for histidine near the heme iron, stabilizing the iron in the ferric state and producing permanent methemoglobinemia. Methemoglobin cannot combine with oxygen.

Mutations at the subunit interaction site, α_1, β_2, may affect the allosteric properties of the molecule leading to increased or decreased oxygen affinity. There is considerable movement in the α_1, β_2, interface region upon oxygenation, which triggers the allosteric interactions. Other substitutions affecting oxygen affinity occur in the binding site for 2,3-BPG and in the C-terminal end of the β-chain, which are sites involved in the stability of the deoxygenated state. High oxygen affinity hemoglobin variants produce congenital erythrocytosis, whereas decreased oxygen affinity variants produce anemia and cyanosis.

ALTERED STABILITY

Amino acid substitutions in the internal residues may prevent the hemoglobin molecule from folding into its normal conformation. Normal folding of the molecule places the hydrophilic residues on the surface, whereas hydrophobic residues are oriented toward the interior of the molecule. Substitution of polar for nonpolar internal residues can disrupt this conformation. Other substitutions may alter the alpha-helix structure or subunit interaction sites. Mutations in the heme crevice may impair the binding of heme to globin. These various altered properties of the hemoglobin molecule cause hemoglobin instability.

Clinically, the unstable variants are known as *congenital Heinz body hemolytic anemias*. The unstable hemoglobin denatures in the form of Heinz bodies. Heinz bodies attach to the cell membrane causing membrane injury and premature cell destruction. In addition to altering the molecule's stability, disruption of normal conformation also may affect the molecule's function. The unstable hemoglobins have a tendency to spontaneously oxidize to methemoglobin.

● Sickle cell anemia

Sickle cell anemia is the most common worldwide, symptomatic hemoglobinopathy with greatest prevalence in Africa. Heterozygotes in certain regions of Africa may reach as high as 40%. The sickle cell gene also is common in northern Mediterranean countries; North, Central, and South America; the Middle East; and in India.[8] The heterozygote condition is found in 8% to 10% of American blacks, while 0.3% to 1.3% have homozygous disease.

It is interesting to note that geographic areas with the highest frequency of sickle cell genes also are areas where infection with *Plasmodium falciparum* is common. This correlation strongly suggests that HbS confers a selective advantage against fatal malarial infections. By this mechanism, the gene frequency builds up. Children with sickle cell trait are readily infected with the malarial parasite, but parasite counts remain low. It has been suggested that resistance to malaria occurs because parasitized cells sickle more readily, leading to sequestration and phagocytosis of the infected cell by the spleen. Other, as yet undefined, factors also may contribute to reduced malarial susceptibility in individuals with HbS.[9] Similar resistance has been noted in thalassemia trait and HbE trait.[10]

PATHOPHYSIOLOGY

Hemoglobin S is the mutant hemoglobin produced when nonpolar valine is substituted for polar glutamic acid at the sixth position, in the A3 helix of the β-chain ($\beta6$ (A3) Glu → Val). This substitution is on the surface of the molecule, producing a change in the net charge; hence, it changes the electrophoretic mobility of the molecule. The solubility of hemoglobin S in the deoxygenated state is markedly reduced, producing a tendency for deoxyhemoglobin S molecules to polymerize into rigid aggregates. After polymerization, the cells assume a crescent shape.

There is a delay between deoxygenation and the formation of HbS polymers. The length of delay is highly dependent on temperature, mean corpuscular hemoglobin concentration (MCHC) of HbS, pH, ionic strength, and oxygen tension. Hypoxia, acidosis, hypertonicity, and temperatures more than 37° C promote deoxygenation and the formation of HbS polymers. The spleen, kidney, retina, and bone marrow provide a sufficiently hypoxic, acidotic, and hypertonic microenvironment to promote HbS polymerization and sickling.

Sickling also depends on HbS concentration within the erythrocyte (MCHC) and intracellular hemoglobin composition (% HbA, % HbS, % HbA$_2$, % HbF). HbA and oxyhemoglobin S are equally soluble at concentrations about the normal MCHC of 34%. The more concentrated the hemoglobin S is within the cell, however, the higher the MCHC and the greater the potential for HbS aggregates to form. Using this concept, attempts have been made to treat the disease by hydrating the cells, which decreases the MCHC and prevents sickling. The presence of other hemoglobins such as HbA also inhibits polymerization and decreases sickling.

Polymerization of deoxyhemoglobin S begins when the oxygen saturation of hemoglobin falls below 85% and is complete at about 38% oxygen saturation. The HbS aggregates cause the erythrocyte to become stiff and less deformable. The aggregates also damage the erythrocyte membrane, leading to increased fragility of the cell.

The polymerization process of hemoglobin S occurs in three stages. The time it takes for the total process is related to the clinical severity of the disease. The first stage, nucleation, begins with the aggregation of about 15 hemoglobin molecules into clusters. This is also known as the lag phase; during this time, the erythrocyte behaves in a normal fashion with no apparent changes. The time for this stage to occur varies considerably with the environment of the molecule (pH, oxygen tension, deoxyhemoglobin concentration, temperature) from a few milliseconds to hours. The second stage, polymerization, increases the viscosity of the intracellular contents as deoxyhemoglobin S polymerizes into 14-strand fibers using the nuclei aggregates of the first stage as starting points. This stage takes only a few seconds. The third stage, alignment, takes minutes as the fibers align into bundles. It is at this stage that the cell acquires its crescent shape.

Irreversibly sickled cells   The sickled erythrocyte may return to a normal biconcave shape upon reoxygenation of the hemoglobin; however, with repeated sickling events, the erythrocyte membrane undergoes changes that cause it to become leaky and rigid. After repeated sickling episodes, the cells become irreversibly sickled cells (ISC) and are removed by phagocytes in the spleen, liver, or bone marrow. The ISC also may initiate or increase the severity of vaso-occlusive crises because of impaired cell deformability and increased cell adherence to vascular endothelium. The mechanism for this interaction between sickled cells and the endothelium is unknown but may be related to changes in the surface properties of sickled cells and endothelial cells as well as plasma factors.[11,12]

The ISC is the result of a permanent deformation of the submembrane skeletal lattice.[13] The spectrin dimer-dimer association is the primary site of skeletal rearrangement. The intracellular polymerization of HbS also may decouple the lipid bilayer from the membrane skeleton. From 5% to 50% of the circulating erythrocytes in patients with sickle cell anemia are ISCs. These cells have a very high MCHC and low MCV. These cells are ovoid or boat-shaped with a smooth outline. They lack the spicules characteristic of deoxygenated sickled cells (Fig. 7-2).

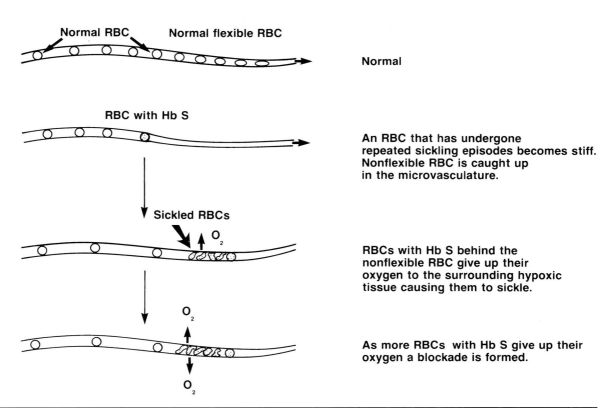

FIGURE 7-2. How sickle cells blockade a vessel and precipitate a vaso-occlusive crisis.

Sickled cells have difficulty changing their shape enough to squeeze through the small capillaries. Consequently, the rigid cells aggregate in the microvasculature. More erythrocytes behind the blockage release their oxygen to the surrounding hypoxic tissue and consequently form rigid intracellular inclusions increasing the size of the plug (Fig. 7-3). Erythrocytes from nearby capillaries are forced to give up more oxygen than they normally would to feed the oxygen starved tissue around the blockage. These cells then form rigid aggregates of deoxyhemoglobin, expanding the blockaded region. Lack of oxygen, in turn, causes local tissue necrosis. Most of the signs and symptoms of the disease are related to this process of microvasculature blockage and tissue necrosis.

Cause of anemia The primary cause of anemia in sickle cell anemia is extravascular hemolysis of the rigid sickled cells. The lifespan of circulating erythrocytes may decrease to as few as 14 days. The hypoglycemic, hypoxic environment of the spleen promotes blood sickling, slows blood circulation in the cords, and enhances phagocytosis of erythrocytes containing HbS. Early in childhood, however, the spleen loses its function as repeated ischemic crises lead to splenic tissue necrosis and atrophy. With splenic atrophy, other cells of the mononuclear phagocyte system in the liver and bone marrow take over the destruction of these abnormal cells.

Sickle cell trait Sickle cell trait is not as severe a disorder as sickle cell anemia since the presence of HbA or other β-chain structural variant of hemoglobin interferes with the process of polymerization. Although hemoglobins other than HbS can be assembled into the polymer of deoxyhemoglobin S, the presence of these alternate β-chains with the β-chains of HbS creates a weakened structure and decreases the degree of polymerization. The poorer the fit, the less polymerization of deoxyhemoglobin S. If, however, the alternate β-chains from another β-chain mutant increase the strength of the intertetramer bonds of the polymer, then sickling is enhanced.

Oxygen affinity of Hbs The oxygen affinity of HbS differs from that of HbA, resulting in important physiologic changes in vivo. HbS has decreased oxygen affinity. The 2,3-DPG (also referred to as 2,3-BPG.) levels of homozygotes is increased. This shift to the right in the oxygen dissociation curve facilitates the release of more oxygen to the tissues. On the other hand, this phenomenon also increases the concentration of deoxyhemoglobin S, promoting the formation of sickle cells.

CLINICAL FINDINGS

The first clinical signs of sickle cell anemia appear at about 6 months of age when the concentration of HbS predominates over HbF. Clinical manifestations result from chronic hemolytic anemia, vaso-occlusion of the microvasculature, overwhelming infections and acute splenic sequestration.

Anemia A moderate to severe chronic anemia as the result of extravascular hemolysis is characteristic of the disease. Gallstones, a complication of any chronic hemolytic disorder, are a common finding due to cholestasis and increased bilirubin turnover. Folate deficiency due to increased erythrocyte turnover may further exacerbate the anemia producing megaloblastosis.

Hemodynamic changes occur in an attempt to compensate for the tissue oxygen deficit; as a result, symptoms of cardiac overload, including cardiac hypertrophy, cardiac enlargement, and eventually congestive heart failure, are frequent complications of the disease.

Hyperplastic bone marrow caused by chronic hemolysis is accompanied by bone changes, such as thinning of cortices and hair-on-end appearance in x-rays of the skull. Hyperplasia results from a futile attempt by the marrow to compensate for premature erythrocyte destruction. Conversely, aplastic crises may accompany or follow viral, bacterial, and mycoplasmal infections. This temporary cessation of erythropoiesis in the face of chronic hemolysis leads to a worsening of the anemia. The aplasia may last from a few days to a week. Increasing evidence suggests that many cases of aplasia occur as a result of infection with parvovirus. Parvovirus also will cause a cessation of erythropoiesis in normal individuals, but normal blood cell production in these individuals is restored before any noticeable changes in erythrocyte concentration take place.

Vaso-occlusive crisis The blockage of microvasculature by rigid sickled cells accounts for the majority of the clinical signs of sickle cell anemia. The occlusions do not occur continuously but rather occur spontaneously, causing acute signs of distress. These episodes are called *vaso-occlusive crises*. The crises may be triggered by infection, decreased atmospheric oxygen pressure, dehydration, or slow blood flow, but frequently they occur without any known cause. The occlusions are accompanied by pain, low grade fever, organ dysfunction, and tissue necrosis. The episodes last 1 to 2 weeks and subside spontaneously.

Recurrent occlusive episodes lead to infarctions of tissue of the genitourinary tract, liver, bone, lung, and

---

FIGURE 7-3. Erythrocytes from a patient with sickle cell anemia examined with scanning beam electron microscopy. **A**, Oxygenated blood. Erythrocytes appear normal except for one microspherocyte. Three leukocytes are evident in the field. **B**, Oxygenated irreversibly sickled cells are smooth in texture and outline, but are ovoid or boat-like in shape. **C**, Partial deoxygenation causes the cells to assume bizarre shapes with spike, spicules, and filaments that protrude from the cells. **D**, More complete deoxygenation causes the cells to assume sickled shapes with longitudinal surface striations. **E**, Higher magnification. Cells have a sculptured texture. Multiple spike-like protrusions are seen at the polar ends of one cell. **F**, Complete deoxygenation of acanthocytic sickle cells produces numerous short protrusions and occasional long filaments. (From: Lee, R.G., Bithell, T.C., Foerster, J., Athens, J.W., Lukens, J.N.: Wintrobe's Clinical Hematology. Philadelphia: Lea & Febiger, 1993).

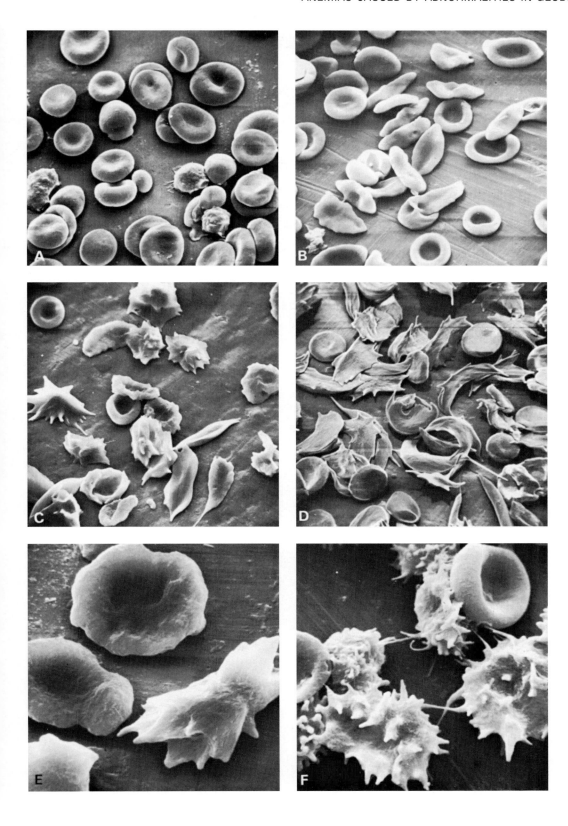

spleen. The chronic organ damage is accompanied by organ dysfunction. Although splenomegaly is present in early childhood, repeated splenic infarctions eventually result in splenic fibrosis and calcifications (usually by age 4 or 5). This organ damage, secondary to infarction, is known as *autosplenectomy*. As a result, splenomegaly is rare in adults with this disease. Aseptic necrosis of the head of the femur is common. Dactylitis, a painful symmetrical swelling of the hands and feet (hand–foot syndrome) caused by infarction of the metacarpals and metatarsals, is often the first sign of the disease in infants. Recurrent priapism is a characteristic, painful complication that occasionally requires surgical intervention.

The slow flow of blood in occlusive areas may lead to thrombosis. Thrombosis of the cerebral arteries resulting in stroke is common. Magnetic resonance imaging shows evidence of subclinical cerebral infarction in 20% to 30% of children with sickle cell anemia. If the arterioles of the eye are affected, blindness can occur. Chronic leg ulcers, also found in other hemolytic anemias, may occur at any age. The ulcers appear without any known injury. These painful sores do not readily respond to treatment and may take months to heal.

Placental infarctions in pregnant women with sickle cell disease can be a hazard to the fetus. Anemia often becomes more severe during pregnancy. In addition, other clinical findings may be exacerbated during pregnancy, endangering the life of both the mother and the fetus.

Bacterial infection   Overwhelming bacterial infection is a common cause of death in young patients. There is an extremely high risk of septicemia from encapsulated microorganisms. Bacterial pneumonia is the most common infection, but meningitis also is prevalent. Infections are primarily due to *Streptococcus pneumoniae* and *Hemophilus influenzae*. The reasons for this increased susceptibility to infection are not fully understood but may be related to functional asplenia, impaired opsonization, and abnormal complement activation.[14] The spleen is important to host defense in the young. There also is significant impairment of in vivo neutrophil adherence to vascular endothelium in HbS disease. This may prevent neutrophils from rapidly relocating to areas of inflammation.[14] Prophylactic penicillin is now advocated for all children with sickle cell anemia to reduce morbidity and mortality from infection.

Acute splenic sequestration   In young children, sudden splenic pooling of sickled erythrocytes may cause a massive decrease in erythrocyte mass within a few hours. Thrombocytopenia also may occur. Hypovolemia and shock follow. At one time, this was the leading cause of death in infants with sickle cell anemia. Early diagnosis, instruction of parents to detect an enlarging spleen, and rapid intervention with transfusion have served to decrease morbidity and mortality associated with splenic sequestration.[15]

Chest syndrome   This illness resembling pneumonia is one of the most common causes of hospitalization and death in children with sickle cell disease.[15] Clinical findings include cough, fever, chest pain, dyspnea, and pulmonary infiltrates. Hemoglobin concentration also decreases. The etiology of chest syndrome is not clear. In some cases, an infectious agent can be identified. Other possible causes include pulmonary edema from overhydration, fat embolism from infarcted bone marrow, hypoventilation due to pain from rib infarcts or from narcotic analgesics used to combat pain. The long-term effects of recurrent episodes of chest syndrome are unknown.

LABORATORY FINDINGS

Peripheral blood (fig. 7-4)   A normocytic, normochromic anemia is characteristic of sickle cell anemia; however, with marked reticulocytosis, the anemia may appear macrocytic. Reticulocytosis from 10% to 20% is typical. The hemoglobin ranges from 6 to 10 g/dL, and the hematocrit from 0.18 to 0.30 L/L. A calculated hematocrit from an electronic cell counter is more reliable than a centrifuged microhematocrit because excessive plasma, trapped by sickled cells in centrifuged specimens, falsely elevates the hematocrit.

The Cooperative Study of Sickle Cell Disease revealed that individuals with HbSS have higher steady-state leukocyte counts than normal, especially in children younger than 10 years of age.[16] Platelet counts also are frequently higher than normal. After the age of 40 the hemoglobin concentration, reticulocyte count, leukocyte count, and platelet count decrease.[17]

The blood smear shows variable anisocytosis with polychromatophilic macrocytes and variable poikilocytosis with the presence of sickled cells and target cells. Nucleated erythrocytes can usually be found. The RDW is increased. During hemolytic crisis, the RDW increases linearly with increases in reticulocytes.[18] If the patient is not experiencing a crisis, sickled cells may not be present.

In older children and adults, signs of splenic hypofunc-

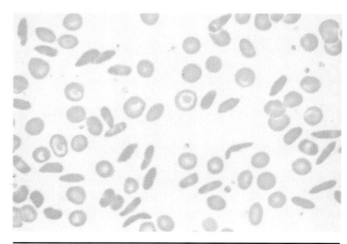

FIGURE 7-4. Hemoglobin S disease (sickle cell anemia). Note abnormal boat-shaped sickled and ovoid erythrocytes. (PB; 250 × original magnification; Wright-Giemsa stain.)

tion are apparent on the peripheral blood smear with the presence of basophilic stippling, Howell-Jolly bodies, siderocytes, and poikilocytes.

Bone marrow Bone marrow aspiration shows erythroid hyperplasia, reflecting the attempt of the bone marrow to compensate for chronic hemolysis. Erythrocyte production increases to four to five times normal. If the patient is deficient in folic acid, megaloblastosis may be seen. Iron stores are most often increased but may be diminished if hematuria is excessive. Bone marrow examination is not usually performed because it yields no definitive diagnostic information.

Hemoglobin electrophoresis The presence of HbS is confirmed by hemoglobin electrophoresis. Electrophoresis on cellulose acetate at a pH of 8.5 shows 85% to 100% HbS. HbS appears as a band about midway between HbA and HbA$_2$ (Fig. 7-1). HbF is usually not greater than 15%. Higher levels of HbF (25% to 35%) may signify double heterozygousity for HbS and for hereditary persistence of fetal hemoglobin. HbA$_2$ is normal. There is no HbA. Newborns have 60% to 80% HbF with the remainder HbS. In infants younger than 3 months of age with small amounts of HbS, electrophoresis on citrate agar gel at a pH of 6.2 permits more reliable separation of HbF from both HbA and HbS. Citrate agar gel electrophoresis also is useful in separating HbD and HbG from HbS. Both of these nonsickling hemoglobins migrate with HbS on alkaline electrophoresis with paper or starch gel, but migrate like HbA on agar gel electrophoresis at acid pH.

Solubility test The solubility test is a rapid confirmatory test for HbS in the heterozygous or homozygous state. HbS liberated from the erythrocyte by a lysing agent is deoxygenated with dithionite. This causes the HbS to polymerize. The presence of insoluble, reduced HbS is indicated by opacity of the solution. In severe anemia, the amount of HbS may be too low to give opacity. Increasing the amount of blood in the test solution may overcome this problem. Unstable hemoglobins may give a false-positive test if many Heinz bodies are present. Other rare hemoglobin variants also may give positive tests (e.g., HbC Harlem, HbI). False-positive tests also occur with elevated plasma proteins and lipids.

Sickling test Another confirmatory test, performed less often, is the sodium metabisulfite slide test for sickling. In this test, the blood is deoxygenated, with the reducing substance sodium metabisulfite placed on a glass slide and sealed with a coverslip to prevent reoxygenation of the cells. After 30 minutes, the blood is examined under the microscope for the presence of sickle-shaped cells. This test is positive in both sickle cell anemia and sickle cell trait.

Other diagnostic tests Isoelectric focusing in agar gels and high performance liquid chromatography are used to identify abnormal hemoglobins such as HbS. Preferred methods for prenatal screening and diagnosis use DNA-based analysis (polymerase chain reaction) to detect point mutation in globin gene sequences.[19] The molecular techniques are discussed in Chapter 21.

Other laboratory findings Other laboratory findings are less specific. The hemolytic nature of the disease causes indirect bilirubin to increase, haptoglobin to decrease, and uric acid and serum lactic dehydrogenase to increase. Osmotic fragility may be decreased due to the presence of target cells. These tests offer no diagnostic information on sickle cell anemia, but may be performed to evaluate complicating conditions.

THERAPY

At present, there is no known effective long-range therapy for sickle cell anemia. Preventive therapy is aimed at eliminating situations that are known to precipitate vaso-occlusion, such as dehydration and infection. Transfusion of packed erythrocytes or whole blood is required in aplastic crises or splenic sequestration. Preoperative transfusion is helpful in preventing the complications of anesthesia-induced sickling. Long-term transfusion therapy may be useful in preventing complications of sickle cell anemia. This therapy is aimed at suppressing the formation of new HbS by the patient's bone marrow. Complications of transfusion therapy includes transmission of blood-borne diseases, alloimmunization, expense, inconvenience, and iron overload.[15]

A therapeutic approach that is receiving much attention is the use of pharmacologic agents to reduce intracellular sickling.[20] Hydroxyurea and butyrate compounds are the drugs currently being used for this purpose. These agents elevate HbF in most HbS-containing erythrocytes. This decreases intracellular polymerization of HbS.

Bone marrow transplantation or gene therapy, in which normal genes are inserted into a patient's defective cells, show promise of long-term therapy but are controversial due to feasibility and ethical issues.[15]

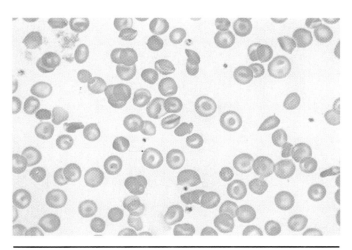

FIGURE 7-5. Hemoglobin C disease. Note the cell in the center with HbC crystal, target cells and folded cells. (PB).

SICKLE CELL TRAIT

Sickle cell trait is the heterozygous β^S state. The patient has one normal β-gene and one β^S-gene. Since HbA constitutes more than 50% of the total hemoglobin in these individuals, there are no clinical symptoms, and results of physical examination appear normal. However, the condition is important to diagnose, because statistically, one of four children born to parents who each have the trait will have sickle cell anemia and two of four will have the trait.

Complications of splenic infarction and renal papillary necrosis have been reported in affected individuals subjected to extreme and prolonged hypoxia such as after flying at high altitude in unpressurized aircraft or after general anesthesia.

Hematologic parameters are normal. No anemia or sickled cells are found in routine blood counts and differentials. Sickling can be induced with the sodium metabisulfite test, however, and the solubility test is also positive. Hemoglobin electrophoresis results show 50% to 65% HbA, 35% to 45% HbS, normal HbF, and normal or slightly increased HbA$_2$. If HbA constitutes less than 50% of the total hemoglobin in sickle cell trait, the patient is probably heterozygous for another hemoglobinopathy such as thalassemia.

● Hemoglobin C disease (fig. 7-5)

Hemoglobin C, the second hemoglobinopathy to be recognized, is the second most prevalent hemoglobin variant. The first cases of HbC were discovered in the heterozygous state with HbS; this is not surprising because both hemoglobinopathies are prevalent in the same geographical area. It is found predominantly in West African blacks, where the incidence of the trait may reach 17% to 28% of the population. Between 2% and 3% of blacks in the United States carry the trait, while 0.02% have the disease.

Hemoglobin C is produced when lysine is substituted for glutamic acid at the sixth position (A3) in the β-chain (β6 (A3) Glu → Lys). Since the nonpolar lysine amino acid substitution is in the same β-chain position as the substitution for HbS, a decrease in hemoglobin solubility can be expected. Deoxyhemoglobin C, like deoxyhemoglobin S, has a decreased solubility, forming intracellular crystals when cells are dehydrated or in hypertonic solutions. Erythrocytes with crystals become rigid and are trapped and destroyed in the spleen. Erythrocyte lifespan is decreased to 30 to 55 days.

Hemoglobin C disease (β^c/β^c), is usually asymptomatic, but patients may experience joint and abdominal pain. In contrast to sickle cell anemia, the spleen is most often enlarged. Variable hemolysis results in a mild to moderate anemia.

The hemoglobin ranges from 8 to 12 g/dL and the hematocrit from 0.25 to 0.35 L/L. The anemia is accompanied by a slight to moderate increase in reticulocytes. The stained blood smear contains small cells that appear to be folded, irregularly contracted, and many target cells. Intracellular hemoglobin crystals may be found if the smear has been dried slowly (Fig. 7-6). Microspherocytes are occasionally present. Osmotic fragility is decreased.

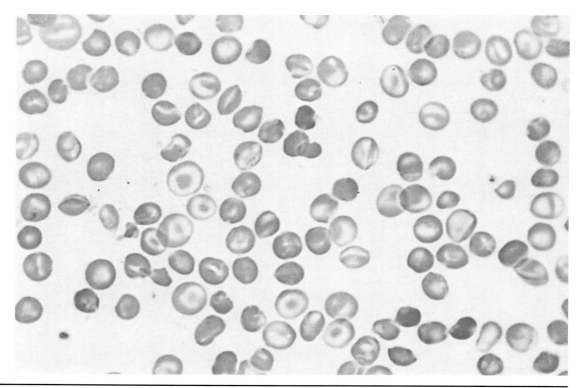

FIGURE 7-6. A blood film from a patient with HbC disease (PB; 250 × original magnification; Wright-Giemsa stain).

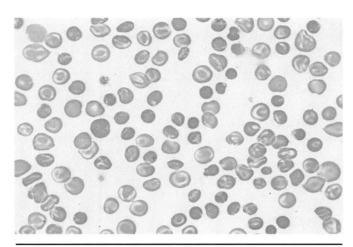

FIGURE 7-7. Hemoglobin C/β-thalaassemia (PB). Note the microspherocytes and target cells. This patient had 94% HbC and 6% Hb F. (250 × original magnification; Wright-Giemsa stain.)

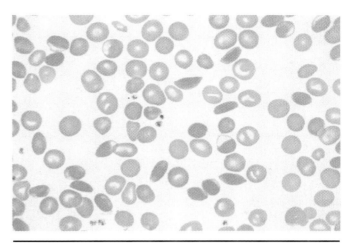

FIGURE 7-8. Hemoglobin S/C disease. Notice the elongated cells and boat-shaped cells. The small contracted cells are typical of those seen in hemoglobin C disease. Target cells are also present. (PB; 250 × original magnification; Wright-Giemsa stain.)

Hemoglobin electrophoresis on citrate agar gel at acid pH demonstrates greater than 90% HbC with a slight increase in HbF (not more than 7%). On cellulose acetate at an alkaline pH, HbC migrates with HbA$_2$. HbE and HbO-Arab also migrate with HbC at alkaline pH but can be separated by agar gel electrophoresis at an acid pH.

Hemoglobin C trait (β^c/β) is symptomless. No hematologic abnormalities are produced except that target cells are readily noted on blood smears. Mild hypochromia may be present. About 60% to 70% of the hemoglobin is HbA, and 30% to 40% is HbC. Higher levels of HbC and microcytosis are found when HbC is associated with β-thalassemia (β^c/β^{thal}) (Fig. 7-7).

There is considerable heterogeneity in the clinical and hematologic features of HbC/β^{thal}, which appears to be dependent on the particular variety of β^{thal} gene interacting with HbC. HbC/β^+ thalassemia is characterized by mild anemia similar to that found in heterozygous β-thalassemia. There is 65% to 80% HbC, 2% to 5% HbF, and the remainder HbA. In HbC/β^othalassemia, there is more severe anemia and an absence of Hb A. Hemoglobin electrophoresis reveals only HbC, HbA$_2$ and HbF. HbF ranges from 3% to 10%.

● Hemoglobin S/C disease

In hemoglobin S/C disease, both β-chains are abnormal. One β-gene codes for β^S chains, and the other gene codes for β^c chains (β^S/β^c). Thus, HbA is absent. This heterozygous state for HbS and HbC results in a disease almost as severe as homozygous HbS. The concentration of hemoglobin in individual erythrocytes is increased (MCHC increased), and the concentration of HbS is greater than in sickle cell trait. The increased MCHC contributed by HbC makes the SC cells more prone to sickling than cells that contain HbA/HbS. HbC also enhances the polymerization of HbS. Increased erythrocyte rigidity is noted at oxygen tensions less than 50 mmHg. Additionally, there

is evidence that cells containing HbSC have intracellular HbC crystals.[21] Thus, in HbSC disease, both sickling and crystal formation contribute to the pathophysiology of the disease.

The clinical signs and symptoms of the disease are similar to those of a mild sickle cell anemia. Patients develop vaso-occlusive crises leading to the complications associated with this pathology. A notable difference from sickle cell anemia, however, is that in HbS/C disease splenomegaly is prominent.

A mild to moderate normocytic, normochromic anemia is present. The hematocrit is above 0.25 L/L, and the hemoglobin concentration is between 10 and 14 g/dL. The higher hemoglobin concentration does not necessarily mean that hemolysis is less severe than in sickle cell anemia; it may be that the higher oxygen affinity of HbS/C cells stimulates higher erythropoietin levels. Peripheral blood smears reveal a large number of target cells (up to 85%), folded cells, and boat-shaped cells, in addition to sickled forms (Fig. 7-8). HbC crystals are found in some patients. Some erythrocytes contain a single eccentrically located, densely stained, round mass of hemoglobin, which makes part of the cell appear empty. These cells have been referred to as "billiard-ball" cells.[21] Anisocytosis and poikilocytosis range from mild to severe. Small, dense, misshapen cells, some with crystals of various shapes jutting out at angles, have been referred to as HbSC poikilocytes.[22] Hemoglobin electrophoresis shows nearly equal amounts of HbS and HbC. HbF may be increased up to 7%. No HbA is found due to the absence of normal β-chains.

● Hemoglobin D

Hemoglobin D has several variants of which the identical variants HbD Punjab and HbD Los Angeles (β 121 (GH4) Glu → Gln) are the most common in American blacks

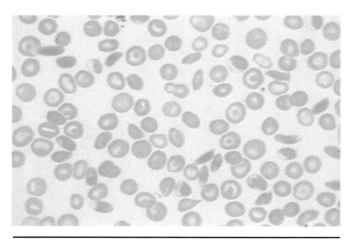

FIGURE 7-9. A blood film from a patient with HbS/D. Homozygous Hb D does not usually cause anemia but when combined with HbS it potentiates the aggregating of deoxyhemoglobin and the sickling of erythrocytes, producing a mild sickle cell anemia. Notice the sickled cells and target cells. (250 × original magnification; Wright-Giemsa stain.)

(<0.02%). The heterozygous and homozygous states are both asymptomatic. Although there are no hematologic abnormalities, the homozygous state may occasionally have an increase in target cells and a decrease in osmotic fragility. Although rare, the heterozygous state of HbD with HbS exists. HbD interacts with HbS, producing aggregates of deoxyhemoglobin (Fig. 7-9). This produces a relatively mild form of sickle cell anemia.

In homozygous HbD, electrophoresis on cellulose acetate at pH 8.5 demonstrates 95% HbD, which has the same electrophoretic mobility as HbS. However, HbD is a nonsickling, soluble hemoglobin. Electrophoresis on citrate agar at pH 6.0 allows separation of HbS and HbD. At this acid pH, HbD migrates with HbA.

Hemoglobin E

Hemoglobin E is the third most prevalent hemoglobinopathy worldwide. It is most often encountered in individuals from southeast Asia. The trait has reached frequencies of almost 50% in areas of Thailand. It is estimated that 15% to 30% of southeast Asian immigrants in North America have HbE. The highest frequencies occur in Cambodians and Laotians. Although found mainly in Asians, the HbE trait also may occur in blacks.

Hemoglobin E is the result of a substitution of lysine for glutamic acid in the β-chain (β26 (B8) (Glu → Lys). The hemoglobin is slightly unstable with oxidant stress. The oxygen dissociation curve is shifted to the right, indicating that HbE has decreased oxygen affinity.

Homozygous HbE is characterized by the presence of a mild, asymptomatic, microcytic anemia with decreased erythrocyte survival. Target cells are prominent, and osmotic fragility is decreased. Electrophoresis demonstrates mostly HbE (90% or more) with the remainder HbA$_2$ and HbF. On alkaline electrophoresis, HbE migrates with

HbA$_2$, HbC, and HbO-Arab. On agar gel at an acid pH, HbE migrates with HbA.

HbE trait is symptomless, and hematologic parameters are normal except for slight microcytosis. Hemoglobin electrophoresis at alkaline pH shows about 27% HbE, the remainder is HbA with normal HbA$_2$ and HbF.

HEMOGLOBIN E/THALASSEMIA

Double heterozygosity for HbE and β-thalassemia causes a moderate to severe thalassemia-like anemia. This is a common combination in southeast Asians, where both genes have a high frequency. The most severe type (β^E/$\beta^{o\text{-thal}}$) reveals only HbE and HbF. The amount of HbE, however, is less than that expected for homozygous HbE, and the HbF is increased proportionally. A more moderate anemia may result if the $\beta^{+\text{thal}}$ gene is inherited together with HbE. In this form of the disease, there is HbE, HbA, HbF, and HbA$_2$. The HbA, however, is less than what would be expected in HbE trait and the anemia is more severe. When the β^{thal} gene is inherited with the β^E gene, the result is microcytic, hypochromic anemia with significant poikilocytosis and nucleated erythrocytes.

Hemoglobin E also may be found in combination with α-thalassemia (Fig. 7-10). This combination produces a more severe anemia than HbE alone. The amount of HbE is dependent on whether the patient is heterozygous or homozygous for HbE and the α-thalassemia genotype inherited (see section on α-thalassemia).

Unstable hemoglobin variants

Unstable hemoglobins result from structurally abnormal globin chains. The abnormal chains contain amino acid mutations in critical internal portions of the chains; these mutations affect the molecular stability.[23] The disorders are characterized by precipitation of the abnormal hemo-

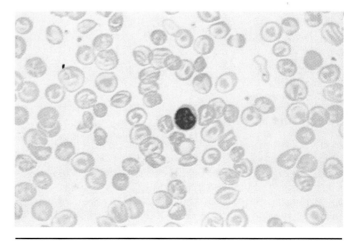

FIGURE 7-10. A Blood film from a splenectomized patient with homozygous HbE and α-thalassemia. The erythrocytes are microcytic, hypochromic with many target cells and poikilocytosis. The patient was from Southeast Asia and had a life-long history of anemia. (250 × original magnification; Wright-Giemsa stain.)

globin in the form of Heinz bodies; this precipitation causes cell rigidity, membrane damage, and subsequent erythrocyte hemolysis. Although hemoglobin denaturation and hemolysis may occur spontaneously, symptoms associated with acute hemolysis usually occur only after drug administration, infection, or other event that changes the normal environment of the hemoglobin molecule. Those variants that cause symptoms are known collectively as *congenital Heinz body hemolytic anemias.*

PATHOPHYSIOLOGY

The many symptomatic variants of unstable hemoglobins discovered so far are all heterozygous. The homozygous condition is probably incompatible with life. Most are autosomal-dominant inherited disorders, but a large number appear to arise from spontaneous mutations with no evidence of hemoglobin instability in parents or other family members.

Unstable hemoglobin variants may be the result of a variety of amino acid substitutions or deletions that disrupt the stability of the globin subunit or hemoglobin tetramer. Substitutions described have included substitutions near the heme-globin link, in the α-helices and near the α-β chain contacts. Amino acid deletions that involve both the inter and intra subunit interactions have a marked effect on the overall conformation of the molecule. Amino acid insertions, truncated or extended chains have occasionally been described.

Unstable hemoglobin denatures and precipitates out of solution as Heinz bodies. Heinz bodies attach to the inner surface of the membrane, thereby decreasing cell deformability. The inclusions are pitted by macrophages in the spleen, leaving the cell with less hemoglobin and decreased membrane. This process leads to rigid cells and their premature destruction in the spleen.

Many of the unstable hemoglobins, in addition to having decreased stability, also have altered oxygen affinity. If the amino acid substitution is strategically located to affect the oxygen binding site, oxygen affinity may be increased or decreased.

CLINICAL FINDINGS

Congenital hemolytic anemia is indicative of an unstable hemoglobin disorder and demands further investigation to establish a definitive diagnosis. Family history is extremely important in defining the hereditary nature of the disease. Patient history may also provide information about the nature of events that precipitate acute hemolytic episodes, such as infection or drug administration.

The severity of the anemia is dependent on the degree of instability and change, if any, in oxygen affinity. Hemoglobins with a high oxygen affinity (Hb Koln) are usually accompanied by erythrocytosis. With increased oxygen affinity, the hemoglobin–oxygen dissociation curve is shifted left, decreasing the amount of oxygen released to the tissues and increasing erythropoietin levels. Thus, there is an increase in erythrocytes. This compensates for hemolysis due to hemoglobin instability and results in normal hemoglobin levels. Conversely, unstable hemoglobins with decreased oxygen affinity (Hb Hammersmith) may be asymptomatic because the hemoglobin–oxygen dissociation curve is shifted right, increasing the amount of oxygen delivered to the tissue. When the oxygen affinity of an unstable hemoglobin is altered, the reticulocyte count is not increased as much as would be expected with an uncomplicated hemolytic anemia.

Most clinical findings occur as the result of increased erythrocyte hemolysis. Jaundice and splenomegaly are common because of chronic extravascular hemolysis. Cyanosis results from the formation of sulfhemoglobin and methemoglobin, which accompany hemoglobin denaturation. Weakness and jaundice frequently follow the administration of oxidant drugs, which increase the instability of the hemoglobin. Acute hemolysis also may be accompanied by the excretion of dark urine due to the presence of dipyrroles in the urine.

LABORATORY FINDINGS

Peripheral blood The anemia of congenital Heinz body hemolytic anemia is usually normocytic and normochromic. It may occasionally have a slightly decreased MCH and MCHC because of the removal of hemoglobin from erythrocytes as Heinz bodies in the spleen. The reticulocyte count is typically increased. The blood film may show basophilic stippling, pitted cells (bite cells), and small contracted cells. Osmotic fragility is usually abnormal after 24 hours of incubation.

Heinz bodies formed in vivo may be demonstrated in the peripheral blood following splenectomy; however, this finding is not specific for unstable hemoglobin disorders. Heinz bodies also can be demonstrated in erythrocyte enzyme abnormalities, which permit oxidation of hemoglobin, in thalassemia, and after administration of oxidant drugs in normal individuals. Heinz bodies of unstable hemoglobins can be generated in vitro by incubation of the erythrocytes with brilliant cresyl blue or other redox agent. These intracellular inclusions cannot be demonstrated with Wright's stain.

Hemoglobin electrophoresis Most unstable hemoglobins have the same charge and electrophoretic mobility as normal hemoglobin. Only about 45% can be diagnosed by electrophoresis. Hemoglobin A_2 and HbF are sometimes increased. This may provide a clue to the presence of an abnormal hemoglobin when it is not dectectable by its electrophoretic pattern.

Heat instability test The heat instability test is always positive in unstable hemoglobin disorders. When an erythrocyte lysate in TRIS buffer is heated to 50° C for 60 minutes, the presence of a fine precipitate is specific for unstable hemoglobins.

Isopropanol stability test The unstable hemoglobin is precipitated in 20 minutes by the presence of nonpolar isopropanol. Nonpolar solvents weaken the internal hemoglobin bonds and decrease stability. Normal hemoglobin remains solvent for 30 to 40 minutes.

THERAPY

Most patients with these disorders do not require any therapy. Splenectomy may be performed if hemolysis is severe. Patients are advised to avoid oxidizing drugs, which may precipitate a hemolytic episode.

● Hemoglobin variants with altered oxygen affinity

Amino acid substitutions in the globin chains close to the heme pocket may affect the ability of hemoglobin to carry oxygen by preventing binding of heme to the globin chain or by stabilizing iron in the oxidized ferric state. Other substitutions that affect oxygen affinity include substitutions near the α, β contacts, substitutions at the C-terminal end of the β-chain, and substitutions near the 2,3-DPG binding site. These are critical sites that are involved in the allosteric properties of hemoglobin and/or in the physiologic regulation of hemoglobin affinity for oxygen. Either the α- or β-chain may be affected but most substitutions are associated with the β-chain. Decreased hemoglobin affinity is characterized by permanent methemoglobin formation and cyanosis. Increased oxygen affinity results in congenital polycythemia, a compensatory mechanism for the inability of the hemoglobin to unload oxygen to the tissues.

DECREASED OXYGEN AFFINITY

Methemoglobin is hemoglobin with iron oxidized to the ferric state ($Fe+++$). Oxygen cannot be carried by methemoglobin, resulting in cyanosis. Normally, the amount of methemoglobin produced under normal physiologic conditions is maintained at concentrations less than 1% through the NADH dependent enzyme, methemoglobin reductase. This system is capable of reducing methemoglobin to deoxyhemoglobin at a rate 250 times the rate at which heme is normally oxidized.

Methemoglobinemia is a clinical condition that occurs when methemoglobin encompasses more than 1% of the hemoglobin. This condition can occur when the methemoglobin reductase system is overwhelmed (acquired) or deficient (congenital) and when a structurally abnormal globin chain stabilizes methemoglobin by rendering the molecule poorly susceptible to reduction (congenital) (Table 7-2).

Acquired methemoglobinemia may occur in normal individuals when drugs or other toxic substances oxidize hemoglobin in circulation at a rate that exceeds the reducing capacity of the methemoglobin reductase system.

Congenital cyanosis caused by the presence of methemoglobin may be inherited as a dominant or recessive characteristic. Recessive inheritance is usually associated with a defect in the methemoglobin reduction system, NADH-diphorase (reductase, dehydrogenase) deficiency, rather than with an alteration in the structure of the hemoglobin molecule. With defects in the methemoglobin reduction system, the small amount of methemoglobin formed daily cannot be reduced and consequently accumulates within the cell. Dominant inheritance of methemoglobinemia is usually ascribed to the presence of a structural variant of hemoglobin called hemoglobin M (HbM). Many variants of HbM have been described; however, all variants have been found only in the heterozygous state. In the homozygous state, the hemoglobin could not deliver any oxygen to tissues; therefore, the homozygous condition is incompatible with life.

Most HbM variants are produced by a tyrosine substitution for the proximal or distal histidine in the heme pocket of the α- or β-chains. Tyrosine forms a covalent link with heme iron, stabilizing the iron in the ferric state. If the substitution occurs in the α-chain, cyanosis is present from birth because the α-chain is a component of HbF ($\alpha_2\gamma_2$), the major hemoglobin at birth. If the substitution occurs in the β-chain, cyanosis does not occur until about the sixth month after birth when HbA ($\alpha_2\beta_2$) becomes the major hemoglobin.

The presence of methemoglobin imparts a brownish color to the blood. Aside from this abnormal color, no other hematologic abnormality is present.

Hemoglobin M will not always separate from HbA at an alkaline pH. Hemoglobin electrophoresis on agar gel at pH 7.1 of a blood sample that contains HbM, reveals a brown band (HbM) running anodal to a red band (HbA). The pattern may appear sharper with gel electrofocusing. Oxidizing the erythrocyte hemolysate with ferricyanide before electrophoresis reveals a sharp separation of congenital HbM and methemoglobin formed from HbA during the oxidizing step. Methemoglobin formed from HbA by oxidation of iron with ferricyanide has no change in molecular charge and therefore has the same electrophoretic mobility as HbA.

TABLE 7-2 *CAUSES AND CHARACTERISTICS OF METHEMOGLOBINEMIA*

Cause	Electrophoretic Pattern	NADH-Diaphorase Activity	Reduction with Methylene Blue
Acquired	Normal	Normal	Yes
Hemoglobin oxidized at a rate exceeding capacity of methemoglobin reductase system			
Congenital			
1. Defect in methemoglobin reductase system (recessive)	Normal	Decreased	Yes
2. Structural abnormality of hemoglobin—HbM (dominant)	HbM variant	Normal	No

The presence of HbM may be detected by spectral abnormalities of the hemoglobin whereas methemoglobin formed in NADH-diaphorase deficiency has a normal absorption spectrum. In addition, methemoglobin formed as the result of NADH-diaphorase deficiency can be readily reduced by incubation of blood with methylene blue, whereas methemoglobin caused by a structural hemoglobin variant such as HbM does not reduce with the methylene blue. To confirm NADH-diaphorase deficiency, a quantitative assay of the enzyme activity is necessary.

Congenital methemoglobinemia resulting from NADH-diaphorase deficiency and acquired toxic methemoglobinemia may be treated by administration of ascorbic acid or methylene blue. Conversely, there is no treatment for the HbM structural variants because the abnormal hemoglobin cannot be reduced.

INCREASED OXYGEN AFFINITY

The first hemoglobin variant with increased oxygen affinity was noted in an 81-year-old patient at Johns Hopkins Hospital. The patient had polycythemia for no apparent reason. Subsequent studies demonstrated a hemoglobin variant with high oxygen affinity. This hemoglobin, which had a leucine substituted for arginine in the α-chain ($\alpha2(FG4)Arg \rightarrow Leu$) was called Hb Chesapeake.

High affinity hemoglobins are inherited as autosomal-dominants. All such hemoglobins discovered have been in the heterozygous state. The variants result from amino acid substitutions which involve the $\alpha_1\beta_2$ contacts. These contacts are involved in considerable intramolecular movement as hemoglobin goes from the oxygenated to deoxygenated state. Other substitutions affect the C-terminal end of the β-chain, which is important in maintaining the stability of the deoxygenated form. A few substitutions affect the 2,3-DPG binding sites.

The abnormal hemoglobin results in a shift to the left of the oxygen dissociation curve. The P50 of the hemoglobin is decreased to 12 to 18 mmHg. This means less oxygen is given up to tissues where the P50 is about 26 mmHg. The resulting tissue hypoxia stimulates erythropoietin production and, subsequently, formation of a compensatory increased erythrocyte mass. In addition to the primary effect of increasing oxygen affinity, secondary effects of the mutations also may occur, including instability of the protein, reduced Bohr effect, and reduced cooperativity of the oxygen binding.[24]

Individuals with these hemoglobin variants are asymptomatic. A ruddy complexion may occasionally be apparent.

The erythrocyte count and hematocrit level are increased, and hemoglobin levels are increased to about 20 g/dL. Other hematologic parameters are normal. About half of the hemoglobin variants have an altered electrophoretic mobility enabling diagnosis by starch gel or cellulose acetate electrophoresis. Diagnosis is established by measuring oxygen affinity.

● THALASSEMIA

The first clinical description of thalassemia was offered by Thomas Cooley in Detroit in 1925.[25] Dr. Cooley suggested the hemolytic nature of the disease, but it was not until after 1940 that enough information was gathered to begin to clarify the pattern of inheritance. By 1960, it was apparent that the thalassemias were a heterogenous group of genetic disorders.

The severe chronic hemolytic anemia of thalassemia is accompanied by bony deformities. Bones expand from within to compensate for the increased erythropoietic activity of the marrow. The bones of the skull are especially involved in this expansion, resulting in characteristic facial deformities. These deformities include a flattened nose, wideset eyes, bossing of the skull, prominent molar eminences, and hypertrophy of the upper maxillae. Evidence exists that suggests that hemoglobinopathies may have occurred in historic or even prehistoric times. Skulls unearthed in Sicily, Sardinia, and other sites exhibit bony changes similar to those seen in the skulls of children with thalassemia. Anthropologists call the bone changes "porotic hyperostosis," which means an increase in porous bony tissue. Although some students of paleontology believe that a few ancient populations may have become extinct due to a hemolytic blood disease, the controversy as to whether the disease was thalassemia remains unsolved. Other chronic anemias can produce bone changes similar to those of thalassemia, including sickle cell anemia.

When first described in 1925, thalassemia was believed to be a rare disorder restricted to the Mediterranean races. The disease was probably seen by physicians before this time, but it was not characterized as a specific hematologic entity. Thalassemia, which produces hematologic abnormalities similar to those seen in severe iron deficiency anemia, can be easily misdiagnosed as such. In the times before laboratory testing was used for diagnosis, it was difficult, if not impossible, to specifically diagnose the pathophysiology of clinically similar hematologic disorders. With the advent of molecular biology, thalassemias have been widely studied by many groups of researchers. Methods developed in the last 25 years enable researchers to measure the quantity of globin chains synthesized and identify specific genetic mutations.

Thalassemia is now recognized as one of the most common genetic disorders affecting the world's population. Evidence indicates that heterozygotes for thalassemia are protected from the severe effects of malaria caused by *Plasmodium falciparum*. Hence, natural selection of these heterozygotes has greatly increased the frequency of thalassemia throughout the tropical and subtropical regions of the world. It is estimated that between 100,000 and 200,000 individuals are born worldwide each year with severe forms of thalassemia. In North America, about 20% of southeast Asian immigrants and 6% to 11% of African-Americans have detectable α-thalassemia. Many more are silent carriers. About 6% of individuals with Mediterranean origin, 5% of southeast Asians, and 0.8% of African-Americans have β-thalassemia.

Studies of family pedigrees have revealed that thalassemias are inherited in a Mendelian autosomal-dominant fashion. Individuals with the homozygous form are severely affected and without treatment die in childhood from complications of severe anemia. Heterozygous thalassemia is a disorder of varying severity. Some heterozygous individuals show no signs of the disease while others exhibit signs and symptoms similar to those seen in the homozygous individuals. This variability of genetic expression is probably related to the many different mutations that lead to thalassemia and to the interaction of the thalassemia gene with other genetic or acquired modifiers.

● Types of thalassemia

Thalassemias are due to genetic mutations that cause a decrease in the rate of synthesis of one of the constituent globin chains, usually α or β, of hemoglobin. The result is a decrease in total hemoglobin and unbalanced synthesis of α- and β-globin chains. (Normally the amount of α and β chains produced are equal, maintaining a balance.) The degree of inbalance is related to the clinical expression of these disorders. No structurally abnormal hemoglobin can be found. Decreased globin chain synthesis may be due to either structural gene deletions or by mutations in intergene controlling sites that impair or prevent gene expression.

Two main variants of classical thalassemia have been described: α-thalassemia and β-thalassemia. When synthesis of the α-chain is impaired, the disease is α-thalassemia. When synthesis of the β-chain is affected, the disease is β-thalassemia. A third type of thalassemia, δ-thalassemia, has been reported, but its occurrence is rare and is not clinically significant because the δ-chain is a component of the minor hemoglobin, HbA$_2$. Rarely, combinations of gene deletions lead to δ-β-thalassemia or δ-γ-β-thalassemia. The affected chains are all synthesized at a reduced rate.

A variant of β-thalassemia is known as hereditary persistence of fetal hemoglobin (HPFH). In this disorder, there is a failure in the switch of γ-chain production to β-chain production after birth. Consequently, only HbF is produced.

Occasionally, synthesis of a structural hemoglobin variant is decreased, giving the clinical picture of thalassemia. These structural variants include those hemoglobins with abnormally long or short globin chains caused by a mutation in the stop codon or to mutation of a nonstop codon to a stop codon (e.g., hemoglobin Constant Spring). Hemoglobin Lepore is a variant hemoglobin whose non-α globin chains are not only structurally abnormal but are also ineffectively synthesized, partly because of the instability of the globin RNA. Because of their clinical similarity to thalassemias, these particular structural variants will be discussed in this section.

● β-thalassemia

The heterogeneity of β-thalassemia became apparent from studies on individuals heterozygous for both HbS and β-thalassemia (β^s/β^{thal}). In sickle cell trait (β/β^s), HbS normally composes less than 50% of the total hemoglobin; the remainder is HbA. However, those individuals with sickle cell trait who inherit a β^{thal} gene from one parent and a β^s gene from the other may produce no HbA. Others with β^s/β^{thal} have been found to produce some HbA, but the HbA concentration is less than that of HbS. Despite these differences in HbA concentration among individuals heterozygous for β^s/β^{thal}, studies show that affected members of the same family produce similar amounts of HbA. The difference in HbA production in these double heterozygotes suggests that there are two β^{thal} genes differing from one another in the extent to which β-chain synthesis is blocked. The two gene varieties have been termed β^+ and β^0. The β^+ gene mutation causes a partial block in β chain synthesis. The β^0 gene mutation causes a complete absence of β chain synthesis. The existence of two β-thalassemia gene mutations helps explain the variability in HbA and HbS concentrations in patients heterozygous for β^s and β^{thal}. Individuals who have the genotype $\beta^s/\beta^{o\text{-thal}}$ produce Hb S but no HbA, whereas those with the genotype $\beta^s/\beta^{+\text{thal}}$ produce some HbA with HbS.

β-thalassemia is the result of several different molecular defects. Over 100 mutations have been described that result in partial to complete absence of β-gene expression. β-thalassemia is rarely due to deletion of the structural gene. Most defects are point mutations in regions which control β-gene expression. Mutations may affect any step in the pathway of globin gene expression, including gene transcription, RNA processing of m-RNA translation, and post-translational integrity of the protein.[26,27] Within a given population, a few mutations account for most of the β-thalassemia genetic defects. For instance, in Greece, five mutations account for 87% of the gene defects.[27]

Any combination of normal β-genes and β^{thal} genes is possible, producing a wide variety of phenotypic (clinical) variants (Table 7-3). In the past, thalassemias were commonly classified according to the clinical severity of the disease: thalassemia major (or Cooley's anemia), thalassemia intermedia, thalassemia minor, and thalassemia minima. These phenotypic terms do not accurately reflect the genetic description of the disease. Even at similar genetic levels, the disease is phenotypically diverse. For instance, a severe form of β^+/β^+ thalassemia (Mediterranean form) is characterized by an increase in HbF (50% to 90%), and HbA$_2$ is normal or only slightly elevated, whereas a milder form of β^+/β^+ thalassemia (Black form) has 20% to 40% HbF with normal or elevated HbA$_2$ and the remainder HbA. Varying amounts of HbA also may be found with various combinations of the β-thalassemia genes: β^0/β^0 no HbA; β^+/β^+ 24% to 36% HbA, β^0/β^+ 4% to 11% HbA. This variation in HbA and HbF concentration accounts for the diverse anemia and varied clinical findings of thalassemia. To avoid confusion, in subsequent discussions, the genotype classification will be given instead of the phenotype classification.

PATHOPHYSIOLOGY

Normally equal quantities of α- and β-chains are synthesized by the maturing erythrocyte resulting in a β- to α-chain ratio of 1.0. In β-thalassemia, synthesis of β-chains is decreased or absent, resulting in an excess of free alpha chains. In heterozygous thalassemia, the β- to α-chain

TABLE 7-3 *CHARACTERISTICS OF β-THALASSEMIAS*

Genotype	Parental Genotypes	Hemoglobin Pattern	Clinical Severity
β^+/β	At least one parent must have β^+ gene, e.g. $\beta^+/\beta \times$ normal	↑HbA$_2$, slight ↑ HbF	mild
β^+/β^+	Both parents must have at least one β^+ gene, e.g. $\beta^+/\beta \times \beta^+/\beta$	↓HbA, ↑HbF, variable HbA$_2$	variable but usually severe (Cooley's anemia)
β^0/β	At least one parent must have one β^0 gene, e.g., $\beta^0/\beta \times$ normal	↑HbA$_2$, ↓HbA, ↑HbF	mild
β^0/β^0	Both parents must have a β^0 gene e.g. $\beta^0/\beta \times \beta^0/\beta$	No HbA, variable HbA$_2$, remainder HbF	severe (Cooley's anemia)
$(\delta\beta)^{0\text{-thal}}/\delta\beta$ (heterozygous)	At least one parent must have $\delta\beta^0$-thal gene, e.g. $(\delta\beta)^{0\text{-thal}}/\delta\beta \times$ normal	HbA$_2$ normal or slight ↓, 5–20% HbF, ↓HbA,	mild
$(\delta\beta)^{0\text{-thal}}/(\delta\beta)^{0\text{-thal}}$ (homozygous)	Both parents must have $\delta\beta^0$-thal gene, e.g. $(\delta\beta)^{0\text{-thal}}/\delta\beta \times (\delta\beta)^{0\text{-thal}}/\delta\beta$	No HbA or HbA$_2$, 100% HbF	mild to moderate
$\delta^0\beta^0/\delta\beta$, HPFH (heterozygous)	At least one parent must have $\delta^0\beta^0$ gene e.g. $\delta^0\beta^0/\delta\beta \times$ normal	↓HbA, ↓HbA$_2$, 10–30% HbF	normal
$\delta^0\beta^0/\delta^0\beta^0$, HPFH (homozygous)	Both parents must have the $\delta^0\beta^0$ gene e.g. $\delta^0\beta^0/\delta\beta \times \delta^0\beta^0/\delta\beta$	100% HbF	normal

ratio is 0.5 to 0.7, whereas in homozygous thalassemia, the ratio is less than 0.25. This imbalanced synthesis of α and β chains has several adverse effects: (1) a decrease in total erythrocyte hemoglobin production, (2) ineffective erythropoiesis, and (3) a chronic hemolytic process.

The decreased production of β-chains causes a decrease in total erythrocyte hemoglobin production as depicted by small cells (microcytic) poorly filled with hemoglobin (hypochromic). Although an increase in δ- and γ-chain synthesis produces an increase in HbA$_2$ and HbF, this increase is not sufficient to alleviate the severe hemoglobin shortage in the cell.

The free excess α-chains are unstable and precipitate within the cell, causing membrane damage and decreased erythrocyte deformability.[28] Evidence indicates that the excess α-chains are partially oxidized and bind to the cell membrane and its skeleton.[29] This causes decreased membrane stability, and subsequent cell hemolysis. Many precipitate-filled erythrocytes in the bone marrow are destroyed by marrow macrophages before the cells can be released to the peripheral blood, resulting in a large degree of ineffective erythropoiesis. Studies of the cause(s) of intramedullary erythroid death suggest that the excess α-chain aggregates turn on programs that lead to cell death (apoptosis) and interfere with normal synthesis and assembly of the membrane skeletal proteins, spectrin and band 4.1.[29]

In circulating erythrocytes, α-chain precipitates are pitted by the spleen, producing many misshapen cells. Many of the cells with damaged membranes are destroyed prematurely in the spleen. This chronic hemolytic process also contributes to the anemia of thalassemia.

Of the three pathologies, the major factor responsible for the severe anemia of β-thalassemia is probably ineffective erythropoiesis caused by the presence of unpaired α-chains (Fig. 7-11).

HOMOZYGOUS β-THALASSEMIA (β^0/β^0, β^+/β^+, β^0/β^+)

Homozygous β-thalassemia is phenotypically and genetically diverse; most cases, however, have severe symptomatic disease. The disorder is caused by a marked reduction or absence of β-chains. Since the major hemoglobin at birth is HbF ($\alpha_2\gamma_2$), the infant with thalassemia is protected from severe anemia until the second 6 months of life, when HbA ($\alpha_2\beta_2$) normally replaces HbF as the major hemoglobin. Deficient β-chain production at birth can be demonstrated on cord blood. Although normal cord blood contains about 20% HbA, cord blood of infants with homozygous thalassemia has less than 2% HbA and cord blood from heterozygotes has from 6% to 10% HbA.[26] The irritable, pale infant fails to thrive and gain weight. Diarrhea, fever, and an enlarged abdomen are common findings. If therapy is not begun during early childhood, the clinical picture of thalassemia develops within a few years.

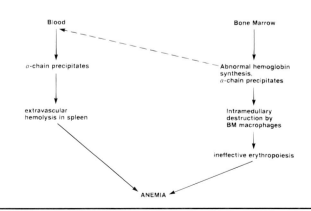

FIGURE 7-11. The chronic anemia in α-thalassemia is primarily the result of the excess α- to β-chain ratio within the erythrocytes.

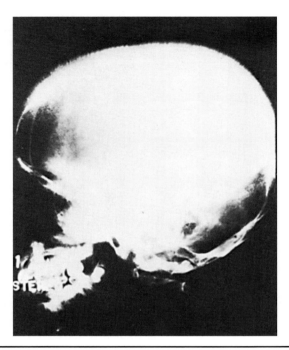

FIGURE 7-12. A skull radiograph of a child with β-thalassemia.

Severe anemia is the clinical disorder responsible for many of the problems these children have. The anemia places a tremendous burden on the cardiovascular system as it attempts to maintain tissue perfusion. Constant high output of blood usually results in cardiac failure in the first decade of life; this is the major cause of death in untreated children. Growth is retarded and a brown pigmentation of the skin is notable. Chronic hemolysis is accompanied by gallstones, gout, and icterus.

The spleen may become massively enlarged. Abnormal erythrocytes become congested within the spleen stimulating the production of more erythrocytes in the marrow. Secondary leukopenia and thrombocytopenia are produced as these components also become trapped in the enlarged spleen.

Bone changes accompany an extremely hyperplastic marrow. Marrow cavities enlarge in every bone, expanding the bone and producing characteristic bossing of the skull, facial deformities, and "hair-on-end" appearance of the skull on X-ray (Fig. 7-12). The thinning bone cortex in long bones also may lead to pathologic fractures.

Extramedullary hematopoiesis in the liver and spleen is an attempt by the body to increase the concentration of peripheral erythrocytes. Occasionally, extramedullary masses of hematopoietic tissue may be found elsewhere in the body.

Other clinical findings are associated with the body's attempt to increase erythrocyte production. Features of the hypermetabolic rate include fever, lethargy, poor musculature, a decrease in body fat, and decrease in appetite. Infection is a common cause of death. Folic acid deficiency may develop as a consequence of its increased utilization by the hyperplastic marrow.

Most children with β-thalassemia major receive regular transfusion therapy, which prolongs life into the second or third decade. The large doses of iron accumulated with these transfusions, however, leads to tissue damage from iron overload similar to that seen in hemochromatosis. Iron-chelating agents are given to decrease the deposition of iron in the tissues. As with other hemolytic anemias, more iron is also absorbed from the gut, exacerbating the iron overload from transfusions. Although the absorbed iron rapidly enters the plasma, it is diverted to the mononuclear phagocyte system for storage because its incorporation into the normoblast is greatly reduced. Usually, in the second decade of life, endocrine disorders and hepatic and cardiac disturbances develop from excessive deposits of iron in these tissues. Diabetes is a common complication of excessive pancreatic iron deposits. Hepatic disturbances may result in cirrhosis. The mode of death in these transfused children is primarily cardiac complications from cardiac siderosis.

Laboratory findings

PERIPHERAL BLOOD The hemoglobin level may be as low as 2 or 3 g/dL in homozygous thalassemia. The anemia is markedly microcytic, hypochromic with an MCV of less than 67 fL.[30] The MCH and MCHC are also markedly reduced. The peripheral blood smear shows marked anisocytosis and poikilocytosis with schistocytes, ovalocytes, dacryocytes, and target cells (Fig. 7-13). Precipitates of α-chains may be visualized with methyl violet stain. Variable basophilic stippling and polychromasia are noted. The reticulocyte count is usually less than 10%. Reticulocytes are not increased to the degree expected for the severity of the anemia because of the high degree of ineffective erythropoiesis. Nucleated erythrocytes are almost always found. The RDW may be increased.[31]

Thalassemia may be confused with severe iron deficiency anemia, thus, the free erythrocyte protoporphyrin

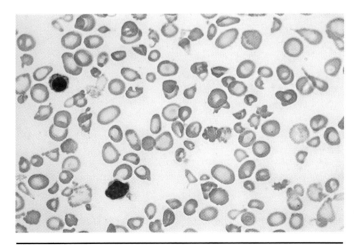

FIGURE 7-13. A blood film from a patient with homozygous β-thalassemia who has been transfusion dependent for 17 years. (250 × original magnification; Wright-Giemsa stain.)

TABLE 7-4   *IRON STUDIES HELPFUL IN DIFFERENTIATING THALASSEMIA FROM IRON DEFICIENCY*

Disease	Serum Iron	Serum Ferritin	TIBC	Percent Saturation	Storage Iron	FEP
Thalassemia	N to ↑	N to ↑	N to ↓	↑	↑	N
Iron Deficiency	↓	↓	↑	↓	Absent	↑

N = normal
↑ = increased
↓ = decreased
TIBC = Total iron binding capacity
FEP = Free erythrocyte protoporphyrin

(FEP) level (or zinc protoporhyrin, ZPP, level) or other index of iron metabolism should be determined to differentiate the two conditions (Table 7-4). The FEP level is normal in thalassemia and increased in iron deficiency. The FEP level may, however, be increased if lead poisoning coexists with thalassemia. Ferrochelatase is inhibited by lead and causes an increase in FEP. Other iron studies are helpful to differentiate thalassemia and iron deficiency. In thalassemia, serum iron and serum ferritin are normal to increased; total iron binding capacity is normal to low with increased transferrin saturation; storage iron is increased. In iron deficiency, serum iron and serum ferritin are low, total iron binding capacity is increased with decreased transferrin saturation, and storage iron is absent. Iron deficiency may, however, coexist with thalassemia, complicating diagnosis.

Chronic hemolysis is reflected by increased unconjugated bilirubin. Urine may appear dark brown from the presence of dipyrroles. Osmotic fragility is decreased due to the large number of target cells but has no diagnostic value.

BONE MARROW   Bone marrow studies are not usually necessary for diagnosis, but when performed, show marked erythroid hyperplasia with an M:E ratio of 0.1 or less. Normoblasts appear abnormal with very little cytoplasm, uneven cytoplasmic membranes, and striking basophilic stippling. Prussian blue stain reveals an abundance of iron. Occasionally, a few ringed sideroblasts are noted. Phagocytic foam cells similar to Gaucher cells have been reported. The "foam" is probably the result of partially digested red cell membrane lipids associated with intense ineffective erythropoiesis. Precipitates from α-chains in developing normoblasts can almost always be demonstrated with methyl violet stain.

HEMOGLOBIN ELECTROPHORESIS   Hemoglobin electrophoresis shows variable results depending on the thalassemia genes inherited. Absence of HbA; 90% HbF and low, normal or increased HbA$_2$ is characteristic of β^o/β^o thalassemia.[32] The other homozygous thalassemias, β^o/β^+, β^+/β^+, show some HbA (4% to 11%, 24% to 36%, respectively) on electrophoresis, but the majority of the hemoglobin is HbF with normal to increased HbA$_2$.[33] The milder form of homozygous thalassemia, β^+/β^+ (Black form) has greater than 50% HbA, 2% to 5% HbA$_2$, and

20% to 40% HbF. The HbF increase in thalassemia is believed to be due to the expansion of a subpopulation of erythrocytes that have the ability to synthesize γ-chains. The distribution of HbF among erythrocytes is heterogeneous.

Definitive diagnosis of β-thalassemia may be made by demonstration of a reduced β- to α-chain ratio of less than 0.25. To determine this ratio, small amounts of peripheral blood are incubated with a radioactively labeled amino acid. The labeled acid is then incorporated into the newly synthesized chains. The chains are separated by chromatographic techniques, and their relative production is estimated by determining radioactivity. Molecular techniques demonstrating specific genetic mutations also may define the presence of thalassemia.

Therapy   Regular blood transfusions from an early age in an attempt to maintain normal hemoglobin levels will prevent the hyperstimulation of the bone marrow and resultant complications. However, as mentioned, this therapy leads to complications arising from iron overload. Administration of iron chelators such as desferrioxamine to help remove excess iron may diminish, but may not prevent, iron overload. Splenectomy is performed in an attempt to decrease hemolysis and prolong erythrocyte survival.

Within the last several years, bone marrow transplants have been attempted in an effort to provide the individual with normal stem cells capable of producing normal erythrocytes. Although bone marrow transplantation is an option for thalassemia patients with a suitable donor, this technology is not widely used at this time.[34] Correction of the molecular defect with gene therapy may be achieved in the future.

HETEROZYGOUS β-THALASSEMIA (β^+/β) OR (β^o/β)

The heterozygous state of β-thalassemia (thalassemia minor) results from the inheritance of either a β^+ or β^o thalassemia gene. One normal β-gene is present. There is mounting evidence that there is no major clinical difference in the expression between the two thalassemia genes in the heterozygous state. The normal β-gene directs synthesis of β-chains and the erythrocyte survival is nearly normal. The heterozygote disorder appears to be symptomless except in periods of stress or during pregnancy when a moderate microcytic anemia develops. The condi-

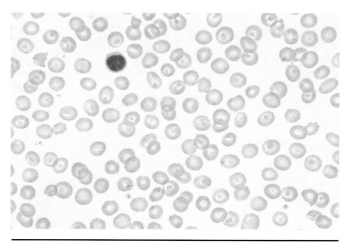

FIGURE 7-14. Blood smear from a patient with β-thalassemia minor. The cells are microcytic and there are target cells. The MCV is 61 fL, MCH 20.2 pg, MCHC 33 L/L, erythrocyte count 5.2 x 10¹²/L, Hb 11.1 gm/dL. (250 × original magnification; Wright-Giemsa stain.)

tion is usually discovered incidently during testing for unrelated symptoms. About 1% of American Blacks are heterozygous for β-thalassemia.

In heterozygous thalassemia, the anemia is mild with hemoglobin values from 9 to 11 g/dL, but the number of erythrocytes nearly doubles for what is expected at that hemoglobin concentration (erythrocyte count greater than 5×10^{12}/L). The cells are microcytic (MCV 55 to 70 fL) and hypochromic (Fig. 7-14) or sometimes normochromic. The MCH is usually less than 22 pg. Heterozygous β-thalassemia patients have higher MCVs than homozygous β-thalassemia patients. The degree of microcytosis as indicated by the MCV is directly related to the degree of anemia.[30] Although the anemia is mild, the peripheral blood smear shows variable anisocytosis and poikilocytosis with target cells and basophilic stippling. Nucleated cells are not usually found. Bone marrow shows slight erythroid hyperplasia and normoblasts poorly filled with hemoglobin.

Hemoglobin electrophoresis demonstrates an increase in HbA_2 from 3.5% to 7%, with a mean of 5.5%. HbF may be normal or increased.[37] If HbF exceeds 5%, however, the individual has probably inherited a HPFH gene in addition to the β-thalassemia gene. Newborns have a normal HbA_2 concentration of 0.27 ± 0.02%.[32]

Heterozygous thalassemia is frequently confused with iron deficiency anemia since the hematologic morphology is similar in these two conditions.[35,36] There are, however, a few parameters that, taken together, may be helpful in differentiation (Table 7-5). Diagnosis may be more difficult if iron deficiency is present concurrently with heterozygous β-thalassemia as the β-thalassemia may be masked by iron deficiency. Successful treatment of the iron deficiency accompanied by persistent microcytosis suggests the presence of thalassemia. Further investigation to help determine the cause of the persistent microcytosis is suggested (Fig. 7-15A and B).

HbS/β-THALASSEMIA (β^S/β^{THAL})

Occasionally, an individual is doubly heterozygous for a structural hemoglobin variant and thalassemia. When an individual inherits one sickle cell gene (β^s) and one β-thalassemia gene, the resulting condition is HbS/β-thalassemia disease. The severity of the clinical and laboratory findings of the heterozygous HbS/β^{thal} state depend on the thalassemia gene inherited (Table 7-6). As already noted, the β^o thalassemia gene produces no β-chains while the β^+-thalassemia gene directs the synthesis of decreased quantities of β-chains. Therefore, the clinical signs of this condition may vary from symptomless with a mild decrease in β-chain synthesis (β^+) to moderately severe with total absence of normal β-chain synthesis (β^o). Some of the findings in the symptomatic disorders include palpable spleen, enlargment of the liver and lymph nodes, and mild episodes of skeletal pain and fever.

The degree of abnormal hematologic findings ranges from a blood picture similar to sickle cell anemia to one similar to heterozygous β-thalassemia. A microcytic, hypochromic anemia with decreased MCV, MCH, and MCHC is typical. This is in contrast to the normocytic, normochromic anemia of sickle cell anemia. Hemoglobin concentration varies from 5 to 10 g/dL. Reticulocytosis from 10% to 20% is present. Peripheral blood smears show erythrocytes with anisocytosis, poikilocytosis, and target cells. Leukocyte and platelet counts are within normal ranges.

Hemoglobin electrophoresis provides a clue to diagnosis and allows differentiation of HbS/β-thalassemia disease from sickle cell anemia or sickle cell trait. In HbS/β-thalassemia disease the concentration of HbS is equal to or more than the concentration of HbA: HbS composes 50% to 95% of the total hemoglobin while HbA ranges

TABLE 7-5 *TYPICAL HEMATOLOGIC PARAMETERS HELPFUL IN DIFFERENTIATING WELL-DEVELOPED IRON DEFICIENCY ANEMIA FROM β-THALASSEMIA TRAIT. IRON DEFICIENCY ANEMIA IS CHARACTERIZED BY A MORE SEVERE ANEMIA WITH MORE MARKED HYPOCHROMIA THAN β-THALASSEMIA TRAIT*

	RDW	RBC	MCV	MCH	MCHC	HbA₂	FEP
β-thalassemia trait	usually N	N or ↑	↓↓	↓↓	↓	↑	N
Iron deficiency anemia	↑	↓↓	↓	↓	↓↓	N	↑

* Usually increased in homozygous β-thalassemia (↓ = decreased; ↓↓ = more decreased; ↑ = increased; N = normal; FEP = free erythrocyte protoporphyrin; RDW = red cell distribution width; RBC = erythrocyte count; MCV = mean corpuscular volume; MCH = mean corpuscular hemoglobin; MCHC = mean corpuscular hemoglobin concentration)

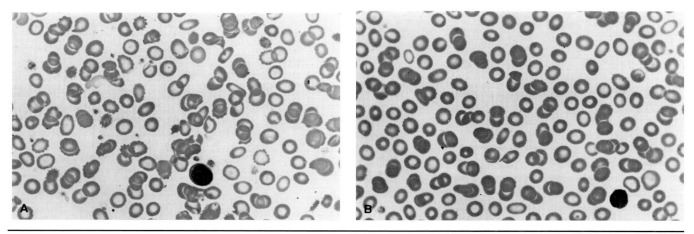

FIGURE 7-15. A, The blood film of a patient with heterozygous β-thalassemia and iron deficiency. **B,** The blood film of the patient in (a) after treatment with iron. Note the persistent microcytosis although the degree of hypochromia, anisocytosis, and poikilocytosis appears improved.

from 0% to 50%. HbF varies from 2% to 30% and HbA$_2$ is > 3.5%. Family studies will also help to establish the HbS/β^{thal} disorder.

Hemoglobin Lepore

Hemoglobin Lepore was first described in 1958 as a structural hemoglobin variant with hematologic changes and clinical manifestations resembling those of thalassemia.[38] The disorder is widely distributed throughout the world but is especially common in middle and eastern Europe.

In Hb Lepore, the non-α-chain is a δ-β-globin hybrid in which the N-terminal end of a δ-chain is fused to the C-terminal end of a β-chain (Fig. 7-16). The variant hybrid chains are believed to arise during meiosis from aberrant recombination of misaligned δ- and β-genes on separate

chromosomes. Two of these hybrid β-chains combine with two α-chains to form Hb Lepore. Hb Lepore is stable and has normal functional properties, except for a slight increase in oxygen affinity.

The pathophysiology is similar to that of β-thalassemia. The Hb Lepore gene is under the influence of the δ-promoter gene, which limits synthesis of the δ-chain gene to 2.5% that of the β-chain. Thus, the abnormal hybrid globin chains are ineffectively synthesized, leading to an excess of α-chains. The excess α-chains precipitate leading to cell membrane damage and inflexibility. As a consequence, erythrocytes are prematurely destroyed. In an attempt to meet the need for peripheral blood erythrocytes, the erythroid marrow expands, producing more abnormal cells. Ineffective erythropoiesis contributes to the anemia as the abnormal cells are destroyed in the bone

TABLE 7-6 *THE GENOTYPIC AND PHENOTYPIC POSSIBILITIES OF CHILDREN BORN TO PARENTS WHO ARE HETEROZYGOUS FOR β-THALASSEMIA AND FOR HbS*

	Mother	Father	Mother	Father
Genotype	$\beta^S\beta$	$\beta^{+thal}\beta$	$\beta^S\beta$	$\beta^{othal}\beta$
Hemoglobin pattern	Hb S 35% Hb A 65% Hb A$_2$ normal Hb F normal	Hb A normal Hb A$_2$ increased Hb F increased	Same as mother at left	Hb A normal to decreased Hb A$_2$ increased Hb F increased
Phenotype	Sickle cell trait	Heterozygous thal	Sickle cell trait	Heterozygous thal

Children								
Genotype	$\beta^S\beta^{+thal}$	$\beta^S\beta$	$\beta^{+thal}\beta$	$\beta\beta$	$\beta^S\beta^{othal}$	$\beta^S\beta$	$\beta\beta^{othal}$	$\beta\beta$
Hemoglobin pattern	Hb S 50% Hb A 50% Hb A$_2$ increased Hb F increased	Hb A 65% Hb S 35% Hb A$_2$ normal Hb F normal	Hb A normal Hb A$_2$ increased Hb F increased	Hb A normal Hb A$_2$ normal Hb F normal	Hb A absent Hb S 70% Hb A$_2$ increased Hb F increased	Hb A 65% Hb S 35% Hb A$_2$ normal Hb F normal	Hb A normal to decreased Hb A$_2$ increased Hb F increased	Hb A normal Hb A$_2$ normal Hb F normal
Phenotype	Mild sickle cell anemia	Sickle cell trait	Heterozygous thalassemia	Normal	Sickle cell anemia	Sickle cell trait	Heterozygous thalassemia	Normal

The percentage of hemoglobin is approximate and given for comparison purposes only.

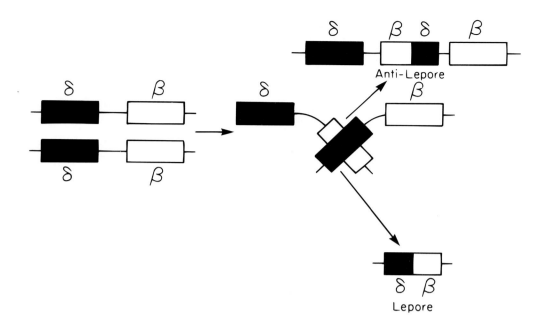

FIGURE 7-16. Schematic drawing of how the Hb Lepore gene is produced during meiosis. It is believed that unequal crossing over of the δ- and β- genes produces the $\delta\beta$ gene (Lepore). This abnormal crossing over also gives rise to a chromosome that contains normal δ and β-genes and a fused $\beta\delta$-gene (anti-Lepore). The rate of synthesis of the abnormal $\beta\delta$ chain is intermediate between that of the δ chain and the β chain.

marrow. The homozygous and heterozygous states of Hb Lepore are clinically similar to those of β-thalassemia.

HOMOZYGOUS Hb LEPORE

Homozygous Hb Lepore is characterized by a variable anemia and a variable clinical course in different racial groups. Clinical manifestations have been reported that are as severe as those seen in homozygous β-thalassemia or as mild as those in heterozygous β-thalassemia. Thalassemia-like abnormalities develop in patients within the first 5 years of life. Anemia ranges from severe to mild. Hepatosplenomegaly is significant. Depending on the degree of ineffective erythropoiesis, skeletal abnormalities similar to those of β-thalassemia may be noted. Growth may be retarded, and mongoloid facies may be prominent. The more severely affected children may become transfusion-dependent and develop complications of hemosiderosis.

Hemoglobin levels range from 4 to 11 g/dL. The peripheral blood picture is similar to that of β-thalassemia, with a microcytic hypochromic erythrocyte population. Anisocytosis, poikilocytosis with target cells, and basophilic stippling is noted on blood films. After splenectomy, nucleated erythrocytes and erythrocytes with α-chain precipitates may be found in peripheral blood. The bone marrow exhibits erythroid hyperplasia.

Because of the absence of normal β and δ globin chains, hemoglobin electrophoresis shows no HbA or HbA$_2$, from 8% to 30% Hb Lepore, with the remainder HbF. Hemoglobin Lepore migrates with HbS on cellulose acetate electrophoresis at alkaline pH but migrates with HbA on citrate agar at acid pH.

The severely anemic cases of Hb Lepore require a regular transfusion protocol from early childhood. Splenectomy also is performed in an attempt to lessen the degree of anemia.

HETEROZYGOUS Hb LEPORE

Heterozygous Hb Lepore is asymptomatic. However, several cases of splenomegaly have been reported. The blood picture is similar to that seen in heterozygous β-thalassemia. The hemoglobin is slightly decreased with a mean of 12.2 g/dL. The erythrocytes are microcytic and hypochromic with a mean MCV of 72 fL. Hemoglobin analysis reveals a mean Hb Lepore concentration of 10%, HbA$_2$ is decreased with a mean of 2%, and HbF is usually slightly elevated to 2% to 3%. The remainder is HbA.

● Hereditary persistence of fetal hemoglobin

Hereditary persistence of fetal hemoglobin (HPFH) is actually a group of heterogenous disorders in which the absence of α- and β-chain synthesis is compensated for by increased γ-chain production into adult life. The result is an absence of HbA and HbA$_2$. Only HbF is synthesized. HbF production continues at high levels throughout life, preventing the clinical symptoms associated with thalassemia. There are no significant hematologic abnormalities. The condition occurs in 0.1% of American Blacks.

This abnormality was first recognized in 1955, when two separate cases were reported in which a healthy adult who appeared to be homozygous for HbS, because only HbS and HbF were detected, had a child with no HbS but high levels of HbF.[39] If these adults were truly homozygous for the β^s gene, they should have passed one β^s gene to each of their children and each child should have some HbS. It was later realized that the parent was not homozygous for β^s but rather was a double heterozygote for β^s and for HPFH. The child in both cases inherited the HPFH rather than the β^s gene from the heterozygous parent and a normal β-gene from the normal parent. This meant the child could synthesize some HbA from the normal β-gene but at the same time synthesized increased amounts of the

TABLE 7-7 *CHARACTERISTICS OF TYPES OF HPFH VARIANTS*

HPFH Type	Type of γ Chains Produced	Distribution of HbF in Erythrocytes
Black	$^G\gamma$ and $^A\gamma$	Homogeneous—"cell-wide"
Swiss	$^G\gamma$ and $^A\gamma$	Heterogeneous
Greek	primarily $^A\gamma$	Homogeneous

γ-chain, producing high HbF levels.[40] Similar cases have been described since these first studies.

HPFH is characterized by either deletion or inactivity of the β- and δ-structural gene complex. In the deletion variants both $^G\gamma$ and $^A\gamma$ are synthesized in increased quantities. In the nondeletion variants, only one of the two γ chains are overexpressed.[26] Most nondeletion variants are due to mutations in gene promoter regions. The γ-chain continues to be produced in increased quantity throughout life, compensating for the lack of β- and δ-chain production. Consequently, there is no accumulation and no precipitation of excess α-chains. Most α-chains combine with the available γ-chains to produce HbF.

A typical finding in HPFH is the "cell-wide" uniform distribution of HbF in erythrocytes, a feature that helps distinguish this disorder from other disorders associated with an increase in HbF. In normal adults and in diseases other than HPFH that are characterized by an increase in HbF, the HbF is restricted to a few erythrocytes called F-cells (heterogeneous HbF distribution).

Several different types of HPFH have been described: the Black type; the Greek type; the Swiss type. In the Black and Swiss types, both $^G\gamma$ and $^A\gamma$ chains are produced in approximately equal amounts. The Greek form is characterized by production of both $^G\gamma$ and $^A\gamma$ chains, but most HbF is made up of the $^A\gamma$-chains. Both the Black type and Greek type have the characteristic "cell-wide" distribution of HbF in erythrocytes. However, the Swiss form has a heterogeneous distribution of HbF. This heterocellular distribution results from an inherited increase in the number of F cells[27] (Table 7-7)

It has been suggested that the various categories of HPFH are actually a continuum of a spectrum of β-thalassemias with homozygous β^o-thalassemia at one end where the lack of β-chain synthesis is poorly compensated for by γ-chain production, and with HPFH at the other end where lack of β-chain synthesis is almost completely compensated for by γ-chain production.

HOMOZYGOUS HPFH

Homozygous HPFH is asymptomatic. There are no clinical findings suggestive of thalassemia including no abnormal growth patterns and no splenomegaly.

Erythrocytosis occurs as the result of the high oxygen affinity of HbF. High hemoglobin levels from 14.8 to 18.2 g/dL are typical of HPFH. Erythrocytes are microcytic and slightly hypochromic with a mean MCV of 75 fL and a mean MCH of 25.0 pg. The erythrocyte count is high, from 6×10^{12}/L to 7×10^{12}/L. There is a mild degree of anisocytosis and poikilocytosis. The reticulocyte count is from 1% to 2%. It is doubtful that there is any significant degree of hemolysis in this disorder since the reticulocyte count, bilirubin, and haptoglobin levels are normal. Electrophoresis demonstrates 100% HbF. Both $^G\gamma$ and $^A\gamma$ chains are present.

HETEROZYGOUS HPFH

Heterozygous HPFH is usually found incidentally through family studies. There is an increase in HbF from 10% to 30%. Hemoglobin A_2 is decreased to 1% to 2%, and the remainder is HbA. In the presence of iron deficiency, HbF levels are lower.

Individuals heterozygous for sickle cell and HPFH exhibit a mild form of sickle cell trait with no occurrence of crises or anemia. This benign form of the disorder is believed to be related to the distribution of HbF in erythrocytes. The peripheral blood smear shows anisocytosis and target cells. The sodium metabisulfite test is positive. Hemoglobin electrophoresis produces a pattern that is easily confused with that of sickle anemia. Only HbS, HbF, and HbA$_2$ are present, with HbF levels ranging from 15% to 35%. Hemoglobin A_2 is normal or reduced.

$\delta\beta$-thalassemia

A rare thalassemia in which β- and δ-chain production is absent is known as $\delta\beta$-thalassemia. Like HPFH, the absence of β- and δ-chains is most often due to deletion of the structural β- and δ-gene complex. This thalassemia is frequently confused with HPFH because both disorders have 100% HbF. However, unlike HPFH, increased γ-chain production fails to fully compensate for the loss of β-chain production. It appears that in $\delta\beta$-thalassemia, there is less compensation of γ-chain synthesis than in HPFH but more than in homozygous β-thalassemia. Thus, most patients with $\delta\beta$-thalassemia have a mild anemia with hemoglobin levels ranging from 10 to 12 g/dL. Microcytosis and hypochromia are seen on peripheral blood smears. The $\delta\beta$-thalassemia patients have slight hepatosplenomegaly and some bone changes associated with chronic erythroid hyperplasia. Hemolysis probably contributes to the anemia since both reticulocytes and bilirubin are elevated.

The heterozygous form of $\delta\beta$-thalassemia is not identified with any specific clinical findings. There is no anemia or splenomegaly. The hematologic picture, however, is similar to that of heterozygous β-thalassemia with microcytic, hypochromic erythrocytes. Hemoglobin A_2 is normal or slightly decreased while HbF is increased to 5% to 20%. HbA is usually less than 90%.

$\gamma\delta\beta$-thalassemia

This rare form of thalassemia has several variants and is characterized by deletion or inactivation of the entire β-gene complex. Only the heterozygous state has been encountered. Although neonates have severe hemolytic anemia, as the child grows, the disease evolves to a mild form of β-thalassemia.

● α-THALASSEMIA

α-thalassemia is a group of disorders characterized by decreased synthesis of α-chains. This form of thalassemia has been the most difficult thalassemia to identify clinically as well as genetically. The mild forms in adults are difficult to identify, because although they may have the typical thalassemia erythrocyte morphology, there is no anemia and hemoglobin electrophoresis usually demonstrates normal HbA$_2$ and HbF. Diagnosis at birth is possible because of the hematologic findings of neonatal microcytosis and Hb Bart's on electrophoresis. There are very few causes of an MCV less than 94 fL in conjunction with normal HbA$_2$ levels at birth other than α-thalassemia. In some areas and ethnic groups, α-thalassemia is as common as β-thalassemia. In particular, it is commonly seen in Blacks, Indians, Chinese, and Middle Eastern people.

The genetic mutation is most commonly a deletion of one or more α-genes. Less frequently the mutation is a functionally abnormal α-gene. Unlike the single β- and δ-gene per haploid genotype, the α-gene is duplicated on chromosome 16, producing two genes per haploid and four genes per diploid. Depending on the number of α-gene mutations (from one to four), α-thalassemia may occur in several different clinical forms.

In 1955, HbH, a symptomatic but nonfatal type of α-thalassemia, was the first type to be described.[41] Many reports of the disease followed this first description, with most occurring in southeast Asia. The configuration of HbH was found to consist of four β chains (β^4). This finding suggested the possibility of a deficiency of α-chains to combine with available β-chains. Subsequently, another abnormal hemoglobin, Hb Bart's, was found in infants who had hematologic findings suggestive of thalassemia. Hb Bart's was discovered to have the configuration of four γ chains ($\gamma 4$). This finding again suggested a deficiency of α-chains. It seemed probable then that Hb Bart's was the fetal equivalent of HbH.

By 1970, the accumulation of information on the hereditary nature of thalassemias and advances in molecular genetics permitted a description of the genetics of α-thalassemia. Disorders had been found in which from one to four genes were deleted; hence, four different clinical types of α-thalassemia could occur ranging from a silent asymptomatic type to one that is fatal. Mutation of one α-gene is clinically silent while mutations of the two α-genes result in microcytic, hypochromic erythrocytes. When three α-genes are abnormal, hemoglobin H is present and there is a hemolytic anemia present. When all four α-genes are abnormal, no α-chains are produced. This results in the syndrome hydrops fetalis with Hb Bart's.

The normal haploid genotype for α-globin genes is designated α,α. In α-thalassemia, depending on whether one or both α-genes are missing from chromosome 16, two haplotypes are possible: one α-gene deletion (-,α), also called α-thal-2; two α-gene deletions (-, -), also called α-thal-1. Four different diploid genotypes are possible by heterozygous or homozygous combination of α-thal-2 and/or α-thal-1 (Table 7-8). The clinical disorders resulting from these genotypes each bear a separate name descriptive of the clinical findings observed.[43] The various α-thalassemias can be found together in the same individual with β-thalassemia.

SILENT CARRIER (α-THAL-2/NORMAL)

The silent carrier of α-thalassemia (α-thal-2 trait) is missing only one of four functioning α-genes. The three remaining α-genes direct the synthesis of an adequate number of chains for normal hemoglobin synthesis. This carrier state is totally benign. In affected infants, 1% to 2% Hb Bart's may be found. Hb Bart's, however, cannot be detected after 3 months of age. The only way to make a definitive diagnosis in the one or two gene deletion thalassemias in adults is by globin gene analysis. It has been estimated that as many as 25% of American Blacks may be missing one α-gene.[43]

α-THALASSEMIA TRAIT (α-THAL 2/α-THAL 2, OR α-THAL-1/NORMAL)

The α-thalassemia trait (homozygous α-thal-2 or α-thal-1 trait) occurs when two of the four α-genes, either on the same or on opposite chromosomes, are missing. The condition is found in all geographic locations but occurs more commonly in the Mediterranean area, West Africa, and in southeast Asia. It also occurs in approximately 2% of American Blacks. The trait is asymptomatic with a mild

TABLE 7-8 *CHARACTERISTICS OF THE FOUR TYPES OF α-THALASSEMIA*

Genotype	Phenotype	Hematologic Finding	Severity	Hemoglobin Patterns
-α/αα (α-thal2/normal)	silent carrier	normal or slight microcytosis	normal	normal
-α/-α (α-thal2/α-thal2) —/αα (α-thal1/normal)	α-thalassemia trait	mild anemia, microcytic hypochromic RBC, target cells, basophilic stippling, poikilocytosis	mild to moderate	Newborns: Hb Bart's Adults: normal or some HbH
—/-α (α-thal1/α-thal2)	Hemoglobin H disease	moderate to marked anemia, microcytic hypochromic RBC, target cells, basophilic stippling, poikilocytosis	chronic, moderately severe hemolytic anemia	Newborns: Hb Bart's Adults: HbH
—/—(α-thal1/α-thal1)	Hydrops fetalis with hemoglobin Bart's	marked anemia, macrocytic hypochromic RBC, marked anisopoikilocytosis, numerous NRBC	fatal	Hb Bart's Hb Portland

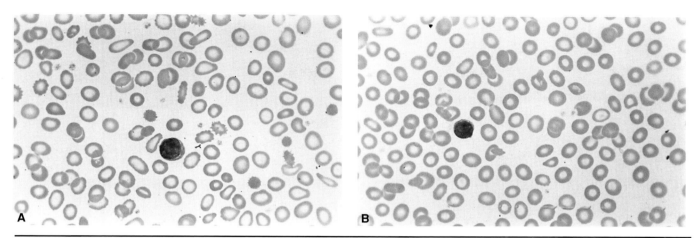

FIGURE 7-17. A, This blood film is from a patient with α-thalassemia trait and iron deficiency. Note the microcytic (MCV 49 fL), hypochromic erythrocytes. There is also poikilocytosis with elliptocytes and anisocytosis. **B,** This is the blood from the patient in (a) after iron therapy. The erythrocytes are now more homogeneous with some hypochromia. The cells, however, are still microcytic with an MCV of only 59 fL. Alpha-thalassemia was not diagnosed until the iron deficiency was treated. Further investigation determined the cause of the persistent microcytic cells to be thalassemia. (250 × original magnification.)

anemia. Hemoglobin levels range from 10 to 12 g/dL, and the erythrocyte count is above 5×10^{12}/L. The peripheral blood film demonstrates significant microcytosis with an MCV of 60 to 70 fL (Fig. 7-17A and 17-B). Mean corpuscular hemoglobin is decreased (MCH 20 to 25 pg), and erythrocytes may appear slightly hypochromic. The imbalance in α- and β-chain synthesis creates an excess in β-chains, which join in tetrads to form HbH. Occasional cells may exhibit HbH inclusions after incubation with brilliant cresyl blue. The presence of 5% to 6% Hb Bart's in neonates may be helpful in diagnosing this condition.[45] However, as in the silent carrier type, Hb Bart's decreases to undetectable levels after 3 months of life and hemoglobin electrophoresis is normal. The only persistent hematologic abnormality is microcytic hypochromic anemia.

As in β-thalassemia trait, the α-thalassemia may be masked by iron deficiency anemia. Successful treatment of iron deficiency but persistence of microcytosis is suggestive of thalassemia (Fig. 17A and 17-B). Further investigation is suggested.

HEMOGLOBIN H (α-THAL-1/α-THAL-2) (FIGURES 7-18A AND 7-18B)

Hemoglobin H disease is the disorder produced when three of four α-genes are deleted. The disease occurs most frequently in southeast Asia. The decreased synthesis of α-chains creates a relative excess of β-chains, which unite to form tetrads of four β-chains. The hemoglobin produced from these β-tetrads is HbH.

Pathophysiology Hemoglobin H is an unstable, thermolabile protein with an oxygen affinity 10 times that of HbA. Its high oxygen affinity is attributed to the lack of heme-heme interaction and absence of the Bohr effect. As a result of these properties, 2,3-DPG binds equally to the oxygenated or deoxygenated forms because HbH does not change quartenary structure after oxygenation. The oxygen dissociation curve of purified HbH would have a rectangular hyperbola shifted to the extreme left. In HbH disease, however, the patient has some HbA mixed with HbH, which produces a sigmoid-shaped dissociation curve shifted left.

In addition to its high oxygen affinity, HbH is unstable precipitating chronic hemolytic anemia. Hemoglobin H is particularly sensitive to oxidation, forming intracellular precipitates in older cells where there is an increase in methemoglobin formation. The erythrocyte lifespan is shortened as these inclusions injure the cell membrane and lead to cell sequestration in the spleen and phagocytosis by mononuclear phagocytes. Erythrocytes appear poorly hemoglobinized because of the decreased α-chain synthesis and decreased HbA production. Ineffective erythropoiesis is not as severe in HbH disease as in β-thalassemia probably because HbH does not readily form precipitates in young intramedullar erythrocytes. With these concepts in mind, it can be seen that tissue hypoxia is the result of both high oxygen-affinity HbH and anemia of chronic hemolysis due to the presence of unstable HbH.

Hemoglobin H also occurs as an acquired defect in erythroleukemia and other myeloproliferative disorders. However, the clinical manifestations and hematologic abnormalities of these acquired disorders make it possible to distinguish them from HbH disease. Acquired HbH is probably due to a defect that prohibits the transcription of the α-gene.

Clinical findings Like β-thalassemia, HbH disease shows a wide variation in the degree of anemia, from mild to severe. The anemia often worsens during pregnancy, in infectious states, and during administration of oxidant drugs. Splenomegaly is usually seen, but hepatomegaly occurs less often. As with other hemolytic anemias, there may be an increase in respiratory infections, leg ulcers, and gallstones.

Less than half of affected patients exhibit skeletal changes similar to those found in β-thalassemia; extra-

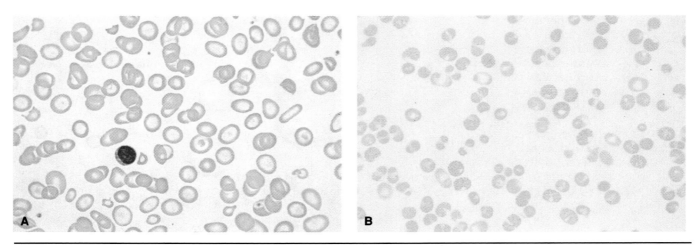

FIGURE 7-18. A Hemoglobin H disease. Note hypochromia. (PB; 250 × original magnification; Wright-Giemsa stain.)
B Hemoglobin H disease (brilliant cresyl blue stain), note the numerous small inclusions in erythrocytes. This is precipitated Hb H (PB; 250 × original magnification).

medullary hematopoietic tissue masses are not seen. Intramedullary iron deposits are not as prominent as in β-thalassemia, and serum iron levels are normal. Survival into adulthood is common, but data are not available on the lifespan of affected individuals.

Laboratory findings A microcytic hypochromic anemia with hemoglobin levels from 8 to 10 g/dL and decreased MCV, MCH, and MCHC is the typical picture of HbH disease (Fig. 7-18A). However, hemoglobin levels as low as 2.6 g/dL have been reported. The erythrocyte count is high, and reticulocytes are moderately increased from 5% to 10%. There is variable poikilocytosis and anisocytosis. Hemoglobin H inclusions are easily found on incubation of blood with brilliant cresyl blue (Fig. 7-18B). The α- to β-chain ratio is about 0.4. Bone marrow exhibits erythroid hyperplasia with normoblasts that have a scant supply of hemoglobin.

Hemoglobin electrophoresis of affected neonates shows about 25% Hb Bart's. As β-chains begin to replace γ-chains, HbH eventually replaces Hb Bart's. HbH, a fast migrating hemoglobin at alkaline pH, makes up from 2% to 40% of the hemoglobin of adults with HbH disease. HbA$_2$ is decreased to a mean of 1.5%, but HbF is normal. A trace of Hb Bart's can be demonstrated even in adults. The remainder of the hemoglobin is HbA.

HYDROPS FETALIS WITH HEMOGLOBIN BART'S

Hydrops fetalis, seen almost exclusively in southeast Asia, is the clinical manifestation of a genetic disorder in which no α-chains are synthesized.[46,47] In the fetus, the excess free γ-chains unite to form a tetrad of γ-chains, producing the abnormal hemoglobin, Hb Bart's.

Infants with hydrops fetalis are either stillborn or die within hours of birth. Hb Bart's has a very high oxygen affinity and no Bohr effect. Therefore, this hemoglobin cannot supply the tissue with oxygen, and the fetus dies of hypoxia. The babies are underweight and edematous with a distended abdomen. The liver and often the spleen are enlarged. On autopsy, other pathologies become evident, including petechial hemorrhages in organs, extramedullary hematopoiesis in the liver and spleen, and massive bone marrow hyperplasia. Hemolysis in the fetus is probably severe, as there is extensive deposition of hemosiderin.

A macrocytic hypochromic anemia with an MCV from 110 to 119 fL and decreased MCH is found in this disorder. Hemoglobin is low, ranging from 3 to 10 g/dL. Reticulocytes are usually increased. There is marked poikilocytosis and anisocytosis with numerous nucleated erythrocytes. Hemoglobin consists of 80% to 90% Hb Bart's with 10% to 20% HbH and Hb Portland. HbA is absent.

HbS/α-THALASSEMIA (HBS/α-THAL)

The sickle cell genes could occur in either the homozygous β^s/β^s state or the heterozygous β^s/β state with α-thalassemia since α-thalassemia affects the α-chain, not the β-chain. Thus, all four thalassemia α-gene combinations are possible with the HbS gene(s).

The wide variety of clinical severity reported in sickle cell anemia may be related to the high incidence of α-thalassemia within the same population, which probably occurs with sickle cell anemia. The clinical state of sickle cell anemia with α-thalassemia is moderate to symptomless.[48–50] The decreased synthesis of chains means that less HbS is synthesized in HbS/α-thal than in sickle cell trait or sickle cell anemia without α-thalassemia. This lesser amount of HbS (decreased MCHC) decreases the tendency of HbS to polymerize and consequently decreases hemolysis.

Although anemia is variable, the erythrocytes are most often hypochromic, microcytic with some degree of poikilocytosis. In sickle cell anemia, the erythrocytes are typically normochromic, normocytic. Microcytosis with hypochromia in sickle cell anemia or sickle cell trait is a clue to the presence of thalassemia.

Hemoglobin electrophoresis reveals variable concentrations of HbS dependent on the number of α-genes affected. In sickle cell trait with α-thalassemia, HbS constitutes about 35% of the hemoglobin when one α-gene is missing; HbS constitutes about 28% of the hemoglobin when two α-genes are missing; and HbS constitutes about 20% of the hemoglobin when three α-genes are missing. The amount of HbA_2 is intermediate between normal and that found in β-thalassemia. In neonates with HbS and α-thalassemia, variable amounts of Hb Bart's also can be detected. Electrophoretic patterns in adults with sickle cell anemia (homozygous) and α-thalassemia are the same as those with sickle cell anemia without α-thalassemia. Family studies, in addition to hemoglobin electrophoresis, are needed to establish the pedigree pattern.

OTHER COMBINATIONS OF STRUCTURAL HEMOGLOBIN MUTANTS WITH α-THALASSEMIA

α-thalassemia also may occur with any of the other β-chain structural mutants and affect the clinical picture of these hemoglobinopathies. Although HbE is a relatively mild, microcytic anemia, when combined with α-thalassemia, a moderate to severe hemolytic anemia occurs (Fig. 7-10).

HEMOGLOBIN CONSTANT SPRING

Hemoglobin Constant Spring (HbCS) is a hemoglobin formed from combination of two structurally abnormal α-chains, each elongated by 31 amino acids at the carboxy-terminal end, and two normal β-chains. This genetic mutation is common in Thailand. The chromosome with the CS gene presumably carries one normal α-gene (α,α^{cs}); thus, the homozygous Hb CS carrier has two normal α-genes, one on each chromosome ($\alpha,\alpha^{cs}/\alpha,\alpha^{cs}$), and the heterozygous Hb CS carrier has three normal α-genes ($\alpha,\alpha/\alpha,\alpha^{cs}$).

The elongated α-chains of HbCS are probably the result of a mutation of the chain termination codon by a single base substitution.[51] The abnormal α-chains are inefficiently synthesized due to reduced stability of the mRNA translation apparatus. Synthesis of HbCS has been demonstrated to decrease significantly during maturation of the normoblasts in the bone marrow. The result is an overall deficiency of α-chain synthesis producing an α-thalassemia-like phenotype.

Clinical findings   The homozygous state is phenotypically similar to mild α-thalassemia. A mild anemia accompanied by mild jaundice, and splenomegaly is typical. Heterozygotes show no clinical abnormalities.

Laboratory findings   In homozygotes, hematologic findings are similar to those of the carrier state of α-thalassemia. A mild microcytic hypochromic anemia with decreased MCV, MCH, and MCHC is characteristic. Hemoglobin concentration varies from 9 to 11 g/dL. Slight reticulocytosis from 3.5% to 7.5% is usually present. Variable anisocytosis and poikilocytosis with target cells is seen on peripheral blood films. Osmotic fragility is slightly increased. Haptoglobin is decreased or absent signifying the presence of a hemolytic component.

Hemoglobin electrophoresis demonstrates the presence of Hb Bart's at birth. In homozygous adults, HbCS makes up 5% to 7% of the hemoglobin. Hemoglobin A_2 and HbF are normal. The remainder is HbA. Neonates have small amounts of Hb Bart's.

Heterozygotes show no hematologic abnormalities but a small amount of HbCS (0.2% to 1.7%) can be found on electrophoresis. HbA_2 and HbF are normal. The remainder is HbA.

In some areas, the occurrence of HbCS with HbH disease is a rather common finding. The patient is heterozygous for α-thal-1 and HbCS ($—/\alpha\alpha^{CS}$). The clinical findings are similar to those of HbH disease, except that hemoglobin levels are lower because of a decrease in HbA. Hemoglobin electrophoresis characteristically shows HbA, HbH, HbBart's, HbA_2, and from 1.5% to 2.5% HbCS.[52]

THERAPY OF α-THALASSEMIA

Silent carrier α-thalassemia, α-thalassemia trait, and HbCS usually require no therapy due to the mild degree of expression of the thalassemia. However, HbH phenotypically resembles homozygous β-thalassemia, and treatment by long-term transfusion and splenectomy is the most common therapy. Hemosiderosis, a complication of chronic transfusion therapy, may be decreased somewhat by administration of iron chelators such as desferrioxamine. Early treatment is necessary to prevent the typical clinical manifestations of thalassemia.

Hydrops fetalis with hemoglobin Bart's is a fatal disorder. Exchange transfusion at birth has been attempted, but the affected infant died within hours of birth.

● Differential diagnosis of thalassemias

The symptomatic homozygous thalassemias are usually diagnosed through a combination of clinical examination and hematologic evaluation. The erythrocyte morphology changes are substantial, and hemoglobin electrophoresis reveals distinct abnormal patterns. Inclusion bodies of precipitated excess globin chains can be demonstrated in developing bone marrow normoblasts. Conversely, heterozygous thalassemia (minor) may be confused with nonthalassemic conditions, most often iron deficiency anemia. Both conditions have similar microcytic, hypochromic erythrocytes. Basophilic stippling, however, is present in thalassemia but not iron deficiency. Hemoglobin electrophoresis reveals increased HbA_2 in thalassemia but normal levels in iron deficiency. In thalassemia, the erythrocyte count is usually elevated in consideration of the low hemoglobin concentration. In iron deficiency, the erythrocyte count is low as expected for given hemoglobin concentrations. Family studies are helpful in identifying the hereditary nature of the anemia in thalassemia.

Although precise identification of the genetic defect in thalassemia is possible with advances in molecular biology techniques, this is generally unnecessary for diagnosis or treatment.

SUMMARY

The hemoglobinopathies are a group of chronic hemolytic anemias caused by either qualitative or quantitative defects in the globin chains of hemoglobin.

Qualitative defects are due to genetic mutations that cause a structural change in the globin chain. Although the mutation may affect any of the globin chain classes, most clinically significant mutations affect the β-chain. The mutation may affect the solubility, stability, and/or oxygen affinity of the hemoglobin molecule. Hemoglobin electrophoresis may be used to detect those mutants in which amino acid mutations cause a change in the electrophoretic mobility of the hemoglobin molecule. Not all variants can be detected by electrophoresis. Other tests detect alterations in hemoglobin solubility and/or stability. The most common structural variants are HbS and HbC. Both are characterized by decreased hemoglobin solubility and can be detected electrophoretically. HbS has decreased solubility when doxygenated, forming rigid aggregates and reduced erythrocyte deformability. The rigid cells aggregate in the microvasculature causing a blockage of blood flow resulting in tissue hypoxia. In HbC disease, the erythrocytes become trapped and destroyed in the spleen when intracellular crystals of HbC form. Generally, these variants produce a normocytic, normochromic anemia with anisocytosis and poikilocytosis characteristic for the specific hemoglobinopathy. The blood smear in HbS disease may show sickled forms and target cells. In HbC disease, there are numerous target cells, irregularly contracted cells, and occasionally the erythrocytes contain HbC crystals.

Thalassemias are genetic defects that affect the production of globin chains. Any of the globin chains may be affected, but the most clinically significant are β- and α-chain defects. The clinical severity of the disease is related to the genetic defect. There are two β-thalassemia gene defects, one that causes a complete absence of β-chain production (β^0-thalassemia), and the other that causes decreased synthesis of β-chain production (β^+-thalassemia). There are normally four α-genes per diploid genotype. In α-thalassemia, from one to four of the α-genes may be deleted. If only one gene is affected, the condition is not clinically or hematologically apparant, but if two or more are affected, there are both clinical and hematologic abnormalities.

The thalassemias generally produce a microcytic, hypochromic anemia with increased concentrations of HbF and/or HbA_2 and decreased concentrations of HbA. In α-thalassemia, HbH (β^4) and Hb Bart's (γ^4) may be detected. The thalassemias have hematologic morphology similar to that of iron deficiency anemia. Iron studies, however, will assist in differentiation of these two entities.

Some structural hemoglobin variants are synthesized in decreased quantities (i.e., Hb Lepore). These variants have morphologic similarities to thalassemias.

Molecular techniques are now available to help definitively diagnose hemoglobinopathies but are not always necessary for diagnostic purposes.

REVIEW QUESTIONS

A 40-year-old white, married mother of three was scheduled for an abdominal hysterectomy. Presurgical blood testing revealed that the patient was anemic. Laboratory results were: Hb 9.5 gm/dL, Hct 0.29 L/L and erythrocyte count 4.6×10^{12}/L. Surgery was deferred and she was given oral and parenteral iron therapy. Three weeks later her blood count results were:

Hb 9.4 gm/dL	Reticulocyte count 2.5%
Hct 0.30 L/L	Bilirubin 0.5 mg/dL total with 0.1 mg/dL conjugated
Erythrocyte count 5.0×10^{12}/L	Serum iron 67 μg/dL
Leukocyte count 7.3×10^9/L	TIBC 294 μg/dL
Differential count normal	Stool guiac negative

She told her physician that she had a history of anemia with many courses of iron therapy, but that to her knowledge, she had never had a normal hematocrit. There was no history of chronic illness, nothing to suggest malabsorption and no known gastrointestinal bleeding. Her ancestry was Northern European. Her father and two sisters were anemic, and a niece was being evaluated for anemia.

1. Calculate the erythrocyte indices. Which of the following best describes this patient's cells morphologically?
   a. macrocytic, normochromic
   b. normocytic, normochromic
   c. microcytic, hypochromic
   d. microcytic, normocytic

2. Hemoglobin electrophoresis was performed on this patient and the following results were obtained: Hb A_2 4.7%, HbF, 1.1%, HbA 94.2%. Based on these results and the above history, what diagnosis should be considered?
   a. iron deficiency anemia
   b. sideroblastic anemia
   c. silent carrier α-thalassemia
   d. heterozygous β-thalassemia

3. What is the pathophysiology of β-thalassemia?
   a. decreased synthesis of α-chains
   b. decreased synthesis of β-chains
   c. synthesis of structurally abnormal β-chains
   d. abnormal heme synthesis

4. If the mother was heterozygous for Hb S and Hb B^0 thalassemia, how much Hb A would you expect to find on hemoglobin electrophoresis?
   a. >50%
   b. about 45%
   c. >10% but <50%
   d. none

5. What primary effect does the amino acid substitution in the β-chain of Hb S have on the hemoglobin molecule?

a. increases its oxygen affinity
b. alters its stability
c. decreases its solubility
d. increases its solubility

6. Congenital Heinz body hemolytic anemias are characterized by:
   a. decreased synthesis of β-chains and increased synthesis of γ-chains
   b. structurally abnormal hemoglobin chains with decreased stability
   c. intravascular hemolysis associated with an abnormal cell membrane
   d. insoluble hemoglobin molecules in the deoxyhemoglobin state

7. Which of the following hemoglobin electrophoresis results is most typical of sickle cell trait?
   a. 85% Hb and 15% Hb A
   b. 85% Hb F and 15% Hb S
   c. 45% Hb S and 55% Hb A
   d. 55% Hb F and 45% Hb S

8. Both deoxyhemoglobin S and deoxyhemoglobin C have a substitution in the same β-chain position. This substitution causes:
   a. decreased hemoglobin stability
   b. increased oxygen affinity
   c. increased hemoglobin stability
   d. decreased hemoglobin solubility

9. Which laboratory test is more appropriate to screen for unstable hemoglobin disorders?
   a. heat instability test
   b. hemoglobin electrophoresis
   c. osmotic fragility
   d. serum bilirubin

10. In hereditary persistence of fetal hemoglobin (HPFH) there is:
    a. increased production of γ-chains
    b. decreased production of γ-chains
    c. increased production of β-chains
    d. increased production of α-chains

● REFERENCES

1. Ohene-Frempong, K., Schwartz, E.: Clinical features of thalassemia. Pediatr. Clin. North. Am., 27:403, 1980.
2. Ranney, H.M.: The spectrum of sickle cell disease. Hosp. Prac., 27: 133, 1992.
3. Steinberg, M.H.: Prospects of gene therapy for hemoglobinopathies. Am. J. Med. Sci., 302:298, 1991.
4. Herrick, J.B.: Peculiar elongated and sickle-shaped red blood corpuscles in a case of severe anemia. Trans. Assoc. Am. Phys., 25: 553, 1910.
5. Pauling, L., Itano, H.A., Singer, S.J., Wells, I.C.: Sickle cell anemia, a molecular disease. Science, 110:543, 1949.
6. Camaschella, C., Saglio, G.: Recent advances in diagnosis of hemoglobinopathies. Crit. Rev. Oncol. Hematol., 14:89, 1993.
7. Fairbanks, V.F.: Coping with chaos. Diagn. Med., 1980.
8. Williams, W.J., Beutler, E., Erslev, A.J., Lichtman, M.A.: Hematology, 3rd Ed. New York: McGraw-Hill Book Co., 1983.
9. Bunyaratvej, A., et al.: Reduced deformability of thalassemic erythrocytes and erythrocytes with abnormal hemoglobins and relation with susceptibility to *Plasmodium falciparum* invasion. Blood, 79: 2460, 1992.
10. Lubin, B., Vinchinsky, E.: Sickle cell disease. In Hematology: Basic Principles and Practice. Edited by R. Hoffman, E.J. Benz, Jr., S.J. Shattil, B. Furie, and H.J. Cohen. New York: Churchill Livingstone, 1995.
11. Ballas, S.K., Smith, E.D.: Red blood cell changes during the evolution of the sickle cell painful crisis. Blood, 79:2154, 1992.
12. Mackie, L.H., Hochmuth, R.M.: The influence of oxygen tension, temperature and hemoglobin concentration on the rheologic properties of sickle erythrocytes. Blood, 76:1256, 1990.
13. Liu, S.C., Derick, L.H., Palek, J.: Dependence of the permanent deformation of red blood cell membranes on spectrin dimer-tetramer equilibrium: Implication for permanent membrane deformation of irreversibly sickled cells. Blood, 81:522, 1993.
14. Boghossian, S.H., Hash, G., Dormandy, J., Bevan, D.H.: Abnormal neutrophil adhesion in sickle cell anaemia and crisis: Relationship to blood rheology. Br. J. Haematol., 78:437, 1991.
15. Buchanan, G.R.: Sickle cell disease: Recent advances. Curr. Prob. Pediatr. 23:219, 1993.
16. West, M.S., Wethers, D., Smith, J., Steinberg, M., The Cooperative Study of Sickle Cell Disease: Laboratory profile of sickle cell disease: A cross-sectional analysis. J. Clin. Epidemiol., 45:893, 1992.
17. Morris, J., et al.: The haematology of homozygous sickle cell disease after the age of 40 years. Br. J. Haematol., 77:382, 1991.
18. el Sayed, H.L., Tawfik, Z.M.: Red cell profile in normal and sickle cell diseased children. J. Egypt. Soc. Parasitol., 24:147, 1994.
19. Wood, N., et al.: Diagnosis of sickle-cell disease with a universal heteroduplex generator. Lancet, 342:1519, 1993.
20. Noguchi, C.T., Schechter, A.N., Rodgers, G.P.: Sickle cell disease pathophysiology. Baillieres Clin. Haematol., 6:57, 1993.
21. Lawrence, C., Fabry, M.E., Nagel, R.L.: The unique red cell heterogeneity of SC disease: Crystal formation, dense reticulocytes, and unusual morphology. Blood, 78:2104, 1991.
22. Bain, B.: Blood film features of sickle cell-haemoglobin C disease. Br. J. Haematol., 83:516, 1993.
23. Williamson, D.: The unstable hemoglobins. Blood Reviews, 7:146, 1993.
24. Rodgers, G.P., Schecter, A.N.: Molecular pathology of the hemoglobin molecule. In Hematology: Basic Principles and Practice. Edited by R. Hoffman, E.J. Benz, Jr., S.J. Shattil, B. Furie, H.J. Cohen. New York: Churchill Livingstone, 1995.
25. Cooley, T.B., Lee, P.: A series of cases of splenomegaly in children with anemia and peculiar bone changes. Trans. Am. Pediatr. Soc., 37:29, 1925.
26. Schwartz, E., Benz, E.J., Jr.: The thalassemia syndromes. In Hematology: Basic Principles and Practice. Edited by R. Hoffman, E.J. Benz, Jr., S.J. Shattil, B. Furie, H.J. Cohen. New York: Churchill Livingstone, 1995.
27. Kattamis, C., et al.: Molecular characterization of beta-thalassemia in 174 Greek patients with thalassemia major. Br. J. Haematol., 74: 342, 1990.
28. Scott, M.D., et al.: Alpha- and beta- haemoglobin chain induced changes in normal erythrocyte deformability: Comparison to beta thalassaemia intermedia and Hb H disease. Br. J. Haematol., 80: 519, 1992.
29. Schrier, S.L.: Thalassemia: Pathophysiology of red cell changes. Ann. Rev. Med., 45:211, 1994.
30. Rund, D.: Mean corpuscular volume of heterozygotes for beta-thalassemia correlates with the severity of mutations. Blood, 79: 238, 1992.
31. Bagar, M.S., Khurahid, M., Molla, A.: Does red blood cell distribution width (RDW) improve evaluation of microcytic anemias? J. Pak. Med. Assoc., 43:149, 1993.
32. Steinberg, M.H., Coleman, M.B., Adams, J.G.: Beta-thalassemia with exceptionally high hemoglobin A^2. Differential expression of the delta-globin gene in the presence of beta-thalassemia. J. Lab. Clin. Med., 100:548, 1982.
33. Weatherall, D.J. (ed): The Thalassemias. In Methods in Hematology, Vol. 6. New York: Churchill Livingstone, 1983.
34. Lucarelli, G., Weatherall, D.J.: For debate: Bone marrow transplantation for severe thalassemia. Br. J. Haematol., 78:300, 1991.

35. Johnson, C.S., Tegos, C., Beutler, E.: Thalassemia minor: routine erythrocyte measurements and differentiation from iron deficiency. Am. J. Clin. Pathol., 80:31, 1983.

36. Steinberg, M.H., Dreiling, B.J.: Microcytosis: Its significance and evaluation. JAMA, 249:85, 1983.

37. Metaxotou-Mavromati, A.D., et al.: Developmental changes in hemoglobin F levels during the first two years of life in normal and heterozygous beta-thalassemia infants. Pediatr., 69:734, 1982.

38. Gerald, P.S., Diamond, L.K.: The diagnosis of thalassemia trait by starch block electrophoresis of the hemoglobin. Blood, 13:61, 1958.

39. Edington, G.M., Lehmann, H.: Expression of the sickle-cell gene in Africa. Br. Med. J. i, 1308, 1955.

40. Edington, G.M., Lehmann, H.: Expression of the sickle-cell gene in Africa. Br. Med. J., ii, 1328, 1955.

41. Rigas, D.A., Koler, R.D., Osgood, E.E.: New hemoglobin possessing a higher electrophoretic mobility than normal adult hemoglobin. Science, 121:372, 1955.

42. Lukens, J.N.: The thalassemias and related disorders: Quantitative disorders of hemoglobin synthesis. In G.R. Lee, T.C. Bithell, J. Foerster, J.W. Athens, J.N. Lukens (eds). Wintrobe's Clinical hematology 9th ed. Philadelphia: Lea & Febiger, 1993.

43. Lehmann, H., Carrell, R.W.: Nomenclature of the alpha-thalassemias. Lancet, 1:552, 1984.

44. Graham, E.A.: The changing face of anemia in infancy. Ped. Rev., 15:175, 1994.

45. Na-Nakorn, S., Wasi, P.: Alpha thalassemia in Northern Thailand. Am. J. Hum. Genet., 22:645, 1970.

46. Taylor, J.M., et al.: Genetic lesion in homozygous thalassemia (hydrops fetalis). Nature, 251:392, 1974.

47. Ottolenghi, S., et al.: The severe form of thalassemia is caused by a haemoglobin gene deletion. Nature, 251:389, 1974.

48. Embury, S.H., Clark, M.R., Monroy, G., Mohandas, N.: Concurrent sickle cell anemia and alpha-thalassemia. Effect on pathological properties of sickle erythrocytes. J. Clin. Invest., 73:116, 1984.

49. de Ceulaer, K., et al.: Alpha-thalassemia reduces the hemolytic rate in homozygous sickle-cell disease (letter). N. Engl. J. Med., 309:189, 1983.

50. Higgs, et al.: The interaction of alpha-thalassemia and homozygous sickle-cell disease. N. Engl. J. Med., 306:1441, 1982.

51. Clegg, J.G., Weatherall, D.J., Milner, P.F.: Haemoglobin Constant Spring—a chain termination mutant? Nature, 234:337, 1971.

52. Weatherall, D.J., Clegg, J.B.: Thalassemia Syndromes. 3rd Ed. Oxford: Blackwell Scientific Publications, 1981.

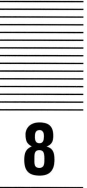

Megaloblastic and nonmegaloblastic macrocytic anemias

8

CHAPTER OUTLINE

KEY TERMS

megaloblastosis
intrinsic factor
pernicious anemia
nuclear-cytoplasmic
asynchrony

179

INTRODUCTION

Macrocytic anemias are characterized by large erythrocytes (average MCV [mean corpuscular volume] more than 100 fL) that usually have a normal hemoglobin content in relation to their size. This is an important group of anemias since macrocytosis is frequently a sign of a disease process that can result in significant morbidity if left untreated.

Macrocytosis is found in 2.5% to 4% of adults who have a routine complete blood count.[1] In up to 60% of cases, macrocytosis is not accompanied by anemia;[2] however, isolated macrocytosis should always be investigated. Macrocytosis without anemia may be an indication of early folate or cobalamin deficiency, as macrocytosis precedes development of anemia.

Macrocytosis detected by automated cell counters may not always be detected microscopically on stained blood smears. In some cases, the erythrocyte size on automated counters is falsely elevated because of hyperglycemia, cold agglutinins, and extreme leukocytosis (Table 8-1). The most common cause of macrocytosis is alcoholism, followed by folate and cobalamin deficiencies, drugs, including chemotherapy, reticulocytosis due to hemolysis or bleeding, myelodysplasia, liver disease, and hypothyroidism.[2]

CLASSIFICATION

These anemias are generally classified as *megaloblastic* or nonmegaloblastic depending on morphologic characteristics of erythroid precursors in the bone marrow Table 8-2). The megaloblastic anemias are the result of abnormal DNA synthesis (a nuclear maturation defect). The basis for the nonmegaloblastic anemias is not as well-defined but may be related to an increase in membrane lipids. Often, in nonmegaloblastic macrocytic anemia, the macrocytes are round while in megaloblastic anemia the macrocytes are oval. A flow chart for laboratory analysis to

TABLE 8-1   *CAUSES OF ARTIFACTUAL MACROCYTOSIS WHEN BLOOD IS ANALYZED ON AUTOMATED INSTRUMENTS*

Cause	Mechanism
Cold agglutinins	Erythrocyte clumping and clumps are sized & counted as single erythrocytes
Hyperglycemia	Intracellular hyperosmolality causing the cell to swell in solution
Marked leukocytosis (ie, chronic lymphocytic leukemia)	Leukocytes are counted as red blood cells

(Adapted from: Colon-Ontero G, Menke D, Hook CC: A practical approach to the differential diagnosis and evaluation of the adult patient with macrocytic anemia. Med Clinics of North Amer, 76:581, 1992)

TABLE 8-2   *CLASSIFICATION OF MACROCYTIC ANEMIAS*

Megaloblastic	Nonmegaloblastic
Vitamin B_{12} or folate deficiency	Alcoholism
Chemotherapy effects	Liver diseases
Myelodysplasia or other primary marrow disorders	Hemolysis or bleeding
	Hypothyroidism

(With permission from: Colon-Ontero G, Menke D, Hook CC: A practical approach to the differential diagnosis and evaluation of the adult patient with macrocytic anemia. Med Clinics of North Amer, 76:581, 1992)

help distinguish causes of macrocytic anemia is shown in Figure 8-1.

MEGALOBLASTIC ANEMIA

Only a few human tissues have cells that rapidly divide to replace those lost through normal aging or sloughing. These include the gastrointestinal epithelium, hematopoietic cells, epidermis, and the germinal epithelium of the testis. All these cells require continual DNA synthesis for cell replication, thus they are sensitive to disruptions in DNA synthesis. In the hematopoietic system, if DNA synthesis is disrupted, the result is megaloblastosis.

Megaloblastic anemia is the result of a nuclear maturation defect with anemia primarily attributed to a large degree of ineffective erythropoiesis. The anemia was called megaloblastic in an attempt to describe the giant abnormal appearing erythroid precursors (megaloblasts) in the bone marrow. Other nucleated cells of the marrow also are typically abnormal.

About 95% of megaloblastic anemias are caused by either cobalamin (vitamin B12) deficiency or folic acid deficiency, vitamins necessary as coenzymes for nucleic acid synthesis. In the majority of cases, cobalamin deficiency is due to a deficiency of intrinsic factor, a factor necessary for absorption of cobalamin, rather than to a nutritional deficiency of the vitamin. Folic acid deficiency, however, is most often due to an inadequate dietary intake. Inherited disorders affecting DNA synthesis are a rare cause of megaloblastosis.

Although very little was known about the function or origin of blood cells before the twentieth century, some perceptive individuals began to make associations between anemia and other clinical signs of the patient. In 1822, J. S. Coombe, a Scottish physician, made the initial clinical description of a patient who appeared to have megaloblastic anemia. He was the first to suggest that this anemia might be related to dyspepsia.[3] In 1855, Thomas Addison reported his description of megaloblastic anemia, but he made no reference to the typical microscopic blood findings.[4] The discovery and description of the abnormal erythroid precursors in the bone marrow associated with this anemia was made possible by the advent of triacid stains. Paul Ehrlich is credited with coining the term "megaloblast" used to describe the large abnormal precursors.[5]

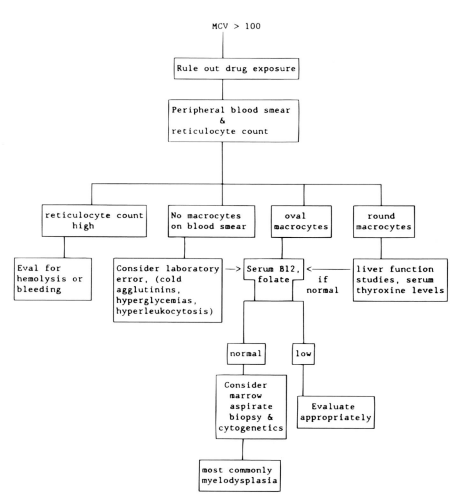

FIGURE 8-1. A flow diagram to help differentiate the cause of macrocytic anemia in the adult patient. Macrocytosis determined by automated instruments should be evaluated microscopically. Oval macrocytes are an indication of megaloblastic anemia, while round macrocytes are usually due to nonmegaloblastic causes. Many polychromatophilic erythrocytes are an indication of reticulocytosis. Young reticulocytes are usually macrocytic. If no macrocytes are found, causes of artificial macrocytosis should be considered. (With permission from: Colon-Ontero, G., Menke, D., Hook, C.C.: A practical approach to the differential diagnosis and evaluation of the adult patient with macrocytic anemia. Med. Clin. North. Am., 76:581, 1992.)

Clinical findings

The onset of megaloblastic anemia is usually insidious with typical anemic symptoms of lethargy, weakness, and a yellow or waxy pallor. Dyspeptic symptoms are common. Glossitis with a beefy red tongue or more commonly a smooth pale tongue is characteristic. Loss of weight and loss of appetite are common complaints. Atrophy of the gastric parietal cells causes decreased secretion of intrinsic factor and hydrochloric acid. Bouts of diarrhea may be the result of epithelial changes in the gastrointestinal tract.

Neurologic disturbances occur only in cobalamin deficiency, not in folic acid deficiency. These are the most serious and dangerous clinical signs because neurologic damage may be permanent if the deficiency is not treated promptly. Occasionally, the patient's initial complaints are related to neurologic dysfunction rather than to anemia. Neurologic damage has been reported to occur even before anemia or macrocytosis develops in some cases of cobalamin deficiency. The bone marrow, however, always reveals megaloblastic changes. Tingling, numbness, and weakness of the extremities reflect peripheral neuropathy. Loss of vibratory and position (proprioceptive) sensibilities in the lower extremities may cause an abnormal gait in the patient. Mental disturbances such as loss of memory, depression, and irritability are sometimes noted by the patient's relatives. "Megaloblastic madness" is a term used to describe severe psychotic manifestations of cobalamin deficiency.

Occasionally, a patient with severe anemia may be asymptomatic, which is probably a reflection of a very slow-developing anemia.

Laboratory findings

PERIPHERAL BLOOD

Megaloblastic anemia is typically a macrocytic, normochromic anemia. The MCV is usually greater than 100 fL and may reach a volume of 140 fL. The Mean corpuscular hemoglobin (MCH)is increased because of the large cell volume, but the MCHC is normal. In cobalamin deficiency, a macrocytosis may precede the development of anemia by months to years.[6-8] Epithelial changes in the gastrointestinal tract may cause iron absorption to be impaired. If an iron deficiency that characteristically produces a microcytic, hypochromic anemia coexists with megaloblastic anemia, macrocytosis may be masked and the MCV may be in the normal range.[9] Other conditions

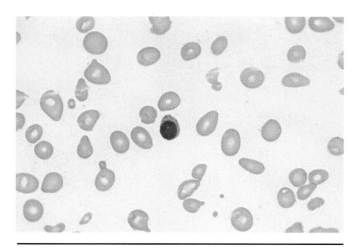

FIGURE 8-2. Macroovalocytes in the peripheral blood from a case of pernicious anemia (PA) (250× original magnification; Wright-Giemsa stain).

that have been shown to coexist with megaloblastic anemia in the absence of an increased MCV include thalassemia, chronic renal insufficiency, and chronic inflammation or infection.[8] Sometimes these coexisting causes of anemia are not recognized until after the megaloblastic anemia has been treated.

Hematologic parameters vary considerably. The hemoglobin and erythrocyte count range from normal to very low. Occasionally, the erythrocyte count may be less than 1×10^{12}/L. In cobalamin deficiency, anemia is not always evident. In one study of 100 patients with confirmed cobalamin deficiency, only 29% had a hemoglobin less than 12 g/dL.[10] Unlike other anemias that typically involve only erythrocytes, the megaloblastic anemias involve all three blood cell lines: erythrocytes, leukocytes, and platelets. The leukocyte count may be decreased due to an absolute neutropenia. Platelets also may be decreased but do not usually fall below 100×10^9/L. The relative reticulocyte

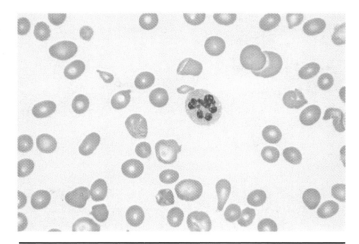

FIGURE 8-3. Hypersegmented neutrophil in the peripheral blood from a case of (PA) (250× original magnification; Wright-Giemsa stain).

TABLE 8-3 *TRIAD OF DISTINGUISHING FEATURES OF MEGALOBLASTIC ANEMIA*

* Oval macrocytes
* Howell-Jolly bodies
* Hypersegmented Neutrophils

count (percentage) is usually normal; however, because of the severe anemia, the reticulocyte production index (RPI) is less than 2.

On the stained blood smear, the distinguishing features of megaloblastic anemia include the triad of oval macrocytes (macro-ovalocytes), Howell-Jolly bodies, and hypersegmented neutrophils (Figures 8-2 and 8-3 (Table 8-3). Anisocytosis is moderate to severe with normocytes and a few microcytes in addition to the macrocytes. Poikilocytosis is striking and is usually more severe when the anemia is severe. Polychromatophilia and nucleated erythrocytes indicate the futile attempt of the bone marrow to increase peripheral erythrocyte mass. Erythrocytes may contain Cabot rings.

Granulocytes and platelets also may show changes evident of abnormal hematopoiesis. Hypersegmented neutrophils (more than five lobes) may be found in megaloblastic anemia even in the absence of macrocytosis. Therefore, hypersegmented neutrophils may be an important clue to megaloblastic anemia in the face of a coexisting disease that tends to keep erythrocyte volume below 100 fL. One study showed that most (94%) patients with renal disease, iron deficiency, or chronic disease who had a normal or decreased MCV but 1% hypersegmented neutrophils, had cobalamin or folic acid deficiency.[8] If 5% hypersegmented neutrophils were counted, the incidence of the cobalamin or folic acid deficiency increased to 98%. Hypersegmented neutrophils tend to be larger than normal neutrophils. A mild shift-to-the-left with large hypogranular bands also may be noted. Platelets may be large, especially when the platelet count is decreased.

BONE MARROW

If physical examination, patient history, and peripheral blood findings are suggestive of megaloblastic anemia, a bone marrow examination will help establish a definitive diagnosis. In megaloblastic states, the bone marrow is hypercellular with an increase in erythroid precursors and a decreased myeloid to erythroid (M:E) ratio. In longstanding anemia, red marrow may expand into the long bones. About half the erythroid precursors show megaloblastic changes. Megaloblasts are large nucleated erythroid precursors with nuclear maturation lagging behind cytoplasmic maturation (Fig. 8-4). The nucleus of the megaloblast contains loose open chromatin that stains poorly. This gives the nucleus a younger than normal appearance for the apparent, more mature stage, of the cytoplasm. Cytoplasmic development continues on in a relatively normal fashion; thus, the term, "nuclear-cytoplasmic asynchrony" is used. Nuclei may fragment in later stages of

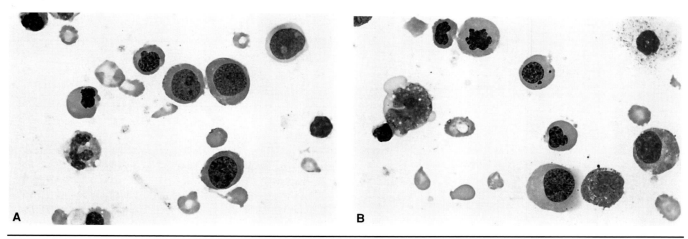

FIGURE 8-4. Bone marrow films of a patient with megaloblastic anemia. **A,** Notice the nuclear/cytoplasmic asynchrony in the three polychromatophilic megaloblasts located in the center and lower center. The nuclear chromatin is open and lacy, typical of a younger cell, but the cytoplasm is characteristic of the polychromatophilic stage of development. The cells also are very large, which is how they earn their name of megaloblasts. The megaloblasts to the left of the polychromatophilic megaloblasts are orthochromatic normoblasts. Notice the irregular contour of the nuclei. **B,** Several of these orthochromatic megaloblasts show irregular nuclear configerations and another has two Howell-Jolly bodies. There is a polychromatophilic megaloblast at the bottom (250× original magnification; Wright-Giemsa stain).

megaloblast development giving rise to Howell-Jolly bodies in erythrocytes (Fig. 8-5).

The megaloblastic features are more easily noted in later stages of erythroid development, especially at the polychromatophilic stage (Fig. 8-6). At this stage, the presence of hemoglobin mixed with RNA gives the cytoplasm the greyish-blue color typical of a more mature erythroid precursor, but the megaloblast nucleus still has an open (lacy) chromatin pattern more typical of a younger stage of development.

Leukocytes and platelets also show typical features of a nuclear maturation defect. Giant metamyelocytes and bands with loose, open chromatin in the nuclei are diagnostic. The myelocytes show poor granulation, as do more mature stages. Megakaryocytes may be decreased, normal, or increased. Maturation, however, is distinctly abnormal. Some larger than normal forms can be found with separation of nuclear lobes and nuclear fragments.

OTHER LABORATORY FINDINGS

The large degree of ineffective erythropoiesis results in an increase in plasma iron turnover, serum iron, indirect bilirubin, and urobilinogen. The characteristic marked increase in fractions 1 and 2 of serum lactic dehydrogenase (LDH) is partially caused by destruction of megaloblasts rich in LDH. The increase is roughly proportional to the degree of anemia. Haptoglobin, uric acid, and alkaline phosphatase are decreased. Due to a block in the metabolism of histidine to glutamic acid in folic acid deficiency, urinary excretion of formiminoglutamic acid (FIGLU), an intermediate metabolite, is increased after administration of histidine. Specific diagnosis of cobalamin or folic acid deficiency necessitates assays for serum cobalamin levels

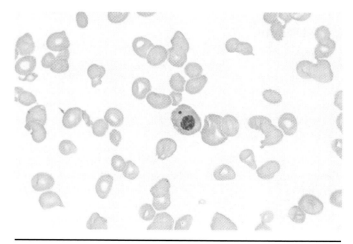

FIGURE 8-5. Orthochromatophilic megaloblast with a Howell-Jolly body in the bone marrow from a case of PA. (250× original magnification; Wright-Giemsa stain.)

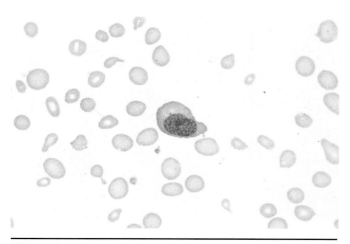

FIGURE 8-6. Polychromatophilic megaloblast in the bone marrow from a case of PA. (250× original magnification; Wright-Giemsa stain.)

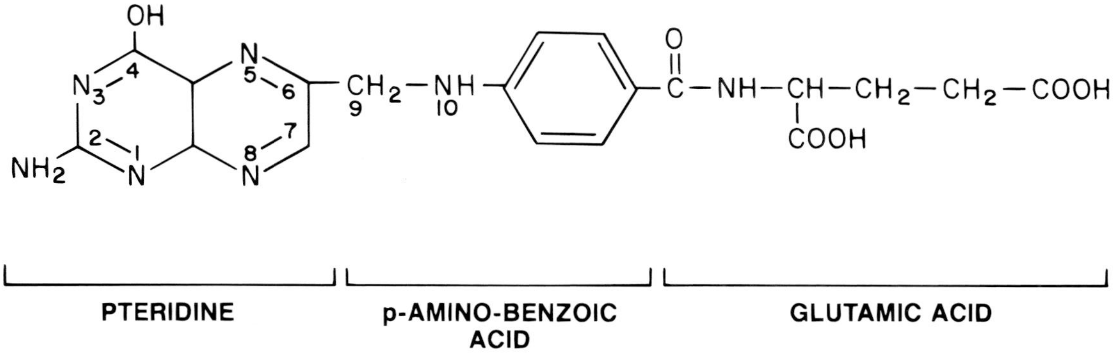

$$PTERIDINE \quad\quad p\text{-}AMINO\text{-}BENZOIC\ ACID \quad\quad GLUTAMIC\ ACID$$

FIGURE 8-7. Folic acid molecule.

and erythrocyte and serum folate levels. These and additional tests will be discussed in the following sections.

Folic acid

STRUCTURE AND FUNCTION

Folic acid (MW 441) is the parent substance of a large group of compounds known as folates. Chemically, folate is known as pteroylglutamic acid. Structurally, folate is composed of three parts: (1) pteridine, a nitrogen containing ring; (2) a ring of p-amino-benzoic acid; and (3) a chain of glutamic acid residues (Fig. 8-7). This structure composes the inert form of folate. Tetrahydrofolate (THF), the active form of folate, is produced by a four hydrogen reduction of the pteridine ring.

The function of THF is to transfer carbon units from donors to acceptors. In this capacity, folate serves a vital role in the metabolism of nucleotides and amino acids:

(1) The main carbon transfer reaction occurs when the carbon side chain of serine is transferred to THF to form $N^{5,10}$-methylene THF (Fig. 8-8A). The carbon of $N^{5,10}$-methylene THF is then transferred to the uracil of deoxyuridilate (dUMP) to form deoxythymidylate (dTMP), a pyrimidine of DNA. This reaction in turn produces dihydrofolate (DHF), an inactive form of folate. DHF is reduced back to the active form, THF, by the enzyme dihydrofolate reductase (DHF reductase). Alternately, the $N^{5,10}$-methylene THF may be oxidized to THF for purine biosynthesis. No clinical manifestations have resulted, however, from a block in this metabolic pathway. In folic acid deficiency, it appears that a block in the conversion of dUMP to dTMP results in defective DNA synthesis.

(2) The metabolism of histidine to glutamic acid also requires THF (Fig. 8-8B). The intermediate metabolite of this reaction is FIGLU, which requires THF for conversion to glutamic acid. A deficiency of folate blocks this reaction resulting in an increase in FIGLU excretion.

METABOLISM

Folic acid is present in most foods, including eggs, milk, yeast, and liver, but is especially abundant in green leafy vegetables (from which it gets its name). It also is synthesized by microorganisms. The vitamin is destroyed by heat; thus, when food is overcooked, much of the folate is destroyed. Ascorbate protects folates from oxidation and when present may protect folate to some extent from heat degradation. Most folic acid in food is in the conjugated polyglutamate form. It is deconjugated in the intestine to the monoglutamate form by a deconjugate enzyme. Absorption takes place throughout the small intestine but especially in the proximal jejunum. Once absorbed into the intestinal epithelial cell, the folate is reduced to N^5-methyl THF. This is the primary circulating form of THF in the blood stream. N^5-methyl THF is distributed throughout the body via the blood and attaches to cells by means of specific receptors. Once inside the cell, N^5-methyl THF must be demethylated and conjugated to keep it from leaking out again. Demethylation is a reaction that requires cobalamin. Thus, a deficiency of cobalamin will trap folate in its methylated form, blocking the formation of conjugated THF. Consequently, the cells are unable to retain their folate leading to tissue folate depletion.

The recommended daily dietary allowance of folic acid for adults is 200 μg. (Approximately 50% to 80% of the folic acid ingested is absorbed in the intestine.) This is adequate to provide the minimum daily requirement of 50 μg/day needed to sustain normal metabolism. The liver stores between 5 and 10 mg of folate, which is enough to provide the daily requirement for 3 to 6 months if folic acid is omitted from the diet.

The need for folate increases in pregnancy, during lactation, and in conditions where there is an increased turnover of cells. It has been suggested that pregnant women need an intake of about 800 μg/day. Folic acid can quickly become depleted in hematologic disorders associated with a rapid cell turnover (i.e., sickle cell anemia).

PATHOPHYSIOLOGY OF FOLIC ACID DEFICIENCY

Folic acid deficiency results in a decrease in synthesis of $N^{5,10}$-methylene THF, the coenzyme in the conversion of uridylate to thymidylate, a pyrimidine component of DNA. Consequently, there is a marked slowing of DNA synthesis.

Evidence indicates that, in folic acid deficiency, the individual steps in DNA synthesis are normal, but there is a great increase in erroneous DNA copying. Normally,

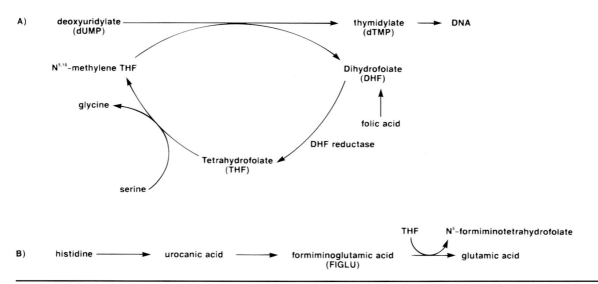

FIGURE 8-8. A and B, Biochemical reactions using folic acid and its derivatives.

the nucleoside monophosphates are interconverted to diphosphates and triphosphates by kinases using ATP as a phosphoryl donor.

$$UMP + ATP \rightarrow UDP + ADP$$

$$UDP + ATP \rightarrow UTP + ADP$$

In folic acid deficiency, however, dUMP (uridylate) is converted to dUTP at a rate that exceeds the ability of UTP pyrophosphatase enzyme to convert dUTP back to dUMP, the precursor of dTMP (thymidylate). As a result, the dUTP accumulates, and thymidylate becomes scarce. The DNA polymerase cannot distinguish between the uridylate residue and the thymidylate residue, thus, the abundant uridylate is erroneously incorporated into the DNA copy. The DNA error correcting mechanism must then remove the uridylate residue and replace it with thymidylate. This correcting mechanism may be prolonged because of the scarcity of dTTP.

All rapidly dividing cells are affected by a folate deficiency, namely, erythrocytes, leukocytes, platelets, and intestinal epithelium. Hematopoietic cells show characteristic megaloblastic changes. Bone marrow erythroid precursors show visible nuclear chromatin patterns related to changes in chromatin structure. The chromosomes, long, slender, and less tightly coiled, are visualized as loose open chromatin on stained blood smears. Macrocytosis accompanies the nuclear changes and may be related to the decrease in mitotic divisions. Cellular RNA continues to synthesize protein at a normal rate, but nuclear development is delayed. Therefore, the cytoplasmic volume continues to expand. The bone marrow indicates a three-fold increase in erythropoiesis, but the peripheral blood reticulocyte count is low, indicating a large degree of ineffective erythropoiesis. Premature cell death is probably a result of an arrest in DNA synthesis. Survival of the

erythrocytes in the peripheral blood also is significantly decreased. This abnormal maturation and survival of erythrocytes results in anemia. Platelets and leukocytes also proliferate and mature abnormally; thus, there may be peripheral blood pancytopenia with morphologically abnormal cells. As mentioned, the most typical leukocyte abnormality associated with megaloblastic anemia is hypersegmentation of neutrophils.

The clinical findings of folate deficiency develop sequentially. Serum folate decreases within 1 to 2 weeks of a folic acid deficiency. Hypersegmented neutrophils are the first morphologic change and occur at 11 weeks. The urinary excretion of FIGLU increases next at about 13 weeks of inadequate folic acid intake, and anemia appears last at about 19 to 20 weeks.

CAUSES OF FOLATE DEFICIENCY

Folate deficiency may occur as the result of an inadequate dietary intake, an increased requirement, malabsorption in the small intestine, or impaired utilization caused by drugs or enzyme deficiencies (Table 8-4).

Inadequate diet The most common cause of folate deficiency is an inadequate dietary intake of folic acid. This is seen most often in the poor and the elderly, who, for financial reasons, lack of motivation, physical disabilities, or lack of knowledge concerning nutrition, fail to obtain enough food to maintain adequate folic acid intake. Alcoholics, whose diet consists mainly of large quantities of ethanol, have a deficiency of many vitamins in addition to folic acid deficiency. Complicating the folate deficiency in alcoholics, the ethanol appears to impair release of folate from the liver and may be toxic to erythroid precursors. (Erythroid precursors in alcoholism are frequently vacuolated.) In alcoholics who have liver disease but who

TABLE 8-4   *CAUSES OF FOLATE DEFICIENCY*

I. Inadequate dietary intake
   Infancy
   Institutional diets
   Goat's milk and special diets
   Cooking techniques (folate destroyed)
   Poverty
   Chronic debilitating disease

II. Malabsorption
   Tropical sprue
   Nontropical sprue
   Regional enteritis
   Intestinal bypass
   Blind loop syndrome
   Steatorrhea
   Drugs
   Congenital folate malabsorption

III. Drug-induced
   Phenytoin
   Primidone
   Phenobarbital
   Sulfasalazine
   Cholestyramine
   Oral contraceptives
   Folate antagonist therapy (methotrexate)

IV. Inherited enzyme deficiencies
   Dihydrofolate reductase
   N^5-methyl tetrahydrofolate transferase
   Formiminotransferase

V. Increased requirement
   Pregnancy
   Lactation
   Chronic hemolysis
   Prematurity
   Neoplasms
   Chronic inflammation
   Hyperthyroidism

also have an adequate diet, the anemia is macrocytic but not megaloblastic.

Increased requirement   In individuals with increased cell replication, the normal daily intake of folic acid may not be sufficient to maintain normal DNA synthesis. Without folate supplements, folate stores are rapidly depleted. This occurs in hemolytic anemias such as sickle cell anemia and thalassemia, and in myeloproliferative diseases such as leukemia, in pregnancy, and in metastatic cancers. Anemia in pregnancy is common and may be caused by deficiencies of iron, folic acid, or both. The deficiency of folic acid is related to the limited reserves of this nutrient and a 5 to 10 times increased demand for its use created by the growing fetus. Prophylactic folic acid supplements are usually prescribed to prevent anemia during pregnancy. Supplements also are recommended before conception in an effort to decrease neural tube defects in the fetus.[11]

Malabsorption   Intestinal diseases affecting the upper small intestine, which interfere with the absorption of nutrients, may cause a folate deficiency. The most common conditions of this type include ileitis, tropical sprue, and nontropical sprue. The blind loop syndrome associated with an overgrowth of bacteria may cause a folate deficiency because the bacteria preferentially use the folate.

Drug inhibition   Megaloblastic anemia also has been associated with certain drugs, including oral contraceptives, long-term anticoagulant drugs, phenobarbital, primidone, and phenytoin. Occasionally, anemia may not be present even though serum and erythrocyte folate is depressed. Although rare, inherited deficiencies of enzymes involved in folate metabolism may cause congenital megaloblastic anemia.

LABORATORY ANALYSIS OF FOLATE DEFICIENCY

The normal serum folate level varies with the method used to determine its concentration. Two methods are in general use: the microbiologic assay and the radioimmunoassay. The microbiologic assay uses bacteria whose growth and replication require folic acid. The most common microorganism used for this purpose is *Lactobacillus casei*. Antibiotic therapy must be discontinued at least 1 week before the blood is drawn for this assay. The reference range is 3 to 25 ng/mL. Radioimmunoassays are more rapid and convenient than microbiologic assays and are not affected by antibiotics. The reference range for serum folate in this radioimmunoassay is from 2 to 10 ng/mL.

Both serum and erythrocyte folate levels must be decreased to diagnose folate deficiency.[1] Serum folate reflects the folic acid intake over the last several days, whereas erythrocyte folate is a reflection of the folate available when the red cell was maturing in the bone marrow. Erythrocyte folate then is a better indication of folate stores. Low serum folate usually indicates an imminent folic acid deficiency and precedes erythrocyte folate deficiency. Normal erythrocyte folate is 140 to 960 ng/mL of packed erythrocytes.

Neither serum nor erythrocyte folate is a good indicator of folate stores in the presence of cobalamin deficiency because cobalamin is necessary to keep the conjugated form of folate within the cells. Thus, serum folate may be falsely increased and erythrocyte folate falsely decreased in cobalamin deficiency (Table 8-5). In approximately two thirds of cobalamin-deficient patients, erythrocyte folate is decreased.[12] In addition, epithelial changes in the gastrointestinal tract, which accompany cobalamin defi-

TABLE 8-5   *SERUM COBALAMIN AND FOLATE LEVELS IN COBALAMIN AND FOLATE DEFICIENT STATES*

	Serum Cobalamin	Serum Folate	Erythrocyte Folate
Cobalamin deficiency	low	low, normal or increased	low
Folate deficiency	*normal	low	low
Combined cobalamin and folate deficiency	low	low	low

* may be falsely decreased.

TABLE 8-6 *CONDITIONS IN WHICH ERYTHROCYTE FOLATE MAY BE FALSELY INCREASED OR FALSELY DECREASED*

FALSE INCREASE

Early folate deficiency

Reticulocytosis

Recent erythrocyte transfusion

FALSE DECREASE

Cobalamin deficiency

Recent alcohol intake

(With permission from: Scates, S., and Glaspy, J.: The macrocytic anemias. *Laboratory Medicine*, 21:736, 1990.)

ciency, may lead to malabsorption of folic acid, in which case both serum and erythrocyte folate will be decreased. Care must be taken in interpreting the folate results, as both serum and erythrocyte folate may be falsely increased or decreased in a variety of other conditions (Tables 8-6 and 8-7).

● Cobalamin

By the early 1900s, megaloblastic anemia was recognized as a unique anemia of adults with typical symptoms and clinical findings. The disease was called pernicious anemia because of the certainty of a fatal outcome. The average survival after the onset of the disease was between 1 and 3 years. It is now recognized that pernicious anemia is a specific form of megaloblastic anemia characterized by a deficiency of cobalamin that is secondary to an absence of intrinsic factor.

In 1925, George Minot, a Boston physician, became interested in the dietary habits of these anemic patients. He found that most had a selective, limited diet; he advised them to include meat and liver in their daily diet. Subsequently, it was noticed that patients who ate a half pound of liver a day had a corresponding reticulocyte response and a conversion to normoblastic erythropoiesis.[13] Nearly 25 years later, in 1948, Karl Folkers and a group of investigators at Merck and Co. discovered that the source of

TABLE 8-7 *CONDITIONS IN WHICH SERUM FOLATE MAY BE FALSELY INCREASED OR FALSELY DECREASED*

FALSE INCREASE

Recent increase in dietary intake

Hemolysis of sample

Coexisting cobalamin deficiency

FALSE DECREASE

Recent low dietary intake

Gallium or technetium administration

(With permission from: Scates S, and Glaspy J.: The macrocytic anemias. *Laboratory Medicine*, 21:736, 1990.)

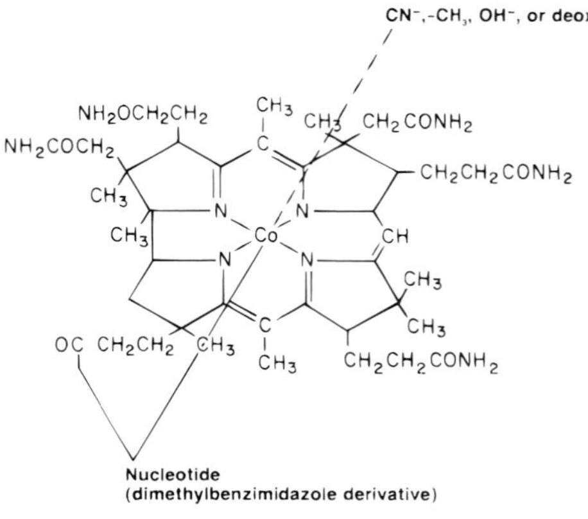

FIGURE 8-9. Cobalamin molecule.

activity in liver responsible for this remarkable erythropoietic activity was cobalamin, which was named vitamin B12.[14]

Shortly after the discovery of the benefits of liver in pernicious anemia, the question arose as to why pernicious anemia patients needed such large quantities of liver to maintain normal hematopoiesis. This led to the idea that perhaps there was a substance present in normal gastric juice responsible for digesting meat and increasing absorption of the potent antipernicious factor (cobalamin) present in liver. In 1929, Castle and Locke reported results of an experiment in which the gastric juice of a normal man taken 1 hour after a meal of meat was administered to pernicious anemia patients.[15] This caused a reticulocyte response in 8 out of 10 anemic patients. Subsequently, Castle determined that there was an intrinsic factor present in normal gastric juice but absent from the gastric juice of pernicious anemia patients.[16] Today it is recognized that this intrinsic factor is essential for absorption of cobalamin.

STRUCTURE AND FUNCTION

Vitamin B12 is commonly used as a generic term for a family of cobalamin vitamins in which ligands may be chelated to cobalt. The more accurate terminology when referring to this family of vitamins is cobalamin, because vitamin B12 refers specifically to the form of cobalamin that contains the ligand, cyanide, forming cyanocobalamin, a form not naturally found in the body but a crystalline form used for treating cobalamin deficiency.

Cobalamin is structurally classified as a corrinoid, a family of compounds with a corrin ring. The corrin ring is formed by the joining of four reduced pyrrole subrings, which are linked to a central cobalt. The cobalamin molecule is composed of three portions: (1) a corrin ring with four pyrrole groups and a cobalt at the center; (2) a nucleotide, which lies perpendicular to the ring and attached to the ring and to cobalt; (3) a β group attached to cobalamin on the opposite side of the ring from the nucleotide (Fig. 8-9). The β group in cobalamins may be of four

A. Biochemical reaction using methylcobalamin as a cofactor. A deficiency of methylcobalamin causes a failure of methylation of homocysteine which leads to a reduction in THF and trapping of the folate as N^5methyl-THF. This causes a deficiency of $N^{5,10}$ methylene THF, a coenzyme needed in the synthesis of dTTP.

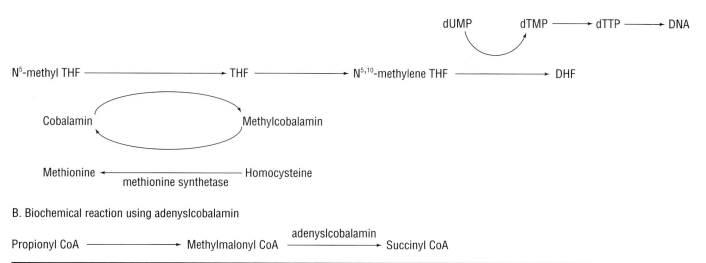

B. Biochemical reaction using adenyslcobalamin

FIGURE 8-10. Biochemical reactions using cobalamin.

types: cyanide, methyl, adenosyl, and hydroxyl. The methyl and adenosyl forms act as coenzymes. Hydroxyl and cyanide forms are not active forms but can be converted to the active methyl and adenosyl forms by tissue enzymes.

Cobalamin is necessary for synthesis of methionine, the central reaction in DNA synthesis (Fig. 8-10A). For this reaction, cobalamins must be converted to the methylcobalamin form. Methylcobalamin functions as a coenzyme with methionine synthetase to convert homocysteine to methionine. Cobalamin accepts a methyl group from N^5-methyl THF and transfers it to homocysteine. The significance of the reaction is primarily that THF is formed from the demethylation of N^5-methyltetrahydrofolate. THF is then converted to $N^{5,10}$ methylene-THF, the folate form necessary for thymidylate synthesis. A deficiency of cobalamin means that folate is trapped in the N^5-methyl THF form. This is commonly referred to as the "folate trap." Thus, cobalamin deficiency leads to a functional deficiency of folic acid activity needed for DNA synthesis.

It has been observed that the DNA synthesis defect in cobalamin deficiency can be corrected by methionine but not by demethylated THF. These observations have led to an alternative hypothesis for the primary defect in cobalamin deficiency. The alternative hypothesis proposed to explain the effect of cobalamin deficiency is the formate starvation hypothesis.[17] In this hypothesis, methionine is the pivotal compound of cobalamin-folate function. When methionine is in excess, its methyl group can be oxidized to formate, which can then be linked to THF to form formyl-THF. Studies with animals show that this folate analogue, formyl-THF, can be used by cobalamin deficient animals to bypass the effects of cobalamin deficiency, whereas folate, THF, and methyl-THF cannot be used.[18] This suggests that the primary problem in cobalamin deficiency is related to the lack of methionine, which is necessary for production of formate.

Although both hypotheses may be contributory to the DNA synthesis defect, neither hypothesis explains the reversal of megaloblastic hematopoiesis in patients receiving pharmacologic doses of folic acid.[19]

Adenyslcobalamin also is required for only one mammalian reaction: the conversion of methylmalonyl CoA to succinyl CoA (Fig. 8-10B). Adenosylcobalamin acts as a coenzyme with methylmalonyl CoA mutase in this reaction. Methylmalonyl CoA is formed from the carboxylation of propionyl-CoA, which is produced from the combustion of valine to isoleucine. Increased excretion of methymalonyl CoA and propionic acid in the urine is a diagnostic aid in cobalamin deficiency.

METABOLISM

Absorption   Cobalamin is present in most foods of animal origin, including milk, eggs, and meat. The vitamin complex is released from food by peptic digestion at a low pH in the stomach and binds to an R-binder, a cobalamin-binding protein secreted in the saliva and in the stomach. R-binding protein, named because it migrates rapidly on electrophoresis, is the preferred binding protein for cobalamin released from food. In the duodenum, pancreatic proteases degrade the R-binding proteins, releasing cobalamin. The released cobalamin quickly binds to intrinsic factor, which is resistant to pancreatic degradation. Intrinsic factor is a glycoprotein secreted by parietal cells in the stomach in response to food and it binds cobalamin in a 1:1 stoichiometry. The intrinsic factor-cobalamin complex passes through the jejunum into the ileum, where it binds to specific intrinsic factor receptors on the microvilli of mucosal cells (Fig. 8-11). Since the ileal receptors are

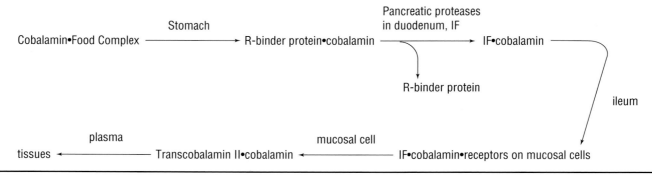

FIGURE 8-11. Assimilation of cobalamin.

specific for intrinsic factor and not R-binding protein, a lack of pancreatic proteases would tie up the cobalamin in a form that could not be absorbed (R-binder:cobalamin) and precipitate cobalamin deficiency. It is not clear as to whether the entire intrinsic factor-cobalamin complex is absorbed into the cell or just the cobalamin portion of the complex.

Transport Cobalamin leaves the mucosal cell and appears in the plasma attached to the transport protein transcobalamin II. Transcobalamin II is a β globulin, MW about 40,000, produced in the liver, the ileum, and by macrophages. It is only about 5% to 10% saturated and accounts for 10% to 30% of plasma cobalamin. This transport complex disappears rapidly from blood (T ½ of 6 to 9 minutes), as it is taken up by cells in the liver, bone marrow, and by other dividing cells that have specific receptors for transcobalamin II. Inside the cell, cobalamin is released and used. The transcobalamin is degraded. Congenital deficiency of transcobalamin II produces a severe megaloblastic anemia in infancy. However, serum cobalamin concentration in this condition is normal.

The plasma cobalamin not bound to transcobalamin II is bound to cobalophilins, including transcobalamin I and transcobalamin III. The functions of transcobalamin I and transcobalamin III are less well understood but they do not serve as transport proteins. Transcobalamin I has an electrophoretic mobility of alpha-1 globulin and is produced in part by granulocytes. Although it binds 75% of circulating cobalamin in fasting plasma, it is only about 50% saturated, its turnover is slow (T ½ of 10 days). It has been suggested that it serves as a passive reservoir of cobalamin, which is in equilibrium with liver stores of the vitamin. Lack of transcobalamin I produces no megaloblastosis or anemia but results in a decreased serum cobalamin. Transcobalamin III has an electrophoretic mobility of the alpha-2 globulins. It appears to be released from granulocytes during the clotting process and does not bind significant portions of cobalamin. Both transcobalamin I and III are increased in myeloproliferative disorders, presumably due to proliferation of granulocytes that produce the proteins.

Other cobalamin binder proteins are present in plasma, saliva, gastric juice, pancreatic juice, amniotic fluid, and milk.

REQUIREMENTS

Approximately 3 to 5 μg of cobalamin per day is needed to maintain normal biochemical functions. It is estimated that only about 70% of cobalamin intake is absorbed, which suggests that the diet should include from 5 to 7 μg of the vitamin per day. This amount is available in a regular mixed diet but will not be provided by strict vegetarian diets. Cobalamin stores (5000 μg) are sufficient to provide the normal daily requirement for about 1000 days. Therefore, it takes several years to develop a deficiency of the vitamin if no cobalamin is absorbed from the diet. About half of this storage vitamin is in the liver.[18] The rest is located in the heart and kidneys.

PATHOPHYSIOLOGY OF COBALAMIN DEFICIENCY

Deficiency of cobalamin is reflected by (1) impaired DNA synthesis and (2) defective fatty acid degradation.

Impaired DNA synthesis As previously mentioned, cobalamin deficiency leads to a lack of methionine synthesis and THF, a precursor of thymidylate. Thus, a lack of THF leads to a defect in thymidylate synthesis and ultimately to a defect in DNA synthesis. All dividing cells are affected, including the hematopoietic cells in the bone marrow. This produces pathologies identical to folic acid deficiency, including a megaloblastic anemia and columnar and squamous epithelial cell abnormalities.

Defective fatty acid degradation Adenyslcobalamin is a cofactor in the conversion of methylmalonyl CoA to succinyl CoA. In cobalamin deficiency, demyelination of nerve fibers appears to be the result of a defect in degradation of propionyl CoA to methylmalonyl CoA and, finally, to succinyl CoA. As propionyl CoA accumulates, it is used as a primer for fatty acid synthesis, replacing the usual primer acetyl CoA. This results in fatty acids with an odd number of carbons. These odd chain fatty acids are incorporated into neuronal membranes, causing disruption of membrane function. It is probable that demyelination is a result of this erroneous fatty acid synthesis.

A critical feature of demyelination in cobalamin deficiency is neurologic disease. Peripheral nerves are most often affected, presenting as motor and sensory neuropathy. The brain and spinal cord also may be affected, leading to dementia, spastic paralysis, and other serious neurologic disturbances. Occasionally, demyelination has been known to occur without any sign of anemia or macrocytosis, making accurate diagnosis difficult but critical. The bone marrow, however, always will show megaloblastic hematopoiesis.[23] Neurologic disease may not be totally reversible but, if treated early, may be partially resolved. Neurologic disease does not occur in folic acid deficiency. Administration of folic acid will correct the anemia of cobalamin deficiency but will not halt or reverse neurologic disease. Therefore, it is essential to differentiate between folate and cobalamin deficiency.

Gastritis and abnormalities of the gastrointestinal epithelium, secondary to cobalamin deficiency, may interfere with the absorption of folic acid and iron, complicating the anemia.

CAUSES OF COBALAMIN DEFICIENCY

There are many causes of cobalamin deficiency (Table 8-8), including lack of intrinsic factor (pernicious anemia), nutritional deficiency, malabsorption, impaired utilization by tissues due to defective or absent transport proteins or enzyme deficiencies, and increased demand.

Pernicious anemia Pernicious anemia is a specific term used to define the megaloblastic anemia caused by an absence of intrinsic factor secondary to gastric atrophy. An absence of intrinsic factor leads to cobalamin deficiency, as the vitamin cannot be absorbed without it. This is the

TABLE 8-8 *CAUSES OF COBALAMIN DEFICIENCY*

I. Nutritional deficiency
   Malnutrition
   Strict vegetarian diets
   Breast-fed infants of strict vegetarian diets
II. Malabsorption
   A. Decreased availability of intrinsic factor
      Pernicious anemia
      Congenital intrinsic factor deficiency
      Abnormal intrinsic factor molecule
      Gastrectomy
      Gastric destruction secondary to ingestion of caustic substances (lye)
   B. Failure of intestinal absorption for causes other than decreased availability of intrinsic factor
      Ileal resection
      Crohn's disease, tuberculosis, other granulomatous diseases
      Celiac disease
      Infiltrative disorders of the ileum or small intestine (lymphoma)
      Bacterial overgrowth syndromes
      Pancreatic malabsorption
      Drugs
III. Impaired utilization
   Nitrous oxide inhalation
   Transcobalamin II deficiency
   Inborn errors of metabolism
IV. Increased demand
   Pregnancy
   Chronic hemolytic anemia
   Neoplasms
   Myeloproliferative disorders
   Hyperthyroidism

most common cause of cobalamin deficiency, accounting for 85% of all deficiencies. Total atrophy of gastric parietal cells is demonstrated by the finding of achlorhydria of gastric juice after histamine stimulation, since these cells also produce hydrochloric acid (HCl). It is a disease of older adults, usually occurring after 40 years of age. This anemia is seen more commonly among people of Northern Europe, especially Great Britain and Scandinavia, but can be found in all racial groups. More women are affected than men. Although no particular genetic abnormality has been identified, some patients have premature graying or whitening of the hair. A positive family history of pernicious anemia increases the risk of developing pernicious anemia 20-fold. There also is an increased incidence of gastric carcinoma in these patients.[21]

Pernicious anemia frequently occurs with other autoimmune diseases, including Grave's disease and Hashimoto's thyroiditis. This association between pernicious anemia and autoimmune diseases has led researchers to suggest that pernicious anemia may develop as the result of a hereditary autoimmune disease. Indeed, up to 90% of pernicious anemia patients have antibodies against parietal cells.[20] However, these antibodies are not specific for patients with pernicious anemia. They also are found in patients with gastritis, thyroid disease, and Addison's disease. Conversely, serum antibodies against intrinsic factor are specific for pernicious anemia patients and can be found in 56% of these patients. Antibodies against intrinsic factor also have been found in the gastric secretions of 75% of pernicious anemia patients. These specific antibodies are of two types: blocking and binding. Blocking antibodies prevent formation of the intrinsic factor-cobalamin complex. Binding antibodies react with the intrinsic factor-cobalamin binding site, preventing absorption of the complex in the ileum. This raises the question whether the intrinsic factor antibodies are pathogenic or merely accompany the development of pernicious anemia.

Pernicious anemia is rare in children. Juvenile pernicious anemia is a term used to describe the anemia accompanying a congenital deficiency of intrinsic factor. There are at least two types of juvenile pernicious anemia. The most common type is characterized by a lack of intrinsic factor, but otherwise normal gastric secretion and no antibodies against parietal cells. A less common type is more typical of the pernicious anemia found in adults. In this type, there is absence of intrinsic factor together with gastric atrophy, decreased gastric secretion, and antibodies against intrinsic factor and parietal cells.

Laboratory diagnosis of pernicious anemia usually involves gastric analysis and/or the Schilling test and serum cobalamin assay. The cobalamin assay establishes the fact that a deficiency exists but does not provide a distinction of pernicious anemia from other causes of cobalamin deficiency. Gastric analysis and the Schilling test are most useful in establishing the specific diagnosis of pernicious anemia.

GASTRIC ANALYSIS Since atrophy of the parietal cells is a universal feature of pernicious anemia, positive diagnosis must indicate an absence of free HCl in gastric juice after histamine stimulation. The parietal cells secrete both HCl and intrinsic factor. Therefore, an absence of HCl is indirect evidence for lack of intrinsic factor. After histamine stimulation in patients with pernicious anemia, the pH fails to fall below 3.5, and gastric volume, pepsin, and rennin are decreased.

SCHILLING TEST The Schilling test is a definitive test useful in distinguishing cobalamin deficiency due to malabsorption, dietary deficiency, or absence of intrinsic factor. The test measures the amount of an oral dose of radioactively labeled crystalline cobalamin that is absorbed in the gut and excreted in the urine. The patient is given 0.5 to 1 μg of ^{57}Co-labeled cobalamin orally. This is given with or followed within 2 hours by an intramuscular injection of 1000 μg of unlabeled cobalamin. The injection is termed the flushing dose, the purpose of which is to saturate all cobalamin receptors in the tissue and plasma. Thus, any of the labeled oral dose absorbed in the gut and passing into the blood will be in excess of available receptors in the tissue and plasma. This excess is filtered by the kidney and appears in the urine. Urine is collected for 24 hours, and the radioactivity of the urine is determined. If more than 7.5% of the standard oral dose is excreted, absorption is said to be normal. In pernicious anemia and in malabsorption, excretion is less than 7.5% because the labeled oral cobalamin is not absorbed.

If excretion is less than 7.5%, part II of the Schilling test is performed to distinguish between pernicious anemia and other causes of malabsorption. In part II, the oral dose of labeled cobalamin is accompanied by a dose of intrinsic factor. The rest of the test is the same as in part I. If part II shows greater than 7.5% excretion, the diagnosis is pernicious anemia. If part II is abnormal, the patient may have another malabsorption defect such as sprue (Table 8-9).

TABLE 8-9 *CONDITIONS ASSOCIATED WITH AN ABNORMAL SCHILLING'S TEST*

ABNORMAL PART I AND NORMAL PART II

Pernicious anemia

Congenital intrinsic factor deficiency

Abnormal intrinsic factor molecule

Gastrectomy

Gastric atrophy secondary to caustic material

ABNORMAL RESULTS IN BOTH PART I AND PART II
Ileal disorders

Bacterial overgrowth of small intestines

Pernicious anemia and other disorders listed above (some cases prior to cobalamin replacement)

Pancreatic disorders

Inadequate urinary collection

Renal failure

Fish tapeworm infestation

(With permission from: Colon-Ontero, G., Menke, D., Hook, C.C.: A practical approach to the differential diagnosis and evaluation of the adult patient with macrocytic anemia. *Med. Clinics of North Amer.*, 76:581, 1992)

Several points must be considered when interpreting the results of a Schilling test. First, the test results are not valid with renal disease. The patient may have been able to absorb the vitamin but, due to abnormal kidney function, cannot filter the excess vitamin efficiently. Second, incomplete collection of urine will invalidate the results. Incontinence or inability to empty the bladder will give false low values even in normal absorption. Third, some patients with hypochlorhydria, achlorhydria, or after gastric surgery cannot absorb cobalamin in food because it requires digestion before absorption. However, these patients may be able to absorb the crystalline form of vitamin B_{12} given in the Schilling test. This may lead to puzzling results when attempting to interpret the test.[22] This problem may be overcome by using labeled cobalamin bound to egg yolk as the oral dose of cobalamin. Spuriously low urinary excretion in part II also may be due to inability to absorb cobalamin-intrinsic factor because of megaloblastoid epithelial changes in the gut.

Other causes of malabsorption Pernicious anemia is only one specific cause of cobalamin malabsorption. Malabsorption also may be caused by a loss of intrinsic factor secondary to gastrectomy or to diseases that prevent binding of the cobalamin-intrinsic factor complex in the ileum. An iron deficiency usually preceeds cobalamin deficiency in patients who have had a gastrectomy. Diseases that can affect the absorption of the cobalamin-intrinsic factor complex in the ileum include Crohn's disease, tropical sprue, celiac disease, and surgical resection of the ileum. In Imerslund-Grasbeck disease, the intrinsic factor receptors are missing or abnormal, causing a form of juvenile pernicious anemia. In patients with severe pancreatic insufficiency, there is a lack of absorption of the cobalamin because the cobalamin cannot be released from the R-proteins and transfered to intrinsic factor. Normally pancreatic protease is responsible for degrading the R-binding proteins. Certain medications may interfere with intestinal absorption. In addition, conditions that allow a build-up of bacteria in the small bowel may cause a cobalamin deficiency. The bacteria preferentially take up the vitamin before it reaches the ileum. This situation occurs in the blind-loop syndrome and in diverticulitis. Infestation with the fish tapeworm, *Diphyllobothrium latum*, may cause a deficiency as the worm accumulates the vitamin avidly.

Nutritional deficiency Dietary deficiency of cobalamin is rare in the United States. Food from animal sources, especially liver, is rich in cobalamin. Strict vegetarian diets, however, do not supply cobalamin, and these individuals (vegans) may develop a deficiency over a period of years. Occasionally, pregnant women with a poor diet may develop a deficiency presumably due to an increased demand by the developing fetus. However, folic acid deficiency is a more common cause of megaloblastic anemia in pregnancy due to the lower stores of this nutrient.

Other causes Transcobalamin II deficiency is the only transcobalamin deficiency that produces megaloblastic anemia. In transcobalamin II deficiency, cobalamin is absorbed normally and serum cobalamin is normal, even though this transport protein is deficient. Tissue cobalamin deficiency develops, however, including megaloblastic anemia.

Nitrous oxide, N_2O ("laughing gas"), abuse has been reported to result in a cobalamin deficiency and megaloblastic anemia. N_2O rapidly inactivates methionine synthase of which cobalamin is a coenzyme. Cobalamin cleaves N_2O and at the same time cobalamin is oxidized to an inert form.[17] This leads to a rapid cobalamin deficiency.

LABORATORY ANALYSIS OF COBALAMIN

Cobalamin in serum is a reflection of vitamin stores. Cobalamin can be measured by the conventional microbiologic assay or the simpler radio-isotope dilution assay. The microbiologic assay uses bacteria that require cobalamin for growth. The two most common micro-organisms used are *Lactobacillus leichmannii* and *Euglena gracilis*. These bacteria normally grow in defined media with specific amounts of cobalamin added. Bacterial growth in media without supplemental cobalamin but with patient serum sample is compared with the bacterial growth curve on defined media with known concentrations of cobalamin. This is a time-consuming method. As in folic acid assays using the microbiologic method, antibiotics must be discontinued for at least 1 week before the blood is drawn.

Radioimmunoassay is the preferred and most accurate method for determining cobalamin levels. Radioimmunoassay gives slightly higher results than the microbiologic assay and is quicker and easier to perform. The higher results are due to the nature of the cobalamin-binding agents. If purified intrinsic factor is used as the binding protein, only cobalamin is bound and measured, and the results are similar to those of microbiologic assays. If, however, a mixture of pure intrinsic factor and R proteins are used as the binding proteins, both cobalamin and cobalamin analogues bind to the mixture, and results are higher than the microbiologic assays. The clinical significance of this is that cobalamin deficient patients may show normal serum cobalamin levels if the binder mixture is used rather than pure intrinsic factor.[23]

Even with purified intrinsic factor, however, patients with laboratory or clinical evidence of cobalamin deficiency may have normal serum cobalamin levels. The normal range of serum cobalamin is 200 to 1000 pg/mL and for newborns the reference range is 160 to 1000 pg/mL. In men, the concentration is highly dependent on age. In men between 20 and 30 years of age, cobalamin ranges from 281 to 1079 pg/mL, and between 70 and 79 years of age the normal range is from 152 to 630 pg/mL.[24] As a group, the older adults (older than 60 years of age) have a lower reference range, 110 to 770 pg/mL. Serum cobalamin may appear falsely decreased (no actual cobalamin deficiency) in folic acid deficiency, in pregnancy, with oral contraceptive use, with antibiotic therapy (using the microbiologic assay), and in multiple myeloma (Table 8-10). Cobalamin deficiency can be masked by folate therapy.

Although not often used, a specific test that measures the excretion of methylmalonic acid (MMA) in the urine

TABLE 8-10   *CONDITIONS IN WHICH THE PLASMA COBALAMIN ASSAY MAY GIVE FALSELY INCREASED OR FALSELY DECREASED VALUES*

FALSE INCREASE

Chronic myelogenous leukemia

Polycythemia rubra vera

Transcobalamin II deficiency

Nitrous oxide anesthesia

Recent parenteral cobalamin

Liver disease

FALSE DECREASE

Severe folate deficiency

Third-trimester pregnancy

Multiple myeloma

Elderly

Technetium or gallium administration

R-protein deficiency

Transcobalamin I deficiency

Vegetarian diet

(With permission from: Scates S, and Glaspy J.: The macrocytic anemias. Lab Med, 21:736, 1990.)

indirectly indicates cobalamin concentration. Up to 40% of patients may have increased MMA levels in the urine but normal serum cobalamin levels.[25] These patients, however, show laboratory and clinical evidence of cobalamin deficiency. The only condition in which MMA is increased in addition to cobalamin deficiency is in congenital methylmalonic aciduria. In the congenital condition, however, there is no megaloblastic anemia. Thus, determination of MMA concentration is useful in distinguishing a cobalamin deficiency from folate deficiency.

THERAPY

Therapeutic trials in megaloblastic anemia using physiologic doses of either cobalamin or folic acid will only produce a reticulocyte response if the specific vitamin that is deficient is being administered. For instance, small doses ($1 \mu g$) of cobalamin given daily will produce a reticulocyte response in cobalamin deficiency but not in folic acid deficiency. Conversely, large therapeutic doses of cobalamin or folic acid may induce a partial response to the other vitamin deficiency, as well as the specific deficiency.

Generally, it is best to determine which deficiency exists and treat the patient with the specific deficient vitamin. Large doses of folic acid are proven to correct the anemia in cobalamin deficiency but will not correct or halt demyelination. This makes diagnosis and specific therapy critical in cobalamin deficiency. Specific therapy will cause a rise in the reticulocyte count after the fourth day of therapy. Reticulocytosis peaks at about 5 to 8 days and returns to normal after 2 weeks. The degree of reticulocytosis is proportional to the severity of the anemia, with more striking reticulocytosis in patients with severe anemia. The hemoglobin rises about 2 to 3 g/dL every 2 weeks until normal levels are reached. The marrow responds quickly to therapy. Normal pronormoblasts appear within 4 to 6 hours. There is nearly complete recovery of erythroid abnormalities within 2 to 4 days. Granulocyte abnormalities disappear more slowly. Hypersegmented neutrophils can usually be found for 12 to 14 days after therapy is begun.[13]

In cobalamin deficiency, specific therapy may reverse the peripheral neuropathy, but spinal cord damage is irreversible.

Pernicious anemia must be treated with lifelong monthly parenteral doses of hydroxycobalamin because of the inability of these patients to absorb oral cobalamin. Recently it was reported that orally administered cobalamin therapy may be feasible if the patient is compliant.[20] The rationale behind oral therapy is that a small amount (from 1% to 3%) of the vitamin is absorbed without intrinsic factor. The optimal dose has not been determined.

● Other megaloblastic anemias

Occasionally, a megaloblastic anemia is associated with drugs, with congenital enzyme deficiencies, or with other hematopoietic diseases (Table 8-11).

DRUGS

A large number of drugs that act as metabolic inhibitors may cause megaloblastosis (Table 8-12). Some of these drugs are used in chemotherapy for malignancy. Although aimed at eliminating rapidly proliferating malignant cells, these drugs are not selective for malignant cells. Any normal proliferating cell also is affected, including hematopoietic cells. These drugs include cytosine arabinoside, hydroxyurea, and methotrexate. Methotrexate is a folate antagonist.

CONGENITAL DEFICIENCIES

Orotic aciduria Inborn defects in enzymes required for pyrimidine synthesis or folate metabolism may result in meg-

TABLE 8-11 *MISCELLANEOUS CAUSES OF MEGALOBLASTIC ANEMIAS NOT DUE TO COBALAMIN OR FOLATE DEFICIENCY*

I. Congenital disorders of DNA synthesis
   Orotic aciduria
   Lesch-Hyhan syndrome
   Methionine synthase deficiency
   Congenital dyserythropoietic anemia
   Homocystinuria and methylmalonic aciduria
   Thiamine-responsive megaloblastic anemia

II. Acquired disorders of DNA synthesis
   Myelodysplastic syndromes
   Acute erythroblastic leukemia
   Refractory sideroblastic anemias: pyridoxine-responsive
   Metabolic inhibitor drugs

III. Other
   Early fetal life

TABLE 8-12 *METABOLIC INHIBITORS THAT MAY CAUSE MEGALOBLASTOSIS*

PURINE
Acyclovir
Gancyclovir
Azathioprine
Mercaptopurine
Thioguanine
Vidarabine
Adenosine arabinoside

PYRIMIDINE
Azauridine

THYMIDYLATE SYNTHETASE
Fluorouracil
Fluorocytidine

DEOXYRIBONUCLEOTIDE
Hydroxyurea
Cytosine arabinoside
Severe iron deficiency

OTHER
Cyclophosphamide
Azacytidine
Zidovudine

(With permission from: Scates, S., and Glaspy, J.: The macrocytic anemias. *Laboratory Medicine,* 21:736, 1990.)

aloblastic anemia. Orotic aciduria is a rare autosomal recessive disorder in which there is a failure to convert orotic acid to uridylic acid. The result is excessive excretion of orotic acid. Children with this disorder also fail to grow and develop normally. The condition responds to treatment with oral uridine.

Congenital dyserythropoietic anemia Congenital dyserythropoietic anemia (CDA) is actually a heterogeneous group of refractory, congenital anemias, characterized by both abnormal erythropoiesis and ineffective erythropoiesis. There are three types: CDA I, CDA II, and CDA III. Types I and II are inherited as autosomal recessive and type III is inherited in an autosomal dominant fashion. Red cell multinuclearity in the bone marrow and secondary siderosis is recognized in all types; however, megaloblastic erythroid precursors are present only in types I and III.

CDA I Marrow erythroblasts are megaloblastic and binucleate with incomplete division of nuclear segments. The incomplete nuclear division is characterized by internuclear chromatin bridges.

CDA II (Fig. 8-12) Bone marrow precursors are not megaloblastic but are typically multinucleated with up to seven nu-

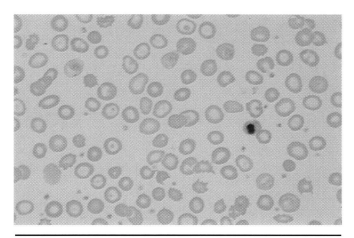

FIGURE 8-12. Peripheral blood film from a case of congenital dyserythropoietic anemia type II. There is anisocytosis with microcytic, hypochromic cells as well as macrocytes and normocytes. Cabot's rings are visible. The nucleated cell is a nucleated erythrocyte showing lobulation of the nucleus. (250× original magnification; Wright-Giemsa stain).

clei. Type II is distinguished by a positive acidified serum test (Ham's test) but a negative sucrose hemolysis test. In the Ham's test, only about 30% of normal sera are effective in lysing CDA II cells. This type also has been termed "hereditary erythroblastic multinuclearity with positive acidified serum test" (HEMPAS). CDA II is the most common of the three types of CDA.

CDA III This type of CDA is morphologically distinct from types I and II because of the presence of giant erythroblasts (up to 50 μm) containing up to 16 nuclei. Sometimes the erythrocytes are agglutinated by anti-I and anti-i antibodies.

OTHER HEMATOPOIETIC DISEASES

The myelodysplastic syndromes are a group of stem cell disorders characterized by peripheral cytopenias and dyshematopoiesis. Erythroid precursors in the bone marrow frequently exhibit megaloblastic-like changes. Occasion-

ally there is a nonmegaloblastic macrocytic anemia. These diseases will be discussed in Chapter 16.

● MACROCYTIC ANEMIA WITHOUT MEGALOBLASTOSIS

The typical findings of megaloblastic anemia are not evident in other macrocytic anemias (Table 8-13). The macrocytes in macrocytic anemias without megaloblastosis are not usually as pronounced as the macrocytes in megaloblastic anemia. In addition, these macrocytes are usually round rather than oval as seen in megaloblastic anemia. Hypersegmented neutrophils are not present, and leukocytes and platelets are variable. There is an absence of glossitis and neuropathy, the typical clinical findings in megaloblastosis. The cause of the macrocytosis without megaloblastosis is unknown in most cases. It has been suggested that macrocytes may be due to an increase in membrane lipids or to a delay in blast maturation. Some diseases associated with nonmegaloblastic macrocytic anemia are listed in Table 8-14. Three of the most common are discussed in this section: alcoholism, liver disease, and reticulocytosis (stimulated erthropoeisis).

● Alcoholism

Alcohol abuse is one of the most common causes of non-anemic macrocytosis. It has been suggested that all patients with macrocytosis should be questioned about their alcohol consumption.[26] The macrocytosis associated with alcoholism is usually multifactorial and may be megaloblastic. Macrocytosis is probably the result of one or more of four causes: (1) folate deficiency due to decreased dietary intake; (2) reticulocytosis associated with hemolysis or gastrointestinal bleeding; (3) associated liver disease; (4) macrocytosis related to alcohol intoxication.

Folate deficiency associated with a megaloblastic anemia is the most common cause of the macrocytosis found in hospitalized alcoholics. The deficiency probably results from poor dietary habits, although ethanol also appears to interfere with folate metabolism.

TABLE 8-13 *DIFFERENTIATION OF MEGALOBLASTIC ANEMIA FROM NON-MEGALOBLASTIC MACROCYTIC ANEMIA*

	Megaloblastic	*Liver Disease (Without Folic Acid Deficiency)*	*Reticulocytosis (Uncompensated Hemolytic State)*
MCV (fl)	120 ± 30	105 ± 10	110 ± 20
Anisocytosis (RDW)	↑	N	↑
Poikilocytosis	↑	N or ↑	N
Erythrocytes	Oval macrocytes	Leptocytes; target cells; acanthocytes	Shift reticulocytes, polychromasia
RPI	<2	<2	>2
Leukocytes & Platelets	Decreased; hypersegmented neutrophils	Variable	May be increased or normal
Bone marrow	Megaloblastic erythroid hyperplasia	Nonmegaloblastic; normal, decreased or increased erythropoiesis	Nonmegaloblastic erythroid hyperplasia

TABLE 8-14 *CAUSES OF MACROCYTOSIS WITHOUT MEGALOBLASTOSIS*

Liver disease

Alcoholism*

Reticulocytosis

Myxedema

Respiratory failure

Myeloproliferative and myelodysplastic syndromes*

Hypoplastic anemia

Acquired sideroblastic anemia**

Obstructive jaundice

Post-splenectomy

Hypothyroidism

Physiologic macrocytosis of the newborn

Pregnancy

Myeloma

Macroglobulinemia

Laboratory artifacts-cold agglutinins, hyperglycemia

Leukocytosis

* may be megaloblastic/megaloblastoid

** may be megaloblastic in alcoholism

The reduced erythrocyte survival with a corresponding reticulocytosis has been associated with chronic gastrointestinal bleeding secondary to hepatic dysfunction (decreased coagulation proteins) or thrombocytopenia, hypersplenism from increased portal and splenic vein pressure, pooling of cells in splenomegaly, and altered erythrocyte membranes caused by abnormal blood lipid content in liver disease (spur cell anemia discussed in Chapter 12). Stomatocytes are associated with acute alcoholism, but there appear to be no cation leaks, and hemolysis of these cells is not significant.

Liver disease is common in alcoholics; typical hematologic findings associated with this disease are discussed in the following section.

Even when anemia is absent, most alcoholics have mild macrocytosis (100 to 110 fL) that is unrelated to liver disease or folate deficiency. This may be caused by a direct toxic effect of the ethanol on developing erythroblasts. Vacuolization of red cell precursors, similar to that seen in patients taking chloramphenicol, is a common finding after prolonged alcohol ingestion. If alcohol intake is eliminated, the cells gradually assume their normal size, and the bone marrow changes disappear. The association of a sideroblastic anemia and alcoholism is discussed in Chapter 6.

The multiple pathologies of this type of anemia result in the possibility of a variety of abnormal hematologic findings. Thus, it is possible to have a blood picture resembling that of megaloblastic anemia, of chronic hemolysis, of chronic or acute blood loss, of liver disease, or (more than likely) of a combination of these conditions.

● **Liver disease**

The most common disease associated with a nonmegaloblastic macrocytic anemia is liver disease (including alcoholic cirrhosis). The causes of this anemia are multifactorial and include hemolysis, impaired bone marrow response, folate deficiency, and blood loss (Table 8-15). Although macrocytic anemia is the most common form of anemia in liver disease, occurring in more than 50% of the patients with the disease, normochromic or microcytic anemia also may be found, depending on the predominant pathologic mechanism.

Erythrocyte survival appears to be significantly shortened in alcoholic liver disease, infectious hepatitis, biliary cirrhosis, and obstructive jaundice. The reason for this is unknown. Cross-transfusion studies in which patient cells are infused into normal individuals demonstrate an increase in cell survival. These studies suggest an extracorpuscular factor is probably responsible for cell hemolysis. The spleen is believed to play an important role in sequestration and hemolysis in individuals with splenomegaly or hypersplenism. In some cases, hemolysis is well compensated for by an increase in erythropoiesis, and there is no anemia. In some patients with alcoholic liver disease, a heavy drinking spree produces a brisk but transient hemolysis. These patients also show abnormal liver function and have markedly increased levels of plasma triglycerides.

Abnormalities in erythrocyte membrane lipid composition is a common finding in hepatitis, cirrhosis, and obstructive jaundice. There is an increase in both cholesterol and phospholipid, resulting in cells with an increased surface-to-volume ratio. This abnormality is not believed to cause decreased cell survival. In contrast, in severe hepatocellular disease, erythrocyte membranes have an excessive

TABLE 8-15 *CLASSIFICATION AND CAUSES OF ANEMIA IN LIVER DISEASE*

Anemia	Possible Causes
Macrocytic anemia	—Abnormal liver function; thin, round macrocytes with increased cell diameter but normal MCV; associated with increased membrane cholesterol and phospholipids in a normal ratio (Probably not a cause of decreased red cell life span.) Association with anemia is likely from multifactorial causes or complications. —Folic acid deficiency; thick oval macrocytes with increased cell diameter and increased MCV. —Stimulated erythropoiesis associated with hemolysis (reticulocytosis).
Normocytic anemia	—Hemolysis; unknown extravascular cause or associated with a marked increase in membrane cholesterol (spur cell anemia); Zieve's syndrome. —Hypersplenism associated with portal hypertension. —Bone marrow hypoproliferation; absence of erythropoietic factor or direct alcohol suppression.
Microcytic anemia	—Blood loss from gastrointestinal tract resulting in iron deficiency.

amount of cholesterol relative to phospholipid, which decreases the erythrocyte deformability. This is associated with the formation of spur cells in which the erythrocyte exhibits spike-like projections. These cells have a pronounced shortened lifespan, leading to an anemia termed "spur cell anemia" (Chapter 12).

Kinetic iron studies have revealed that the bone marrow response in liver disease may be impaired. It has been proposed that liver disease may affect the production of erythropoietin because this organ has been shown to be an important extrarenal source of the hormone in rats.[27] In alcoholic cirrhosis, the alcohol may have a direct suppressive effect on the bone marrow.

Clinical findings and symptoms in liver disease are secondary to the abnormalities in liver function. The liver is involved in many essential metabolic reactions and in the synthesis of many proteins and lipids. Therefore, anemia is only a minor finding among the abnormalities associated with dysfunction of this organ.

The anemia is usually mild with an average hemoglobin concentration around 12 g/dL. With complications, the anemia may be severe. The erythrocytes may appear normocytic, macrocytic (usually not greater than 115 fL MCV), or microcytic. Often there is a discrepancy between the MCV and the appearance of the cells microscopically. In these cases, thin, round macrocytes (as determined by diameter) with target cell formation are found on the blood smear but the MCV is within normal limits. The reticulocyte count may be increased but the RPI is usually less than two, unless hemolysis is a significant factor. Thrombocytopenia is a frequent finding and platelet function may be abnormal. A variety of nonspecific leukocyte abnormalities have been described including neutropenia, neutrophilia, and lymphopenia.

The bone marrow is either normocellular or hypercellular, often with erythroid hyperplasia. The precursors are qualitatively normal, unless folic acid deficiency is present. In this case, megaloblastosis is apparent with the typical associated blood abnormalities.

Other laboratory tests of liver function are variably abnormal, including increased serum bilirubin and increased hepatic enzymes. Tests for carbohydrate and lipid metabolites are frequently abnormal, depending on the degree of liver disease.

Stimulated erythropoiesis

Increased erythropoietin (stimulation) in the presence of an adequate iron supply (e.g., autoimmune hemolytic anemia) can result in the release of shift reticulocytes from the bone marrow. These cells are larger than normal with an MCV that may be as high as 130 fL. A reticulocyte count and examination of the blood smear will allow distinction of this macrocytic entity from megaloblastic anemia. In the presence of large numbers of shift reticulocytes, there is a marked increase in polychromasia. In addition, the oval macrocycytes typical to megaloblastic anemia are not present in conditions associated with increased erythropoietin stimulation.

SUMMARY

The macrocytic anemias are characterized by erythrocytes that have an MCV greater than 100 fL but that are usually normochromic. This group of anemias may be classified into megaloblastic and nonmegaloblastic, depending on specific hematologic characteristics. The megaloblastic macrocytic anemias are characterized by nuclear/cytoplasmic asynchrony and are usually due to cobalamin or folic acid deficiency. The triad of peripheral blood features include oval macrocytes, Howell-Jolly bodies, and hypersegmented neutrophils. Folic acid and cobalamin are necessary for DNA synthesis. Thus, a deficiency of either interferes with normal cell development. Cobalamin deficiency is usually due to malabsorption of the vitamin due to an absence of intrinsic factor. The intrinsic factor is normally secreted by parietal cells in the stomach and complexes with cobalamin so the vitamin can be absorbed in the gastrointestinal tract. The anemia caused by absence of intrinsic factor is known as pernicious anemia. The Schilling test is a defintive test useful in distinguishing cobalamin deficiency due to absence of intrinsic factor. Folic acid deficiency is usually due to an inadequate dietary intake. Both erythrocyte and serum folate levels should be measured to diagnose folate deficiency. Serum folate reflects the folic acid intake over the last several days, whereas erythrocyte folate is a reflection of the folate available when the erythrocyte was maturing in the bone marrow. Erythrocyte folate is a better indication of folate stores. Low serum folate precedes low erythrocyte folate. Neither erythrocyte or serum folate are good indicators of folate stores in the presence of cobalamin deficiency because cobalamin is necessary to keep the conjugated form of folate within the cells. Thus, in cobalamin deficiency, serum folate may be increased and erythrocyte folate decreased.

Macrocytic anemias without megaloblastosis are most commonly associated with alcoholism, liver disease, and reticulocytosis. The macrocytes are usually round rather than oval as is typical of the macrocytes in megaloblastic anemia. Macrocytes in alcoholism may be due to folic acid deficiency, liver disease, or reticulocytosis associated with reduced erythrocyte survival. Even when anemia is absent, most alcoholics have a mild macrocytosis. Liver disease is the most common disease associated with macrocytosis. The causes of anemia are multifactorial and include blood loss, hemolysis, folate deficiency, and impaired bone marrow response. When erythropoiesis is stimulated, the bone marrow may release large numbers of reticulocytes. These cells are generally larger than more mature erythrocytes and may result in an MCV as high as 130 fL. The reticulocytes can be identified on stained blood films as polychromatophilic erythrocytes.

REVIEW QUESTIONS

A 38-year-old woman came to the family practice clinic because of weakness and shortness of breath of 2 months' duration. During the patient interview, it was noted that she had a 15-year history of seizures, which have been controlled by dilantin. Results of physical examination showed a middle-aged woman with very pale and sallow skin color. There was no lymphadenopathy or organomegaly.

Initial Laboratory Data:

RBC	1.52×10^{12}/L
Hb	6.2 gm/dL
Hct	0.18 L/L
PLT	132×10^9/L
WBC	5.2×10^9/L

Differential

Segmented Neutrophils	72%
Lymphocytes	19%
Monocytes	5%
Eosinophils	3%
Basophils	1%

Laboratory Data for Anemia Work-up:

Reticulocyte count:	4.8%
Serum Iron:	176 µg/dL
Total Iron-binding capacity (TIBC):	324 µg/dL
Serum Folate:	0.4 ng/mL
Red cell Folate:	96 ng/mL
Serum Cobalamin:	465 pg/mL
Indirect bilirubin:	3.0 mg/dL
Urine urobilinogen:	increased
LDH:	532 IU/L

1. Based on the patient's reticulocyte production index (RPI) and other laboratory data, what is the functional classification of this anemia?
   a. survival defect
   b. proliferation defect
   c. maturation defect

2. Which type of hemolysis is most likely occurring in this patient?
   a. intravascular hemolysis
   b. extravascular hemolysis

3. If a bone marrow aspiration was performed, which description would best fit this patient's diagnosis?
   a. normoblastic hypocellular
   b. megaloblastic hyperplasia
   c. megaloblastic hypocellular
   d. normoblastic hypercellular

4. What is the most likely cause of this patient's anemia?
   a. Drug-induced
   b. Malabsorption
   c. Inadequate dietary intake
   d. Lack of intrinsic factor

5. Asynchronous development of hematopoietic cells within the bone marrow is the result of:
   a. inadequate levels of RNA
   b. decreased production of erythropoietin
   c. defective stem cells
   d. impaired DNA synthesis

6. Given the laboratory data and patient history, what is the most likely cause of the anemia?
   a. cobalamin deficiency
   b. folate deficiency
   c. stem cell disorder
   d. liver disease

7. What features would you expect to find on this patient's stained blood film?
   a. Howell-Jolly bodies, Pappenheimer bodies, microcytes
   b. Pappenheimer bodies, macrocytes, hypersegmented neutrophils
   c. Oval macrocytes, hypersegmented neutrophils, Howell-Jolly bodies
   d. Round macrocytes, hypersegmented neutrophils, Howell-Jolly bodies

8. Is a Schilling's test indicated in this case?
   a. no
   b. yes

9. Which of the following best describes this patient's erythrocyte population?
   a. microcytic, hypochromic
   b. normocytic, normochromic
   c. macrocytic, normochromic
   d. macrocytic, hypochromic

10. If a bone marrow aspiration on this patient revealed hypercellularity and a low M:E ratio, why is there peripheral blood anemia?
    a. There is significant ineffective hematopoiesis.
    b. The dilantin is toxic to more mature erythrocytes in the blood.
    c. The erythrocytes are being sequestered in the spleen.
    d. There is an acute drug-induced hemolysis.

REFERENCES

1. Hoggarth, K.: Macrocytic anemias. Practitioner, 237(1525):331, 1993.
2. Colon-Otero, G., Menke, D., Hook, C.C.: A practical approach to the differential diagnosis and evaluation of the adult patient with macrocytic anemia. Med. Clin. North. Am., 76:581, 1992.
3. Kas, L.: Pernicious Anemia. Philadelphia: W. B. Saunders, Co., 1976.
4. Addison, T.: On the Constitutional and Local Effects of Disease of the Suprarenal Capsules. London: Sam Highley, 1855.
5. Ehrlich, P.: Farbenanalytische Untersuchungen zur Histologie und Klinik des Blutes. Berlin: A. Hirschwald, 1891.
6. Carmel, R.: Macrocytosis, mild anemia, and delay in the diagnosis of pernicious anemia. Arch. Intern. Med., 139:47, 1979.
7. Hall, C.A.: Vitamin B12 deficiency and early rise in mean corpuscular volume. JAMA, 245:1144, 1981.
8. Spivak, J.L.: Masked megaloblastic anemia. Arch. Intern. Med., 142(12):2111, 1982.
9. Carmel, R., Weiner, J.M., Johnson, C.S.: Iron deficiency occurs frequently in patients with pernicious anemia. JAMA, 257:1081, 1987.
10. Pruthi, R.K., Tafferi, A.: Pernicious anemia revisited. Mayo. Clin. Proc., 69:144, 1994.

11. MRC Vitamin Study Group: Prevention of Neural Tube Defects: results of the MRC vitamin study. Lancet, 238:131, 1991.
12. Henry, J.B.: Clinical Diagnosis and Management by Laboratory Methods. 16th Ed. Philadelphia: W. B. Saunders Co., 1979.
13. Minot, G.R., Murphy, W.: Observations on patients with pernicious anemia partaking of a special diet. A. Clinical aspects. Trans. Assoc. Am. Phys., 41:72, 1926.
14. Rickes, E.L., et al.: Crystalline vitamin B12. Science, 107:396, 1948.
15. Castle, W.W.: I. The effect of the administration to patients with pernicious anaemia of the contents of the normal human stomach after ingestion of beef muscle. Am. J. Med. Sci., 178:748, 1929.
16. Castle, W.B., Townsend, W.C., Heath, C.W.: III. The nature of the reaction between normal human gastric juice and beef muscle leading to clinical improvement and increased blood formation similar to the effect of liver feeding. Am. J. Med. Sci., 180:305, 1930.
17. Chanarin, I.: Megaloblastic anaemia, cobalamin, and folate. J. Clin. Pathol., 40:978, 1987.
18. Chanarin, I., Deacon, R., Lumb, M., Perry, J.: Cobalamin and folate: Recent developments. J. Clin. Pathol., 45:277, 1992.
19. Tefferi, A., Pruthi, R.K.: The biochemical basis of cobalamin deficiency. Mayo. Clin. Proc., 69:181, 1993.
20. Pruthi, R.K., Tefferi, A.: Subspecialty clinics: Hematology. pernicious anemia revisited. Mayo. Clin. Proc., 69:144, 1994.
21. Hsing, A.W., et al.: Pernicious anemia and subsequent cancer: a population-based cohort study. Cancer, 71:745, 1993.
22. Carmel, R., Sinow, R.M., Siegel, M.E., Samloff, I.M.: Food cobalamin malabsorption occurs frequently in patients with unexplained low serum cobalamin levels. Arch. Intern. Med., 148:1715, 1988.
23. Antony, A.C.: Megaloblastic anemias. In: Hematology. Edited by W.J. Williams, E. Beutler, A.J. Erslev, M.A. Lichtman. New York: McGraw-Hill Book Company, 1991.
24. Fairbanks, V.F., Elveback, L.R.: Tests for pernicious anemia: serum vitamin B12 assay. Mayo. Clin. Proc., 58(2):135, 1983.
25. Norman, E.J., Morrison, J.A.: Screening elderly populations for cobalamin (vitamin B12) deficiency using the urinary methylmalonic acid assay by gas chromatography mass spectrometry. Am. J. Med., 94:589, 1993.
26. Seppa, K., Sillanaukee, P., Saarni, M.: Blood count and hematologic morphology in nonanemic macrocytosis: differences between alcohol abuse and pernicious anemia. Alcohol, 10(5):343, 1993.
27. Katz, R., et al.: Studies on the site of production of erythropoietin. Ann. N.Y. Acad. Sci., 149:120, 1968.

Hypoproliferative anemia

9

KEY TERMS

INTRODUCTION

The hypoproliferative anemias are a heterogeneous group of acquired and constitutional disorders in which there is a normocytic or macrocytic, normochromic anemia associated with chronic bone marrow hypocellularity (Table 9-1). Much of the area in bone marrow normally occupied by hematopoietic tissue is replaced by fat. The terms *aplastic*, *aplasia*, and *hypoplastic* refer to a bone marrow with an overall decrease in hematopoietic cellularity. If there is hypoplasia of only one of the cellular elements, the terms erythroid, myeloid, or megakaryocytic hypoplasia should be used to define the specific entity.

The hematopoietic defect is usually due to depletion, damage, or inhibition of stem cells. Either the unipotent erythroid stem cell or the pluripotential stem cell may be affected. The peripheral blood findings provide important clues to help identify the bone marrow abnormality. If only the erythroid stem cells are affected, platelets and leukocytes remain normal, and the diagnosis is *pure red cell aplasia*. More commonly, the pluripotential stem cell is defective, resulting in pancytopenia (decrease of all three cell lines) and a diagnosis of *aplastic anemia*.

APLASTIC ANEMIA

Aplastic anemia is a pluripotential stem cell disorder characterized by peripheral pancytopenia and accompanied by a hypocellular bone marrow. The blood cells are usually intrinsically normal with normal survival. The first description of aplastic anemia was provided by Ehrlich in 1888.[1] He reported a case of a young man who died of a combination of anemia and neutropenia. Results of autopsy showed a yellow, hypocellular marrow. Chaufford, however, is credited with coining the term aplastic anemia 16 years later to describe the typical clinical condition of this disorder.[2]

Before the 1930s, bone marrow examination was performed only during autopsy. Patients with pancytopenia were usually found (by autopsy) to have had hypocellular bone marrows. As a result of this discovery, the hematologic finding of pancytopenia in living patients automatically led to a diagnosis of aplastic anemia. Aplasia of the bone marrow is now recognized as only one of several possible causes of peripheral blood pancytopenia. The term aplastic anemia should be reserved to describe the pancytopenia that is associated with a hypocellular bone marrow.

The diagnosis of aplastic anemia is generally made when the bone marrow is less than 25% cellular and there is a combination of any two of the following findings in peripheral blood: granulocytes less than 0.5×10^9/L, platelets less than 20×10^9/L, and corrected reticulocyte count less than 1%.[3] With progression of the disease, all three cell lines eventually become decreased.

Epidemiology

These anemias are rare, but they are encountered more frequently now than they were at the beginning of the century. Approximately one fourth of all cases occur in individuals younger than 20 years of age, and one third occur in individuals older than 60 years of age.[4] Younger individuals are affected more commonly by the idiopathic form, whereas older individuals are typically affected by the secondary form.[5] There is a geographic variation in incidence, with more cases in Asia than in western countries.[6] It is believed that this variation is related to environmental rather than genetic factors. Individual susceptibility also plays a probable role.

Pathophysiology

The etiologic hypothesis for aplastic anemia has been referred to as the seed, the soil, and the worm hypothesis.[7] A fourth component could be added, the fertilizer. For a viable seed to grow, it must be planted in an environment (soil) conducive to growth, protected from antagonists (worms), and nourished with fertilizer. A deficiency in any of these elements will inhibit the growth of the seed. Likewise, the production of blood cells by the bone marrow depends on the presence of adequate numbers of functionally normal stem cells (the seed). The stem cells must be able to proliferate and differentiate into normal progeny. In many cases, aplastic anemia is believed to be due to deficient or defective stem cells. However, aplastic anemia also may result from abnormalities in growth factors (the

Table 9-1 CLASSIFICATION OF HYPOPROLIFERATIVE ANEMIAS

I. Aplastic Anemia
  A. Acquired
    1. Idiopathic
    2. Drugs: chloramphenical, trimethodione, phenylbutazone, gold compounds, sulfa drugs, antihistamines, antithyroid, tetracyclines, penicillin, methylphenylethylhydantoin
    3. Chemical agents: benzene, insecticides, hair dyes, carbon tetrachloride, chemotherapeutics (vincristine, busulfan, etc.), arsenic
    4. Ionizing radiation
    5. Biological agents: parvo virus, infectious mononucleosis, infectious hepatitis, measles, influenza, errors of amino acid metabolism, starvation
    6. Pregnancy
    7. Paroxsymal Nocturnal Hemoglobinuria
  B. Constitutional
    1. Fanconi's anemia
    2. Familial aplastic anemia
    3. Dyskeratosis congenita
    4. Shwachman-Diamond syndrome
II. Pure Red Cell Aplasia
  A. Transitory Infections
  B. Acquired Pure Red Cell Aplasia
    1. acute
      Infections, transient erythroblastopenia of childhood (TEC), drugs
    2. chronic
      thymoma, autoimmune disorders
  C. Diamond-Blackfan Syndrome
III. Other Hypopoliferative Anemias
  A. Anemia of Chronic Renal Disease
  B. Anemia Associated with Endocrine Abnormalities

fertilizer), from a defective bone marrow microenvironment (the soil), or from cellular or humoral immunosuppression of hematopoiesis (the worm).

BONE MARROW MATRIX DEFECTS

There is substantial evidence to support the importance of the marrow matrix or microenvironment in the proliferation and maturation of blood cells. For example, maintenance of stem cells in long-term cultures depends on the presence of marrow stromal cells.[8] In vivo stromal damage or microvascular injury to the marrow appears to inhibit the seeding of viable stem cells. In a small number of aplastic anemia cases, it has been demonstrated that the bone marrow is unable to support growth of normal hematopoietic cells.

IMMUNOLOGIC SUPPRESSION

Recently, attention has been focused on the immunologic suppression of hematopoiesis in aplastic anemia. Studies reveal that only 50% of all twins with aplastic anemia respond to bone marrow transplants from their normal twin. The other 50% recovered only when the transplant was preceded by immunosuppression.[4]

The immune mechanism responsible for aplastic anemia may involve the suppression of stem cell growth and differentiation by a group of suppressor T-lymphocytes. Immunosuppression with antilymphocyte globulin (ALG), antithymocyte globulin (ATG), or cyclosporine results in improvement in up to 77% of patients, but only one third of these responders achieve a complete remission. Immunosuppression presumably serves to eliminate an abnormal population of activated T-lymphocytes, which produce suppressive substances such as interferon-gamma and tumor necrosis factor.[9] Cell culture studies of peripheral blood T-lymphocytes from patients with aplastic anemia suggest that abnormal interferon-gamma production accounts for inhibition of hematopoiesis under a wide variety of experimental conditions.[10] In addition to eliminating the abnormal lymphocyte population, ALG also can exert a mitogenic effect on other lymphocytes and induce them to produce hematopoietic growth factors.[11]

Experimental studies using lymphocytes from patients with aplastic anemia tend to support this immunosuppression hypothesis. Flow cytometric analysis of lymphocyte subpopulations in aplastic anemia has revealed a marked increase in activated suppressor lymphocytes.

In other cases, stem cell inhibition may be the result of antibodies to hematopoietic precursors or (less commonly) antibodies to the growth factors, erythropoietin, granulopoietin, or thrombopoietin.

In Epstein-Barr viral infection as well as other viral infections, the virus may infect the hematopoietic stem cell, triggering an immune response. The stem cell is then destroyed by cytotoxic lymphocytes. Other mechanisms of stem cell damage in viral infections have been postulated, including direct cytotoxicity of the virus and inhibition of cellular proliferation and differentiation.[6]

DEFICIENT GROWTH FACTORS

Deficient hormonal stimulation of stem cell growth and differentiation by growth factors as the primary event in the development of aplastic anemia is probably an unlikely cause. Patients with aplastic anemia show variable response to treatment with hematopoietic growth factors. Treatment with specific cell growth factors such as CSF-G usually is not effective.[12] When, however, preceded by treatment with IL-3, a multicolony stimulating factor, to prime residual hematopoiesis, the specific cell growth factor may be effective in stimulating cell proliferation.[13] Growth factor therapy may be used to stimulate granulopoiesis after immunosuppressive therapy with ALG.

ABNORMAL OR DEFICIENT STEM CELLS

The success of bone marrow transplants in many patients with aplastic anemia suggests that the bone marrow deficit can be corrected by repopulation of the marrow with normal stem cells; thus, defective or deficient stem cells are apparently a common cause of this anemia. This is supported by the results of long-term bone marrow culture assays in which bone marrow cells from patients with aplastic anemia exhibit defective hematopoiesis when grown on normal bone marrow stroma.[14,15] Aplastic anemia bone marrow cells grow significantly lower numbers of colonies compared with normal marrow. The stem cell abnormality may either be acquired or hereditary in nature.

● Classification and etiology of aplastic anemia

Aplastic anemia may be classified into two groups: acquired and constitutional (Table 9-1). The causes of acquired types of anemia are not always clear, making the diagnosis of *idiopathic* aplastic anemia appropriate. Sometimes, it is possible to identify previous exposure to drugs, chemicals, radiation, infectious agents, or other environmental factors that could potentially cause harm to the bone marrow stem cells. When environmental factors are identified and linked to aplastic anemia, the anemia is considered secondary to this environmental exposure. The exposure may cause temporary or permanent aplasia. Constitutional aplastic anemia is a chronic failure of the bone marrow with a congenital disposition. It may be associated with other congenital anomalies. These forms are rare and less understood than the acquired forms. The defect may be a quantitative or qualitative abnormality of stem cells.

ACQUIRED FORMS OF APLASTIC ANEMIA

Idiopathic Approximately 50% to 70% of cases of aplastic anemia cannot be linked to any cause; however, there may be some previously unrecognized toxic agent responsible for stem cell damage.

Drugs Drugs are responsible for about one third of the acquired cases of aplastic anemia. The most probable mode of action of the drug is direct stem cell injury. It has been proposed that some drugs are not easily metabolized by the marrow; as a result, the drug accumulates, causing injury to stem cells.[16] It also is possible that drugs may induce an antibody-mediated suppression of the marrow. With drug injury, neutropenia usually develops before anemia or thrombocytopenia because of the relatively short lifespan of the neutrophil. Within 7 days after stem cell injury, the neutrophil bone marrow reserve is exhausted and neutropenia develops. The longer lifespan of erythrocytes and platelets provides a buffer for a limited time until stem cell differentiation can resume, if it does.

Chloramphenicol, a broad spectrum antibiotic, is a well-known drug associated with aplastic anemia. This drug is associated with two types of bone marrow failure. Most commonly, a dose- and time-dependent pancytopenia may develop during drug administration; however, blood counts return to normal after discontinuing use of the drug. During treatment, the reticulocyte count is low, and the serum iron increased. Anemia is followed by a decrease in leukocytes and platelets. Bone marrow normoblasts are characteristically vacuolated. In this type of reaction to chloramphenical, bone marrow suppression is most likely caused by inhibition of mitochondrial protein synthesis, especially involving the enzymes in heme synthesis.

More rarely, a severe, irreversible bone marrow depression follows even small doses of chloramphenicol. The aplasia may occur weeks or months after drug treatment. There is permanent destruction of the bone marrow, which results in a severe, often fatal, aplasia. Because aplasia develops in some individuals after exposure to certain drugs and chemicals while in others it does not, there is probably a genetic or acquired defect in drug elimination or detoxification. Perhaps also, some individuals have stem cells that are more vulnerable to damage or inhibition by drugs and chemicals than others.

Chemical agents The widespread use of toxic chemical agents in industry and agriculture is probably responsible for the increased incidence of toxic bone marrow aplasia.[16] Benzene derivatives are well established as a cause of bone marrow depression. Most cases develop within a few weeks after exposure, but some occur months or years after chronic exposure. Although stem cells may be damaged, the main toxic effect of benzene is expressed on transient stages of committed proliferating blood cells.

Most of the chemicals used in chemotherapy of malignant diseases kill rapidly proliferating cells. However, the chemicals do not distinguish between malignant and normal cells. Therefore, all proliferating cells are damaged, including normal cells of the hematopoietic compartment. Although resting stem cells are spared, repeated doses of the chemical over a long period of time will eventually deplete the remaining stem cells as they enter the proliferating pool.

Ionizing radiation Aplastic anemia due to x-irradiation is encountered in persons exposed in industrial accidents, to military nuclear tests, and therapeutic regimens for malignancy. The effects of irradiation are dose-dependent. Small doses affect all cells but are especially destructive to rapidly dividing cells. The bone marrow can recover from sublethal doses of irradiation because dormant stem cells become active after exposure. In high doses, more than 4000 rads, there is usually a permanent bone marrow aplasia and peripheral blood pancytopenia. The aplasia appears to be caused by damage of the supporting marrow matrix. Thus, the seeding of the marrow with normal stem cells (bone marrow transplant) is usually unsuccessful in alleviating pancytopenia in these cases.

Infectious agents Viral and bacterial infections may be followed by a transient cytopenia. The aplasia may be limited to the erythroid elements or may include all three cell lines. Aplasia has been described in patients after recovery from infectious mononucleosis and infectious hepatitis. A particularly severe aplasia occurs occasionally in young males a few months after infection with a non-A, non-B type hepatitis virus. This aplasia has a poor prognosis. Aplastic anemia also can occur in disseminated tuberculosis with or without tubercles in the bone marrow. In patients with hereditary hemolytic anemias, aplastic crisis is commonly associated with human parvovirus infection.[17] This aplasia, however, is limited to the erythroid cell line.

Metabolic The rare inborn errors of amino acid metabolism, which result in accumulation of ketones and glycine, have been associated with aplastic anemia.

Starvation or protein deficiency results in hypoproliferative anemia after about 3 months of deprivation. Starvation that is not self-induced usually occurs in areas where other endemic pathologies also are present, such as parasitic infection and blood loss. Thus, the causes of this anemia may be multifactorial.

Decreased hormonal or growth factor stimulation of hematopoietic stem cells is important primarily as a factor in erythroid hypoplasia. Renal disease and endocrine diseases are examples of hypoproliferation caused by a decrease in erythropoietin.

Rarely, a life-threatening pancytopenia occurs during pregnancy. The condition remits after delivery or abortion. It has been suggested that the aplasia may be related to estrogen inhibition of stem cell proliferation.[18]

Paroxysmal nocturnal hemoglobinuria *Paroxysmal nocturnal hemoglobinuria* (PNH) is an acquired stem cell disease in which a blood cell membrane abnormality exists, making the cells susceptible to in vivo complement hemolysis. Although there is considerable variation in clinical manifestations, the typical picture is pancytopenia and marrow hypoplasia. Occasionally, a patient with an initial diagnosis of aplastic anemia develops an erythrocyte population typical of that seen in PNH with a positive acidified serum test (Ham test). This is an especially prominent, later complication in aplastic anemia patients who have received immunosuppressive ALG therapy.[19,20]

Other diseases Aplastic anemia also has been found associated with preleukemic syndromes, hypogammaglobulinemia, and carcinoma.

CONSTITUTIONAL APLASTIC ANEMIA

Fanconi's anemia *Fanconi's anemia* (FA) is an autosomal recessive disorder characterized by chromosomal instability. It has a prevalence of about 1 in 350,000 in North America with a heterozygote frequency of about 1 in 200. Patients have a complex assortment of congenital anomalies in addition to a progressive bone marrow hypoplasia. The congenital defects include dysplasia of bones, renal abnormalities, and other organ malformations, as well as mental retardation, dwarfism, microcephaly, hypogonadism, and skin hyperpigmentation.

The hematologic abnormalities are progressive from birth. Peripheral blood lymphocytes in metaphase preparations exhibit an increase in chromosome breaks, gaps, rearrangements, exchanges, and reduplications. Bone marrow preparations may show these abnormalities but to a lesser extent. The addition of a mutagenic agent such as diepoxybutane to a bone marrow sample of a patient with this disorder, however, will cause chromosome breaks even in patients who have not yet developed aplasia. Thus, it is a good diagnostic test for this disorder. Care should be used in interpreting the results from chromosomal breakage tests, however, since some patients' breakage rate varies with time and in others the breakage may only occur in a particular clone of cells. The chromatid breaks in FA cells occur in cells from different lineages. Chromosome exchanges occur primarily between nonhomologous chromosomes.[21]

Two theories have been proposed to explain the defect in FA: first, that the cell is unable to overcome oxidative stress and the oxygen causes chromosome damage; second, that there is a defective DNA repair protein. There is evidence to support both theories. Thus, it has been suggested that in FA cells there is a DNA repair protein that is particularly sensitive to oxidative stress.

Research to identify the genes involved in FA has revealed that the molecular defect is heterogeneous. There are at least four genetic mutations as identified by functional complementation studies.[22] In these studies, isolated sequences of DNA from normal cells are transfected into FA cells. The transfected FA cells are selected based on their ability to overcome the increased sensitivity to chromosomal breakage agents. Genes from normal cells that correct the hypersensitivity are probably the genes that are mutated in FA patients (FA genes). Using this technique, one of the FA genes has been cloned and localized to chromosome 9q22.3. This gene is referred to as the FACC gene (Fanconi anemia complementation group C). Not much is known, however, about the function of the protein product of this gene. Cloning and characterization of other FA genes will help define the molecular basis for the phenotypic heterogeneity of this disorder.

Aplastic anemia occurs in about 90% of FA patients. The hematologic manifestations develop slowly. Usually clinical signs of pancytopenia occur between the ages of 5 and 10 years, with the median age of 7 at diagnosis. Anemia is usually macrocytic, with macrocytosis often preceding anemia. Leukopenia primarily involves the granulocytes. Thrombocytopenia often precedes anemia

and leukopenia. Bone marrow transplant may be used to treat the bone marrow failure, but the risk for developing other tumors is high. Androgen therapy may reverse the pancytopenia for several years (in about 50% of FA patients). Acute nonlymphocytic leukemia is a common complication. This leukemia is difficult to treat, and survival is poor. Other malignancies, particularly gastrointestinal and gynecologic tumors, also are major risks. The median survival for FA patients is now about 25 years of age.

Familial aplastic anemia *Familial aplastic anemia* is a subset of Fanconi's anemia with no congenital abnormalities. It is interesting to note that some patients with this familial form have a relative with Fanconi's anemia. The familial disease may manifest itself anywhere between 1 to 77 years of age. The typical characteristics of aplastic anemia, including pancytopenia and bone marrow hypoplasia, are present. Young children with aplastic anemia should be screened for this subgroup of Fanconi's anemia because these patients do not respond to ALG therapy. Bone marrow transplant is the only effective treatment.

Other familial disorders associated with aplasia include dyskeratosis congenita, Shwachman-Diamond syndrome, amegakaryocytic thrombocytopenia, and Aase-Smith syndrome.

● Clinical findings

The onset of symptoms in aplastic anemia is usually insidious and related to the cytopenias. The most common initial sign is bleeding acompanied by petechial and fundal hemorrhages. Anemia and infection may occur separately, or in combination with the bleeding. Hepatosplenomegaly and lymphadenopathy are absent. Splenomegaly has been noted occasionally in later stages of the disease, but, if found in the early stages, the diagnosis of aplastic anemia should be questioned.

● Laboratory findings

PERIPHERAL BLOOD

Pancytopenia is typical. Although the degree of severity may vary, it is good practice to question the diagnosis of aplastic anemia unless the leukocyte count, erythrocyte count, and platelet count are all below the reference ranges. Hemoglobin is usually less than 7 g/dL. Erythrocytes appear normocytic and normochromic or they may be slightly macrocytic. There is mild to moderate anisocytosis and poikilocytosis. The presence of nucleated erythrocytes and teardrops is not typical of aplastic anemia but rather suggest marrow replacement, myelophthisic anemia. The relative reticulocyte count alone may be misleading due to the severe anemia. Therefore, the reticulocyte count should always be determined in absolute numbers or be corrected for the anemia before interpretation. The absolute reticulocyte count is less than 25 $\times 10^9$/L. The corrected count is less than 1%. Most often, thrombocytopenia is present at the time of diagnosis. Neutropenia precedes leukopenia; initial lymphocyte and

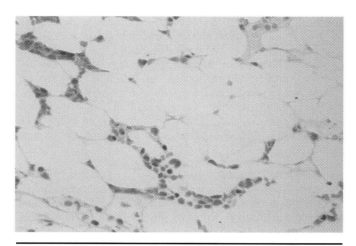

FIGURE 9-1. Bone marrow preparation from a patient with aplastic anemia shows marked hypocellularity (10%). The patches of cells remaining are primarily composed of lymphocytes. (100× original magnification.)

monocyte counts are normal. Because of the neutropenia, the differential count reflects a relative lymphocytosis. When the leukocyte count is below $1.5 \times 10^9/L$, an absolute lymphocytopenia also is present. There is an increase in the band to segmented neutrophil ratio, and occasionally more immature forms are found. Neutrophil granules are frequently larger than normal and stain a dark red; these granules should be distinguished from toxic granules, which are bluish-black.

BONE MARROW

Examination of the bone marrow is necessary to differentiate aplastic anemia from other diseases accompanied by pancytopenia. In aplastic anemia, the bone marrow is hypocellular, with more than than 70% fat (Fig. 9-1). This sometimes makes aspiration difficult. In addition, bone marrow infiltration with granulomas or cancer cells can lead to fibrosis, resulting in a hypocellular dry tap on aspiration. Thus, both aspiration and biopsy are needed for a correct diagnosis. It is recommended that several different sites be aspirated because spot sampling of an organ as large as the marrow may be misleading.[23] Some areas of acellular stroma and fat are infiltrated with clusters of lymphocytes, plasma cells, and reticulum cells. Areas of focal hyperplasia termed "hot spots" are found predominately in early remission but also can be found in severe refractory cases. Iron stain reveals many iron granules in macrophages, but granules rarely are seen in normoblasts.

OTHER LABORATORY FINDINGS

Other abnormal findings are not specific for aplastic anemia but are frequently found associated with the disease. Hemoglobin F may be increased (up to 1.5 g/dL), especially in children. Erythropoietin is often increased, particularly when compared with the erythropoietin levels in patients with similar degrees of anemia. Serum iron is increased with greater than 50% saturation of transferrin reflecting erythroid suppression. The clearance rate of iron from the plasma is decreased because of the decrease in

iron utilization by a hypoactive marrow. Coagulation tests that reflect platelet activity (bleeding time and clot retraction) are abnormal in relation to the degree of thrombocytopenia.

Prognosis and therapy

The prognosis in aplastic anemia is poor, with complete recovery occurring in only 10% of cases. Approximately 70% of patients die within 5 years of diagnosis. Clinically, patients whose anemia is related to exposure to a toxin do better than those with idiopathic aplastic anemia or those in whom aplastic anemia develops a lengthy time after exposure to the toxin. In general, the worse the pancytopenia and marrow hypoplasia, the worse the prognosis.

The first goal in management of acquired aplastic anemia is removal of the causative agent. This may involve withdrawal of drugs or removal of the patient from a hazardous environment. Because aplastic anemia is not a malignant disease, the mode of treatment is supportive. This requires multiple transfusions of erythrocytes, platelets, and leukocytes. Splenectomy in some patients has reduced the need for transfusions. Androgen has been used with limited success, inducing remission in some patients.

Bone marrow transplants have become a relatively common procedure for aplastic anemia. Although replacement of needed stem cells is successful in most cases, some transplants, even some performed between twins, do not induce remission. These unsuccessful transplants suggest that either the microenvironment of the recipient's bone marrow is unsupportive of cell growth or stem cell growth is immunosuppressed.

Immunosuppressive therapy has been advocated in patients unresponsive to bone marrow transplants.[4] Immunosuppressive therapy with ALG or ATG is effective in some patients. More than 50% of patients who receive this therapy improve, but only one third achieve complete remission.[9] Within 8 years of remission, secondary disorders or relapse develop in up to 57% of patients who receive immunosuppressive therapy.[19,20] Thus, this therapy does not appear to cure the underlying cause. Long-term complications of immunosuppressive therapy include the development of marrow clonal disorders such as PNH, leukemia, and myelodysplasia.

Factors considered when selecting bone marrow transplant or immunosuppressive therapy are listed in Table 9-2.

Differentiation of aplastic anemia from other causes of pancytopenia

Pancytopenia is associated with anemias other than aplastic anemia, but these anemias differ from aplastic anemia in that the pancytopenia is not the result of a defect in stem cell proliferation. Rather, the bone marrow is normocellular, hypercellular, or infiltrated with abnormal cellular elements. These anemias are mentioned here to help the laboratory scientist differentiate them from true hypoproliferative anemias.

TABLE 9-2 *FACTORS CONSIDERED WHEN SELECTING BONE MARROW TRANSPLANT OR IMMUNOSUPPRESSIVE THERAPY FOR PATIENTS WITH APLASTIC ANEMIA*

	Bone Marrow Transplantation	**Immunosuppressive Therapy**
Pretreatment patient factors		
Important	Age ≤20 HLA-matched sibling Fanconi's anemia	Age >40 No HLA-matched sibling
Relatively important	ANC <200/mm³ No or minimal prior blood product transfusions No serious medical disorders No uncontrolled infection	ANC >200/mm³
Treatment-related effects/outcome	Morbidity and mortality of chronic GVHD; chronic GVHD occurs in 10–40%	Incomplete hemopoietic recovery in ⅔ of responders; Late relapse of aplasia or occurrence of leukemia, PNH, or myelodysplastic syndrome in 5–57%

ANC = absolute neutrophil count, PNH = paroxysmal nocturnal hemoglobinuria. (From: Stewart, F.M.: Hypoplastic/aplastic anemia. *Med. Clin. N. Amer.,* 76:683, 1992.)

MYELOPHTHISIC ANEMIA

Myelophthisic is a term used to signify marrow replacement or infiltration by fibrotic, granulomatous, or neoplastic cells. The abnormal replacement cells reduce normal hematopoiesis and disrupt the normal bone marrow architecture, allowing release of immature cells into the peripheral blood. Anemia may be accompanied by normal, increased, or decreased leukocyte and platelet counts. The most characteristic findings are a leukoerythroblastic reaction and a moderate to marked poikilocytosis. Dacryocytes are commonly found as are large bizarre platelets. By contrast, nucleated erythrocytes and significant morphologic changes are almost never found in the peripheral blood in aplastic anemia. Myelophthisic anemia is associated with diffuse cancer of the prostate, breast, and stomach. It also is typical of myelofibrosis and lipid storage disorders.

MYELODYSPLASTIC SYNDROMES

This is a group of hematologic disorders that have a propensity to terminate in acute leukemia (Chapter 16). The principal peripheral blood findings are pancytopenia, bicytopenia, or isolated cytopenias with reticulocytopenia. The bone marrow, however, is normocellular or hypercellular with various degrees of qualitative abnormalities of one or more cell lines *(dyshematopoiesis).* Signs of dyshematopoiesis also are reflected in morphologic abnormalities of one or more cell lineages in the peripheral blood. Peripheral blood erythrocytes are either normocytic or macrocytic with poikilocytosis and basophilic stippling. Nucleated erythrocytes may be found. Dysgranulopoiesis is reflected by peripheral blood granulocyte abnormalities such as hypogranulation, pseudo Pelger-Huet anomaly, and giant granules. Dysmegakaryopoiesis may produce hypogranular and/or abnormally large platelets. These qualitative abnormalities of peripheral blood cells are useful in differentiating cytopenias due to true hypoproliferation of stem cells (aplastic anemia) from cytopenias due to dyshematopoiesis (ineffective erythropoiesis).

CONGENITAL DYSERYTHROPOIETIC ANEMIA

Congenital dyserythropoietic anemia is a rare familial refractory anemia characterized by both abnormal erythropoiesis and ineffective erythropoiesis. The bone marrow is normocellular or hypercellular, but the peripheral blood is pancytopenic. In contrast to aplastic anemia, erythrocyte precursors in the bone marrow exhibit multinuclearity, and myeloblasts and promyelocytes are increased. The anemia may be normocytic, but most often it is macrocytic. The three types of congenital dyserythropoietic anemia are discussed in Chapter 8.

HYPERSPLENISM

Hypersplenism from a variety of causes may result in a lack of one or more cellular elements of the blood, as these elements become pooled and sequestered in the spleen. In this condition, the bone marrow is hyperplastic, corresponding to the peripheral blood cytopenia. Anemia is accompanied by a reticulocytosis, as opposed to the reticulocytopenia found in the true hypoproliferative anemias. Granulocytopenia may be accompanied by a shift to the left. From a clinical standpoint, splenomegaly and other findings of the underlying disease are important in diagnosing this disorder. Splenectomy, although not always advisable, corrects the cytopenias.

OTHER

Deficiency of cobalamin or folic acid may be accompanied by pancytopenia. The bone marrow in these cases, however, reveals normocellularity or hypercellularity with megaloblastic changes. In the peripheral blood, hypersegmented neutrophils and Howell-Jolly bodies are typical. In contrast, these are not found in aplastic anemia.

● PURE RED CELL APLASIA

Pure red cell aplasia is characterized by a selective decrease in erythroid precursor cells in the marrow and peripheral blood anemia. The disease is believed to occur due to selective hypoproliferation of the unipotent erythroid stem cell. The term aplastic anemia should be avoided in describing this disease, because there is no disturbance of granulopoiesis or thrombopoiesis. Reticulocytes may be present but are less than 1% when corrected for the degree of anemia. Pure red cell aplasia may be acquired (acute or chronic) or congenital. Acquired pure red cell aplasia is seen in thymoma, with administration of certain drugs, in autoimmune disorders, and in infection. Transient erythroblastopenia of childhood (TEC) is an acquired, self-limited form of erythroid hypoplasia found in children.

Acquired acute pure red cell aplasia

Viral (parvovirus, Epstein-Barr virus, and viral hepatitis) and/or bacterial infections are associated with a temporary depression of erythropoiesis. Transient erythroblastopenia of childhood is a form of acquired acute pure red cell aplasia, but because of the importance of distinguishing this pediatric anemia from Diamond Blackfan anemia (DBA), it will be discussed with DBA.

In individuals with a normal erythrocyte lifespan and hemoglobin level, temporary erythroid hypoproliferation is not noticed. However, if the erythrocyte lifespan is decreased, the complication of erythroid hypoproliferation may be life-threatening (aplastic crises). These aplastic crises are most frequently noted in hemolytic anemias, including sickle cell anemia, paroxysmal nocturnal hemoglobinuria, and autoimmune hemolytic anemias.

The aplastic crises cases that are brought to the attention of a physician probably represent only a minor fraction of the actual occurrence of temporary erythroid aplasia. The aplastic crises often are preceded by fever with upper respiratory and intestinal complaints. Several members of the same family are frequently affected with the illness. Patients with concurrent hemolytic anemia have a rapid onset of lethargy and pallor. Patients without hemolytic anemia usually seek medical attention because of the primary illness, and anemia is only an incidental finding.

Laboratory findings include decreased erythrocyte count, hematocrit, and hemoglobin with absence of reticulocytes. Leukocytes and platelets usually are normal and sometimes increased. Serum bilirubin is low or normal. If the patient is seen early enough, the bone marrow will reveal an absence of erythroid cells. Usually, however, the patient is seen after the marrow has begun to recover. In these cases, there is an increase in young erythroid cells, which may be mistaken for an erythroid maturation arrest. If the patient is followed, however, these cells show normal maturation and differentiation.

If the anemia is severe, supportive therapy of packed erythrocyte transfusions may be necessary until spontaneous recovery occurs. Pure red cell aplasia associated with viral hepatitis has a poor prognosis.

Acute erythroid hypoplasia also occurs with administration of some drugs and chemicals. After removal of the drug, normal erythropoiesis usually resumes.

Acquired chronic pure red cell aplasia

An acquired selective, chronic depression of erythroid precursors is a rare disorder encountered in middle-aged adults. Thymoma has been diagnosed in 30% to 60% of these cases. However, only 5% to 10% of thymoma patients have pure red cell aplasia. After removal of the thymus, about 29% enter remission of the anemia. This disease also occurs in association with autoimmune hemolytic anemia, systemic lupus erythematosus, rheumatoid arthritis, and hematologic neoplasms. The high incidence of autoimmune disorders in this anemia suggest that an immunologic mechanism may be responsible for the red cell aplasia. Cytotoxic antibodies to erythropoietin-sensitive cells in the marrow and to erythropoietin have been demonstrated in some cases.

Pallor usually is the only physical finding. Anemia and reticulocytopenia with normal concentrations of leukocytes and platelets are characteristic laboratory findings. The marrow reveals normal myelopoiesis and thrombopoiesis with marked erythroid hypoplasia.

Therapies include transfusion with packed erythrocytes, thymectomy if the thymus is enlarged, immunosuppression, and steroids to stimulate erythrocyte production. In drug-induced red cell aplasia, withdrawal of the drug is indicated. Approximately 80% of patients with pure acquired red cell aplasia will have a spontaneous remission or remission induced by immunosuppression. About half will relapse but with additional immunosuppression; 80% will enter a second remission. By retreating relapsing patients or continuing maintenance immunosuppression, many can be maintained transfusion-free for years.[25]

Diamond-blackfan syndrome

Diamond-Blackfan syndrome (also called erythroblastic hypoplasia, erythroblastopenia, erythroid hypoplasia, red cell agenesis, aregenerative anemia, and hypoplastic anemia) is a congenital progressive erythrocyte aplasia that occurs in very young children. Symptoms of the anemia are usually apparent in the first year of life but may occur as late as 6 years of age. There is no leukopenia or thrombocytopenia.

There is evidence for both autosomal dominant and autosomal recessive modes of inheritance. Chromosomal karyotype is normal, but approximately 25% of cases have a wide range of congenital defects. These are usually minor aberrations that are significantly different from the major aberrations found in Fanconi's anemia. Many cases have no familial pattern, suggesting spontaneous mutations or acquired disease. It is now generally agreed that Diamond-Blackfan syndrome is actually a diverse family of diseases with a common hematologic phenotype.

The disease is not due to a deficiency of erythropoietin (EPO), since EPO levels are consistently increased and higher than expected for the degree of anemia. The EPO is active, and there are no antibodies directed against this hormone. The most probable defect in Diamond-Blackfan syndrome is an intrinsic defect of erythroid progenitor

TABLE 9-3 *DIAGNOSTIC CRITERIA FOR DBA*

1. macrocytic-normochromic anemia in first year of life
2. reticulocytopenia
3. normocellular marrow with marked erythroid hypoplasia
4. increased serum erythropoietin
5. normal or slightly decreased leukocyte count
6. normal or increased platelet count

cells. In vitro studies suggest that the defect may be a disorder of receptor-ligand interaction between erythroid precursors and one or more growth factors.[26] The defective interaction may occur at one or more steps in the proliferation and differentiation pathway of erythroid progenitors.

Physical findings and symptoms are those associated with the underlying anemia. Anemia is severe with erythroid hypoplasia in the bone marrow.

Diagnostic criteria for all cases of DBA are included in Table 9-3.[26] Vitamin B12 and folate levels are normal. Hemoglobin F is increased from 5% to 25%, and the i antigen is increased on erythrocytes. Serum iron and serum ferritin are increased, and transferrin is 100% saturated.

Therapy includes transfusions and administration of adrenal corticosteroids. Up to half of these patients develop prolonged remission, but most eventually require additional therapy. Most deaths are due to complications of therapy such as hemosiderosis.

Diamond-Blackfan anemia must be distinguished from TEC, a temporary suppression of erythropoiesis that frequently occurs after a viral infection in children. The age of onset of TEC ranges from 1 month to 10 years. Progressive pallor in a previously healthy child is the primary clinical finding. Key points in differentiating these two childhood diseases are included in Table 9-4. The fetal characteristics of erythrocytes seen in Diamond-Blackfan anemia are not found in TEC. The presence of fetal-like erythrocytes is not particularly useful, however, in diagnosing Diamond-Blackfan anemia in children younger than 1 year of age because children in this age group normally possess erythrocytes with fetal characteristics. The pathophysiology in TEC is believed to be either a virus-associated, antibody-mediated or T-cell–mediated suppression/inhibition of erythroid precursors. Therapy involves only supportive care. It is important that the distinction be made between DBA and TEC since DBA requires treatment that is unnecessary and potentially harmful to children with TEC.[27] Patients with TEC recover within 2 months of diagnosis. Therapy involves only supportive care.

OTHER HYPOPROLIFERATIVE ANEMIAS

Other hypoproliferative anemias, due primarily to defective hormonal stimulation of erythroid stem cells, include the anemia associated with renal disease and the anemias associated with endocrine disorders. In most cases, these anemias can be traced to a decrease in erythropoietin production.

Renal disease

Chronic renal disease is a common cause of anemia. Anemia, however, is only an incidental finding; the patient primarily seeks medical attention for symptoms related to

TABLE 9-4 *DIAMOND-BLACKFAN ANEMIA VS. TRANSIENT ERYTHROBLASTOPENIA OF CHILDHOOD*

	Diamond-Blackfan Anemia	**Transient Erythroblastopenia of Childhood**
Pure red cell aplasia	Present	Present
Age at onset	25% at birth; 90% by one year	0–4 years
Mode of inheritance	Autosomal dominant and recessive	Not inherited
Associated anomalies	At least one in 30% of patients	Absent
Fetal hemoglobin	Elevated	Normal
i antigen	Present	Absent
MCV	Elevated (30%) at diagnosis	Normal
Fetal pattern of red cell glycolytic and HMP shunt enzymes	Present	Absent
Adenosine deaminase activity (ADA)	Elevated in the vast majority of patients	Normal
Responses to corticosteroid therapy	Frequent (~70%)	Spontaneous recovery without therapy
Prognosis	Long periods of control; potential iron overload for those dependent on red cell transfusion requiring Desferal chelation; in long-term survivors, development of leukemia	Excellent for total recovery without sequelae

(With permission: Lipton JM: Congenital Pure Red Cell Aplasia. IN *Hematology: Basic principles and practice*. ED. R. Hoffman, EJ. Benz, SJ. Shattel, B. Furie, HJ Cohen. Churchill-Livingstone Inc. New York, 1995.)

TABLE 9-5 *POSSIBLE CAUSES OF ANEMIA IN CHRONIC RENAL DISEASE*

1. Decreased erythropoietin production
2. Presence of a dialyzable inhibitor of erythropoiesis
3. Decreased erythrocyte survival
4. Blood loss
5. Folate deficiency

TABLE 9-6 *HEMOSTATIC ABNORMALITIES IN CHRONIC RENAL DISEASE*

Platelet Abnormalities
  Abnormal platelet aggregation with adenosine diphosphate, epinephrine, collagen
  Decreased platelet adhesiveness
  Decreased platelet factor 3 availability
  Decreased clot retraction
  Prolonged bleeding time
  Thrombocytopenia

Coagulation Abnormalities
  Decreased factors XII, XI, prothrombin
  Increased factors VII, X, and fibrinogen
  Factor XIII deficiency or inhibitor
  Decreased fibrinolytic activity
  Decreased antithrombin III
  Decreased protein C

(With permission from Hacking, W.F.: Hematologic abnormalities in patients with renal diseases. Hem. Onc. Clin. North Am., 1(2):229, 1985).

renal failure. The hemoglobin begins to decrease when the blood urea nitrogen level increases to greater than 30 mg/dL. Anemia is slow-developing, and most patients tolerate the low hemoglobin levels well.

PATHOPHYSIOLOGY
Due to the complexity of the clinical settings in uremia, anemia is frequently the result of several different pathophysiologies (Table 9-5): (1) the most important and consistent factor is bone marrow hypoproliferation, attributed to a decrease in erythropoietin production by the diseased kidney; (2) in some cases, the erythropoietin level is normal, but the bone marrow does not respond. The unresponsiveness may be caused by the presence of a low molecular weight dialyzable inhibitor of erythropoiesis present in the serum of uremic patients. Improvement in hemoglobin levels is seen after dialysis; (3) in addition to hypoproliferation, decreased erythrocyte survival compounds the anemia. One factor responsible for the shortened survival is related to an unknown extracorpuscular cause—perhaps an unfavorable metabolic environment or mechanical trauma. Another cause of hemolysis may be related to an acquired abnormality in erythrocye metabolism that involves the pentose phosphate shunt. This abnormality causes impaired generation of NADPH and reduced glutathione.[28] Thus, when exposed to oxidants, the erythocytes develop Heinz bodies, inducing acute hemolysis. Hemolysis also may be related to a reversible defect in erythrocyte membrane sodium-potassium ATPase. (4) The anemia may be related to blood loss from the gastrointestinal tract because of a decrease in platelets and/or platelet dysfunction. Blood also is lost during priming for dialysis. Patients receiving dialysis lose about 5 to 6 mg of iron daily. Thus, an anemia associated with iron deficiency is common. (5) In addition, patients receiving dialysis may become folate-deficient because folate is dialyzable. Without folate supplements, megaloblastic anemia may develop.

LABORATORY FINDINGS
A normocytic and normochromic anemia is typical in renal disease, except when the patient is deficient in folate or iron; then a macrocytic anemia or microcytic anemia prevails. Moderate anisocytosis with some degree of microcytosis may be present. Hemoglobin levels are reduced to 5 to 8 g/dL, and the reticulocyte production index (RPI) is about 1. There is moderate to severe poikilocytosis with burr cells and schistocytes. The number of burr cells corre-

lates roughly with the severity of azotemia. Spherocytes are associated with hypersplenism. Nucleated erythrocytes are noted in the peripheral blood. Leukocytes and platelets are usually normal. The bone marrow reveals erythroid hypoproliferation, especially when compared with the degree of anemia.

Serum ferritin levels are higher than normal in chronic renal failure, even if iron deficiency is present. Therefore, it has been suggested that if the serum ferritin level is below 40 to 105 ng/mL, iron deficiency should be considered. Increased iron binding capacity may be a useful predictor of iron deficiency in these cases.

Other laboratory findings vary depending on the severity of renal impairment. Blood urea nitrogen is more than 30 mg/dL, and serum creatinine is increased. Electrolytes are abnormal. Hemostatic abnormalities found in chronic renal disease are listed in Table 9-6.

THERAPY
Therapy for chronic renal disease includes renal transplantation, hemodialysis, or continuous ambulatory peritoneal dialysis. All treatments tend to ameliorate the anemia, but hemodialysis exposes the patient to additional causes of anemia. These additional causes include blood loss, iron and folate deficiency, and hemolysis. Thus, iron and folic acid supplements are frequently given in conjunction with hemodialysis. The isolation and cloning of the human EPO gene and subsequent production of EPO by recombinant technology has allowed its use in therapeutic applications. Intermittent doses of EPO three times a week causes improvement in 1 to 2 weeks. In some cases, a normal hemoglobin is achieved, and, in all cases, the patients remain transfusion-independent.

● Endocrine abnormalities

Endocrine deficiencies are associated with a decrease in erythropoietin. The resulting anemia is usually normocytic, normochromic with normal erythrocyte morphology. The bone marrow findings suggest erythroid hypoproliferation.

A slow-developing normocytic normochromic anemia is characteristic of hypothyroidism. Erythrocyte survival is normal, and reticulocytosis is absent. The anemia is most likely a physiologic response to a decrease in tissue demands for oxygen. With hormone replacement therapy, the anemia slowly remits.

Hypopituitarism is associated with an anemia more severe than that of hypothyroidism, and the leukocyte count may be decreased. However, anemia is a minor component of the other manifestations of hypopituitarism. The pituitary has an effect on multiple endocrine glands, including the thyroid and adrenals. In males, a decrease in androgens may be partly responsible for the anemia, since androgens stimulate erythropoiesis. In addition, a decrease in the growth hormone may have a trophic effect on the bone marrow.

● SUMMARY

The hypoproliferative anemias include a group of acquired and constitutional disorders in which there is marrow hypocellularity. If only the erythrocytes are affected, the term pure red cell aplasia is appropriate. More commonly, there is a hypocellularity affecting all cell lines, and the diagnosis is aplastic anemia.

The hypocellularity in aplastic anemia may be due to defective or deficient stem cells, immune suppression, a defective bone marrow microenvironment, or deficient hormonal stimulation of hematopoiesis. Acquired aplastic anemia may be idiopathic or secondary to drugs, chemical agents, ionizing radiation, or infectious agents. Constitutional aplastic anemia has a congenital disposition and may be associated with other anomalies. Fanconi's anemia is a form of constitutional anemia with progressive bone marrow hypoplasia and other congenital defects. The disorder is characterized by chromosomal instability. A subset of Fanconi's anemia is familial aplastic anemia. This form does not have congenital abnormalities.

The laboratory findings in aplastic anemia reveal pancytopenia. The erythrocytes are usually normocytic, normochromic but may be macrocytic. The reticulocyte count is low and the RPI is less than 2. The bone marrow is less than 30% cellular.

Pure red cell aplasia is characterized by a selective decrease in erythroid cells. This disorder may be acquired or congenital. The acquired forms are seen in thymoma, with administration of certain drugs, in autoimmune disorders, and in infection, especially viral infections. Diamond-Blackfan syndrome is a congenital progressive erythrocyte aplasia occurring in young children. This congenital form of aplasia must be differentiated from TEC, a temporary aplasia occurring after viral infection.

Other hypoproliferative anemias are due primarily to defective hormonal stimulation of erythroid stem cells. These include anemia associated with renal disease and with endocrinopathies. The laboratory findings reflect not only anemia but also pathologies of the primary disorder.

● REVIEW QUESTIONS

A 13-year-old girl was admitted to the hospital with complaints of progressive weakness and shortness of breath with minimal physical effort. She has experienced recurrent fevers reaching 102° F. For the past 3 months, her physician has been following her recovery from viral hepatitis. Her recovery was uneventful with her liver enzyme levels returning to normal within 2 months. She has no other relevant medical history, and family history is noncontributory.

Results of physical examination show a well-developed adolescent with good nutritional status and no acute distress. There is no lymphadenopathy or organomegaly. Many petechial hemorrhages cover her chest and legs. Several bruises were found on her legs.

Initial Laboratory Data:

Erythrocyte count	2.42×10^{12}/L
Hb	7.1 g/dL
Hct	0.22 L/L
Platelet count	8.0×10^9/L
Leukocyte count	1.2×10^9/L
Differential:	
Segmented Neutrophils	2%
Lymphocytes	94%
Monocytes	4%
Reticulocyte count:	0.4%

1. What is the morphologic classification of this anemia?
   a. hypochromic microcytic
   b. normochromic normocytic
   c. normochromic macrocytic
   d. hypochromic macrocytic

2. What follow-up test should be performed?
   a. serum iron
   b. hemoglobin electrophoresis
   c. bone marrow aspiration
   d. direct antiglobulin test (DAT)

3. What term best describes this peripheral blood picture?
   a. pancytopenia
   b. bicytopenia
   c. granulocytopenia
   d. pure red cell aplasia

4. What is the possible cause of this patient's anemia?
   a. drug-induced
   b. decreased production of beta-globin chains
   c. viral-induced
   d. ionizing radiation

5. What is the absolute reticulocyte count?
   a. 4×10^9/L
   b. 40×10^9/L
   c. 97.0×10^9/L
   d. 10.0×10^9/L

6. What is the most likely diagnosis?
   a. aplastic anemia
   b. beta thalassemia minor
   c. anemia of chronic disease
   d. autoimmune hemolytic anemia

7. Which of the following features is helpful in differentiating Diamond-Blackfan anemia from transient erythroblastopenia of childhood?
   a. bone marrow erythroid hypoplasia
   b. erythrocytes with fetal characteristics
   c. age of onset
   d. pancytopenia

8. Which of the following is most characteristic of the peripheral blood picture in pure red cell aplasia?
   a. pancytopenia
   b. granulocytopenia and thrombocytopenia
   c. leukocytosis
   d. anemia

9. Autoimmune disorders are frequently associated with:
   a. aplastic anemia
   b. Diamond-Blackfan anemia
   c. pure red cell aplasia
   d. Fanconi's anemia

10. The bone marrow in pure red cell aplasia can be best described as:
    a. erythroid hypoplasia
    b. erythroid hyperplasia
    c. hypocellular
    d. hypercellular

● REFERENCES

1. Ehrlich, P.: Uber einen Fall von Anamie mit Bemerkungen iiberregenerative Veranderungen des Knochenmarks. Charite. Ann., 13: 300, 1888.
2. Chaufford, M.: Un Cas d'anemie pernicieuse aplastique. Bull. Soc. Med. Hop., Paris 21:313, 1904.
3. Henry, J.B. (ed.): Clinical Diagnosis and Management by Laboratory Methods. 17th Ed. Philadelphia: W.B. Saunders Co., 1984.
4. Gale, R.P., Champlin, R.E., Feig, S.A., Fitchen, J.H.: Aplastic anemia: biology and treatment. Ann. Intern. Med., 95:477, 1981.
5. Hassan, K., et al.: Severe aplastic anemia—an aetiological correlation. J. Pak. Med. Assoc., 44:43, 1994.
6. Young, N.S.: The pathogenesis and pathophysiology of aplastic anemia. IN Hematology: Basic Principles and Practice. Ed. R. Hoffman, E.J. Benz, S.J. Shattel, B. Furie, H.J. Cohen. New York: Churchill-Livingstone Inc., 1995.
7. Shumacher, M.D., Garvin, D.F., Triplett, D.A.: Introduction to Laboratory Hematology and Hematopathology. New York: Alan R. Liss, Inc., 1984.
8. Young, N.S., Levine, A.S., Humphines, R.K. (eds.): Aplastic Anemia Stem Cell Biology and Advances in Treatment. New York: Alan R. Liss Inc., 1984.
9. Stewart, F.M.: Hypoplastic/aplastic anemia. Med. Clin. North. Am., 76:683, 1992.
10. Zoumbos, N., Raefsky, E., Young, N.: Lymphokines and hematopoiesis. Prog. Hematol., 14:201, 1986.
11. Abe, T., et al.: Correlation of response of aplastic anemia patients to antilymphocyte globulin with in vitro lymphocyte stimulatory effect: predictive value of in vitro test for clinical response. Blood, 77:2225, 1991.
12. Marsh, J.C., et al.: Haemopoietic growth factors in aplastic anemia: a cautionary note. European Bone Marrow Transplant Working Party for Severe Aplastic Anemia. Lancet, 344:172, 1994.
13. Geissler, K., et al.: Effect of interleukin-3 on responsiveness to granulocyte-colony-stimulating factor in severe aplastic anemia. Ann. Intern. Med., 117:223, 1992.
14. Marsh, J.C., et al.: The hematopoietic defect in aplastic anemia assessed by long-term marrow culture. Blood, 76:1748, 1990.
15. Marsh, J.C., et al.: In vitro assessment of marrow 'stem cell' and stromal cell function in aplastic anemia. Br. J. Haematol., 78:258, 1991.
16. Levere, R.D., Ibraham, M.G.: The bone marrow as a metabolic organ. Am. J. Med., 73:615, 1982.
17. Smith, J.C., et al: Clinical characteristics of children with hereditary hemolytic anemias and aplastic crisis: a 7-year review. South. Med. J., 89:702, 1994.
18. Baker, R.I., Manoharan, A., de Luca, E., Begley, C.G.: Pure red cell aplasia of pregnancy: a distinct clinical entity. Br. J. Haematol. 85: 619, 1993.
19. de Planque, M.M.: Haematopoietic and immunologic abnormalities in severe aplastic anemia patients treated with antithymocyte globulin. Br. J. Haematol., 71:421, 1989.
20. Tichelli, A., et al.: Late haematological complications in severe aplastic anaemia. Br. J. Haematol., 69:413, 1988.
21. dos Santos, C.C., Gavish, H., Buchwald, M.: Fanconi anemia revisited: old ideas and new advances. Stem Cells, 12:142, 1994.
22. Alter, B.P.: Fanconi's anemia and its variability. Br. J. Haematol., 85:9, 1993.
23. Freedman, M.H.: Erythropoiesis in Diamond-Blackfan anemia and the role of interleukin 3 and steel factor. Stem Cells, 11 (Suppl 2): 98, 1993.
24. Erslev, A.J.: Erythrocyte disorders—anemias related to disturbance of erythroid precursor cell proliferation or differentiation. In: Hematology. Edited by W. J. Williams, E. Beutler, A. J. Erslev, M. A. Lichtman. New York: McGraw-Hill, 1990.
25. Krantz, S.B.: Acquired pure red cell aplasia. In: Hematology: Basic Principles and Practice. Edited by R. Hoffman, E. J. Benz, S. J. Shattel, B. Furie, H. J. Cohen. New York: Churchill Livingstone, 1995.
26. Freedman, M.H.: Pure red cell aplasia in childhood and adolescence: pathogenesis and approaches to diagnosis. Br. J. Haematol., 85:246, 1993.
27. Miller, R., Berman, B.: Transient erythroblastopenia of childhood in infants <6 months of age. Am. J. Ped. Hematol. Onc., 16:246, 1994.
28. Hocking, W.G.: Hematologic abnormalities in patients with renal diseases. Hem. Onc. Clin. North. Am., 1:229, 1987.

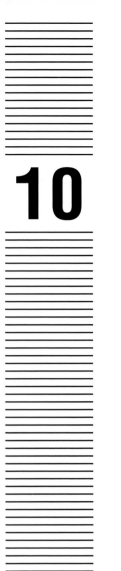

10

General aspects and classifications of hemolytic anemias

KEY TERMS

hemolysis
compensated hemolytic
   disease
jaundice

●
OVERVIEW OF HEMOLYTIC ANEMIA

●
Definition

The hemolytic anemias are a heterogenous group of normocytic, normochromic anemias in which the erythrocyte is prematurely destroyed. This premature destruction is referred to as *hemolysis*. Hemolysis may occur when erythrocytes are intrinsically abnormal. These abnormalities include defects in the cell membrane, structurally abnormal hemoglobins, defects in globin synthesis (thalassemia), or deficiencies/defects of cell enzymes. Hemolysis also may occur in the presence of abnormalities extrinsic to the erythrocyte, such as when antibodies are formed against the cell's antigens. Intrinsic abnormalities are generally genetically determined, while extrinsic abnormalities are acquired.

Reticulocytosis is a constant feature of all hemolytic anemias reflecting the increased activity of the bone marrow as it attempts to maintain erythrocyte mass in the peripheral blood. If the bone marrow is able to increase erythropoiesis enough to compensate for the decreased erythrocyte lifespan, anemia does not develop. In this case, cells are being produced at the same or nearly the same rate as they are hemolyzed. This condition is called *compensated hemolytic disease*. Compensated hemolytic disease may rapidly develop into anemia if one of the following occurs: (1) erythrocyte destruction accelerates beyond the compensatory capacity of the marrow (hemolytic crisis); (2) the marrow suddenly stops producing erythrocytes (aplastic crisis). Normal bone marrow can compensate for decreased erythrocyte survival by increasing production until the erythrocyte lifespan drops to one eighth of normal or about 15 to 18 days. If the lifespan decreases to less than 15 days, anemia develops.

●
LABORATORY FINDINGS

Hematologic characteristics of hemolytic anemia reflect the increased activity of the bone marrow and the increased erythrocyte destruction (Table 10-1). In hemolytic anemia, erythroid hyperplasia of the bone marrow with decreased amounts of fat is more pronounced than in any of the nonhemolytic anemias. Consequently, the myeloid to erythroid ratio (M:E) is decreased. Increased plasma iron turnover reflects the increased erythrocyte destruction and increased utilization of iron by erythroid precursors in the bone marrow.

Peripheral blood reticulocytosis, marked polychromasia, and nucleated erythrocytes in the peripheral blood are clues to the presence of increased erythropoietic activity in the bone marrow. The hemolytic anemias are the only anemias with a reticulocyte production index (RPI) greater than 2 (except in acute hemorrhage). Thus, the RPI is useful in differentiating hemolytic anemias from other normocytic, normochromic anemias in which the bone marrow is not increasing effective erythropoiesis (e.g.,

TABLE 10-1   *COMMON LABORATORY FINDINGS IN HEMOLYTIC ANEMIAS*

Laboratory Findings Reflecting Increased Bone Marrow Activity

Reticulocytosis (RPI > 2)

Leukocytosis

Nucleated erythrocytes in the peripheral blood

Polychromasia of erythrocytes on stained blood smears

Normoblastic erythroid hyperplasia of the bone marrow

Laboratory Findings Reflecting Increased Erythrocyte Destruction

Anemia

Presence of spherocytes, schistocytes, and/or other poikilocytes

Positive AHG** test

Decreased haptoglobin and hemopexin

Decreased glycosylated hemoglobin

Increased fecal and urine urobilinogen

Increased bilirubin (unconjugated)

*Hemoglobinemia

*Hemoglobinuria

*Hemosiderinuria

*Methemoglobinemia

Increased serum LDH

Increased expired CO

* Associated only with intravascular hemolysis.
** AHG = antihuman globulin.

pure red cell aplasia). Occasionally, the degree of reticulocytosis is great enough to cause an increased MCV.

The blood smear may exhibit poikilocytosis depending on the pathophysiologic cause of the hemolysis; when present, the specific poikilocytes may provide important clues to the underlying disease process. For example, spherocytes indicate hereditary spherocytosis or an immune hemolytic anemia, whereas schistocytes usually indicate mechanical damage to the cell.

Results of laboratory tests that are used to evaluate heme catabolism are usually abnormal. Unconjugated/indirect bilirubin is often increased, but the conjugated/direct fraction is usually normal unless hepatic or biliary dysfunction is present. A significant number of patients with hemolytic disease have normal serum bilirubin levels suggesting that serum bilirubin is not a reliable index of erythrocyte destruction. Bilirubin levels over 5 mg/dL are unusual in hemolytic disease except in neonates and in those with coexisting liver dysfunction. Urine and fecal urobilinogen is elevated. Heme binding plasma proteins, haptoglobin and hemopexin, often are decreased as a result of increased consumption.

Although haptoglobin levels less than 250 mg/L are highly specific for hemolytic anemia, levels also may be decreased in liver disease due to decreased synthesis of the protein and in hereditary deficiency of haptoglobin.

TABLE 10-2 *CLINICAL FINDINGS ASSOCIATED WITH HEMOLYTIC ANEMIA*

- jaundice
- gallstones
- dark or red urine
- symptoms of anemia
- thinning of cortical bone
- extramedullary hematopoietic masses
- splenomegaly

Caution should be used in interpretation of haptoglobin levels because it is an acute-phase reactant and may be increased in the presence of inflammation, infection and malignancy. Haptoglobin functions as an intravascular heme-binding protein but it also may be decreased in association with extravascular hemolytic diseases.

CLINICAL FINDINGS

Clinical signs of hemolytic anemia are associated with increases in both heme catabolism (erythrocyte destruction) and erythropoiesis (Table 10-2). *Jaundice* is a reflection of an increase in bilirubin production. Gallstones consisting primarily of bilirubin are common in congenital hemolytic anemias. Dark or red urine due to excretion of plasma hemoglobin may be noted in intravascular hemolysis.

The primary symptoms are those associated with anemia, including pallor, fatigue, and cardiac symptoms. Chronic severe hemolytic anemias stimulate the expansion of bone marrow, consequently thinning cortical bone and widening spaces between inner and outer tables of bone. In children, this expansion is evident in skeletal abnormalities. These bone changes may result in spontaneous fractures and a type of arthritis termed osteoarthropathy.[1] Extramedullary hematopoietic masses may be found. Some of these masses are believed to represent extrusions of the marrow cavity through thinned out bone cortex. Small colonies of erythrocytes also may be found in the spleen, liver, lymph nodes, and perinephric tissue. The hematopoietic tumor masses may cause pressure symptoms on adjacent organs.[1] In extravascular hemolysis, splenic hypertrophy is a constant finding.

SITES OF DESTRUCTION

Hemolysis may occur within the circulation (intravascular) or within the macrophages of the spleen, liver, or bone marrow (extravascular). In some cases, depending on the degree of damage to the cell, destruction may occur both intravascularly and extravascularly. The results of laboratory tests may provide important clues to the hemolytic process. To correlate laboratory results with the pathophysiology of the anemia, an understanding of intravascular and extravascular hemolysis is essential. Refer to Chapter 3 for a full review of these processes.

Intravascular hemolysis

In intravascular hemolysis, the erythrocyte is destroyed within the blood vessels. In summary, when the erythrocyte is hemolyzed, free hemoglobin is released into the plasma. The hemoglobin is bound to the plasma protein haptoglobin, transported as a complex to the liver, where it is metabolized to bilirubin, and excreted to the intestinal tract via the bile duct. Normally the concentration of hemoglobin in plasma is less than 5 mg/dL. However, in severe intravascular hemolysis, synthesis of haptoglobin may not be sufficient to replace that being used and free hemoglobin accumulates in the plasma. It should be remembered, however, that haptoglobin is an acute phase reactant and may be normal or even increased in individuals with infections, inflammation or malignant disease despite an increase in intravascular hemolysis. Another plasma protein, hemopexin, complexes with heme when haptoglobin is depleted. This complex also may be cleared from the plasma by the liver faster than it can be synthesized and is quickly depleted. A decrease in hemopexin, however, is secondary to a reduction in haptoglobin.

Hemoglobin bound to haptoglobin or hemopexin forms complexes that are too large to pass through the glomerulus of the kidney. When these two transport proteins are depleted, free hemoglobin circulates in the plasma. Some of this hemoglobin is removed directly by the liver, but some dissociates into dimers small enough to be filtered by the glomerulus. Filtered hemoglobin may be reabsorbed in the proximal renal tubules, but when the rate of filtration exceeds the tubular reabsorption capabilities, free hemoglobin appears in the urine. The presence of free hemoglobin in the urine is a sign of rapid and severe intravascular hemolysis.[2] Depending on the degree of hemolysis, the urine may be pink, red, or brownish-black.

Some renal tubular cells may become laden with hemoglobin iron and when sloughed off into the urine, hemosiderin granules may be visualized. Hemosiderin in the urine is a sign that a significant amount of hemoglobin has been filtered by the kidney.[2] With chronic intravascular hemolysis, hemosiderin granules may appear in the urine even in the absence of hemoglobinuria.

Free hemoglobin not bound to either of the two transport proteins or not excreted by the kidney is quickly oxidized to methemoglobin. Methemoglobin dissociates into hemin (oxidized form of heme) and globin. Hemin may bind to hemopexin if it is available or to albumin, forming methemalbumin. Methemalbumin is not excreted in the urine but can be detected in the plasma by Schumm's test.

Laboratory findings of intravascular hemolysis include hemoglobinemia, hemoglobinuria, hemosidernuria, methemoglobinemia, decreased haptoglobin, and decreased hemopexin. In addition, the serum lactic dehydrogenase may increase to as much as 800 IU/L (upper normal 207 IU/L). Lactic dehydrogenase is released from the erythrocyte into the plasma in intravascular hemolysis, and it is cleared from plasma even more slowly than hemoglobin.

TABLE 10-3 *ANEMIAS CHARACTERIZED BY INTRAVASCULAR HEMOLYSIS*

1) Activation of complement on the erythrocyte membrane
   - Paroxysmal nocturnal hemoglobinuria
   - Paroxysmal cold hemoglobinuria
   - Some transfusion reactions
   - Some autoimmune hemolytic anemias

2) Physical or mechanical trauma to the erythrocyte
   - Microangiopathic hemolytic anemia
   - Abnormalities of the heart and great vessels
   - Disseminated intravascular coagulation

3) Toxic microenvironment
   - Bacterial infections
   - *Plasmodium falciparum* infection
   - Venoms
   - Arsine poisoning
   - Acute drug reaction in G-6PD deficiency
   - Intravenous administration of distilled water

Erythrocytes must be severely damaged to undergo intravascular destruction. Minimally or moderately damaged erythrocytes are removed by phagocytes in the spleen or liver. Intravascular hemolysis may be caused by: (1) activation of complement on the erythrocyte membrane; (2) physical or mechanical trauma to the erythrocyte; or (3) the presence of soluble toxic substances in the erythrocyte's environment (Table 10-3).

Extravascular hemolysis

If the premature erythrocyte destruction is the result of extravascular hemolysis, the erythrocytes are removed from circulation by phagocytes in the spleen, liver, or bone marrow. This type of hemolysis is more common than intravascular hemolysis. There is no hemoglobinemia, hemoglobinuria, or hemosidinuria, as hemoglobin is not released directly into the plasma. Instead, the hemoglobin is degraded within the phagocyte to heme and globin. The heme is further catabolized to iron, biliverdin, and carbon monoxide. The biliverdin then enters the plasma as bilirubin, binds to albumin, and is excreted by the liver.

Significant laboratory findings in hemolytic anemias associated with extravascular hemolysis are measurements of the products of heme catabolism. These findings include an increase in expired carbon monoxide, an increase in carboxyhemoglobin, an increase in serum bilirubin (especially in the indirect fraction), and an increase in both urine and fecal urobilinogen. In severe or chronic extravascular hemolysis, haptoglobin and hemopexin levels also may be decreased.

Extravascular hemolysis may occur in phagocytes of the spleen, liver, or bone marrow. The type and degree of erythrocyte damage determines the primary site of erythrocyte destruction. The spleen is more efficient at removing slightly damaged erythrocytes because of the unique circulation pattern in the splenic cords. In this relatively static environment, erythrocytes are susceptible to fine scrutiny by splenic macrophages. The liver blood flow exceeds blood flow in the spleen and is an important site

for the removal and phagocytosis of extensively damaged erythrocytes.

Antibody and complement attached to the cell membrane make the erythrocyte a target for removal from the circulation by phagocytes. The sites and extent of extravascular hemolysis are dependent on the class of antibody attached to the erythrocyte as well as to whether complement is present. Thus, it is sometimes helpful to determine the specific class of antibody present. Erythrocytes sensitized with both complement and IgM are readily removed in the liver by hepatic macrophages, which have receptors for the complement component, C3b. Conversely, IgM sensitized cells without attached complement components appear to survive normally, since macrophages lack Fc receptors for IgM. Clearance of IgM-sensitized cells is thus completely dependent on activation of complement. If the terminal complement components are activated on the cell membrane, hemolysis is intravascular. Erythrocytes sensitized with IgG may or may not activate complement since it takes many molecules of IgG on the erythrocyte membrane to bind one molecule of complement. However, cells sensitized with IgG can be removed by macrophages even in the absence of complement. IgG-sensitized erythrocytes are cleared primarily in the spleen by macrophages, which have Fc receptors for IgG in addition to C3b receptors.[3] The clearance of erythrocytes sensitized by both IgG and complement is accelerated since phagocytosis is mediated by two receptors.

Bone marrow macrophages are responsible for the removal of maturing precursor cells that are intrinsically abnormal. Cytoplasmic or nuclear maturation abnormalities are associated with this type of hemolysis, resulting in a high degree of ineffective erythropoiesis. Many of the abnormal cells never enter the peripheral blood. Thalassemias and megaloblastic anemias are examples of anemias with a significant degree of ineffective erythropoiesis.

Many of the hemolytic anemias that are associated with inherited defects of the erythrocyte membrane, of hemoglobin, and of intracellular enzymes have some degree of ineffective erythropoiesis. In most cases, however, a significant number of the defective cells gain access to the peripheral blood. These cells are not physiologically equipped to withstand the assaults of the peripheral circulation and are damaged. The damaged cells are then removed by liver or splenic macrophages. Anemias associated with extravascular hemolysis are listed in Table 10-4.

Erythrocyte survival studies

Erythrocyte survival studies are helpful in defining a hemolytic process in which erythrocyte survival is only mildly decreased. In mild hemolysis, laboratory findings typical of extravascular or intravascular hemolysis may be absent. Survival studies give insight into the rate and mechanism of hemolysis.

To study erythrocyte survival, a sample of patient's blood is removed and labeled in vitro with tracer amounts of radionuclide. The most common random label for erythrocytes and that recommended by the International

TABLE 10-4 *ANEMIAS CHARACTERIZED BY EXTRAVASCULAR HEMOLYSIS*

1) Inherited erythrocyte defects
   • Thalassemia
   • Hemoglobinopathies
   • Enzyme deficiencies
   • Membrane disorders

2) Acquired erythrocyte defects
   • Megaloblastic anemia
   • Spur cell anemia
   • Vitamin E deficiency in newborns

3) Immunohemolytic anemias
   • Autoimmune
   • Drug-induced

TABLE 10-5 *ASHBY'S CROSS-TRANSFUSION STUDIES FOR DIFFERENTIATING INTRINSIC FROM EXTRINSIC ERYTHROCYTE ABNORMALITIES IN HEMOLYTIC ANEMIA*

		Erythrocyte Survival	
Donor	*Recipient*	Intrinsic Abnormality	Extrinsic Abnormality
Patient	Normal subject	Reduced	Normal
Normal subject	Patient	Normal	Reduced

(From: Lee, G.R., Bithell, T.C., Foerster, J., Athens, J.W., Lukens, J.N.: Wintrobe's Clinical Hematology. Philadelphia: Lea & Febiger, 1993.)

Committee for Standardization in Hematology is radioactive chromium (^{51}Cr).[4] The chromium penetrates the erythrocyte and remains trapped there. This labeled sample is injected intravenously into the patient. To determine the erythrocyte survival pattern, small samples of patient's blood are assayed at specified time intervals for radioactivity levels. The erythrocyte lifespan is expressed as the time it takes for blood radioactivity to decrease by one-half ($T\frac{1}{2}$^{51}Cr) starting 24 hours after injection. About 1% of the ^{51}Cr is normally eluted from surviving cells daily. In addition, only 1% of the labeled cells can be expected to have a lifespan of 100 to 120 days, since only 1% of the total erythrocyte mass is replaced each day. The remaining labeled cells have expected lifespans from 0 to 100 days. Taking these facts into consideration, the normal $T\frac{1}{2}$ with this method has been determined to be 25 to 35 days. A steady state is necessary for accurate interpretation of erythrocyte survival studies, as blood loss or transfusions can alter the data significantly. Labeled erythrocytes in this method also are useful in determining the sites of erythrocyte destruction. The amount of radioactivity taken up by an organ can be measured by scanning the body for ^{51}Cr deposition and is proportional to the number of erythrocytes destroyed there.

Before the development of radioisotope studies, a method to differentiate intrinsic from extrinsic erythrocyte abnormalities was Ashby's cross-transfusion erythrocyte survival studies. Normal erythrocytes from a compatible donor are transfused to the patient. At appropriate intervals, blood samples are tested with potent antisera to determine the rate of disappearance of donor cells. In patients with an intrinsic erythrocyte abnormality, only the patient's cells are abnormal and have shortened survival; donor erythrocytes survive normally. However, if the abnormality is extrinsic, the transfused donor erythrocytes will have a shortened survival similar to that of the patient because the hemolytic agent is likely to attack both the donor and the patient's own cells. The technique can be carried a step further by transfusing patient blood into a normal compatible donor. If the patient cells survive normally in the donor, the patient cells are probably intrinsically normal. If, however, the infused patient cells have a shortened survival, similar to that in the patient, the patient's cells are abnormal. This method is still valuable in theory in explaining the pathophysiology of some hemolytic anemias (Table 10-5).

● SOURCE OF DEFECT

Hemolytic anemias may be classified as intrinsic or extrinsic according to the cause of the shortened erythrocyte survival (Table 10-6). Intrinsic refers to an abnormality

TABLE 10-6 *CLASSIFICATION OF HEMOLYTIC ANEMIAS*

Intrinsic (Inherited)

Membrane defects
   Hereditary spherocytosis
   Hereditary elliptocytosis
   Hereditary pyropoikilocytosis
   Hereditary stomatocytosis
   Hereditary xerocytosis
   PNH (acquired)

Enzyme disorders
   G6PD deficiency
   Pyruvate kinase deficiency

Abnormal hemoglobins
   Thalassemia
   Structural hemoglobin variants

Extrinsic (Acquired)

Antagonistic plasma factors
   Chemicals, drugs
   Animal venoms
   Infectious agents
   Plasma lipid abnormalities

Traumatic physical cell injury
   Microcirculation lesions
   Thermal injury
   March hemoglobinuria

Immune mediated cell destruction
   Autoimmune
   Alloimmune
   Drug-induced

of the erythrocyte itself. The abnormality may be in the membrane, in the cell enzymes, or in the hemoglobin molecule. Extrinsic refers to an antagonist in the cell's environment that causes injury to the erythrocyte. Contrary to intrinsic defects, in extrinsic defects the erythrocyte is normal.

● Intrinsic defects

With a few exceptions, intrinsic defects are hereditary. Using Ashby's technique, normal tranfused donor erythrocytes will survive normally in the patient, whereas patient cells transfused into a normal donor will have a shortened lifespan similar to that in the patient. The site of hemolysis in intrinsic defects is usually extravascular.

In some cases, intrinsic defects render the cell more susceptible than normal cells to damage by environmental (extracorpuscular) factors. Although extracorpuscular factors may be involved, the initiating event in hemolysis is considered to be the intrinsic abnormality. For example, a patient with the glucose-6-phosphate dehydrogenase (G6PD) enzyme deficiency may not be able to produce enough glutathione to handle the oxidation products that accompany the administration of some drugs. Consequently, the erythrocytes suffer oxidant injury precipitated by the drug, leading to hemolysis. Intrinsic defects causing hemolysis include the following:

DEFECTS OF THE ERYTHROCYTE MEMBRANE
Structural defects of the erythrocyte membrane may cause the membrane to become abnormally permeable, rigid, or unstable and easily fragmented. In most cases, the defect is in one or more of the cytoskeletal proteins under the membrane lipid bilayer causing abnormal interaction between the lipid bilayer and the cytoskeleton. In other cases, the membrane is abnormally permeable to cations because of defects in integral proteins and/or lipids. These hereditary membrane disorders include hereditary spherocytosis, hereditary elliptocytosis, hereditary pyropoikilocytosis, hereditary xerocytosis, and hereditary stomatocytosis. In paroxysmal nocturnal hemoglobinuria, the erythrocyte membrane lacks a protein that serves a critical role in controlling complement attachment and activation on the cell membrane. As a result, the cell is abnormally sensitive to complement. The defective membrane is an acquired abnormality.

DEFECTS OF HEMOGLOBIN STRUCTURE OR PRODUCTION
Structurally abnormal hemoglobins that cause hemoglobin insolubility or instability may cause erythrocyte rigidity and, ultimately, hemolysis. Examples include sickle cell anemia and the unstable hemoglobin disorders. Thalassemias also contain a hemolytic component. In thalassemia, precipitates of excess globin chains cause erythrocytes to become rigid, and severe hemolytic anemia develops.

DEFECTS OF ERYTHROCYTE ENZYMES
Deficiencies of erythrocyte enzymes necessary for maintaining hemoglobin and membrane sulfhydryl groups in the reduced state or for maintaining adequate levels of adenosine triphosphate (ATP) for cation exchange may result in hemolytic anemia. The enzyme disorders may be divided into two groups: (1) deficiencies in enzymes of the Embden-Meyerhoff pathway (e.g., pyruvate kinase); and (2) deficiencies in enzymes of the hexose-monophosphate shunt (e.g., G6PD).

● Extrinsic defects

Extrinsic defects are usually acquired. The erythrocytes, as innocent bystanders, are damaged by chemical, mechanical, or physical agents. Hemolysis may be either intravascular or extravascular. Normal cells transfused into the patient have a shortened lifespan similar to that of the patient's own erythrocytes. The external factors causing hemolysis are:

PLASMA OR SOLUBLE FACTORS IN THE ERYTHROCYTE'S ENVIRONMENT
These factors include antibodies directed against the erythrocyte antigens or immune complexes absorbed onto the erythrocyte membrane (immune hemolytic anemias), animal venoms, chemicals, drugs, toxins, and altered plasma lipid concentrations.

PHYSICAL OR MECHANICAL TRAUMA
Trauma to the erythrocyte in peripheral circulation may cause the erythrocyte to fragment, producing striking abnormalities on the blood smear. These anemias include the microangiopathic hemolytic anemias, intracellular parasitic infections, and anemia due to thermal injury. In addition, splenomegaly may cause anemia by hypersequestration of erythrocytes.

SUMMARY

Hemolytic anemias are chacterized by decreased erythrocyte survival. Hemolysis may be due to an intrinsic erythrocyte abnormality or an abnormality extrinsic to the cell. Intrinsic abnormalities are generally inherited and include defects in the cell's membrane, hemoglobin, or enzymes. Extrinsic abnormalities are acquired. These include hemolysis due to factors in the erythrocyte environment such as drugs, toxins, and physical or mechanical trauma to the erythrocyte.

Laboratory findings in hemolytic anemia reflect increased bone marrow production as well as increased erythrocyte destruction. Reticulocytosis, erythroid hyperplasia of the bone marrow, and increased iron turnover are signs of increased bone marrow activity. Findings associated with increased erthrocyte destruction include decreased haptoglobin, hemosidinuria, hemoglobinuria, increased serum bilirubin and increased urine and fecal urobilinogen. Hemolysis may occur intravascularly or extravascularly or both.

Erythrocyte survival studies give insight into the rate and mechanism of hemolysis. An erythrocyte sample from the patient is radioactively labeled and infused back into the patient. The erythrocyte lifespan is the time it takes for the radioactivity to decrease by one half (T ½) starting 24 hours after injection. The reference range for T ½ is 25 to 35 days.

REVIEW QUESTIONS

1. Which of the following is characteristic of severe intravascular hemolysis?
   a. decreased bilirubin
   b. increased hemopexin
   c. decreased urobilinogen
   d. decreased haptoglobin

2. Hemolytic anemias caused by intrinsic erythrocyte abnormalities include:
   a. immune hemolytic anemia
   b. hereditary spherocytosis
   c. microangiopathic hemolytic anemia
   d. thermal injury anemia

3. Which of the following reticulocyte counts is typical of a hemolytic anemia?
   a. 40×10^9/L
   b. 1%
   c. 10%
   d. 10×10^9/L

4. A 2-year-old child was seen by his physician for pallor and an enlarged abdomen. Results of laboratory tests showed a severe anemia. Family history revealed a mother and maternal uncle who had lifelong anemia. Further testing revealed the child had thalassemia. This anemia is an example of:
   a. an extrinsic erythrocyte defect
   b. an erythrocyte enzyme defect
   c. an intrinsic erythrocyte defect
   d. an acquired hemolytic anemia

5. Which of the findings below are characteristic of the bone marrow in a hemolytic anemia?
   a. erythroid hyperplasia
   b. increased M:E ratio
   c. increased amount of fat
   d. hypoplasia

REFERENCES

1. Papavasiliou, C.: Clinical expressions of the expansion of the bone marrow in the chronic anemias: The role of radiotherapy. Int. J. Rad. Oncol. Biol. Phys., 28:605, 1994.
2. Tabbara, I.A.: Hemolytic anemias. Diagnosis and Management. Med. Clin. North. Am., 76:649. 1992.
3. Schreiber, A.D.: Autoimmune Hemolytic Anemia. Pediatr. Clin. North. Am., 27:253, 1980.
4. DeVries, R.A., DeBruin, M., Marx, J.J.M., Van De Wiel, A.: Radioisotopic labels for blood cell survival studies: A review. Nucl. Med. Biol., 20:809, 1993.

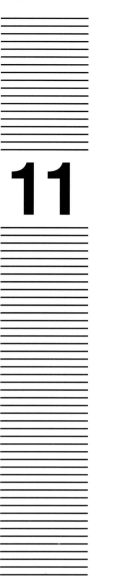

Hemolytic anemia caused by intrinsic erythrocyte defects

11

TABLE 11-1 *INTRINSIC ERYTHROCYTIC DEFECTS THAT MAY RESULT IN A HEMOLYTIC ANEMIA*

- Defects in the erythrocyte membrane
- Hemoglobinopathies
  - Structurally abnormal hemoglobins
  - Defects in globin synthesis (thalassemia)
- Deficiency or defect of erythrocytic enzymes

INTRODUCTION

Erythrocyte lifespan may be significantly shortened if the cell is intrinsically defective (intracorpuscular defect). Hemolytic anemia has been associated with defective erythrocyte membranes, structually abnormal hemoglobins or defective globin synthesis (hemoglobinopathies), and deficiencies of erythrocyte enzymes (Table 11-1). Almost all of these defects are hereditary in nature. The hemoglobinopathies, which have a significant hemolytic component, have been discussed previously (Chapter 7). This chapter will include the hemolytic anemias due to membrane defects and enzyme deficiencies.

The intrinsic nature of the erythrocytic defect can be demonstrated by transfusing normal cells into the patient. These transfused erythrocytes will have a normal lifespan. Conversely, if patient erythrocytes are transfused into a normal individual, the patient erythrocytes will have a shortened lifespan.

MEMBRANE DEFECTS

An erythrocyte membrane that is normal in both structure and function is essential to the survival of the cell. (The reader is referred to Chapter 3 for a discussion of the normal erythrocyte membrane.) Composed of proteins and lipids, the membrane is responsible for maintaining stability and the normal discoid shape of the cell, for preserving cell deformability, and for retaining selective permeability. Hemolytic anemia may result from abnormalities in constituent membrane proteins or lipids, both of which may alter the stability, shape, deformability and/or permeability of the membrane. Most hemolysis associated with abnormal membranes is extravascular, occurring primarily in the splenic cords.

Defects in membrane affecting cell stability, shape and deformability

Inherited abnormalities in the erythrocyte's membrane proteins may result in decreased membrane stability. Membrane instability may cause loss of portions of the lipid bilayer or disrupt the organization and interaction of the cell's cytoskeleton proteins. These membrane changes may cause the erythrocyte to assume abnormal shapes or fragment. Erythrocytes with abnormal membrane lipid may form acanthocytes. Abnormally shaped erthrocytes

are generally less deformable than normal biconcave, discoid erythrocytes. These abnormal cells are particularly susceptible to entrapment in the splenic cords. Anemia results when the rate of hemolysis is increased to the point in which the bone marrow cannot adequately compensate.

SKELETAL PROTEIN ABNORMALITIES

The membrane protein and lipid interactions associated with abnormal erythrocyte membranes can be divided into two categories, vertical and horizontal[2] (Fig. 11-1)(Table 11-2).

Vertical interactions Vertical interactions are perpendicular to the plane of the erythrocyte membrane and include interactions between the skeletal lattice on the cytoplasmic side of the membrane and its attachment to the integral proteins and lipids of the membrane. These interactions stabilize the lipid bilayer membrane. Defects in verticle contacts between the skeletal lattice proteins and the membrane integral proteins and lipids causes uncoupling of the lipid bilayer from the underlying skeletal lattice. This causes a selective loss of portions of the lipid bilayer. The net loss of cell membrane results in formation of a spherocyte and eventual hemolysis of the cell. The skeletal lattice, however, is not disrupted, and the cell is mechanically

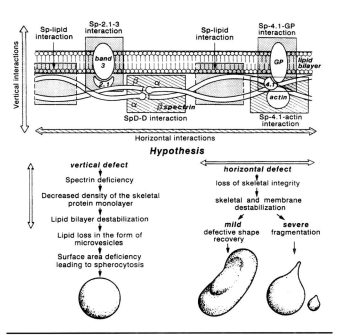

FIGURE 11-1. Pathobiology of the red cell lesion in hereditary spherocytosis (HS), hereditary elliptocytosis (HE), and hereditary pyropoikilocytosis (HPP). Partial deficiency in spectrin due to a defect of spectrin or to a defective spectrin ankyrin binding leads to a reduced density of the skeletal monolayer. This vertical interaction defect leads to a loss of the lipid bilayer and spherocytosis. Defects of spectrin self-association are horizontal defects of protein associations. These defects lead to a disruption of the membrane skeletal lattice and cell destabilization. Depending on the severity of the destabilization, either HE or HPP results. (With permission from: Palek, J. The red cell skeleton and haemolytic anemias. Br. J. Haematol., 82:260, 1992.)

TABLE 11-2 *PROTEIN ABNORMALITIES IN THE ERYTHROCYTE MEMBRANE THAT RESULT IN VERTICAL OR HORIZONTAL INTERACTION DEFECTS AND CAUSE HEMOLYTIC ANEMIA*

A. Vertical interaction defects may be caused by:
1. primary spectrin deficiency
2. secondary spectrin deficiency due to defects or deficiencies in:
- protein 4.2
- ankyrin
- band 3
- spectrin structure

B. Horizontal interaction defects may be caused by defects or deficiencies in:
1. actin
2. protein 4.1
3. adducin

Horizontal interactions Horizontal interactions are parallel to the plane of the membrane and are important in the formation of the stress-supporting skeletal protein lattice. This lattice provides mechanical stability to the membrane. Horizontal interactions include spectrin heterodimer head-to-head association to form spectrin tetramers as well as skeletal protein interactions in the junctional complexes at the distal ends of spectrin tetramers (spectrin, actin, protein 4.1, and adducin contacts). Horizontal defects characterized by defects of the skeletal protein interactions beneath the lipid bilayer lead to disruption of the skeletal lattice and consequently membrane destabilization. This causes cell fragmentation with formation of poikilocytes.

Disorders associated with vertical and horizontal skeletal protein abnormalities include hereditary spherocytosis (HS), hereditary elliptocytosis (HE), and hereditary pyropoikilocytosis (HPP) (Table 11-3).

LIPID COMPOSITION ABNORMALITIES

Disorders that affect the composition of the membrane lipid bilayer lead to the formation of acanthocytes. Normally, the erythrocyte membrane contains equal amounts of free cholesterol and phospholipids. In patients with excess free plasma cholesterol, the excess free cholesterol

stable. One type of verticle protein interaction defect is caused by a primary deficiency of spectrin. The degree of spectrin deficiency correlates with the severity of clinical expression of hemolysis. Other types of verticle interaction defects are caused by defects or deficiencies of protein 4.2, ankyrin (band 2.1), band 3, and with abnormal spectrin that binds poorly to protein 4.1.

TABLE 11-3 *HEMOLYTIC ANEMIAS ASSOCIATED WITH ERYTHROCYTE MEMBRANE DEFECTS*

Disorder	Inheritance Pattern	Membrane Defect	Abnormal Membrane Function	Erythrocyte Morphology
Hereditary spherocytosis	Usually autosomal dominant; rarely autosomal recessive; spontaneous mutation in 25%	Primary deficiency of spectrin or secondary deficiency of spectrin due to defective interaction with other skeletal proteins	Defective vertical protein interaction with lipid; loss of lipid bilayer and subsequent formation of a spherocyte with decreased deformability	Spherocytes
Hereditary elliptocytosis	Autosomal dominant except in Melanesian variant which is autosomal recessive	1. Defective spectrin 2. Deficiency or defect in band 4.1 3. Abnormal integral proteins	Defect in horizontal protein interactions resulting in membrane instability; also may be a defect in permeability	Elliptocytes
Hereditary pyropoikilocytosis	Autosomal recessive	Two defects: deficiency of α-spectrin and presence of a mutant spectrin	Defect in horizontal and vertical interactions resulting in membrane instability	Schistocytes
Hereditary stomatocytosis	Autosomal dominant	Unknown	Abnormally permeable to Na+ and K+; decreased deformability	Stomatocytes
Hereditary xerocytosis	Autosomal dominant	Unknown	Abnormally permeable resulting in loss of K+; decreased deformability	Xerocytes
Acanthocytosis (abetalipoproteinemia)	Autosomal recessive	Increase in sphingomyelin which may be secondary to abnormal plasma lipid composition	Expansion of outer lipid layer causes abnormal shape; increased membrane viscosity and decreased fluidity/deformability	Acanthocytes
Paroxysmal nocturnal hemoglobinuria	Acquired	Deficiency of DAF and C8bp	Increased sensitivity to complement lysis	Normocytic or macrocytic; microcytic, hypochromic if iron deficient

(DAF = decay accelerating factor; C8bp = C8 binding protein) accumulates in the outer bilayer of the erythrocyte. It is hypothesized that preferential expansion of the outer face of the lipid bilayer in comparison to the inner face leads to formation of acanthocytes as the spleen attempts to remodel the cell. Acanthocytes are more spheroidal cells with sharp irregular projections. These cells are poorly deformable and readily trapped in the spleen. There are a variety of conditions that lead to acanthocytosis.

● Defects in membrane affecting cell permeability

Often erythrocyte membrane defects not only alter the flexibility, stability, and shape of the cell but also may affect membrane permeability. Erythrocyte membranes that are abnormally permeable to Na + and K + result in cells with either an increased osmotic resistance or an increased osmotic fragility. Normal plasma Na + concentration is 140 mmoles/L and the K + plasma concentration is 4 mmoles/L, whereas the erythrocyte concentrations of Na + and K + are 6 mmoles/L and 100 mmoles/ L, respectively. Although the erythrocyte has low permeability to these cations, this difference in Na + and K + concentration gradients across the membrane passively drives Na + into the cell and K + out. The membrane enzyme, Na +/K + ATPase, is responsible for counteracting this tendency to equilibration by actively pumping Na + out of the cell in exchange for K +. This active pumping process requires ATP and accounts for the majority of erythrocyte ATP consumption.

Erythrocytes derive their ATP from glycolysis. If cells with abnormally permeable membranes are incubated for several hours in vitro without glucose, structural and biochemical changes begin, leading to eventual cell hemolysis. This in vitro phenomenon is analogous to what happens in vivo when these cells enter the hostile environment of the splenic cords. Here the cells are deprived of glucose; consequently, they are unable to maintain osmotic homeostasis. At first, a net increase in Na + causes the cells to swell (at this stage they are called hydrocytes). As the barrier to cations is progressively lost, there is prominent K + loss, the cells shrink (xerocytes), and eventually hemolyze.

Calcium concentration within the cell is normally very low. Most intracellular calcium is associated with the membrane. Calcium extrusion from the cell also requires ATP. If Ca + + is allowed to build up within the cell, the cell changes shape to form an echinocyte. With loss of the spiny membrane projections, the echinocyte eventually becomes a spherocyte.

Abnormal membrane permeability has been implicated in the pathogenesis of hereditary stomatocytosis and hereditary xerocytosis (Table 11-3).

● Hereditary spherocytosis

Hereditary spherocytosis (HS) is a common inherited membrane disorder that affects 1 in 5000 northern Europeans. It is usually inherited in an autosomal-dominant fashion; although, rarely, it may be autosomal recessive.

It also may result from spontaneous mutation. In about 25% of the cases neither parent is affected.[2]

PATHOPHYSIOLOGY

Hereditary spherocytosis is a clinically heterogeneous disorder characterized by mild to moderate hemolysis.

The membrane defect is a disorder of *verticle* protein interactions most often characterized by a deficiency of spectrin. The spectrin deficiency may be a primary deficiency of spectrin or a secondary deficiency due to defective attachment of the skeleton to the lipid bilayer. Defective attachment may occur as a result of a decrease in protein 4.2, ankyrin, band 3 protein, or the presence of an abnormal spectrin molecule that is unable to bind to protein 4.1.[4-7] The severity of hemolysis is directly related to the degree of spectrin deficiency.

These defects in spectrin and its interactions with other skeletal proteins result in a weakening of the vertical connections between the skeletal proteins and lipid bilayer membrane. It is hypothesized that uncoupling between the inner membrane skeleton and outer lipid bilayer leads to loss of the lipid bilayer in the form of microvesicles.[1] Secondary to membrane loss, the cell has a decreased surface area to volume ratio, changing the morphology of the cell from a discocyte to a spherocyte. The most spheroidal cells have a greatly increased cytoplasmic viscosity. The spheroidal shape and increased viscosity result in reduced cellular flexibility. Reticulocytes in HS are normal in shape, emphasizing the fact that erythrocytes lose their membrane fragments after encountering the stress of the circulation.

In addition to the abnormal cytoskeleton of HS erythrocytes, other membrane abnormalities may be present. The HS erythrocyte membrane has a decrease in total lipids both before and after splenectomy. Although the organization of lipids in the membrane is known to affect membrane fluidity, an association between abnormal fluidity and HS erythrocytes has not been established. The HS erythrocytes also are abnormally permeable to sodium, causing an influx of Na + at 10 times the normal rate. The leak may be compensated for by an increase in the activity of the cation pump, if adequate glucose is available for ATP production. The increased permeability is probably related to a functional abnormality of the membrane proteins.

The spherocytic shape, increased cytoplasmic viscosity, and increased membrane permeability account for the eventual destruction of HS cells in the spleen. Spherocytes lack the flexibility of normal cells, causing them to become trapped in the splenic cords. In this environment of very low glucose concentration, the cell quickly runs out of the ATP needed to pump out excess Na +. As energy production ceases, the metabolically stressed cells are destroyed by splenic macrophages.

CLINICAL FINDINGS

The clinical severity of HS varies between families and even between patients in the same family. About 25% of the patients have compensated hemolytic disease, no anemia, little or no jaundice, and only slight splenomegaly. In contrast, a few patients are severely anemic; neonatal jaundice is common in this group. Most patients, however, develop a partially compensated hemolytic anemia in childhood and appear asymptomatic. The HS in some asymptomatic individuals may only be detected when family studies are done on patients with more severe forms of the disease. Anemia is mild to moderate with intermittent jaundice. The jaundice appears especially with viral infections. Splenomegaly is present in about 50% of affected infants and increases to 75% to 95% in older children and adults. Aplastic crisis is a life-threatening complication that may occur in childhood during or after a viral infection. Untreated older patients commonly develop pigment bile stones from excess bilirubin catabolism (cholelithiasis). These patients also are predisposed to cholelithiasis and cholecystitis.

LABORATORY FINDINGS

Hemoglobin levels may be normal or decreased, varying inversely with the age of the individual upon presentation of symptoms. Infants have the lowest values, 8 to 11 g/dL. Older children usually have concentrations above 10 g/dL. The reticulocyte count is usually greater than 8%. The diagnosis of hereditary spherocytosis is suspected with the finding of many densely stained spherocytic cells with a decreased diameter (Fig. 11-2) and increased polychromasia on the blood smear. Small, dense microspherocytes with a decreased MCV and increased MCHC also may be found. The number of microspherocytes varies considerably, and in 20% to 25% of patients, microspherocytes may not be prominent. In mild forms of HS, the changes in erythrocyte morphology may be too subtle to detect, even by experienced hematologists. Nucleated red cells may be found in children with severe anemia.

In cases where the inheritance pattern of HS cannot be established, HS must be distinguished from other conditions causing spherocytosis. Spherocytes also may be found in acquired immune hemolytic anemia (AIHA), but in HS the spherocytes are more uniform in size and shape than in AIHA.

Usually, the MCV is normal or only slightly decreased (77 to 87 fL). If reticulocytosis is marked (more than 50%), the MCV may be increased. The MCH is normal but the MCHC is generally greater than 36 g/dL. Spherocytes are the only erythrocytes with an increased MCHC. The H-1 Technicon, a flow cytometer, was recently shown to be extremely sensitive in detecting erythrocytes with a MCHC more than 41 g/dL (hyperhemoglobin).[8] These erythrocytes are typically spherocytes. With this technology, even the mild forms of HS are detectable. It is important to remember that the indices may vary depending on iron and folate stores. Folate frequently becomes depleted in chronic hemolytic states. As in other hemolytic states, the bone marrow demonstrates normoblastic erythroid hyperplasia with an increase in storage iron.

Osmotic fragility test for HS The osmotic fragility test is the principal confirmation test in the diagnosis of HS. This test is a measure of the erythrocyte's resistance to hemolysis by osmotic stress, which depends primarily on the volume of the cell, the surface area, and its membrane function. The erythrocytes are incubated in hypotonic sodium chloride (NaCl) solutions of varying concentrations. As the NaCl concentration decreases, the erythrocytes take in water in an effort to achieve osmotic equilibrium. The cell swells until a spherocyte is formed. Further uptake of water leads to a porous membrane that permits the release of hemoglobin (hemolysis). Normal cells begin to hemolyze at NaCl concentrations of about 0.50%. Hemolysis is complete at about 0.30% NaCl. Because of their decreased surface to volume ratio, spherocytes are unable to expand as much as normal discoid-shaped cells. Very little fluid needs to be absorbed before the cells hemolyze. The spherocytes also may have increased membrane permeability, contributing to their increased fragility. Lysis of HS erthrocytes, therefore, begins at higher NaCl concentrations and is completed between 0.5% to 0.4% NaCl. These HS cells are said to exhibit increased osmotic fragility.

The osmotic fragility test will not be abnormal unless spherocytes contitute from 1% to 2% of the erythrocyte population; thus, patients with mild HS may have a normal osmotic fragility. These cells will, however, show marked abnormal hemolysis if the blood is incubated overnight (24 hours) at 37° C before it is added to the NaCl solution. Because of its increased sensitivity, this incubated osmotic fragility test is the most reliable diagnostic test for hereditary spherocytosis.

In most laboratories, the osmotic fragility test results are graphed to depict the degree of fragility in comparison to normal (Fig. 11-3). A shift to the left of normal in the curve indicates increased osmotic fragility, whereas a shift to the right indicates decreased osmotic fragility. Decreased osmotic fragility occurs in thalassemia, sickle cell anemia, and conditions associated with target cells.

Autohemolysis test for HS The autohemolysis test also is used in the diagnosis of HS but does not have an advantage

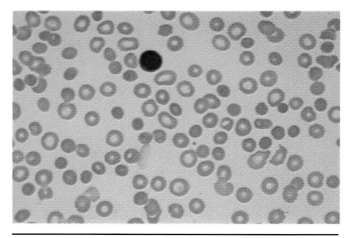

FIGURE 11-2. A blood smear from a patient with hereditary spherocytosis shows the presence of many densely staining spherocytes (peripheral blood, 250× original magnification; Wright-Giemsa stain).

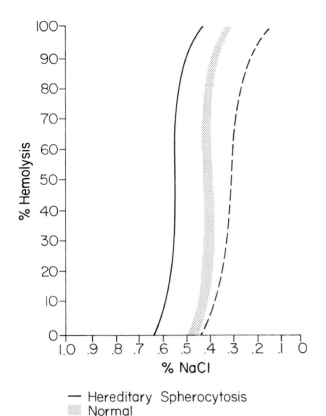

FIGURE 11-3. A graph depicting the osmotic fragility of normal cells, spherocytes, and cells from a patient with thalassemia. Spherocytes show an increased fragility with a shift to the left in the osmotic fragility curve and the thalassemia cells show a decreased fragility with a shift to the right in the osmotic fragility curve. In thalassemia, the decreased fragility is caused primarily by the presence of target cells.

over the osmotic fragility test. It is of more value in differentiating various types of congenital, nonspherocytic hemolytic anemias. This test measures the degree of spontaneous hemolysis of blood incubated at 37° C. The degree of hemolysis is dependent on the integrity of the cell membrane and on the adequacy of cell enzymes involved in glycolysis. Incubation of blood in vitro probably causes alteration of membrane lipids. This alteration leads to a change in cell permeability and an increase in the utilization of both glucose and ATP. In enzyme deficiencies, increased autohemolysis is probably caused by defective cation transport and/or loss of reducing power. Hemolysis is minimal in normal blood at 24 hours; in some hemolytic anemias, however, spontaneous lysis is increased. The addition of glucose or ATP to the incubation medium can sometimes reduce the degree of hemolysis.

In this test, sterile defibrinated blood is incubated at 37° C for 24 to 48 hours. Normal blood will show 0.2% to 2.0% spontaneous hemolysis during this period. When glucose or ATP is added to the blood before incubation, hemolysis decreases to 0% to 0.9%. Two abnormal pat-

terns of hemolysis may be identifed with the autohemolysis test.

TYPE I Autohemolysis is mildly to moderately increased (2% to 6%), and there is incomplete but significant correction when glucose is added to the incubating medium. This type of reaction is found in paroxsymal-nocturnal hemoglobinuria and glucose-6-phospho-dehydrogenase deficiency.

TYPE II Autohemolysis is greatly increased (8% to 44%). Glucose has no effect on the hemolysis. This type of reaction is found in pyruvate kinase deficiency.

HS is characterized by a third pattern of hemolysis where autohemolysis is increased to between 5% and 25% at 24 hours and may increase to 75% at 48 hours. If glucose is added to the blood before incubation, hemolysis is significantly decreased. If large numbers of microspherocytes are present, hemolysis may not be corrected with glucose.

Autohemolysis also is increased in the immune spherocytic anemias, but glucose does not usually affect the test results.

OTHER LABORATORY TESTS

Other laboratory tests reflect the usual findings of increased intravascular hemolysis, including increased indirect serum bilirubin, increased fecal urobilinogen, and increased LDH. Haptoglobin levels are often decreased. The antihuman globulin (AHG) test is negative, a finding helpful in distinguishing HS from immune hemolytic anemias in which large numbers of spherocytes also are found. Immune hemolytic anemias are usually associated with a positive AHG test.

THERAPY

Mild forms of HS do not require therapeutic intervention. Splenectomy is the standard treatment in patients with symptomatic hemolysis. Splenectomy corrects the anemia and hemolysis. The basic membrane defect, however, remains, and spherocytes can still be found in peripheral blood. Fragments of the unstable membrane are probably removed in the liver.

● Hereditary elliptocytosis

Hereditary elliptocytosis (HE) is inherited as an autosomal-dominant trait except for a rare Melanesian type that is inherited as a recessive trait. The disorder occurs in all racial groups with an occurrence of 0.02% to 0.05%. The disease is heterogeneous in the degree of hemolysis and in clinical severity. As its name indicates, the most prominent peripheral blood finding is an increase in oval and elongated erythrocytes (elliptocytes).

A classification has been proposed that is based on erythrocyte morphology[9]: (1) common HE; (2) spherocytic HE (hemolytic ovalocytosis); (3) stomatocytic HE or

TABLE 11-4 *CLASSIFICATION OF HEREDITARY ELLIPTOCYTOSIS (HE) BASED ON ERYTHROCYTE MORPHOLOGY*

Type of HE	Hemolysis	Erythrocyte Shape
Common HE	Variable; minimal to severe	Elliptocytes
Spherocytic HE (hemolytic ovalocytosis)	Present	Spherocytes and fat elliptocytes
Southeast Asian ovalocytosis (SAO) (stomatocytic HE; Melanesian ovalocytosis)	Mild or absent	Roundish elliptocytes that are also stomatocytic

Melanesian ovalocytosis, or Southeast Asian ovalocytosis (SAO) (Table 11-4).

PATHOPHYSIOLOGY

The abnormal erythrocyte shape in hereditary elliptocytosis is the result of a defect in one of the skeletal proteins in the membrane. It is interesting to note that reticulocytes and nucleated erythrocytes in this disorder are normal in shape; therefore, the elliptical erythrocyte form is acquired in the circulation. In the microcirculation, erythrocytes are subjected to shear stress and normally acquire an elliptical shape, but normal erythrocytes recover their biconcave shape in the absence of the circulatory stress. It is possible that the disruption of skeletal protein contacts in the membrane of HE erythrocytes due to this stress in microcirculation is followed by formation of new protein contacts that prevent recovery of the normal erythrocyte biconcave shape.

The principal defect involves horizontal membrane protein interactions. Evidence indicates that several different membrane molecule defects may be linked to this disease: (1) Decreased association of spectrin dimers to form tetramers due to defective spectrin chains.[1] (2) A deficiency or defect in band 4.1, which aids in binding spectrin to actin.[1,10] (3) Abnormalities of the integral proteins also have been identified, including deficiency of glycophorin C and abnormal anion transport protein (band 3) with increased affinity to ankyrin.[9]

Each of these defects can lead to skeletal disruptions that can cause the cell to become elliptical in shape and/or fragment under the stresses of circulation depending on the extent of the defect. Mildly dysfunctional proteins cause only elliptocytosis; whereas, severely dysfunctional proteins cause membrane fragmentation in addition to elliptocytosis. Alteration in shape only does not appear to affect cell deformability, and cells have a nearly normal lifespan. Elliptocytosis with membrane fragmentation, however, causes a decrease in cell surface area and a reduced cell deformability. The lifespan of these cells is severely shortened.

In addition to membrane instability, HE erythrocytes are abnormally permeable to Na+. This altered permeability demands an increase in ATP to maintain osmotic equilibrium. Cells detained in the spleen may quickly deplete their ATP and become osmotically fragile.

The defect in the SAO variant of HE is an abnormal band 3 protein rather than a defect in the cytoskeletal proteins under the lipid bilayer. There is a deletion of nine amino acids near the boundary of the membrane and cytoplasmic domains of the protein. This is associated with a tighter binding of band 3 to ankyrin, a lack of transport of anions, and a restriction in the lateral and rotational mobility of band 3 protein within the membrane. These erythrocytes are very rigid.[1,11]

CLINICAL FINDINGS

Ninety percent of patients with HE show no overt signs of hemolysis. Although erythrocyte survival may be decreased, the hemolysis is usually mild and well compensated for by the bone marrow (compensated hemolytic disease). Anemia is not characteristic.

Common HE is rare in western populations but more common in blacks, particularly in equatorial Africa. The severity ranges from asymptomatic to severe clinical disease. There may be minimal hemolysis and only mild elliptocytosis (15%) or severe hemolysis with cell fragmentation and formation of poikilocytes.

A variant of common HE noted in black infants is associated with moderately severe anemia at birth and neonatal jaundice. The peripheral blood smear exhibits erythrocytes similar to those seen in hereditary pyropoikilocytosis with budding and fragile bizarre poikilocytes. Variable numbers of elliptocytes are noted. Between the ages of 6 and 12 months, the infant's hemolysis decreases, and the number of elliptocytes increases. In affected infants, one of the parents has mild hereditary elliptocytosis.

The spherocytic HE variant constitutes a relatively rare form of HE characterized by the presence of hemolysis despite minimal changes in erthrocyte morphology. The erthrocytes have characteristics of both HS and HE cells: some are spherocytic and others are fat elliptocytes.

The Southeast Asian variant of HE (SAO, stomatocytic HE) is characterized by a mild or absent hemolytic component. Erythrocyte cation permeability appears to be increased, and the expression of blood group antigens is muted. The elliptocytes are roundish and stomatocytic with one or two transverse bars or a longitundinal slit. Evidence indicates these cells may have more stable cytoskeletons than normal.[10]

The high prevalence of the SAO variety of HE in some parts of the world is related to the resistance of the HE erythrocytes to invasion by malarial parasites.[2] The resistance may be due to the abnormal rigidity of the erythrocyte membrane. This protection against malaria has led to natural selection of individuals with HE in areas of the world where malaria is endemic and, thus, increased incidence of HE.

HE cells are poorly agglutinable with antisera against erythrocyte antigens. This is presumably due to defective lateral movement and clustering of surface antigens associated with an abnormal band 3 protein. The laboratory scientist should be aware of this problem since it may interfere with testing of patients' cells in the blood bank.

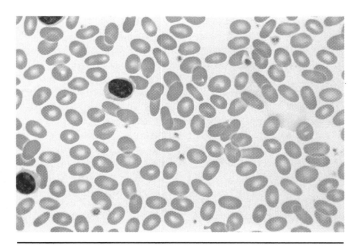

FIGURE 11-4. Hereditary elliptocytosis. Almost all cells are abnormally elongated. (PB; 250× original magnification; Wright-Giemsa stain.)

LABORATORY FINDINGS

The most consistent and characteristic laboratory finding in all variants is prominent elliptocytosis (Fig. 11-4). Elliptocytes also can be found in association with other diseases, but elliptocytes in these conditions usually constitute less than 25% of the erythrocytes. Acquired elliptocytosis is seen in megaloblastic anemias and in iron deficiency anemia. In contrast, in HE, the elliptocytes comprise more than 25% of the erythrocytes and usually more than 60%. In the asymptomatic variety of HE, elliptocytes may be the only morphologic clue to the disease. Hemoglobin levels are usually greater than 12 g/dL. Reticulocytes are mildly elevated, up to about 4%.

In the hemolytic HE variants, hemoglobin concentration is 9 to 10 g/dL, and reticulocytes are elevated to as high as 20%. Microelliptocytes, bizarre poikilocytes, schistocytes, and spherocytes are usually evident (Fig. 11-5). The bone marrow shows erythroid hyperplasia with normal maturation.

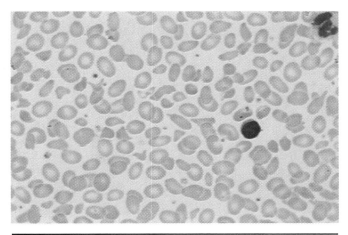

FIGURE 11-5. A blood smear from a patient with the hemolytic hereditary elliptocytosis. There are schistocytes as well as elliptocytes present. (250× original magnification; Wright-Giemsa stain.)

The incubated and unincubated osmotic fragility tests and autohemolysis tests are usually abnormally increased in the overt hemolytic variants. However, the obvious blood picture suggests that there should be no need to perform these tests.

THERAPY

The hemolytic variants of HE respond well to splenectomy. As in HS, splenectomy prevents hemolysis and protects the patient from complications of chronic hemolysis. The membrane defect, however, remains, and elliptocytes are still present. The asymptomatic variants require no therapy.

● Hereditary pyropoikilocytosis (hpp)

Hereditary pyropoikilocytosis, a rare autosomal-recessive disorder, is closely related to HE. It occurs primarily in blacks. The disease presents in infancy or early childhood as a severe hemolytic anemia with extreme poikilocytosis. The morphologic similarities of erythrocytes in HPP and that of erythrocytes associated with thermal injury led investigators to examine the thermal stability of HPP cells. In contrast to normal erythrocytes that fragment at 49° to 50° C, HPP cell membranes fragment when heated to 45° to 46° C. In addition, pyropoikilocytes disintegrate when incubated at 37° C for more than 6 hours.

PATHOPHYSIOLOGY

The HPP cells have two defects, one inherited from each parent. One is related to a deficiency of α-spectrin (a defect of vertical interaction) and the other to the presence of a mutant spectrin that prevents self-association of heterodimers to tetramers (defect of horizontal interaction).[2] The parent carrying the mutant spectrin trait either has mild HE or is asymptomatic. The other parent, with the deficiency of spectrin trait, is hematologically normal. The HPP phenotype also is found in patients who are homozygous or doubly heterozygous for one or two spectrin mutations found in HE. The defects lead to a disruption of the membrane skeletal lattice and membrane cell destabilization, followed by erythrocyte fragmentation and poikilocytosis.[12] Poikilocytes are removed in the spleen. Patients show improvement after splenectomy, but the membrane defect remains and fragmented erythrocytes are still present.

CLINICAL FINDINGS

Clinical features consistent with a hemolytic anemia are present at birth. Hyperbilirubinemia requiring exchange transfusion or phototherapy is present.[13] Laboratory serologic studies for hemolytic disease of the newborn (HDN), however, are negative.

LABORATORY FINDINGS

Stained blood smears exhibit striking erythrocyte morphologic abnormalities including budding, fragments, microspherocytes (2 to 4 fL), elliptocytes, triangulocytes, and other bizarre erythrocyte shapes. The MCV is decreased (25 to 55 fL), most likely as a result of the many erythro-

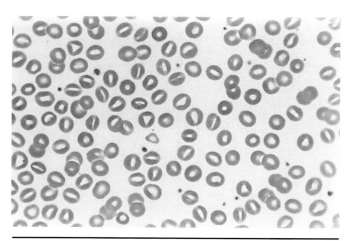

FIGURE 11-6. This peripheral blood picture from a patient with hereditary stomatocytosis reveals erythrocytes red cells with slit-like or mouth-like (stoma = mouth) areas of pallor (250× original magnification).

cyte fragments. The osmotic fragility is abnormal, especially after incubation. Autohemolysis is increased, and the hemolysis is not corrected with glucose.

Hereditary stomatocytosis

Hereditary stomatocytosis is a rare autosomal-dominant hemolytic anemia in which the erythrocyte membrane is abnormally permeable to both Na+ and K+. The net gain of Na+ ions is greater than net loss of K+ ions as the capacity of the cation pump to maintain normal intracellular osmolality is exceeded. As a result, the intracellular concentration of cations increases, water enters the cell, and the overhydrated cells take on the appearance of stomatocytes. Stomatocytes (hydrocytes) on dried, stained blood films are erythrocytes with a slit-like (mouth-like) area of pallor (Fig. 11-6). These cells are uniconcave and appear bowl-shaped on wet preparations. The MCHC of stomatocytes is decreased, and the MCV may be increased.

PATHOPHYSIOLOGY
The specific membrane abnormality has not been identified. Abnormalities of erythrocyte lipids have been demonstrated to induce stomatocytosis with impaired sodium transport. However, stomatocytosis also occurs when membrane lipids are normal. In these cases, membrane proteins may be abnormal. Although membrane proteins are usually electrophoretically normal, there may be an alteration in their conformation. A deficiency in band 7 proteins has been described.

From the variability of clinical findings, laboratory results, and the response to splenectomy, it appears the disease may be caused by several different membrane defects. Some patients have marked stomatocytosis but no abnormal sodium transport. Up to one third of patients with stomatocytosis do not have overt hemolysis.[14] Rh null disease also is associated with the presence of stomatocytes.

The association between a lack of the Rh complex and the membrane abnormality has not been explained.

The stomatocytic cells of hemolytic stomatocytosis are osmotically fragile and less deformable than normal cells and as a result the cells are sequestered in the spleen where glucose supplies are readily exhausted. As the ATP levels fall, the cation pump is unable to maintain osmotic equilibrium, causing cell lysis or phagocytosis.

Anemia is usually mild to moderate with hemoglobin concentration between 8 and 10 g/dL. Bilirubin is increased, and reticulocytosis is moderate. The blood smear is remarkable for 10% to 50% stomatocytes. Osmotic fragility and autohemolysis are increased. Autohemolysis is partially corrected with glucose and ATP.

Splenectomy results in variable responses. In some cases, hemolysis is completely ameliorated; in others, there is only a partial improvement in erythrocyte lifespan.

Inherited stomatocytosis must be differentiated from acquired causes of stomatocytosis. Stomatocytes also are seen as an acquired defect in acute alcoholism, liver disease, and cardiovascular disease. However, in these acquired conditions, there are no cation leaks, and little hemolysis is present.

Hereditary xerocytosis

In direct contrast to hereditary stomatocytosis is a permeability disorder called hereditary xerocytosis (HX). This autosomal-dominant disorder is characterized by a net loss of intracellular K+ that exceeds the passive Na+ influx and net Na+ gain. Consequently, the cell dehydrates as reflected by the increased MCHC, and the cell appears either targeted or contracted and spiculated.[3] As the MCHC of the cell increases beyond 37%, the cytoplasmic viscosity increases, and cellular deformability decreases. The rigid cells become trapped in the spleen. The pathophysiology is unknown.

Acanthocytosis

Acanthocytosis is most often associated with acquired or inherited abnormalities of the membrane lipids. This occurs in liver disease and a rare inherited condition, abetalipoproteinemia.

Abetalipoproteinemia is an autosomal-recessive disease characterized by a defect in betalipoprotein particle assembly and secretion in the intestine and liver.[15] As a result, there are decreased levels of apoprotein B and individual lipoprotein fractions that contain this apoprotein (chylomicrons, very low density lipoproteins, and low density lipoproteins). Plasma cholesterol and phospholipids are decreased leading to a relative increase in sphingomyelin. There is defective absorption and transport of fat-soluble vitamins A, D, E, and K to the tissues. Major clinical symptoms appear to be due to vitamin E deficiency. The erythrocytes in this disease have a striking increase in sphingomyelin. It is hypothesized that preferential expansion of the outer face of the erythrocyte lipid bilayer (primarily phosphatidylcholine and sphingomyelin) in comparison to the inner face leads to acanthocytosis. This expansion probably mirrors the alterations in composition of the plasma lipids.

The rare forms of acanthocytosis associated with abnormalities of membrane proteins include the McLeod phenotype with a deficiency of Kx substance and the K antigen, chorea-acanthocytosis syndrome, and acanthocytosis with band 3 protein abnormalities.

● Paroxysmal nocturnal hemoglobinuria (PNH)

All the erythrocyte membrane disorders discussed so far are hereditary in nature. *Paroxysmal nocturnal hemoglobinuria* is a rare acquired disorder of the erythrocyte membrane characterized by its abnormal sensitivity to complement. The disease derives its name from the classic pattern of intermittent bouts of intravascular hemolysis and nocturnal hemoglobinuria. The condition is exacerbated during sleep and remits during the day. However, many patients have chronic hemolysis that is not associated with sleep and with no obvious hemoglobinuria.

PATHOPHYSIOLOGY

PNH is an intrinsic erythrocyte disorder. Transfusion studies show that PNH cells are short lived in healthy individuals, and normal cells have normal survival in PNH patients. PNH is the result of a stem cell somatic mutation that leads to an abnormal clone of differentiated hematopoietic cells. The abnormal stem cell clone produces erythrocytes, platelets, and neutrophils that bind abnormally large amounts of complement and that are abnormally sensitive to complement lysis. The susceptibility of PNH cells to complement induced lysis is related to deficient regulation of complement activation after initial attachment of the C3bBb complex (formed via the alternate pathway) or the C4b2a complex (formed via the classic pathway) to the cell membrane. These complexes serve as C3/C5 convertases. Without controlling factors, this C3 convertase activity is amplified, leading to cleavage of C5, which produces the C5b fragment. Fragment C5b is a protein in a multistep process that results in assembly and activation of the terminal complement complex, C5b, C6, C7, C8, C9. Attachment and activation of this terminal complex on the cell membrane culminates in lysis of the cell.

At least two regulatory proteins found on normal hematopoietic cell membranes are responsible for preventing this amplification of complement activation. The first, *decay accelerating factor* (DAF), accelerates decay (dissociation) of membrane-bound C3bBb and blocks the ability of C4b to catalyze the conversion of C2 to the enzyme C2a. Thus, DAF prevents amplification of C3/C5 convertase activity. The second regulating protein, *C8 binding protein* (C8bp), interferes with the terminal stages of complement activation that causes lysis of the cell. These two regulating factors help normal cells avoid lysis by autologous complement. Lack of DAF and C8bp on PNH cells is causally related to excessive sensitivity of these cells to complement.

TABLE 11-5 *GPI-LINKED PROTEINS THAT ARE DEFICIENT IN PNH BLOOD CELLS*

A. GPI-Linked Proteins Deficient in PNH Erythrocytes
1. CD 55 (DAF)
2. CD 59 (thought to control later stages of complement activation by binding C 8)
3. Acetyl cholinesterase (function unknown)
4. CD 58 (LFA-3; cell adhesion molecule of immunoglobulin superfamily; acts as ligand for CD 2 on T-lymphocytes; function in erythrocyte unknown)
5. C 8 binding protein (HRF 60, MIP)
6. Dombrock protein
7. JMH Protein

B. Other GPI-Linked Proteins Deficient in Blood Cells in PNH
1. Alkaline Phosphatase (leukocytes)
2. Urokinase receptor
3. 5¹-Ectonucleotidase (lymphocytes)
4. Folate receptor
5. Endotoxin binding protein receptor (CD 14)
6. CD 48 (lymphocytes)
7. CD w52 (lymphocytes, some monocytes)
8. CD 24
9. CD 66
10. CD 67
11. P-50-80 (granulocytes)

Evidence suggests that deficiency of DAF and C8bp in PNH is not due to lack of production of these proteins but rather to the absence of a membrane glycolipid that serves as an anchor for DAF and C8bp and that attaches the proteins to the cell membrane. Other proteins anchored to the cell membrane in a similar manner also are deficient in PNH cells.[16] It appears that the common link to these membrane protein deficiencies is the lack of the glycolipid anchoring structure.[17] This anchor has been identified as glycosyl-phosphatidyl inositol (GPI), a molecule embedded in the cell membrane that is important for the covalent linkage of a wide variety of proteins to the cell membrane.[18] These GPI linked proteins vary in structure and function. They include adhesion molecules, hydrolases, and receptors[18] (Table 11-5).

Recently, it was found that the GPI-anchoring deficiency is due to a defect in the phosphatidylinositol glycan Class A (PIG-A) gene, although different mutations are responsible among different patients.[19] Analysis of stem cells in the bone marrow indicate that hematopoietic progenitor cells are affected by the genetic defect. Although not understood, this mutated cell(s) has a proliferative advantage in the bone marrow. Previous to the genetic mutation discovery, evidence that PNH was a clonal disease came from the finding that all blood cell lines are deficient in DAF activity in PNH.[20] This explains why many patients with PNH are not only anemic but also granulocytopenic and thrombocytopenic.[17] The abnormal clone may appear after damage to the marrow or it may appear spontaneously (idiopathic). A significant number of patients with PNH have or eventually develop another clonal blood disorder such as acute nonlymphocytic leukemia, chronic lymphocytic leukemia, myeloproliferative disorders, or myelodysplastic syndromes.[21]

PNH cells vary in their sensitivity to complement-induced lysis. Based on this variability, PNH cells have been classified as:[22]

1. Type I: little or no hemolysis by complement.
2. Type II: moderately sensitive to complement lysis.
3. Type III: highly sensitive to complement lysis.

This variability in complement sensitivity is related to the degree of DAF deficiency on cell membranes.

The increased sensitivity of PNH cells to complement can be demonstrated to occur in vitro whether the complement is activated by the classic or alternative pathway. In vivo activation is probably by the alternate pathway.

CLINICAL FINDINGS

PNH occurs most often in adults but may occasionally be found in children. The four basic disease mechanisms are hyperhemolysis, venous thrombosis, infection, and bone marrow hypoplasia.[18] The disease begins insidiously with irregular brisk episodes of acute intravascular hemolysis accompanied by hemoglobinuria. The patient usually seeks medical attention when reddish-brown urine is noted. In some patients, the irregular exacerbations of hemolysis are associated with sleep, hence the name nocturnal paroxysmal hemoglobinuria. In others, these hemolytic episodes may follow infections, transfusions, vaccinations, surgery, or ingestion of iron salts. In a large number of patients, hemolysis is unrelated to any specific event. Iron deficiency anemia may occur due to chronic blood loss through the kidneys. Folic acid deficiency may occur due to increased demand for this nutrient. Abdominal and lower back pain, eye pain, and headaches may occur during hemolytic episodes. Even with moderate thrombocytopenia, venous thrombosis is a prominent and severe complication. Thrombosis is a common cause of death. Thrombotic events may be related to abnormal platelet or neutrophil function due to lack of GPI-anchored proteins. Renal functions may become abnormal due to chronic iron deposition. When leukopenia is present, infections are a common complication. Proneness to infection also may be related to absence of granulocyte glycoproteins and altered response of granulocytes. Immunologic abnormalities also may be present.

LABORATORY FINDINGS (TABLE 11-6)

In most patients, there is severe anemia with a hemoglobin concentration between 8 to 10 g/dL. The erythrocytes are normocytic or macrocytic but may appear microcytic and hypochromic if iron deficiency develops. Reticulocytes are increased (5% to 10%) but not to the extent expected for a hemolytic anemia. Nucleated red blood cells may be found on the blood smear. Often, isolated development of leukopenia and/or thrombocytopenia may occur during the course of the disease. Neutrophil alkaline phosphatase and erythrocyte acetylcholinesterase are decreased.

The bone marrow usually exhibits normoblastic hyperplasia but may be hypocellular. In some cases, marrow failure develops during the course of the disease. Interestingly, aplastic anemia may be the initial diagnosis with an abnormal clone of PNH cells developing during the course of the disease. Rarely, PNH may precede aplastic anemia. PNH should be considered as a diagnosis when hypoplastic anemia is found in association with hemolysis.[23] Iron is decreased or absent.

The osmotic fragility is normal. Autohemolysis is increased after 48 hours, and when glucose is added the hemolysis may even increase more. The direct AHG test is negative for imunoglobulin (Ig) but may be positive for complement given the fact that PNH cells have a propensity to bind C3b.

Although hemoglobinuria may be intermittent or even mild, hemosidinuria is a constant finding, indicating chronic intravascular hemolysis. When hemoglobin passes into the glomerular filtrate, some is reabsorbed into the renal tubules. Here iron is released from heme and remains in the renal tubular cells. When these cells are exfoliated, they are washed into the urine. The iron within these exfoliated cells in the urine can be visualized by staining the urine sediment with Prussian blue. Iron granules appear blue or bluish-green.

The *sucrose hemolysis test* (sugar-water test) is a screening test that is useful in identifying erythrocytes that are abnormally sensitive to complement lysis. Patient's blood is incubated in a sucrose solution. The sucrose provides a low ionic strength medium that promotes the binding of complement to the erythrocytes. PNH cells will show hemolysis in this medium.

The *Ham test* (acid-serum lysis test) is a more specific test for PNH cells (Fig. 11-7). Patient's erythrocytes are incubated with acidified serum (pH 6.5 to 7.0). The acidified serum serves to activate the alternate complement pathway. As the complement components are deposited on the erythrocytes, the PNH cells lyse (10% to 50% of total erythrocytes). Care should be used in interpreting the test as spherocytes or antibody sensitized cells also may cause hemolysis. If it is suspected that hemolysis may be due to the presence of these cells rather than PNH cells, the test is repeated using heat-inactivated serum (inactivating complement). If the lysis is still present with the inactived serum, the diagnosis is not PNH. In this case, the blood smear and osmotic fragility test may verify the presence of spherocytes, and the direct AHG test will detect antibody sensitized cells. The Ham test also may be positive in CDA-II (congenital dyserythropoietic anemia) but only with 30% of normal sera and not with the patient's own serum. Immunophenotyping blood cells for selected GPI-linked molecules by flow cytometry may be helpful in identifying PNH cell populations. A suggested diagnostic

TABLE 11-6 *LABORATORY FINDINGS IN PNH*

Anemia

Granulocytopenia, thrombocytopenia

Hemoglobinuria

Hemosidinuria

Decreased leukocyte alkaline phosphatase (LAP)

Positive sucrose hemolysis test

Positive Ham test

Acidified-Serum Lysis Test (Ham Test)

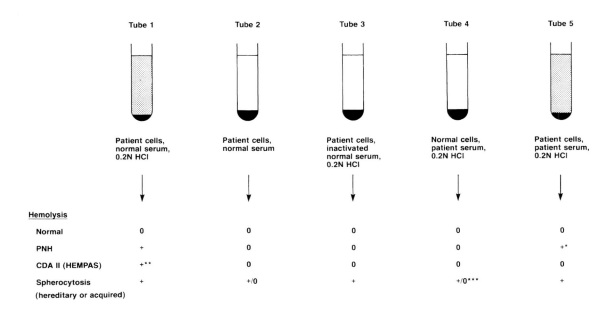

Hemolysis	Tube 1 Patient cells, normal serum, 0.2N HCl	Tube 2 Patient cells, normal serum	Tube 3 Patient cells, inactivated normal serum, 0.2N HCl	Tube 4 Normal cells, patient serum, 0.2N HCl	Tube 5 Patient cells, patient serum, 0.2N HCl
Normal	0	0	0	0	0
PNH	+	0	0	0	+*
CDA II (HEMPAS)	+**	0	0	0	0
Spherocytosis (hereditary or acquired)	+	+/0	+	+/0***	+

Key: PNH–Paroxysmal nocturnal hemoglobinuria; CDA–Congenital dyserythropoietic anemia; + = hemolysis;
0 = no hemolysis;
*May be negative if complement has been depleted.
**Hemolysis occurs with only 30% of normal compatible sera.
***Hemolysis may occur if immune hemolysins are present.

FIGURE 11-7. The Ham test is useful in diagnosing paroxysmal nocturnal hemoglobinuria (PNH). When PNH erythrocytes are incubated in acidified serum, the cells hemolyze. The test results should be interpreted carefully. Anemias with considerable numbers of spherocytes and CDAII also may give positive results.

panel for a PNH immunophenotype screen is summarized in Table 11-7.

THERAPY

Treatment is primarily supportive in the form of transfusions, antibiotics, and anticoagulants. In patients with PNH-induced marrow aplasia, bone marrow transplantation may be indicated.

TABLE 11-7 *PANEL FOR PNH IMMUNOPHENOTYPING. PNH CELLS SHOW LOW STAINING INTENSITY FOR THESE ANTIGENS AS COMPARED TO NORMAL CELLS*

Cell Type	Antigen
Erythrocytes	CD 59
Granulocytes	CD 67
Monocytes	CD 14
Platelets	CD 59
B-Lymphocytes	CD 24
T-Lymphocytes	CD 59

● ERYTHROCYTE ENZYME DEFICIENCIES

As reticulocytes mature, they lose their mitochondria and microsomes. Consequently, they also lose their ability to synthesize protein. Due to the absence of mitochondria, the erythrocyte is critically dependent on anaerobic glucose metabolism for its metabolic needs. All erythrocyte enzymes for intracellular metabolism are present in a fixed concentration and must remain active for the entire lifespan of the erythrocyte. An inherited deficiency in one of these enzymes may compromise the integrity of the cell membrane or hemoglobin and cause hemolysis. The more common hereditary enzyme deficiencies known to cause a hemolytic anemia are listed in Table 11-8.

● Hexose-monophosphate (HMP) shunt

Glucose, the cell's primary metabolic substrate, enters the cell in a carrier-mediated, energy-free, transport process and is catabolized via the Embden-Meyerhof (EM) pathway or the hexose-monophosphate shunt (HMP). Approximately 10% of the glucose is catabolized by the HMP shunt, which is essential for maintaining adequate concentrations of reduced glutathione (GSH), the major

TABLE 11-8 *ERYTHROCYTE ENZYME DEFICIENCIES THAT ARE ASSOCIATED WITH CONGENITAL NONSPHEROCYTIC HEMOLYTIC ANEMIA*

Metabolic Pathway	Enzyme Deficiency
Embden-Meyerhof	Pyruvate kinase (PK) Glucose phosphate isomerase (GPI) Hexokinase (HK) Phosphoglycerate kinase (PGK) Triosephosphate isomerase (TPI)
Hexose-Monophosphate	Glucose 6-Phosphate dehydrogenase Shunt (G6PD) Glutathione synthetase Glutamylcysteine synthetase
Nucleotide	Pyrimidine 5'-nucleotidase (P5N)

cellular antioxidant, through the production of NADPH (Fig. 11-8). Glutathione maintains hemoglobin in the reduced functional state and preserves vital cellular enzymes from oxidant damage. When the cell is exposed to an oxidizing agent, the production of NADPH increases. If enzymes in this pathway are lacking or missing, the reducing power of the cell is compromised, and oxidized hemoglobin accumulates, subsequently denaturing in the form of Heinz bodies. Heinz bodies damage the cell membrane, leading to premature extravascular hemolysis. The most

common enzyme deficiency of the HMP shunt is glucose-6-phosphate dehydrogenase deficiency.

Embden-Meyerhof pathway

Most of the energy of the cell is produced via glycolysis in the EM pathway. About 90% of the glucose is used by this pathway as one mole of glucose is catabolized to lactic acid with a net production of two moles of ATP. ATP is needed for active cation transport of $Na+$, $K+$, and $Ca++$, for maintaining membrane deformability, and for maintaining normal erythrocyte shape. Deficiencies in enzymes of the EM pathway decrease ATP production and lead to hemolysis, but Heinz bodies are not formed since the reducing power of the cell is primarily linked to the HMP shunt. The mechanism of hemolysis is unclear, but decreased ATP may lead to impaired cation pumping and increased osmotic fragility. The osmotically fragile cells are trapped in the hostile splenic environment and phagocytosed.

The Rapoport-Luebering shunt of the EM pathway provides the erythrocyte with 2,3-DPG. If this shunt is used, there is no net gain of ATP from glycolysis. The activity of this shunt is stimulated in hypoxia. When 2,3-DPG combines with hemoglobin, the oxygen affinity of hemoglobin is decreased, making more oxygen available to the tissues.

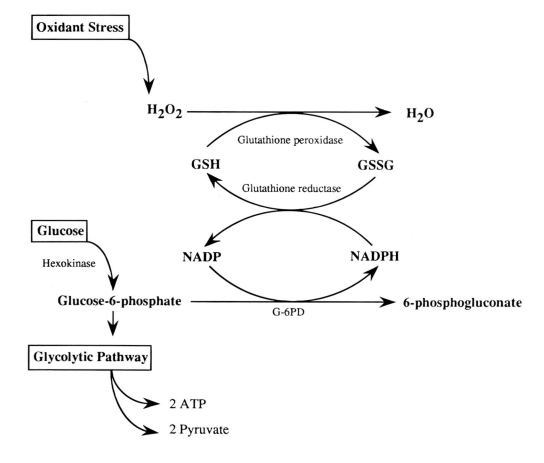

FIGURE 11-8. G6PD is needed for maintaining adequate quantities of glutathione (GSH), an important buffer to oxidants within the erythrocyte. As GSH reduces H_2O_2 to H_2O, it is oxidized (GSSG). G6PD generates NADPH in the conversion of glucose-6-phosphate to 6-phosphogluconate. NADPH, in turn, serves to regenerate reduced glutathione from oxidized glutathione.

Clinical and laboratory findings in erythrocyte enzyme deficiencies

Most erythrocyte enzyme deficiencies are inherited as autosomal-recessive traits. However, the most common enzyme deficiency, G6PD deficiency, is inherited as an X-linked (sex-linked) disorder. Patients with the homozygous autosomal-recessive enzyme deficiencies and males with X-linked G6PD deficiency have a chronic normocytic, normochromic anemia (sometimes no anemia is present or hemolysis is sporadic), reticulocytosis, hyperbilirubinemia, and neonatal jaundice. The direct AHG test is negative indicating an absence of autoantibodies, and there is no evidence to suggest a defect in either the erythrocyte membrane or hemoglobin. These anemias are often collectively referred to as *chronic nonspherocytic hemolytic anemias*. Although the anemias are not life-threatening, they can be disabling and lead to debilitating complications.[24]

Diagnosis

Definitive diagnosis of enzyme deficiencies requires spectrophotometric measurement of the enzyme. The time of testing and interpretation of results is important for accurate diagnosis. Sometimes the abnormal cells are selectively removed from circulation in vivo, and the enzyme activity of the remaining cells is normal. Some abnormal enzymes have normal activity in the reticulocytes, but enzyme activity decreases as the cell ages. Thus, depending on the degree of reticulocytosis, the enzyme content may appear normal. For these reasons, it is important to delay testing of the patient immediately after a hemolytic attack when most of the enzyme deficient cells have been hemolyzed and there is a reticulocytosis. Sometimes it may be helpful to centrifuge the blood and test the erythrocytes at the bottom of the column. These cells are usually the older erthrocytes. If a patient has been transfused, testing should be delayed until the transfused cells have outlived their lifespan.[24] The parents should be tested as well as the patient.

Glucose-6-phosphate dehydrogenase deficiency (G6PD)

G6PD deficiency is the most common erythrocyte enzyme disorder. It was first recognized during the Korean War when 10% of black American soldiers who were given the antimalarial drug, primaquine, developed a self-limited hemolytic anemia. G6PD deficiency is found worldwide in whites, blacks, and Asians. It occurs most frequently in the Mediterranean area, Africa, and China. The geographic distribution coincides with that of malaria, suggesting that G6PD-deficient cells may be more resistant to malarial parasites than normal cells. The disease is a sex-linked disorder carried by a gene on the X chromosome that is fully expressed only in males (Fig. 11-9). Carrier females appear to have two populations of cells, one deficient in G6PD and one normal. The disease is heterogeneous with differences in severity among races and sexes. The majority of people with G6PD deficiency have

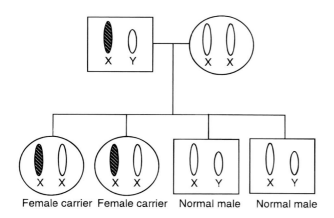

Female carrier   Female carrier   Normal male   Normal male

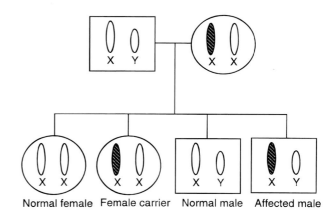

Normal female   Female carrier   Normal male   Affected male

 X chromosome carrying G-6PD Deficiency gene

Normal X chromosome

FIGURE 11-9. Glucose-6-phosphate dehydrogenase (G6PD) deficiency is a sex-linked disorder that is carried by a gene on the X chromosome. The disease is fully expressed in males who carry the affected X-chromosome. Females who carry one affected X-chromosome (female carrier) and one normal X-chromosome have two populations of cells, one deficient in G6PD and one with normal G6PD. This is due to random inactivation of one X-chromosome in each cell of the female embryo. The chromosome remains inactive throughout subsequent divisions of the cell. This figure illustrates the expected progeny from G6PD deficient males or females.

TABLE 11-9 *COMPOUNDS ASSOCIATED WITH HEMOLYTIC ANEMIA IN G6PD DEFICIENCY*

Antimalarials	Primaquine
	Pamaquine
	Pentaquine
Sulfonamides	Sulfanilamide
	Sulfacetamide
	Sulfapyridine
	Sulfamethoxazole
Sulfones	Thiazolesulfone
	Diaphenylsulfone (DDS, Dapsone)
Nitrofurans	Nitrofurantoin (Furadantin)
Analgesic	Acetanilid
Miscellaneous	Methylene blue
	Nalidixic acid (Negram)
	Naphthalene
	Niridazole (Ambilhar)
	Phenylhydrazine
	Toluidine blue
	Trinitrotoluene (TNT)

(From: Wintrobe GE: Clinical Hematology, 9th Ed. Philadelphia, Lea & Febiger, 1993.)

no clinical expression of the deficiency unless they have neonatal jaundice, are exposed to chemicals or drug oxidants, or have severe infection. Compounds that have been associated with hemolytic anemia in G6PD deficiency are listed in Table 11-9.

PATHOPHYSIOLOGY

As mentioned, glutathione is the most important erythrocyte buffer to oxidants, preventing oxidant damage to hemoglobin. Glutathione (GSH)-mediated oxidant detoxification occurs spontaneously but is enhanced by glutathione peroxidase (GSSG-Px). In the process of GSH-mediated detoxification, GSH itself is oxidized. The oxidized form is commonly referred to as GSSG to differentiate it from the reduced form, GSH. In the regeneration of GSH, glutathione reductase (GSSG-Rx) catalyzes the NADPH-dependent reduction of GSSG to GSH and produces NADP +. In turn, G6PD is necessary for the regeneration of NADPH (Fig. 11-8). Normally, G6PD activity is highest in young cells, decreasing as the cell ages; however, under normal conditions, even older cells retain enough G6PD activity to maintain adequate GSH levels.

In G6PD deficiency, the production of NADPH is impaired. Thus, GSSG cannot be regenerated to GSH, and cellular oxidants accumulate. The buildup of cellular oxidants lead to erythrocyte injury and hemolysis. Hemoglobin is oxidized to methemoglobin, which precipitates in the form of Heinz bodies. Heinz bodies attach to the erythrocyte membrane, causing increased membrane permeability to cations, osmotic fragility, and cell rigidity. Heinz bodies are removed from the erthrocytes by splenic macrophages producing, "bite" cells, and blister cells. With progressive membrane loss, spherocytes may be formed. These cells, less deformable than normal, become trapped and hemolyzed in the spleen.

Oxidant stress also may oxidize membrane lipids and proteins. This disruption of the membrane structural integrity results in removal of the cell from circulation by splenic macrophages. It also is likely that membrane damage may account for the acute intravascular hemolysis seen in G6PD deficiency.

It has been shown that normal erythrocytes only use 0.1% of their maximum G6PD enzyme capacity.[25] This explains why even G6PD-deficient cells can maintain normal function, and hemolysis is sporadic. Only in situations that create excessive oxidant stress is there inadequate G6PD activity to maintain normal metabolic function. Those cells that are most deficient undergo oxidant damage and are rapidly removed from circulation. This accounts for the sporadic hemolysis that accompanies oxidant stress in G6PD deficiency. In most G6PD variants, hemolysis is self-limited. Self-limited refers to the fact that hemolysis stops after a time, even if the oxidant stress continues. This occurs because initially the older, most G6PD-deficient erythrocytes are destroyed, but the younger cells remain. The reticulocytes released from the bone marrow in response to the hemolytic episode have enough enzyme activity to maintain metabolic activity even under oxidant stress.

It is important to recognize that under the stress of severe oxidants (drugs, chemicals) even normal cells may experience oxidant damage and hemolyze.

G6PD variants More than 350 variants (isoenzymes) of the G6PD enzyme have been identified.[24] Many of these variants differ in their activity, stability, and electrophoretic mobility (Table 11-10). The mutant enzymes have

TABLE 11-10 *CHARACTERISTICS OF THE MOST COMMON VARIANTS OF G6PD ENZYME IN COMPARISON TO THE NORMAL ISOENZYME (B)*

G6PD Isoenzyme	Half-Life	Clinical Severity	Favism	Class	Electrophoretic Mobility
G6PD-B	62 days	normal	−	IV	normal
G6PD-A⁺	—	normal	−	IV	fast
G6PD-A⁻	13 days	mod to severe hemolysis after oxidant exposure; self-limiting	−	III	fast (about the same as A⁺)
G6PD-Mediterranean	hours	severe hemolysis after oxidant exposure; not self-limiting	+	II	normal (same as B)
G6PD-Canton	—	severe hemolysis after oxidant exposure; may not be self-limited	?	III	fast

TABLE 11-11 *CLASSES OF MUTANT G6PD ISOENZYMES*

Class	G6PD Activity	Hemolysis
I	Severely deficient	Chronic
II	Severely deficient	Acute, episodic
III	Moderately to mildly deficient	Acute, episodic
IV	Mildly deficient to normal	Absent
V	Increased	Absent

been classified into five classes according to the degree of deficiency and hemolysis (Table 11-11). Most of the variants have normal activity. Only the most common variants will be discussed here. G6PD-B is the most common worldwide normal isoenzyme. All variants except G6PD-B, G6PD-A +, and G6PD-A- are given geographic or other types of names.

G6PD-A+ The isoenzyme G6PD-A+ (Class IV) is found in 20% of American black males. This isoenzyme has normal enzymatic activity. The A+ isoenzyme has the same mobility as G6PD-A on electrophoresis.

G6PD-A- G6PD-A- (Class III) is found in 10% of American blacks. The minus sign denotes deficient enzyme activity. This variant has only 5% to 15% of the enzymatic activity of G6PD-B and the same electrophoretic mobility as G6PD-A+. Individuals with this variant are susceptible to hemolytic episodes after administration of oxidant drugs or during infections. In G6PD-A-, the older cells are markedly deficient in enzyme activity and are preferentially destroyed, but young cells have enough activity to maintain GSH levels. The reticulocytosis that accompanies hemolytic episodes causes the hemolysis to be self-limited. However, if either the drug is withdrawn or the infection subsides, older cells will once again accumulate and hemolysis could occur again if the cell is stressed with oxidants.

G6PD MEDITERRANEAN G6PD Mediterranean (Class II) is the most common abnormal variant in whites, especially in those living in the Mediterranean area. This isoenzyme has the same electrophoretic mobility as G6PD-B but it has a marked decrease in enzyme stability and activity. Thus, it was formerly referred to as G6PD-B-. In contrast to G6PD-A-, all erythrocytes, even reticulocytes, are grossly deficient in enzyme activity; therefore, hemolysis is more severe than in G6PD-A- and it is not self-limited.

G6PD CANTON G6PD Canton (Class III) is the most common abnormal variant among Asians. Its activity is similar to that of G6PD Mediterranean. Hemolysis is usually severe and may not be self-limited. Persons with this variant may be susceptible to a wider variety of drugs than those with G6PD-A-.

Females with G6PD deficiency Female heterozygotes for G6PD deficiency always have two populations of cells—one normal and one with G6PD deficiency. In affected males, all cells are G6PD-deficient. The dual population in females is caused by random inactivation of one X chromosome in a given stem cell. If the X chromosome with the normal G6PD gene is inactivated, the stem cell progeny will be deficient in G6PD, whereas, if the X chromosome coding for G6PD deficiency is inactivated, the stem cell progeny will have normal enzyme activity. Depending on the proportion of abnormal erythrocytes, females may have no clinical expression of the deficiency or they may be affected as severely as males.[26] Females may theoretically be homozygous if they inherit a deficient gene from both parents, but this condition has not been reported.[24]

CLINICAL FINDINGS
Most persons with G6PD deficiency have no clinical symptoms and are not anemic. Diagnosis usually occurs during or after infectious illnesses or after exposure to certain drugs, because these conditions commonly precipitate hemolytic attacks. Hemolysis is variable and is dependent on the degree of oxidant stress, the G6PD isoenzyme, and sex of the patient. The symptoms are those of acute intravascular hemolytic anemia. Drug-induced hemolysis usually occurs within 1 to 3 days after exposure to the drug. Sudden anemia develops with a 3- to 4-g/dL drop in hemoglobin. Jaundice is not prominent. The patient may experience abdominal and low back pain. Urine is dark or black because of hemoglobinuria. In one study of 35 G6PD-deficient children in India, the most common important complication, occurring in more than 50% of cases, was renal failure.[27] Hemoglobinemia is prominent. Often, however, hemolysis is less striking and is not accompanied by hemoglobinuria or conspicuous symptoms.

Favism *Favism* is a peculiar disorder in which some individuals with G6PD deficiency develop a sudden severe hemolytic episode after the ingestion of fava beans. This complication is often believed to be associated with severe G6PD deficiency, especially the G6PD Mediterranean variant. It is now clear, however, that other forms of G6PD deficiency also are associated with favism, including G6PD-A- and G6PD Aureo, a type identified in Algerian subjects.[28]

The hemolysis is similar to the acute hemolytic episodes that occur after primaquine administration in individuals with the G6PD-A- variant. Consumption of fava beans (broad beans) is widespread in the Mediterranean area and the Middle East. The first signs of favism are malaise, severe lethargy, nausea, vomiting, abdominal pain, chills, tremor, and fever.[24] Hemoglobinuria occurs a few hours after ingestion of the beans. Persistent hemoglobinuria usually prompts the individual to seek medical attention. Jaundice may be intense. Severe favism usually affects children between the ages of 2 and 5 years. The age distribution of favism is changing in some countries, however, due to neonatal screening and parental education. Here the children are not affected as much as adults. Even though favism occurs more often in males due to the X-linked nature of the disease, females also may be affected

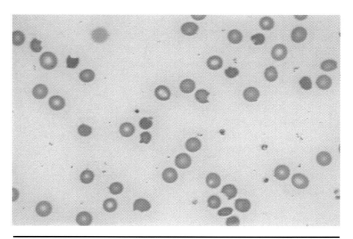

FIGURE 11-10. Heinz body hemolytic anemia. Peripheral blood from a patient with G6PD deficiency during a hemolytic episode. There are erythrocytes with a portion of the cell missing. These are known as "bite" cells. The spleen pits the Heinz body with a portion of the cell producing these misshapen erythrocytes. Some of the cells reseal and become spherocytes. (250× original magnification; Wright-Giemsa stain.)

depending on the proportion of enzyme-deficient erythrocytes present.

LABORATORY FINDINGS

There is no anemia or abnormal peripheral blood findings except during hemolytic attacks. Rarely patients may exhibit chronic hemolysis. During or immediately after a hemolytic attack, polychromasia, occasional spherocytes, small hypochromic cells, erythrocyte fragments, and bite cells may be seen on the blood smear. Bite cells, which have a chunk of the cell removed from one side (Fig. 11-10), are frequently believed to be typical of G6PD deficiency. However, bite cells are more characteristic of drug-induced oxidant hemolysis in individuals with normal hemoglobin and enzyme activity.[29]

A peculiar cell, referred to by a variety of descriptive terms, including irregularly contracted cell, eccentrocyte, erythrocyte hemighosts, double-colored erythrocytes, and cross-bonded erythrocytes, has been described in G6PD deficiency after oxidant-related hemolysis. These cells are rigid with decreased volume and increased MCH. The hemoglobin is confined to one side of the cell while the other side is transparent. The transparent side often contains Heinz bodies. The transparent part of the cell has flattened membranes in which the opposing membrane sides are interconnected. This crossbonding of the membrane appears to decrease deformability and destine the cell for phagocytosis by macrophages.

Reticulocytosis from 8% to 12% is typical within 5 to 15 days after the hemolytic episode.[30] Leukocytes may be increased during hemolytic attacks. Platelets are normal. Indirect bilirubin and serum LDH may be increased. Haptoglobin is commonly decreased during the acute hemolytic phase. Absence of haptoglobin in the recovery stage indicates chronic hemolysis.

Definitive diagnosis depends on the demonstration of a decrease in erythrocyte G6PD enzyme activity. In blacks, the enzyme activity may appear normal during and after a hemolytic attack because older cells with less G6PD are preferentially destroyed during the attack, and reticulocytes have normal activity. A reticulocytosis of greater than 7% is associated with a normal enzyme screen after hemolysis.[31] For this reason, assays for G6PD should be performed 2 to 3 months after a hemolytic episode in blacks. In G6PD Mediterranean, however, even young cells have gross deficiencies of G6PD, and enzyme activity appears abnormal even with reticulocytosis. Both severe and mild types of G6PD deficiency are detected with measurement of the enzyme if the patient is not undergoing hemolysis.

Fluorescent spot test
The fluorescent spot test is a reliable and sensitive screening test for G6PD deficiency. Whole blood is added to a mixture of glucose-6-phosphate (G6P), NADP, and saponin. A drop of this mixture is placed on a piece of filter paper and examined under ultraviolet light for fluorescence. Normally, the G6PD enzyme present in erythrocytes metabolizes G6P producing NADPH:

$$G6P + NADP \xrightarrow{G6PD} \text{6-Phosphogluconate} + NADPH$$

NADPH fluoresces but NADP does not. Lack of fluorescence indicates G6PD deficiency.

Dye reduction test
In the dye reduction screening test, a hemolysate of patient's blood, G6P, NADP, and the dye brilliant cresyl blue are incubated together. If the hemolysate contains G6PD, the NADP will be reduced to NADPH, which in turn reduces the blue dye to its colorless form. The time it takes for this change to occur is inversely proportional to the amount of G6PD present. Normal blood is used in this test for comparison. The test is specific and is available in commercial kits.

Ascorbate cyanide test
The ascorbate cyanide test is the most sensitive screening test for detecting heterozygotes and for detecting G6PD deficiency during hemolytic attacks in blacks. The test is not specific for G6PD deficiency but also will detect defects or deficiencies in the HMP shunt. The test also is positive in PNH, pyruvate kinase deficiency, and in unstable hemoglobin disorders. The principle of the test is based on the failure of G6PD-deficient cells to reduce hydrogen peroxide. Patient's blood is incubated with sodium ascorbate, sodium cyanide, and glucose. Hydrogen peroxide is generated by the interaction of ascorbate with hemoglobin. The sodium cyanide inhibits the activity of normal erythrocyte catalase, an inhibitor of the formation of hydrogen peroxide. With inhibition of catalase, hydrogen peroxide is formed. Using glucose through the HMP shunt, the erythrocytes are able to reduce the peroxide to water. However, erythrocytes deficient in G6PD cannot reduce the peroxide, and hemoglobin is oxidized to methemoglobin. Methemoglobin imparts a brown color to the solution.

Definitive test   The definitive test for G6PD deficiency requires quantitation of the enzyme. An erythrocyte hemolysate is incubated with G6P and NADP, and the rate of reduction of NADP to NADPH is measured at 340 nm in a spectrophotometer.

THERAPY

The majority of patients with G6PD deficiency are asymptomatic and do not experience chronic hemolysis; thus, no therapy is indicated. Patients, however, should avoid exposure to the oxidant drugs and foods that may precipitate hemolytic episodes. In acute hemolytic episodes, supportive therapy, including blood transfusions, treatment of infections, and removal of the precipitating agent, is used. Exchange transfusion may be necessary in severe neonatal jaundice. Dialysis is indicated in patients with oliguria and severe azotemia.[27]

Other defects and deficiencies of the HMP shunt and GSH metabolism

Erythrocytes synthesize about 50% of their total glutathione every 4 days. Deficiencies in the enzymes needed for glutathione synthesis (glutathione synthetase and glutamylcysteine synthetase) have been reported to be associated with a decrease in GSH and a nonspherocytic congenital hemolytic anemia. Hemolysis increases during administration of certain drugs. Glutathione reductase is an enzyme that catalyzes the reduction of GSSG to GSH. Deficiencies in this enzyme are not associated with a hematologic disorder. Glutathione peroxidase catalyzes the detoxification of hydrogen peroxide by GSH. Deficiencies in this enzyme, although common, are not a cause of hemolysis. This might be explained by the fact that peroxide reduction by GSH occurs nonenzymatically at a significant rate.

Pyruvate kinase deficiency

Pyruvate kinase (PK) deficiency is the most common enzyme deficiency in the Embden-Meyerhof pathway and the second most common erythrocyte enzyme deficiency. There are many pyruvate kinase enzyme mutants, which probably explains the variety of clinical manifestations of the disorder. The more severe types are noted in infancy, whereas milder types may not be detected until adult life. Inheritance is autosomal-recessive. Clinically significant hemolytic anemias of PK deficiency are limited to the homozygous state or double heterozygosity for two mutant enzymes. Acquired PK deficiency is seen in some leukemias and myelodysplastic disorders.

PATHOPHYSIOLOGY

A number of different mutations in the PK gene that affect the enzyme's activity have been identified.[32] PK catalyzes the conversion of phosphoenol-pyruvate (PEP) to pyru-

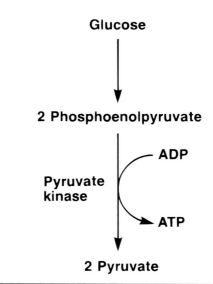

FIGURE 11-11. Glucose is metabolized to pyruvate in the Embden-Meyerhof pathway. ATP is generated as phosphoenolpyruvate is converted to pyruvate. There is a net gain of two ATP at this step. Two molecules of pyruvate are formed from one mole of glucose. In pyruvate kinase deficiency, this reaction is slowed, resulting in deficient production of ATP.

vate-producing ATP (Fig. 11-11). In PK deficiency, this energy-producing reaction is prevented, resulting in a loss of two ATP molecules per mole of glucose catabolized. The inability of the cell to maintain normal ATP levels results in alterations of the erythrocyte membrane, causing potassium loss and dehydration (echinocytes). The decrease in echinocyte deformability enhances erythrocyte sequestration in splenic cords and phagocytosis by macrophages.

CLINICAL FINDINGS

There is mild to moderate anemia with splenomegaly. The anemia is well tolerated because of the increase in 2,3-DPG that accompanies the distal block in glycolysis. The two to three times normal increase in 2,3-DPG enhances the release of oxygen to the tissues. Jaundice may occur with intermittant hemoglobinuria. Gallstones are a common complication.

LABORATORY FINDINGS

Patients with PK deficiency have a normocytic, normochromic anemia with hemoglobin levels from 6 to 12 g/dL. Reticulocytosis ranges from 2% to 15% and increases even more after splenectomy, often above 40%. The blood smear exhibits irregularly contracted cells and occasional echinocytes before splenectomy (Fig. 11-12). After splenectomy, these abnormal cells are a more conspicuous finding. In contrast to G6PD deficiency, Heinz bodies and spherocytes are not found in PK deficiency. Serum indirect bilirubin and LDH are increased. Haptoglobin is decreased or absent.

Osmotic fragility is normal, but cells demonstrate increased hemolysis when incubated at 37° C. Autohemo-

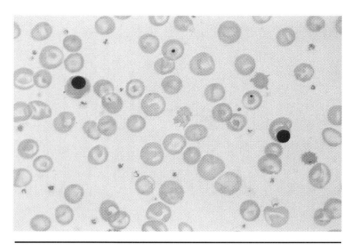

FIGURE 11-12. This is a blood smear from a patient with pryuvate kinase deficiency. Note the echinocyte, acanthocyte, target cells and irregularly contracted cells. There are also Howell-Jolly bodies present. (250× original magnification; Wright-Giemsa stain.)

lysis is increased at 48 hours, is not corrected with the addition of glucose, but is corrected with addition of ATP.

In performing enzyme tests for PK, the erythrocytes are separated from leukocytes because leukocytes contain more PK than erythrocytes. In PK deficiency, only the erythrocytes are deficient; leukocytes are normal. In the screening procedure developed by Bentler, erythrocytes are incubated with phosphoenol-pyruvate (PEP), NADH, LDH and ADP. As PK catalyzes the formation of PEP to pyruvate, one mole of ATP is generated from ADP. Pyruvate is then reduced to lactate by NADH producing NAD:

$$\text{Phosphoenolpyruvate} + \text{ADP} \xrightarrow{\text{PK}} \text{Pyruvate} + \text{ATP}$$

$$\text{Pyruvate} + \text{NADH} + \text{H}^+ \xrightarrow{\text{LDH}} \text{Lactate} + \text{NAD}^+$$

NADH fluoresces under ultraviolet light, whereas NAD does not. With normal erythrocytes, all fluorescence disappears within 30 minutes. Persistence of fluorescence for 45 to 60 minutes indicates PK deficiency. Some mutant PK enzymes have normal activity at high PEP concentrations and abnormal activity at low PEP concentrations. A modification of this procedure has been developed to improve the interpretation of the endpoint.[33] In this modification, patient blood is frozen and thawed to ensure complete hemolysis of the specimen before testing.

The quantitative test for PK deficiency is performed in the same manner as the screening test, except that the rate of disappearance of fluorescence is measured in a spectrophotometer at 340 nm. A rapid new potentiometric method in which enzymatic activity is measured by monitoring the change in pH in a reaction buffer during the conversion of PEP to pyruvate has been developed.[34]

THERAPY

There is no specific therapy for PK deficiency. Transfusions help maintain the hemoglobin above 8 to 10 g/dL. Splenectomy may improve the hemoglobin level and de-

crease the need for transfusions in some affected individuals; however, hemolysis continues.

Other enzyme deficiencies in the Embden-Meyerhoff pathway

When associated with anemia, other enzyme deficiencies in the Embden-Meyerhoff pathway have clinical manifestations and laboratory findings that resemble those of PK deficiency.

GLUCOSE PHOSPHATE ISOMERASE DEFICIENCY (GPI)

This is the second most common disorder of the EM pathway. Almost all GPI mutants are unstable, causing hemolytic anemia. Affected individuals show a partial response to splenectomy.

HEXOKINASE (HK) DEFICIENCY

Hexokinase is the first enzyme in the glycolytic pathway and, thus, is responsible for priming the glycolytic pump. There are two types of HK deficiency. One is associated with hemolytic anemia that responds to splenectomy. The other is associated not only with hemolytic anemia but also with an array of other abnormalities. A deficiency in this enzyme interferes with production of 2,3-DPG, and patients tolerate the anemia poorly.

PHOSPHOGLYCERATE KINASE (PGK) DEFICIENCY

This is a sex-linked disorder that causes hemolytic anemia and mental retardation in males. Females have a milder form of the disorder.

TRIOSEPHOSPHATE ISOMERASE (TPI) DEFICIENCY

A deficiency of TPI causes severe abnormalities in erythrocytes resulting in severe hemolysis. Abnormalities also are noted in striated muscle and the central nervous system. Death in infancy is common.

Abnormal erythrocyte nucleotide metabolism

Pyrimidine 5'-nucleotidase (P5N) contributes to the degradation of nucleic acids by cleaving pyrimidine nucleotides into small substances that can diffuse out of the cell. P5N deficiency is an autosomal-recessive disorder that leads to a severe hemolytic anemia unresponsive to splenectomy. Partially degraded mRNA and rRNA accumulate within the cell and are visualized as basophilic stippling in stained smears. Lead inhibits this enzyme, which may explain the similar coarse basophilic stippling seen in lead poisoning.

SUMMARY

The erythrocyte lifespan may be significantly shortened if the erythrocyte has intrinsic defects such as an abnormal membrane, structurally abnormal hemoglobin, defective globin synthesis, or deficient erythrocyte enzymes. These abnormalities are almost always inherited defects. When the bone marrow is unable to compensate, hemolytic anemia results.

Erythrocyte membrane defects may be caused by abnormalities of membrane proteins or lipids. These abnormalities may affect cell deformability, stability, and/or permeability. The abnormal erythrocytes become trapped in splenic cords and are removed from circulation. Interactions between the skeletal lattice proteins and integral proteins and lipids of the membrane are vertical interactions that, when disrupted, cause a reduced density of spectrin and uncoupling of the lipid bilayer. This causes selective loss of lipid bilayer and formation of spherocytes. Skeletal lattice proteins also interact horizontally to form the stress-supporting skeletal protein lattice. Defects in these proteins result in mechanical instability and fragmentation of the cell. Inherited defects in membrane proteins produce the hereditary hemolytic anemias including hereditary spherocytosis, or hereditary elliptocytosis, and hereditary pyropoikilocytosis. Abnormally permeable membranes may cause hereditary stomatocytosis, hereditary xerocytosis. The specific abnormality of the membrane in these two disorders has not been definitively identified.

Paroxysmal nocturnal hemoglobinuria (PNH), a stem cell disorder, is an acquired membrane abnormality in which there is complement-mediated destruction of the cell. The defect is due to a lack of decay-accelerating factor (DAF) and C8 binding protein (C8bp) on the erythrocytes. The lack of these proteins is due to the absence of a membrane glycolipid, glycosyl-phosphatidyl inositol (GPI), to anchor these proteins to the cell membrane. Hemolysis is intravascular resulting in hemoglobinuria and decreased haptoglobin. Leukopenia and thrombocytopenia are common, as these cells also are susceptible to complement destruction. The sucrose hemolysis test is a screening test for PNH. The Ham test is a more specific test in which patient cells are incubated with acidified serum. A positive test shows hemolysis.

Erythrocyte enzyme deficiencies may compromise the integrity of the cell membrane or hemoglobin and cause hemolysis. These hemolytic anemias are known as congenital nonspherocytic hemolytic anemia. The HMP shunt provides the cell with reducing power, protecting it from oxidant damage. Defects in this shunt allow hemoglobin to be oxidized and denatured to Heinz bodies. The Heinz bodies damage the cell membrane. The finding of bite cells on the blood smear are evidence that Heinz bodies have been pitted from the cells. The most common deficiency in this pathway is G6PD deficiency, a sex-linked disorder. There are many different variants of this enzyme, some of which cause severe hemolysis and others mild hemolysis. In most cases, hemolysis is sporadic, occurring during infections or with administration of certain drugs and is self-limited. In these variants, the younger cells have adequate enzyme activity, but the older cells are severely deficient and are selectively hemolyzed. Testing for the enzyme should be delayed until 2 months after the hemolytic episode when reticulocytes are normal and the erythrocytes produced after the hemolytic episode have aged. Screening tests for the enzyme include the fluorescent dye test, dye reduction test, and ascorbate cynanide test. Definitive testing requires quantitation of the enzyme.

Deficiencies of enzymes in the EM pathway decrease ATP production and lead to hemolysis. There may be impaired cation pumping and increased osmotic fragility. PK is the most common enzyme abnormality in this pathway. There are many PK enzyme mutants, resulting in a diverse array of clinical and laboratory findings. There is significant reticulocytosis. The blood film is remarkable for the presence of irregularly contracted cells and echinocytes. Heinz bodies and bite cells are not found. Screening and definitive tests for the enzyme are based on the conversion of phosphoenol-pyruvate to pyruvate catalzyed by PK and subsequent reduction of pyruvate to lactate by NADH producing NAD. Since NAD does not fluoresce but NADH does, a lack of fluorescence indicates the presence of PK.

● REVIEW QUESTIONS

A 1-month-old boy with a history of bilirubinemia since birth is seen by his pediatrician for a routine follow-up examination.

Postnatal Laboratory Data:

Total bilirubin:	12.0 gm/dL at birth, 19.7 gm/dL 2 days postnatal, 10.2 gm/dL at discharge
Indirect AHG test	negative
Direct AHG test	negative
Blood Type	Group B, Rh negative

Mother's Post-partum Laboratory Data:

Blood Type	Group B, Rh negative
Antibody screen	negative
Direct AHG	negative

Laboratory data of infant at 1 month of age:

Erythrocyte count	2.31×10^{12}/L
Hb	7.4 gm/dL
Hct	0.20 L/L
Platlet count	378×10^9/L
Leukocyte count	9.2×10^9/L

Differential:

Segmented neutrophils	16%
Band neutrophils	2%
Lymphocytes	78%
Monocytes	4%

Erythrocyte morphology: The erythrocytes were normochromic with slight polychromasia. There was mild anisopoikilocytosis. Numerous spherocytes were present.

Reticulocyte count:	10.2%
Serum bilirubin:	7.3 gm/dL
Serum LDH:	325 IU/L

1. Based on the patient's reticulocyte production index (RPI), what is the functional classification of this anemia?
   a. survival defect
   b. proliferation defect
   c. maturation defect

2. If an erythrocyte osmotic fragility test were performed on this baby's blood, what results would you expect?
   a. normal osmotic fragility
   b. increased osmotic fragility
   c. decreased osmotic fragility

3. What is this patient's most likely anemia?
   a. G6PD deficiency
   b. Hereditary spherocytosis
   c. Warm immune hemolytic anemia
   d. Paroxysmal nocturnal hemoglobinuria

4. What is the most common erythrocyte membrane defect in this disorder?
   a. spectrin deficiency
   b. DAF deficiency
   c. band 4.1 deficiency
   d. deficiency of membrane phosphatidylcholine

5. How would you classify this anemia morphologically?
   a. normocytic, hypochromic
   b. microcytic, hypochromic
   c. normocytic, normochromic
   d. normocytic, hyperchromic

Additional questions

6. What disorder is associated with erythrocytes that are thermally unstable and fragment when heated to 45° to 46°C.
   a. hereditary spherocytosis
   b. hereditary elliptocytosis
   c. PNH
   d. hereditary pyropoikilocytosis

7. A positive sucrose hemolysis test was followed by a Ham test. There was hemolysis of the patient's cells in acidified serum. These results are indicative of:
   a. G6PD deficiency
   b. hereditary spherocytosis
   c. pyruvate kinase deficiency
   d. PNH

8. A 20-year-old black man was suspected of having G6PD deficiency when he experienced hemolytic anemia after administration of primaquine. An erythrocyte G6PD analysis, performed on blood taken 2 days after symptoms appeared, was normal. A reticulocyte count revealed 12% reticulocytes at this time. These results suggest:
   a. the patient definitely does not have G6PD deficiency but may have pyruvate kinase deficiency
   b. another G6PD test should be done in several months when the reticulocyte count returns to normal
   c. leukocytes may be contaminating the sample and giving a false result
   d. the patient probably has the G6PD Mediterranean variant

9. Bite cells are associated with:

a. pyruvate kinase deficiency
b. PNH
c. G6PD deficiency
d. hereditary pyropoikilocytosis

10. The principal confirmation test in the diagnosis of hereditary spherocytosis is:
   a. Autohemolysis test
   b. Ham test
   c. Osmotic fragility test
   d. Thermal stability test

REFERENCES

1. Palek, J., Jarolim, P.: Clinical expression and laboratory detection of red blood cell membrane protein mutations. Semin. Hematol., 30:249, 1993.
2. Palek, J.: The red cell skeleton and haemolytic anaemias. Br. J. Haematol., 82:260, 1992.
3. Beck, W.S.: Hematology, 3rd Ed. Cambridge: The Massachusetts Institute of Technology, 1981.
4. Ideguchi, H., Nishimura, J., Nawata, H., Hamasaki, N.: A genetic defect of erythrocyte band 4.2 protein associated with hereditary spherocytosis. Br. J. Haematol., 74:347, 1990.
5. Iolascon, A., et al.: Ankyrin deficiency in dominant hereditary spherocytosis: a report of three cases. Br. J. Haematol., 78:551, 1991.
6. Duru, F., et al.: Homozygosity for dominant form of hereditary spherocytosis. Br. J. Haematol., 82:596, 1992.
7. Peters, L.L., Lux, S.E.: Ankyrins: Structure and function in normal cells and hereditary spherocytes. Semin. Hematol., 30:85, 1993.
8. Gilsanz, F., Ricard, M.P., Millan, I.: Diagnosis of hereditary spherocytosis with dual-angle differential light scattering. Am. J. Clin. Pathol., 100:119, 1993.
9. Palek, J., Lambert, S.: Genetics of the red cell membrane skeleton. Semin. Hematol., 27:290, 1990.
10. Conboy, J.G.: Structure, function and molecular genetics of erythroid membrane skeletal protein 4.1 in normal and abnormal red blood cells. Semin. Hematol., 30:58, 1993.
11. Wang, D.N.: Band 3 protein: structure, flexibility and function. FEBS Letters, 346:26, 1994.
12. Liu, S.C., Derick, L.H., Agre, P., Palek, J.: Alteration of the erythrocyte membrane skeletal ultrastructure in hereditary spherocytosis, hereditary elliptocytosis, and pyropoikilocytosis. Blood, 76:198, 1990.
13. DePalma, L., Lubon, N.L.C.: Hereditary poikilocytosis. AJDC, 147:93, 1993.
14. Kanzaki, A., Yawata, Y.: Hereditary stomatocytosis: phenotypical expression of sodium transport and band 7 peptides in 44 cases. Br. J. Haematol., 82:133, 1992.
15. Rader, D.J., Brewer, H.B.: Abetalipoproteinemia. JAMA, 270:865, 1993.
16. Yeh, E.T.H., Rosse, W.F.: Paroxysmal nocturnal hemoglobenuria and the glycosylphosphatidylinostol anchor. J. Clin. Invest., 93:2305, 1994.
17. Schultz, D.R.: Erythrocyte membrane protein deficiencies in paroxysmal nocturnal hemoglobinuria. Am. J. Med., 87:22N, 1989.
18. Rotoli, B., Bessler, M., Alfinito, F., del Vecchiu, L.: Membrane proteins in paroxysmal noctural hemoglobinuria. Blood Rev., 7:75, 1993.
19. Schubert, J., Ostendorf, T., Schmidt, R.E.: Biology of GPI anchors and pathogenesis of paroxysmal nocturnal hemoglobinuria. Immunol. Today, 15:299, 1994.
20. Okuda, K., et al.: Membrane expression of decay-accelerating factor on neutrophils from normal individuals and patients with paroxysmal nocturnal hemoglobinuria. Blood, 75:1186, 1990.
21. Graham, D.L., Gastineau, D.A.: Paroxysmal nocturnal hemoglobinuria as a marker for myelopathy. Am. J. Med., 93:671, 1992.

22. Rosse, W.F., Parker, C.J.: Paroxysmal nocturnal haemoglobinuria: an acquired membrane disorder. Clin. Haematol., 14:105, 1985.

23. Desforges, J.F.: Paroxsymal nocturnal hemoglobinuria. In Hematology Principles and Practice. Edited by R. Hoffman, E.J. Benz, Jr., S.J. Shattil, B. Furie, H.J. Cohen. New York: Churchill Livingstone, 1995.

24. Jaffe, E.R.: Chronic nonspherocytic hemolytic anemia and G6PD deficiency. Hosp. Prac., 26:57, 1991.

25. Arese, P., DeFlora, A.: Pathophysiology of hemolysis in glucose-6-phosphate dehydrogenase deficiency. Semin. Hematol., 27:1, 1990.

26. Babior, B.M., Stossel, T.P.: Hematology, A Pathophysiological Approach. New York: Churchill Livingstone, 1984.

27. Sarkar, S., et al.: Acute intravascular haemolysis in glucose-6-phosphate dehydrogenase deficiency. Ann. Trop. Paediatr., 13:391, 1993.

28. Mafa, L., et al.: G6PD Aures: a new mutation (48 Ile Thr) causing mild G6PD deficiency is associated with favism. Hum. Mol. Gen., 2:81, 1993.

29. Ward, P.C.J., Schwartz, B.S., White, J.G.: Heinz-Body anemia: "bite cell" variant—a light and electron microscopic study. Am. J. Hem., 15:135, 1983.

30. Berner, J.J.: Effects of Diseases on Laboratory Tests. Philadelphia: J.B. Lippincott, 1983.

31. Shannon, K., Buchanan, G.R.: Severe hemolytic anemia in black children with glucose-6-phosphate dehydrogenase deficiency. Pediatr., 70:364, 1982.

32. Lenzner, C., et al.: Mutations in the pyruvate kinase L gene in patients with hereditary hemolytic anemia. Blood, 83:2817, 1994.

33. Tsang, S.S., Feng, C-S.: A modified screening procedure to detect pyruvate kinase deficiency. Am. J. Clin. Pathol., 99:128, 1993.

34. Mosca, A., et al.: Rapid determination of erythrocyte pyruvate kinase activity. Clin. Chem., 39:512, 1993.

Hemolytic anemias due to extrinsic factors

12

CHAPTER OUTLINE

KEY TERMS

Blackwater fever
microangiopathic hemolytic anemia
immune hemolytic anemia
drug-induced hemolytic anemia
alloimmune hemolytic anemia
autoimmune hemolytic anemia
incomplete antibodies
complete antibodies
zeta potential
immune tolerance
Evan's syndrome
acrocyanosis
Raynaud's phenomenon
Donath-Landsteiner antibody
erythroblastosis fetalis

TABLE 12-1 *CAUSES OF PREMATURE DESTRUCTION OF INTRINSICALLY NORMAL ERYTHROCYTES*

- antagonists in the cells' environment
- abnormal plasma lipid concentrations
- physical or mechanical trauma
- antibodies and/or complement

INTRODUCTION

Premature erythrocyte destruction initiated by factors extrinsic to the cell (extracorpuscular defect) are classified as extrinsic hemolytic anemias. The erythrocytes are intrinsically normal in that they have normal membranes, enzymes and hemoglobin. The extrinsic nature of the hemolysis can be demonstrated by transfusing normal, compatible donor erythrocytes into the patient. These donor cells will have a shortened lifespan, similar to that of the patient's erythrocytes. This premature destruction of normal erythrocytes may be precipitated by antagonistic factors in the cells' environment (i.e., toxins, infectious agents); by exposure to abnormal lipid concentrations in the circulation; physical or mechanical factors in plasma (i.e., intravascular fibrin deposition); or antibodies and/or complement deposited on the erythrocyte membrane (i.e., immune hemolytic anemias) (Table 12-1). Hemolysis may be either intravascular or extravascular depending on the type and extent of erythrocyte injury.

HEMOLYTIC ANEMIAS CAUSED BY ANTAGONISTS IN THE BLOOD OR ABNORMALITIES OF PLASMA LIPIDS

Erythrocyte hemolysis may be due to the presence of antagonistic substances in the environment of the cell (Table 12-2). This type of hemolysis is caused by either injury to the erythrocyte membrane or to denaturation of hemoglobin.

TABLE 12-2 *HEMOLYTIC ANEMIAS CAUSED BY NONIMMUNE ANTAGONISTS IN THE ERYTHROCYTE ENVIRONMENT*

Category	Antagonist	Mode of Hemolysis
CHEMICALS AND DRUGS		
	Water	Osmotic lysis
	Oxidants	Hemoglobin denaturation
	Arsine gas	?
	Lead	Erythrocyte membrane damage
ANIMAL VENOMS		
	Snake bites	Mechanical cell damage due to disseminated intravascular coagulation
	Spider bites	Venom?
	Bee stings	Venom?
INFECTIOUS AGENTS		
	Malarial parasite	Direct parasitization; hypersplenism; acute intravascular hemolysis may occur in *P. falciparum* infection
	Babesiosis parasite	Direct parasitization
	Bartonellosis	Red cell membrane attachment
	Clostridium	Hemolytic toxins
ABNORMAL PLASMA LIPID COMPOSITION		
Spur cell anemia	Excess membrane cholesterol	Decreased membrane deformability; membrane loss; sequestration in the spleen
Abetalipoproteinemia	Plasma hyperlipidemia; membrane lecithin decreased and sphingomyelin increased	Membrane fluidity decreased
LCAT deficiency	Increase in plasma and membrane cholesterol	Same as in spur cell
MICROANGIOPATHIC HEMOLYTIC ANEMIA		
HUS, TTP, DIC	Thrombi in microcirculation	Physical damage to erythrocytes by microthrombi
Malignant hypertension	?	Physical damage to erythrocytes
OTHER PHYSICAL TRAUMA		
March hemoglobinuria	External force	Fragmentation of erythrocytes due to excessive external force as they pass through microcapillaries
Thermal injury	Heat	Thermal damage to erythrocyte membrane proteins
Traumatic cardiac	Physical stress	Erythrocyte fragmentation

Chemicals and drugs

A variety of chemicals and drugs have been identified that may cause erythrocyte hemolysis; many of these are dose-dependent. In addition to causing erythrocyte hemolysis, chemicals and drugs also may produce methemoglobinemia and cyanosis or, in some instances, aplasia of the bone marrow.

Water can enter the vascular system during transurethral resection producing hemoglobinemia and hemoglobinuria as a result of osmotic lysis of erythrocytes.

Some drugs known to cause hemolysis in G6PD deficient persons also can cause hemolysis in normal persons if the dose is sufficiently high. The mechanism of hemolysis is similar to that in G6PD deficiency with hemoglobin denaturation and Heinz body formation due to strong oxidants. Drugs also may cause immune-mediated destruction of erythrocytes. This will be discussed later in this chapter.

Inhalation of arsine gas from industrial processes may cause hemolysis.

The anemia of lead poisoning is usually classified with sideroblastic anemias since the pathophysiologic and hematologic findings are similar. Lead inhibits heme synthesis causing an accumulation of iron within mitochondria. However, it is apparent that lead also damages the erythrocyte membrane. This damage is manifested by an increase in osmotic fragility and mechanical fragility. Progressive anemia in lead poisoning is accompanied by coarse basophilic stippling, reticulocytosis, and leukocytosis. Erythrocyte inclusions, in addition to basophilic stippling, usually are present, including Howell-Jolly bodies and Cabot's rings. Nucleated erythrocytes can be found in the peripheral blood.

Animal venoms

Venoms injected by bees, wasps, spiders, and scorpions may cause hemolysis in some susceptible individuals. Although snake bites only rarely cause hemolysis directly, they may cause hemolysis secondary to disseminated intravascular coagulation.

Infectious agents

MALARIAL PARASITES

The anemia accompanying malaria is indirectly due to the intracellular malarial parasites (Fig. 12-1). The spleen may remove the entire parasitized cell or splenic macrophages may pit the parasite from the erythrocyte, damaging the cell membrane. Anemia also may result from an immune-mediated process whereby antimalarial antibodies and complement react with malarial antigens on the erythrocyte membrane. This results in removal of the sensitized cell by splenic macrophages. The anemia is mild but can be severe in some cases of infection with *P. falciparum*.

Blackwater fever is a complication of infection with *P.*

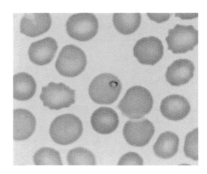

FIGURE 12-1. Ring form of trophozoite of malaria (PB; 250× original magnification, Wright-Giemsa stain).

falciparum malaria. Acute intravascular hemolysis with hemoglobinemia, methemalbuminemia, hyperbilirubinemia, hemoglobinuria, and renal failure is characteristic of this disorder. What precipitates the hemolytic episode is unclear, but among Europeans it is associated with those who have taken quinine irregularly.

BABESIOSIS

Babesiosis is a protozoan infection of rodents and cattle that may be transmitted to humans by ticks. The parasites appear as intracellular pleomorphic ring-like structures on Romanowsky-stained smears. This parasitic infection is associated with hemolysis.

BARTONELLOSIS

Bartonellosis, an infection by *Bartonella bacilliformis*, is characterized by a severe febrile hemolytic anemia (Oroya fever). The disease, which is restricted to Columbia, Peru, and Ecuador, is transmitted by sandflies. The organism is readily visualized on or within erythrocytes on Wright- or Giemsa-stained peripheral blood smears. The organisms are rod- or round-shaped, appearing singly, in pairs, or in chains.

CLOSTRIDIUM WELCHII

Rapid hemolysis develops from *Clostridium welchii* (also *Clostridium perfringes*) infections due to the release of potent hemolysins. The hemolytic toxin is a phospholipiase C that hydrolyzes sphingomyelin and lecithin of the erythrocyte membrane. Hemoglobinuria and eventually anuria develops. The peripheral blood smear shows many microspherocytes and erythrocyte fragments accompanied by thrombocytopenia.

Abnormal plasma lipid composition (acquired membrane disorders)

The erythrocyte membrane structure is a phospholipid–protein complex with almost equal quantities of lipids and proteins. The mature cell has no capacity for de novo synthesis of lipids or proteins; however, the lipids of the membrane are in continual exchange with plasma lipids. Thus, plasma lipids and lipoproteins are closely associated with the erythrocyte membrane. Erythrocytes may acquire excess lipids when the concentration of plasma lipids increase. Excess membrane lipids expand the membrane surface area and cause the cell to acquire abnormal shapes, including target cells (codocytes), leptocytes, or acanthocytes. If portions of the membrane are lost due to "grooming" of excess lipids in the spleen or if the lipid viscosity of the membrane increases, the cells lose their ability to deform and are sequestered in the spleen.

SPUR CELL ANEMIA

Spur cell anemia is associated with severe hepatocellular disease, in which there is an increase in serum lipoproteins, which leads to an excess of erythrocyte membrane cholesterol. The total phospholipid content of the membrane, however, is normal. As the membrane ratio of cholesterol to phospholipid increases, the cell becomes flattened (leptocyte) with a scalloped edge. The increased cholesterol to phospholipid ratio also causes a decrease in membrane fluidity and an associated decrease in cell deformability. Through repeated splenic conditioning, membrane fragments are lost, and the cell acquires irregular spike-like projections typical of acanthocytes (spur cells). Spherocytes also may be found as a result of this membrane loss. Eventually, the cell is hemolyzed. Hemolysis is enhanced by congestive splenomegaly in cirrhosis. Acanthocytes must be distinguished from echinocytes (burr cells) and keratocytes. Echinocytes have regular, small, spiny projections throughout the cell membrane, while keratocytes have just a few large surface projections.[5]

Transfusion studies have established that spur cells acquire their characteristic shape as innocent bystanders.[1] When normal cells are transfused into the patient, they acquire the abnormal shape and are hemolyzed as fast as the patient's cells.[2]

The peripheral blood shows a moderate to severe normocytic, normochromic anemia with hemoglobin concentration between 5 and 10 g/dL. Reticulocytes are increased to 5% to 15%. Approximately 20% to 80% of the erythrocytes are acanthocytes (Fig. 12-2). Echinocytes and spherocytes also may be found. Evidence of liver disease is reflected by an increase in indirect bilirubin and in liver enzymes. Serum albumin is decreased.

Biliary obstruction is commonly associated with the presence of normocytic or slightly macrocytic target cells, which result from an acquired excess of lipids on the cell membrane. However, in contrast to the acanthocytes found in severe hepatocellular disease, the excess lipid on target cells associated with biliary obstruction includes an increase in both cholesterol and phospholipids in a ratio similar to that of normal cells. As a result, lipid viscosity is normal, and membrane deformability is normal. These target cells have a normal survival.

ABETALIPOPROTEINEMIA (HEREDITARY ACANTHOCYTOSIS)

This is a rare autosomal recessive disorder characterized by the absence of serum β-lipoprotein, low serum cholesterol, low triglyceride, and low phospholipid and an increase in the ratio of cholesterol to phospholipid. The primary abnormality is defective synthesis of apoprotein B, which normally transports triglyceride. Acanthocytes are typically found, but hemolysis is negligible with little or no anemia. Reticulocytes usually are normal but may be slightly increased. The acanthocytes have normal cholesterol levels, but lecithin is decreased and sphingomyelin is increased. This is in contrast to spur cells found in severe liver disease, which have increased membrane cholesterol. Membrane fluidity is decreased, presumably because of the increase in sphingomyelin, which is less fluid than

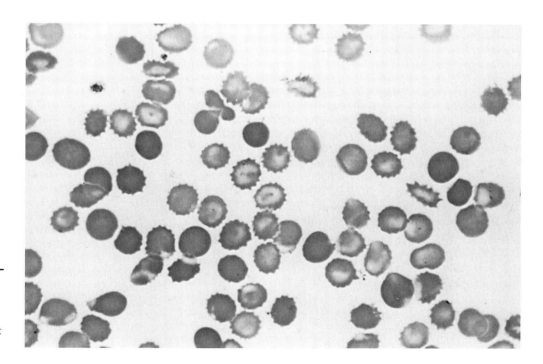

FIGURE 12-2. Spur cell anemia in a patient with alcoholic cirrhosis; note the numerous echinocytes, acanthocytes (spur cells) and spherocytes (peripheral blood, 250× original magnification).

other phospholipids. The degree of distortion of erythrocytes increases with cell age. The acanthocytes have normal membrane permeability, normal glucose metabolism, and normal osmotic fragility. Autohemolysis at 48 hours is increased and only partially corrected by glucose. In addition to hypolipidemia, the disorder is characterized by steatorrhea, retinitis pigmentosa, and neurologic abnormalities.

LECITHIN–CHOLESTEROL ACYL TRANSFERASE (LCAT) DEFICIENCY

This is a rare autosomal-recessive disorder with onset in young adulthood. It is characterized by a deficiency of LCAT, the enzyme that catalyzes the formation of cholesterol esters from cholesterol. As a result, cholesterol, phospholipids, and triglycerides accumulate in the blood. Since erythrocyte membrane cholesterol is in a comparative rapid equilibrium with unesterified plasma cholesterol, the activity of LCAT indirectly regulates the amount of free cholesterol in the cell. The most characteristic hematologic findings include a mild hemolytic anemia marked by the presence of numerous target cells. The target cells are loaded with cholesterol.

● HEMOLYTIC ANEMIA CAUSED BY PHYSICAL INJURY TO THE ERYTHROCYTE

Hemolytic anemia caused by traumatic physical injury to the erythrocytes in the vascular circulation is characterized by intravascular hemolysis and striking erythrocyte abnormalities, including fragments and helmet cells.

● Microangiopathic hemolytic anemia

Microangiopathic hemolytic anemia is an inclusive term that describes a hemolytic process caused by microcirculatory lesions. Microcirculatory lesions are found in a variety of disorders, including disseminated cancer, eclampsia, pre-eclampsia, hemolytic uremic syndrome, thrombotic thrombocytopenic purpura, and malignant hypertension. The blood smear reveals evidence of erythrocyte fragmentation with the presence of schistocytes and keratocytes. Hemolysis is usually extravascular with a mild to moderate decrease in haptoglobin. Severely damaged cells may be destroyed intravascularly. Depending on the underlying pathology, platelets may be decreased, and evidence of coagulation and fibrinolysis may be present.

HEMOLYTIC UREMIC SYNDROME

Hemolytic uremic syndrome (HUS) is a disorder of childhood with a tetrad of clinical findings, including hemolytic anemia with erythrocyte fragmentation, acute renal failure, thrombocytopenia, and variable central nervous sys-

TABLE 12-3 *TETRAD OF CLINICAL FINDINGS ASSOCIATED WITH HUS*

1. Hemolytic anemia with red cell fragmentation
2. Acute renal failure
3. Thrombocytopenia
4. Variable central nervous system symptoms

tem symptoms (Table 12-3). This syndrome usually begins a few days or weeks after an episode of gastroenteritis (especially with *Shigella* or *E. coli*), an upper respiratory infection, urinary tract infection, or viral disease such as varicella or measles.[3] The disease also may occur in young women with complications of pregnancy, after normal delivery, or with the use of oral contraceptives. HUS also has been associated with immunosuppressive therapy used in renal and bone marrow transplantation.[4]

Pathophysiology Most cases of HUS (more than 90%) have been associated with damage to the renal glomerular capillary endothelium by toxins (Shiga toxin and Shiga-like toxins I and II) produced by bacterial pathogens, in particular *Shigella dysenteriae* and *E. coli*. It has been suggested that in *S. pneumoniae* infections, the enzyme neuraminidase, produced by the bacteria, is the responsible agent for capillary damage. Neuraminidase cleaves cell membrane glycoproteins and glycolipids, facilitating tissue invasion by the bacteria. It has been proposed that this cleavage exposes the normally hidden T-antigen (Thomsen-Friedenreich antigen) on capillary walls, platelets, and erythrocytes. Circulating anti-T antibodies cause agglutination of cells and platelets, leading to thrombosis in the small vessels.[3] Leukocytes also may play a role in capillary endothelial cell damage. Catabolic enzymes released from the granules of neutrophils, especially leukocyte elastase, have been implicated in causing endothelial damage. In addition, activated neutrophils generate oxidative products that cause cell membrane damage.

Endothelial damage has been linked to the release of vasoactive and platelet-aggregating substances causing platelet activation with subsequent formation of thrombi, primarily in the renal microvasculature, although other organ systems (central nervous system, heart, liver, gut) can be affected. This thrombotic microangiopathy is responsible for the clinical findings associated with HUS.

HUS can be subdivided into two groups, based on the presence or absence of a bloody diarrheal prodrome (Table 12-4).[3] The diarrhea-associated (D+) HUS is the most common form and is responsible for acute renal failure in children. The D+ HUS is usually associated with verocytotoxin producing *E. coli* (VTEC) infections. Cases have been traced to the ingestion of incompletely cooked beef contaminated with VTEC. About 2% to 4% of individuals with this infection will develop HUS. The other organism associated with D+ HUS is *S. dysenteriae* type I. Mild to moderately severe cases of D+ HUS have the best prognosis for recovery (more than 80%). The non-

TABLE 12-4 *GROUPS OF HUS*

Groups	Percentage of Occurrence
I. Diarrhea-related (classical) HUS (D+)	85–95
II. Non-diarrhea-related HUS (D−)	5–15
A. Postinfectious	5–10
B. Immunosuppression-related	<5
1. Chemotherapy	
2. Complement deficiency	
3. Transplant immunosuppression	
C. Pregnancy or oral-contraceptive related	Rare
D. Hereditary	Rare

diarrhea-associated (D-) HUS has been reported in both children and adults. Various causes have been attributed to D- HUS (Table 12-5).[3]

The age of onset of D+ HUS tends to occur between the ages of 6 months and 1 year, while D- HUS does not appear to show an age predilection.

Clinical findings The disease occurs in previously healthy children, with the highest incidence in the first year of life. The onset is acute, with sudden pallor, abdominal pain, vomiting, bloody diarrhea, and macroscopic hematuria. The most important and/or serious complication of HUS is acute renal failure. The duration of oliguria and anuria is variable, with the longest reported period of anuria being 75 days.[4] The disorder may be widespread, affecting the gut, liver, heart, and central nervous system. Regardless of the organ system involved, the pathology is the same (i.e., thrombosis of the microcirculation). About 50% of patients experience hypertension. Central nervous system symptoms may result directly from microangiopathy of the central nervous system or from hypertension. Seizures are the most common symptom and occur in 20%

TABLE 12-5 *CLINICAL CONDITIONS THAT MAY BE PRECIPITATING FACTORS IN HUS. (D+ : DIARRHEA-ASSOCIATED; D− : NON-DIARRHEA-ASSOCIATED)*

D+ HUS

E. coli infection

Shigella dysenteriae serotype I infection

D− HUS

Post-partum

Oral contraceptives

Drugs

Viral infections

Kawasaki disease

Acute rhabdomyolysis

Acute bromate poisoning

Renal and bone marrow transplantation

TABLE 12-6 *LABORATORY FINDINGS IN HUS AND TTP*

EVIDENCE OF HEMOLYSIS

Decreased hemoglobin

Increased reticulocytes

Leukocytosis with shift-to-the-left

Schistocytes and polychromasia on the blood smear

EVIDENCE OF INTRAVASCULAR HEMOLYSIS

Hemoglobinemia

Hemoglobinuria

Decreased haptoglobin

Increased serum bilirubin

EVIDENCE OF THROMBOTIC MICROANGIOPATHY

Thrombocytopenia

Normal or only mildly abnormal prothrombin time and partial thromboplastin time

Fibrin degradation products normal to increased

Factors I, V, VIII normal to increased

to 50% of children. Hepatosplenomegaly may be present. Hyperglycemia is common in children due to pancreatic damage secondary to HUS.

Laboratory findings (Table 12-6) A moderate to severe normocytic, normochromic anemia is typical with hemoglobin levels as low as 3 to 4 g/dL (median values, 7 to 9 g/dL). The peripheral blood smear shows fragmented and deformed cells (schistocytes, burr cells, helmet cells, spherocytes), with the degree of morphologic change correlating directly with the degree of anemia. Polychromasia and an occasional nucleated erythrocyte may be seen (Fig. 12-3). A leukocytosis with a shift to the left is common. Platelet counts vary from low normal to markedly decreased,

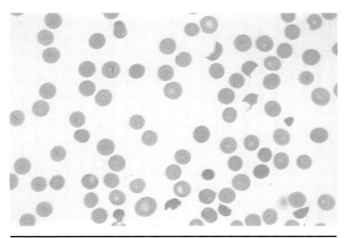

FIGURE 12-3. A blood smear from a patient with hemolytic uremic syndrome. The platelets are markedly decreased. There are schistocytes and spherocytes present. (250× original magnification; Wright-Giemsa stain).

with a median value of $50 \times 10^9/L$. The duration of thrombocytopenia is 1 to 2 weeks.

Hemoglobinemia with an increase in serum bilirubin and a decrease in serum haptoglobin reflects chronic intravascular hemolysis. The serum bilirubin is increased to 2 to 3 mg/dL. Fibrin split products are elevated, although a consumptive coagulopathy or DIC is rare. The prothrombin time may be prolonged, but the partial thromboplastin time is usually normal. The direct and indirect antiglobulin test are usually negative unless the HUS is due to infection with *S. pneumoniae*.[4]

Urinalysis reveals gross abnormalities, including moderate to massive amounts of protein (1 to 2 g/24 hours to 10 g/24 hours), gross and microscopic hematuria, pyuria, casts (hyaline, granular, and epithelial), and hemosiderin.[5] Blood urea nitrogen and creatinine levels are increased, reflecting the renal failure. Metabolic acidosis, hyponatremia, and hypokalemia are common. Serum lactate dehydrogenase is markedly elevated, and cardiac enzymes may be elevated due to myocardial damage.

Therapy With improvement in early diagnosis and supportive care, the mortality of the disease has been reduced to 5% to 15%. Supportive care includes close observation, blood transfusion (if hematocrit is less than 20%), control of electrolyte and water imbalances, control of hypertension, and peritoneal dialysis in anuria. The beneficial use of fresh frozen plasma infusions in HUS remains unclear. It has not been shown to be efficatious in patients with D + HUS. In contrast, D- HUS patients may benefit from plasma infusion or plasmapheresis. Plasma infusions are contraindicated in patients with HUS who have a positive direct antiglobulin test or who are infected with *S. pneumoniae*.

THROMBOTIC THROMBOCYTOPENIC PURPURA

Thrombotic thrombocytopenic purpura (TTP) is an acute disorder of unknown cause that affects young adults. It is characterized by the same tetrad of clinical findings as HUS (thrombocytopenia, microangiopathic hemolytic anemia, neurologic abnormalities, and renal dysfunction) with the addition of fever (Table 12-7). Neurologic findings are more prominent in TTP than HUS.

TTP is a rare disorder that occurs more often in females than in males. Although it is a disorder of unknown cause, a variety of clinical events have been identified as possible

TABLE 12-7 *PENTAD OF CLINICAL FINDINGS ASSOCIATED WITH TTP*

1. Microangiopathic hemolytic anemia with a negative DAT
2. Thrombocytopenia
3. Central Nervous System abnormalities
4. Fever
5. Renal dysfunction

TABLE 12-8 *CLINICAL CONDITIONS THAT MAY BE PRECIPITATING FACTORS IN TTP. INFECTIONS ARE THE FACTOR IN UP TO 40% OF PATIENTS AND PREGNANCY IN 10–25%*

CATEGORIES

Pregnancy or oral-contraceptive related

Infections
  Bacterial
    Shigella sp.
    Escherichia coli
    Salmonella sp.
    Campylobacter jejuni
    Yersinia sp.
    Pneumococcus
    Legionella sp.
    Mycoplasma sp.
  Viral
    Coxsackie B
    EBV
    HIV
    Influenza
    Echovirus
    Herpes Simplex

Surgery

Myocardial infarction

Lymphomas and carcinomas

Drugs
  Penicillin
  Sulfonamides
  Penicillamine
  Iodine
  Ticlopidine
  Chemotherapeutic agents

Connective Tissue Diseases
  Systemic lupus erythromatosus (SLE)
  Rheumatoid arthritis (RA)
  Ankylosing spondylitis
  Polymyositis
  Sjogren's syndrome
  Polyarteritis nodosa

Miscellaneous
  Bee sting
  Dog bite
  Carbon monoxide poisoning

precipitating factors (Table 12-8). Infections are the most common precipitating factor (40%), followed by pregnancy (10% to 25%).

Without treatment, TTP has a mortality rate in excess of 90% due to multi-organ failure.

Pathophysiology Autopsy findings in TTP reveal multiple small hyaline-like thrombi occluding capillaries and arterioles in a variety of organs, most frequently the kidneys, brain, pancreas, heart, spleen, and adrenal glands. Immunohistochemical stains have shown that the thrombi contain platelets and fibrin and frequently immunoglobin and complement.[6]

The primary stimulus for the vascular deposits is unknown but is probably due either to damage of the endothelial lining of small blood vessel walls, resulting in enhanced platelet aggregation, or to platelet activation and subsequent endothelial damage. Several possible causes of TTP have been suggested and include:[6] (1) a von Willebrand factor anomaly in which platelet aggregation occurs as a response to a platelet aggregating agent released into the circulation. One of the agents implicated is unusually large von Willebrand's factor (ULvWF) multimers, not typically found in normal plasma or in TTP plasma during remission but found in plasma during TTP episodes.[7] These multimers are very effective in binding to glycoproteins (Ib and IIb/IIIa) on the endothelial cell surface and inducing platelet aggregation. These ULvWF multimers may be the agents responsible for inducing platelet aggregation in HUS. (2) Defect in prostaglandin I_2 (PGI_2) synthesis. PGI_2 has important thromboresistant properties because of its potent inhibition of platelet activation. It has been reported that plasma from patients with TTP depresses the synthesis of PGI_2 in the vessel wall and also rapidly degrades PGI_2 in the plasma. (3) Depressed fibrinolysis. Fibrinolytic activity is depressed at the site of microthrombin formation. Decreased tissue plasminogen activator activity and decreased levels of protein C also have been reported in TTP plasma. Impaired fibrinolysis may contribute to the stability of the platelet plug and enhance tissue injury.

Clinical findings The disease is similar to HUS except that it occurs most often in young adults, involves more organ systems, neurologic symptoms are prominent, renal dysfunction is less severe, and the mortality rate is higher.

A variety of manifestations due to damage of multiple organs is present. Central nervous system damage is the most constant finding. Headaches, confusion, seizures, and coma reflect cerebral lesions. Symptoms may be reversible if treated early, although some patients recovering from TTP may have permanent manifestations of hematuria, proteinuria, and increased blood urea nitrogen. Some patients require dialysis, and, in rare cases, chronic renal failure occurs. Jaundice reflects both hemolysis and liver damage. The widespread thrombotic process results in visual defects, heart failure, abdominal pain, and damage to the pancreas and adrenal glands.

Four different types of TTP have been recognized.[6] These include: (1) single-episode TTP (most common); (2) relapsing TTP, which is characterized by episodes that recur after healthy periods of months or years; (3) chronic TTP, which is characterized by very frequent recurrent episodes. These individuals have ULvWF in their plasma even between episodes; and (4) childhood/familial TTP, which is very rare. Only a few cases have been reported. In this type, TTP begins very early in life (6 months of age) with multiple relapses continuing through adult life. Reports of families with multiple siblings with recurrent childhood TTP have been described.

Laboratory findings Results are shown in Table 12-6. The hemoglobin is usually less than 10.5 g/dL (average, 8 to 9 g/dL). The MCV may be normal; decreased, if there is marked erythrocyte fragmentation; or increased, depending on the degree of reticulocytosis. The MCH and

MCHC are normal. Reticulocytes are increased, and nucleated erythrocytes are found in the peripheral blood, reflecting the bone marrow response to hemolysis. Increased polychromasia is indicative of the reticulocytosis. The most striking blood finding is the abundance of shistocytes. Thrombocytopenia is often severe (8 to 44 × 10^9/L) due to consumption of platelets in the formation of microthrombi. Megakaryocytes are abundant in the bone marrow. The bleeding time may be prolonged if the platelet count is less than 100 × 10^9/L. Leukocytosis with counts of more than 20 × 10^9/L occur in 50% of patients. Leukocytosis is usually accompanied by a shift to the left.

Hemoglobinemia, hemoglobinuria, decreased haptoglobin levels, and increased serum bilirubin are direct evidence of intravascular hemolysis.

Coagulation tests are usually normal or only mildly disturbed in TTP, which helps differentiate TTP from disseminated intravascular coagulation (DIC). In DIC, there is a consumption of coagulation factors and an increase in fibrin degradation products, which may cause a prolonged prothrombin time, activated partial thromboplastin time, and thrombin time.

Biopsy of affected tissue to demonstrate the vascular lesion typical of TTP is sometimes done but not considered necessary. Inguinal nodes have been recommended as the biopsy site because vessels in lymph node capsules contain typical lesions, and bleeding can be controlled with pressure.

Therapy TTP is a rare disorder, making the establishment of treatment protocols difficult. With early diagnosis and new modes of therapy, more than 50% of TTP patients survive. Plasma exchange and plasma infusion have become the treatment of choice for TTP. Patients undergoing plasma exchange have shown a higher response rate and lower mortality rate than those given only plasma infusions. Antiplatelet agents such as aspirin and dipyridamole have widespread use as platelet-inhibitor drugs. Vincristine, in combination with corticosteroids and plasma, also has been used. Splenectomy has been reported to have beneficial effects in the absence of other treatment modalities. It is not considered to be the treatment of choice except for patients resistant to or dependent on plasma therapy.

MALIGNANT HYPERTENSION

The hemolytic anemia associated with malignant hypertension is characterized by a low platelet count and erythrocyte fragmentation. The mechanism of hemolysis is unknown. It has been suggested that it may be caused by fibrinoid necrosis of arterioles or deposition of fibrin fed by thromboplastic substances released from membranes of lysed erythrocytes. Hemolysis disappears when the blood pressure is lowered.

DISSEMINATED INTRAVASCULAR COAGULATION

Activation of the coagulation mechanism in vivo by thromboplastic substances results in deposition of fibrin in the microvasculature. Erythrocyte fragmentation oc-

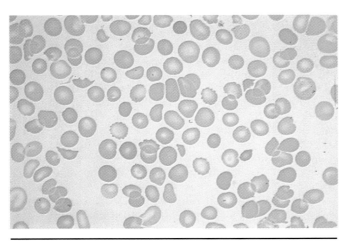

FIGURE 12-4. Peripheral blood from a patient with disseminated intravascular coagulation. Notice the schistocytes and thrombocytopenia. (250× original magnification; Wright stain).

curs as the erythrocytes become entangled in the fibrin meshwork as they circulate through capillaries (clothesline effect). Hemolysis is not usually severe, but the effects of consumptive coagulopathy (consumption of various coagulation proteins) may cause serious bleeding complications and occasionally thrombosis. Pathologic activation of coagulation may be caused by infection, neoplasm, or trauma. The typical laboratory findings include the presence of schistocytes, thrombocytopenia, (Fig. 12-4), and abnormal coagulation tests, including prolonged prothrombin time, activated partial thromboplastin time, and thrombin time, as well as an increase in fibrin degradation products (FDP) and a decrease in fibrinogen. If the prothrombin time, fibrinogen, and platelet count are all abnormal, DIC may be diagnosed with greater than 90% certainty. If only two of the three are abnormal, but FDP titres are high, diagnostic accuracy remains greater than 90%. (For a more detailed discussion of DIC, see Chapter 25.)

Traumatic Cardiac Hemolytic Anemia

This type of hemolytic anemia follows surgical insertion of prosthetic heart valves. Excessive turbulence of blood flow around the valve tears the erythrocytes apart from sheer stress. The term "Waring blender syndrome" has been used to describe this disorder because of the localized turbulent blood flow. Many erythrocyte fragments are apparent on the blood smear. Some of the severely traumatized cells are removed in the spleen, but most undergo intravascular hemolysis.

March hemoglobinuria

March hemoglobinuria is a descriptive term for a transient hemolytic anemia occurring after strenuous exercise that involves contact with a hard surface (e.g., running, tennis). However, it is not seen in every individual participating in these activities. The hemolysis is presumably due to the physical injury of erythrocytes as they pass through the capillaries of the feet. At least two cases of March hemoglobinuria have been reported in individuals with varicosity of the long saphenous veins.[9] After crossectomy of the vein and resection of the convolutes, the episodes of hemoglobinuria ceased.

No erythrocyte fragments are seen on the peripheral blood smear, but the hallmarks of intravascular hemolysis are present: hemoglobinemia and hemoglobinuria. The passage of red colored urine immediately after exercise and for several hours thereafter is usually the only complaint from affected individuals. Anemia is uncommon, as less than 1% of the erythrocytes are hemolyzed during an attack. Iron deficiency may occur if exercise and hemolysis are frequent. Osmotic and mechanical fragility tests are normal.

Thermal injury

Hemolytic anemia occurs 24 to 48 hours after extensive thermal burns. The degree of hemolysis depends on the body surface area burned. Hemolysis probably results from the direct effect of heat on spectrin in the erythrocyte membrane. If erythrocytes are heated to 48° C in vitro, they lose elasticity and deformability because of degradation of spectrin. Peripheral blood smears show erythrocyte budding, schistocytes, and spherocytes. After 48 hours, signs of hemolysis are not prominent. Thermal injury to erythrocytes also has occurred during hemodialysis when the dialysate is overheated.

IMMUNE HEMOLYTIC ANEMIAS

When erythrocytes are destroyed prematurely by an immune-mediated process, the disorder is known as *immune hemolytic anemia* (IHA). The individual may or may not be anemic, depending on the ability of the bone marrow to compensate for erythrocyte loss, but other laboratory findings provide clues of a hemolytic process. These include an increase in reticulocytes, an increase in indirect bilirubin, and a decrease in serum haptoglobin. Since hemolysis is mediated by immunoglobulin (antibody) and/or complement, diagnosis is confirmed by the demonstration of antibodies and/or complement attached to the patient's erythrocytes.

Classification of immune hemolytic anemias

Immune hemolytic anemia may be classified according to the stimulus for antibody production into three broad categories (Table 12-9): (1) autoimmune hemolytic anemia; (2) drug-induced hemolytic anemia and (3) alloimmune hemolytic anemia.

Autoimmune hemolytic anemia (AIHA) is characterized by an immune reaction against self. Individuals produce antibodies against their own erythrocyte antigens (autoantibodies). Most autoantibodies react with high in-

TABLE 12-9 *CLASSIFICATION OF IMMUNE HEMOLYTIC ANEMIAS*

1. Autoimmune
   A. Warm-reactive antibodies
      1. Primary or idiopathic
      2. Secondary
         —Systemic lupus erythematosus and other autoimmune disorders
         —Chronic lymphocytic leukemia
         —Hodgkin's disease
         —Viral infections
         —Neoplastic disorders
         —Chronic inflammatory diseases
   B. Cold-reactive antibodies
      1. Primary or idiopathic
      2. Secondary
         —Mycoplasma pneumoniae
         —Viral infections
         —Lymphoproliferative disorders
      3. Paroxysmal cold hemoglobinuria
2. Drug-induced
   1. Drug adsorption (hapten type)
   2. Immune complex formation (innocent bystander type)
   3. Membrane modification
   4. Autoantibody induction
3. Alloimmune
   A. Hemolytic transfusion reaction
   B. Hemolytic disease of the newborn

cidence antigens (e.g., I, Rh system) and will agglutinate, lyse, or sensitize the erythrocytes of most individuals.

Autoimmune hemolytic anemias are further classified as warm or cold hemolytic anemia based on optimal temperature for antibody reactivity and on clinical symptoms (Table 12-10). Some antibodies react best at temperatures between 35° and 40° C, and the anemia they produce is termed warm hemolytic anemia. About 70% of the AIHA are of the warm type. There are two types of warm autoantibodies, incomplete autoantibodies and autohemolysins. Warm incomplete autoantibodies are almost always associated with an IgG antibody (primarily of the IgG1 subclass). Rarely the antibody may be IgM or IgA. However,

TABLE 12-10 *CHARACTERISTICS OF AGGLUTININS IN HEMOLYTIC ANEMIA*

Property of Agglutinin	Warm Antibodies	Cold Antibodies
Immunoglobulin (Ig) class	IgG; rarely IgM or IgA	IgM (except PCH-IgG)
Optimal reactivity	37°C	<30°C
Mechanism of hemolysis	Attachment of membrane bound Ig or C3b to macrophage receptors (extravascular)	Complement lysis (intravascular), or attachment of membrane bound C3b to macrophage receptors (extravascular)
Specificity	Usually anti-Rh	Usually anti-I (PCH-anti-P)

warm autohemolysins are IgM antibodies that cause hemolysis through activation of complement.

Cold hemolytic anemias are usually due to the presence of an IgM antibody with an optimal thermal reactivity below 30° C. Hemolysis with cold reacting antibodies results from the binding and activation of complement by IgM, which becomes attached to erythrocytes in the cold. After warming, the cold-reacting antibody dissociates from the cell, but the complement remains, causing direct cell lysis or initiating extravascular hemolysis.

Drug-induced hemolytic anemia may occur by several mechanisms. Drugs may act as antigens when combined with plasma proteins. Subsequently, the drug–protein complex may be adsorbed to the erythrocyte membrane. Alternatively, the drug may induce alteration of the erythrocyte membrane in such a way that proteins nonspecifically adsorb to the membrane. This is a nonimmune adsorption. These drug-induced membrane alterations may stimulate the production of antibodies, which bind to the erythrocyte membrane. Some drugs adsorb directly to the erythrocyte membrane. If an individual has formed antibodies to the drug, these antibodies will react with the drug bound to the erythrocyte. Thus, the cell becomes coated with antibody. Sensitized erythrocytes, those with antibody or complement attached, have a shortened lifespan.

Alloimmune hemolytic anemia is generated when blood cells from one person are infused into another individual. Antigens on the infused donor cells may be recognized as foreign by the recipient's lymphocytes, stimulating the production of antibodies. In vitro autologous controls made from mixtures of patient's serum and patient's cells show no reaction, but mixtures of patient's serum and donor's cells produce agglutination or hemolysis. (If the autologous control is made from serum and cells taken after the transfusion, mixed field agglutination may occur because of the presence of both patient and donor cells.) This type of isosensitization is seen in hemolytic disease of the newborn (HDN), in which the mother has become sensitized to the erythrocyte antigens of her fetus, and in hemolytic transfusion reactions.

Sites of hemolysis

Hemolysis may be either intravascular or extravascular, depending on the class of antibody involved and whether the complement cascade has been completely activated. Most immune mediated hemolysis is extravascular. Erythrocytes sensitized with antibody or complement components become attached to macrophages in the spleen or liver via macrophage receptors for the Fc of immunoglobulin or the C3b component of complement and are phagocytosed (Fig. 12-5). Intravascular hemolysis may occur if terminal complement components C5 to C9 are deposited on the erythrocyte membrane.

Mechanisms of hemolysis

IgG-MEDIATED HEMOLYSIS

IgG mediates erythrocyte destruction by attaching to erythrocyte membrane antigens through the Fab portion

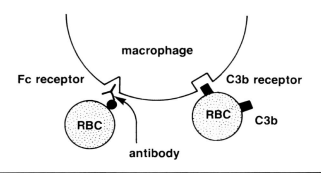

FIGURE 12-5. Immune mediated extravascular hemolysis. Red cells sensitized with antibody or complement (C3b) attach to macrophages via specific cell receptors for these immune proteins.

of the Ig molecule. The Fc portion of IgG is exposed to the environment. The cell becomes trapped in the red pulp of the spleen when the Fc fragment of attached IgG is exposed to macrophage Fc receptors. After binding, the macrophage pits the antigen-antibody (Ag/Ab) complex, fragmenting the cell membrane. The erythrocyte reseals itself. With repeated splenic passage, the erythrocyte continues to lose membrane and gradually assumes a spherocytic shape. Eventually, the cell becomes more spherocytic, rigid and less deformable, and is phagocytosed by splenic macrophages. Alternatively, the antibody sensitized cell may be entirely engulfed by the macrophages. Killer or null cells and neutrophils also have receptors for the Fc portion of IgG. However, the role of these cells in immune-mediated hemolysis is controversial.

As the spleen becomes saturated with more antigen sensitized cells, the liver assists in filtering. The liver also may be of some importance in removing heavily sensitized cells. Lightly opsonized cells are more efficiently removed in the spleen because of the sluggish blood flow there. The spleen tissue proliferates in response to an increase in erythrocyte sequestration accounting for splenic enlargement (splenomegaly) in warm immune hemolytic anemias. In the majority of immune hemolytic anemias, complement is activated, and complement and IgG can be detected on the erythrocyte membrane. This complement binding enhances the phagocytosis of sensitized cells by increasing the likelihood of the cell binding to the Fc and C3b receptors of macrophages.

COMPLEMENT-MEDIATED HEMOLYSIS

The complement system consists of at least 20 serum proteins. The proteins are designated numerically (i.e., C1, C2, C3, etc.) or by letters or historic names. This system of proteins is responsible for a number of diverse biologic activities, including the mediation of acute inflammatory responses and destruction of cells and micro-organisms. The most important roles of complement in immune hemolytic anemias are sensitization or the lysis of erythrocytes.

Normally, complement proteins circulate in an inactive state. Under certain circumstances, the proteins become sequentially enzymatically active (in a cascade-like fashion), similar to the components of the coagulation cas-

cade. An activated component is identified by placing a bar over the component ($\overline{C5}$).

The complement cascade may be initiated by two separate mechanisms called the classic and the alternate pathways (Fig. 12-6). The classic complement pathway may be initiated by an antigen–antibody reaction. Only anti-

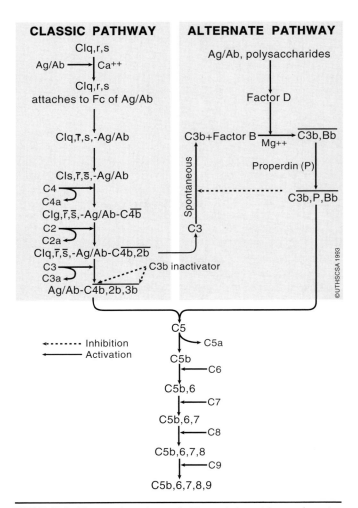

FIGURE 12-6. The complement cascade. The central event in complement activation is the activation of C3 by C3 convertases. This may occur by two separate but interrelated mechanisms, the classic and alternate pathways. The classic complement pathway may be initiated by an antigen-antibody reaction. The antigen-antibody complex activates the C1q,r,s complex which in turn activates C4 by proteolytic cleavage to C4a and C4b. C2 binds to C4b and is proteolytically cleaved by C1s to form C2a and C2b. The C4b2b complex serves as C3 convertase. This convertase has commonly been referred to as C4b2a but recently it was suggested that C2a should be renamed to C2b to be consistent with the terminology of the larger fragments of C4, C3 and C5 which are all "b" fragments. This cascade shows this newer terminology, C4b2b not C4b2a. In the alternate pathway, C3b serves as the cofactor of the C3-cleaving enzyme complex (C3b, P, Bb), also known as C3 convertase. Thus, the C3b serves to prime its own activation. The C3b formed through the classic pathway can directly initiate the assembly of the alternate pathway C3 convertase. C3 can also be activated by spontaneous hydrolysis. The C3b complexes formed by the classic and alternate pathways activate C5 to C5a and C5b. Membrane damage is initiated by the assembly of C5b with C6, 7, 8, 9.

bodies of the IgG1 and IgG3 (IgG2 less efficiently) subclasses of IgG and IgM can activate this pathway. The sequence is activated by binding of the first complement component, C1, to the Fc portion of IgG or IgM. This attachment initiates activation of the other complement components. The alternate pathway of activation can be initiated by aggregated IgG, IgA, and IgE, as well as by a number of polysaccharides and liposaccharides. In this pathway, C3 is activated directly, bypassing C1, C2, and C4 activation. The terminal complement components (C5 to C9) are responsible for the lytic attack on the erythrocyte membrane and are common to both pathways. The activation of these terminal components is initiated by C3b. Membrane leakage begins at the C8 stage but is greatly enhanced by C9, resulting in osmotic lysis.

If complement activation on the erythrocyte membrane is complete (C1-C9), intravascular hemolysis will occur. However, activation of complement is not always complete and thus does not always lead to direct cell lysis. More commonly, only C1 to C3 is activated on the erythrocyte membrane, and the cell is not lysed. Instead, the sensitized cell with attached C3b is totally or partially engulfed by binding to the C3b receptor of macrophages in the liver. Most complement-coated cells are removed in this organ.[9] Because of the enzymatic action of C3b inactivator in serum, C3b on erythrocytes may be cleaved to form C3d and C3c before the cell encounters macrophages. C3c dissociates from the membrane, but C3d remains attached. Erythrocytes coated with C3d have a normal survival rate because macrophages have no receptors for this complement component. Thus, the balance between C3b deposition on the membrane and C3b inactivation determines the susceptibility of erythrocytes to phagocytosis by macrophages via the C3b receptor.

In addition to C3b inactivator, other inhibitors of complement activation on the erythrocyte membrane include: (1) decay-accelerating factor (DAF), which prevents the assembly of the C3 convertases of the classic and alternate pathways (C4b,2b and C3b,Bb respectively); (2) C-8 binding protein, which inhibits the C8-C9 interaction and thus prevents lysis; and (3) P18/CD59 protein, which inhibits the incorporation of C9 into the C5b-9 complex.

The attachment of the first complement component to antibody requires two antibody binding sites in close proximity. Thus, the attachment of complement is highly dependent on the concentration of antibody molecules and on their spatial arrangement on the cell surface. The IgG molecule is much less efficient than IgM in providing these side by side antibody Fc regions. Therefore, IgM is much more likely to activate complement than IgG. Thus, the nature of the antibody is an important determinant of the extent of erythrocyte destruction by complement.

IgM-MEDIATED HEMOLYSIS

In cold hemolytic anemia, IgM becomes attached to the erythrocyte membrane. IgM-sensitized cells are not removed from circulation because macrophages do not have receptors for the Fc portion of IgM. However, IgM is an efficient activator of complement. Cells may be lysed intravascularly if complement activation is complete. If activation is incomplete and only C3b coats the cells, the cells may be hemolyzed extravascularly via adherence to C3b complement receptors on macrophages. Adherence of the cell to macrophages via complement receptors and subsequent phagocytosis, however, is less efficient than immune adherence and phagocytosis via Fc macrophage receptors. It has been estimated that greater than 100,000 molecules of the complement component C3b are required on the cell surface to induce phagocytosis by macrophages via complement. C3b also is inefficient in promoting adherence to macrophages because much of the C3b is inactivated to C3d. As mentioned previously, cells coated with C3d have a normal survival time. Thus, hemolysis of cells sensitized with complement is not as severe as hemolysis of cells sensitized with IgG.

In addition to activating complement, IgM antibodies agglutinate cells. It is possible that agglutinated cells are trapped in organs rich in phagocytes and subsequently are removed from the circulation. This mechanism, however, is probably not the major mechanism of destruction. Conversely, agglutination in vitro is a useful phenomenon for detecting the presence of cold agglutinins.

● Factors affecting hemolysis

The rate of hemolysis in hemolytic anemia is related to several factors (Table 12-11):

First, the class of Ig coating the erythrocyte is important in determining if and at what rate hemolysis will occur. Macrophages have three different Fc receptors (FcR) for IgG: FcR I, FcR II, and FcR III.[10] These receptors have varying affinities for different subclasses of IgG and for monomeric IgG. All three receptors bind IgG1 and IgG3 (IgG3 > IgG1) most avidly but have little or no affinity for IgG2 and IgG4. The FcR I receptor has a high affinity for monomeric forms of IgG1 and IgG3, whereas FcR II and FcR III bind only IgG dimers. It is believed that the FcR I receptor on macrophages is normally occupied by monomers of plasma IgG. Thus, it is likely that the FcR II and FcR III receptors that bind dimeric IgG1 and IgG3 are responsible for initially binding the erythrocytes coated with IgG. This differential affinity of Fc receptors for IgG subclasses explains the different rates of erythro-

TABLE 12-11 *FACTORS THAT AFFECT THE RATE OF HEMOLYSIS IN IMMUNE HEMOLYTIC ANEMIAS*

1. Class of immunoglobulin (Ig) coating the erythrocytes. For the IgG subclasses, the affinity of macrophage receptors and rate of hemolysis is greatest for IgG3 and IgG1.

2. The number of Ig molecules per erythrocyte. High density antigens bind more Ig per cell than low density antigens.

3. Ability of the Ig to activate complement. IgM and IgG (IgG1 and IgG3) can activate complement. IgG2 is less efficient and IgG4 is unreactive with complement.

4. Thermal amplitude of the antibody. Warm (37°C) reacting antibodies may cause hemolysis but cold (0–4°C) reacting antibodies do not.

5. The activity level of macrophages.

cyte survival based on the subclass of IgG bound to the cell. It has been shown that IgG2 and IgG4 antibodies have little effect on erythrocyte survival, and 35% of individuals with IgG1-sensitized erythrocytes have no signs of decreased cell survival.[10] Thus, the class of antibody coating the erythrocyte is important in determining the severity of hemolysis.

A macrophage receptor for IgA has recently been cloned.[11] Although unusual, IgA may be responsible for decreased erythrocyte survival by a mechanism similar to that for IgG.

It is controversial as to whether IgM can cause immune-mediated hemolysis other than through complement activation. Macrophages do not have receptors for IgM. It is possible, however, that IgM can act synergistically with IgG to destroy erythrocytes.[12]

Second, the amount of antibody bound to the erythrocyte and its avidity for the erythrocyte antigen is important in determining the rate of hemolysis. It has been shown that a certain number of IgG molecules per erythrocyte are needed for hemolysis to occur.[10,13] If the density of the antigens on the erythrocyte membrane is increased, more antibodies can be bound. Thus, autoantibodies specific for high density antigens are more likely to cause hemolysis than autoantibodies to low-density antigens.

Third, antibodies that are able to activate complement may increase the rate of hemolysis. Complement activation opsonizes the sensitized cell and leads to an increase in the rate of removal by macrophages via complement receptors. The classes of immunoglobulin that have the ability to activate complement are IgM and IgG. The subclasses of IgG have differing potencies for complement activation as follows: IgG1 > IgG3 > IgG2 > IgG4.[13]

Fourth, the thermal amplitude of the antibody is the maximum temperature at which the antibodies exhibit activity. Most warm-reacting IgG antibodies will cause clinical symptoms of hemolytic anemia because optimal reactivity of the antibody is 37° C (body temperature). Cold-reacting antibodies may cause hemolysis, depending on the thermal range of reactivity. Cold-reacting antibodies bind to antigens better at 4° C. However, pathologic cold agglutinins have a reactivity up to 32° C. When the peripheral circulation cools to this temperature, the antibody attaches to the cell and activates complement.[14] After warming to 37° C, the antibody dissociates, but the complement remains fixed to the cell membrane (Fig. 12-7). Naturally occurring cold reactive antibodies with a thermal amplitude of 20° to 25° C cause no in vivo destruction.

Fifth, the activity of macrophages also is involved with hemolytic anemia. The ability of the individual's macrophages to sequester and remove sensitized cells is probably an important determinant in the rate of hemolysis. In most patients receiving glucocorticoids, hemolysis is dramatically slowed. This response is most likely mediated by a suppression in macrophage activity.

● Laboratory identification of sensitized erythrocytes

Whenever immune hemolytic anemia is suspected, tests to detect and identify the causative antibody are indicated.

IgM antibodies can be detected by agglutination reactions between test sera and appropriate erythrocytes suspended in saline. These IgM antibodies are referred to as *complete antibodies*. IgG antibodies do not agglutinate saline-suspended cells and are referred to as *incomplete antibodies*. Detection of these IgG antibodies requires a technique using antisera to human IgG. This difference in the ability of IgG and IgM to cause agglutination can be explained on the basis of the difference in size of the two antibodies. The erythrocyte *zeta potential* is an electrostatic potential created by a difference in the charge density of the inner and outer layers of the ionic cloud of the erythrocyte when cells are suspended in saline. This force tends to keep the erythrocytes about 25 nm apart in solution. Thus, any antibody that causes agglutination of saline- or plasma-suspended cells must be large enough to span the 25 nm gap between cells. The maximum span of the IgG molecule is about 14 nm, and it cannot reach antigens on two separate cells to cause agglutination. On the other hand, the IgM is a pentamer with a possible span of 35 nm; therefore, it can overcome the electrostatic forces separating the cells (Fig. 12-8).

The antihuman globulin (AHG) test, sometimes referred to as the Coombs test, is the specific laboratory procedure designed to detect erythrocytes sensitized with IgG and/or complement. The AHG test has two applications: direct and indirect.

DIRECT ANTIHUMAN GLOBULIN TEST

The direct antihuman globulin test (DAT or direct Coombs test) detects erythrocytes that have been sensitized with antibody and/or complement in vivo. This test should always be performed in suspected cases of AIHA, as it will differentiate AIHA from all other types of hemolytic anemia. The procedure involves mixing polyspecific broad spectrum antisera (anti-IgG and anticomplement), Coombs' serum, or antihuman globulin (AHG), with saline-washed patient cells. The washing of cells removes any traces of plasma proteins not actually attached to the cell membrane. The AHG antiserum contains divalent antibodies that are capable of attaching to the Fc region of the immunoglobulins on two separate cells, thus bridging the gap between cells and leading to the lattice formation known as agglutination (Fig. 12-9). Agglutination of patient cells or hemolysis by this antisera is considered positive evidence for the presence of IgG (incomplete antibodies) and/or complement components on the cells.

A positive test with polyspecific AHG antiserum should be followed by a DAT with antiserum that reacts specifically with either immunoglobulin or complement (monospecific antiserum to IgG or complement) to determine the type of protein bound to the erythrocyte. IgG antibodies may be found with or without complement attached. Therefore, if the DAT with anti-IgG is positive, the test with anticomplement (anti-C3d and anti-C4) may be positive or negative. If the anti-IgG test is positive, the antibody can be eluted from the cell by an elution process and the eluate reacted with a panel of cells of known antigenic makeup to identify the specificity of the antibody.

If an autoantibody is IgM, only complement will be

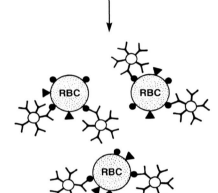

RBC's with attached
IgM at temperatures
<37°C
(Probably occurs
in circulation in
extremities)

+

Complement

Complement in serum

37° C

RBC's with both IgM
and complement
attached

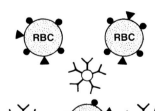

RBC's with only
complement attached;
IgM elutes from the cell

FIGURE 12-7. Cold reacting IgM antibodies attach to the cell and activate complement on the cell membrane at temperatures below 37° C. As the cell enters the warm circulation, the antibody detaches from the cell but the complement (C3b) remains. These complement-coated cells are said to be sensitized cells and are removed by liver macrophages.

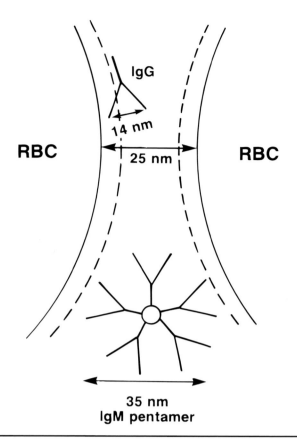

FIGURE 12-8. The zeta potential of red cells keep the cells about 25 nm apart when suspended in saline. IgG antibodies have a span of about 14 nm, not enough to bridge the gap between cells and cause agglutination. IgM antibodies, however, are pentamers with a span of about 35 nm, a distance sufficient to bridge the space between cells and cause agglutination.

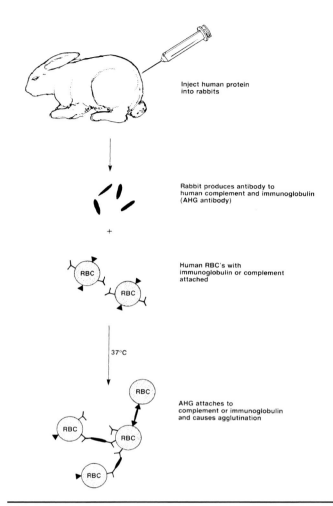

FIGURE 12-9. The direct antihuman globulin test involves mixing antihuman globulin (AHG) serum with patient's red blood cells (RBC). If the cells are sensitized in vivo with either antibody or complement, the antibodies in the AHG serum will attach to neighboring cells resulting in agglutination.

detected on the erythrocytes as the IgM dissociates from the cells in the warmer part of the circulation. The anti-C3 component of the AHG antisera reacts with the C3-sensitized erythrocyte, resulting in a positive DAT.

INDIRECT ANTIHUMAN GLOBULIN TEST

The indirect antihuman globulin test is used to detect antibodies in the patient's serum (as opposed to antibodies on patients' cells in the DAT) that will react with defined erythrocyte antigens. A patient serum sample is reacted with erythrocytes that contain the defined specific antigens. After a specified incubation period, the cells are washed free of excess serum, and the AHG antiserum is added. If antibody reacts with the corresponding erythrocyte antigen during the initial incubation period, the cells will agglutinate with AHG (Fig. 12-10). A positive indirect AHG test is indicative of either isoimmunization (immunization to antigens from another individual) or of the presence of free autoantibody in the patient's serum. Free autoantibody may be present when there are large amounts of autoantibody with a low erythrocyte-binding affinity or when the cells' antigenic sites are saturated with antibody.

Specimens collected in tubes with ethylenediaminetetra-acetate (EDTA) are preferred to clotted specimens for AHG testing. The reason for this is that EDTA chelates $Ca++$ and $Mg++$, preventing the in vitro binding of complement to erythrocytes mediated by naturally occurring cold reactive antibodies (anti-H and anti-I). However, in vivo-bound complement will be detected when using an EDTA specimen.

NEGATIVE DAT IN AIHA

In some cases, antibody cannot be detected on the erythrocytes, even though erythrocyte survival is markedly decreased. In these cases, the antibody may be present on the cell, but there may be an insufficient number of antibodies to be detected with the DAT. The DAT will detect concentrations as low as 100 to 500 molecules of IgG per cell, but the in vivo removal of sensitized cells by macrophages may occur at much lower concentrations. Thus, the in vivo lifespan of the sensitized cell may be significantly shortened, as evidenced by the clinical findings of

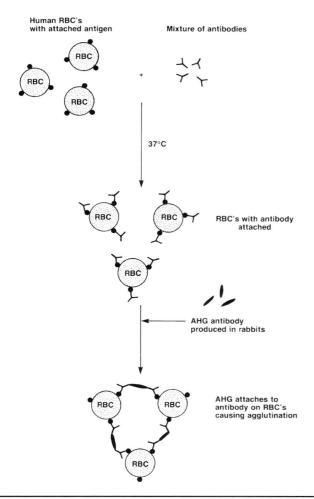

Human RBC's with attached antigen

Mixture of antibodies

+

37°C

RBC's with antibody attached

AHG antibody produced in rabbits

AHG attaches to antibody on RBC's causing agglutination

FIGURE 12-10. The indirect antiglobulin test is primarily used to detect antibodies in the patient's serum. In this test, the patient's serum is incubated with red blood cells (RBC) of known antigenic makeup. This incubation is followed by reaction of the washed cells with AHG serum. If antibody from patients serum reacted with the corresponding antigen on the red blood cells, the AHG serum will cause agglutination of the cells.

a typical hemolytic anemia, but the concentration of antibodies on the cell may be insufficient to give a positive DAT.[10] More sensitive techniques, such as enzyme-linked DAT, may detect antibodies not detected by the conventional DAT technique.

POSITIVE DAT IN HEALTHY INDIVIDUALS

In contrast, some patients test positive for DAT but show no evidence of hemolytic anemia. The reason some individuals have autoantibody coating their erythrocytes and no evidence of hemolytic disease is not clear. Several factors may be responsible for this phenomenon:

1. The individual's macrophages may not be as active in removing sensitized cells as the macrophages in individuals with hemolytic disease.
2. Patients with hypergammaglobulinemia may have a positive test result for DAT because of nonspecific

binding of immunoglobulins to the erythrocytes. This also may occur in patients receiving high-dose intravenous gamma globulin.

3. The thermal amplitude of the antibody may be less than 37° C.
4. The amount of antibody bound to cells may not be sufficient to cause decreased erythrocyte lifespan.
5. The subclass of antibody sensitizing the cell may not be recognized by macrophages. The macrophage Fc receptors have low affinity for the IgG2 and IgG4 subclasses. Erythrocytes coated with these immunoglobulins will give a positive direct DAT because the DAT antiserum contains anti-IgG to all subclasses. However, survival of the cells in vivo will be normal.
6. Patients taking certain drugs (i.e., α-methyldopa) may have a positive DAT but normal erythrocyte survival.
7. The positive DAT may be due to the presence of complement on erythrocytes. Increased amounts of C3d may be found on the erythrocytes of individuals who are ill. C3d, however, does not cause decreased erythrocyte survival.

● Autoimmune hemolytic anemias (AIHA)

The immune system normally ignores self-antigenic determinants such as occur on an individual's erythrocytes preventing autoimmunization. These antigens may, however, stimulate an immune response if injected into another individual. The mechanisms that prevent autoimmunization but permit alloimmunization are collectively known as *immune tolerance*.[13]

The mechanism of antibody formation in AIHA is unknown. It is generally accepted that autoimmune diseases occur because of a defect in the mechanism regulating immune tolerance. Suppressor T-lymphocytes normally induce tolerance to self-antigens by inhibiting the antibody producing activity of B-lymphocytes to these antigens. Loss of this suppressor cell activity could result in the formation of antibodies against self. The cause of this defect is unknown, but since many cases of AIHA are associated with microbial infection, neoplasia, or drug administration, these agents may be involved in the immune system dysfunction.

WARM AUTOIMMUNE HEMOLYTIC ANEMIA

Warm AIHA is the most common form of AIHA (70% of cases).[15] Warm AIHA is mediated by IgG antibodies with maximal reactivity at 37° C. Rarely, the antibody may be IgM or IgA. In a majority (87%) of warm AIHA cases, erythrocytes are sensitized with IgG and complement or IgG alone. Only 13% of cases are sensitized with complement alone.[15] Most often, the antibody involved is IgG1 or IgG3.

Hemolytic anemia that is associated with no apparent underlying cause is termed primary or idiopathic hemolytic anemia. About 60% of cases of warm AIHA are idiopathic.

The idiopathic type may occur acutely, with severe anemia developing over 2 to 3 days. In most individuals with this type of anemia, the hemolysis is self-limited with a duration of several weeks to several years. In others, the hemolysis is chronic and unabating.

Those AIHA that are associated with underlying disorders are referred to as secondary hemolytic anemias. These underlying disorders include: (1) lymphoproliferative disease, including chronic lymphocytic leukemia, and Hodgkin's disease (many children with idiopathic AIHA will eventually develop a lymphoproliferative disease, especially Hodgkin's disease)[16]; (2) neoplastic diseases; (3) other autoimmune disorders, including systemic lupus erythematosus and rheumatoid arthritis; (4) certain viral and bacterial infections (e.g., viral hepatitis); (5) some chronic inflammatory diseases (e.g., ulcerative colitis).[7]

Pathophysiology The warm autoantibody in AIHA is reactive with antigens on the patient's erythrocytes. Even after the hemolytic episode has abated, serum taken during the active form of the disease will react with the patient's erythrocytes. This suggests the antigen is not transiently expressed on the cell membrane. Most often (70%), the specificity of the antibody is directed against the Rh system, although other antigen systems may be involved. When directed against the Rh system, the antibody may be specific for a single antigen such as auto-anti-D, or, more commonly, the antibody will react with all erythrocytes except Rh null cells.[10] Some antibodies may appear to have specificity against a particular antigen such as anti-E, but the antibody can be absorbed from patient serum with erythrocytes that lack the corresponding antigen. The patient also is negative for the antigen. The epitope against which these mimicking antibodies are directed has not been defined.[10]

Most hemolysis is extravascular. The Fc portion of the IgG antibody on the erythrocyte mediates the attachment of the cell to splenic macrophages via Fc receptors. Most often, this process results in erythrocyte membrane fragmentation as the antibody–antigen complex is pitted from the cell. This is followed by sphering, as the membrane reseals itself. Alternatively, the whole cell may be engulfed upon initial attachment to macrophages. Although complement is not needed for cell destruction, if both antibody and complement are on the cell membrane, phagocytosis is enhanced. If erythrocyte destruction exceeds the compensatory capacity of the bone marrow to produce new cells, anemia develops. Direct complement-mediated intravascular hemolysis associated with IgM antibodies in warm AIHA is rare.

Clinical findings The most common presenting symptoms in idiopathic AIHA are related to anemia. Progressive weakness, dizziness, and jaundice are common. Secondary AIHA may present with signs and symptoms of the underlying disorder obscuring the features of the hemolytic anemia. Mild to modest hepatosplenomegaly may be present, but massive splenic enlargement is suggestive of an underlying lymphoproliferative disorder.

Laboratory findings

PERIPHERAL BLOOD Moderate to severe normocytic, normochromic anemia is typical, but, in well-compensated he-

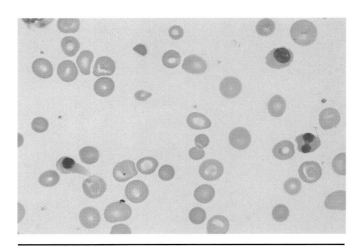

FIGURE 12-11. A blood smear from a patient with warm autoimmune hemolytic anemia. There is marked anisocytosis due to the presence of spherocytes and large polychromatophilic erythrocytes. The nucleated cells are normoblasts (250× original magnification; Wright stain).

molytic disease, anemia may be mild or absent. In well-compensated hemolytic disease, the only abnormal parameters may be a positive DAT and an increase in reticulocytes. Depending on the degree of reticulocytosis, macrocytosis may be present. Reticulocytes are invariably increased in uncomplicated hemolytic disease. The reticulocyte production index may be as high as 6 or 7.

The blood smear frequently shows erythrocyte abnormalities suggestive of a hemolytic process. Spherocytes, schistocytes, and other poikilocytes, polychromasia, and nucleated erythrocytes are characteristic (Fig. 12-11). The spherocytes of AIHA are usually more heterogeneous than the spherocytes associated with hereditary spherocytosis. This anisocytosis is readily noted when examining the blood smear and also is indicated by an increase in red cell distribution width (RDW) on automated hematology analyzers. Erythrophagocytosis by monocytes may be seen. The engulfed erythrocyte is readily detected within the monocyte if the cell still contains its pink staining hemoglobin. If the hemoglobin has leaked out of the cell, however, only colorless vacuoles within the monocyte may be seen. Leukocyte counts are normal or increased with neutrophilia. Platelet counts are usually normal or slightly decreased. When severe thrombocytopenia accompanies warm AIHA, the disease is called *Evan's syndrome*.

BONE MARROW The bone marrow shows erythroid hyperplasia. Erythrophagocytosis by macrophages may be seen. Compensatory bone marrow response may be less than expected in concomitant folic acid deficiency. In chronic hemolysis, the folic acid requirement increases two to three times normal; without folic acid supplements, the stores of this vital nutrient are quickly depleted. If the patient contracts certain viral infections, bone marrow suppression may occur, leading to life-threatening anemia (aplastic crisis).

OTHER LABORATORY TESTS The DAT is a useful test to distinguish the immune nature of this hemolytic anemia from nonimmune-mediated hemolytic anemias. The test is usually positive with polyspecific and anti-IgG monospecific antiserum. Reaction with anti-C3d is positive in about half the cases of warm AIHA.

Other laboratory findings are nonspecific but reflect the hemolytic component of the condition. Osmotic fragility is increased in the presence of spherocytosis. Total serum bilirubin is increased up to 5 mg/dL, with the unconjugated fraction constituting most of the increase. Urine and fecal urobilinogen are increased. Respiratory excretion of carbon monoxide is increased.

Serum haptoglobin is often decreased, especially when hemolysis is severe, but hemoglobinemia, hemoglobinuria, methemoglobinemia, and hemosiderinuria are unusual findings. These indicators of intravascular hemolysis are seen only in hyperacute hemolytic episodes.

Reaction of patients' serum with screening cells typically shows no agglutination at room temperature or at 37° C, but agglutination is observed with the DAT. The autocontrol using patient serum and patient erythrocytes shows similar reactions.

Differential diagnosis Warm AIHA, with the presence of spherocytes, may be differentiated from hereditary spherocytosis by the DAT. Antibodies are not responsible for the formation of spherocytes in hereditary spherocytosis (HS); therefore the DAT in this condition is negative. The autohemolysis test is abnormal in both HS and in AIHA with spherocytes. In HS, autohemolysis is significantly corrected by the addition of glucose. However, glucose does not correct hemolysis in AIHA.

Therapy In self-limiting hemolytic disorders without life-threatening anemia, transfusion therapy is not necessary. In those instances when transfusion is indicated, cross-matching to find a suitable donor is difficult since the patient's autoantibody is usually directed against a high incidence antigen. If serologically compatible blood cannot be found, donor cells with the least incompatibility are usually chosen. The problem arises, however, that donor cells may be destroyed as rapidly as the patient's own erythrocytes.

Glucocorticoids have been administered to patients with this disorder in an attempt to suppress macrophage sequestration of sensitized cells and to produce immunosuppression.[17] About 20% of patients undergo complete remission with this therapy, and many more show significant improvement.

Splenectomy may be indicated when severe anemia is unresponsive to glucocorticoid therapy. If, however, the antibody concentration remains high, sensitized erythrocytes may be removed in the liver.

Immunosuppressive drugs are reserved for treatment of patients unresponsive to glucocorticoids or splenectomy. The drugs may suppress synthesis of autoantibody.

Plasma exchange and plasmapheresis have been successful in an effort to dilute or remove the antibody in some cases.

TABLE 12-12 *AUTOIMMUNE HEMOLYTIC ANEMIA CAUSED BY COLD-REACTING ANTIBODIES*

Cold hemagglutinin disease (CHD)
Primary   —idiopathic
Secondary—*Mycoplasma pneumoniae*
infectious mononucleosis
lymphoproliferative diseases
Paroxysmal cold hemoglobinuria

In patients with secondary AIHA, treatment of the underlying disease is important.[17]

COLD AUTOIMMUNE HEMOLYTIC ANEMIA

The AIHAs caused by cold-reacting antibodies are listed in Table 12-12. Cold AIHA is associated with an IgM (rarely IgG or IgA) antibody that fixes complement and is reactive below 37° C. The disorder, also termed cold hemagglutinin disease (CHD), is less common (occurring in about 16% of all immune hemolytic anemias) than anemia associated with warm antibodies.

Cold AIHA like warm AIHA may be either idiopathic or secondary. Idiopathic cold agglutinin disease is usually a chronic disease, occurring after age 50[18]; the antibody is usually a monoclonal kappa light chain IgM antibody. The antibody in secondary cold AIHA is usually a polyclonal IgM antibody.[10] The secondary form is associated with *Mycoplasma pneumoniae* infections and infectious mononucleosis (an acute, self-limiting type) and lymphoproliferative disorders (a chronic form typically found in older individuals).

A more severe type of cold AIHA, paroxysmal cold hemoglobinuria (PCH) is associated with a biphasic cold-reacting IgG antibody and is discussed in the next section.

Pathophysiology The extent of CHD is related to the thermal range of the antibody. Those cold-reacting antibodies with a wide range of activity up to 32° C can cause problems when the peripheral circulation cools to this temperature. In the cool environment, IgM complement-fixing antibody binds to the erythrocyte and activates complement. As the cell enters the warm circulation, the antibody dissociates from the cell, but complement remains attached. Complement-mediated lysis accounts for most of the erythrocyte destruction. Complement injury may be caused by direct lysis (intravascular hemolysis) if the complement sequence proceeds through C8 and C9. More commonly, complement activation is only partial (through C3b), opsonizing the cell for sequestration by macrophages via C3b receptors (extravascular hemolysis).

The cold-reacting antibody is usually directed against the I antigen, although in CHD associated with infectious mononucleosis and lymphoproliferative disease, the antibody has anti-i specificity.[19] The I-antigen is expressed on the erythrocytes of almost all adults, whereas the i-antigen is expressed on the erythrocytes of infants (younger than 2 years old). The I-antigen specificity of the antibody may be defined by reactivity of the patient's serum with all adult erythrocytes but minimal or no reactivity with infant cells.

The second most common specificity for cold autoagglutinins is the Pr antigens. These antigens are O-linked sialylated oligosaccharide structures residing within the N-terminal amino acid residues of glycophorins A, B, and C.[14] These antigens are sensitive to protease and neuraminidase and are expressed on both adult and infant erythrocytes. Other specificities are anti-Gd, anti-Sa, anti-Lud, anti-F1, anti-Vo, anti-A$_1$, anti-Type II H, anti-IA, anti-Ju, anti-IP$_1$, anti-D, and anti-M-like.[10,14]

Clinical findings The disease may be associated with a chronic hemolytic anemia with or without jaundice. In others, hemolysis is episodic and associated only with chilling. The agglutination of erythrocytes occurs in areas of the body that cool to the thermal range of the antibody, causing sludging of the blood flow within capillaries. The skin turns white, then blue, and, on rewarming, red. Discoloration is frequently accompanied by numbness, tingling, and pain. These vascular changes are referred to as *acrocyanosis* or *Raynaud's phenomenon*. The condition primarily affects the extremities, especially the fingers and toes. Hemoglobinuria accompanies the acute hemolytic attacks. Splenomegaly may be present.

Laboratory findings Blood counts are difficult to perform unless both the blood and diluting reagents are kept warm. Often, the first indication of the presence of unsuspected cold agglutinins is from blood counts performed on electronic cell counters. The erythrocyte count is inappropriately decreased for the hemoglobin content, and the MCV is falsely elevated. These erroneous values occur when erythrocyte agglutinates are sized and counted as individual cells. The hematocrit calculated from this erroneous erythrocyte count and MCV is falsely low. The MCH and MCHC, calculated from the erythrocyte count, and hematocrit are falsely elevated. The hemoglobin assay is accurate as the cells are lysed to determine this parameter. Accurate cell counts may be obtained by warming blood and all diluting reagents to 37° C. Visible autoagglutination can be observed in anticoagulated blood as the blood cools to room temperature.

When blood counts are performed at 37° C, the results indicate a mild to moderate normocytic, normochromic anemia. Reticulocytes are increased. The blood film shows polychromasia, some spherocytes, rouleaux, or clumps of erythrocytes, and, sometimes, nucleated erythrocytes (Fig. 12-12). Erythrophagocytosis may be seen but is more typical on smears made from buffy coats after the blood has incubated at room temperature. Leukocyte and platelet counts are usually normal. Leukocytosis may occur during acute hemolysis as the result of a bone marrow stress response. The bone marrow exhibits normoblastic hyperplasia.

The serum bilirubin is increased up to 3 mg/dL, with most of the increase caused by indirect bilirubin. Haptoglobin is decreased or absent. Acute hemolytic attacks are accompanied by hemoglobinemia and hemoglobinuria. Hemosiderinuria may be found in patients who have had chronic hemoglobinuria.

The Ehrlich finger test is used to demonstrate hemolysis in the microcirculation at cold temperatures. The venous

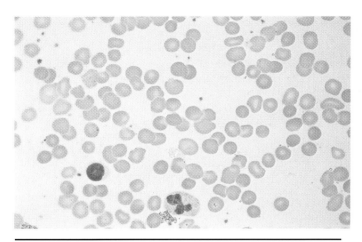

FIGURE 12-12. Cold autoimmune hemolytic anemia from a patient with chronic lymphocytic anemia. Some of the erythrocytes are in small clumps. There are also spherocytes present. (PB; 250× original magnification; Wright stain).

blood flow is stopped on two fingers (one on each hand) with a rubber band. One finger is immersed in cold water (20° C) and the other in warm water (37° C). Using capillary tubes, blood is taken from each finger, and the tubes are centrifuged in a microhematocrit centrifuge. The plasma layer is examined for hemolysis. A positive test shows hemolysis in the blood from the finger incubated in cold water, but no hemolysis in the blood from the finger incubated in warm water.

Differentiation of CHD agglutinins from benign cold agglutinins (Table 12-13) The serum of most normal individuals exhibit the presence of cold autoantibodies when the serum and cells are incubated at 4° C. These antibodies are termed benign cold autoagglutinins because their thermal

TABLE 12-13 *DIFFERENTIATION OF PATHOLOGIC COLD AGGLUTININS FOUND IN CHD FROM BENIGN COLD AGGLUTININS FOUND IN NORMAL INDIVIDUALS*

Characteristic of Agglutinin	Pathologic Agglutinins	Benign Agglutinins
Antibody class	IgM	IgM
Antibody specificity	Usually anti-I but in secondary CHD may be anti-i	Anti-I
Antibody clonality	Monoclonal in idiopathic type; polyclonal in secondary type	Polyclonal
Thermal amplitude	0°–31°	0°–4°
Agglutination at room temperature	Significant	Not present
Agglutination in albumin	Enhanced	No effect
Titer	Usually >1:1,000	<1:64
DAT	Positive with polyspecific AHG and monospecific anti-complement	Negative

TABLE 12-14 *CLINICAL CRITERIA FOR THE DIAGNOSIS OF COLD AGGLUTININ SYNDROME*

1. Clinical signs of an acquired hemolytic anema, with a history of acrocyanosis and hemoglobinuria upon exposure to the cold.
2. A positive DAT result using polyspecific antisera
3. A positive DAT result using monospecific C3 antisera
4. A negative DAT result using monospecific IgG antisera
5. The presence of reactivity in the patient's serum due to a cold autoantibody
6. A cold agglutinin titer of 1000 or greater in saline at 4°C, with visible autoagglutination of anticoagulated blood at room temperature.

(From: Harmening, DM: *Clinical hematology and fundamentals of hemostasis.* 2nd edition. Philadelphia: FA Davis. 1992).

amplitude and concentration is not high enough to cause clinical problems. Whenever pathologic cold agglutinins are suspected as the cause of anemia, laboratory tests should be performed to differentiate the harmless cold agglutinins from the pathologic ones. The DAT with polyspecific AHG and monospecific anticomplement antiserum is positive in pathologic cold agglutinin disease but negative or only weakly positive with benign cold agglutinins. The DAT, using monospecific IgG antisera, is negative in both CHD and with benign cold agglutinins.

The cold agglutinin test should be performed whenever a diagnosis of cold AIHA is suspected. This test demonstrates the ability of the pathologic antibody to agglutinate the patient's cells at temperatures from 0° to 20° C in saline and up to 32° C in albumin suspensions. The reaction is reversible with agglutinates dispersing at 37° C. With benign cold antibodies, agglutination occurs at 0° to 4° C and may occur up to 20° C. Agglutination is not enhanced, however, in albumin suspensions. Titers of benign cold agglutinins reach 1:64 in normal individuals; in cold agglutinin disease, the titer is usually 1:1000 to 1:30,000. Titers of 1:256 or more, with a positive DAT using monospecific anti-C3 antisera, and a negative DAT using monospecific anti-IgG antisera, are highly suggestive of cold agglutinin disease.

The criteria for a diagnosis of CHD are summarized in Table 12-14.

Therapy Effective relief is usually achieved by keeping the extremities warm. Difficult cases with chronic hemolysis may require more aggressive treatment such as chlorambucil or plasma exchange. Splenectomy is not usually effective.

PAROXYSMAL COLD HEMOGLOBINURIA

Paroxysmal cold hemoglobinuria (PCH) is a rare disorder that may occur at any age. This form of AIHA is characterized by massive, intermittent, acute hemolysis and hemoglobinuria after cold exposure. It was more common at the turn of the century, probably as a result of its association with syphillis.

Pathophysiology PCH was the first hemolytic anemia for which a mechanism of hemolysis was established. This

hemolytic anemia is distinct from the other cold AIHA because of the nature of the offending antibody. It is not caused by IgM antibody but rather by a biphasic IgG antibody, the *Donath-Landsteiner* (D-L) antibody. Biphasic refers to the two incubation temperatures necessary for optimal lysis of the erythrocytes. The antibody reacts with erythrocytes in the capillaries at temperatures less than 15° C, where it avidly binds the early-acting complement components. Upon warming to 37° C, the terminal complement components are activated on the cell membrane, causing cell lysis. The antibody disperses from the cell at 37° C. The PCH antibody is specific for the P-antigen.

The disease was previously associated with congenital or tertiary syphilis. It is now also seen in children with viral infections (e.g., measles, mumps). It is usually a transient disorder resolving after recovery from the infectious process. The disease also may be idiopathic.

Clinical findings After cold exposure, the patient experiences sudden onset of chills, back and leg pain, and fever, followed by hemoglobinuria. Raynaud's phenomenon may occur during acute episodes followed by jaundice.

Laboratory findings Between attacks, the peripheral blood is relatively normal except for anemia. The degree of anemia depends on the frequency and severity of hemolytic attacks. During the attack, there is a sharp drop in hemoglobin concentration accompanied by hemoglobinemia, methemalbuminemia, and hemoglobinuria. Leukopenia caused by abrupt neutropenia, a shift to the left, erythrophagocytosis, and spherocytes accompany erythrocyte lysis. Serum bilirubin is elevated. Serum complement and haptoglobin are decreased.

A weakly positive DAT with anticomplement antisera may appear and persist for several days after the hemolytic episode. Antibodies on the cells are not usually detected by the DAT since the D-L antibody elutes at warm temperatures. The indirect AHG test may be positive, if performed in the cold. Normal erythrocytes incubated with patient serum reacts more positively in the indirect AHG test than patient cells.

D-L antibodies are not usually present in high titers, but their presence may be verified by the biphasic reaction noted in the D-L test (Table 12-15). In this test, the pa-

TABLE 12-15 *DONATH-LANDSTEINER (D-L) TEST FOR DETECTING THE PRESENCE OF D-L ANTIBODIES. TWO TUBES OF PATIENT'S BLOOD IS USED, ONE TUBE SERVES AS THE CONTROL AND THE OTHER AS THE TEST*

Procedure	Control	Test
1. Incubate for 30 min. at	37° C	4°
2. Incubate for 30 min. at	37° C	37°
3. Centrifuge and observe plasma for presence of hemolysis		
4. Interpretation		
D-L antibodies present	No hemolysis	Hemolysis
No D-L antibodies present	No hemolysis	No hemolysis

tient's blood is collected in two clot tubes; one is incubated at 4° C for 30 minutes and the other at 37° C for 30 minutes. This is followed by an incubation of both tubes at 37° C. The antibody, if present, causes intense hemolysis in the tube initially incubated at 4° C upon warming. No hemolysis is present in the tube kept at 37° C. Hemolysis in this test also may occur in cold hemagglutinin disease, but the hemolysis occurs very slowly. Table 12-16 compares PCH and CHD.

Therapy PCH associated with acute infections terminates spontaneously upon recovery from the infection. The chronic form of the disease is best treated by avoiding exposure to the cold.

DRUG-RELATED HEMOLYTIC ANEMIAS

Drug-related immune hemolytic anemia is the result of an immune-mediated hemolysis precipitated by ingestion of certain drugs. The drug does not cause erythrocyte injury by itself.

Drugs also may cause immune destruction of other blood cells. Anemia, thrombocytopenia, and agranulocytosis may occur together or separately. It has been proposed that the ability of a drug to precipitate the production of antibodies against different cell lines is related to the affinity of the drug to the cells.[20] The greater the affinity, the more likely sensitization against the drug–cell complex will occur.

Many drugs have been found that induce an immune-

TABLE 12-16 *COMPARISON OF COLD HEMAGGLUTININ DISEASE (CHD) AND PAROXYSMAL COLD HEMOGLOBINURIA (PCH)*

	CHD	PCH
Patient	Usually adults >50 years of age	Usually children after viral infection
Clinical findings	Acrocyanosis	Chills, fever, hemoglobinuria
DAT	Positive with polyspecific AHG and monospecific C3	Postiive with polyspecific AHG and monospecific C3
Donath-Landsteiner test	negative	positive
Antibody class	IgM	Biphasic IgG (Donath-Landsteiner)
Antibody specificity	Anti-I	Anti-P
Thermal amplitude of antibody	Up to 31° C	Under 20° C
Hemolysis	Chronic extravascular/ intravascular	Acute, intravascular
Therapy	Avoid the cold	Supportive; treatment of underlying illness

TABLE 12-17 *DRUGS THAT MAY INDUCE IMMUNE HEMOLYTIC ANEMIA*

Mechanism	Drug
Hapten	Penicillin Cephalasporin Tetracycline
Immune Complex Formation (innocent bystander)	Stibophen P-Anunosalicyclic acid Quinidine Aminopyrine Anhistine Cefotaxime Ceftazidime Ceftriaxone Chlorambucil Chlorpromazine Dipyrone Doxepin Fluorouracil Insecticides Isoniazid Nomifensine Sulfonamides Sulfonylurea Suprofen Teniposide Thiazides Tolmetin Phenacetin Quinine Rifampicin
Membrane Modification	Cephalosporin
Autoantibody (α-methyldopa-type)	α-methyldopa Levodopa Mefenamic acid Procainamide

(Adapted from Wintrobe's Clinical Hematology, Lee GR, et al., 1993)

mediated hemolytic anemia (Table 12-17). This type of hemolysis must be distinguished from both drug-induced, nonimmune hemolysis that occurs secondary to erythrocyte metabolic defects (G6PD deficiency) and from spontaneous autoimmune disorders. The distinction is important because drug induced, immune hemolytic anemias are the result of a normal immune response to drug-induced alteration of the erythrocyte antigenicity. The hemolytic anemia is considered benign because a "cure" involves only withdrawal of the drug and primarily supportive treatment.

Four mechanisms have been hypothesized to explain drug-induced immune hemolysis (Table 12-18): (1) drug adsorption; (2) immune complex formation; (3) autoantibody induction; and (4) membrane modification. Each of these mechanisms will cause a positive DAT with polyspecific AHG and with one or more monospecific antisera (Table 12-18).

Drug adsorption (hapten-type) In this type of drug-induced hemolysis, it is proposed that the offending drug or its metabolites bind to proteins on the erythrocyte mem-

TABLE 12.18 *REACTIONS IN DRUG-INDUCED HEMOLYTIC ANEMIA*

Type of Reaction	Role of Drug/Drug Metabolite	Nature of Attachment of Antibody to Erythrocyte	Direct Antiglobulin Test	Mechanism of Cell Destruction
Hapten	Cell-bound hapten	Binds to cell-bound drug	Positive (reaction to Ig)	Adhesion to macrophages via Fc and phagocytosis
Immune Complex (innocent bystander)	Drug combines with a plasma protein to form an antigenic complex in plasma; antigen-antibody-complement complex forms in plasma.	Adsorption of antigen-antibody-complement complex to cell membrane	Positive (usually reaction to complement)	Complement lysis
Membrane Modification	Modification of cell membrane	Nonspecific attachment of proteins as well as IgG and complement (non-immune)	Positive (to a variety of proteins)	No hemolysis
Autoantibody induction (α-methyldopa-type)	Triggers formation of anti-erythrocyte antibody	Binds to native antigens on erythrocyte	Positive (reaction to Ig)	Adhesion to macrophages via Fc and phagocytosis

(Adapted from: Lee, G. R., et al.: Wintrobe's Clinical Hematology. Philadelphia, Lea & Febiger, 1993).

brane, creating an immunogenic complex on the cell membrane. If antibodies are produced against the drug–cell complex, they will react with the complex on the erythrocyte membrane. Thus, the cell becomes coated with antibody (Fig. 12-13). The DAT is usually positive. Both IgG and IgM antibodies may be formed, but only the IgG antibody causes hemolysis. Complement activation does not usually occur. Penicillin and cephalosporin are the two most common drugs associated with the formation of haptenic groups on erythrocytes. Only patients receiving high doses of intravenous penicillin have the penicillin coating on their cells. Only a small portion of these individuals will have a positive DAT; even fewer develop hemolysis. Hemoglobinemia and hemoglobinuria do not occur, indicating intravascular hemolysis is not prominent. Hemolysis is extravascular, mediated by Fc receptors on splenic macrophages. The hemolytic anemia usually develops over a 7- to 10-day period. Spherocytes may be present. The reticulocyte count is usually elevated.

A high titer of the IgG penicillin antibody can be detected in the serum. This can be done by incubating the patient's serum with normal donor erythrocytes in the presence and absence of penicillin (indirect AHG test). If antibodies to the penicillin-protein membrane complex are present in the patient's serum, the AHG test with the "penicillinized" erythrocytes is positive and negative with cells without penicillin.

Immune complex formation (innocent bystander)   In this mechanism, the drug or drug metabolite combines with a plasma protein to form a new antigenic plasma complex (neoantigen). Either IgM or IgG antibodies are formed to the new plasma complexes. The antigen–antibody complex (immune complex) formed in the plasma is adsorbed on to the erythrocyte in a nonimmune-mediated reaction (Fig. 12-14). The drug itself has a low affinity for the cell membrane. The attached immune complex usually has the

ability to activate complement. Complement-mediated hemolysis occurs as the C3b-coated erythrocytes are cleared from circulation by macrophages, or the cells may be lysed, if the terminal complement components are activated.

After the immune complex activates complement on the cell membrane, it can dissociate from the membrane and attach to another cell. The immune complex also may bind to leukocytes and platelets and shorten the lifespan of these cells. Most often the hemolytic episode is acute, with signs of intravascular hemolysis (hemoglobinuria, hemoglobinemia). Spherocytes may be present on the blood smear. The DAT with anti-C3 is positive but with anti-IgG is often negative as the antibody complex may dissociate from the membrane. The anti-C3 DAT may remain positive for several months after the hemolytic episode because of the persistence of inactivated complement components (C3d) on the erythrocyte.

Unlike the hemolysis associated with penicillin, only small amounts of the drug are needed to induce immune hemolysis by immune complex formation. Although there are a large number of drugs that can cause this type of reaction, the incidence of drug-induced immune hemolysis by this mechanism is low.

In the laboratory, the antibody is detected only if the drug and complement are present in the test system. Diagnosis is confirmed by incubating the patient's serum with normal erythrocytes in the presence of the offending drug (indirect AHG test). If the antibody is present in the patient's serum, it will combine with the drug–protein complex and the erythrocytes. Subsequently, complement is activated. Specific antiserum to complement is used to demonstrate the deposition of complement on the cell membrane.

Membrane modification   Cephalosporins are capable of modifying the erythrocyte membrane so that normal

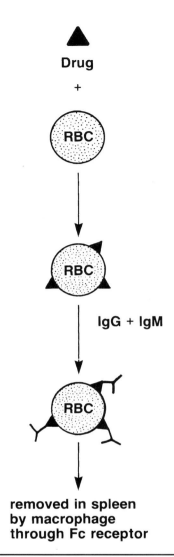

FIGURE 12-13. The mechanism of immune-mediated hemolysis when drug is adsorbed to the red blood cell (RBC) membrane (Hapten-type). The drug combines with the RBC membrane proteins creating a new antigenic complex. Antibodies are formed to the complex precipitating extravascular hemolysis.

plasma proteins (e.g., albumin, globulins) as well as IgG and complement can bind to the membrane in a nonspecific manner. The adsorption of proteins to the membrane is not the result of an immunologic mechanism. The DAT is positive with polyspecific antisera, anti-IgG, and anti-C3, and may be positive with monospecific reagents such as antifibrinogen, antiglobulin, and antialbumin. This nonspecific adsorption is not associated with a hemolytic anemia.

Cephalosporins also can induce a positive DAT through the drug-adsorption mechanism. In this mechanism, anticephalosporin antibodies react with the cephalosporin adsorbed onto the erythrocyte and cause hemolysis. These antibodies can cross-react with penicillin-coated erythrocytes.

Autoantibody induction In approximately 10% to 20% of patients receiving the antihypertensive drug, Aldomet (α-methyldopa), a positive DAT develops after 3 to 6 months. However, hemolytic anemia develops in only 1%. The DAT is dose-dependent: the larger the dose of Aldomet, the more likely the patient is to have a positive DAT. Those in whom hemolytic anemia develops also have a positive indirect AHG test using patient serum and normal erythrocytes. This is because the drug induces the formation of IgG autoantibodies against native erythrocyte antigens. The antibody does not react with the drug itself in vitro. Complement is rarely activated, and the DAT using anti-C3 is usually negative. The mechanism by which antibody production is induced is unknown; however, it has been suggested that α-methyldopa may suppress or alter the function of T suppressor cells, allowing the production of antibody by B cells against self-antigens, or that the drug alters normal erythrocyte antigens so they are no longer recognized as self.[21] Erythrocyte destruction is extravascular, and anemia develops gradually. Serologically, the antibodies are indistinguishable from those of warm autoimmune hemolytic anemia. If the drug is withdrawn, the antibody production gradually stops, but the DAT may remain positive for years.

●
Alloimmune (isoimmune) hemolytic anemia

Hemolytic anemia induced by immunization of an individual with erythrocyte antigens from another individual is known as alloimmune hemolytic anemia. The recipient's erythrocytes lack the antigen(s) present on donor cells. Therefore, the donor's cells are recognized as foreign, inducing the recipient to form antibodies. The antibodies react with donor cells. This type of immunologic destruction of erythrocytes is characteristic of transfusion reactions and HDN.

HEMOLYTIC TRANSFUSION REACTIONS

Transfusion of blood may cause an acute or delayed hemolytic transfusion reaction. The acute reaction is usually the result of laboratory or clerical error in which the patient is given the wrong blood. In these cases, the blood of the donor and recipient are not compatible. Blood that is crossmatched compatible also may stimulate an immune reaction. This type of reaction results in a delayed hemolytic transfusion reaction. The delayed reaction is usually the result of an anamnestic response whereby the donor erythrocytes contain an antigen to which the patient has been previously sensitized. In contrast to AIHA, the antibodies produced in transfusion reactions do not react with the erythrocytes of the person making the antibody. The antibodies cause immunologic destruction of only donor cells. The clinical signs of the patient are the first clue to the adverse reaction taking place in vivo. When an acute transfusion reaction is suspected, the transfusion must be stopped immediately. Laboratory investigation of the reaction then follows.

Pathophysiology Hemolysis of donor cells may be mediated by either IgM antibodies or IgG antibodies. IgM

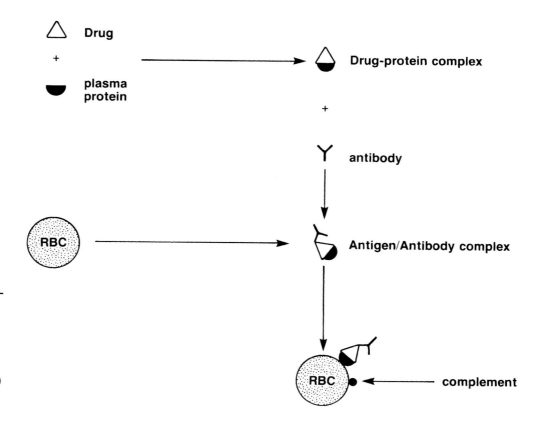

FIGURE 12-14. Immune complex formation may occur when a drug combines with a plasma protein. If antibodies are made to the complex, a hemolytic anemia develops if the drug-protein-antibody complex is adsorbed to the red blood cell (RBC) membrane. The hemolysis is usually complement mediated.

antibodies mediate hemolysis through complement activation. Acute intravascular hemolysis with hemoglobinuria is the result of binding of IgM antibodies to erythrocytes and complete sequential activation of complement components. Subsequently, the release of thromboplastic-like substances from the erythrocyte membrane into the blood may initiate the coagulation cascade. The resulting consumptive coagulopathy (disseminated intravascular coagulation) may damage the kidney by deposition of fibrin in the microvasculature. Specific antibodies, which have been identified to cause this type of hemolysis, are anti-A, anti-B, anti-I, and anti-P_1 and less often anti-Jk^a, anti-K, and anti-Fy^a.

Extravascular hemolysis in the spleen, typical of a delayed hemolytic transfusion reaction, occurs when erythrocytes are coated with IgG antibodies. Although complement is not usually involved, complement, when present, enhances phagocytosis. The speed of the removal depends on the amount of antibody on the cell.

Delayed transfusion reactions occur 2 to 14 days after a transfusion. Hemolysis occurs when the transfused erythrocytes possess an antigen to which the patient has been previously sensitized (through pregnancy or previous transfusion). The antibody to this antigen may not be detected in pretransfusion testing if it is present at concentrations below the sensitivity threshold of the crossmatch test. The antigens on infused donor cells induce a secondary antigenic stimulus. The antibody produced to this stimulus is usually IgG, and hemolysis is extravascular. The first indication of a reaction is a sharp drop in the hemoglobin concentration several days after the transfusion. Intravascular hemolysis also may occur but is less pronounced than in acute reactions. Laboratory investigation reveals a positive DAT because of antibody-coated donor cells in the patient's circulation. Antibodies characteristically associated with a delayed transfusion reaction are in the Kidd System (anti-Jk^a, anti-Jk^b) and Rh system, especially anti-E, anti-c, and anti-D. Others such as anti-K and anti-Fy^a have been reported.

Clinical findings Symptoms of an immediate transfusion reaction begin within minutes to hours after the transfusion is begun. A variety of nonspecific symptoms may occur, including fever, low back pain, sensations of chest compression, hypotension, nausea, and vomiting. Without immediate termination of the transfusion, shock may occur. Anuria, due to tubular necrosis secondary to inadequate renal blood flow, and bleeding are both common complications. The severity of the reaction and extent of organ damage is directly proportional to the amount of blood infused. Transfusions of less than 200 mL do not usually cause severe reactions.

Most delayed transfusion reactions cause few signs or symptoms. The most common sign is unexplained fever several days after the transfusion.

Laboratory findings The laboratory findings will vary depending on whether the transfusion reaction is acute or delayed. The acute reaction is usually accompanied by intravascular hemolysis, and the delayed reaction is usually accompanied by extravascular hemolysis. The DAT is usually positive in both types of reaction but may only be detected 12 or more hours after transfusion in the delayed type of reaction.

ACUTE TRANSFUSION REACTION If an acute transfusion reaction is suspected, blood samples should be drawn immediately after terminating the transfusion. The post-transfusion specimen is centrifuged and the plasma checked for pink, red, or brown discoloration. Subtle changes are more apparent if the pretransfusion and post-transfusion specimens are compared. Discoloration after transfusion indicates the presence of free hemoglobin or its derivatives in the plasma (hemoglobinemia). The post-transfusion specimen also is tested for the presence of cell-bound immunoglobulin and/or complement by the DAT. Often the DAT is only weakly or transiently positive if the antibody-coated cells are rapidly destroyed. A mixed field positive DAT may be seen because only donor cells are coated by immunoglobulin or complement and are agglutinated by AHG, not the patient's cells.

If the DAT is positive and/or there is evidence of hemolysis and/or clerical error, the following procedure is generally followed. The specimens taken before and after transfusion are typed for ABO and Rh blood groups to assure that the pretranfusion specimen was identified and tested correctly. Crossmatches also are repeated. Post-transfusion specimens drawn several hours after the reaction may not contain free hemoglobin, but hemoglobinuria can usually be detected if intravascular hemolysis occurred. Free erythrocytes (hematuria) in the urine are not associated with intravascular or extravascular hemolysis.

DELAYED TRANSFUSION REACTION In a delayed transfusion reaction, the post-transfusion specimen will show a positive DAT.[19] In many cases, the clinical signs of a delayed transfusion reaction are so mild that the positive DAT is only discovered if the patient is crossmatched again several days later for another transfusion. If the DAT is positive, an eluate should be performed to determine the specificity of the antibody. If, however, the DAT is only weakly or transiently positive, there may not be sufficient antibody on the erythrocytes to prepare an eluate. After several days, the antibody level may be increased enough to allow identification of its specificity. Hemoglobinemia and hemoglobinuria are not usually found. Other laboratory tests such as haptoglobin and bilirubin analyses may be helpful. If a reaction has occurred, the haptoglobin may be decreased and serum bilirubin increased.

Therapy The most important immediate action taken when an acute transfusion reaction occurs is prompt termination of the transfusion. A major effort is made to maintain urine flow to prevent renal damage. Shock and bleeding require immediate attention.

HEMOLYTIC DISEASE OF THE NEWBORN

HDN is an alloimmune disease of the newborn associated with fetal erythrocyte destruction during fetal and neonatal life caused by fetomaternal blood group incompati-

TABLE 12-19 *A COMPARISON OF HEMOLYTIC DISEASE OF THE NEWBORN CAUSED BY ABO AND Rh₀ INCOMPATIBILITY*

	Rh	*ABO*
Antibody	Immune IgG	Non-immune or immune IgG
Blood group	Mother Rh negative, Baby Rh positive	Mother O, Baby A or B
Obstetric history	Only pregnancies after the first are affected	First pregnancy and subsequent pregnancies may be affected
Clinical findings	Moderate to severe anemia and bilirubinemia	Mild anemia, if present. Mild to moderate bilirubinemia with a peak 24–48 hours after birth
Laboratory findings	DAT positive, no spherocytes	DAT weakly positive or negative; spherocytes present
Therapy	Exchange transfusion, if severe	Phototherapy

bility. *Erythroblastosis fetalis* is another term used to describe this condition. This name relates to the presence of large numbers of nucleated erythrocytes found in the baby's peripheral blood. Antibody specificity is usually directed to the ABO or Rh blood group systems (Table 12-19).

Pathophysiology Four conditions must be met for HDN to occur: (1) the mother must be exposed (sensitized) to an erythrocyte antigen that she lacks; (2) the mother must produce antibodies to the foreign antigens; (3) the mother's antibody must be able to cross the placenta and enter the fetal circulation; (4) the fetus must possess the antigen to which the mother is sensitized.

The mother may have been exposed to (nonself) foreign erythrocyte antigens by previous pregnancy or transfusion. Normally, the placenta does not allow free passage of erythrocytes from fetal to maternal circulation, but small amounts of erythrocytes may enter the maternal circulation. Additionally, during delivery, small amounts of fetal blood can enter the mother's circulation. The risk of sensitization increases as the volume of the fetal bleed increases. If the fetal-maternal bleed is sufficient to stimulate the production of maternal antibodies, subsequent pregnancies may be at risk for HDN.

More than 95% of HDN cases are due to Rh₀(D) or ABO antibodies. Although HDN caused by ABO antibodies is more common than HDN caused by Rh₀ antibodies, Rh₀ incompatibility causes more severe disease. The most common antibodies associated with the remaining 5% of HDN are anti-C, anti-E, and anti-Kell.

Three classes of immunoglobulins may be produced during immunization of the mother—IgG, IgM, and IgA—but only IgG has the ability to cross the placenta and cause HDN. The IgG antibody is actively transported across the placenta via its Fc portion and causes destruction of fetal erythrocytes.

The fetus becomes anemic and may develop complications as a result of the anemia. The most serious complication is cardiac failure. As compensation for the anemia, extramedullary hematopoiesis occurs in the liver and spleen, enlarging these organs. Because of hemolysis, the unconjugated (indirect) bilirubin concentration increases. In the fetus, this bilirubin traverses the placenta and is excreted by the mother. After birth, however, the newborn must conjugate and excrete the bilirubin on its own. In the neonate, albumin levels for bilirubin transport are limited, and liver glucuronidase for bilirubin conjugation is low; therefore, considerable amounts of toxic unconjugated bilirubin may accumulate after delivery. Unconjugated bilirubin is toxic because, in this form, it is lipid-soluble and can easily cross cell membranes. This form of bilirubin has a high affinity for basal ganglia of the CNS. Thus, the excess unconjugated bilirubin may lead to kernicterus, an irreversible form of brain damage. The conjugated form of bilirubin is water-soluble but lipid-insoluble and cannot cross cell membranes.

About 7% to 8% of Rh_o-negative women develop antibodies to Rh_o positive cells after the birth of an Rh_o-positive ABO-compatible infant. The routine use of Rh_o immune globulin (RhIG, which contains increased levels of anti-D) in Rh_o-negative women during gestation (antepartum) and after the birth (postpartum) of an Rh_o-positive child has decreased the incidence of HDN considerably. The majority of women (92%) who develop anti-D during pregnancy do so at 28 weeks gestation or later. Thus, antepartum administration of RhIG is given prophylactically between weeks 28 and 30 of gestation.[15] The RhIG acts as an immunosuppressant, depressing the production of immune IgG. The RhIG binds to fetal cells in maternal circulation, mediating their removal in the spleen, thereby preventing the possibility of maternal sensitization to the Rh antigen.

Most ABO incompatibilities occur in Group A or Group B infants of Group O mothers. The Group O mother produces sufficient anti-A and anti-B IgG, without fetal antigenic stimulation, which may cross the placental barrier to destroy fetal cells. In contrast to Rh_o HDN, in ABO HDN the first baby may be affected because the mother has an IgG anti-A,B antibody in her circulation.

Clinical findings Anemia is the greatest risk to the infant with HDN in the first 24 hours of life, and bilirubinemia is the greatest risk thereafter. In Rh incompatibility, the cord blood hemoglobin may be low normal at birth (normal hemoglobin at birth is 14 to 20 g/dL), and the baby does not appear jaundiced. However, significant hemolysis, occurring in the first 24 hours of life outside the womb, results in anemia with pallor and jaundice. In severe cases, hepatosplenomegaly may be present. Severe anemia may be accompanied by heart failure and edema. As the level of unconjugated bilirubin rises, kernicterus may occur, causing irreversible brain damage. With premature infants, the risks of hyperbilirubinemia are even greater be-

cause of the inability of the premature liver to excrete the excess bilirubin.

ABO incompatibility is not as severe as Rh incompatibility. Within 24 to 48 hours after birth, the infant appears jaundiced but kernicterus is extremely rare. Anemia is mild, and pallor is uncommon. Hepatosplenomegaly is mild, if present.

Laboratory findings

Rh_o INCOMPATIBILITY About 50% of affected infants have a cord blood hemoglobin concentration less than 14 g/dL. Capillary blood hemoglobin may be up to 4 g/dL higher due to placental transfer of blood at birth. The cord blood hemoglobin concentration is useful as an indicator of anemia at birth and as a baseline to follow destruction of erythrocytes after birth. There is a direct relationship between the initial cord blood hemoglobin level and the severity of the disease. Lower cord blood hemoglobin levels at birth are associated with a more severe clinical course. After birth, hemoglobin levels may fall at the rate of 3 g/dL/day. Lowest hemoglobin values are present at 3 to 4 days. The erythrocytes are macrocytic and normochromic. Reticulocytes are markedly increased, sometimes reaching 60%. Nucleated erythrocytes are markedly increased in the peripheral blood (10 to 100 $\times$ 10^9/L), reflecting the rapid formation of cells in response to erythrocyte destruction. Normal infants also have nucleated erythrocytes in the peripheral blood, but their concentration is much lower (0.2 to 2 $\times$ 10^9/L).

The blood smear shows marked polychromasia, mild or absent poikilocytosis, and few, if any, spherocytes. The leukocyte count is increased to 30 $\times$ 10^9/L or more due to an increase in neutrophils reflecting the marrow response to stress. Often, there is a significant shift to the left. The normal leukocyte count at birth is 15 to 20 $\times$ 10^9/L. The platelet count is usually normal, but thrombocytopenia may develop with an increase in disease severity.

Cord blood bilirubin is elevated but is usually less than 5.5 mg/dL. However, cord blood bilirubin does not accurately reflect the severity of hemolysis since bilirubin readily crosses the placenta. The serum bilirubin peaks on the third or fourth day and may reach 40 to 50 mg/dL if the baby is not treated. Most is in the unconjugated form. Full-term infants with bilirubin concentrations more than 10 mg/dL are at increased risk for brain damage. Premature infants may develop kernicterus with levels as low as 8 to 10 mg/dL.

Only the unconjugated bilirubin not bound to albumin is toxic to the CNS. Therefore, the potential risks of bilirubin toxicity can be determined by measuring the amount of bilirubin binding reserve of albumin. One such test uses the ability of the infants' albumin to bind a dye, hydroxybenzeneazobenzoic acid (HBABA) or phenolsulfonphthalein (PSP). An inverse relationship between the dye-binding capacity of albumin and serum bilirubin levels has been established.

The DAT is positive with polyspecific antiserum and monospecific anti-IgG sera. An eluate is performed to determine the specificity of the antibody coating the baby's cells. The baby's and mother's blood is typed. The erythrocyte-typing results of an infant's cells must be interpreted with care. Sometimes baby cells, coated with a large amount of anti-D antibody, will type as an Rh negative. This is due to the blocking of Rh antigenic sites by maternal antibody.

ABO INCOMPATIBILITY In ABO incompatibility, the cord blood hemoglobin is usually normal. If anemia is present, it is minimal. Reticulocytes are increased. The peripheral blood smear exhibits polychromatophilia, nucleated erythrocytes, and striking spherocytosis (not seen in Rh_o incompatilibity). The unconjugated bilirubin, although increased, is less elevated, and the increased bilirubin concentration is of shorter duration than in Rh_o incompatibility. The osmotic fragility is increased due to the presence of spherocytes.

A weakly positive DAT is found in the cord blood, but it becomes negative after 12 hours. The weak reaction is due to the small number of anti-A or anti-B antibody molecules attached to the erythrocyte. In addition, the A and B antigens are present on cells other than erythrocytes in the fetus. Eluates demonstrate the antibody specificity. Complement is not attached to the cells.

Therapy The major efforts of therapy are prevention of hyperbilirubinemia and anemia. In less severe cases, the infant is treated with phototherapy, which slowly lowers the toxic bilirubin level. Infusion of albumin to bind more unconjugated bilirubin is used less often. If the bilirubin level reaches 19 to 20 mg/dL, exchange transfusion is performed. The transfusion has several beneficial effects: (1) it dilutes the concentration of antibodies causing the hemolysis; (2) it removes some of the antibody-coated erythrocytes; (3) it lowers the level of bilirubin; and (4) it corrects the anemia and reverses congestive heart failure in hydropic infants.

Methods for detecting in utero hemolysis have allowed decisions to be made on whether an intrauterine transfusion with Group O Rh-negative, washed, irradiated cells should be given. The antigen-negative cells lack the specific binding site for antibody and, therefore, have a normal lifespan. This permits the fetus to remain in the womb longer to help ensure survival after delivery.

The widespread use of RhIG has dramatically reduced the incidence of HDN in the last 20 years. As mentioned, the passive injection of anti-Rho IgG prevents isoimmunization of the mother.

● SUMMARY

HA may be caused by factors extrinsic to the erythrocyte. Hemolysis may be precipitated by factors in the cells' environment, by physical or mechanical trauma to the cell, or by antibodies or complement. The hemolysis may occur intravascularly or extravascularly, depending on the type and extent of injury.

If the bone marrow can compensate for the decreased erythrocyte survival, there is no anemia. In most cases,

however, there is a normocytic, normochromic anemia with pronounced reticulocytosis. The peripheral blood smear may give clues to the pathophysiologic process. The presence of spherocytes, acanthocytes, and schistocytes is indicative of cell damage. In hemolytic anemias mediated via antibodies and/or complement, the AHG test is helpful. The bone marrow generally shows erythrocyte hyperplasia. Other laboratory tests may be helpful in determining the presence and extent of hemolysis. These include serum bilirubin and haptoglobin concentrations and evaluation for hemosidinuria and hemoglobinuria.

Microangiopathic hemolytic anemia is caused by microcirculatory lesions or mechanical trauma in the vessels. These anemias include two similar disorders, TTP and HUS. They are characterized by the tetrad of clinical findings of thrombocytopenia, microangiopathic hemolytic anemia, neurologic abnormalities, and renal dysfunction. In TTP, there is fever, and neurologic findings are more prominent. HUS occurs more frequently in children and is associated with viral infections.

Immune hemolytic anemias are mediated by antibodies and/or complement. There are three broad categories: alloimmune, autoimmune, and drug-induced. The alloimmune hemolytic anemias occur in transfusion reactions and in HDN. In these diseases an individual is sensitized to antigens from another individual either through transfusions or pregnancy. The patient produces antibodies against donor erythrocytes causing hemolysis. These are self-limited reactions. Laboratory testing involves demonstrating the presence of antibody on the erythrocytes with the DAT and identifying the antibody specificity. Autoimmune HA are a reaction against self. Autoimmune HA may be classified as warm or cold HA with the majority being warm HA. Warm refers to the fact that the antibodies react optimally at 37° C, whereas cold antibodies react best at 0° to 20° C. In warm HA the offending antibodies are usually IgG antibodies directed against antigens on the patient's erythrocytes. Most hemolysis is extravascular. Laboratory findings include a positive DAT, reticulocytosis and anemia with poikilocytes, usually spherocytes. Cold agglutinin disease and PCH are two types of cold autoimmune HA. In cold agglutinin disease, the antibody is usually an IgM complement-fixing antibody, whereas in PCH the antibody is a biphasic IgG antibody, the DL antibody. The DL antibody reacts with erythrocytes in capillaries at less than 15° C and binds complement. Upon warming to 37° C, the terminal complement components are activated and lyse the cell. Laboratory findings are typical of those found in intravascular hemolysis.

Drug-related HA are caused by an immune-mediated hemolysis precipitated by ingestion of certain drugs. Four hypotheses have been offered to explain drug-induced HA, some of which are associated with specific drugs. In the drug adsorption mechanism, the drug binds to erythrocyte membrane proteins, and antibodies are produced against the drug-cell complex. In the immune bystander mechanism, the drug combines with plasma proteins to form new antigenic complexes that are adsorbed onto the erythrocyte. Some drugs are able to modify the cell membrane so normal plasma proteins bind to the membrane.

This nonspecific adsorption mechanism is not associated with HA. A few drugs (Aldomet) can induce the formation of antibodies against self erythrocyte antigens.

REVIEW QUESTIONS

An 81-year-old white man with chest pain was brought to the emergency room. The pain was not relieved with nitroglycerin. He was admitted to CCU for testing and observation. Results of physical examination showed a moderately obese, alert, and congenial man in relatively good health for his age.

Admission laboratory data:

Erythrocyte count	3.05×10^{12}/L
Hb	8.6 gm/dL
Hct	0.26 L/L
Platelet count	234×10^9/L
Leukocyte count	8.8×10^9/L

Differential:

Segmented Neutrophils	68%
Band Neutrophils	5%
Lymphocytes	23%
Monocytes	4%

8 nucleated erythrocytes per 100 leukocytes

Erythrocyte morphology: The erythrocytes are normochromic with moderate polychromasia. There is slight anisocytosis and moderate poikilocytosis with spherocytes.

Reticulocyte count:	7.8%
Serum LDH:	212 IU/L
Total bilirubin:	5.2 mg/dL
Direct bilirubin:	1.9 mg/dL
Urine urobilinogen:	5 EU
Cardiac enzymes:	normal

Over the next two days, the patient's hemoglobin continued to drop and two units of packed red cells were ordered. All units were found to be incompatible. Initial serological testing showed that he was group B, Rh positive. The antibody screen and autocontrol were positive at 37° C and AHG. The patient had no history of transfusion. Further tests revealed a positive DAT with polyspecific antihuman globulin (AHG) and a most probable Rh genotype of CDe/cde. Antibody panels demonstrated auto-anti-e in both the serum and eluate.

1. Which of the following is not detected by the DAT with polyspecific AHG?
   a. erythrocyte sensitization with antibodies "in vivo"
   b. erythrocyte sensitization with incomplete antibodies "in vivo"
   c. erythrocyte sensitization with complement "in vivo"
   d. erythrocyte sensitization with antibodies "in vitro"

2. What is this patient's most likely diagnosis?
   a. Hereditary spherocytosis
   b. Cold autoimmune hemolytic anemia
   c. Paroxysmal nocturnal hemoglobinuria
   d. Warm autoimmune hemolytic anemia

3. What is the most likely mechanism of hemolysis?
   a. Phagocytosis of IgG-coated erythrocytes
   b. Increased sensitivity to complement
   c. Complement fixation of IgM-coated erythrocytes
   d. Increased membrane instability with progressive membrane loss

4. From the laboratory data given, how would you classify the source of the defect?
   a. intrinsic, hereditary
   b. extrinsic, hereditary
   c. extrinsic, acquired
   d. intrinsic, acquired

5. What is this patient's RPI?
   a. 1.8
   b. 2.2
   c. 3.0
   d. 5.0

6. Based on your calculations of the erythrocyte indices, how would you classify this patient's erythrocytes morphologically?
   a. microcytic, hypochromic
   b. macrocytic, hypochromic
   c. normocytic, normochromic
   d. macrocytic, normochromic

7. In warm AIHA the offending antibody is usually:
   a. IgG
   b. IgM
   c. IgA
   d. a mixture of IgG and IgM

8. The Donath-Landsteiner test is positive in:
   a. PNH
   b. CHD
   c. PCH
   d. warm AIHA

9. In an acute hemolytic transfusion reaction, hemolysis is usually mediated by:
   a. IgG
   b. IgM and complement
   c. IgA
   d. antibodies directed toward the Rh system

10. The rate of hemolysis in hemolytic anemia is related to all of the following **except**:
    a. the age of the patient
    b. the class of the offending antibody
    c. the amount of antibody bound to the erythrocytes
    d. the thermal amplitude of the antibody

REFERENCES

1. Cooper, R.A.: Anemia with spur cells: a red cell defect acquired in serum and modified in the circulation. J. Clin. Invest., 48:1820, 1969.

2. Doll, D.C., Doll, N.J.: Spur cell anemia. South. Med. J., 75(10): 1205, 1982.

3. Parsonnet, J., Griffin, P.M.: Hemolytic uremic syndrome: Clinical picture and bacterial connection. Curr. Clin. Top. Infec. Dis., 13: 172, 1993.

4. Robson, W.L.M., Leung, A.K.C., Kaplan, B.S.: Hemolytic-uremic Syndrome. Curr. Prob. Pediatr., 23:16, 1993.

5. Neild, G.H.: Haemolytic-Uraemic syndrome in practice. Lancet, 343:398, 1994.

6. Rose, M., Rowe, J.M., Eldor, A.: The changing course of thrombotic thrombocytopenic purpura and modern therapy. Haemostasis Thromb., 9(2):94, 1993.

7. Moake, J.L.: Thrombotic thrombocytopenic purpura and the hemolytic uremic syndrome. In Hematology: Basic Principles and Practice. Edited by R. Hoffman, E.J. Benz, S.J. Shattil, B. Furie, H.J. Cohen. New York: Churchill Livingstone, 1995.

8. Rubin, R.N., Colman, R.W.: Disseminated intravascular coagulation. Drugs, 44:963, 1992.

9. Schwurman, A.H., Breederveld, R.S., Rauwerda, J.A.: Exertional (March) hemoglobinuria. Neth. J. Surg., 43(2):39, 1991.

10. Engelfriet, C.P., Overbeeke, M.A.M., von dem Borne, A.E.G.Kr.: Autoimmune hemolytic anemia. Sem. Hematol., 29:3, 1992.

11. Moleszewski, C.R., et al.: Expression cloning of a human Fc receptor for IgA. J. Exp. Med., 172:1665, 1990.

12. Sokol, R.J., Booker, D.J., Stamps, R.: The pathology of autoimmune hemolytic anaemia. J. Clin. Pathol., 45:1047, 1992.

13. Schwartz, R.S., Berkman, E.M., Silberstein, L.E.: The autoimmune hemolytic anemias. In Hematology: Basic Principles and Practice. Edited by R. Hoffman, E.J. Benz, S.J. Shattil, B. Furie, H.J. Cohen. New York: Churchill Livingstone, 1995.

14. Silberstein, L.E.: Natural and pathologic human autoimmune responses to carbohydrate antigens on red blood cells. Springer Semin. Immunopathol., 15:139, 1993.

15. Walker, R.H. (ed.): Technical Manual. 10th Ed. Arlington, Virginia, American Association of Blood Banks, 1990.

16. Carpentieri, U., Dalscher III, C.W., Haggard, M.E.: Immunohemolytic anemia and Hodgkin's disease. Pediatrics, 70:320, 1982.

17. Collins, P.W., Newland, A.C.: Treatment modalities of autoimmune blood disorders. Sem. Hematol., 29:64, 1992.

18. Hadnagy, C.: Agewise distribution of idiopathic cold agglutinin disease. Z. Gerontol., 26:199, 1993.

19. Harmening, D.: Modern blood banking and transfusion practices. 2nd Ed. Philadelphia, F.A. Davis, 1989.

20. Salama, A., Mueller-Eckhardt, C.: Immune-mediated blood cell dyscrasias related to drugs. Sem. Hematol., 29:54, 1992.

21. Petz, L.D.: Drug-induced autoimmune hemolytic anemia. Transf. Med. Rev., 7:242, 1993.

13

Nonmalignant granulocyte and monocyte disorders

INTRODUCTION

It is well-recognized that changes in leukocyte concentration and morphology are a normal response of the body to various disease processes and toxic challenges. Most often, one type of leukocyte is affected by the disease or challenge more than others, providing an important clue to diagnosis. The type of cell affected depends in a large part on the function of that cell (i.e., bacterial infection commonly results in an absolute neutrophilia, viral infections are characterized by an absolute lymphocytosis, and certain parasitic infections cause an eosinophilia). Thus, determination of absolute concentrations of cell types in hematologic evaluation aids in differential diagnosis especially when the total leukocyte concentration is abnormal.

Leukocytosis refers to a condition in which the total leukocyte count is more than $11.0 \times 10^9/L$. Although this condition is usually due to an increase in neutrophils, it also may be related to an increase in lymphocytes or less often in monocytes, and rarely in eosinophils or basophils.

Quantitative variations of different types of leukocytes are evaluated by performing a total leukocyte count and a differential count. The absolute concentration of each type of leukocyte can be calculated from these two values as described in Chapter 1 (total leukocyte count/L × percentage of cell type from differential = cells/L).

Leukopenia refers to a decrease in leukocytes below $3.5 \times 10^9/L$. This condition is usually due to a decrease in neutrophils, but lymphocytes, monocytes, eosinophils, and basophils also may be decreased.

Morphologic variations of leukocytes are noted by examination of the stained blood smear. Variations in the appearance of the cell together with its concentration may give the physician specific clues to the pathologic process.

NEUTROPHIL DISORDERS

Quantitative disorders

Quantitative abnormalities of neutrophils may occur because of a malignant or benign disorder. The malignant disorders are caused by neoplastic transformation of hematopoietic stem cells and will be discussed in Chapters 15-19. Benign disorders are usually acquired and may cause neutrophilia or neutropenia, but neutrophilia is more common. Some benign disorders affecting neutrophils are hereditary or familial. These disorders are characterized by neutropenia.

Peripheral blood neutrophil concentration is affected by three interrelated mechanisms: (Table 13-1) (1) bone

TABLE 13-1   *FACTORS AFFECTING NEUTROPHIL CONCENTRATION IN PERIPHERAL BLOOD*

1. Bone marrow production and release.
2. Rate of egress to tissue or survival time in blood.
3. Ratio of marginating to circulating neutrophils in peripheral blood.

marrow production and release; (2) rate of neutrophil egress to the tissues or survival time in the blood; (3) proportion of marginating to circulating leukocytes.

NEUTROPHILIA

Neutrophilia (neutrophilic leukocytosis) refers to an increase in the total circulating mass (absolute concentration) of neutrophils. The normal concentration varies with age, so it is important to evaluate the count based on reference values for specific age groups. In adults, neutrophilia occurs when the concentration of neutrophils exceeds $7.0 \times 10^9/L$. The reference ranges for neutrophil concentrations of different age groups are listed in table B on the inside cover.

Benign neutrophilia most often occurs as a result of a reaction to a physiologic or pathologic process (reactive neutrophilia). *Reactive neutrophilia* may be immediate, acute, or chronic, and involve any or all of the three mechanisms mentioned above.

Immediate neutrophilia   Immediate neutrophilia may occur without tissue damage or other pathologic stimulus. It is probably produced by a simple redistribution of the marginated granulocyte pool (MGP) to the circulating granulocyte pool (CGP). The circulating pool is measured by the leukocyte count. The neutrophil increase is immediate but transient (lasting about 20 to 30 minutes) and appears to be independent of bone marrow input and tissue egress. This type of neutrophilia is also referred to as *pseudoneutrophilia* because there is no real change in the number of neutrophils within the vasculature. Most circulating granulocytes are mature cells, and there is no change in the band to segmented neutrophil ratio. This mechanism of redistribution is responsible for the physiologic neutrophilia that accompanies active exercise, epinephrine administration, anesthesia, convulsions, and states of anxiety. It also has been referred to as *"shift" neutrophilia.*

Acute neutrophilia   Acute neutrophilia occurs within 4 to 5 hours of a pathologic stimulus (e.g., bacterial infection, toxin). This type of neutrophilia results from an increase in the flow of neutrophils from the bone marrow storage pool to the blood. The neutrophilia is more pronounced than in pseudoneutrophilia, and the proportion of immature neutrophils may increase. The normal band to segmented neutrophil ratio in peripheral blood is from 0.1 to 0.3, but the ratio will increase (more bands present) if the tissue demand for neutrophils creates an acute shortage of segmented neutrophils in the storage pool. Continued demand may result in the release of metamyelocytes and myelocytes. As the bone marrow production increases and the storage pool is replenished, the band to segmented neutrophil ratio in the peripheral blood will return to normal.

Chronic neutrophilia   Chronic neutrophilia follows acute neutrophilia. If the stimulus for storage pool neutrophil release continues beyond a few days, the pool will become depleted. The mitotic pool will then increase production in an attempt to meet the demand for neutrophils. In this

TABLE 13-2 *CONDITIONS ASSOCIATED WITH NEUTROPHILIA*

1. Acute infections, local or generalized: especially coccal but also those due to certain bacilli, fungi, spirochetes, parasites, and some viruses; in diseases usually not associated with neutrophilia when complications develop
2. Other inflammation: tissue damage resulting from burns or after operations; ischemic necrosis as in myocardial infarction, gout, collagen vascular disease, hypersensitivity reactions, and other similar inflammatory processes
3. Intoxication: Metabolic, including uremia, diabetic acidosis, and eclampsia Poisoning by chemicals and drugs: lead, digitalis, insect venoms, and foreign protein
4. Acute hemorrhage, internal, external
5. Acute hemolysis
6. Malignant neoplasms
7. Physiologic neutrophilia: during strenuous exercise, after epinephrine injection, in association with convulsions or paroxysmal tachycardia, and in the newborn
8. Myelocytic leukemia, polycythemia vera, myelofibrosis, and myeloid metaplasia
9. Other causes: chronic idiopathic neutrophilia, hereditary neutrophilia, and adrenocorticosteroids

(From: Lee, GR, et al.: Wintrobe's Clinical Hematology, 9th ed. Philadelphia, Lea & Febiger, 1993.)

state, the marrow will show increased numbers of early neutrophil precursors, including myeloblasts, promyelocytes, and myelocytes. The blood will contain increased numbers of bands, metamyelocytes, myelocytes, and (very rarely) promyelocytes and myeloblasts. An increase in the concentration of immature forms of leukocytes in the circulation is termed a *"shift to the left."*

Conditions associated with reactive neutrophilia (Table 13-2)
Neutrophilia caused by benign or toxic conditions are usually characterized by total leukocyte counts less than 50×10^9/L and a shift to the left (Fig. 13-1). The imma-

ture cells present are usually bands and metamyelocytes, but myelocytes and promyelocytes may be seen occasionally. Toxic granulation may be present, even if the neutrophil count is not increased. Döhle bodies are frequently present. Vacuolization of neutrophils is common in septicemia. The leukocyte alkaline phosphatase score may be increased.

INFECTION The most common cause of neutrophilia is bacterial infection, especially infection with pyogenic organisms such as staphylococci and streptococci. Depending on the virulence of the microorganism, the extent of infection, and the response of the host, the neutrophil count may range from 7.0×10^9/L to 70×10^9/L or, in unusual cases, may increase even more. Usually, the count is in the range of 10 to 20×10^9/L. As the demand for neutrophils at the site of infection increases, the early response of the bone marrow is an increase of its output of storage neutrophils to the peripheral blood, causing a shift to the left. The increased flow of neutrophils from the bone marrow to the blood continues until it exceeds the neutrophil outflow to the tissues, causing an absolute neutrophilia (transient overshoot). In very severe infections, the storage pool of neutrophils may become exhausted, the mitotic pool may be unable to keep up with the demand, and a neutropenia develops. Neutropenia in overwhelming infection is a very poor prognostic sign. Chronic bacterial infection may lead to chronic stimulation of the marrow, whereby the production of neutrophils remains high and a new steady state of production develops (Fig. 13-2).

The body's response to infection involves a gradual transformation of the blood picture. Eosinopenia accompanies the progressive neutrophilia and shift to the left. When the infection subsides and the fever drops, monocytosis occurs. After monocytosis, there is a slight lymphocytosis and eosinophilia.

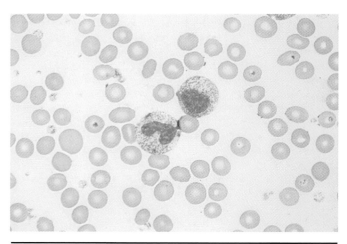

FIGURE 13-1. A shift to the left in granulocytic cells. The band and metamyelocyte have toxic granulation. (Peripheral blood; 250× magnification; Wright-Giemsa stain)

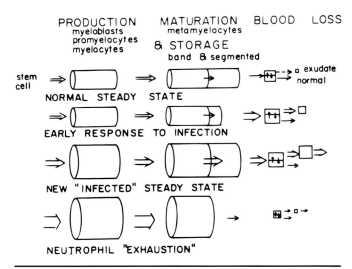

FIGURE 13-2. Neutrophil kinetics in response to infection change over a period of time depending on demand and duration of stimulus. (From Boggs, D.R. and Winkelstein A.: A white cell manual, 4th ed. Philadelphia: F.A. Davis, 1983).

Neutrophilia is not a unique nor absolute finding in bacterial infections. Infections with other organisms such as fungi, rickettsia, spirochetes, and parasites may cause a neutrophilia. Some bacterial infections are characterized by a neutropenia rather than a neutrophilia (e.g., typhoid fever, paratyphoid fever, and brucellosis). In a few types of infection, lymphocytosis, rather than neutrophilia, is typical (e.g., tuberculosis, undulant fever, whooping cough).[1] Viral infections are typically accompanied by a lymphocytosis, but neutrophilia may be present in the early phases of some infections.

TISSUE DESTRUCTION/INJURY, INFLAMMATION, METABOLIC DISORDERS Conditions other than infection that may result in a neutrophilia include those conditions involving tissue necrosis, inflammation, and metabolic or drug intoxication. All these conditions produce neutrophilia by increasing neutrophil input from the bone marrow in response to increased egress to the tissue. Examples of these conditions include rheumatoid arthritis, tissue infarctions, burns, neoplasms, uremia, and gout.

Leukocytes, although defenders of the body, also are responsible for a significant part of the continuing inflammatory process. In gout, for example, depositions of uric acid crystals in joints attract neutrophils to the area. In the process of phagocytosis and death, the leukocytes release toxic intracellular enzymes (granules) and oxygen metabolites. These toxic substances mediate the inflammatory process by injuring other body cells and propagating the formation of chemotactic factors, which attract more leukocytes. This mechanism is responsible for the tissue destruction in many diseases such as glomerulonephritis and rheumatoid arthritis. Recently, it was proposed that leukocytes adhering to veins in response to local injury may contribute to development of deep vein thrombosis.[2]

LEUKEMOID REACTION Extreme neutrophilic reactions to severe infections or necrotizing tissue may produce a *leukemoid reaction* (Fig. 13-3). A leukemoid reaction is a benign leu-

TABLE 13-3 *LABORATORY RESULTS IN LEUKEMOID REACTIONS AND CHRONIC MYELOCYTIC LEUKEMIA (CML)*

	Leukemoid Reaction	CML
Leukocyte Count	Increased	Increased
Differential	Shift-to-the-left	Shift-to-the-left
Erythrocyte Count	Normal	Usually decreased
Platelets	Usually normal	Often increased or decreased
LAP	Increased	Decreased
Philadelphia Chromosome	Absent	Present

LAP: leukocyte alkaline phosphatase

kocyte proliferation characterized by a total leukocyte count usually greater than 30×10^9/L with many circulating immature leukocyte precursors. The leukemoid response may be lymphocytic, or eosinophilic as well as neutrophilic, especially in viral infections. In a neutrophilic-leukemoid reaction, the blood contains many bands and metamyelocytes in addition to a number of myelocytes and occasionally promyelocytes and blasts.

Leukemoid reactions may produce a blood picture indistinguishable from that of chronic myelocytic leukemia. Generally, anemia and thrombocytopenia or thrombocytosis, typically found in leukemia, are not present in a leukemoid reaction, but when present may make differential diagnosis more difficult. When this situation occurs, chromosome studies and leukocyte alkaline phosphatase (LAP) scores may help to distinguish the two pathologies (Table 13-3). Leukemoid reactions are accompanied by normal karyotypes and increased LAP scores, whereas chronic myelocytic leukemia is characterized by the presence of abnormal karyotypes (Philadelphia chromosome) and decreased LAP scores. Contrary to leukemia, a leukemoid reaction is transient, disappearing when the inciting stimulus is removed (e.g., excising tumor, controlling infection). A leukemoid reaction may be seen in tuberculosis, chronic infections, malignant tumors, acute alcoholic hepatitis, and other infectious and noninfectious processes.

LEUKOERYTHROBLASTIC REACTION A *leukoerythroblastic reaction* (Fig. 13-4) is characterized by the presence of nucleated erythrocytes and a shift to the left in neutrophils in the peripheral blood. The total neutrophil count may be increased, decreased, or normal. Usually, mature erythrocytes in this condition exhibit poikilocytosis and anisocytosis. A leukoerythroblastic reaction is most often associated with *myelophthisis*, a proliferation of abnormal elements in the bone marrow. This blood picture also is seen in severe hemorrhagic or hemolytic anemias such as erythroblastosis fetalis.

STIMULATED BONE MARROW STATES In reactive states such as hemorrhage or hemolysis when the bone marrow is stimulated

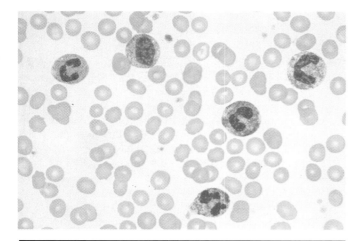

FIGURE 13-3. A leukemoid reaction. There is a shift to the left and an increase in granulocytic cells. The cells have heavy toxic granulation which suggests an infectious or toxic state may be the cause of the reactive leukocytosis. (Peripheral blood; 250× magnification; Wright-Giemsa stain)

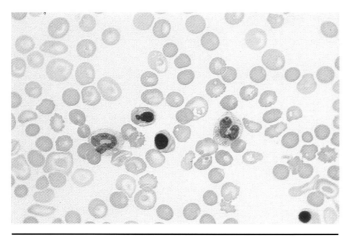

FIGURE 13-4. A leukoerythroblastic reaction with a shift to the left in neutrophilic cells and nucleated red cell (peripheral blood; 250× original magnification; Wright-Giemsa stain).

to produce erythrocytes in response to a decreased erythrocyte survival, neutrophils also may become caught up in the process, resulting in neutrophilia. This is often accompanied by a shift to the left. Internal hemorrhages usually stimulate a greater leukocytosis than external hemorrhages. The leukocytosis associated with external hemorrhages appears to be dependent on the rate and amount of blood lost.[3]

CORTICOSTEROID THERAPY Corticosteroid therapy produces a neutrophilia that occurs as a result of increased bone marrow output accompanied by a decreased migration of neutrophils to the tissues. This corticosteroid inhibition of neutrophil migration to the tissues may, in part, explain the increased incidence of bacterial infection in patients receiving steroid therapy even though the blood neutrophil count is increased. Steroids also inhibit macrophage function.

PHYSIOLOGIC LEUKOCYTOSIS Physiologic leukocytosis and neutrophilia are present at birth and for the first few days of life. In the newborn, the normal leukocyte count ranges from 10 to 25 × 10^9/L with 60% neutrophils. The leukocytosis is accompanied by a shift to the left. A gradual decrease in leukocytes is seen during childhood, until adult values are reached at about 14 years of age. Physiologic stress, including exposure to extreme temperatures, emotional stimuli, exercise, and labor during delivery may cause neutrophilia.

NEUTROPENIA (TABLE 13-4)

Neutropenia occurs when the neutrophil count falls below 2 × 10^9/L in whites and below 1.3 × 10^9/L in blacks. *Agranulocytosis* is a term that refers to a neutrophil count below 0.5 × 10^9/L. Basophils and eosinophils also are commonly depleted in severe neutropenia. At neutrophil concentrations less than 0.5 × 10^9/L, the probability of infection is great.

Neutropenia may occur because of the following: (1)

TABLE 13-4 *CAUSES OF LEUKOPENIA AND/OR NEUTROPENIA*

1. Certain infections
   Bacterial
   Viral
   Rickettsial
   Protozoal
2. All types of overwhelming infections: e.g., miliary tuberculosis, septicemia, especially in debilitated patients with poor resistance
3. Effect of physical agents, chemicals, and drugs
   Chemical and physical agents that produce marrow hypoplasia and aplasia in all subjects if given in sufficient dose, e.g., ionizing radiation, benzene, nitrogen mustards, urethane, antimetabolites (e.g., folic acid antagonists, purine and pyrimidine analogues), periwinkle alkaloids (e.g., vinblastine), colchicine, anthracyclines
   Chemical and drugs that occasionally produce leukopenia apparently as a result of individual sensitivity: e.g., aminopyrine, phenothiazines, sulfonamides, antithyroid drugs, anticonvulsants, antihistamines, tranquilizers, antimicrobial agents, etc. (see section on Agranulocytosis)
4. Certain hematologic disorders and other conditions of unknown or poorly defined etiologic basis
   Those that may be related to decreased or ineffective production, e.g., pernicious anemia, aplastic anemia, chronic hypochromic anemia
   Those that may be related to increased utilization, destruction or sequestration, e.g., cirrhosis of the liver with splenomegaly, lupus erythematosus, Felty's sysndrome, Banti's syndrome, Gaucher's disease, hemodialysis
5. Cachexia and debilitated states (alcoholism, etc.)
6. In anaphylactoid shock and in early stages of reaction to foreign protein
7. Certain are hereditary, congenital, or familial and miscellaneous disorders (cyclic neutropenia, chronic hypoplastic neutropenia, infantile genetic agranulocytosis, primary splenic neutropenia)

decreased bone marrow production or ineffective production; (2) increased cell loss (mechanical or immune destruction, increased neutrophil egress to the tissue); or (3) pseudoneutropenia (alterations in the MGP to CGP) (Fig. 13-5).

Decreased bone marrow production Neutropenia may develop as a result of decreased bone marrow production. In this case, the bone marrow shows myeloid hypoplasia, and the myeloid to erythroid ratio (M:E) is decreased. With defective production, the bone marrow storage pool is decreased, neutrophil egress to tissues is decreased, and both the peripheral blood circulating pool and marginal pool decrease. Immature cells may enter the blood in an attempt to alleviate the neutrophil shortage; bands may marginate, egress, and phagocytose. Cells younger than bands, however, are less motile, less deformable, and less efficient in phagocytosis. The end result is a lack of neutrophils at inflammatory sites, precipitating overwhelming infections. Decreased bone marrow production may occur with stem cell failure, radiotherapy, chemotherapy, or in myelophthisis.

Neutropenia is a characteristic finding in megaloblastic anemia and dysmyelopoietic syndromes. In these cases, however, the marrow is usually hyperplastic. Neutropenia results not from marrow failure but from dysmyelopoiesis. The abnormal myeloid cells are destroyed before being

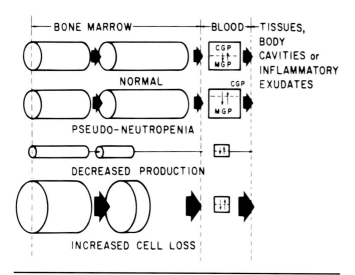

FIGURE 13-5. Various kinetic mechanisms responsible for neutropenia (From Boggs, D.R., Winkelstein, A.: White cell manual. 4th ed. Philadelphia, FA Davis, 1983).

TABLE 13-5 *INFECTIONS ASSOCIATED WITH NEUTROPENIA*

Viral
  Influenza
  Measles
  Chicken pox
  Colorado tick fever
  Dengue
  Infectious mononucleosis
  Poliomyelitis
  Psittacosis
  Sand-fly fever
  Smallpox
  Rubella
  Infectious hepatitis

Bacterial
  Typhoid
  Bacillary dysentery
  Paratyphoid
  Brucellosis
  Ehrlichiosis

Rickettsial
  Rickettsial pox
  Typhus
  Rocky Mountain spotted fever

Protozoal
  Malaria
  Kala-azar
  Relapsing fever

released to the blood (ineffective granulopoiesis). Increased levels of serum muramidase and LDH in these conditions are evidence of increased granulocyte turnover.

A wide variety of drugs and chemicals are associated with leukopenia and neutropenia if given in sufficient dosage (Table 13-4). Many of these agents are used in chemotherapy for malignant disease. Their mode of action is primarily interference of bone marrow cell production. The degree of neutropenia is usually dose-related, and the onset is variably delayed.[4] The time it takes for neutropenia to develop is related to the size of the neutrophil reserve pool before therapy and the rate of consumption of neutrophils after therapy is initiated. Generally, in a healthy person with a normal reserve pool and normal consumption, it takes 8 to 14 days for neutropenia to develop after therapy begins.

Increased cell loss Neutropenia may occur as the result of increased neutrophil egress from the blood. In severe infection or early infection, the bone marrow may not produce cells as rapidly as they are being used, resulting in neutropenia. A wide variety of viral, bacterial, rickettsial, and protozoal infections produce leukopenia and neutropenia (Table 13-5). Leukopenia in viral infections begins within 24 to 48 hours of the onset of illness and remains depressed for 3 to 6 days. The leukopenia is a result of neutropenia and lymphocytopenia, with one cell type being more prominently depressed than the other depending on the viral infection. It is believed that viral-induced tissue damage results in an increased demand and utilization of neutrophils. In this type of neutropenia, toxic changes may appear in peripheral blood neutrophils.

Ehrlichia species has become a major tick-borne pathogen in humans over the last decade. Ehrlichiosis was previously known as a disease that occured only in animals. The infection was first described in a human in the United

States in 1986. The disease is characterized by fever, leukopenia, thrombocytopenia, and elevated liver enzymes.[5,6] The leukopenia is a result of a decrease in neutrophils and lymphocytes. The leukocyte count reaches a nadir in the first week of illness and then gradually rises.[6] Most cases of ehrlichiosis occur in the months in which ticks are most active—April through September. *Ehrlichia* species are small, obligate intracellular, coccobacilli bacteria. They infect leukocytes where they grow within membrane-bound vacuoles (phagosomes). The intracellular organisms are pleomorphic, appearing as amphophilic or basophilic, condensed or loose aggregates of bacteria. The intracellular microcolony of *Ehrlichia* is called a *morula* and is easily observed in leukocytes on Romanowsky stained blood films (Fig. 13-6). The leukocyte eventually ruptures and releases the organisms which then infect other leukocytes. There are at least two species of *Ehrlichia* that infect humans. *E. chaffeensis* infects monocytes and is the causative agent of human monocytic ehrlichiosis (HME). An organism closely related to *E. equi* infects granulocytes and is the causative agent of human granulocytic ehlichiosis (HGE). Confirmation of infection is made through serologic determination of antibody titers to *E. equi* or *E. chaffeensis* or by identification of DNA sequences of *Ehrlichia* by polymerase-chain-reaction assay. More severe disease and a poorer outcome may occur if diagnosis and therapy are delayed. The pathogenesis of ehrlichiosis may be related to direct cellular injury by the bacteria or a cascade of inflammatory or immune events. Peripheral blood cytopenia is probably the result of sequestration of infected cells in the spleen, liver, and lymph nodes.[7] The bone marrow is usually hypercellular.

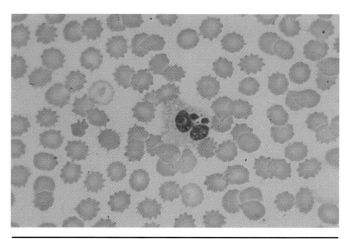

FIGURE 13-6. This segmented neutrophil contains two dense, basophilic inclusions called morulae. This blood came from a patient with human granulocytic ehrlichiosis (HGE). (Courtesy from: Cindy Johnson, St. Mary's Medical Center, Duluth, MN).

Neutropenia also may occur due to an immune mechanism, whereby antileukocyte antibodies are produced or complement is activated, destroying the cells (similar to immune hemolytic anemia). In a pregnant female sensitized to leukocyte antigens by previous pregnancy or transfusion, leukoagglutinins may cross the placenta and destroy fetal leukocytes, producing neutropenia of the newborn. The total leukocyte count is usually normal and monocytosis is common, but neutropenia is severe and lasts from 2 to 17 weeks.

In some cases, drugs may precipitate an immunologic, hypersensitivity reaction accompanied by the sudden disappearance of cells from the circulation. The immunologic mechanism is not clear, but several types of immune damage are possible, including direct cell lysis, agglutination, and sequestration and destruction in the spleen.[4] Cells sensitized with antibody in this manner are removed from circulation by macrophages in the spleen. Drugs may cause leukopenia and/or neutropenia by other mechanisms, including damage to stem cells in the marrow. A wide variety of drugs are associated with leukopenia and neutropenia (Table 13-6). Leukopenia is a complication of hemodialysis when activated complement induces neutrophil aggregation and adhesion to vessel walls. Neutropenia also develops in anaphylactoid shock through a mechanism similar to that in hemodialysis.

Hypersplenism may result in a selective splenic culling of neutrophils producing mild neutropenia. The bone marrow in this case exhibits neutrophilic hyperplasia. Hypersplenism also may be accompanied by thrombocytopenia and, occasionally, anemia. Felty's syndrome is a complication of rheumatoid arthritis accompanied by splenomegaly, neutropenia, and frequent infections. Although the exact cause of the neutropenia in this syndrome has not been definitely established, the spleen, in some cases, may be responsible for decreased neutrophil survival. Normal neutrophil levels appear in up to 80% of patients after splenectomy.[8]

TABLE 13-6 *AGENTS OCCASIONALLY ASSOCIATED WITH GRANULOCYTOPENIA AND LEUKOPENIA*

1. Analgesics, sedatives and anti-inflammatory agents
   *aminopyrine** and compounds containing it (Pyramidon, aminopyrine, Allonal, Amidophen, Cibalgin, Veramon, Amytal compound, Corosedine, Optalidon, Somnosal, Veropyron, antipyrine, Causalin, Neonal compound, Neurodyne, Peralga, Pyraminol, Yeast vite, etc.)
   dipyrone, a sulfonated aminopyrine, and compounds containing it (Novalgin, Novaldin, Migesic, Pyralgin, etc.) phenactin (acetophenetiden, acetanilid, allylisopropyl barbituric acid (New Allonal), other barbiturates
   phenybutazone (Butazolidin), oxyphenbutazone, indomethacin, acetylsalicylic acid, carbamazepine (Tegretol), ibuprofen (Motrin), tolmetin (Tolectin)

2. Phenothiazines and other tranquilizers
   chlorpromazine (Thorazine), mepazine (Pacatol), promazine (Sparine), thioridazine (Mellaril), prochlorperazine (Compazine), imipramine (Tofranil), diazepam, etc.
   meprobamate (Miltown, Equanil), thiothixene (Navane), haloperidol (Haldol)

3. Sulfonamides (antibacterial)
   sulfanilamide, sulfisoxazole (Gantrisin), sulfamethoxypryridazine (Kynex), salicylazosulfapyridine (Azulfidine), sulfapyridine, sulfathiazole, sulfadizine, sulfadiazine silver (Silvadene), succinyl sulfathiazole, sulfasalazine (Salazopyrin), sulfaguanidine, trimethoprim-sulfamethoxazole (Bactrim)

4. Sulfonamides (nonantibacterial)
   chlorothiazides (Diuril), *carbutamide*, tolbutamide (Orinase), chlorpropamide (Diabinese), chlorthalidone (Hygroton), acetazolamide (Diamox)

5. Antithyroid drugs
   thiouracil, propylthiouracil, methimazole (Tapazole), carbimazole

6. Anticonvulsants
   diphenylhydantoin sodium (Dilantin), trimethyloxazolidine (Tridione), methylpenylethyl hydantoin (Mesantoin), phethenylate

7. Antihistamines and H2 blockers
   tripelennamine (Pyribenzamine), methapheniline (Diatrin), thenalidine (Sandostene), possibly chlorpheniramine, ranitidine, cimetidine (Tagamet)

8. Antimicrobial agents
   chloramphenicol, thiosemicarbazone (Tibione), ristocetin (Spontin), methicillin (Staphcillin), ampicillin, novobiocin, vancomycin, organic arsenicals, nitrofurantoin (Furadantin), para-aminobenzoic acid, metronidazole (Flagyl), cephalothin (Keflin), isonicotinic acid hydrazide (INH), levamisol, oxacillin, penicillin, augmentin, norfloxacin

9. Miscellaneous agents
   dinitrophenol, phenindione, penicillamine, thioglycolic acid (cold wave), mercurial diuretics, DDT, ethacrynic acid, procainamide, diethazine, cinchophen, dapsone, antimony (Neostibosan), pyrithyldione (Presidon), quinine, plasmochin, gold salts, rauwolfia (ajmaline)

* Drugs in italics are those associated most frequently with leukopenia.

(From: Lee, GR et al.: Wintrobe's Clinical Hematology, 9th ed. Philadelphia, Lea & Febiger, 1993.)

Pseudoneutropenia *Pseudoneutropenia* is similar to pseudoneutrophilia in that it is produced by alterations in the circulating and marginal pools. Pseudoneutropenia results from the transfer of an increased proportion of circulating neutrophils to the marginal neutrophil pool with no change in the total peripheral blood pool. This temporary shift is characteristic of some viral infections, bacterial infections with endotoxin production, and hypersensitivity. Because of the selective margination of neutrophils, the total leukocyte count drops, and a relative lymphocytosis develops.

Periodic or cyclic neutropenia

Periodic or cyclic neutropenia is a curious form of neutropenia that begins in infancy or childhood and occurs in regular 21- to 30-day cycles. This rare disorder is believed to be inherited as an autosomal-dominant trait but with variable expression. The neutrophil count drops to below 0.2×10^9/L. The neutropenic period lasts for several days and is marked by frequent infection, mucosal ulcers, fever, and malaise. During the neutropenic period, lymphocytosis, monocytosis, eosinophilia, and thrombocytopenia may develop. The total leukocyte count may vary with the neutrophil count or may remain constant in the low normal range.[4] Between the neutropenic attacks, the patient is asymptomatic. The marrow becomes hypoplastic shortly before neutropenia develops, and neutrophil precursors reappear in the bone marrow before the neutropenia in the peripheral blood abates.

The basic mechanism underlying the cyclic neutropenia is unknown. Recent studies have focused on the responsiveness of neutrophil precursors to hematopoietic growth factors. In one study, patients given G-CSF experienced a reduction in the frequency of infections and inflammation.[9] The neutrophil count increased, the duration of neutropenia decreased, and neutrophil nadir counts increased. The cyclic fluctuation however persisted. A more recent study revealed that bone marrow cells from patients with cyclic neutropenia require higher concentrations of G-CSF than normal bone marrow cells to stimulate granulocyte colony growth.[10] It has been demonstrated that the number of G-CSF binding sites (receptors) and the affinity of binding sites for recombinant human G-CSF are similar to controls.[11] These results suggest there may be a defective response mechanism to G-CSF.

Familial neutropenia

Another rare disorder marked by neutropenia is familial neutropenia, a benign, chronic anomaly. The total leukocyte count in these patients is usually normal with an absolute decrease in neutrophils and a relative increase in monocytes and lymphocytes. The platelets and erythrocytes are normal. The bone marrow is of normal cellularity with a shift to the left in neutrophil precursors. The disorder is transmitted as an autosomal-dominant trait and is usually detected by chance. Clinical symptoms are not always present but if so are usually mild.

Severe congenital neutropenia

Severe congenital neutropenia (SCN), also known as infantile genetic agranulocytosis or Kostmann's syndrome, is a rare, often fatal disorder marked by neutropenia. It is inherited as an autosomal-recessive trait, but sporadic cases have been reported. The neutrophil count is extremely low (less than 0.5×10^9/L) and accompanied by eosinophilia, monocytosis, and anemia. The total leukocyte count is often in the normal range. Evidence indicates the neutropenia is due to defective bone marrow production rather than shortened neutrophil survival. The marrow shows a maturation arrest with almost no development of the neutrophils past the myelocyte stage. Decreased production is probably the result of an intrinsic myeloid cell defect. Patients treated with pharmacologic doses of recombinant human G-CSF demonstrate an increase in neutrophil concentration.[12] The number of G-CSF binding sites on neutrophils is increased and the receptors' affinity for G-CSF is normal.[11] These findings suggest that the defect may be decreased responsiveness to G-CSF. Recent studies indicate that the combination of stem cell factor and G-CSF therapy lead to more normal neutrophil precursor growth and maturation.[13]

Immune neutropenia

Immune neutropenia is associated with the presence of antibodies directed against neutrophil-specific antigens (NA). These antigens include NA1, NA2, NB2, and 9a.

ALLOIMMUNE NEONATAL NEUTROPENIA This immune process is similar to that found in erythroblastosis fetalis. Alloimmune (isoimmune) neonatal neutropenia occurs when there is transplacental transfer of maternal alloantibodies directed against antigens on the infant's neutrophils. However, in contrast to erythroblastosis fetalis, the first born child is commonly affected. Infection may develop in affected infants until the neutropenia is resolved.

AUTOIMMUNE NEUTROPENIA Two forms of autoimmune neutropenia (AIN) are recognized: primary and secondary.

PRIMARY AUTOIMMUNE NEUTROPENIA Primary AIN is not associated with other diseases or disorders, and neutropenia is the only hematologic abnormality.[14] It occurs predominantly in children younger than 3 years. Diagnosis is usually made when the children are brought to the physician because of fever and recurrent infections. Infections are not usually life-threatening and are treated with routine antibiotic therapy. Median duration of neutropenia is from 13 to 20 months. Remission is usually spontaneous.

Neutropenia probably develops as a result of sequestration and destruction of antibody-coated neutrophils in the spleen. Phagocytosis of mature neutrophils by bone marrow macrophages also has been reported. In some cases, there also appears to be interference of myelopoiesis.

The etiology of the disorder is unknown. A variety of factors may contribute to AIN, including infections, drugs, dysfunction of the helper/suppressor T-lymphocyte mechanism, and heredity.

Laboratory findings are variable. The total leukocyte count may range from normal to decreased, but the neutrophil count is 0.25×10^9/L or lower. Monocytes often are increased, especially during periods of infection. Lymphocytes are relatively increased, but their absolute value is normal. The bone marrow is hypercellular or normal, but there is a decrease in mature neutrophils and bands. This gives the appearance of a maturation arrest.

Antineutrophil antibodies can almost always be detected.[11] The ability to detect these antibodies, however, varies among laboratories.[15] This variation appears to be due to the different techniques used to detect the antibod-

TABLE 13-7 *CAUSES OF FALSE LOW NEUTROPHIL COUNTS IN CLINICAL LABORATORY TESTING*

1. EDTA induced neutrophil adherence to erythrocytes. This may occur when blood is collected and mixed with the anticoagulant EDTA.
2. Distintegration of neutrophils due to delayed testing after the blood is drawn from the patient.
3. Disruption of abnormally fragile leukocytes during preparation of the blood for testing.
4. Neutrophil aggregation

ies. Neutrophil antibodies react differently in different serologic tests. Optimal sensitivity is dependent on using a combination of techniques. It has been suggested that laboratories use the combination of granulocyte agglutinatin test (GAT) and granulocyte immunofluorescence test (GIFT) as well as a typed granulocyte panel. Autoantibodies against most of the neutrophil-specific surface antigens have been detected.[15] Most cases demonstrate specificity against the NA-1 antigen located in the low affinity receptor for the Fc region of IgG (FcR III). GIFT is more sensitive than GAT for most neutrophil antibodies except antibodies to NB2 antigen. These antibodies are strong agglutinins and reportedly do not react in GIFT.[14]

Treatment is usually supportive. Antibiotic agents are used to control infections. Intravenous doses of immunoglobulin may be used in severe cases. Steroids are not generally recommended because of side effects.

SECONDARY AUTOIMMUNE NEUTROPENIA Secondary autoimmune neutropenia is generally found in older patients, many of whom have been diagnosed with other autoimmune disorders. Drug-induced immune neutropenia is often suspected but usually not confirmed by in vitro assays. Therapy depends on the cause but is usually similar to the therapy used in primary AIN.

False neutropenia It is important for the laboratory scientist to recognize when neutropenia is a result of laboratory in vitro manipulations of blood. There are at least four in vitro causes of a low neutrophil count (Table 13-7):

1. Erroneously low neutrophil counts may occur when blood is drawn in EDTA as neutrophils may adhere to erythrocytes. This phenomenon can be observed on stained blood smears. To obtain accurate cell counts, blood is obtained from a fingerstick to make manual dilutions and blood smears without using EDTA.
2. Neutrophils disintegrate faster than other white cells, and, when blood is left to stand for long periods before the count is performed, the neutrophil count will be erroneously decreased.
3. In some pathologic conditions, the white cells are more fragile than normal and may rupture with the manipulations of preparing blood for testing in the laboratory.
4. The neutrophil count may be falsely decreased if the neutrophils clump together, as occurs in the presence of some paraproteins (Fig. 13-7).

●
Morphologic abnormalities of neutrophils

Morphologic abnormalities of neutrophils may be identified by observation of cells on stained blood smears (Table 13-8). Cytoplasmic abnormalities are more common than nuclear abnormalities. Most of these cytoplasmic changes (Döhle bodies, toxic granulation, and vacuoles) are reactive transient changes accompanying infectious states.

DÖHLE BODIES
Döhle bodies (Fig. 13-8) are light gray-blue oval staining areas in the cytoplasm of neutrophils and eosinophils. They are usually found near the periphery of the cell. These bodies are composed of aggregates of rough endoplasmic reticulum. They were first described in 1911 by H. Döhle in patients with scarlet fever. They are seen in

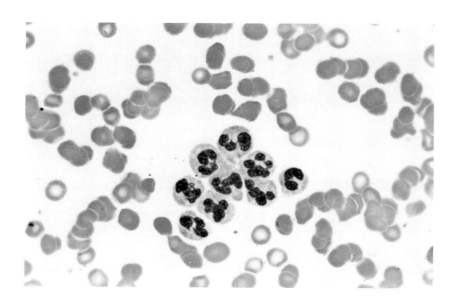

FIGURE 13-7. Aggregation or clumping of neutrophils. This blood smear was made from an immunosuppressed liver transplant patient. The clumping could be observed in blood smears made from blood collected in EDTA anticoagulant as well as in smears made from a fingerstick where blood did not come into contact with an anticoagulant. Accurate white blood cell counts could not be made. (250× original magnification.)

TABLE 13-8 *CYTOPLASMIC INCLUSIONS FOUND IN NEUTROPHILS IN INFECTIOUS CONDITIONS*

Inclusion	Morphologic Characteristics	Composition	Associated Conditions
Döhle body	Light grey-blue oval areas near periphery of cell	Aggregate of rough endoplasmic reticulum	Bacterial infections, pregnancy, burns, cancer, aplastic anemia, toxic states
Toxic granules	Large blue-black granules	Primary granules; peroxidase positive	Same as Döhle body
Cytoplasmic vacuole	Clear, unstained circular area	End stage of digestion of phagocytosed material or fat	Same as Döhle body
Morulae	Basophilic, granular, irregularly shaped	Tightly packed clusters of rickettsial organism from genus Ehrlichia	Ehrlichiosis

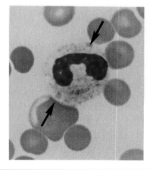

FIGURE 13-8. Döhle bodies (see arrows). (250× original magnification; Wright stain.)

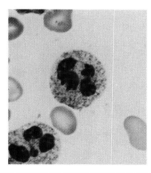

FIGURE 13-9. Neutrophil with toxic granulation (PB; 250× original magnification; Wright stain).

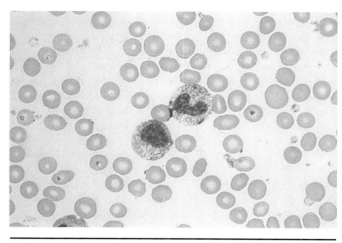

FIGURE 13-10. Band and metamyelocyte (shift to the left) with toxic granulation (PB; 250× original magnification).

severe bacterial infections, pregnancy, burns, cancer, aplastic anemia, and toxic states. Döhle bodies should be looked for whenever toxic granulation or other reactive morphologic changes are present, as they are frequently noted to occur together. Döhle bodies are similar in morphologic appearance to the neutrophilic inclusions found in May-Hegglin anomaly.

TOXIC GRANULES

Toxic granules (Figs. 13-9 and 13-10) are large, blue-black granules in the cytoplasm of segmented neutrophils and sometimes in band neutrophils and metamyelocytes. Histochemical stains (peroxidase) and electron microscopy indicate that these granules are primary (azurophilic) granules. Primary granules usually lose their basophilia as the cell matures; therefore, although about one third of the granules in the mature neutrophil are primary granules, their presence is obscured. In contrast, toxic primary granules retain their basophilia in the mature neutrophil, perhaps because of a lack of maturation, and they are easily observed on stained smears. Toxic granulation is seen in the same conditions in which Döhle bodies are seen. Care should be taken in reporting toxic granulation, as toxic-like granules may appear as an artifact with increased staining time or decreased pH of the buffer used in the staining process.

CYTOPLASMIC VACUOLES

Cytoplasmic vacuoles appear as clear, unstained areas in the cytoplasm. Vacuoles may represent the end stage of digestion of phagocytosed material, or they may represent fat or other stored substances. They are usually seen in the same conditions as toxic granulation and Döhle bodies. Although not specific, cytoplasmic vacuoles in neutrophils are a highly sensitive parameter for the presence of septicemia Figure 13-11. When this parameter is combined with the finding of an increased band count or granulocyte count, the sensitivity for the presence of septicemia is even greater (>97%).[16]

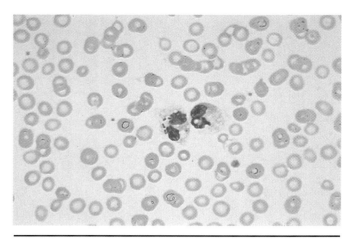

FIGURE 13-11. Bacteria and vacuoles in segmented neutrophil (PB; 250× original magnification; Wright-Giemsa stain).

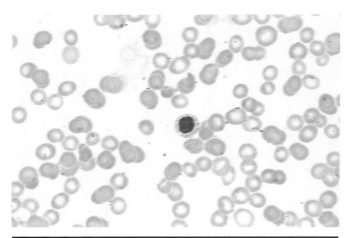

FIGURE 13-13. Pseudo-Pelger-Huet cell from a patient with a myelodysplastic syndrome. This neutrophil has a single round nucleus and the chromatin is condensed. (Peripheral blood; 250× original magnification; Wright-Giemsa stain).

Vacuoles also may appear as an artifact in blood smears made from blood that has been collected and stored in EDTA. The artifact can be eliminated by making smears from fresh blood without anticoagulant.

PELGER-HUET ANOMALY

Pelger-Huet anomaly (Fig. 13-12) is a benign, inherited, autosomal-dominant trait occurring in about 1 of 5000 individuals. The neutrophil nucleus in the heterozygous state does not segment beyond the two-lobed stage. It also may appear round with no segmentation. In the rare homozygote, the nuclei of all neutrophils are round or oval. Nuclear clumping of chromatin is intense, aiding in the differentiation of bi-lobed cells from true bands. The bi-lobed nucleus has a characteristic dumbbell shape with the two lobes connected by a thin strand of chromatin. Cells with this appearance are called "pince-nez" cells. Rod-shaped and peanut-shaped nuclei also are found. The cell is functionally normal. The significance of recognizing

this anomaly lies in differentiating the hereditary defect from a shift to the left occurring with infections.

Acquired or pseudo-Pelger-Huet (Fig. 13-13) anomaly can be seen in myeloproliferative disorders and myelodysplastic states. It also is found after chemotherapy for acute or chronic myelocytic leukemia. The acquired form is frequently accompanied by hypogranulation because of a lack of secondary granules, and the nuclei acquire the round rather than dumbbell shape. The chromatin shows intense clumping, aiding in differentiation of these mononuclear cells from myelocytes.

● Inherited qualitative (functional) abnormalities of neutrophils

Functional neutrophil abnormalities are almost always inherited and may or may not be accompanied by morphologic abnormalities. It is suggested that granulocyte function abnormalities be suspected in patients with recurrent, severe infections, abscesses, delayed wound healing, and in antibiotic-resistant sepsis. Special laboratory procedures are usually used to identify functional disorders.

ALDER-REILLY ANOMALY

Alder-Reilly anomaly, inherited as a recessive trait is characterized by the presence of large purplish granules in the cytoplasm of all leukocytes or, if incompletely expressed, in only one cell type. The granules stain metachromatically with toluidine blue. The inclusions in lymphocytes tend to occur in clusters in the shape of dots or commas and are surrounded by vacuoles (Gasser's cells) Fig. 13-14. This abnormal granulation accompanies the inherited group of mucopolysaccharide disorders such as Hurler's syndrome and Hunter's syndrome.[17] Frequently, the inclusions are seen only in cells of the bone marrow and not in the peripheral blood. The defect in these diseases is an incomplete breakdown of mucopolysaccharides due to various inherited enzyme deficiencies in the cells. Conse-

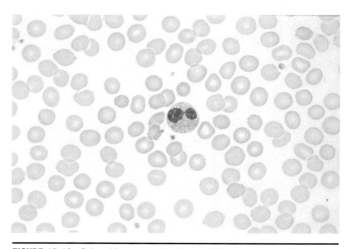

FIGURE 13-12. Pelger-Huet anomaly. A typical bilobular neutrophil (pince-nez cell) (peripheral blood ×800).

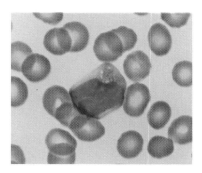

FIGURE 13-14. Lymphocyte from Hurler's disease (mucopolysaccharidoses), note the halo around the granules (PB).

quently, the partially degraded protein-carbohydrate accumulates in the liposomes of all body cells.

CHEDIAK HIGASHI ANOMALY

Chediak Higashi anomaly (Fig. 13-15) is a rare autosomal-recessive disorder in which death usually occurs in infancy or childhood because of serious pyrogenic infection. Giant gray-green peroxidase-positive bodies are found in the cytoplasm of leukocytes as well as in most granule-containing cells of all other tissues. In neutrophils, the bodies are formed by aggregation and fusion of primary azurophilic and specific granules. In monocytes, the granules are formed from fusion of granules. In lymphocytes and plasma cells, the abnormal granules may be primary granules. The histochemical reaction of the abnormal granules is similar to that seen in normal granules of the particular cell type. Neutrophils have abnormal fusion of cytoplasmic membranes. Neutrophil locomotion is impaired, decreasing the cell's activity in tissues. Defective chemotaxis is due to a defect at the membrane receptor level. These abnormal cells are ineffective in killing microorganisms. Neutropenia and thrombocytopenia are frequent complications as the disease progresses. The patients have skin hypopigmentation, silvery hair, and photophobia, from an abnormality of melanosomes. Lymphadenopathy and hepatosplenomegaly are characteristic.

MAY-HEGGLIN ANOMALY

May-Hegglin anomaly is a rare, inherited, autosomal-dominant trait in which granulocytes contain large baso-

philic and pyroninophilic inclusions. The inclusions are similar to Döhle bodies and consist mainly of RNA. Also characteristic of this disorder are giant platelets that contain a few granules and have a short survival. Thrombocytopenia and leukopenia are variable. Patients may have bleeding disorders because of platelet deficiencies, but no other clinical symptoms are apparent.

CHRONIC GRANULOMATOUS DISEASE

Chronic granulomatous disease (CGD) is an inherited disorder characterized by defects in the respiratory burst oxidase system. The morphology of the neutrophil is normal. Affected children suffer from recurrent infections with low-grade pathogens (micro-organisms that do not usually cause infections in normal individuals such as *Serratia marcescens,* enterobacteriacae, or staphylococci). The infections affect many tissues, producing recurrent pneumonia, osteomyelitis, and lymphadenitis. Granulomas are found in affected tissues. Although CGD occurs primarily in the pediatric population, it is now apparent that CGD also should be considered in the older population when persistent, recurrent infections occur.[18]

The abnormal neutrophils phagocytose the microorganisms but do not kill them because of a lack of respiratory burst and superoxide production. Catalase-positive microorganisms are not killed because they are capable of destroying the H_2O_2 of their own metabolism. They continue to grow intracellularly, protected from antibiotics. Catalase-negative organisms, however, kill themselves by generating H_2O_2, which they cannot break down.

CGD may be caused by a variety of defects that affect the leukocyte's ability to kill bacteria. Some defects are inherited in a sex-linked fashion and others are autosomal-recessive. Four subgroups of CGD are recognized, each due to an abnormal oxidase protein (Table 13-9).[15] Two subgroups are due to defective membrane-associated cytochrome b (composed of subunits gp 91 and p22), which serves as an electron carrier in the oxidase system. The more common sex-linked CGD is the result of a defect in the cytochrome subunit gp 91 phagocyte oxidase (gp 91^{phox}). A rare form of autosomal-recessive CGD is due to a defect in the cytochrome subunit p22 phagocyte oxidase

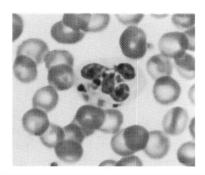

FIGURE 13-15. Neutrophil from Chediak-Higashi syndrome (PB).

TABLE 13-9 *CHARACTERISTICS OF CHRONIC GRANULOMATOUS DISEASE SUBGROUPS AND FREQUENCY AMONG SUBGROUPS*

Defect Site	Abnormal Protein	Inheritance/Site of Genetic Defect	Frequency
Membrane	Cytochrome b (gp 91 component)	Sex-linked X p21.1	56–65%
Membrane	Cytochrome b (p 22 component)	Autosomal recessive 16q24	5–6%
Cytosol	p 47	Autosomal recessive 7q11.23	25–33%
Cytosol	p 67	Autosomal recessive 1q25	5%

TABLE 13-10 *PERCENTAGE OF NEUTROPHILS POSITIVE IN THE NITROBLUE TETRAZOLIUM DYE TEST (NBT) ON BOYS WITH CHRONIC GRANULOMATOUS DISEASE (CGD), THEIR MOTHERS, GRANDMOTHERS AND SISTERS WHO ARE CARRIERS OF THE DISEASE, THEIR FATHERS, BROTHERS AND SISTERS WHO DO NOT CARRY THE GENE FOR THE DISEASE AND NORMAL CONTROLS. A POSITIVE CELL IS CAPABLE OF INITIATING AN INCREASE IN OXYGEN METABOLISM AFTER PHAGOCYTOSIS*

	Number	*% NBT-Positive Cells*
Patients (hemizygotes)	7	9.9 ± 4.2
Mother and grandmothers (heterozygote)	9	49.8 ± 5.4
Carrier sisters	7	51.3 ± 6.6
Fathers, brothers and normal sisters	18	74.4 ± 5.4
Normal subjects	12	89.5 ± 5.4

(From: Windhost, DB, et al: The pattern of genetic transmission of the leukocyte defect in fatal granulomatous disease of childhood. Journal of Clinical Investigations, 47, 1026, 1968)

($p22^{phox}$). The other two subgroups are due to defective soluble cytosol proteins (p 47 and p 67), whose function in the respiratory burst is not clear. These two proteins are inherited in an autosomal-recessive fashion.

Laboratory findings The peripheral blood neutrophil count is normal and increases in the presence of infection. Monocytosis may be present. Immunoglobulin levels are often increased because of chronic infection.[19]

The nitroblue tetrazolium dye test (NBT) is useful in detecting the abnormal oxygen metabolism of neutrophils. Neutrophils are mixed with the yellow dye, nitroblue tetrazolium, and microorganisms. In normal individuals, the leukocytes phagocytose the microorganisms, initiating an increase in oxygen uptake and a shift of glucose metabolism to the HMP shunt. This leads to accumulation of H_2O_2 and O_2-. These oxygen metabolites reduce the yellow NBT to formazan, a blue compound. Neutrophils from individuals with CGD cannot metabolize oxygen, there is insignificant accumulation of H_2O_2 and O_2-, and the NBT solution retains its yellow color. The test also is helpful in detecting female carriers of the sex-linked subgroup, who have about half normal and half abnormal neutrophils (Table 13-10). The depth of color may be read spectrophotometrically. The test also may be performed histochemically. In the histochemical procedure, individual cells on blood smears are evaluated for the presence of the blue formazen.

Treatment Treatment involves the use of prophylactic antibiotics and early treatment of infections.

MYELOPEROXIDASE DEFICIENCY

Myeloperoxidase deficiency is a benign, autosomally recessive inherited disorder. The disorder is characterized by an absence of myeloperoxidase in neutrophils and monocytes. Although this enzyme is needed to potentiate the effect of H_2O_2 by catalyzing the formation of the highly reactive oxidizing radical, HOCl, an increase in infections is not usually a complication of myeloperoxidase deficiency even in homozygous individuals. Therefore, the neutrophil must have other important mechanisms for killing microorganisms other than the myeloperoxidase reaction. In patients with concomitant diseases, however, there may be an increase in bacterial and fungal infections.[20] The peroxidase-deficient cells can be demonstrated with peroxidase stain (Figs. 13-16A and 13-16B). Peroxidase-deficient cells demonstrate a lack of peroxidase activity with this stain.

The Technicon H.1 automated hematology analyzer has very distinct cytograms in myeloperoxidase deficiency.[21] This cell counting system uses two leukocyte cytograms to enumerate and classify leukocytes: the peroxidase and the BASO/lobularity cytograms. The peroxidase cytogram clusters leukocytes based on size and peroxidase content. The BASO/lobularity cytogram clusters leuko-

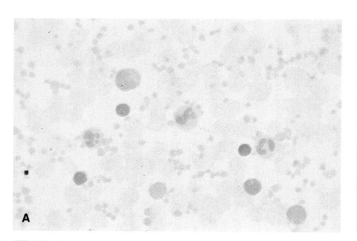

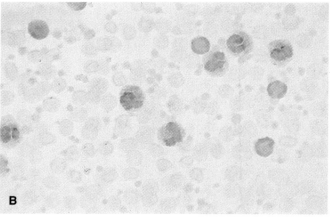

FIGURE 13-16. (A) Peripheral blood neutrophils from a patient with myeloperoxidase deficiency showing a lack of reactivity with peroxidase stain (PB); (B) Peripheral blood neutrophils from a normal individual showing reactivity with peroxidase stain (brown granules in cytoplasm) (PB).

cytes on nuclear shape and chromatin density. In myeloperoxidase deficiency, the peroxidase cytogram reveals a lack of cells with peroxidase activity, which results in a decreased neutrophil count. The BASO/lobularity cytogram, however, reveals a normal distribution of neutrophils. This discrepancy causes the instrument to flag the results. The discrepancy can be resolved by reviewing the stained blood smear. The neutrophils are present on the stained smears and appear morphologically normal.

An acquired form of myeloperoxidase deficiency occurs in some patients with acute myeloid leukemia, myelodysplastic syndromes, and chronic myelocytic leukemia. The myeloperoxidase-deficient cells may be derived from an abnormal stem cell and may function abnormally.

LEUKOCYTE ADHESION DEFICIENCY

Leukocyte adhesion deficiency (LAD) is a rare, autosomal-recessive disorder characterized by the absence of the leukocyte cell-surface adhesion proteins (integrins), the CD11/CD18 complex. The CD11/CD18 complex is composed of three proteins that share an identical β-chain (CD18) but possess distinct α-chains (CD11a, CD11b, CD11c). In LAD, there is a deficiency of the CD18 molecule. The CD11/CD18 molecules are important in cell motility, transendothelial migration, and serve as receptors for complement fragment C3bi, an important trigger for phagocytosis and respiratory burst activity. Neutrophils from patients with LAD have multiple defects in adhesion-related functions, including adhesion to endothelial cells, chemotaxis, C3bi mediated phagocytosis, particle-triggered respiratory burst activation, and degranulation.[20]

Clinical features of LAD include frequent bacterial and fungal infections, lack of pus formation, and delayed separation of the umbilical cord. There is persistent leukocytosis with granulocytosis (20 to 100 $\times$ 10^9/L).[22] The leukocytosis is believed to be due to increased stimulation of bone marrow related to recurrent infection. Because of defective adhesion proteins, the neutrophils cannot adhere to endothelial cells of the blood vessel walls and exit the circulation. Diagnosis can be made by flow cytometric analysis of neutrophil CD11b/CD18 levels using a monoclonal antibody.[12] Severity of the disease is related to the level of CD11/CD18 expression, which may be from 0% to 10% of normal.

Treatment includes prophylactic antibiotics, maintenance of oral hygiene, and early, aggressive treatment of infections. Mortality rate in childhood is high, and bone marrow transplantation is recommended in severe cases.

● EOSINOPHIL DISORDERS

Eosinophilia refers to an increase in eosinophils above 0.45 $\times$ 10^9/L. A slight physiologic eosinophilia occurs in the first 3 months of life. The normal eosinophil count for a newborn is up to 0.85 $\times$ 10^9/L.

● Reactive eosinophilia

Reactive eosinophilia appears to be induced by substances secreted from T-lymphocytes. A variety of conditions associated with the cellular immune response (mediated by T-lymphocytes) are characterized by eosinophilia including: (1) infection with metazoic parasites; (2) allergic conditions; (3) hypersensitivity reactions; (4) cancer; (5) chronic inflammatory states. In one study, parasitism and/or atopy (hypersensitivity or allergic response with a genetic predisposition) explained the eosinophilia in 92% of patients.[23] When the eosinophil concentration is high and immature forms are present, the blood picture may resemble that seen in chronic eosinophilic leukemia. This condition is referred to as an eosinophilic leukemoid reaction. The conditions associated with eosinophilia are listed in Table 13-11.

Tissue invasion by parasites produces an eosinophilia more pronounced than parasitic infestation of the gut or blood. Eosinophilia may disappear when the parasite encysts. Eosinophils are especially effective in fighting tissue larvae of parasites. Once the larvae become coated with IgG, IgE, and/or complement, the eosinophil becomes aggressive and begins its attack on the parasite. Products secreted by mast cells enhance eosinophil migration and increase the density of eosinophil receptors for chemotaxins. The larva is too large for the eosinophil to phagocytose; instead, the cell molds itself around the larva. Intracellular eosinophilic granules fuse with the eosinophil membrane and expel their contents into the space between the cell and the larva. The granular substances attack the larva wall, partially digesting it. The eosinophil continues its attack by sending cellular processes into the larva through the damaged area and expelling more of its granules into the larva.[24]

Eosinophils may play a major role in the formation of hepatic granulomas in schistosomiasis. A granuloma is a nodular aggregate of macrophages and lymphocytes that are involved in a cell-mediated immune response. The cellular aggregate is accompanied by fibroblasts and collagen tissue. An eosinophilic granuloma is distinguished by the presence of mature eosinophils within the aggregate of

TABLE 13-11 *CONDITIONS ASSOCIATED WITH EOSINOPHILIA*

Parasitic infection

Allergic disorders
  Hay fever
  Asthma
  Drug reactions

Infections
  Leprosy
  Brucellosis
  Tuberculosis
  Fungal infections
  Scarlet fever

Dermatitis

Malignancies

Collagen disease

Idiopathic hypersinophilic syndromes

Leukemia

Gastrointestinal disorders

cells. In the granulomatous reaction to hepatic schistosomiasis, the activity of the eosinophils contributes to the formation of the tissue-damaging granuloma and also kills some of the schistosome eggs.

Idiopathic eosinophilic esophagitis and idiopathic eosinophilic grastroenteritis occurring alone or concurrently are accompanied by peripheral blood eosinophilia. Cutaneous disorders (e.g., mycosis fungoides) or disorders associated with cutaneous rash (e.g., scarlet fever) are frequently accompanied by eosinophilia, especially in children. Inflammatory infectious diseases characterized by neutrophilia are not usually associated with an increase in eosinophils.

Various neoplasms and occult malignant tumors are associated with eosinophilia, which persists until the neoplasm is removed or reduced. Hodgkin's lymphoma is occasionally associated with a marked eosinophilia. In some myeloproliferative disorders, especially chronic myelogenous leukemia, eosinophilia is common. Sezary T-cell leukemia with hypereosinophilia and elevated IgG has been described. It is suspected that production of IL-4 and IL-5 by the malignant T-cells is responsible for these abnormalities.

Allergic disorders are characterized by a moderate increase in eosinophils. Large numbers also can be found in nasal discharges and sputum of allergic individuals. Eosinophilia may be found in a response to drug hypersensitivity.

● Hypereosinophilic syndrome

Hypereosinophilic syndrome (HES) is a catchall term used to describe a persistent blood eosinophilia more than 1.5 $\times$ 10^9/L with tissue infiltration and no apparent cause. Males are affected more frequently than females. Hepatosplenomegaly is common. If an increased serum IgE is found to accompany the idiopathic eosinophilia, HES may be the result of an immune response. Chronic eosinophilia may cause extensive tissue damage as the granules are released from disintegrating eosinophils. In many cases of HES, the heart is damaged by large numbers of circulating eosinophils. Charcot-Leyden crystals, which are formed from either eosinophil cytoplasm or granules, may be found in exudates and tissues where large numbers of eosinophils migrate and disintegrate.

Treatment with corticosteroids, hydroxyurea, and/or α-interferon is sometimes effective in reducing the eosinophil count.

The probability of whether the patient has eosinophilic leukemia should be considered in HES. In eosinophilic leukemia, there are usually increased numbers of myeloblasts and eosinophilic myelocytes, whereas in HES, the eosinophils are mature (Fig. 13-17). An abnormal chromosome karyotype suggests eosinophilic leukemia rather than HES.

Loffler's syndrome is a benign, self-limiting pulmonary form of HES, which subsides in a few weeks. The pulmonary tissue is infiltrated with eosinophils, but damage to the tissue is minimal or absent. Clinical manifestations include malaise, fever, and cough. Sputum usually con-

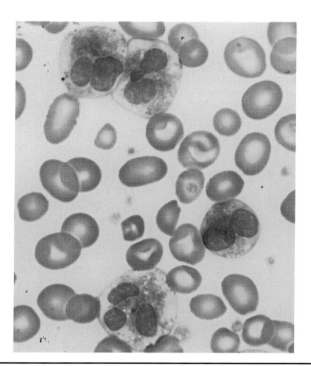

FIGURE 13-17. Eosinophils from a case of hypereosinophilic syndrome (HES); note that all cells are mature forms (PB; 250× original magnification; Wright stain).

tains eosinophils. It has been suggested that Loffler's syndrome may be caused by an allergic reaction to parasitic helminths, drugs, or inhaled antigens.

● Pulmonary infiltrate with eosinophilia syndrome

A more severe type of pulmonary eosinophilic infiltrate is known as pulmonary infiltrate with eosinophilia (PIE) syndrome. The syndrome consists of asthma, pulmonary infiltrates, central nervous system involvement, peripheral neuropathy, periateritis nodosa, and local or systemic eosinophilia. This syndrome may be produced by parasitic or bacterial infections, allergic reactions, or collagen disorders. In some cases, no cause can be found.

● Tropical eosinophilia

Tropical eosinophilia is a debilitating disease that occurs predominantly in males from India and Southeast Asia. The disease is most likely a hyperimmune response to microfilariae found in lung and lymph node tissues or other parasitic infection. This form of eosinophilia is associated with paroxysmal cough and bronchospasms. The disease can be cured with appropriate therapy to eliminate the parasite.

● Eosinopenia

Eosinopenia is difficult to establish because of the low normal levels of these cells. Although no eosinophils may be counted in a 100 leukocyte cell differential, a scan of the blood smear under 100 to 400 × magnification should reveal the presence of a few eosinophils. If no eosinophils are noted after scanning the smear, eosinopenia is probably present. Eosinopenia may be seen in acute stressful situations, inflammatory reactions, and with the administration of glucocorticosteroids, ACTH, epinephrine, and prostaglandins. Glucocorticosteroids and epinephrine inhibit eosinophil release from the bone marrow and increase margination. Bacterial infection may cause a decrease in eosinophils due to increased margination and migration of these cells to tissues, but recovery may be associated with a slight eosinophilia.

BASOPHIL DISORDERS

Basophilia refers to an increase in basophils above 0.15 $\times$ 10^9/L. Basophilia is associated with immediate hypersensitivity reactions. Basophils have receptors for IgE, the major immunoglobulin of hypersensitivity states. When the IgE binds to the basophil, the cell degranulates and releases histamine and other inflammatory mediators. Many of these cells can be found in tissues during hypersensitivity reactions.

Basophilia is associated with chronic myeloproliferative disorders, including myelofibrosis with myeloid metaplasia, polycythemia vera, and chronic myelogenous leukemia (CML). The basophil count in CML varies from 2% to 20%. The count reaches even higher levels late in the disease, often preceding the terminal phase. The basophil in CML is derived from the neoplastic stem cell clone because the basophil contains the abnormal Philadelphia chromosome, a chromosome found in the hematopoietic cells in CML. An absolute basophilia is often helpful in distinguishing CML from a leukemoid reaction or other benign leukocytosis. In benign leukocytosis, the basophil count is usually decreased. When the basophil count exceeds 80% of the total leukocyte population and the Philadelphia chromosome is not present, some hematologists prefer to call the disease basophilic leukemia, an extremely rare condition. Recently, a variant of acute promyelocytic leukemia was described, which showed basophil-like differentiation.[25] The leukemic promyelocyte granules showed metachromatic staining when stained with toluidine blue.

Basophilia also is seen in inflammatory bowel diseases, myxedema, and after radiation exposure.

Basophilopenia, a decrease in basophils, is even more difficult than eosinopenia to establish. Scanning a blood smear with 100$\times$ magnification will reveal a rare basophil in normal individuals. Decreases in basophils are seen in leukocytosis of infection, urticaria, immediately after anaphylaxis, inflammatory states, immunologic reactions, neoplasia, hemorrhage, and glucocorticoid therapy.

MONOCYTE DISORDERS

Quantitative disorders
MONOCYTOSIS
Monocytosis occurs when the absolute monocyte count exceeds 0.8 $\times$ 10^9/L. When evaluating a patient for mono-

TABLE 13-12 *CONDITIONS ASSOCIATED WITH MONOCYTOSIS*

Myelodysplastic syndromes

Myeloproliferative diseases
   Polycythemia vera
   Chronic myelogenous leukemia
   Acute leukemias
      acute monocytic leukemia
      acute myelomonocytic leukemia
      acute myeloblastic leukemia

Lymphocytic tumors
   Hodgkin's disease
   Lymphoma

Hemolytic anemia

Idiopathic thrombocytopenic purpura

Chronic neutropenia

Postsplenectomy state

Inflammatory disorders
   Collagen diseases
   Immune disorders
   Infections (e.g., TB, syphilis)
   Gastrointestinal disorders

Nonhematologic malignancies

Disorders of the monocyte-macrophage system
   Hand-Schüller-Christian disease
   Letterer-Siwe disease
   Eosinophilic granuloma

cytosis, it is important to take into consideration the age of the patient. In infants and children, the normal monocyte count ranges up to 1 $\times$ 10^9/L. When capillary blood is obtained from a finger puncture in individuals who have peripheral vascular disease (e.g., Raynaud's phenomenon), the monocyte count may be falsely elevated.[26]

Monocytes play an important role in inflammation and immune reactions; hence, an increase in these cells may be noted in a wide variety of conditions (Table 13-12). Monocytosis occurring in the recovery stage of acute infections and in agranulocytosis is considered a favorable sign. Monocytes play an important role in the immune cellular response in tuberculosis. Monocytes are the primary cell in new tubercle formation, which may be reflected in peripheral blood monocytosis.

Unexplained monocytosis has been reported to be associated with as many as 62% of all malignancies. Myelodysplastic states, acute myelocytic leukemia, and chronic myelocytic leukemia are associated with monocytosis. About 25% of Hodgkin's lymphomas are characterized by an increase in monocytes. In these conditions, the monocyte is probably a part of a reactive process to the neoplasm rather than a part of the clonal neoplasm itself. Neoplastic proliferation of monocytes occurs in acute monocytic leukemia and acute and chronic myelomonocytic leukemia.

MONOCYTOPENIA
A monocyte concentration below 0.2 $\times$ 10^9/L is referred to as *monocytopenia*. Monocytopenia is found in stem cell disorders such as aplastic anemia. Decreased monocyte

counts also are seen in hairy-cell leukemia and after gluco-corticosteroid therapy.

●
Qualitative disorders

Most inherited qualitative defects of neutrophils are associated with similar qualitative defects in the monocyte, indicating that the defective cells originate from a common stem cell. Chronic granulomatous disease affects monocytes in the same manner as neutrophils, because the monocytes in this disease also lack oxidase activity. In Chediak-Higashi disease, giant abnormal granules may be seen in the monocytes as well as in the neutrophils.

LIPID STORAGE DISORDERS

Cells or parts of cells are continually being replaced in the normal process of growth, development, and senescence. The breakdown of cellular debris takes place largely in the phagolysosomes of macrophages as a result of sequential enzymatic degradation. Macrophages are associated with a group of lipid storage disorders in which the cells are unable to completely digest phagocytosed material because of a deficiency of a particular enzyme needed for the degradation process. As a result, the undigested substance accumulates within the cell. The type of storage material in the cell and the tissue involved are characteristic for each different disorder (Table 13-13).

Gaucher disease   Gaucher (pronounced gaw-shay) disease is an inherited recessive trait that is characterized by a deficiency of glucocerebrosidase.[27] In this disease, the macrophage is unable to digest the stroma of ingested cells, and glucocerebroside accumulates. The clinical findings of the disease are related to the accumulation of this lipid in macrophages of the lymphoid tissue, spleen, liver, and bone marrow. The macrophages are large (20 to 80 μm) with small eccentric nuclei. The cytoplasm appears

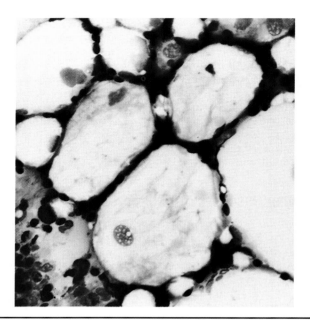

FIGURE 13-18. Gaucher cells from bone marrow. (100× original magnification; Wright stain.)

wrinkled or striated, often filled with debris (Gaucher cell) (Fig. 13-18). The cytoplasm is periodic acid–Schiff (PAS) and Sudan black B positive.[28]

Gaucher cells are present primarily in lymphoid tissue but may be found throughout the body. The spleen and liver become greatly enlarged. The bone marrow also is involved; destructive lesions of the bone may cause severe bone pain. Gaucher cells are demonstrable in bone marrow aspirations. Leukopenia, thrombocytopenia, and anemia may occur as the result of their sequestration by an enlarged spleen. Extravascular hemolysis is relatively mild with hemoglobin levels usually maintained above 8 g/dL. A consistent finding useful in diagnosis of Gaucher disease is an increase in serum acid phosphatase activity.

Three different types of Gaucher disease have been described, Types 1, 2, and 3. Type 1, the nonneurologic, chronic adult type, and Type 2, the infantile neuronopathic type, are genetically and clinically distinct. Type 3 (juvenile type) is considered a subacute neuronopathic disease with onset of symptoms between 6 months and 1 year of age. Death occurs in the first few years of life in Types 2 and 3. Type 1 has a better prognosis, with most patients living until adulthood or even into old age.

Cells similar to Gaucher cells may be found in the marrow of individuals with a rapid granulocyte turnover, especially in chronic myelocytic leukemia. The accumulation of lipid in these disorders does not result from a deficiency of an enzyme but rather to the inability of the macrophage to keep up with the flow of globoside into the cell. Gaucher disease may be confirmed by measuring the leukocyte β-glucosidase activity. It is decreased in Gaucher disease but normal or increased in myeloproliferative disorders.

Neimann-Pick disease   Neimann-Pick disease is a rare autosomal-recessive disease, more commonly seen in Ashke-

TABLE 13-13   *CHARACTERISTICS OF THE LIPID STORAGE DISORDERS*

Disease	Enzyme Deficiency	Type of Lipid Accumulated
Gaucher	β-glucocerebrosidase	glucocerebroside
Neimann-Pick	sphingomyelinase	sphingomyelin/ phospholipids/ cholesterol
Tay-Sachs	β-hexosaminidase A	gangliosides, glycolipids, mucopolysaccharides
Sandhoff	β-hexosaminidase A and β-hexosaminidase B	gangliosides, glycolipids, mucopolysaccharides
Fabry	α-galactosidase	ceremide trihexose
Wolman's	acid esterase	triglycerides, cholesterol esters
Tangier	HDL	cholesterol esters
Sea-blue histiocytosis	?	lipids containing cerebroside and carbohydrates

nazid Jews. Signs of the disease begin in infancy with poor physical development. The spleen and liver are greatly enlarged. The disease is often fatal by 3 years of age. The defect is a deficiency of sphingomyelinase, resulting in excessive sphingomyelin and ceroid storage.[29]

Foamy macrophages are found in lymphoid tissue and the bone marrow. The foam cells are large (20 to 100 μm) with an eccentric nucleus and globular cytoplasmic inclusions. Peripheral blood lymphocytes and monocytes may show characteristic vacuoles (lipid-filled liposomes). Leukopenia and thrombocytopenia may occur, but anemia is not conspicuous. The disease is confirmed by demonstrating sphingomyelinase deficiency in blood leukocytes.

Tay-Sachs disease and Sandhoff disease   Tay-Sachs disease and Sandhoff disease are autosomal-recessive diseases characterized by a deficiency of β-hexosaminidase. Tay-Sachs disease lacks β-hexosaminidase A, whereas Sandhoff disease lacks both β-hexosaminidase A and β-hexosaminidase B. As a result of these enzyme deficiencies, gangliosides and other glycolipids and mucopolysaccharides accumulate in tissue. The central nervous system is exclusively affected. The onset of symptoms occurs in the first few months of life. Infants fail to develop. The disease is often fatal by 4 years of age.

Fabry disease, Wolman's disease, and Tangier disease   Fabry disease, Wolman's disease, and Tangier disease also are variants of lipid storage diseases. In Fabry disease, the macrophages accumulate ceremide trihexose due to a deficiency of galactosidase. The disease is sex-linked, but heterozygote females usually manifest symptoms of the disease. Death is most commonly attributed to renal failure, which occurs in the third or fourth decades of life.

Wolman's disease is characterized by an increase in macrophage triglycerides and cholesterol esters due to a deficiency of acid esterase. The disease is clinically similar to Niemann-Pick disease, and death occurs early in infancy.

Tangier disease, a recessively inherited disorder, results in an increase of cholesterol esters stored in macrophages because of a deficiency of a high-density lipoprotein (HDL). This leads to hepatosplenomegaly and lymphadenopathy. The disease is benign in childhood, but arterial lipid deposits may precipitate pulmonary stenosis or coronary occlusion in adults. Plasma cholesterol and β-lipoproteins are decreased but pre-β-lipoproteins, chylomicrons, and triglycerides may be increased.

Sea-blue histiocytosis syndrome   Sea-blue histiocytosis syndrome is a primary familial disorder characterized by splenomegaly, thrombocytopenia, and occasionally hepatic cirrhosis.[30] Sea-blue staining macrophages (Fig. 13-19) are found in the spleen and bone marrow. The cell is large (20 to 60 μm in diameter) with a densely stained eccentric nucleus. The cytoplasm contains granules that stain blue or blue-green with Wright's stain. The granules stain positive with Sudan black B and PAS. No specific enzyme deficiency has been identified to account for the storage of lipids containing cerebroside and carbohydrate in these

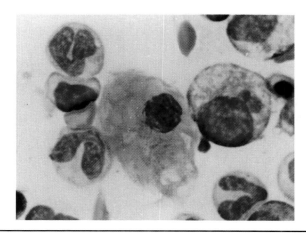

FIGURE 13-19. Sea-blue histiocyte from bone marrow. (250× original magnification; Wright stain.)

cells. Considerable variation in clinical manifestations is present but, in most patients, the course of the disease is benign. A secondary or acquired type of this disease has been described in which the sea-blue histiocytes are found in the spleen but only rarely in the bone marrow. This acquired type has been found in association with idiopathic thrombocytopenic purpura, chronic myelocytic leukemia, hyperlipoproteinemia, thalassemia, polycythemia vera, sickle cell anemia, sarcoidosis, chronic granulomatous disease, and other lipid disorders. It is not clear if the presence of the sea-blue histiocytes in these secondary types is due to lipid overload of the normal enzyme system or if there is a deficiency of an enzyme.

SUMMARY

Leukocytes respond to toxic, infectious, and inflammatory processes to defend the tissues and limit and/or eliminate the disease process or toxic challenge. This may involve a change in leukocyte concentration, most often an increase in one or more leukocyte types. The type of cell affected depends on the cell's function. Thus, a differential count as well as the total leukocyte count aids in diagnosis.

Neutrophilia, an increase in neutrophils, most often occurs as a result of a reaction to a physiologic or pathologic process. The most common cause is bacterial infection. Tissue injury or destruction and inflammation also may cause a neutrophilia.

Neutropenia, a decrease in neutrophils, is less commonly encountered. It may be caused by drugs, immune mechanisms, or by decreased bone marrow production. There are several inherited conditions that are characterized by neutropenia and recurrent infections.

Morphologic abnormalities of neutrophils may be found in infectious states and are important to identify on stained blood smears. These include the acquired abnormalities Döhle bodies, toxic granulation, and cytoplasmic vacuoles. Other morphologic abnormalities include pince-nez cells found in Pelger-Huet anomaly and morulae found in ehrlichiosis.

There are a number of inherited conditions characterized by functional and morphologic abnormalities of neutrophils. Chronic granulomatous disease and myeloperoxidase deficiency are characterized by defects in the generation of oxidizing radicals after phagocytosing bacteria. These two disorders may be identified by specific laboratory tests. The nitroblue tetrazolium dye test is used to detect abnormal oxygen metabolism in CGD. Peroxidase-deficient cells can be demonstrated with peroxidase stain. LAD is identified by the absence of leukocyte cell-surface adhesion proteins, CD11/CD18 complex. Diagnosis can be made by flow cytometric analysis of neutrophil CD11/CD18 levels using monoclonal antibodies. Other rare leukocyte functional abnormalities include Alder-Reilly anomaly, Chediak Higashi anomaly, and May-Hegglin anomaly.

Eosinophils are increased in a variety of conditions, particularly those associated with the cellular immune response. Eosinophilia may be seen in infections with metazoic parasites, allergic conditions, hypersensitivity reactions, cancer, and chronic inflammatory states.

Basophilia is seen in hypersensitivity reactions and chronic myeloproliferative disorders.

Monocytes play an important role in inflammation and immune reactions. Hence, monocytosis is found in a wide variety of conditions, especially malignancies. Qualitative disorders of monocytes are found in many of the inherited neutrophil disorders. Macrophages are associated with a group of lipid storage disorders in which the cells are unable to completely digest phagocytosed material because of a deficiency of a particular enzyme needed for the degradation process.

REVIEW QUESTIONS

A 56-year-old man with abdominal pain and tenderness, vomiting, and moderate fever was brought to the emergency room. The physician ordered a complete blood count. The results were:

Hb	15.2 gm/dL
Hct	0.46 L/L
Erythrocyte count	5.17×10^{12}/L
Leukocyte count	16.6×10^{9}/L
Platelet count	308×10^{9}/L

Differential count:
74%   segmented neutrophils
1%   eosinophils
23%   lymphs
2%   monocytes

Neutrophils have vacuoles and Döhle bodies. The patient was diagnosed with peritonitis.

1. The changes in the neutrophils are indicative of what type of abnormality in the neutrophil?
   a. myeloperoxidase deficiency
   b. intracellular parasites
   c. reactive toxic changes
   d. glucocerebrosidase deficiency

2. Based on the results of this patient's differential and leukocyte count, which of the following best describes the physiology of the neutrophilia?
   a. There is an indication that the bone marrow storage pool of mature neutrophils has been depleted.
   b. The peripheral blood marginal pool has been redistributed to the circulating pool increasing the neutrophil count.
   c. The bone marrow has increased its release of mature neutrophils from the storage pool to the peripheral blood.
   d. The neutrophilia is a reaction to a chronic stimulus for neutrophils, probably related to chronic hemorrhage into the peritoneal cavity.

3. What are Döhle bodies?
   a. Aggregates of rough endoplasmic reticulum
   b. Primary granules
   c. Fat globules
   d. Liposomes containing partially degraded mucopolysaccharides

4. The vacuoles in the neutrophils are indicative of:
   a. fat
   b. digested bacteria
   c. morulae
   d. mucopolysaccharides

5. Which term best describes the results of this blood count?
   a. lymphocytosis
   b. neutropenia
   c. lymphocytopenia
   d. neutrophilia

6. A leukemoid reaction may be distinguished from chronic myelocytic leukemia by:
   a. the total leukocyte count
   b. the presence or absence of immature neutrophils
   c. chromosome studies
   d. the presence or absence of anemia

7. A leukoerythroblastic reaction is characterized by the presence of _____ in the peripheral blood:
   a. immature leukocytes and nucleated erythrocytes
   b. lymphocytosis and neutropenia
   c. leukocytosis and erythrocytosis
   d. pseudo-Pelger Huet cells

8. In leukocyte adhesion deficiency, there is a:
   a. decrease in neutrophils in the peripheral blood
   b. hypoplastic bone marrow
   c. failure of the nucleus to segment in neutrophils
   d. decrease in CD11/CD18 complex on leukocytes

9. An increase in basophils is associated with:
   a. chronic myeloproliferative diseases
   b. parasitic infection
   c. chronic infection
   d. administration of glucocorticoids

10. Lipid storage disorders are characterized by:
    a. a decrease in enzymes needed for the respiratory burst

b. a leukoerythroblastic reaction
c. myeloperoxidase deficiency
d. deficiency of enzymes needed to digest phagocytosed material

● REFERENCES

1. Necheles, T.F.: Quantitative disorders of leukocytes: differential diagnosis. In CRC Handbook Series in Clinical Laboratory Science. Section I: Hematology Volume II. Edited by D. Seligson. Boca Raton, CRC Press Inc., 1980.
2. Stewart, G.J.: Neutrophils and deep venous thrombosis. Haemostasis, 23(suppl1): 127, 1993.
3. Athens, J.W.: Variations of leukocytes in disease. In Wintrobe's Clinical Hematology. Edited by G.R. Lee, T.C. Bithell, J. Foerster, J.W. Athens, and J.N. Lukens. Philadelphia, Lea & Febiger, 1993.
4. Athens, J.W.: Neutropenia. In Wintrobe's Clinical Hematology. Edited by G.R. Lee, T.C. Bithell, J. Foerster, J.W. Athens, J.N. Lukens. Philadelphia, Lea & Febiger, 1993.
5. Bakken, J.S., et al.: Human granulocytic ehrlichiosis in the upper midwest United States. JAMA, 272:212, 1994.
6. Fishbein, D.B., Dawson, J.E., and Robinson, L.E.: Human erlichiosis in the United States, 1985-1990. Ann. Intern. Med., 120:736, 1994.
7. Dumler, J.S., and Bakken, J.S.: Ehrlichial diseases of humans: emerging tick-borne infections. Clin. Infect. Dis., 20:1102, 1995.
8. Spivak, J.L. (ed.): Fundamentals of Clinical Hematology. 2nd Ed. Philadelphia, Harper & Row, 1984.
9. Hammond, W.P., Price, T.H., Souza, L.M., Dale, D.C.: Treatment of cyclic neutropenia with granulocyte-colony stimulating factor. N. Engl. J. Med., 320:1306, 1989.
10. Hammond, W.P., Chatta, G.S., Andrew, R.G., Dale, D.C.: Abnormal responsiveness of granulocyte-committed progenitor cells in cyclic neutropenia. Blood, 79:2536, 1992.
11. Kyas, U., Pietsch, T., Welte, K.: Expression of receptors for granulocyte colony-stimulating factor in neutrophils from patients with severe congenital neutropenia and cyclic neutropenia. Blood, 79:1144, 1992.
12. Bonilla, M.A., et al.: Effects of recombinant human granulocyte colony-stimulating factor on neutropenia in patients with congenital agranulocytosis. N. Engl. J. Med., 320:1574, 1989.
13. Hestdal, K., Welte, K., Lie, S.O., Keller, J.R., Ruscetti, F.W., Abrahamsen, T.G.: Severe congenital neutropenia: abnormal growth and differentiation of myeloid progenitors to granulocyte colony-stimulating factor (G-CSF) but normal response to G-CSF plus stem cell factor. Blood, 82:2991, 1993.
14. Bux, J., Mueller-Eckhardt, C.: Autoimmune Neutropenia. Sem. Hematol., 29:45, 1992.
15. Dinauer, M.C.: Leukocyte function and nonmalignant leukocyte disorders. Curr. Opin. Pediatr., 5:80, 1993.
16. Strand, C.L., Goldstein, D., Castella, A.: Value of cytoplasmic vacuolization of neutrophils in the diagnosis of bloodstream infection. Lab. Med., 22:263, 1991.
17. Reilly, W.A., Lindsay, S.: Gargoylism (lipochondrodystrophy): a review of clinical observation in eighteen cases. Am. J. Dis. Child., 75:595, 1948.
18. Becker, C.E., Graddick, S.L., Roy, T.M.: Patterns of chronic granulomatous disease. J. Ky. Med. Assoc., 91:447, 1993.
19. Athens, J.W.: Qualitative disorders of leukocytes. In Wintrobe's Clinical Hematology. Edited by G.R. Lee, T.C. Bithell, J. Foerster, J.W. Athens, J.N. Lukens. Philadelphia, Lea & Febiger, 1993.
20. Falloon, J., Gallin, J.I.: Neutrophil granules in health and disease. J. Allergy Clin. Immunol., 77:653, 1986.
21. McKenzie, S.B., Metz, J.A.: Hematology Tech Sample No. H-3 (1991). Chicago: American Society of Clinical Pathology, 1991.
22. Yang, K.D., Hill, H.R.: Neutrophil function disorders: Pathophysiology, prevention, and therapy. J. Pediatr., 119:343, 1991.
23. Teo, C.G., et al.: Evaluation of the common conditions associated with eosinophilia. J. Clin. Pathol., 38:305, 1985.
24. Boggs, D.R., Winkelstein, A.: White Cell Manual. 4th Ed. Philadelphia, F.A. Davis Co, 1983.
25. Castoldi, G.L., Liso, V., Specchia, G., Tomasi, P.: Acute promyelocyte leukemia: Morphological aspects. Leukemia, 8:1441, 1994.
26. Czaczkes, J.W., Dreyfuss, F.: Discrepancy of fingertip and ear lobe leukocyte counts in Raynaud's disease. Am. J. Med. Sci., 234:325, 1957.
27. Brady, R.O., Kanfer, J.N., Bradley, R.M., Shapiro, D.: Demonstration of a deficiency of glucocerebroside-cleaving enzyme in Gaucher's disease. J. Clin. Invest., 45:1112, 1966.
28. Athens, J.W.: Disorders involving the monocyte-macrophage system- the "Storage diseases." In Wintrobe's Clinical Hematology. Edited by G.R. Lee, T.C. Bithell, J. Foerster, J.W. Athens, J.N. Lukens. Philadelphia, Lea & Febiger, 1993.
29. Brady, R.O., Kanfer, J.N., Mock, M.B., Fredrickson, D.S.: The metabolism of sphingomylin: II. Evidence of an enzymatic deficiency in Niemann-Pick disease. Proc. Natl. Acad. Sci. USA., 55:366, 1966.
30. Silverstein, M.N., Ellefson, R.D.: The syndrome of the sea-blue histiocyte. Semin. Hematol., 9:299, 1972.

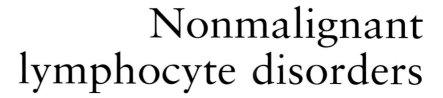

Nonmalignant lymphocyte disorders

14

INTRODUCTION

Laboratory evidence of abnormal concentrations of lymphocytes or the presence of abnormal or reactive lymphocytes often provides the clinician with important information for diagnosis, for directing subsequent workup, and/or for initiating appropriate therapy. Nonmalignant lymphocyte disorders or reactive lymphocyte changes may be acquired or congenital and may affect either T-lymphocytes or B-lymphocytes or both cell populations.

Acquired disorders

In most cases, acquired disorders are quantitative in nature and occur as a self-limited reactive process to infections or inflammatory conditions. Both T- and B-lymphocytes are usually affected. The function of the cells is usually normal. Occasionally, acquired conditions, such as viral infections, may cause a functional impairment of the lymphocytes (qualitative disorder) as well as quantitative changes.

The stimulated lymphocytes in infections and inflammatory conditions are in various states of activation, resulting in a heterogeneous morphologic appearance on stained blood smears (Figs. 14-1 and 14-2). These activated cells may appear large with irregular shapes and cytoplasmic basophilia. The nuclear chromatin usually becomes more disperse. Occasionally, there is intense proliferation of lymphoid elements in the lymph nodes and spleen, causing lymphadenopathy and splenomegaly, respectively.

Acquired quantitative disorders

LYMPHOCYTOSIS

In most acquired quantitative lymphocyte disorders, the lymphocytes are increased. *Lymphocytosis* in adults oc-

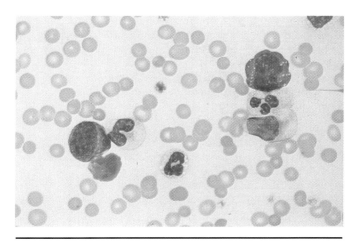

FIGURE 14-2. Two immunoblasts (1 o'clock and 8 o'clock) and a reactive lymph (3 o'clock). These are reactive forms of stimulated lymphocytes and can be found in infectious states, especially viral infections. (Peripheral blood; 250× original magnification; Wright-Giemsa stain).

curs when the absolute lymphocyte count exceeds $4 \times 10^9/L$ and in children when the count exceeds $9 \times 10^9/L$. T-lymphocytes comprise about 60% to 80% of peripheral blood lymphocytes. Thus, changes in the concentration of these lymphocytes are more likely to cause increases or decreases in the relative lymphocyte count than changes in the B-lymphocytes. Absolute lymphocytosis is not usually accompanied by leukocytosis except in infectious mononucleosis, infectious lymphocytosis, *Bordatella pertussis* infection, cytomegalovirus, and lymphocytic leukemia. Relative lymphocytosis, secondary to neutropenia, is more common than absolute lymphocytosis and occurs in a variety of viral infections.

It is important to differentiate benign conditions associated with lymphocytosis from neoplastic lymphoproliferative disorders. The presence of reactive lymphocytes, positive serologic tests, and absence of anemia and thrombocytopenia favor a benign diagnosis.

Infectious mononucleosis *Infectious mononucleosis* is a self-limiting lymphoproliferative disease caused by infection with Epstein-Barr virus (EBV). EBV usually affects young adults, and the peak age for infection is 14 to 24 years. In children from lower-income groups, infection usually occurs before 4 years of age, while in more affluent populations, peak infection incidence occurs during adolescence. The disease rarely occurs in adults. About 80% to 90% of adults have been exposed and possess antibody to the virus. These individuals have a lifelong immunity to infection with EBV.

Cellular immunity is important in limiting the growth potential of EBV-infected B-lymphocytes; those individuals with compromised cellular immunity are at increased risk of serious infection. EBV-associated B-cell tumors and lymphoproliferative syndromes may occur in transplant patients or in patients with acquired immune deficiency syndrome (AIDS).[1] These patients have severe T-lymphocyte immunodeficiency. Male children with a rare x-linked

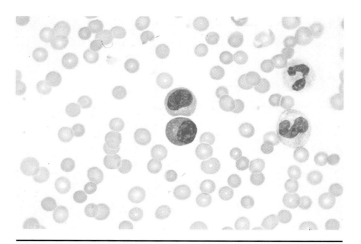

FIGURE 14-1. A reactive lymph (top) and plasmacytoid lymph (bottom). These stimulated cells can be found in infectious states, especially viral infections. (Peripheral blood; 250× original magnification; Wright-Giemsa stain).

lymphoproliferative syndrome are unable to limit EBV infection of B-lymphocytes via a T-lymphocyte response. As a result, there is a fatal B-lymphocyte proliferation (polyclonal).[3]

The disease, not considered to be highly contagious, is usually transmitted through saliva; the most common means of transmission is kissing (hence the nickname "kissing disease").

MECHANISM OF INFECTION WITH EBV The EBV attaches to B-lymphocytes by means of a specific EBV receptor designated CD21 on the lymphocyte membrane surface.[1] This also is the receptor for the C3d complement component. The virus preferentially infects resting B-lymphocytes as well as epithelial cells of the oropharynx and cervix. The binding of the virus to the lymphocyte activates the lymphocyte, causing it to express the activation marker, CD23.[2] CD23 serves as the receptor for a B-lymphocyte growth factor. Once internalized, the virus is incorporated into the B-lymphocyte genome, instructing the cell to begin production of EBV proteins. These viral proteins are expressed on the B cell membrane. Thus, EBV-infected cells express markers of activated B-lymphocytes as well as viral markers. The viral genome is maintained in the lymphocyte nucleus and passed on to the cell's progeny. This results in EBV-immortalized B-lymphocytes and latent infection.

Acute EBV infection is controlled primarily by a complex, mulitfaceted cellular immune response. In the first week of illness, there is a polyclonal increase in immunoglobulins. During the second week, however, the number of immunoglobulin secreting B-lymphocytes decrease presumably due to the action of suppressor T-lymphocytes. Activated cytotoxic cells that resemble activated killer cells are present early in the course of the disease. These cells are neither EBV-specific or HLA-restricted (virus-nonspecific). Cytotoxic T-lymphocytes inhibit the activation and proliferation of EBV-infected B-lymphocytes and also participate in the cell-mediated immune response. The majority of the reactive lymphocytes seen in the peripheral blood are the suppressor-cytotoxic T-lymphocytes.

CLINICAL FINDINGS Prodromal symptoms include lethargy, headache, fever, chills, sore throat, nausea, and anorexia. The classic triad of symptoms at presentation are fever, pharyngitis, and lymphadenopathy.[3] (In children younger than 10 years of age, symptoms may not be present or are mild and nonspecific).[4] The cervical, axillary, and inguinal lymph nodes are commonly enlarged. Splenomegaly occurs in 50% to 75% of these patients, and hepatomegaly occurs in about 25%. Occasionally, jaundice may develop. Ampicillin given to patients with infectious mononucleosis causes rashes in 70% to 100% of the individuals. Hematologic complications that may occur during or immediately after the disease include autoimmune hemolytic anemia, thrombocytopenia, agranulocytosis, and (very rarely) aplastic anemia. The disease is usually self-limited. The convalescence period usually lasts a few weeks, but it can extend into months, especially when complications occur.

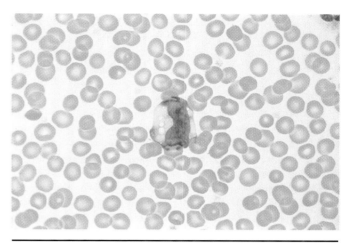

FIGURE 14-3. A reactive (atypical) lymphocyte from a case of infectious mononucleosis. (PB; 250× original magnification; Wright-Giemsa stain.)

LABORATORY FINDINGS

PERIPHERAL BLOOD During active viral infection, there is an intense proliferation of lymphocytes within affected lymph nodes. The leukocyte count is usually increased (12 to 25×10^9/L), primarily because of an absolute lymphocytosis. Lymphocytosis begins about 1 week after symptoms appear, peaks at 2 to 3 weeks, and remains for 2 to 8 weeks.[5] Lymphocytes usually constitute more than 50% of the leukocytes. Various forms of reactive lymphocytes (>20%) in the process of blast transformation can be found in the peripheral blood, and many contain vacuoles (Figs. 14-3 and 14-4). Immunoblasts are usually present, especially early in the disease. Plasmacytoid lymphocytes and an occasional plasma cell also may be found. When present, immunoblasts should be distinguished from leu-

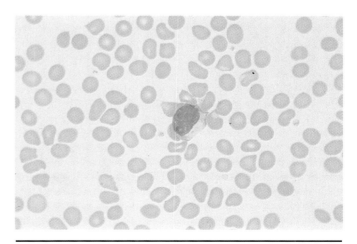

FIGURE 14-4. Lymphocyte from a patient with infectious mononucleosis. Note the large nucleolus and irregular cytoplasmic membrane. This cell must be distinguished from a leukemic lymphoblast. (PB; 250× original magnification; Wright-Giemsa stain.)

kemic lymphoblasts to prevent misdiagnosis. The chromatin pattern of leukemic lymphoblasts is usually finer than the reticular chromatin of immunoblasts. In addition, immunoblasts generally have more abundant, often vacuolated, cytoplasm. Another important criterion that helps differentiate infectious mononucleosis from leukemia is the morphologic heterogeneity of the lymphocyte population characteristic of viral infections in infectious mononucleosis. Other diseases associated with a reactive lymphocytosis may be confused with the blood picture of infectious mononucleosis. These include cytomegalovirus infection, viral hepatitis, and toxoplasmosis.

The platelet count is often mildly decreased, but counts less than 100×10^9/L are rare.

BONE MARROW Bone marrow aspirations in EBV infection are not indicated, but when performed may show hyperplasia of all cellular elements except neutrophils.

SEROLOGIC TESTS Serologic tests are used to differentiate this disease from similar more serious diseases (i.e., diptheria, hepatitis). Paul, in 1932, found that the sera of patients with infectious mononucleosis contained greatly increased levels of antibodies against sheep erythrocytes.[6] He named these antibodies *heterophil antibodies* because the antibodies are directed against a heterologous antigen that did not stimulate their production. Later, it was found that these antibodies also reacted against beef and horse erythrocytes but in different patterns. The IgM heterophil antibodies agglutinate horse erythrocytes and lyse, but do not agglutinate beef erythrocytes.These characteristics of heterophil antibodies were used to develop the Paul-Bunnell serologic test and Davidsohn differential serologic test, tests that are helpful in the diagnosis of infectious mononucleosis. In the Paul-Bunnell serologic test, serial dilutions of the patient's serum are incubated with suspensions of sheep or horse erythrocytes. The highest dilution that agglutinates erythrocytes is noted. The test is positive in infectious mononucleosis after the first week of illness. The peak titer of heterophil agglutinins occurs at 2 to 3 weeks after infection and falls in 6 to 8 weeks.

Other diseases also are associated with production of heterophil antibodies, and these antibodies also may agglutinate sheep erythrocytes. The specificity of the serologic test for infectious mononucleosis is increased when one aliquot of serum is absorbed with beef (ox) erthrocytes and another aliquot is absorbed with guinea pig kidney cells before reacting the serum with sheep erythrocytes (Davidsohn's differential test) (Table 14-1). Heterophil antibodies associated with infectious mononucleosis are absorbed from serum by beef erythrocytes but not by guinea pig kidney cells. Thus, the guinea pig absorbed serum will still agglutinate sheep erythrocytes, but the beef-absorbed serum will not.

Another type of heterophil antibody that occurs in almost all human sera and also agglutinates sheep erythrocytes is called the *Forssman antibody*. Forssman antibodies are produced by a variety of infectious agents and are not associated with infectious mononucleosis. These antibodies can be differentiated from the heterophil antibodies

TABLE 14-1 *THE PATTERN OF ABSORPTION OF DIFFERENT TYPES OF HETEROPHIL ANTIBODIES (ANTI-SRBC) BY GUINEA PIG KIDNEY AND BEEF ERYTHROCYTES*

	Absorbed by*	
Antibody	*Guinea Pig Kidney*	*Beef Erythrocytes*
Infectious mononucleosis antibodies	−	+
Forssman antibodies	+	∓
Serum sickness antibodies	+	+

* + complete absorption; − no absorption; ∓ incomplete absorption

of infectious mononucleosis because they are totally removed from serum by absorption with tissue that contains the Forssman antigen (such as guinea pig kidney cells) but are only partially absorbed by beef erythrocytes. Thus, the guinea pig-absorbed serum will not agglutinate sheep erythrocytes, but there will be some agglutination with the beef erythrocyte-absorbed serum if Forssman heterophil antibodies are present.

Heterophil antibodies that occur in serum sickness can be differentiated from Forssman antibodies and heterophil antibodies of infectious mononucleosis because they are absorbed by both guinea pig kidney cells and beef erythrocytes. With serum sickness, there will be no agglutination of sheep erythrocytes by either absorbed serum.

The ability of serum dilutions to agglutinate sheep erythrocytes before and after absorption with beef erythrocytes and guinea pig kidney cells will help determine the concentration of heterophil antibodies resulting specifically from infectious mononucleosis. Heterophil titers of 1:56 or greater before guinea pig absorption and 1:28 or greater after absorption are considered positive for infectious mononucleosis antibodies.

A rapid, specific, and sensitive slide agglutination test (Monospot) uses the same principles as the original heterophil antibody test. Serum or blood of the patient is mixed with a ground suspension of guinea pig kidney and beef erythrocyte stroma on two separate spots of a glass slide. Horse erythrocytes are then mixed with each suspension and observed for agglutination. A positive test will show agglutination of horse erythrocytes in the guinea pig suspension but not in the beef erythrocyte stroma suspension.

Occasionally, a patient with all the clinical manifestations and peripheral blood findings of infectious mononucleosis may not have an elevated heterophil titer (heterophil-negative mononucleosis). In 10% to 20% of adult cases and in 50% of children younger than 10 years of age, the test is negative in the presence of EBV infection. In other cases, the heterophil-negative syndrome is caused by other viral infections. The most likely causative agent is cytomegalovirus; however, toxoplasmosis, hepatitis, and drug intoxication also should be considered.

A variety of antibodies to EBV antigens are produced by the infected individual. These antibodies are distinct

TABLE 14-2 *ANTIBODIES TO EBV THAT ARE FOUND IN INFECTIOUS MONONUCLEOSIS*

Stage of Infection	Heterophil Antibodies	VCA-IgM (titer)	VCA-IgG (titer)	EBNA (titer)
Acute (0–3 months)	Present	>1:160	>1:60	not detected
Recent (3–12 months)	Present	not detected	>1:160	>1:10
Past (>12 months)	Absent	not detected	>1:40	>1:40

from the transient heterophil antibodies and appear at various stages of infection (Table 14-2). The IgG antibody to the viral capsid antigen (VCA) develops early in the infection and remains with the individual for life. Immunofluorescent techniques are used to test for this antibody. IgM antibodies to the VCA also can be detected in active infection but disappear after a few months. An antibody to EBV nuclear antigen (EBNA) appears after the acute phase of infection and persists for life. Thus, acute infection is best detected using the VCA-IgM titer while recent infection is detected by VCA-IgG titers and past infection by EBNA antibody. Antibody responses may not be detected in immunosuppressed individuals.

Other laboratory tests may be abnormal depending on the presence or absence of complications. A rare complication of infectious mononucleosis is hemolytic anemia. The anemia appears to be due to cold agglutinins directed against the erythrocyte i antigen. Hepatitis of some degree is common and can be a severe complication. An elevation of both bilirubin fractions, direct and indirect, and an increase in serum liver enzymes is a common finding.

THERAPY Since the disease is self-limited, therapy is supportive. Bed rest is recommended if fever and myalgia are present. Strenuous exercise should be avoided for several weeks, especially if splenomegaly is present. Antibiotics are not useful except in the presence of secondary infections.

Toxoplasmosis *Toxoplasmosis* is the result of infection with the intracellular protozoan *Toxoplasma gondii*. This obligate parasite can multiply in all body cells except erythrocytes. The infection may be congenital or acquired. Congenital infection results from placental transmission of organisms from the parasitized mother. Congenital toxoplasmosis infection is most serious and may cause jaundice, hepatosplenomegaly, chorioretinitis, hydrocephalus, microcephaly, cerebral calcification, and mental retardation. The most common hematologic complication is hemolytic anemia, which may be severe. Eosinophilia and thrombocytopenia also may be present in infected newborns.

Infection in children and adults is acquired by ingestion

of oocysts from cat feces or from inadequately cooked meat. Acquired infection may be asymptomatic or may cause symptoms resembling infectious mononucleosis. There is a leukocytosis with a relative lymphocytosis or more rarely an absolute lymphocytosis and an increase in reactive lymphocytes. Most reactive cells are similar to lymphoblasts or lymphoma cells. Splenomegaly is rare, and the heterophil antibody test is negative. Biopsy of lymph nodes shows a reactive follicular hyperplasia and may play an important role in diagnosis. Diagnosis of an active infection is established by confirming a rising titer of toxoplasma antibodies. Disseminated toxoplasmosis is a more severe infection usually seen in immunologically compromised hosts.

Cytomegalovirus Infection with the herpes-group virus, cytomegalovirus, may be the result of congenital or acquired infection. Infection in neonates occurs when organisms from the parasitized mother cross the placenta and infect the fetus. The newborn demonstrates jaundice, microcephaly, and hepatosplenomegaly. Only about 10% of infected infants exhibit clinical evidence of the disease. The most common hematologic findings in neonates are thrombocytopenia and hemolytic anemia.

Acquired infection is spread by close contact and blood transfusions. It can be spread by sexual contact, a mechanism that is important with the advent of AIDS. The disease occurs in immunosuppressed individuals, in patients with malignancy, after massive blood transfusions, or in previously healthy adults. It is the most common viral infection complicating tissue transplants and is a significant cause of morbidity and mortality in immunocompromised patients.[7] Infected adults with acquired infection present with symptoms similar to those of infectious mononucleosis except pharyngitis is absent. Many cytomegalovirus infections are subclinical or cause mild flu-like symptoms.

The virus infects leukocytes, which serve as a means of transporting the virus to other body sites. The virus appears to suppress cell-mediated immune function and induce formation of autoantibodies that have lymphocytotoxic properties.[8] There is a decrease in circulating T-helper lymphocytes and an increase in T-suppressor/cytotoxic lymphocytes.

Laboratory findings include a leukocytosis with an absolute lymphocytosis. Many of the lymphocytes are reactive, but the heterophil agglutinin test is negative. Hepatic enzymes are usually abnormal. Diagnosis is confirmed by demonstrating the virus in the urine or blood or by a rise in the cytomegalovirus antibody titer, except in immunocompromised patients.[9]

Infectious lymphocytosis *Infectious lymphocytosis* is an infectious, contagious disease of young children, which may occur in epidemic form. The etiology of the disease is unknown, but it is probably induced by a virus or bacteria. The incubation period is from 12 to 21 days. Clinical symptoms, if present, are mild and include diarrhea, gastrointestinal distress, respiratory infection, and fever. Patients also exhibit symptoms of central nervous system involvement, such as headache, vertigo, as well as pain and stiffness of the neck. Pharyngitis and lymphadenopathy are absent.

Laboratory findings help establish the diagnosis. The hemoglobin, erythrocyte count, platelet count, and sedimentation rate are normal. The most striking hematologic abnormality is a leukocytosis of 40 to 50 $\times$ 10^9/L with 60% to 97% small, normal-appearing lymphocytes. This is in contrast to the reactive lymphocytes found in most other infectious states that are associated with lymphocytosis. The lymphocytosis occurs in the first week of illness and falls within the next 3 weeks, but may remain elevated for as long as 3 months. The lymphocytosis is primarily due to an increase in T-lymphocytes. As the leukocytosis recedes, the eosinophil count may increase to 2 to 3 $\times$ 10^9/L. Within 4 to 6 weeks, the eosinophil count returns to normal.

Bordetella pertussis Infection with *Bordetella pertussis* (whooping cough) causes a blood picture very similar to that of infectious lymphocytosis. The leukocyte count rises to 15 to 25 $\times$ 10^9/L but may reach 50 $\times$ 10^9/L. The rise in leukocytes is caused by a lymphocytosis, although neutrophils also may be increased. The lymphocytes are small cells with folded nuclei, less condensed chromatin, and indistinct nucleoli. A toxin-promoting factor, produced by the bacteria, appears to block lymphocyte migration into lymphoid tissue causing accumulation of lymphocytes in the blood. Rapid lymphocytosis of the blood is accompanied by decreased cellularity of the lymph nodes. Toxic changes may be present in granulocytes.

Persistent lymphocytosis A rare disorder found in young to middle-aged females who are heavy smokers produces a persistent polyclonal B-cell lymphocytosis.[10] The disorder is often asymptomatic and found by chance on a routine blood analysis. Symptoms may include fever, fatigue, weight loss, recurrent chest infections, or generalized lymphadenopathy. Hematologic findings are normal except for lymphocytosis and the presence of binucleated lymphocytes. There is a polyclonal increase in serum IgM but low IgG and IgA levels. Bone marrow examination reveals lymphocytic infiltrates. Patients have a benign course.

Other disorders associated with lymphocytosis A variety of viral infections are associated with a mild to moderate relative lymphocytosis and, more rarely, an absolute lymphocytosis. Many of the lymphocytes are large reactive cells with deep blue cytoplasm, fine chromatin, and cytoplasmic vacuoles. These reactive cells are usually nonclonal T-lymphocytes and CD8-positive large granular lymphocytes. It is important to differentiate the pleomorphism of reactive lymphocytes in viral infections from the homogeneous lymphocyte populations in lymphocytic leukemias. In some viral infections, lymphocytosis is preceded by lymphocytopenia and neutropenia. As the infection subsides, plasmacytoid lymphocytes may be found. Although a lymphocytosis is commonly used as a clue to

TABLE 14-3 *CONDITIONS ASSOCIATED WITH LYMPHOCYTOSIS*

Non-Neoplastic Conditons	Neoplastic Conditions
Infectious mononucleosis	Acute lymphocytic leukemia
Infectious lymphocytosis	Chronic lymphocytic leukemia
Bordatella pertussis infection	Hairy cell leukemia
Cytomegalovirus infection	Lymphoma
Toxoplasmosis	Heavy chain disease
Persistent polyclonal B-cell lymphocytosis	

Viral infection
  chicken pox
  measles
  mumps
  roseola infantum
  infectious hepatitis	

Chronic infections
  tertiary symphillis
  congenital syphillis
  brucellosis	

Endocrine disorders
  thyrotoxicosis
  Addison's disease
  panhypopituitarism	

Convalescence of acute infections	
Immune reactions	
Inflammatory diseases	

differentiate viral from bacterial infections, it should be recalled that a few bacterial infections also are associated with lymphocytosis (e.g., *B. pertussis*). Other disorders accompanied by a reactive lymphocytosis include inflammatory diseases, drug hypersensitivity reactions, tertiary and congenital syphillis, smallpox, thyrotoxicosis, and Addison's disease (Table 14-3).

Lymphocytic leukemoid reactions *Lymphocytic leukemoid reactions* are characterized by an increased lymphocyte count with the presence of reactive or immature-appearing lymphocytes. In some cases, the condition resembles chronic lymphocytic leukemia. Bone marrow aspirations, however, show minimal, if any, increase in lymphocytes. Adenopathy and splenomegaly are usually absent. In addition, the patients are usually young, whereas, in chronic lymphocytic leukemia, the patients are usually older adults. Lymphocytic leukemoid reactions are associated with whooping cough, chickenpox, infectious mononucleosis, infectious lymphocytosis, and tuberculosis.

Plasmacytosis Plasma cells are not normally found in the peripheral blood. They may be present, however, with intense stimulation of the immune system, such as occurs in some viral and bacterial infections and in disorders associated with elevated serum gamma globulin. They are commonly found in rubeola infection.

Circulating plasma cells also may be found in skin diseases, cirrhosis of the liver, collagen disorders, and sarcoidosis. In the neoplastic diorders, plasma cell leukemia and multiple myeloma, plasma cells are frequently found.

LYMPHOCYTOPENIA

Lymphocytopenia, a decrease in lymphocytes, is a more vague entity than lymphocytosis and has not been as extensively studied. Lymphocytopenia occurs in adults when the lymphocyte count is less than 1.5×10^9/L and in children when less than 2×10^9/L.

Lymphocytopenia may result from decreased production, increased destruction, changes in lymphocyte circulation, or other unknown causes (Table 14-4).[11] Corticosteroid therapy causes a sharp drop in circulating lymphocytes within 4 hours. The drop is caused by sequestration of lymphocytes in the bone marrow. Values return to normal within 12 to 24 hours after cessation of therapy. Acute inflammatory conditions, including viral and bacterial infections, also may be associated with a transient lymphopenia. Disseminated neoplastic disease, connective tissue disease, and Hodgkin's disease may be accompanied by lymphocytopenia. Carcinoma of the breast and stomach with an associated lymphocytopenia is a poor prognostic sign. Systemic lupus erythematosus is frequently associated with a lymphocytopenia presumably caused by autoantibodies produced against these cells. Chemotherapeutic alkylating drugs for malignancy, such as cyclophosphamide, cause the death of T- and B-lymphocytes in both interphase and mitosis. Malnutrition is the most common cause of lymphocytopenia. Starvation causes thymic involution and depletion of T-lymphocytes. Irradiation may cause a prolonged suppression of lymphocyte production. T-helper lymphocytes are more sensitive to radiation than T-suppressor lymphocytes. It appears that small daily fractions of radiation are more damaging to lymphocytes than periodic large doses. During periods of nonradiation, the lymphocytes may be able to renew. Both congenital and acquired immune deficiency may cause lymphocytopenia. AIDS is one of these disorders that has caused much concern in the last decade. This disease will be discussed in the next section of this chapter.

Table 14-4 *CONDITIONS ASSOCIATED WITH LYMPHOCYTOPENIA*

Malnutrition

Disseminated neoplasms

Connective tissue disease (e.g., SLE)

Chemotherapy

Radiotherapy

Corticosteroids

Acute inflammatory conditions

Chronic infection (e.g., TB)

Congenital immune deficiency diseases

Acquired immune deficiency diseases

Acute and chronic renal disease

Stress

Acquired qualitative disorders

Acquired defects of either T- or B-lymphocytes can result in serious clinical manifestations. Some inflammatory states can transiently impede the response of T-lymphocytes to antigen. These include idiopathic granulomatous disorders and malignancy. Sometimes, severe infection by one microorganism impedes the ability of T-lymphocytes to react to other infectious organisms. Starvation or severe protein deficiency can severely affect the functional ability of the T-lymphocyte. Aggressive treatment of hematologic malignancies with chemotherapeutics or ionizing radiation can lead to immunodeficiency by depleting antibody-forming B lymphocytes (short-lived cells).

ACQUIRED IMMUNE DEFICIENCY SYNDROME (AIDS)

In 1981, a new, highly lethal immune deficiency disease was described, *AIDS*.[12] The disease is caused by infection with a retrovirus, human immunodeficiency virus type I (HIV-I). The virus is transmitted through sexual contact and by blood or blood products. The occurrence of the disease is expanding at a rapid rate. About 6000 are infected each day.[13] About 17 million people worldwide have been infected. In 1994, about 75,000 cases of AIDS in adolescents and adults were reported to the Centers for Disease Control and Prevention (CDC) in the United States. In the first 8 months of 1995, about 47,000 cases of AIDS were reported to the CDC.[14]

The patients, with unexplained immunodeficiency, have repeated infections with multiple opportunistic organisms and an increase in malignancies, especially Kaposi's sarcoma. Those infected with HIV progress from an asymptomatic carrier stage to the AIDS-related complex (ARC) stage and finally to symptomatic AIDS. About 50% of men infected with HIV progress to symptomatic AIDS within 7 years.[15]

The disease occurs primarily in certain high-risk groups, among them homosexual and bisexual men, intravenous drug abusers, Haitians, and hemophiliacs. The disease also is found in women who have had sexual relations with someone at high risk of HIV infection and in infants of infected women. In 1994, 18% of new AIDS cases in the United States were in women.[16] Transmission of the virus is through sexual intercourse and blood and blood products. Maternal-infant transmission is not completely understood but may be transplacental or it may occur at birth when the infant comes in contact with cervical secretions.

Disease definition In 1982, the CDC developed a case definition of AIDS for surveillance purposes. This has been revised periodically as more is learned about the virus. The HIV case definition originally required the presence of a disease (clinical condition) indicative of a cell-mediated immune defect in a person without a known cause for diminished resistance to the disease. In 1985, the case definition also required a positive result for serum antibodies to HIV or a positive culture for HIV if available. The 1993 revised case definition is based on monitoring the CD4 + T-lymphocyte counts since this correlates with severity of immune dysfunction and disease progression.[17] Those individuals with CD4 + T-lymphocyte counts less than 200 cells/μL or a CD4 + T-lymphocyte count that composes less than 14% of the total lymphocytes and laboratory confirmation of HIV infection meet the AIDS case definition. The number of HIV-infected persons meeting this case definition is larger than the number of persons with one of the AIDS-defining clinical conditions.[17] There are now 23 clinical conditions indicative of a cell-mediated immune defect (Table 14-5). These diseases are used for AIDS case definition. Patients with milder symptoms, including weight loss, fever, lymphadenopathy, thrush, chronic rash, or intermittent diarrhea, are included in the ARC category.

Mechanism of infection with HIV The etiologic agent of AIDS has been identified as the retrovirus, HIV-1. This virus selectively infects helper T-lymphocytes (CD4 +),

causing rapid, selective depletion of this lymphocyte subset. The CD4 antigen composes the T-lymphocyte cell receptor (TCR) that binds the virus. Once in the cell, HIV sheds its coat and uses reverse transcriptase to make a DNA copy of the viral RNA. A second strand of DNA is made using the first as a template, and the proviral double stranded DNA is integrated into the host cell DNA. The virus replicates within the host cell. CD4 + monocytes and macrophages are also infected but are not destroyed by the virus.

Laboratory findings There are multiple hematologic abnormalities in AIDS, including leukopenia, lymphocytopenia, anemia, and thrombocytopenia. Leukopenia is usually related to lymphocytopenia, although neutropenia also may be present.[18] Lymphocytes may include reactive forms. Mild to moderate normocytic, normochromic anemia is present in the majority of HIV-infected individuals and worsens as the disease progresses.[19] Macrocytosis (>110 fL) occurs in up to 70% of patients 2 weeks after receiving zidovudine.[20] Anti-erythrocyte antibodies may be found in up to 20% of patients with hypergammaglobulinemia. These antibodies react like polyagglutinins and cause a positive antiglobulin test (Coombs' test). Immune thrombocytopenia, indistinguishable from ITP, is common.

The severity of lymphocytopenia and CD4 lymphocytopenia correlate with severity of disease.[15] Lymphocytopenia appears to be due to HIV cytolysis of CD4 lymphocytes. The normal CD4 to CD8 ratio in peripheral blood is about 2. In AIDS, this ratio reverses progressively and permanently. The CD4 T-lymphocyte count is performed at initial diagnosis and every 6 months thereafter until the count is less than 500 CD4 cells/μL. At this time, treatment with zidovudine (azodothymidine, AZT) is recommended. Treatment with zidovudine appears to increase survival, improve performance, decrease the number of opportunistic infections, and transiently increase the number of CD4 T lymphocytes.[15] Benefits of treatment with this drug are temporary.

T-lymphocyte analysis continues every 6 months until the count declines to 200 CD4 T-lymphocytes/μL. At this point, testing is repeated every 3 months until the count falls to less than 200 CD4 T-lymphocytes/μL. Prophylaxis with trimethoprim-sulfamethoxazole is then begun to decrease the risk of infection. When the count reaches less than 200 CD4 T-lymphocytes/μL, there is no recommendation to continue analysis.

Cell-mediated immunity and humoral immunity are abnormal. Cell-mediated immunity declines as CD4 T-lymphocyte helper function for monocytes, macrophages, and other T-lymphocytes declines.[21] Humoral responses are exaggerated with polyclonal B-lymphocyte proliferation and increased immunoglobulin production.[22] The B-lymphocytes, however, are incapable of responding to signals that trigger resting B-lymphocytes.

Therapy There is no cure for AIDS. AZT is the only antiviral drug approved by the United States Food and Drug Administration for treatment of AIDS patients.

Table 14-5 *CLINICAL CONDITIONS INCLUDED IN THE CENTER FOR DISEASE CONTROL 1993 AIDS SURVEILLANCE CASE DEFINITION*

Candidiasis of bronchi, trachea, or lungs

Candidiasis, esophageal

Cervical cancer, invasive*

Coccidioidomycosis, disseminated or extrapulmonary

Crytococcosis, extrapulmonary

Cryptosporidiosis, chronic intestinal (>1 month's duration)

Cytomegalovirus disease (other than liver, spleen, or nodes)

Cytomegalovirus retinitis (with loss of vision)

Encephalopathy, HIV-related

Herpes simplex: chronic ulcer(s) (>1 month's duration); or bronchitis, pneumonitis, or esophagitis

Histoplasmosis, disseminated or extrapulmonary

Isosporiasis, chronic intestinal (>1 month's duration)

Kaposi's sarcoma

Lymphoma, Burkitt's (or equivalent term)

Lymphoma, immunoblastic (or equivalent term)

Lymphoma, primary, of brain

Mycobacterium avium complex or *M. kansasii*, (disseminated or extrapulmonary)

Mycobacterium tuberculosis, any site (pulmonary* or extrapulmonary)

Mycobacterium, other species or unidentified species, disseminated or extrapulmonary

Pneumocystis carinii pneumonia

Pneumonia, recurrent*

Progressive multifocal leukoencephalopathy

Salmonella septicemia, recurrent

Toxoplasmosis of brain

Wasting syndrome due to HIV

* Added in the 1993 expansion of the AIDS surveillance case definition.
(From: Appendix B from MMWR, 41, No. RR-17, December 1992)

TABLE 14-6 *LABORATORY FINDINGS IN SELECTED IMMUNODEFICIENCY DISORDERS*

Disorder	Immunoglobulins	*B-lymphocytes	*T-lymphocytes	Inheritance
Severe combined immunodeficiency (X-linked and autosomal recessive)	Decreased IgG, IgM, IgA	Decreased or normal	Absence of mature T lymphocytes	Sex-linked, autosomal recessive, sporadic
Wiskott-Aldrich syndrome	Decreased IgM; Increased IgA, IgE; Normal IgG	Normal	Progressive decrease	Sex-linked
DiGeorge syndrome	Normal	Normal	Decreased	—
X-linked agammaglobulinemia	Decreased IgG, IgM, IgA	Decreased	Normal	Sex-linked
Hereditary ataxia-telangiectasia	Variable; decreased IgG, IgA, IgE; increased IgM	Normal	Decreased	Autosomal recessive

*concentration; function may be normal or abnormal—see text.

CONGENITAL QUALITATIVE DISORDERS

Congenital disorders are usually characterized by a decrease in lymphocytes and impairment in either cell mediated immunity (T-lymphocytes), humoral immunity (B-lymphocytes) or both (Table 14-6). In contrast to the morphologic heterogeneity of lymphocytes associated with acquired disorders, the lymphocytes in congenital disorders are normal in appearance, and there is no organ enlargement. The functional impairment of the immune response is apparent from birth or from a very young age.

Severe combined immunodeficiency syndrome

A number of other terms have been used to describe this syndrome, including Swiss-type agammaglobulinemia, lymphopenic agammaglobulinemia, thymic alymphoplasia, and Nezelof's syndrome.[22] Severe combined immune deficiency syndrome (SCIDS) is a heterogeneous group of disorders based on diverse genetic origins, different inheritance patterns, and severity of clinical manifestations. This is the most severe immune deficiency disease. The disease may be inherited either as a sex-linked trait or as an autosomal-recessive trait. Sporadic forms of the disorder have been reported. About 75% of individuals with this disease are males. Both the T and B lymphoid systems are profoundly deficient. The total lymphocyte count is usually decreased to less than 0.1×10^9/L, but in infancy, the count may be normal. T-lymphocytes are absent in peripheral blood, but B-lymphocyte numbers may be normal or decreased. Peripheral blood B-lymphocytes are, however, unresponsive to mitogens, and immunoglobulin is decreased. B-lymphocytes will respond normally when incubated with normal T-lymphocytes in vitro.[22]

Lymph node examination reveals a lack of plasma cells, B-lymphocytes, and T-lymphocytes. No lymphoid tissue is found in the spleen, tonsils, or intestinal tract. The bone marrow also is deficient in plasma cells and lymphocyte precursors. Frequent recurrent infections, presence of skin rashes, diarrhea, and a failure to thrive are characteristic findings in infants with this disorder. Death related to overwhelming sepsis usually occurs within the first 2 years of life. Bone marrow transplantation may be the only hope of survival.

X-LINKED SCIDS

The genetic defect in the X-linked form of SCIDS has been mapped to the long arm of the X chromosome (Xq13). Family history is important in determining the mode of inheritance, although a negative family history of the disease does not rule out an X-linked mode of inheritance. Up to one third of the cases show up as spontaneous mutations.[23] X-linked SCIDS accounts for more than 50% of cases.

X-linked SCIDS is characterized by absent or severely reduced T-lymphocytes. The thymus is hypoplastic. The defect appears to reside in the marrow-derived T-precursor cells. T-lymphocytes do not mature. B-lymphocytes are normal or even increased in number but have abnormal function. Immunoglobulin levels are severely depressed. The defect in B-lymphocyte function may be partially due to the lack of T-lymphocyte help. Additional abnormalities intrinsic to B-lymphocytes are probable.

Females who carry the abnormal X-linked SCIDS gene have normal immunity. These carriers can be detected by molecular assays that are used to assess X-chromosome inactivation patterns. Normally, either the maternal or paternal X-chromosome in cells of females is randomly inactivated permanently during embryogenesis. All progeny of this progenitor cell will have the same active X-chromosome. The mature cell population is mosaic with one or the other X-chromosome inactivated. In female SCIDS carriers, however, the normal X-chromosome is the only active X-chromosome found in lymphocytes rather than the mixture of normal and abnormal X-chromosome activation expected. It has been found that random X-chromosome inactivation occurs in these carriers but the gene product of the X-mutant chromosome will not support normal lymphocyte development. This means that the lymphocytes with the X-mutant chromosome fail to develop. Thus, the T-lymphocytes of carriers consist entirely of lymphocytes in which the normal X-chromosome is active.

AUTOSOMAL SCIDS

The autosomal forms of SCIDS exhibit severe deficiencies of T- and B-lymphocytes. The most common form, found in about 50% of autosomal-recessive SCIDS, is due to adenosine deaminase deficiency.[24] The adenosine deaminase gene is located on chromosome 20. Both point mutations and deletions in this gene have been associated with adenosine deaminase deficiency. Another enzyme, purine nucleoside phosphorylase, also is a cause of SCIDS. These enzymes are purine degradation enzymes. A deficiency results in accumulation of deoxyadenosine triphosphate and deoxyguanosine triphosphate, which are toxic to lymphocytes. Other defects include a deficiency of MHC class II gene expression, IL-2 deficiency, and defective assembly of the T-lymphocyte receptor/CD3 complex.[25]

Wiskott-Aldrich syndrome

Wiskott-Aldrich syndrome (WAS) is a sex-linked recessive disease characterized by the triad of eczema, thrombocytopenia, and immunodeficiency. About two thirds of the children have a family history of the disease, while one third reflect a spontaneous mutation. Most children die before 10 years of age due to infection or bleeding. Those who survive longer may develop neoplasms of the histiocytic, lymphocytic, or myelocytic systems.

Laboratory findings play an important role in diagnosis of WAS (Table 14-7). There is a progressive decrease in thymic-dependent immunity and depletion of paracortical areas of lymph nodes. Total circulating lymphocytes and B-lymphocyte concentrations are normal, but there is a decrease in T-lymphocytes. Antibody production by the B-lymphocytes is abnormal.[22] Serum IgM is decreased, but IgE and IgA are increased. IgG is usually normal.

One of the most consistent findings is low or absent levels of circulating antibodies to the blood group antigens.[26] This is due to the inability of these children to produce antibodies to polysaccharide antigens. This is a T-lymphocyte–independent phenomenon, suggesting that there is an intrinsic B-lymphocyte abnormality.

T-lymphocyte function also is abnormal. The absolute numbers of helper and suppressor T-lymphocytes and their ratio is variable but can be normal. A highly glycosylated cell marker, CD43, present on all nonerythroid hematopoietic cells, is abnormal in WAS T-lymphocytes. These T-lymphocytes are not induced to proliferate by anti-CD43 antibodies or periodate, as are normal T-lymphocytes. This is a highly specific finding and is the test of choice when WAS is suspected.[27] Because the gene for CD43 is on chromosome 16 and not the X-chromosome, this is probably not the primary defect in WAS.

TABLE 14-7 *LABORATORY FEATURES IN WISKOTT-ALDRICH SYNDROME*

- Platelets: decreased concentration; small in size
- Lymphocytes: decreased or normal concentration; T-lymphocytes variable; B-lymphocytes usually normal
- Immunoglobulin: IgM decreased; IgE and IgA increased; IgG normal
- Absent antibodies to blood group antigens
- No mitogenic response of lymphocytes to anti-CD43 or periodate

Abnormal bleeding in the neonatal period is one of the first clinical signs of WAS. The bleeding time is abnormal, but the prothrombin time and activated prothrombin time are normal. Platelets are decreased and platelet size (volume) is decreased. Megakaryocytes in the bone marrow are normal or increased in number. Splenectomy usually results in correction of platelet concentration and size.

The genetic defect has been localized to the short arm of the X-chromosome between Xp11.3 and Xp11.22.[27] Molecular analysis using restriction fragment length polymorphisms reveals that female carriers have selective inactivation of the WAS X-chromosome rather than random inactivation of paternal or maternal X-chromosomes. This nonrandom inactivation pattern is found in the carrier's T- and B-lymphocytes, granulocytes, monocytes, and megakaryocytes, indicating all hematopoietic cells in WAS express the defect.

Therapy includes treatment for bleeding and infection. Splenectomy significantly reduces the risk of bleeding complications. Bone marrow transplantation has been used with some success.

DiGeorge syndrome

DiGeorge syndrome is a congenital immunodeficiency marked by the absence or hypoplasia of the thymus, hypoparathyroidism, heart defects, and dysmorphic facies. Hypocalcemia is typical; the presenting symptom may be seizure due to hypocalcemia. There is usually a decrease in peripheral blood T-lymphocytes as well as a decrease in cellularity of the thymic-dependent regions of peripheral lymphoid tissue. The low lymphocyte count is related to the low CD4 lymphocyte level. T-lymphocyte function varies. Those children with a hypoplastic thymus may be able to produce enough T-lymphocytes with normal function to maintain immunocompetence. B-lymphocytes are normal in number and function and immunoglobulin levels are normal. Infants exhibit increased susceptibility to viral, fungal, and bacterial infections that are frequently overwhelming. Death occurs in the first year unless thymic grafts are performed.

Cytogenetic studies on these children reveal a deletion within chromosome 22q11.[28] This defect also is found in a parent of a child with DiGeorge syndrome in 25% of the cases.

X-linked agammaglobulinemia

X-linked agammaglobulinemia (Bruton's disease) is inherited as a sex-linked disease characterized by frequent respiratory and skin infections with extracellular, catalase-negative, pyogenic bacteria. Molecular analysis has revealed that the genetic defect is on the long arm of the X-chromosome (q21.3-22). The genetic mutation results in a block in B-lymphocyte maturation at the pre-B-lymphocyte stage. The variable and constant regions of the IgM immunoglobin chain fail to connect. Peripheral blood lymphocyte counts are normal as are T-lymphocytes; there is, however, a decrease in B-lymphocytes and an absence of plasma cells in lymph nodes. The serum concentrations of IgG, IgM, and IgA are decreased or absent. Cell-mediated immune function is normal. Monthly injections of gammaglobulin are effective in preventing severe infections.

Female carriers of this disease have normal immunity. All their B-lymphocytes carry the paternal, normal X-chromosome. This suggests the normal X-chromosome confers a growth advantage to the normal cells.

Hereditary ataxia-telangiectasia

Hereditary ataxia-telangiectasia is inherited as an autosomal-recessive disease. The disease is characterized by progressive neurologic disease, immune dysfunction, and predisposition to malignancy. Affected individuals are ataxic and develop telangiectasias in childhood or adolescence. Chronic respiratory infection and lymphoid malignancy are the most common causes of death. These patients have a defect in cell-mediated immunity with hypoplasia or dysplasia of the thymus gland and depletion of thymic-dependent areas in the lymph nodes. B-lymphocyte function also is abnormal. There is lymphocytopenia and decreased IgG, IgA, and IgE. IgM levels are increased.

Cytogenetic analysis reveals excessive chromosome breakage and rearrangements in cultured cells and clonal abnormalities of chromosome 7 or 14.[29]

SUMMARY

Lymphocytes may be involved as reactive cells in inflammatory or infectious states. In these states, the lymphocytes will often include various reactive forms such as immunoblasts or plasmacytoid cells. The total lymphocyte concentration may be increased or decreased in reactive states. Although the lymphocyte induces an immune response to eliminate foreign antigens, it also may serve as the site of infection for some viruses that use lymphocyte membrane receptors to attach to the cell.

Infectious mononucleosis is a common self-limiting lymphoproliferative disorder caused by infection with EBV. Laboratory diagnosis of this disorder includes serologic testing for heterophil antibodies and identification of reactive lymphocytes on Romanowsky-stained blood smears.

AIDS is a disease caused by infection of the CD4 lymphocyte with the retrovirus, HIV-I. The virus suppresses the immune response by destroying the CD4 lymphocytes. The progression of the disease is monitored by the level of CD4 lymphocytes. Antiviral treatment is initiated when the count falls below 500 cell/μL. There is no cure for this disease.

Congenital qualitative disorders of lymphocytes include a wide variety of immunodeficiency disorders. Either the T- or B-lymphocyte or both may be affected. These are usually very serious defects with most affected individuals succumbing to the disease in childhood. Bone marrow transplant is the only treatment in many cases.

REVIEW QUESTIONS

A 19-year-old woman is seen at the university student health center with complaints of sore throat and fatigue over the past week. Results of physical examination show anterior cervical lymphadenopathy and swollen exudative tonsils. Slight hepatomegaly is noted.

Laboratory Data:
Erythrocyte count:	4.96 x 10^{12}/L
Hb	14.6 gm/dL
Hct	0.44 L/L
Platelet count	354 x 10^9/L
Leukocyte count	11.8 x 10^9/L

Differential:
Segmented neutrophils	21%
Lymphocytes	79% (55% were reactive)

Erythrocyte morphology: Erythrocytes are normochromic and normocytic.

1. What is the most likely etiology of this patient's reactive lymphocytosis?
   a. Epstein-Barr virus
   b. cytomegalovirus
   c. Toxoplasma gondii
   d. HIV-1

2. What is the major immunologic classification of the reactive lymphocytes?
   a. infected B lymphocytes
   b. activated T-lymphocytes
   c. Natural killer lymphocytes
   d. plasma cells

3. Which laboratory test would you use to confirm this patient's diagnosis?
   a. throat swab for culture
   b. serologic test for heterophil antibody
   c. serum alkaline phosphatase
   d. anti-streptolysin O titer

4. A clue to differentiating the lymphocytes of infectious mononucleosis from those found in neoplastic lymphocytic disorders is that in neoplastic disorders the lymphocytes are:
   a. morphologically similar
   b. heterogeneous morphologically
   c. not increased
   d. reactive

5. The best description of this patient's leukocyte count is:
   a. relative lymphocytopenia
   b. neutropenia
   c. absolute lymphocytosis
   d. absolute neutrophilia

6. In female carriers of the sex-linked severe combined immunodeficiency gene the lymphocytes:
   a. are normal T-lymphocytes
   b. are abnormal T- and B-lymphocytes

   c. carry the mutant X-chromosome in all T-lymphocytes
   d. carry the mutant X-chromosome in 50% of T-lymphocytes

7. The HIV-1 virus infects the _____ lymphocytes.
   a. B-lymphocytes
   b. suppressor T-lymphocytes
   c. helper T-lymphocytes
   d. cytotoxic T-lymphocytes

8. The 1993 AIDS case definition states that for a diagnosis of AIDS the patient must have:
   a. A CD4 lymphocyte count greater than 400 /μL and presence of a disease indicative of a cell-mediated immune defect.
   b. A CD8 lymphocyte count less than 400/μL and a total lymphocyte count less than 5×10^9/L.
   c. A B-lymphocyte count less than 200/μL and a B-lymphocyte count that comprises more than 14% of the total lymphocyte count.
   d. A CD4 lymphocyte count less than 200 /μL and laboratory confirmation of HIV infection.

9. Heterophil antibodies found in infectious mononucleosis are absorbed by:
   a. beef erythrocytes but not guinea pig kidney cells
   b. both beef erythrocytes and guinea pig kidney cells
   c. neither beef erythrocytes or guinea pig kidney cells
   d. guinea pig kidney cells but not beef erythrocytes

10. A 2-year-old child has a total leukocyte count of 10×10^9/L and 60% lymphocytes. The following best describes this blood picture:
   a. absolute lymphocytosis
   b. relative lymphocytosis
   c. normal lymphocyte count for the age given
   d. absolute lymphocytopenia

REFERENCES ●

1. Straus, S.E., Cohen, J.I., Tosato, G., Meier, J.: Epstein-Barr virus infections: Biology, pathogenesis, and management. Ann. Intern. Med., 118:45, 1993.
2. Foerster, J.: Infectious mononucleosis. In Wintrobe's Clinical Hematology. Edited by G.R. Lee, T.C. Bithell, J. Foerster, J.W. Athens, J.N. Lukens. Philadelphia: Lea & Febiger, 1993.
3. Bailey, R.E.: Diagnosis and treatment of infectious mononucleosis. Am. Fam. Phys., 49:879, 1994.
4. Nathwani, D., Wood, M.J.: Herpesvirus infections in childhood:2. Br. J. Hosp. Med., 50:301, 1993.
5. Peterson, L., Hrisinko, M.A.: Benign lymphocytosis and reactive neutrophilia. Clin. Lab. Med., 13:863, 1993.
6. Paul, J.R., et al.: The presence of heterophile antibodies in infectious mononucleosis. Am. J. Med. Sci., 183:90, 1932.
7. Epstein, J., Scully, C.: Cytomegalovirus: a virus of increasing relevance to oral medicine and pathology. J. Oral. Pathol. Med., 22:348, 1993.
8. Mustafa, M.M.: Cytomegalovirus infection and disease in the immunocompromised host. Pediatr. Infect. Dis. J., 13:249, 1994.
9. Landini, M.P.: New approaches and perspectives in cytomegalovirus diagnosis. Prog. Med. Virol., 40:157, 1993.
10. Agrawal, S., Matutes, E., Voke, J., Dyer, M.J.S., Khokhar, T., Catovsky, D.: Persistent polyclonal B-cell lymphocytosis. Leuk. Res., 18:791, 1994.
11. Schoentag, R.A., Cangiarella, J.: The nuances of lymphocytopenia. Clin. Lab. Med., 13:923, 1993.
12. Gottlieb, M.S., et al.: Pneumocystis carinii pneumonia and mucosal candidiasis in previously healthy homosexual men. Evidence of a new acquired cellular immunodeficiency. N. Engl. J. Med., 305:1425, 1981.
13. MMWR. 43:825, Nov. 18, 1994.
14. MMWR. 44:665, Sept. 15, 1995.
15. Gold, J.W.M.: HIV-1 Infection. Med. Clin. North. Am., 76:1, 1992.
16. MMWR. 44:81, Feb 10, 1995.
17. U.S. Department of Health and Human Services: Expansion of the CDC surveillance case definition for AIDS. MMWR, 41/No. RR-17, December 18, 1992.
18. Brynes, R.K., Gill, P.S.: Clinical characteristics, immunologic abnormalities, and hematopathology of HIV infection. In Pathology of AIDS and other manifestations of HIV infection. Edited by V.V. Joshi. New York, Igaku-Shoin, 1990.
19. Doukas, M.A.: Human immunodeficiency virus associated anemia. Med. Clin. North Am., 76:699, 1992.
20. Aboulafia, D.M., Mitsuyasu, R.T.: Hematologic abnormalities in AIDS. Hematol. Oncol. Clin. North. Am., 5:195, 1991.
21. Said, J.W.: Pathogenesis of HIV infection. In Pathology of AIDS and HIV Infection. Edited by G. Nash, J.W. Said. Philadelphia: W.B. Saunders, Co., 1992.
22. Lukens, J.N.: Immune deficiency diseases: Inherited and acquired. In Wintrobe's Clinical Hematology. Edited by G.R. Lee, T.C. Bithell, J. Foerster, J.W. Athens, J.N. Lukens. Philadelphia: Lea & Febiger, 1993.
23. Puck, J.M.: Prenatal diagnosis and genetic analysis of X-linked immunodeficiency disorders. Ped. Res., 33(Suppl) No. 1:529, 1993.
24. Hilman, B.C., Sorensen, R.U.: Management options: SCIDS with adenosine deaminase deficiency. Ann. Allergy., 72:395, 1994.
25. Leonard, W.J., Noguch, M., Russell, S.M., McBride, O.W.: The molecular basis of X-linked severe combined immunodeficiency: The role of the interleukin-2 receptor τ chain as a common τ chain, π. Immunol. Rev., No. 138:61, 1994.
26. Peacocke, M., Siminovitch, K.A.: Wiskott-Aldrich syndrome: New molecular and biochemical insights. J. Am. Acad. Dermatol., 27:507, 1992.
27. Peacocke, M., Siminovitch, K.A.: The Wiskott-Aldrich syndrome. Sem. Dermatol., 12:247, 1993.
28. Wilson, D.I., Burn, J., Scanbler, P., Goodship, J.: DiGeorge Syndrome: Part of CATCH 22. J. Med. Genet., 30:852, 1993.
29. Swift, M., Heim, R.A., Lench, N.J.: Genetic aspects of ataxia telangiectasia. Adv. Neurol., 61:115, 1993.

Myeloproliferative disorders

Key Terms

neoplasm
neoplastic
chloromas
chronic myelocytic leukemia
leukemic hiatus
*myelofibrosis with myeloid
   metaplasia*
myelophthisic anemia
polycythemia vera
essential thrombocythemia

INTRODUCTION

Hematopoiesis is a highly regulated process whereby a normal steady state production of hematopoietic cells in the bone marrow and destruction of senescent cells in the tissue maintains a rather constant peripheral blood cell concentration. Acquired mutations in hematopoietic stem cells that allow them to escape the controls regulating proliferation and/or differentiation in the bone marrow result in hematopoietic neoplasms. *Neoplasm* is a general term used to define an unregulated production of cells. Neoplasms may be benign or malignant.

The *neoplastic* disorders of bone marrow hematopoietic cells can generally be grouped into three main categories: myeloproliferative disorders (MPD), myelodysplastic states or syndromes (MDS), and acute leukemias (Fig. 15-1). Acute leukemias represent the clearly malignant neoplasms with a proliferation of malignant blast cells. The MPD and MDS, although not clearly malignant, are characterized by an autonomous neoplastic proliferation of hematopoietic precursors. Myeloproliferative disorders can generally be distinguished from MDS, because in MPD the peripheral blood shows increases in erythrocytes, leukocytes, and/or platelets. Myelodysplastic states, however, are characterized by peripheral blood cytopenias (except chronic myelomonocytic leukemia). Both MPD and MDS may have a chronic or acute course and have the potential of evolving into acute leukemia.

CLASSIFICATION OF MYELOPROLIFERATIVE DISORDERS

The term myeloproliferative syndrome, coined by Dameshek in 1951, describes a group of disorders that result from an unchecked, autonomous proliferation of one or more types of cellular elements in the bone marrow.[1] The MPDs are characterized by panhypercellularity (panmyelosis) of the bone marrow accompanied by erythrocytosis, granulocytosis, and thrombocytosis in the periph-

TABLE 15-1 *CLASSIFICATION OF MYELOPROLIFERATIVE DISORDERS BY PREDOMINANCE OF CELL TYPES*

Involved Cell Line	Myeloproliferative Disorder
Erythroid	Polycythemia vera
Myeloid	Chronic myelocytic leukemia
Megakaryocytic	Essential thrombocythemia
Fibroblast*	Myelofibrosis

* The fibroblast in myelofibrosis is not a part of the neoplastic process but rather is increased as a part of a reactive process.

eral blood. Although trilineage cell involvement (erythrocytic, granulocytic, thrombocytic) is characteristic of MPDs, one cell line is usually more prominently affected than the others. Hematologic classification is based on the most affected cell line (Table 15-1). The spectrum of MPDs includes *chronic myelocytic leukemia* (CML), *myelofibrosis with myeloid metaplasia* (MMM), *polycythemia vera* (PV), and *essential thrombocythemia* (ET). The classification of these disorders is not always clear because there are overlapping clinical and laboratory features between subgroups at different times during the course of the disease (Table 15-2).

PATHOPHYSIOLOGY

The primary defect in MPD appears to be in the pluripotential stem cell. Studies indicate that there appear to be increased numbers of stem cells, including committed stem cells, in the stem cell compartment.[2] A clone of abnormal pluripotent hematopoietic stem cells preferentially expands until normal polyclonal cell growth is inhibited and all functioning bone marrow is derived from the abnormal clone. Commitment, differentiation, and maturation of the abnormal clone is preserved, leading to increased numbers of mature cells in the peripheral blood. Although all progeny of the abnormal pluripotential stem cell bear

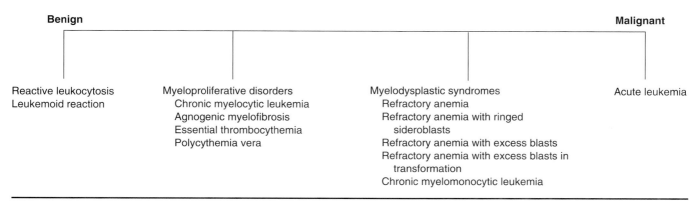

FIGURE 15-1. The spectrum of granulocytic proliferation disorders ranges from benign to malignant processes. Benign granulocyte proliferation is usually a reactive process. Myeloproliferative disorders, myelodysplastic syndromes, and acute myelocytic leukemia (AML) are neoplastic clonal stem cell defects characterized by autonomous proliferation of hematopoietic cells. (With permission from: McKenzie, S.: Chronic myelocytic leukemia. Tech Sample H-4, 1990. Chicago, ASCP.)

TABLE 15-2 *DIFFERENTIAL FEATURES OF MYELOPROLIFERATIVE DISORDERS*

Parameter	CML	MMM	PV	ET
Hematocrit	N or ↓	↓	↑	N or ↓
Leukocyte	↑↑↑	↑ or ↑↑	N or ↑	N or ↑
Platelets	↑ or ↓	N, ↑, ↓	↑	↑↑↑
Immature granulocytes	↑↑↑	↑↑	absent or ↑	rare
LAP	↓	N, ↑, ↓	N or ↑	N or ↑
Philadelphia chromosome	present	absent	absent	absent
Spleen size	N or ↑	↑↑↑	↑	N or ↑
Bone marrow fibrosis	absent or ↑	↑↑↑	absent or ↑	absent or ↑

Key to abbreviations N = Normal; ↓ = decreased; ↑ = increased; CML = chronic myelocytic leukemia; MMM = myelofibrosis with myeloid metaplasia; PV = polycythemia vera; ET = essential thrombocythemia.

identical genetic and biochemical markers, one cell line, erythroid, myeloid, or megakaryocytic, predominates.

The factors that determine the eventual differentiation pathway of the abnormal pluripotential cell are not entirely understood. There is evidence to suggest that hematopoietic growth factors may be involved. Serum CSF-1 levels have been found to be elevated in all MPD phenotypes, but there is no apparant correlation between CSF-1 concentration and levels of circulating erythrocytes, leukocytes, or platelets.[3] This growth factor stimulates the survival, proliferation, and differentiation of mononuclear phagocytes and interacts with other growth factors to stimulate the proliferation and differentiation of earlier cells. Plasma levels of platelet-derived growth factor (PDGF) are significantly elevated in myelofibrosis and essential thrombocythemia.[4] This growth factor is stored in the α-granules of platelets and megakaryocytes and is the major mitogenic factor in serum. PDGF stimulates the growth and cell division of fibroblasts and other cells.

Cell growth also is critically regulated by the cell's receptors for these growth factors, by transducers that help ramify cell signals from the cell membrane receptors to the interior of the cell, and by nuclear-effectors, which respond to mitogenic signals.

Some of these growth regulators are encoded by proto-oncogenes. Interestingly, many of the chromosomal rearrangements associated with neoplastic hematologic disorders occur in the regions of these proto-oncogenes, which can lead to qualitative or quantitative alterations in gene expression and abnormal control of cell growth. For example, follicular lymphoma is associated with a t(14;18) chromosome translocation in the lymphoma cells. This translocation has a unique BCL-2 gene rearrangement that brings the BCL-2 gene from the locus on chromosome 18 to the IgH locus on chromosome 14.[5] At this new locus, the BCL-2 gene escapes its normal regulation and comes under the same regulatory influence as IgH. This results in a high level of BCL-2 protein. The BCL-2 protein's function is blockage of programmed cell death (apoptosis). This leads to an abnormally long lifespan of the lymphoma cells.

The clonal origin of the MPDs is suggested by the finding of uniform biochemical, cytogenetic, or molecular genetic abnormalities in hematopoietic cells from the bone marrow or peripheral blood of patients with MPD. The most useful biochemical marker for demonstrating monoclonality of MPD is the glucose-6-phosphate dehydrogenase enzyme (G6PD). There are two G6PD isoenzymes, A and B, determined by separate genes on the X chromosome. Females heterozygous for isoenzyme A and isoenzyme B will produce both enzymes since there is random inactivation of one X chromosome, and hence, one G6PD gene per cell. Approximately half of the cells will contain isoenzyme A while the remaining cells will contain isoenzyme B. The blood cells of females with a MPD, and who are G6PD heterozygous, however, contain either one isoenzyme or the other in granulocytes, erythrocytes, and platelets, which reflects the clonal origin of the cells. In addition, many individuals with a MPD have identical karyotypic abnormalities in all hematopoietic cell lines, suggesting these cells were derived from a single mutant stem cell. These abnormalities are not present in other somatic cells, indicating the mutations are acquired rather than inherited. The most consistent chromosome abnormality, the Philadelphia chromosome, is found in all types of blood cells in 90 to 95% of the patients with CML. The application of molecular biology to the study of hematopoietic neoplasms has been useful in identifying the specific abnormality at the DNA and protein level. These studies have supported the clonality hypothesis of MPD. Molecular analysis has revealed that the specific gene rearrangement found in Philadelphia chromosome positive CML is also found in many individuals with CML-like disease but a normal chromosome karyotype.

●
GENERAL FEATURES

Myeloproliferative disorders usually occur in the middle aged or the older adult but rarely in children. The onset of the disease is gradual, evolving over a period of months or even years. Clinical findings include hemorrhage, thrombosis, infection, pallor, and weakness.

Anemia or polycythemia, leukoerythroblastosis, leukocytosis, and thrombocytosis with bizarre platelets are common laboratory findings. Anemia is variable and may be caused by ineffective erythropoiesis, marrow fibrosis, or by a shortened survival secondary to splenomegaly.

Decreased bone marrow iron, not reflective of true iron deficiency, is a consistent finding in MPD.[6] For this reason, serum ferritin and serum iron are more reliable estimates of iron deficiency in the presence of MPD than evaluation of bone marrow iron.

Thrombocytosis in MPD is classified as a primary disorder and is believed to result from an autonomous, unregulated proliferation of megakaryocytes. This is supported by the finding of normal interleukin-6 (IL-6) levels (which promotes megakaryopoiesis in vitro and raises the platelet concentration in vivo) in patients with MPD and thrombocytosis.[17] In contrast, IL-6 levels are usually increased in secondary or reactive thrombocytosis. The platelet membrane glycoprotein IIb/IIIa complex, a receptor for von Willebrand factor (VWF), fibrinogen, fibronectin, and vitronectin, on activated platelets are significantly decreased in many patients with MPD.[8,9] Circulating activated platelets and in vitro spontaneous platelet aggregation in whole blood also has been described.[10] The relationship between these findings to hemorrhage and thrombosis in MPD requires further investigation.

The bone marrow is hypercellular but often becomes fibrotic in the course of the disease. Fibrosis in MDP is thought to be a reactive process, secondary to the expansion of hematopoietic cells. As evidence of their benign proliferation, the fibroblasts exhibit normal karyotypes and G6PD mosaicism in female heterozygotes. The reactive fibrosis may result from the intramedullary release of a cytokine from platelets, megakaryocytes, and malignant cells that is mitogenic for fibroblasts. Human PDGF is able to stimulate the growth and cell division of fibroblasts as well as other cells. The concentration of PDGF in platelets of patients with MPD is significantly decreased. Although this could be due to either decreased synthesis or excessive release, assays of circulating PDGF in MPD suggest excessive release. PDGF levels are significantly higher in patients with MMM and ET than in other MPD or in normal controls. Not surprising, MMM and ET are the two MPD with the most significant degree of fibrosis.[4] The increase in fibroblasts leads to an increase in collagen, laminin, and fibronectin in the medullary cavity.

When marrow fibrosis supervenes over the course of the disease, the major sites of hematopoiesis become the extramedullary tissues, particularly the liver and spleen. Hepatosplenomegaly is a common clinical finding. Extramedullary hematopoiesis also occurs in benign diseases, such as chronic hemolytic anemias, but the hematopoiesis in these extramedullary masses is confined to only one cell lineage. In contrast, all cell lineages are present in the extramedullary masses that accompany myeloproliferative syndromes. It has been hypothesized that marrow fibrosis causes distortion of marrow sinusoids, which permits hematopoietic stem cells to leak into the sinusoids and gain entry to the peripheral blood.[11] These stem cells then lodge in extramedullary sites, such as the spleen, and proliferate and differentiate.

Many of the chronic myeloproliferative disorders carry a significant risk of terminating in acute nonlymphocytic leukemia. This transition is most commonly seen in CML. The question has been raised whether leukemia is a natural transition of myeloproliferative disorders or is the result of "leukemogenic" chemotherapy and radiotherapy for the original myeloproliferative disorder.

⬤ CHRONIC MYELOCYTIC LEUKEMIA

Chronic myelocytic leukemia (CML), also known as chronic granulocytic leukemia (CGL), is the most well-defined of the MPD. It is characterized by a neoplastic growth of primarily myeloid cells in the bone marrow with an extreme elevation of these cells in the peripheral blood. Extramedullary, granulocytic proliferation in the spleen

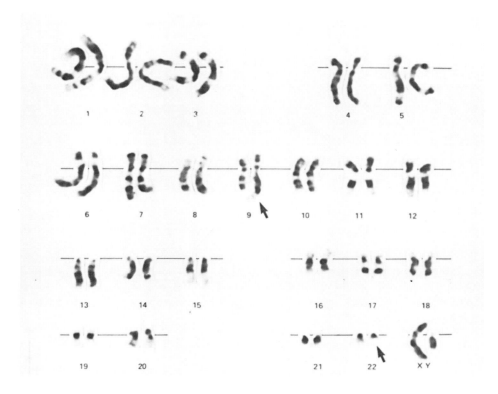

FIGURE 15-2. Karyotype from a patient with CML showing the Philadelphia chromosome translocation, t(9:22)(q34;q11). The Philadelphia chromosome is chromosome number 22.

TABLE 15-3 *CLASSIFICATION OF CHRONIC MYELOCYTIC LEUKEMIA (CML)*

Typical CML-Philadelphia chromosome positive

Atypical CML-Philadelphia chromosome negative

Juvenile CML
-infantile variant
-adult variant

Chronic eosinophilic leukemia

Chronic basophilic leukemia

Chronic neutrophilic leukemia

and liver is progressive. Erythrocyte and megakaryocyte masses also may expand.

There are two phases to the disease: the chronic phase and the blast crisis phase. The initial chronic phase responds well to therapy; normal health can usually be restored and maintained for months or years. About 75% of cases, however, eventually enter a gradual transformation to a blast crisis that is hematologically and clinically indistinguishable from acute myeloblastic leukemia. Management of this stage is difficult with complications commonly intervening. After progression to blast crisis, the prognosis is poor with a survival of less than 6 months.

Several variants of CML have been identified. These variants are listed in Table 15-3.

● Pathophysiology

EVIDENCE OF CLONALITY

Evidence of the clonal nature of CML comes from demonstration of both cytogenetic and biochemical abnormalities in hematopoietic cells of patients with the disease. When females who are normally heterozygous for G6PD isoenzymes are diagnosed with CML, their hematopoietic cells reveal only one of the isoenzymes, suggesting the cells were derived from a single abnormal hematopoietic precursor cell.

An acquired chromosome abnormality, the Philadelphia chromosome, is present in all hematopoietic cells, except T-lymphocytes and sometimes B-lymphocytes, in about 90% to 95% of patients with a morphologic diagnosis of CML (Fig. 15-2). This was the first chromosome abnormality to be found consistently in a malignant disease. It is not found in somatic cells or fibroblasts.

In some cases, the Philadelphia chromosome has been detected months before the diagnosis of CML. Once the chromosome abnormality is present, it rarely disappears, even in remission. Because all hematopoietic cells are involved in the neoplastic process, the original neoplastic cell is most likely a progenitor cell common to all cell lines, the pluripotential cell (Fig. 15-3). The presence of the Philadelphia chromosome in some, but not all, lymphocytes suggests that either the lymphoid stem cell is suppressed or only selective progeny of pluripotential stem cells are stimulated to proliferate.

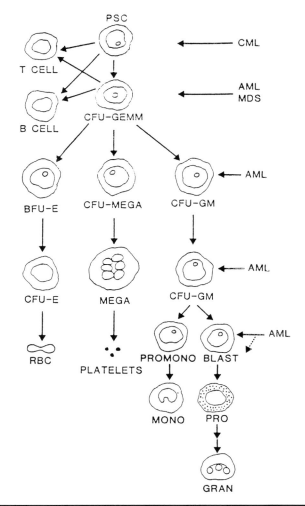

FIGURE 15-3. The possible cells of origin of chronic myeloid leukemia, acute myeloid leukemia, and myelodysplastic syndrome. (From: Griffin J.D., Lowenberg, B.: Clonogenic cells in acute myeloblastic leukemia. Blood, 68: 1185, 1986.)

ROLE OF THE PHILADELPHIA CHROMOSOME

Molecular biology has dramatically increased our understanding of the role of the Philadelphia chromosome in this disease. The Philadelphia chromosome is a chromosome that results from a reciprocal translocation between chromosomes 9 and 22, t(9;22)(q34;q11). This involves the movement of a segment of the Abelson proto-oncogene, ABL, from the long arm of chromosome 9 to the major breakpoint cluster region (M-BCR) on chromosome 22 and the movement of a piece of chromosome 22 to chromosome 9 (Fig. 15-4). The resulting chromosomes are labeled 22q− because part of the long arm is missing and 9q+ because the long arm is longer than normal. The M-BCR is a 5.8 kb region of the BCR gene and is divided into five subregions. There is variability in the possible breakpoints within the M-BCR but this variation does not appear to be associated with any clinical differences of the disease. The translocation results in the fusion of the 5′

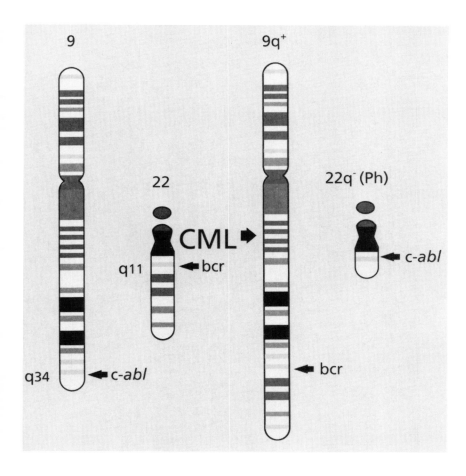

FIGURE 15-4. The Philadelphia translocation in CML. Arrows indicate the chromosome breakpoints at 9q34 and 22q11 and the genes directly involved in the translocation. The translocation results in a 9q + chromosome and a 22q − chromosome (Philadelphia chromosome). (With permission: Crisan, D., Carr, E.R. BCR/abl gene rearrangement in chronic myelogenous leukemia and acute leukemias. Laboratory Medicine, 23, 730; 1992.)

BCR and the 3' ABL genes in a head to tail fashion. The fusion BCR/ABL gene is under the control of the promoter region of the BCR gene and transcribes an 8.5 kb chimeric mRNA.[12,13] This RNA produces a specific protein of 210,000 daltons (P210) (Fig 15-5). The BCR/ABL fusion gene, 8.5 kb mRNA and P210 are tumor-specific markers of CML. The characteristics of the abl and BCR genes, as well as the BCR/ABL fusion oncogene, are described in Table 15-4.

The abnormal protein, P210, has increased tyrosine kinase activity. Tyrosine kinase proteins are important in the regulation of metabolic pathways and some serve as receptors for growth factors. In addition, altered ABL proteins or P210 have been shown to confer growth-factor

TABLE 15-4   *CHARACTERISTICS OF THE ONCOGENES INVOLVED IN THE BCR/ABL GENE REARRANGEMENTS IN CML*

Gene	ABL	BCR	BCR/ABL fusion
Size	>230 kb	>100 kb	variable
No. exons	11	20	variable
Breakpoint	5' of exon II (100–200 kb)	bcr (5.8 kb)	fusion BCR exon 2 or 3-ABL exon II
Transcript(s)	6 kb; 7 kb	4.5 kb; 6.7 kb	8.5 kb
Protein	p145	p160	p210
Size	145 KDa	160 KDa	210 KDa
Location	nucleus	unknown	plasma membrane
Enzymatic activity	tyrosine kinase	unknown	tyrosine kinase (abnormally high)
Expression	hematopoietic cells (predominantly)	constitutive	increased in CML cells
Function	unknown (probable growth control)	unknown	signal transducer (transmembrane tyrosine kinase); transforming activity

(From Crisan D, and Carr ER: BCR/abl gene rearrangement in chronic myelogenous and acute leukemias. Lab Med, 23:733, 1992)

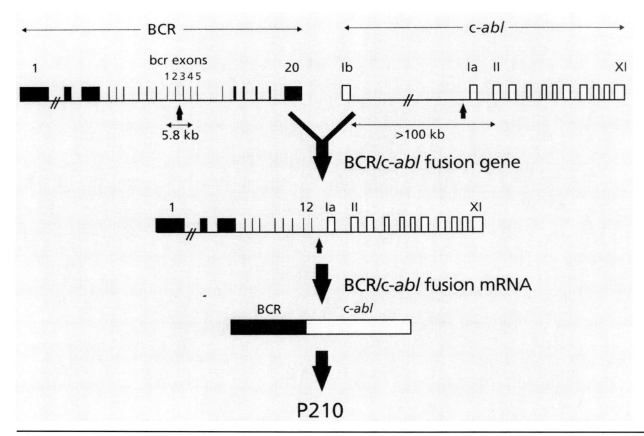

FIGURE 15-5. Exon maps of the normal BCR and c-abl genes, and the BCR/abl gene rearrangement in the Philadelphia translocation of CML. Upward arrows indicate examples of breakpoints in the bcr region, in intron 1 of the c-abl gene, and the fusion site in the BCR/c-abl fusion gene. (With permission: Crisan, D., Carr, E.R.: BCR/abl gene rearrangement in chronic myelogenous leukemia and acute leukemias. Laboratory Medicine, 23, 730; 1992.)

independence to various cells. This suggests that P210 may play a central role in oncogenesis.

Other molecular defects on chromosome 22 outside the M-BCR in Philadelphia positive hematologic diseases have been reported. It is controversial whether these disorders are distinct diseases separate from CML.[14-16]

Molecular analysis to detect the BCR gene rearrangement has several clinical uses in diagnosing and prognosing CML.5 (Table 15-5). About 5% to 10% of patients with CML lack the Philadelphia chromosome. In about 50% of these cases, the translocation is masked at the

TABLE 15-5 *CLINICAL USES OF MOLECULAR ANALYSIS FOR THE BCR GENE REARRANGEMENT*[5]

1. Diagnosis of CML when the Philadelphia chromosome is absent.
2. Confirmation of a CML diagnosis when the Philadelphia chromosome is present.
3. Confirmation of a diagnosis of CML when the patient presents in the blast crisis phase of CML
4. Differentiation of CML from other myeloproliferative diseases and myelodysplastic syndromes when overlapping features are present.
5. Monitoring of CML patients on therapy.

karyotypic level, but the molecular BCR/abl rearrangement has still occurred and can be detected by molecular analysis (Table 15-6). The malignant cells in these cases express the 8.5 kb chimeric mRNA and the P210 protein. The clinical course and response to treatment of these Philadelphia-negative cases is the same as for the Philadelphia-positive cases. Of the remaining Philadelphia-negative CML cases that do not express the BCR/abl rearrangement at the molecular level, many are cases of CMML or another myelodysplastic syndrome. The term atypical CML (aCML) has been used to describe Philadelphia-negative CML that has hematologic features intermediate between typical CML and CMML, but that is distinct from both.[17] Many aCML cases show numerical and structural chromosome aberrations other than the Philadelphia chromosome.[15]

DISEASE PROGRESSION AND ADDITIONAL CHROMOSOME ABNORMALITIES

Progression of CML is marked by an accelerated or acute phase (blast crisis) for most patients. In more than 75% of patients, this progression is preceded or accompanied by development of additional chromosomal abnormalities, including additional Philadelphia chromosomes[15,18,19] (Table 15-7). Thus, following patients with

TABLE 15-6 *THE MOLECULAR GENETIC REARRANGEMENTS AND THE RELATED PROTEINS FOUND IN PHILADELPHIA CHROMOSOME POSITIVE AND NEGATIVE CML AND ALL*

Clinical Condition	Involvement of Ph/BCR	TPK
Normal	Ph −, BCR −	145 kD
CML	Ph +, BCR +	210 kD
	Ph −, BCR +	210 kD
	Ph −, BCR −	145 kD (aCML, Myelodysplasia)
ALL	Ph +, BCR +	210 kD
	Ph +, BCR −	190 kD (?*de novo* ALL)
	Ph −, BCR −	145 kD (*de novo* ALL)

TPK = tyrosine protein kinase; CML = chronic myelocytic leukemia; ALL = acute lymphocytic leukemia; Ph + = Philadelphia chromosome positive; Ph − = Philadelphia chromosome negative; BCR + = rearrangement within the 5.8 kb BCR region; BCR − = no rearrangement in the BCR region. (Adapted from: Hoffbrand, A. V. and Pettit, J.E. *Clinical Hematology*. 1988. New York: Gower Medical Publishing)

repeated chromosome analysis may be helpful in predicting impending blast crisis.

At the molecular level, mutations in the P53 gene, a tumor suppressor anti-oncogene, are found in at least 30% of patients in the blast crisis, especially myeloid and megakaryocytic blast crisis.[20] Mutations/alterations of this gene in the chronic state of CML are rare. The P53 gene normally functions as an anti-oncogene by preventing proliferation of DNA-damaged cells, promoting apoptosis of these damaged cells, and preventing unwanted DNA amplification.[20] When mutated, the gene may lose its tumor-suppressive effect.

Mutations in the n-RAS proto-oncogene are found in megakaryocytic and Philadelphia-negative myeloid blast crises of CML. RAS genes encode proteins that bind gua-

TABLE 15-7 *CHROMOSOMAL CHANGES IN BLAST CRISIS OF CML*

FREQUENT

Additional Ph
Trisomy 8
Isochromosome 17
Loss of Y chromosome

LESS FREQUENT

Trisomy 9

RARE

Translocation (15;17)
Translocation (3;21)(q26;q22)
Translocation (3;3) or inversion (3)

VERY RARE

Loss of chromosome 5(− 5) or the long arm of chromosome 5(5q-)
Loss of chromosome 7(− 7) or the long arm of chromosome 7(7q-)

(From: Hoffbrand AV and Pettit JE: Clinical Hematology. New York: Gower Medical Publishing, 1988)

nosine triphosphate (GTP) and subsequently hydrolyze it to the diphosphate. The RAS proteins are found on the inner surface of plasma membranes, where it is believed that they function as G proteins. The G proteins are involved in signal transduction pathways that are activated when they bind GTP. The oncogenic forms of RAS have a reduced ability to be converted to the inactive state, thus sending inappropriate signals to the cell.

PHILADELPHIA CHROMOSOME IN ACUTE LEUKEMIAS

Approximately 2% to 5% of childhood acute lymphoblastic leukemia (ALL), 25% of adult ALL, and some cases of AML also have the Philadelphia chromosome. The Philadelphia-positive AML cases may actually be CML in blast crisis that were not diagnosed in the chronic phase. In about 50% of the Philadelphia-positive cases of ALL, the molecular defect is identical to that found in CML and the ABL protein, P210, is present. In the remaining 50% of Philadelphia-positive cases of ALL, the breakpoints on chromosome 22 fall 5′ to the M-BCR but are still within the first intron of the BCR gene, referred to as the minor-BCR (m-BCR). These leukemias express a distinct translation product of the mRNA hybrid termed the P190 protein[21] (Figure 15-6). These Philadelphia-positive cases of ALL may actually be de novo acute leukemia cases. Like P210, the P190 protein also shows an increased tyrosine kinase activity but its role in the development of the ALL phenotype is unknown. A comparison of the laboratory features of the Philadelphia-positive ALLs and lymphoid blast crises of CML are illustrated in Table 15-8.

CELL CYCLE KINETICS

The enormous numbers of granulocytic cells in CML lead one to believe that the cell cycle time for granulocytic precursors must be greatly decreased. However, the cell cycle for leukemic myeloblasts appears to be the same as for normal cells or only slightly decreased. The best explanation for the increased number of granulocytic cells in CML is an increase in the number of committed progenitor cells due to a growth advantage of the malignant clone. Further definition of how this growth advantage is derived will probably result from the studies of specific oncogenes involved in the disease.

ETIOLOGY

Normally, random chromosome breaks that occur frequently are repaired by existing nuclear enzymes. Theoretically, abnormal repair of these breaks may cause a t(9:22)(q34;q11) in a stem cell, giving it a proliferative advantage, perhaps due to the resulting P210 protein production. Over a period of several years, the t(9:22) cell line replaces the normal marrow, and CML is expressed. The event precipitating the malignant transformation of the pluripotential stem cell remains unknown. It is known that radiation exposure, toxic chemicals, and viral agents increase the numbers of random chromosome breakage.

●
Clinical findings

CML is a disease of middle age, with a peak incidence at 40 to 49 years of age and almost equal distribution be-

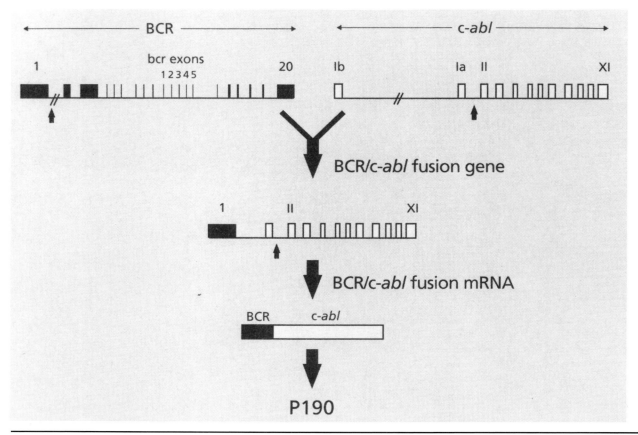

FIGURE 15-6. Exon maps of the normal BCR and c-abl genes and the BCR/abl gene rearrangement in the Philadelphia translocation of de novo acute leukemias. Upward arrows indicate examples of breakpoints in intron 1 of the BCR gene, upstream of the common c-abl exon II, and the fusion site in the BCR/c-abl gene. (With permission: Crisan, D., Carr, E.R.: BCR/abl gene rearrangement in chronic myelogenous leukemia and acute leukemias. Laboratory Medicine, 23, 730; 1992.)

tween sexes. However, it also occurs in young adults, more so than the other MPD. Although rare, CML may occur in childhood and is then referred to as juvenile-type CML (discussed later in this chapter). More advanced countries have been reported to have a higher incidence of CML. The question arises, however, as to whether the higher incidence in these countries reflects the increased availability of advanced medicine.

The disease has an insidious onset with the most common symptoms being increased weakness, loss of stamina, unexplained fever, sweats, weight loss, and feelings of fullness in the abdomen. Bleeding from the gastrointestinal

TABLE 15-8 COMPARISON OF ACUTE LYMPHOCYTIC LEUKEMIA AND PH-POSITIVE LYMPHOID LEUKEMIAS

	Acute Lymphocytic Leukemia	Childhood Ph[1] + ALL	Adult Ph[1] + ALL	CML Lymphoid Blast Crisis
Age	Median 8 years	<14 years	>14 years	Adult
Cell lineage	B Lymphocyte	Pluripotent	Pluripotent	Pluripotent
Ph[1] chromosome	−	+, some marrow cells	+, some marrow cells	+, most marrow cells
Additional chromosomal changes	+	−	−	+
BCR-ABL fusion protein	−	190 KDa	190 or 210 kDa	210 kDa
Prognosis	Fair	Poor	Poor	Very poor
Remission karyotype	Normal	Normal or Ph[1]	Normal or Ph[1]	Ph[1]

(From: Hoffman R, Benz EJ, Shattil SJ, Furie B, and Cohen HJ: Hematology: Basic Principles and Practice. New York: Churchill Livingstone, 1995.)

tract or retinal hemorrhages may occasionally be the first signs of the disease. Physical examination reveals pallor, tenderness over the lower sternum, splenomegaly, and occasionally hepatomegaly. Lymphadenopathy is not typical; when present, it suggests an onset of the acute phase of the disease. Petechiae and ecchymoses reflect the presence of quantitative and/or qualitative platelet abnormalities. CML also may be disguised in an asymptomatic patient being found incidentally to other medical problems or in routine examinations.

Any organ may eventually be infiltrated with myeloid elements, but extramyeloid masses in areas other than the spleen and liver are uncommon findings in the chronic phase. On fresh incision, the extramyeloid masses appear green, presumably due to the presence of the myeloid enzyme, myeloperoxidase. These greenish tumors have been called *chloromas*. The green color fades to a dirty yellow after exposure of the tumor to air.

About 30 to 40 months after diagnosis, a worsening of symptoms and increased debilitation herald the onset of the blast phase. After onset of blast crisis, response to therapy is poor and survival is less than 6 months.

● Laboratory findings

The most striking abnormality in the peripheral blood is the extreme leukocytosis (Table 15-9). The white count is usually greater than 100×10^9/L with a mean of 200 to 500×10^9/L. Counts as high as 1000×10^9/L have been reported. Patients diagnosed in the earlier stages may have a leukocyte count of 25 to 75×10^9/L. Thrombocytosis is found in more than 50% of patients with variation in shape and presence of megakaryocyte fragments. Occasionally, megakaryoblasts and micromakaryocytes can be found in peripheral blood (Fig. 15-7) If thrombocytosis is a new observation, blast crisis is probable to follow. Thrombocytopenia is rare as an initial finding except in Philadelphia-negative CML.[22] In blast crises, thrombocytopenia is a common finding. Platelet function also is frequently abnormal. At the time of diagnosis, a moderate normocytic, normochromic anemia is typical with a hemoglobin concentration in the range of 9 to 13 g/dL. The severity of anemia is proportional to the in-

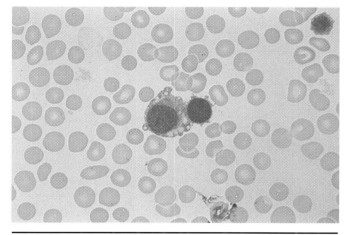

FIGURE 15-7. Micromegakaryocytes in the peripheral blood of a patient with chronic myelocytic leukemia. (250 × original magnification; Wright-Giesma stain).

crease in leukocytes. Erythrocyte morphology is generally normal, but nucleated erythrocytes can usually be found. Reticulocytes are normal or slightly increased.

The blood smear exhibits a shift to the left (Fig. 15-8). Although granulocytes in all stages of maturation are found, the predominant cells are the segmented neutrophils and myelocytes. Promyelocytes and blasts do not usually exceed 20% of the leukocytes and often are less than 10%. Blast concentrations over 20% may indicate blast crises or may occur if the leukocyte count is very high. Eosinophils and basophils often are increased in both relative and absolute terms. Progressive basophilia may herald blast crisis. Monocytes are moderately increased. Signs of myeloid dysplasia can almost always be found, including pseudo Pelger-Huet anomaly and decreased leukocyte alkaline phosphatase (LAP). Low or absent LAP is not specific for CML, but it is characteristic. Monocytosis and myeloid dysplasia are overlapping features found in both CML and chronic myelomonocytic

TABLE 15-9 *PERIPHERAL BLOOD FEATURES OF CML USUALLY FOUND AT THE TIME OF DIAGNOSIS*

Leukocytosis ($100–500 \times 10^9$/L)

Thrombocytosis ($400–500 \times 10^9$/L)

Monocytosis

Basophilia

Eosinophilia

Shift-to-the-left in myeloid cells with predominance of myelocytes and neutrophils

Normocytic, normochromic anemia (Hb 9–13 g/dL)

Occasional nucleated erythrocytes

Decreased leukocyte alkaline phosphatase (LAP)

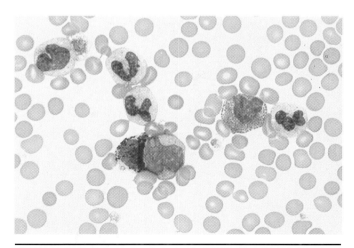

FIGURE 15-8. Chronic myelocytic leukemia (CML) with leukocytosis and a shift to the left. (PB; 250× original magnification; Wright-Giemsa stain).

leukemia, a myelodysplastic syndrome. Other features such as the presence of the Philadelphia chromosome may help differentiate the two disorders, but occasionally specific diagnosis is only possible with disease progression.

The bone marrow is 90% to 100% cellular, with a striking increase in the myeloid to erythroid ratio (10:1 to 50:1). The active red marrow may extend into the long bones. Thinning of the cortex and erosion of the trabeculae may be present. The hematopoietic marrow cells are primarily immature granulocytes with less than 30% blasts, an important characteristic that distinguishes CML from acute leukemia. Often, the marrow differential count of leukocyte precursors is within normal range. The typical *leukemic hiatus* (gap) between immature cells (blasts) and mature cells (segmented neutrophils) characteristic of acute leukemia is not present in CML. Auer rods may be found in the blasts during blast crisis, but this is an unusual finding. Erythropoiesis is normoblastic, but there may be a decrease in normoblasts. Megakaryocytes are usually increased with frequent immature and atypical forms. In contrast to the large megakaryocytes found in other subgroups of MPD, CML typically reveals small megakaryocytes. Gaucher-like cells (histiocytes) have been observed in the bone marrow. However, these cells with the typical wrinkled tissue paper appearance of the cytoplasm are not due to the lack of the β-glucocerebrosidase enzyme as in Gaucher's disease but rather to the overload of cerebrosides caused by increased cell turnover. The histiocytes in CML have normal to increased amounts of the β-glucocerebrosidase, but the cell cannot process the cerebrosides at a rate fast enough to keep them from accumulating in the cell.

The marrow may become fibrotic late in the course of the disease. If the patient is not seen by a physician until the fibrosis is prominent, a diagnosis of MMM may be mistakenly made. At this point, only chromosome analysis can differentiate the diagnosis.

Other nonspecific findings related to the increased proliferation of cells may be present. Total serum cobalamin and the unsaturated cobalamin-binding capacity are increased. Serum transcobalamin I is often elevated. These findings are probably related to the increased number of granulocytes that are thought to synthesize the cobalamin-binding proteins. Secondary to increased cell turnover, uric acid and LDH are elevated. Muramidase is normal or only slightly increased.

● Terminal phase

Approximately 30 to 40 months after the diagnosis of CML, the typical course of the disease is transition to the accelerated stage (Fig. 15-9). This transitional, accelerated stage may occur at any time after the initial diagnosis and often precedes blastic transformation. Transition is heralded by an increase in splenomegaly and a rising leukocytosis refractive to previously effective chemotherapy. Laboratory investigation reveals a worsening of anemia, development of thrombocytopenia, prominent basophilia, an increase in the number of peripheral blood and bone

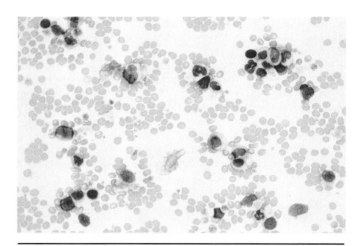

FIGURE 15-9. Peripheral blood from a patient with CML in the accelerated stage. There is an increase in blasts. Micromegakaryocytes and giant platelets are present. (100 X original magnification; Wright-Giemsa stain).

marrow blasts, and an increase in fibrosis of the marrow. Additional chromosomal abnormalities also may be found. Clinical features are reflective of an increase in debilitation, including pyrexia, night sweats, weight loss, increased weakness, malaise, bone pain, and lymphadenopathy. Approximately 30% of patients in the accelerated phase die before a blastic crisis develops.

Although blast crisis develops in most patients with CML after a short accelerated phase, in approximately one third of patients a blastic transformation develops abruptly. After onset of blast crisis, survival is about 1 to 2 months. The clinical features in blast crisis are similar to those of acute leukemia.

The hematologic criteron for identifying a blast crisis is generally accepted as a blast concentration over 30% in either the peripheral blood or the bone marrow in a patient previously diagnosed as having CML. The bone marrow may exhibit an increase in blasts before the peripheral blood. Any type of blast involvement is possible, including myeloid, lymphoid, erythroid, and megakaryocytic cells. Since blast morphology alone is not sufficient to identify the type of blast involved, cytochemical, enzymatic, ultrastructural, and immunologic studies are helpful. About 65% to 75% of the blast crises are myeloblastic, while 25% to 35% of the blast crises are lymphoblastic. The lymphoblasts in blast crises are always immunologically typed as CALLA-positive and demonstrate an elevated terminal deoxynucleotidyl transferase (TdT), findings that indicate these cells belong to the B-lymphocyte lineage. Erythroblastic and megakaryoblastic crises are uncommon.

● Treatment of CML

Therapy for CML is aimed at reducing the leukocyte mass, restoring bone marrow function, reducing splenomegaly, and abolishing symptoms. Busulfan, an alkylating agent, is the agent of choice for treating CML. Other cytotoxic drugs including hydroxyurea, 6-mercaptopurine, and 6-thioguanine also are used. Regular blood counts are necessary in the first months of treatment to monitor the patient's response. Leukophoresis is sometimes used to initially reduce the leukocyte mass. Supportive measures during therapy regimens include transfusion for treatment of severe anemia and antibiotics for treatment of infections. No treatment method has been devised that will prevent eventual blast transformation. Remission generally lasts for 2 to 3 years. The effectiveness of treatment in blast crisis depends on the correct identification of leukemic cells, as the specific sensitivity of various blast populations to selected drugs varies.

A most promising treatment modality for leukemia is bone marrow transplant.[2] High-dose chemoradiotherapy is followed by transplant of hematopoietic stem cells from syngeneic or allogenenic donors. Bone marrow transplant has produced some cures, but the toxicity of the treatment and the limited availability of HLA-compatible donors have limited the application of this approach. It is currently the only treatment that promises long-term, disease-free survival for many patients.

Alpha-interferon, a glycoprotein produced by a variety of cells in response to viral infection, immune stimulation, and chemical inducers, is receiving widespread attention in the treatment of malignancy. Interferons have a myelosuppressive effect, directly inhibiting myeloid progenitor cells.[24] Alpha-interferon is proving to be very effective therapy for CML in early stages of the disease, inducing remission in 55% to 75% of patients.[25,26] It also can suppress and, in some cases, eliminate the Philadelphia-positive clone. In general, however, trials have not indicated that interferon can improve the survival of CML patients beyond that achieved through conventional chemotherapy. Secondary resistance to interferon usually occurs after an average remission of 41 months and the disease progresses.[26] Further studies are underway to determine the therapeutic potential of interferon used in combination with chemotherapy and bone marrow transplantation.

Interferon is given in intramuscular or subcutaneous injection several times per week. Almost all patients experience some toxic side effects similar to flu symptoms. Tolerance to side effects, however, usually occurs within several weeks of therapy.

Differential diagnosis

Many infectious, inflammatory, and malignant disorders, and severe hemorrhage or hemolysis may cause a leukemoid reaction indistinguishable from the picture of CML (Table 15-10). At times, the clinical findings may permit an accurate diagnosis, but in some cases differential diagnosis requires further investigation. In a leukemoid reaction, the leukocytosis is generally accompanied by a predominance of segmented neutrophils and bands on the blood smear. There may be myelocytes and metamyelocytes present but, if so, are few in number compared with CML. Although blasts and promyelocytes are easily found in CML, these cells are rarely present in a leukemoid reaction. Benign toxic leukocytosis due to infection is often accompanied by toxic granulation, cytoplasmic vacuoles, and Döhle bodies in granulocytes. These are not common findings at the time of diagnosis of CML. Monocytes, eosinophils, and basophils are generally not elevated in a leukemoid reaction, whereas they are typically increased in CML.

Other diagnostic tests are helpful in differentiating a leukemoid reaction from CML. In a leukemoid reaction, the LAP score is typically elevated, and the Philadelphia chromosome is absent. Splenomegaly is uncommon in a leukemoid reaction. Rarely, a bone marrow examination is necessary to make a differential diagnosis. In a leukemoid reaction, the marrow may be hypercellular, but there is an orderly maturation of granulocytic cells.

Occasionally, CML resembles myelofibrosis with myeloid metaplasia. Distinguishing features of myelofibrosis include a markedly abnormal erythrocyte morphology with nucleated erythrocytes and immature leukocytes (leukoerythroblastic reaction), an increased LAP score, frank bone marrow fibrosis, and the absence of the Philadelphia chromosome.

TABLE 15-10 *COMPARISON OF PERIPHERAL BLOOD FEATURES OF CML AND LEUKEMOID REACTIONS*

Laboratory Parameter	CML	Leukemoid Reaction
Leukocytes	Blasts and promyelocytes as well as more mature forms in peripheral blood; toxic changes usually absent; absolute basophilia and/or eosinophilia; neutrophils with single lobed nuclei and hypogranular forms may be present.	Blasts and promeylocytes in peripheral blood are rare; toxic granulation, Döhle bodies, cytoplasmic vacuoles present; no absolute basophilia or eosinophilia
Platelets	Often increased with abnormal morphological forms present	Usually normal
Erythrocytes	Anemia usually present, variable anisocytosis, poikilocytosis, NRBC present	Anemia may be present but NRBC not typical
LAP	Low	Increased
Chromosome karyotype	Ph chromosome present	Normal

TABLE 15-11 *A COMPARISON OF THE FEATURES OF TYPICAL CML WITH CML VARIANTS*

Variant	Predominant Age/Sex	Leukocyte Count	Leukocyte Differential	LAP Score	Ph Chromosome	Other
CML	Middle-age; 40–49 peak/ equal sex distribution	100–500 × 10⁹/L	Shift to the left; usually less than 30% blasts	Decreased	Present	
Juvenile 1) infantile (juvenile) type	Less than than 5 years of age	15–100 × 10⁹/L	Shift to the left; less than 10% blasts	Usually decreased	Absent	Erythrocytes have fetal characteristics; urinary and serum muramidase high
2) adult type	Over 5 years of age	Same as CML	Same as CML	Decreased	Present	
Eosinophilic	Middle age/male predominance	More than 30 × 10⁹/L	30–70% eosinophils with immature forms; shift to the left in neutrophils	Normal	Present or absent	Serum cobalamin, uric acid, and muramidase high
Basophilic	Middle age/ slight predominance of males	Normal or increased	40–80% basophils with immature forms present	Normal or decreased	Present or absent	Serum and urine histamine levels high
Neutrophilic	Usually over 50 years of age/ equal between sexes	Markedly increased	Mature cells	Increased	Absent	
Atypical CML	Older adults	Lower than CML	Shift to the left with more blasts in the peripheral blood and bone marrow than CML	Decreased	Absent	Basophils normal to low; granulocytic cells dysplastic with hypogranularity and hypolobulation

●
Variants of chronic myelocytic leukemia (Table 15-11)

ATYPICAL CHRONIC MYELOCYTIC LEUKEMIA

Atypical CML is a disease characterized by a CML-like morphologic picture but it is Philadelphia chromosome-negative and BCR/ABL-negative. There are several peripheral blood features that help differentiate it from typical CML (Table 15-12):[17] (1) some of the myeloid cells have abnormal morphology, including hypogranular or agranular myelocytes, metamyelocytes, bands, and neutrophils. The promyelocytes may lack primary granules. Some neutrophils are mononuclear, bilobed, or have irregular segmentation. (2) Basophils are absent or present in low numbers in contrast to CML. (3) The platelet count is often less than 150 × 10⁹/L.

In patients with a high monocyte count, the disease may be confused with chronic myelomonocytic leukemia (CMML), a myelodysplastic syndrome. In atypical CML however, the sum of promyelocytes, myelocytes, and metamyelocytes accounts for more than 10% of the total leu-

TABLE 15-12 *DIFFERENTIATING CHARACTERISTICS OF PH-POSITIVE AND PH-NEGATIVE CML (ATYPICAL)*

Characteristic	Ph-Positive CML	Atypical CML (Ph-Negative)
Median age, years	42	60
Leukocyte count (×10⁹/L) median	210	75
<100 × 10⁹/L (%)	23	65
Platelet count median (×10⁹/L)	400	170
<100 × 10⁹/L (%)	10	40–50
>450 × 10⁹/L (%)	60	36
Basophils ≥3% (%)	30–50	10–20
Low LAP score (%)	70	70
Remission with therapy (%)	100	30
Median survival (months)	44	15

(Adapted from: Lee GR, et al: Wintrobe's Clinical Hematology 9th ed. Philadelphia, Lea & Febiger, 1993 and Kantarjcan HM, et al: Philadelphia chromosome-negative chronic myelogenous leukemia and chronic myelomonocytic leukemia. Hematol/Oncol Clin North Am, 4:389, 1990)

kocytes, whereas in CMML these myelocytic cells account for less than 10% of the total leukocytes due to the high monocytic cell count.

Prognosis is poorer than Philadelphia-positive CML, with a median survival after diagnosis of less than 1 year.

JUVENILE CHRONIC MYELOGENOUS LEUKEMIA

All forms of chronic leukemias in children are uncommon. The most common (1.3% to 5% of all childhood leukemias) and most important of these disorders is CML. Two variants of CML occur in children: infantile, or juvenile-type, and adult-type.

Infantile variant The infantile type of CML occurs in children younger than 5 years of age, with a peak incidence between 1 and 2 years of age. The children present with prominant lymphadenopathy, mild to moderate splenomegaly, hepatomegaly, dermal infiltrates with an eczematous skin rash, and recurrent infections. The leukocyte count is lower than that seen in adult CML, averaging 30 × 10⁹/L and ranging from 15 to 100 × 10⁹/L. Thrombocytopenia is an early discovery. The Philadelphia chromosome is always absent, and there is no BCR/ABL arrangement; about 20% of the patients have other cytogenetic abnormalities. The LAP is usually decreased. Peripheral blood leukocytosis reveals an absolute increase in all stages of granulocyte and monocyte maturation and less than 10% blasts (Fig. 15-10). An absolute monocytosis is present, and urinary and serum muramidase levels are markedly elevated. There is often a polyclonal increase in immunoglobulins, suggesting that the monocytes are producing high levels of IL-6, which stimulates the maturation of B-lymphocytes. Nucleated erythrocytes also are present. Anemia with evidence of ineffective erythropoiesis is common. The erythrocytes have a variety of metabolic and antigenic characteristics of fetal erythrocytes, including an increase in hemoglobin F and the presence of the i antigen.

There are less than 10% blasts in the bone marrow, megakaryocytes are normal or decreased, and, in contrast to adult CML, there is only a slight increase in the myeloid to erythroid ratio.

The disorder is generally resistant to chemotherapy. Sepsis is the most common cause of death. Blast crisis may occur, but most patients have a progressive steady increase in blasts accompanied by progressive thrombocytopenia and splenomegaly. Some have a terminal phase resembling DiGuglielmo's syndrome with erythroid hyperplasia and circulating normoblasts. Death occurs within 2 years of diagnosis.

Adult variant The adult form of CML in children typically affects children older than 5 years of age, with a mean age of 9 years. Clinical features include marked splenomegaly, mild lymphadenopathy, absent to moderate hepatomegaly, and bone pain. Rarely, priapism, retinopathy, and skin nodules have been reported to occur in association with this disease. The blood and bone marrow findings are similar to those found in the adult form of CML. The Philadelphia chromosome is present, and the LAP is decreased.

Remission can be induced by chemotherapy, but most patients undergo blast transformation and die of acute leukemia or complications within 3 to 5 years after initial diagnosis.

CHRONIC EOSINOPHILIC LEUKEMIA

Chronic eosinophilic leukemia as a distinct entity is questioned by many investigators. It is considered by some to be a variant of CML. Still others classify persistent eosinophilia accompanied by unexplained organ system dysfunction and with no underlying provoking cause, under the broad classification, hypereosinophilic syndrome.

The diagnosis of chronic eosinophilic leukemia is often a diagnosis of exclusion. This means that before a diagnosis of leukemia is considered, all other conditions associated with an eosinophilia are excluded, such as collagen, vascular, and infectious diseases. The criteria suggested for a diagnosis of eosinophilic leukemia include: (1) persistent eosinophilia with immature forms in the peripheral blood and the presence of myeloblasts and other immature neutrophilic cells; immature forms are usually absent in other causes of eosinophilia; (2) less than 5% blasts in the bone marrow, with evidence of disorderly cellular differentiation and maturation; (3) infiltration of tissue by eosinophils; (4) brief clinical course measured in months; (5) associated anemia and thrombocytopenia.[27]

The leukocyte count is usually over 30 × 10⁹/L, with 30% to 70% eosinophils. The bone marrow shows a shift to the left, with many eosinophilic myelocytes. Marrow fibrosis is a common finding. The LAP score is normal, but the serum cobalamin, uric acid, and muramidase are frequently elevated. Occasionally, the Philadelphia chromosome has been demonstrated, which suggests that the disease is sometimes a variant of CML. In other patients, the Philadelphia chromosome is not present, but other clonal chromosmal aberrations can be found, including trisomy for group C chromosomes and isochromosome 17.

Eosinophilic leukemia is most often diagnosed in mid-

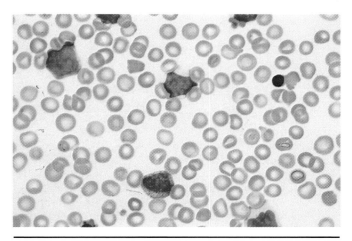

FIGURE 15-10. Peripheral blood from a patient with juvenile CML. There is a shift to the left but the leukocyte count is lower than in the adult CML.

dle-aged men. Presenting symptoms include fever and significant weight loss. Clinical features include CNS irregularities, hepatosplenomegaly, congestive heart failure, pulmonary fibrosis, and, occasionally, lymphadenopathy.

The prognosis is poor, as patients do not respond to therapy. Most patients die within 1 year. Autopsy reveals tissue injury due to the release of substances from disintegrating eosinophils. The major cause of death is congestive heart failure.

CHRONIC BASOPHILIC LEUKEMIA

Chronic basophilic leukemia is the rarest variant of CML; it occurs in middle age, with a slight predominance in males. As with eosinophilic leukemia, many investigators question whether basophilic leukemia is a distinct entity or a variant of CML. The disease needs to be distinguished from the basophilia in CML that commonly precedes blast crisis and from the basophilia found in other myeloproliferative disorders.

The onset of the disease may be insidious or abrupt. Clinical features are similar to those found in CML, including weakness, fatigue, fever, and hepatosplenomegaly. Many patients have symptoms related to hyperhistaminemia, such as wheezing, urticaria, diarrhea, pruritis, and peripheral edema. These symptoms are related to the massive increase in histamine-containing granules derived from basophils.[28] Massive release of basophil granules may occur after effective therapy, resulting in shock or severe disseminated intravascular coagulation (DIC). Patients do not respond well to conventional therapy modalities.

The leukocyte count may be normal but is most often increased. The most striking finding on the blood smear is an extreme increase in the number of basophils, usually between 40% and 80%, with some immature forms present. The basophils are abnormal, resembling tissue mast cells. Fine uniform granules cover most of the nucleus and cytoplasm. Abnormal neutrophils, monocytes, and eosinophils also may be found. The LAP score is normal or low. Serum and urine histamine levels are from 10 to 15 times normal.

CHRONIC NEUTROPHILIC LEUKEMIA

A rare entity included in the myeloproliferative disorders is chronic neutrophilic leukemia. Like the other myeloproliferative disorders, chronic neutrophilic leukemia may evolve into other myeloproliferative syndromes or acute leukemia. There is controversy as to whether this is a variant of CML or a distinct MPD entity. The LAP is increased, and the Philadelphia chromosome is absent. Criteria for diagnosis include sustained leukocytosis without immature myeloid precursors in the peripheral blood, tissue infiltration by neutrophils, increased LAP, and absence of the Philadelphia chromosome.[29] Anemia is often present, and nucleated erythrocytes may be found. Platelets are usually present in normal concentration but may be decreased. Bone marrow examination shows hypercellularity with granulocytic hyperplasia. Granulocyte maturation appears normal, but megakaryocytes may exhibit dysplasia. Patients are usually older than 50 years of age,

with equal sex distribution. It is often symptomatic. Splenomegaly is the primary clinical finding. The disease is slowly progressive and survival is variable.

MYELOFIBROSIS WITH MYELOID METAPLASIA

Myelofibrosis with myeloid metaplasia (MMM) is known by many synonyms. Most of the different names are an attempt to describe the typical blood, bone marrow, and spleen abnormalities. Some of the more common terms include agnogenic myeloid metaplasia, idiopathic myelofibrosis, primary myelofibrosis, aleukemic myelosis, myelosclerosis, splenomegalic myelophthisis, and leukoerythroblastic anemia. Regardless of the synonym used, the disease is considered to be one entity.

Myelofibrosis with myeloid metaplasia is considered to be a clonal hematopoietic stem cell disorder[30] with unchecked proliferation of hematopoietic elements, progressive bone marrow fibrosis, and extramedullary hematopoiesis (myeloid metaplasia).

Pathophysiology

The underlying process of this disorder is controversial. Some believe it to be leukemic in nature, while others consider it to be a neoplastic disorder, closely related to, but different from, CML and PV. Still others believe the disease is a response of the marrow to some type of toxic agent that injures hematopoietic cells.

Studies suggest that MMM is a clonal disorder that originates in an abnormal hematopoietic stem cell. Isoenzyme studies in females with MMM who are heterozygous for G6PD demonstrate only one type of enzyme in granulocytes, erthrocytes, and platelets; however, they show enzyme heterozygosity in other tissue cells, including fibroid cells. Chromosome aberrations, when present, are restricted to those cells with a common hematapoietic progenitor cell. The CFU-GEMM stem cell appears to be affected most often. These cells are found in increased concentration in the peripheral blood of patients with MMM. Some are highly sensitive to or independent of regulation by stimulatory factors. In some cases, the pluripotential stem cell may be the neoplastic cell, since MMM has been reported to terminate in ALL as well as AML.

All three cell lines, erythrocytes, granulocytes, and platelets, may be involved in the disease process. In most cases, however, only one or two cell lines are involved. The typical peripheral blood findings reflect both qualitative and quantitative abnormalities of these cells. The bone marrow exhibits varying degrees of fibrosis. The fibrosis is not considered to be a part of the primary abnormal clonal proliferation but rather is a secondary reactive event. Fibroblasts do not contain the chromosome abnormalities found in hematopoietic cells, and they exhibit heterozygosity rather than homozygosity for the G6PD isoenzyme in heterozygote females.

Understanding of this disease has increased considerably over the last decade, with a better understanding of the composition of the normal and myelofibrotic bone marrow stroma and of the role of growth factors from megakaryocytes as mediators of fibrogenesis.[31] The stroma of normal bone marrow includes collagen types I, III, IV, and V. Myelofibrotic stroma is characterized by an increase in total collagen, especially in types I and III.[31] Myelofibrotic stroma also contains continuous sheets of collagen type IV and laminin, resulting from marked neo-vascularization and endothelial cell proliferation. In normal marrow, collagen type IV and laminin are limited to discontinuous sinusoidal basement membranes. Fibronectin, normally limited to megakaryocytes and walls of blood vessels, is found deposited in the stroma of myelofibrotic marrow. Vitronectin, another adhesive glycoprotein that promotes cell attachment and spreading, also is abnormally deposited in myelofibrotic marrow stroma.

Evidence indicates that megakaryocytes may play an important role in the pathogenic development of this abnormal marrow stroma in MMM. Megakaryocytic hyperplasia, with abnormal or dysplastic forms, is associated with all myeloproliferative disorders but is especially common in MMM. In marrow areas of megakaryocyte necrosis, fibroblast proliferation and collagen deposition is often most prominent.[31] It is believed that the growth factor, PDGF, contained in the α-granules of megakaryocytes and platelets, is largely responsible for stimulating the growth and proliferation of fibroblasts. Reduced platelet PDGF and increased serum PDGF are characteristic of MMM. This condition is believed to represent abnormal release or leakage of the growth factor from the platelet. It is evident, however, that additional growth factors also must be involved in MMM because PDGF does not stimulate synthesis of collagen, laminin, and fibronectin. One of these additional growth factors is probably transforming growth factor-beta (TGF-β), a polypeptide synthesized by megakaryocytes and stored in high concentration in the α-granules. This growth factor is recognized by receptors on all cells and serves as a regulator of extracellular matrix (stroma) synthesis. TGF-β stimulates increased expression of genes for fibronectin, collagens type I, III, and IV, while decreasing synthesis of collagenase-like enzymes. The net result of these interactions is accumulation of bone marrow stromal elements.[31]

Myeloid metaplasia usually occurs in both the spleen and the liver. These organs can become massive in size due to islands of proliferating erythroid, myeloid, and megakaryocytic elements. The extramedullary hematopoiesis is similar to that which occurs in embryonic hematopoiesis.[37]

Clinical findings

MMM generally affects individuals older than 50 years of age. It rarely occurs in childhood. It appears to occur equally between sexes. The onset is gradual, and the disease is very chronic. Early in the disease, there may be no symptoms, making the time of onset impossible to determine. If symptoms are present, they are usually related to anemia or pressure from an enlarged spleen. Occasionally, bleeding may be a presenting symptom. Bleeding may be

trivial (such as petechiae) or life-threatening. Patients experience weakness, weight loss, loss of appetite, night sweats, extremity pain, and discomfort in the upper left quadrant. The major physical findings are splenomegaly, hepatomegaly, pallor, and petechiae.

Myeloid metaplasia is found in the spleen and frequently in the liver but also may be found in the kidney, adrenal glands, peritoneal and extraperitoneal surfaces, skin, and lymph nodes. Osteosclerosis is a frequent finding and, when found in association with splenomegaly, suggests a diagnosis of myelofibrosis.

An atypical acute form of the disease has been described with a rapid and progressive course of a few months to 1 year. Anemia develops rapidly, and the leukocyte count is decreased. The bone marrow in these cases exhibits a proliferation of reticular and collagen fibers.

Patients with systemic lupus erythrematosus (SLE) may present with myelofibrosis morphologically indistinguishable from the myelofibrosis of MMM. These patients also have various peripheral blood cytopenias similar to those found in MMM, but splenomegaly is not found. The myelofibrosis in SLE has been referred to as "autoimmune myelofibrosis." Peripheral blood counts usually normalize with glucocorticoid therapy, but fibrosis persists in most. It has been suggested that all patients with myelofibrosis and an absence of splenomegaly should have an antinuclear antibodies test (ANA) to rule out SLE.[32] Hematologic remission is possible with glucocorticoid therapy in SLE-associated myelofibrosis.

Laboratory findings

PERIPHERAL BLOOD

Although peripheral blood findings are variable, a moderate leukoerythroblastic anemia, with striking anisocytosis and poikilocytosis, is characteristic of this disease (Table 15-13) (Fig 15-11A and 11B). The anemia is usually normocytic, normochromic, but hypochromia may be found after a history of hemorrhage. Folic acid deficiency may develop as a result of increased utilization. Folic acid deficiency is associated with a macrocytic anemia. Anemia uncomplicated by iron deficiency or folic acid deficiency correlates directly with the extent of bone marrow fibrosis and the effectiveness of extramedullary hematopoiesis. The anemia becomes more severe with progression of the disease. The anemia is aggravated in some patients by a combination of splenomegaly, which causes sequestration of erythrocytes and expanded plasma volume, which dilutes the erythrocytes.

Fifteen percent of patients have major hemolytic episodes during the course of their disease.[33] Decreased haptoglobin and hemosidinuria found in about 10% of patients suggest intravascular hemolysis. The cause of hemolysis may be hypersplenism, PNH-like defective erythrocytes, and anti-erythrocyte antibodies. Some patients have a positive Ham's test and/or sucrose hemolysis test.

Hemostatic abnormalities suggestive of disseminated intravascular coagulation (DIC) may be present, including

TABLE 15-13 *HEMATOLOGIC FINDINGS IN MYELOFIBROSIS WITH MYELOID METAPLASIA*

TYPICAL:

Anemia

Anisocytosis

Poikilocytosis with prominent dacryocytes

Nucleated erythrocytes

Leukocytosis or leukopenia

Shift-to-the-left in granulocytic cells

Increased or normal leukocyte alkaline phosphatase (LAP) unless leukocyte count is low

Basophilic stippling

Thrombocytopenia or thrombocytosis

Giant, bizarre platelets

Micromegakaryocytes or naked nuclei

Abnormal platelet aggregation

Increased uric acid

Increased lactate dehydrogenase (LDH)

Bone marrow fibrosis with reticulin in early stages, collagen in late stages

OTHER:

Positive Ham's test and/or sucrose hemolysis test

Increased fibrin split products

Low concentration of Factors V and VIII

decreased platelet count, decreased concentration of Factors V and VIII, and increased fibrin split products.[33] Usually DIC in these patients produces no symptoms and may only become apparent after surgery.

The appearance of the erythrocytes is an important feature in this disease. The most typical poikilocyte is the dacryocyte, although elliptocytes and ovalocytes also are present (Fig. 15-12). A few nucleated erythrocytes are usually found; sometimes they are numerous. Basophilic stip-

pling is a common finding. Reticulocytosis is typical ranging from 2% to 15%. The majority of patients have an absolute reticulocyte count more than $60 \times 10^9/L$.

The leukocyte count is usually elevated but may be normal, or less often, decreased. The count generally ranges from 15 to $30 \times 10^9/L$, and it is rare to find a leukocyte count above 60 to $70 \times 10^9/L$ before splenectomy. The leukocyte concentration is rather constant and does not decrease with progression of the disease, as is typical of erythrocytes and platelets. An orderly progression of immature granulocytes is characteristically found. Blasts generally compose less than 5% of circulating leukocytes. Other common findings include basophilia, eosinophilia, and pseudo Pelger-Huet anomaly. The LAP is elevated or normal but occasionally may be decreased. A low LAP correlates with leukopenia. When elevated, the LAP score helps to differentiate this disease from CML. The Philadelphia chromosome is not present.

Platelets may be low, normal, or increased. Higher counts are associated with early disease stages, whereas thrombocytopenia is usually found in the latter stages. Thrombocytopenia is often attributed to excessive splenic pooling. The platelets are typically giant, bizarre, and frequently hypogranular. Circulating megakaryocyte fragments, mononuclear micromegakaryocytes, and naked megakaryocyte nuclei may be found (Fig. 15-13). The micromegakaryocytes may present a problem in identification as they frequently resemble mononuclear leukocytes. However, an important differentiating feature is the presence of demarcation membranes with bull's eye granules in the cytoplasm, characteristic of megakaryocytes. Qualitative platelet abnormalities, including abnormal aggregation, adhesiveness, and defective platelet factor-3 (PF3) release on exposure to collagen, are consistent findings.

Other laboratory tests are frequently abnormal in this disease. Serum uric acid and LDH are elevated in most patients. Serum cobalamin may be slightly increased but is usually normal.

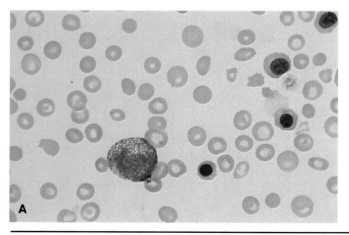
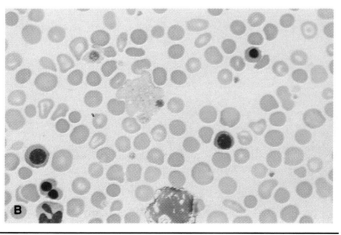

FIGURE 15-11. **A,** Promyelocyte and nucleated erythrocytes from a case of myelofibrosis with myeloid metaplasia. (PB). **B,** Giant platelet, nucleated erythrocytes and dacryocytes from a case of myelofibrosis with myeloid metaplasia (PB). (250× original magnification; Wright-Giemsa stain).

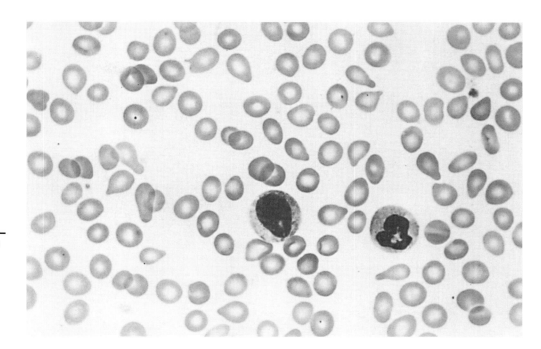

FIGURE 15-12. A blood smear from a patient with myelofibrosis with myeloid metaplasia. There is a shift to the left as indicated by the myelocyte and band here. Notice also the numerous dacryocytes (teardrops) (Peripheral blood, 250 × original magnification).

BONE MARROW

The bone marrow is difficult to penetrate and, during aspiration, frequently yields a dry tap. If aspiration is successful, smears made from aspirates may show no abnormalities. Biopsy specimens are needed to reveal fibrosis. In most cases, the marrow is hypercellular, with varying degrees of diffuse fibrosis and focal aggregates of megakaryocytes.

The following three bone marrow histologic patterns have been described: panhyperplasia with absence of myelofibrosis, but a slight increase in reticulin fibers; myeloid atrophy with fibrosis, prominent collagen and reticulin fibers, and cellularity less than 30%; and myelofibrosis and myelosclerosis with bony trabeculae occupying 30% of the biopsy and extensive fibrosis.

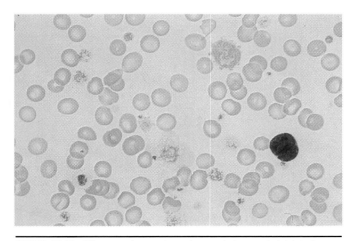

FIGURE 15-13. Micromegakaryocyte nucleus and abnormal platelets from a case of myelofibrosis with myeloid metaplasia. (PB; 250× original magnification).

Cytogenetics

Cytogenetic analysis may be important to differentiate myelofibrosis from other myeloproliferative disorders, particularly from CML, which may have some degree of fibrosis. The Philadelphia chromosome is not present. Although no specific cytogenetic abnormality is diagnostic, a trisomy or deletion of Group C chromosomes is associated with myelofibrosis. These same abnormalities may be seen in PV. Complete or partial loss of chromosomes, especially chromosomes 5 and 7, is associated with MMM cases that are treated with chemotherapy.

Prognosis and therapy

The average survival time after diagnosis is 4 to 5 years. The main causes of death are infection, hemorrhage, thrombosis, and cardiac failure. About 10% to 15% of patients die with an acute myeloid leukemia and some with acute lymphoid leukemia.

There is no cure or specific treatment for this disorder. Corticosteroids and androgens have been used to stimulate erythropoiesis, but most patients require periodic transfusions. When anemia cannot be controlled, splenectomy may be considered. Splenectomy, however, gives inconsistent results and is a controversial procedure. The benefit is temporary, and the mortality rate is high. Irradiation has been suggested to decrease spleen size in an attempt to relieve symptoms or to decrease excessive erythrocyte destruction. Alkylating agents have been used, but they have the potential of causing severe pancytopenia. Drugs to control hyperuricemia have been used to prevent or decrease problems with gout and nephropathy.

TABLE 15-14 *CONDITIONS ASSOCIATED WITH MARROW FIBROSIS*

Myelofibrosis with myeloid metaplasia

Chronic granulocytic leukemia

Polycythemia vera

Essential thrombocythemia

Megakaryocytic leukemia

Metastatic carcinoma

Miliary tuberculosis

Fungus infection

Hairy cell leukemia

Lymphoma

Hodgkin's disease

Granulomas

Marrow damage by radiation or chemicals

Differential diagnosis

Differentiation of MMM from other conditions associated with fibrosis is essential to assure appropriate therapy regimens (Table 15-14). Splenomegaly, anemia, and a leukoerythroblastic blood picture are significant findings in both myelofibrosis and CML. In myelofibrosis, the leukocyte count is generally lower, less than 50×10^9/L, while in CML the count is expected to be higher. In myelofibrosis, a shift to the left is less pronounced, and poikilocytosis is striking. The bone marrow in myelofibrosis is fibrous, with large numbers of megakaryocytes. In leukemia, the bone marrow also may exhibit some fibrosis, but the most abnormal finding is myeloid hyperplasia. The serum cobalamin level is not as elevated in myelofibrosis as it is in CML. The LAP score in myelofibrosis is variable, but when elevated, it is strong evidence against CML. The most reliable test to differentiate CML and MMM is cytogenetic analysis. Up to 95% of patients with CML demonstrate the Philadelphia chromosome.

Differentiation of myelofibrosis from PV, especially in the latter stages, is more difficult. The latter stages of PV may be accompanied by increased marrow fibrosis or actual transformation to myelofibrosis.

When thrombocytosis is a principle initial hematologic finding, myelofibrosis may be confused with essential thrombocythemia. A bone marrow biopsy, however, aids in the differentiation, revealing a frank fibrosis in myelofibrosis.

Myelophthisic anemia and leukoerythroblastosis are nonspecific terms that have been used to describe the finding of nucleated erythrocytes and immature myeloid cells in the peripheral blood. This may be accompanied by bone marrow fibrosis and extramedullary hematopoiesis. A variety of disease processes that results in replacement of bone marrow are associated with myelophthisic anemia, including bone marrow tumors. Although myelophthisic anemia may have a very similar morphologic peripheral blood picture to myelofibrosis, the leukocyte count is usually normal or decreased in myelophthisic anemia. Bone marrow examination from more than one site may be necessary to rule out such a secondary reaction due to tumor, granulocytes, etc., replacing the marrow.

POLYCYTHEMIA VERA

The term polycythemia means literally an increase in the cellular blood elements. However, it is most commonly used to describe an increase in erythrocytes, exclusive of leukocytes and platelets. *Polycythemia vera* (PV) is a myeloproliferative disorder characterized by an unregulated proliferation of the erythroid elements in the bone marrow and an increase in erythrocyte concentration in the peripheral blood. In addition to erythroid cells, other progeny of the pluripotential stem cell also may be simultaneously or sequentially involved in the autonomous proliferation, resulting in a pancytosis in the blood. Polycythemia vera has several synonyms, including polycythemia rubra vera, primary polycythemia, erythremia, and Osler's disease.

Classification

Polycythemia is a general term used to describe erythrocytosis with an increase in both hemoglobin concentration and packed cell volume (hematocrit). Hemoglobin, hematocrit, and erythrocyte counts are parameters that are measured in relative terms (e.g., the ratio of hemoglobin or erythrocytes to blood volume), not in absolute concentrations. When evaluating a patient for polycythemia, it is important to differentiate whether these blood parameters are elevated because of an absolute increase in total erthrocyte mass (absolute erythrocytosis) or to a decrease in plasma volume (relative erythrocytosis) (Fig. 15-14). Although an absolute erythrocytosis suggests a diagnosis of polycythemia vera, polycythemia secondary to tissue hypoxia also should be considered.

In an attempt to clarify the pathogenesis of the disorder,

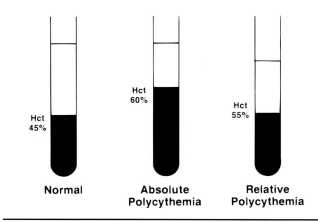

FIGURE 15-14. The hematocrit may be increased due to an absolute increase in erythrocyte mass, absolute polycythemia (center), or to a decrease in plasma volume, relative polycythemia (right).

TABLE 15-15 *CLASSIFICATION OF POLYCYTHEMIA*

I. Polycythemia vera (primary)
II. Secondary polycythemia
  A. Appropriate erythropoietin production (tissue hypoxia)
    1. High altitude
    2. Chronic obstructive pulmonary disease
    3. Obesity (Pickwickian syndrome)
  B. Inappropriate erythropoietin production
    1. Tumors (e.g., hepatoma, uterine fibroma, renal carcinoma)
    2. Renal ischemia
  C. Familial erythrocytosis
    1. Hemoglobins with high oxygen affinity
    2. Congenital decrease in erythrocyte 2,3-DPG
III. Relative polycythemia
  A. Gaisböck's syndrome (stress polycythemia, spurious polycythemia, pseudopolycythemia)
  B. Dehydration

TABLE 15-16 *POSSIBLE MECHANISMS FOR INCREASED ERYTHROPOIESIS IN POLYCYTHEMIA VERA*

1. Erythropoietin-independent proliferation of neoplastic stem cells.
2. Hypersensitivity of erythroid stem cells to erythropoietin.
3. Hypersensitivity of erythroid stem cells to growth factors other than erythropoietin.
4. Presence of abnormal growth factors that act on normal stem cells.

polycythemia is classified into three different groups (Table 15-15): polycythemia vera, secondary polycythemia and relative polycythemia.

Polycythemia vera and secondary polycythemia are both results of an absolute increase in the total body erythrocyte mass. Secondary polycythemia can be distinguished from polycythemia vera by a distinct although not always apparent, explanation for the erythrocytosis. Hence, the name "secondary" polycythemia. Conversely, polycythemia vera is caused by a primary unregulated increase in erythrocyte production, with no identifiable inciting cause. Relative polycythemia is characterized by a normal or even decreased erythrocyte mass. It occurs as a result of decreased plasma volume. It is a mild polycythemia due to dehydration, hemoconcentration, or to a condition known as Gaisbock's syndrome.

● Pathophysiology

The panhyperplasia often associated with this disease suggests a clonal stem cell defect. The clonal nature of the disease is confirmed by the finding of only one type of G6PD in erythrocytes, granulocytes, and platelets in women with PV who are heterozygous for the enzyme. This finding persists in cells even during complete remission. Abnormal chromosome karaotypes, when present, are also clonal in nature.

Although all cells in the peripheral blood may be increased in polycythemia vera, an increase in erythropoiesis is the outstanding feature. The cause of the erythrocytosis is unknown, but a number of possible mechanisms have been suggested[34] (Table 15-16). In vitro studies using cell culture systems revealed that PV bone marrow cells could form erythroid colonies without addition of exogenous erythropoietin. This suggests that increased proliferation may be due to an erythroprotein-independent, unregulated neoplastic proliferation of stem cells. Conversely, more recent studies reveal that erythropoietin levels increase in PV patients after phlebotomy and after ascent to high altitudes. In addition, anti-erythropoietin antibodies in PV cultures inhibit erythroid colony formation.

These results suggest that erythropoiesis in PV is responsive to erythropoietin.

Another mechanism for increased erythropoiesis in PV may be increased sensitivity of erythroid stem cells to erythropoietin. This hypersensitivity may give PV cells a growth advantage. Studies using serum-free culture systems, however, have shown that the erythropoietin sensitivity of PV progenitors is the same as normal progenitors. Studies of the erythropoietin receptor on PV cells has failed to reveal a qualitative or quantitative abnormality that could account for the PV phenotype.

The role of growth factors other than erythropoietin has been studied in PV. Evidence reveals that PV progenitor cells are two times more sensitive to insulin-like growth factor-I (IGF-I), a growth factor that stimulates hematopoiesis. Erythropoiesis in PV is not dependent on IGF-I, however, since in its absence a constant baseline of erythroid colony growth is present. It is possible that PV progenitor cells are hypersensitive to IGF-I due to mutations in the IGF-I receptor and/or the IGF-I related signaling pathway. The role of other myeloproliferative growth factors in PV remains to be explained.

Erythroid maturation is normal and erythrocytes function normally. Mature erythrocytes also have a normal lifespan.

● Clinical findings

Polycythemia vera is an uncommon disorder with an annual incidence in the United States of 5 to 17 cases per million population per year. It occurs most often between the ages of 40 and 60 years. The peak incidence is in the sixth decade of life. The disease is rare in children. It occurs more frequently in males than females and is more common in whites than blacks, particularly in those of Jewish descent. The incidence in Japan is extremely low, except for the population exposed to atomic bomb explosions. There are several reports of PV occurring within several members of the same family. These findings indicate that, in some cases, the disease may develop as a result of a genetic predisposition.

The onset of the disease is usually gradual with a history of symptoms for several years. In some cases, PV is found in asymptomatic individuals. When symptoms are present, they are usually related to the increased erythrocyte mass and the associated cardiovascular disease due to sludging of the thickened blood. Headache, weakness, puritis, weight loss, and fatigue are the most common symptoms. Pruritis is attributed to hyperhistaminemia that may be spontaneous or induced by hot showers or baths. Itching is generalized, with absence of rash.

About one third of the patients experience thrombotic or hemorrhagic episodes. Gingival bleeding, menorrhagia, hemoptysis, and gastrointestinal bleeding are common. Myocardial infarctions, retinal vein thrombosis, thrombophlebitis, and cerebral ischemia may occur at any stage of the disease and may occasionally be the first indication of the disease.

Results of physical examination show splenomegaly in approximately 75% of the patients and hepatomegaly in 40% to 50%. Splenomegaly may not be an initial finding but occurs with disease progression. Both the spleen and liver show extramedullary hematopoiesis.

When the hematocrit exceeds 60%, the blood viscosity increases steeply, decreasing blood flow, and increasing peripheral vascular resistance. These interactions produce hypertension in about 50% of the patients with PV. Phlethora, especially on the face but also on the hands, feet, and ears, is a common finding on physical examination. Optical examination reveals engorgement of the fundus veins and conjunctional phlethora.

After a period of 2 to 10 years, bone marrow failure may develop, accompanied by an increase in splenomegaly. At this time, anemia and bleeding may be the primary clinical findings, secondary to a decreased platelet count and decreasing hematocrit. This is known as the spent phase. Myelofibrosis develops in about 30% of PV cases. Acute leukemia may develop as an abrupt transition in 5% to 10% of patients. Leukemia appears to develop at a higher rate in those patients treated with myelosuppressive drugs than in those treated with phlebotomy alone.

● Laboratory findings

PERIPHERAL BLOOD

The most striking finding of the peripheral blood is an absolute erythrocytosis in the range of 6 to 10 $\times$ 10^{12}/L, with a hemoglobin concentration over 18 g/dL. The hematocrit in females is greater than 0.48 L/L (48%) and in males is greater than 0.52 L/L (52%). The range is usually between 0.55 L/L to 0.60 L/L. The total erythrocyte mass is increased, but the plasma volume may be normal, elevated, or decreased. Early in the disease, the erythrocytes are normocytic, normochromic; however, after repeated therapeutic phlebotomy, iron deficient erythropoiesis results in microcytic, hypochromic cells. Occasionally, patients with PV may present with iron deficiency, as the platelets may not function normally, resulting in occult blood loss. This creates a confusing peripheral blood picture, as the erythrocytes are normal to increased with significant microcytosis, simulating a thalassemia. Nucleated erythrocytes may be found. On the blood smear the erythrocytes typically appear crowded even at the feather edge. The reticulocyte count is normal or slightly elevated. The ESR does not exceed 2 to 3 mm/hour.

Leukocytosis in the range of 12 to 20 $\times$ 10^9/L occurs in about two thirds of the cases because of an increase in granulocytes. Early in the disease there may be a relative granulocytosis and a relative lymphopenia with a normal total leukocyte count. A shift to the left may be found with the presence of myelocytes and metamyelocytes, but it is unusual to find promyelocytes, blasts, or excessive numbers of immature granulocytic cells. Relative and absolute basophilia is common. The LAP score is usually greater than 100.

Megakaryocytic hyperplasia, accompanied by an increase in platelet production, is a consistent finding in PV. The platelet count is above 400 $\times$ 10^9/L in 20% of PV patients and occasionally exceeds 1000 $\times$ 10^9/L. Giant forms may be found on the blood smear. Qualitative platelet abnormalities are reflected by abnormal aggregation to one or more aggregating agents. The most common abnormality is a decreased aggregating response to epinephrine, but the response to ADP, collagen, and thrombin also may be abnormal. In a few cases, the platelets show hyperaggregability to one or more aggregating agents. The prothrombin time and activated partial thromboplastin time are normal. The presence of abnormal multimeric forms of von Willebrand factor in about half of PV patients may lead to a diagnosis of acquired von Willebrand's disease.

Advanced disease is accompanied by striking morphologic changes in erythrocytes. The peripheral blood picture may resemble that seen in myelofibrosis with a leukoerythroblastic anemia, poikilocytosis with dacryocytes, and thrombocytopenia. In cases that advance to acute leukemia, the blood picture exhibits anemia with marked erythrocyte abnormalities, thrombocytopenia, and blast cells.

BONE MARROW

Most patients with PV have a moderate to marked increase in bone marrow cellularity. The hypercellularity is greater than that seen in secondary polycythemia. Hematopoietic marrow may extend into the long bones. There is an increase in myeloid precursors as well as erythroid precursors; consequently, the myeloid to erythroid ratio is usually normal. One of the most significant findings is an increase in megakaryocytes. One study of 175 cases revealed a slight to marked increase in megakaryocytes in 95% of the patients.[35] Eosinophils are often increased. Sometimes bone marrow biopsies reveal a slight to marked increase in reticulin. The amount of reticulin is in direct proportion to the degree of cellularity (e.g., more cellular marrows demonstrating more reticulin fibers). Iron stores are usually absent. This is presumably due to a diversion of iron from storage sites to the large numbers of developing normoblasts.

BLOOD GAS STUDIES

Arterial oxygen saturation studies are helpful to differentiate the different types of absolute polycythemia. In PV, the arterial oxygen saturation levels are normal, whereas in the secondary polycythemias resulting from tissue hypoxia, the arterial oxygen saturation levels are decreased.

The secondary polycythemias caused by an inappropriate increase in erythropoietin may have normal oxygen saturation levels. Further tests are necessary to distinguish these secondary polycythemias from polycythemia vera.

OTHER LABORATORY FINDINGS

Other laboratory tests may be abnormal. Serum uric acid is greater than 7 mg/dL in two thirds of patients and may cause symptoms of gout. The increase probably reflects an increase in the turnover of nucleic acids from blood cells. There is an increase in serum cobalamin-binding capacity in most of the untreated PV patients, primarily due to an increase in transcobalamin III derived from granulocytes. Serum cobalamin also is increased, but not in proportion to the unsaturated binding capacity.

● Cytogenetics

About 25% to 50% of patients show abnormal clonal karyotypes. The abnormalities are nonspecific and varied, including aneuploidy and deletions. The most consistent abnormality is an extra group C chromosome, especially trisomy 8 or trisomy 9. Other abnormal findings include abnormal chromosome 1 with an addition of chromosomal material to the long arms and a partial deletion of the long arms of chromosome 20. The frequency of karyotype abnormalities increases from 15% to 20% at diagnosis, to 35% to 55% after years of treatment, to more than 80% in those in whom acute leukemia develops. Thus, progression from a normal to an abnormal karyotype is an adverse prognostic idicator.

● Prognosis and therapy

There is no known cure for PV, but treatment usually prolongs survival. Two types of therapy are generally used to treat the disease—phlebotomy and myelosuppressive therapy. Phlebotomy is performed at periodic intervals to reduce blood volume and also to reduce iron supplies. It is expected that lack of iron will slow down the production of erythrocytes. Myelosuppressive therapy with chemotherapy and/or radiotherapy also are used to extend the quality and length of the patient's life. Myelosuppressive therapy, however, carries the risk of an increased incidence of transformation to acute leukemia.

Without treatment, 50% of the patients will survive about 18 months. With phlebotomy as the only palliative treatment, survival extends to about 14 years. Thrombosis is the most frequent complication in this group. Those patients receiving myelosuppressive therapy with or without phlebotomy have a mean survival of 9 years with chlorambucil therapy and 12 years with ^{32}P therapy. There is a progressive incidence of malignant complications in this group, especially acute leukemia.

● Differential diagnosis

It is essential that PV be differentiated from the more benign causes of erythrocytosis so that effective therapy can

TABLE 15-17 *NATIONAL POLYCYTHEMIA VERA STUDY GROUP DIAGNOSTIC CRITERIA FOR POLYCYTHEMIA VERA*

Three Criteria for Diagnosis of Polycythemia Vera

Total erythrocyte volume
  male $\geq$ 36 mL/kg
  female $\geq$ 32 mL/kg

Arterial O_2 saturation $\geq$ 92%
Splenomegaly

Absence of Splenomegaly Requires the Presence of Two of the Following

Platelet count > 400 $\times$ 10^9/L
Leukocyte count > 12 $\times$ 10^9/L in the absence of obvious infection or fever
Leukocyte alkaline phosphatase > 100
Serum cobalamin > 900 pg/mL or the serum unsaturated cobalamin binding capacity over 2200 pg/mL.

be initiated. The National Polycythemia Vera Study Group has defined a set of diagnostic criteria for PV that includes determination of erythrocyte mass, arterial oxygen saturation, and the presence of splenomegaly. (Table 15-17).

SECONDARY POLYCYTHEMIA

Secondary polycythemia can be classified into the following three groups:

1. polycythemia due to an increase in erythropoietin as a normal physiologic response to tissue hypoxia;
2. polycythemia due to a nonphysiologic increase in erythropoietin (inappropriate);
3. familial polycythemia associated with high oxygen affinity hemoglobin variants.

Tissue hypoxia A decreased arterial oxygen saturation and subsequent tissue hypoxia is the most common cause of secondary polycythemia. The polycythemia disappears when the underlying cause is identified and effectively removed. Residents of high altitude areas demonstrate a significant increase in hemoglobin and hematocrit that is progressively elevated at higher altitudes. The decrease in barometric pressure at high altitudes decreases the inspired oxygen tension. As a result, less oxygen enters the erythrocytes in the alveoli, and the arterial blood oxygen saturation decreases. The reduced oxygen pressure in the lungs is partially compensated for by a chronic hyperventilation. Compensation at the cellular level involves an increase in 2,3-DPG, facilitating the transfer of oxygen to the tissues. Tissue hypoxia secondary to a decrease in arterial blood oxygen saturation also may occur in severe obstructive lung disease and in obesity. The hematocrit is generally not greater than 0.57 L/L in these cases.

Inappropriate increase in erythropoietin A nonphysiologic increase in erythropoietin (inappropriate) has been described in association with certain tumors that appear to secrete an erythropoietin-like substance. About 50% of these patients have renal tumors. Other tumors that have been associated with erythrocytosis include tumors of liver, cerebellum, uterus, adrenals, ovaries, lung, and thymus. In almost all cases, erythropoietin levels return to normal, and the erythrocytosis disappears after resection of the tumor. Renal cysts also are associated with polycythemia, possibly because of localized pressure and hypoxia to the juxtaglomerular apparatus, resulting in increased erythropoietin secretion. In some patients with hypertension, renal artery disease, and in renal transplants, renal ischemia may occur, resulting in erythrocytosis secondary to increased erythropoietin production.

Familial polycythemia Inherited hemoglobin variants with increased oxygen affinity cause tissue hypoxia and are associated with a secondary erythrocytosis. Less oxygen is released to the tissues, stimulating erythropoietin production. Inherited deficiency of 2,3-DPG also results in decreased oxygen release to tissues. These inherited conditions are usually found in young children and are present in other family members as well.

Neonatal polycythemia Neonatal polycythemia with a hematocrit greater than 0.48 L/L is common. The etiology is usually attributed to placental transfusion that occurs as a result of late cord clamping (7 to 10 seconds after delivery) and/or increased erythropoiesis stimulated by intrauterine hypoxia.[36]

RELATIVE POLYCYTHEMIA

Relative polycythemia is a mild polycythemia due to dehydration, hemoconcentration, or to a condition known as Gaisböck's syndrome. Gaisböck's syndrome is known by several synonyms, including spurious polycythemia, pseudopolycythemia, and stress erythrocytosis. It is diagnosed most frequently in hypertensive, overweight, nervous males who smoke and ingest large amounts of alcohol.[37] The individuals are older than 40 years, with a mean age of 53 years. The erythrocyte mass is essentially normal. High hematocrit and hemoglobin concentrations appear to be the result of a combination of high normal erythrocyte concentrations with a low normal plasma volume. The most common symptoms are lightheadedness, headaches, and dizziness. Plethora is common, but splenomegaly is rare. These patients have a high incidence of thromboembolic complications and cardiovascular disease. Although the hemoglobin, hematocrit, and erythrocyte counts are increased, leukocytes and platelets are normal. Bone marrow cellularity is normal with no increase in megakaryocytes or reticulin. Bone marrow iron stores are absent in 50% of the patients, but serum iron studies are normal. Uric acid is normal, but serum cholesterol may be slightly elevated. Chromosome karyotypes are almost always normal.

LABORATORY DIFFERENTIATION OF POLYCYTHEMIA

Most helpful in the differentiation of polycythemias is a classification scheme using the results of erythrocyte volume studies, arterial oxygen saturation studies, hemoglo-

TABLE 15-18 *DIFFERENTIAL FEATURES OF POLYCYTHEMIA*

	PV	Secondary	Relative
Spleen size	↑	N	N
Red cell volume	♂ ≥ 36 mL/Kg ♀ ≥ 32 mL/Kg	↑	N
Leukocyte count	↑	N	N
Platelet count	↑	N	N
Serum cobalamin	↑	N	N
Arterial O₂ saturation	N	↓	N
Bone marrow	Panhyperplasia	Erythroid hyperplasia	N
Iron stores	↓	N	N
Chromosome studies	Abnormal (50%)	N	N

Key to abbreviations and symbols: N = Normal; ↑ = Increased; ↓ = Decreased

bin-oxygen dissociation determinations, and erythropoietin assays (Fig. 15-15) (Table 15-18). Although the diagnostic process is discussed in a sequential process here, it should be remembered that clinical findings and patient history may eliminate the need for some of these tests. In addition, it is always imperative in any classification scheme to recognize the possibility of two coexisting disease states. For instance, a patient may have both polycythemia vera and a secondary polycythemia such as occurs in chronic obstructive pulmonary disease.

Erythrocyte volume studies The first step in classification of polycythemias is the determination of the erythrocyte volume. This is performed by isotope dilution techniques with ^{51}Cr radioisotopes that tag a sample of the patient's erythrocytes in vitro. The tagged erythrocytes are infused into the patient. After a period of time, a sample of blood is drawn, and the degree of dilution of the tagged erythrocytes is determined. The degree of dilution is proportional to the volume of dilution. Alternatively, a substance that tags the plasma may be used. Whichever compartment is measured, the other is calculated from the hematocrit. A normal erythrocyte volume with an elevated hemoglobin and hematocrit indicates relative polycythemia. An increase in erythrocyte volume greater than 36 mL/kg in men and greater than 32 mL/kg in women is considered an absolute polycythemia.

Arterial oxygen saturation and p50 Once it is established that there is an absolute increase in erythrocytes, arterial oxygen saturation assays will help differentiate some secondary polycythemias from PV. The adequacy of tissue oxygenation is dependent on: (1) hemoglobin concentration; (2) hemoglobin oxygen affinity; and (3) availability of environmental oxygen.

An arterial blood oxygen saturation below 92% indicates a decrease in the oxygen carrying capacity of blood. The polycythemia that occurs in these instances is secondary to tissue hypoxia and an appropriate increase in eryth-

LABORATORY DIFFERENTIATION OF POLYCYTHEMIA

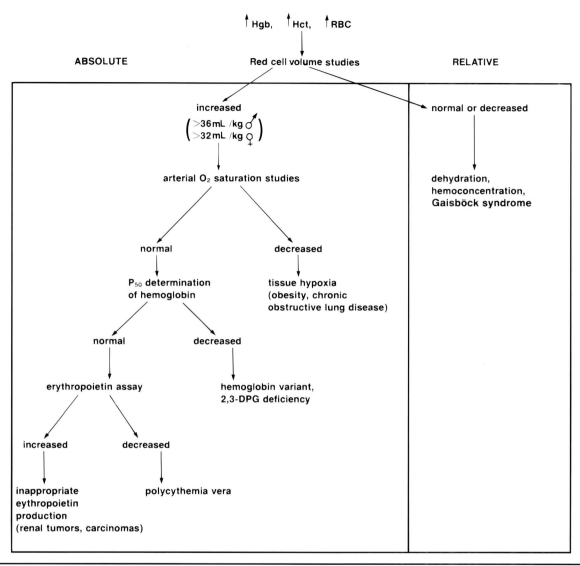

FIGURE 15-15. Laboratory differentiation of polycythemia.

ropoietin production. The most common polycythemias in this group are those associated with chronic lung disease or heavy smoking. A history and physical examination are essential to establishing an accurate diagnosis.

A normal arterial oxygen saturation demands further investigation. Measurement of arterial blood oxygen saturation is a measure of the amount of oxygen brought to the tissues by blood but is no indication of the amount of oxygen actually released. Arterial blood oxygen saturation is normal in the familial high oxygen affinity hemoglobinopathies and in the rare inherited deficiencies of erythrocyte 2,-3-DPG, but the hemoglobin releases very little of this oxygen to the tissues. The best screening test for a high oxygen affinity hemoglobin variant is a determination of the P50 of blood. The P50 is defined as the

partial pressure of oxygen at which the hemoglobin is one-half saturated. The P50 of normal hemoglobin is 26 mmHg under standard conditions of temperature (37° C) and pH (7.4). Abnormal hemoglobins with an increased affinity for oxygen will have a lower P50, meaning that less oxygen is released at a given partial pressure of oxygen. This shifts the oxygen dissociation curve left. This results in a decrease of oxygen released to tissues, an increase in erythropoietin production, and a concomitant increase in erythrocyte production. Although hemoglobin electrophoresis should always be performed when an abnormal hemoglobin is suspected, in some cases the hemoglobinopathies cannot be diagnosed by electrophoretic patterns as the amino acid substitutions in globin chains may not change the charge of the molecule.

Erythropoietin measurement A normal arterial blood oxygen saturation and normal oxygen dissociation should be followed by urinary erythropoietin assays to distinguish PV from those polycythemias due to an inappropriate increase in erythropoietin. Erythropoietin is low or absent in PV but normal or increased in secondary polycythemias that are associated with tumors and renal carcinomas. In these cases, the increased erythropoietin production is considered inappropriate because tissue hypoxia is not responsible for its synthesis.

ESSENTIAL THROMBOCYTHEMIA

Essential thrombocythemia (ET) is a myeloproliferative syndrome affecting primarily the megakaryocytic element. There is an extreme thrombocytosis in the peripheral blood together with thrombocytopathy. There has been considerable controversy over the inclusion of ET as a specific entity in the myeloproliferative disorders since thrombocytosis and other pathologic findings are often a part of CML, MMM, and PV. In these other myeloproliferative disorders, however, the platelet count is usually less than 1000×10^9/L, while in ET, the count is almost always greater than 1000×10^9/L. In addition, there is a predominant occurrence of hemorrhage and thrombosis, which are a common cause of death in patients with ET. These findings are considered justification to treat ET as a distinct entity of the myeloproliferative disorders.

Synonyms for ET include primary thrombocythemia, hemorrhagic thrombocythemia, and megakaryocytic leukemia.

Pathophysiology

Essential thrombocythemia is a stem cell defect that affects all three cell lines but chiefly the megakaryocytes. Studies on women with heterozygosity for G6PD have established it as a clonal disorder of the pluripotent stem cell.

Although it was originally believed that megakaryocyte progenitor cells from ET bone marrow proliferated in the absence of added cytokines (endogenous growth), new in vitro culture assay systems have shown that megakaryocyte colony formation from CFU-Meg is dependent on the addition of cytokines. The formation of endogenous megakaryocyte colonies in previous studies was probably due to trace amounts of cytokines in the serum used in these assays. This may mean that the abnormal progenitor cells in ET are hypersensitive to cytokines giving them a growth advantage over normal cells.

Clinical findings

Essential thrombocythemia is a rare disorder with peak incidence between 40 to 60 years of age and between 20 to 30 years of age. The younger age of incidence occurs predominantly in women. Bleeding or thrombosis occur as the most common presenting feature. These problems appear to be more frequent in patients older than 59 years of age. There is little predictive value of the degree of thrombocytosis to clinical hemostatic complications,[38] but thrombosis appears to be more likely than bleeding at the lower end of platelet increases.[39] Thrombosis is probably related to the hyperaggregability of the platelets. Both venous and arterial thrombosis lead to complications such as stroke, priapism, gangrene in the legs, and splenic infarction.

Due to the frequency of bleeding problems, ET was first described as hemorrhagic thrombocytosis. The types and sites of bleeding are typical of those seen in platelet disorders. Bleeding from the gastrointestinal tract, renal tract, and mucous membranes is common. About half the patients have a palpable spleen, but splenomegaly is usually slight. Occasionally, absence of splenomegaly is due to splenic atrophy, resulting from repeated splenic thrombosis and silent infarctions. About 20% of the patients are initially asymptomatic. In these cases, the disease is discovered incidentally upon the finding of thrombocytosis and, occasionally, splenomegaly.

Most cases of thrombocytosis are not neoplastic but secondary reactive processes and require differentiation from ET. Duration of the thrombocytosis and spleen size are commonly used as practical variables, but occasionally bone marrow examination is necessary. Sustained thrombocytosis and splenomegaly favor a diagnosis of ET.

Laboratory findings

PERIPHERAL BLOOD

The most striking finding in the peripheral blood is extreme and consistent thrombocytosis (Fig. 15-16). The platelet count usually ranges from 1000 to 5000×10^9/L. The peripheral blood smear may show giant, bizarre platelets. Platelets may appear in aggregates. Megakaryocytes and megakaryocyte fragments also may be found. However, in many cases, platelet morphology appears

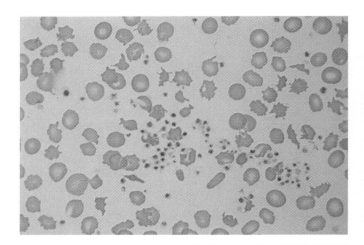

FIGURE 15-16. Essential thrombocythemia. The platelets are markedly increased. Erythrocyte morphology is also markedly abnormal. (PB; 250 × original magnification; Wright-Giemsa stain).

normal. Abnormalities in platelet aggregation and adhesiveness suggest a defect in platelet function.

Anemia, if present, is proportional to the severity of bleeding and is usually normocytic; however, long-standing hemorrhagic episodes may lead to iron deficiency and a microcytic hypochromic anemia. In about one third of patients, slight erythrocytosis is present, which may cause confusion with polycythemia vera. Aggregated platelets may lead to an erroneous increase in the erythrocyte count on automated cell counters. In these cases, the hemoglobin should be used to assess the anemic status of the patient. Histograms may reveal a high take-off on the leukocyte histogram because of platelet clumps. The reticulocyte count may be increased if bleeding is present, and mild polychromatophilia is noted. Peripheral blood abnormalities, secondary to autosplenectomy, may occur if the spleen has been infarcted. These abnormalities include Howell-Jolly bodies, nucleated erythrocytes, and poikilocytosis.

A leukocytosis from 15 to 40 $\times$ 10^9/L is almost always present. A shift to the left is not uncommon with myelocytes and metamyelocytes present. Eosinophilia and basophilia also are observed. The LAP score is normal or increased. Rarely, it may be low.

BONE MARROW

The bone marrow exhibits marked hyperplasia with a striking increase in megakaryocytes often present in clusters. The background of stained slides shows many platelets. The megakaryocytes are large, with abundant cytoplasm and frequently increased nuclear lobulation. Mitotic forms are increased. Erythroid and myeloid hyperplasia also is evident. Stains for iron reveal normal or increased stores, unless chronic hemorrhage has occurred. In some cases, reticulin is increased.

OTHER LABORATORY FINDINGS

Other laboratory tests may be abnormal. Serum cobalamin and the unsaturated cobalamin binding capacity are increased. An increase in cell turnover may cause serum uric acid, LDH, and acid phosphatase to be elevated. Serum potassium may be elevated as a result of in vitro release of potassium from platelets (pseuudohyperkalemia). The spurious nature of this hyperkalemia can be verified by performing a simultaneous potassium assay on plasma, which should be normal. Arterial blood gases may reveal a "pseudo-hypoxia" if the sample is not tested promptly. This is due to the in vitro consumption of oxygen by increased numbers of platelets.

TESTS OF HEMOSTASIS

Laboratory tests alone are unreliable in predicting bleeding or thrombotic complications in ET. The prothrombin time and activated partial thromboplastin time are usually normal, but evidence of low-grade DIC may be present. A variety of qualitative platelet abnormalities have been described in ET and other MPDs, but their relationship to bleeding and thrombosis is uncertain. Although platelet aggregation abnormalities are variable in ET, defective platelet aggregation with epinephrine caused by a loss of platelet α-adrenergic receptors is diagnostic of a MPD and is useful in differentiating ET from secondary thrombocytosis. Spontaneous in vitro platelet aggregation or hyperaggregability is a common finding, and in vivo platelet aggregation is suggested by finding increased levels of β-thromboglobulin (released from platelets). Other platelet abnormalities that have been described in association with ET include a decreased number of receptors for platelet inhibitory prostaglandin D$_2$ (PGD$_2$); increased expression of Fc receptors; reduction of membrane glycoprotein GpIb associated with an increase in GpIIIb and decreased GpIIb; defective coagulant activity; impaired serotonin binding and uptake; changes in the platelet membrane fatty acid composition; abnormal arachidonic acid metabolism; increased glyoxalase I activity; and increased lactate production.[38] A form of acquired von Willebrand's disease has been described in association with ET. There is a reduction of large multimer forms and reduced levels of ristocetin cofactor activity.

● Cytogenetics

The low incidence of clonal cytogenic abnormalities (about 5%) in ET makes cytogenetic studies less useful than in other MPD.[40] Acquired, clonal chromosome aberrations may be identified in the hematopoietic precursors of the bone marrow. There is no diagnostic abnormality reported, but trisomies of the C group are commonly seen.

● Prognosis and therapy

About 50% of patients with ET survive 5 years. The prognosis appears to be better in younger patients. The most common causes of death are thrombosis and bleeding. In some cases, the disease transforms to acute myeloblastic leukemia, PV, or MMM.

There is controversy as to which patients with ET require therapy. It is generally agreed that patients with a history of thrombosis or cardiovascular risk factors require therapy to reduce the platelet count. Plateletpheresis is used to quickly reduce the platelet count below 1000 $\times$ 10^9/L for control of vascular accidents. Anticoagulants and drugs to inhibit platelet function are sometimes necessary to control thrombosis.

The benefit of specific therapy in asymptomatic patients has not been established. Recent therapeutic trials with β-interferon have led to improvement of both hematologic parameters and clinical symptoms in nearly all patients.[41] Withdrawal of interferon, however, leads to recurrence of thrombocytosis. Chronic megakaryocyte suppression is achieved by radiation or chemotherapy. There is concern, however, about the leukemogenic potential of these therapeutic agents. Development of acute leukemia in treated and untreated patients with a history of ET is rare.[40]

● Differential diagnosis

Although the other MPDs have certain diagnostic markers, ET is largely a diagnosis of exclusion. Essential

TABLE 15-19 *CONDITIONS ASSOCIATED WITH THROMBOCYTOSIS*

Essential thrombocythemia
Polycythemia vera
Chronic myelocytic leukemia
Myelofibrosis with myeloid metaplasia
Chronic inflammatory disorders
Acute hemorrhage
Hemolytic anemia
Hodgkin's disease
Metastatic carcinoma
Lymphoma
Post-splenectomy
Post-operative
Iron deficiency

thrombocytosis must be differentiated from a secondary, reactive thrombocytosis (Table 15-19). Secondary thrombocytosis is associated with many acute and chronic infections, inflammatory diseases, carcinomas, and Hodgkin's disease. The platelet count in ET exceeds 1000 × 10^9/L and is persistent over a period of months or years. Secondary thrombocytosis rarely reaches 1000 × 10^9/L and is transitory. In addition, in secondary thrombocytosis, platelet function is normal, leukocytes and erythrocytes are normal, and splenomegaly is absent.

Differentiation of ET from PV may be difficult. However, marked erythrocytosis together with clinical findings suggestive of hypervolemia are more typical of PV.

TABLE 15-20 *THE POLYCYTHEMIA VERA STUDY GROUP DIAGNOSTIC CRITERIA FOR ESSENTIAL THROMBOCYTHEMIA*

Criteria for Essential Thrombocythemia Diagnosis	Helps Differentiate ET From:
1. Platelet count >600 × 10^9/L	Secondary thrombocytosis
2. Hemoglobin ≤13 g/dL or normal erythrocyte mass	Polycythemia vera
3. Stainable iron in the marrow or failure of iron therapy to raise the hemoglobin by at least 1 g/dL after one month of iron therapy.	Polycythemia vera
4. Absence of the Philadelphia chromosome	Chronic Myelocytic Leukemia
5. Absent collagen fibrosis of marrow or collagen fibrosis in >⅓ biopsied area but no splenomegaly or leukoerythroblastic reaction.	Myelofibrosis with myeloid metaplasia
6. No known cause for reactive thrombocytosis	Reactive thrombocytosis

(Adapted from: Murphy S, Iland H, Rosenthal G, Laszlo J: Essential thrombocythemia: An interim report form the polycythemia vera study group. Sem Hematol, 23:177, 1986)

The Polycythemia Vera Study Group has proposed a set of criteria for diagnosis of ET[42] (Table 15-20). The first criterion, a platelet count over 600 × 10^9/L, excludes many cases of secondary thrombocytosis. The second criterion, a hemoglobin less than 13 g/dL, and the third criterion, presence of iron in the bone marrow or failure of response to iron therapy, excludes cases of PV. The fourth criterion, absence of the Philadelphia chromosome, was designed to rule out CML, and the fifth criterion, absence of collagen fibrosis, rules out MMM. The sixth criterion excludes conditions associated with reactive thrombocytosis.

SUMMARY

The MPDs are a group of neoplastic stem cell disorders characterized by excessive production of one or more bone marrow and peripheral blood cell lineages. There are four MPD subgroups: chronic myeloid leukemia (CML), myelofibrosis with myeloid metaplasia (MMM), polycythemia vera (PV), and essential thrombocythemia (ET).

Although all hematopoietic cell lineages may be involved in the unregulated proliferation in MPD, one cell line is usually involved more than the others. In CML, the granulocytic cells are primarily affected; in PV, the erythrocytes are affected; and, in ET, the platelets/megakaryocytes are affected. In MMM, the most characteristic finding is a benign proliferation of fibroblasts in the bone marrow. Splenomegaly, bone marrow fibrosis, and megakaryocytic hyperplasia are findings common to all subgroups. The underlying pathophysiology that allows the cells to escape the regulation of proliferation is unknown but probably differs among the subgroups. It could be related to sensitivity to growth factors, abnormal growth factors or growth factor independent proliferation.

Abnormal karyotypes in hematopoietic cells may be found in any of the subgroups, but the most well-characterized abnormality is the Philadelphia chromosome, found in up to 95% of individuals with CML. The Philadelphia chromosome is the result of a translocation of genetic material between chromosomes 9 and 22 (9;22)(q34;q11). A fusion gene BCR/ABL results that encodes an abnormal protein, p210. This protein may play a role in the pathogenesis of CML.

The survival of MPD patients varies with the subgroup. Patients with PV appear to survive longer than patients with CML, MMM, or ET. Any of the subgroups may evolve into acute leukemia, with or without specific therapy. There is currently no cure for any of the MPD.

REVIEW QUESTIONS

A 45-year-old white woman was admitted to the hospital from the emergency room. She experienced pain in the upper left quadrant and bloating for the last several weeks. She had multiple bruises on her legs and arms. She also stated that her gums bled easily when she brushed her teeth. She had been unusually tired and lost about 10 pounds in the last 2 months. Results of physical examination showed a massive spleen. The following results were noted on blood count on admission.

Hb	7.4 gm/dL
Erythrocyte count	2.9×10^{12}/L
Hct	0.22 L/L
RDW	18.0
Leukocyte count	520×10^9/L
Platelet count	900×10^9/L
Differential:	31% segmented neutrophils
	26% bands
	8% metamyelocytes
	11% myelocytes
	4% promyelocytes
	2% blasts
	4% lymphocytes
	3% monocytes
	5% eosinophils
	6% basophils
	4 nucleated erythrocytes/100 leukocytes
	occasional micromegakaryocytes

There was moderate anisocytosis and poikilocytosis.

A bone marrow aspiration was performed. The marrow was 90% cellular with a myeloid to erythroid ratio of 10:1. The majority of the cells were neutrophilic precursors. There was an increase in eosinophils and basophils. Myeloblasts accounted for 10% of the nucleated cells. Megakaryocytes were increased. (Questions 1–5 relate to this case).

1. What findings suggest that this patient has a defect in the pluripotential stem cell rather than a benign proliferation of hematopoietic cells?
   a. the presence of a leukoerythroblastic blood picture.
   b. the involvement of several cell lineages in the proliferative process, including neutrophilic cells and platelets.
   c. the shift to the left in the neutrophilic cell line.
   d. an increase in the RDW

2. Chromosome analysis revealed the presence of the Philadelphia chromosome. Based on this information, what myeloproliferative disorder is present?
   a. CML
   b. PV
   c. ET
   d. MMM

3. What cytochemical stain is used to help differentiate a leukemoid reaction from CML?
   a. Peroxidase
   b. New methylene blue
   c. Leukocyte alkaline phosphatase (LAP)
   d. Perl's Prussian blue

4. Which of the following terms *most accurately* describes the peripheral blood picture of this patient?
   a. Leukemoid reaction
   b. Leukoerythroblastic
   c. Leukopenia
   d. Myelodysplastic

5. What is the best description of the bone marrow?
   a. Decreased M:E ratio and increased cellularity
   b. Increased M:E ratio and decreased cellularity
   c. Increased M:E ratio and increased cellularity
   d. Decreased M:E ratio and decreased cellularity
   Additional questions

6. Extensive bone marrow fibrosis, leukoerythroblastic peripheral blood and the presence of anisocytosis with dacryocytes are most characteristic of:
   a. CML
   b. PV
   c. ET
   d. MMM

7. A 50-year-old man was admitted to the emergency room for chest pain, and a blood count was ordered. The results showed: erythrocyte count 6.5×10^{12}/L; hematocrit 0.60 L/L; leukocyte count 15×10^9/L; platelet count 500×10^9/L. These results indicate:
   a. the need for further investigation for a possible diagnosis of MPD
   b. normal findings for an adult male
   c. that the patient has experienced a thrombotic episode
   d. an instrument malfunction

8. Which of the following is not typical of a MPD at the time of diagnosis?
   a. hypercellular bone marrow
   b. anemia
   c. leukoerythroblastosis
   d. predominance of blasts in peripheral blood

9. A disease that has hematologic features intermediate between typical CML and CMML and that does not show the Philadelphia chromosome is known as:
   a. juvenile CML
   b. chronic neutrophilic CML
   c. chronic eosinophilic CML
   d. atypical CML

10. The fusion gene, BCR/ABL, produced from translocation between chromosomes 9 and 22, is characteristic of:
    a. all MPD
    b. CML
    c. atypical CML
    d. MMM

REFERENCES

1. Dameshek, W.: Some speculations on the myeloproliferative syndromes. Blood, 6:372, 1951.
2. Dover, D., Fabian, I., Cline, M.J.: Circulating pleuripotent haemo-

poietic cells in patients with myeloproliferative disorders. Br. J. Haematol., 54:373, 1983.

3. Gilbert, H.S., Praloran, V., Stanley, E.R.: Increased circulating CSF-1 (M-CSF) in myeloproliferative disease: association with myeloid metaplasia and peripheral bone marrow extension. Blood, 74:1231, 1989.

4. Gersuk, G.M., Carmel, R., Pattengale, P.K.: Platelet-derived growth factor concentrations in platelet-poor plasma and urine from patients with myeloproliferative disorders. Blood, 74:2330, 1989.

5. Mattson, J.C., Crisan, D., Wilner, F., Decker, D., Burdakin, J.: Clinical problem solving using bcl-2 and bcr gene rearrangement analysis. Lab. Med., 25:648, 1994.

6. Cervantes, F., Salgado, C., Rozman, C.: Assessment of iron stores in hospitalized patients. Am. J. Clin. Pathol., 95:105, 1991.

7. Hollen, C.W., Henthorn, J., Koziol, J.A., Burstein, S.A.: Elevated serum interleukin-6 levels in patients with reactive thrombocytosis. Br. J. Haematol., 79:286, 1991.

8. Landolfi, R., et al.: Increased platelet-fibrinogen affinity in patients with myeloproliferative disorders. Blood, 71:978, 1988.

9. Mazzucato, M., et al.: Platelet membrane abnormalities in myeloproliferative disorders: decrease in glycoproteins Ib and IIb/IIIa complex is associated with deficient receptor function. Br. J. Haematol., 73:369, 1989.

10. Wehmeier, A., et al.: Circulating activated platelets in myeloproliferative disorders. Thromb. Res., 61:271, 1991.

11. Dickstein, J.I., Vardiman, J.W.: Issues in the pathology and diagnosis of the chronic myeloproliferative disorders and the myelodysplastic syndromes. Am. J. Clin. Pathol., 99:513, 1993.

12. Epner, D.E., Roeffler, H.P.: Molecular genetic advances in chronic myelogenous leukemia. Ann. Intern. Med., 113:3, 1990.

13. Guo, J.Q., Wang, J.Y., Arlinghaus, R.B.: Detection of BCR-ABL proteins in blood cells of benign phase chronic myelogenous leukemia patients. Cancer Res., 51:3048, 1991.

14. Saglio, G., et al.: Variability of the molecular defects corresponding to the presence of a Philadelphia chromosome in human hematologic malignancies. Blood, 72:1203, 1988.

15. Hild, F., Fonatsch, C.: Cytogenetic peculiarities in chronic myelogenous leukemia. Cancer Genet. Cytogenet., 47:197, 1990.

16. Mills, K.I., Benn, P., Birnie, G.D.: Does the breakpoint within the major breakpoint cluster region (M-bcr) influence the duration of the chronic phase in chronic myeloid leukemia? An analytical comparison of current literature. Blood, 78:1155, 1991.

17. Wiedemann, L.M., et al.: The correlation of breakpoint cluster region rearrangement and p210 phl/abl expression with morphological analysis of Ph-negative chronic myeloid leukemia and other myeloproliferative diseases. Blood, 71:349, 1988.

18. Tien, H.F., et al.: Chromosome and bcr rearrangement in chronic myelogenous leukaemia and their correlation with clinical states and prognosis of the disease. Br. J. Haematol., 75:469, 1990.

19. Ahuja, H., et al.: The spectrum of molecular alterations in the evaluation of chronic myelocytic leukemia. J. Clin. Invest., 87:2042, 1991.

20. Imamura, J., Miyoshi, I., Koeffler, H.P.: P53 in hematologic malignancies. Blood, 84:2412, 1994.

21. Ponzetto, C., et al.: ABL proteins in Philadelphia-positive acute leukaemias and chronic myelogenous leukemia blast crisis. Br. J. Haematol., 76:39, 1990.

22. Kantarjian, H.M., Kurzrock, R., Talpaz, M.: Philadelphia chromosome-negative chronic myelogenous leukemia and chronic myelomonocytic leukemia. Hematol. Oncol. Clin. North. Am., 4:389, 1990.

23. Delage, R., Ritz, J., Anderson, K.C.: The evolving role of bone marrow transplantation in the treatment of chronic myelogenous leukemia. Hematol. Oncol. Clin. North. Am., 4:369, 1990.

24. Galvani, D.W., Cawley, J.C.: Mechanism of action of alpha interferon in chronic granulocytic leukaemia: evidence for preferential inhibition of late progenitors. Br. J. Haematol., 73:475, 1989.

25. Cole, H.M.: Alpha-interferon and chronic myelogenous leukemia. JAMA, 264:2137, 1990.

26. Talpaz, M., Kantarjian, H., Kurzrock, R., Gutterman, J.U.: Interferon alpha in the therapy of CML. Br. J. Haematol., 79, Suppl. 1: 38, 1991.

27. Rickles, F.R., Miller, D.R.: Eosinophilic leukemoid reaction. J. Pediatr., 80:418, 1972.

28. Youman, J.D., Taddeini, L., Cooper, T.: Histamine excess, symptoms in basophilic chronic granulocytic leukemia. Arch. Intern. Med., 131:560,1973.

29. Zittoun, R., Rea, D., Ngoc, L.H., Ramond, S.: Chronic neutrophilic leukemia. Ann. Hematol., 68:55, 1994.

30. Kreipe, H., et al.: Clonal granulocytes and bone marrow cells in the cellular phase of agnogenic myeloid metaplasia. Blood, 78:1814, 1991.

31. Reilly, J.T.: Pathogenesis of idiopathic myelofibrosis: role of growth factors. J. Clin. Pathol., 45:461, 1992.

32. Paquette, R.L., Meshkinpour, A., Rosen, P.J.: Autoimmune myelofibrosis. Med. 73:145, 1994.

33. Hoffman, R., Silverstein, M.N.: Agnogenic myeloid metaplasia. In Hematology: Basic Principles and Practice. Edited by R. Hoffman, et al. New York: Churchill Livingstone, 1995.

34. Prchal, J.T., Prchal, J.F.: Evolving understanding of the cellular defect in polycythemia vera: implications for its clinical diagnosis and molecular pathophysiology. Blood, 83:1, 1994.

35. Ellis, J.T., Silver, R.T., Coleman, M., Geller, S.A.: The bone marrow in polycythemia vera. Semin. Hematol., 12(4):433, 1975.

36. Danish, E.J.: Neonatal polycythemia. Prog. Hematol., 14:55, 1986.

37. Weinreb, N.J., Shih, C.: Spurious polycythemia. Semin. Hematol., 12(4):397, 1975.

38. Schafer, A.I.: Essential thrombocytemia. Prog. Hemost. Thromb., 10:69, 1991.

39. van Gendersen, P.J.J., Michiels, J.J.: Primary thrombocythemia: diagnosis, clinical manifestations and management. Ann. Hematol., 67:57, 1993.

40. Tefferi, A., Hoagland, H.C.: Issues in the diagnosis and management of essential thrombocythemia. Mayo. Clin. Proc., 69:651, 1994.

41. Gisslinger, H., et al.: Interferon in essential thrombocythemia. Br. J. Haematol., 79, Suppl. 1:42, 1991.

42. Murphy, S., Iland, H., Rosenthal, G., Laszlo, J.: Essential thrombocythemia: an interim report from the Polycythemia Vera Study Group. Semin. Hematol., 23:177, 1986.

Myelodysplastic syndromes

16

INTRODUCTION

The *myelodysplastic syndromes* (MDS) are primary, neoplastic, pluripotential stem cell disorders. They are characterized by one or more peripheral blood cytopenias together with prominent maturation abnormalities (*dyspoiesis* or *dysplasia*) in the bone marrow. These relatively common entities evolve progressively, leading to aggravation of the cytopenias, and, in some cases, transform into a condition indistinguishable from acute leukemia. MDS occurs most commonly in the elderly, although it is being diagnosed with increasing frequency in children.

Before the 1980s there was much confusion and disagreement in the literature concerning the criteria for defining, subgrouping, and naming the MDS. Because of the predisposition of MDS to terminate in leukemia, the term preleukemia has been commonly used to describe these disorders. However, the evolution of MDS to acute leukemia is not obligatory, and, in fact, many patients die of intercurrent disease or complications of the cytopenia before evolving to leukemia.[1] Whether leukemia would have developed in these patients had they survived the cytopenic complications is, of course, unknown. In addition, the diagnosis of preleukemia can only be made in retrospect (i.e., after the leukemia develops). Thus, the term myelodysplasia is more appropriate until overt leukemia actually develops. In the past, MDS also has been described by the terms refractory anemia with excess blasts, chronic erythremic myelosis, refractory anemia with or without sideroblasts, subacute or chronic myelomonocytic leukemia, and smoldering leukemia. Most hematologists currently consider the terms dysmyelopoietic syndrome and myelodysplastic syndrome to be more acceptable than preleukemia or other synonyms in describing these hematologic disorders. In this book, the term myelodysplastic syndrome will be used.

CLASSIFICATION

The French–American–British (FAB) group that proposed criteria for categorizing acute leukemias also has proposed a classification scheme for the myelodysplastic syndromes.[2] This classification defines five subgroups based on the blast count and degree of dyspoiesis in the peripheral blood and bone marrow. Hematologists are cautioned that classification in some difficult cases may not always be possible by morphology alone. Overlap among the groups also occurs, delaying definitive characterization. The five groups include:

1. Refractory anemia (RA)
2. Refractory anemia with ringed sideroblasts (RARS, RA-S)
3. Refractory anemia with excess blasts (RAEB)
4. Chronic myelomonocytic leukemia (CMML)
5. Refractory anemia with excess blasts in transformation (RAEB-t)

PATHOGENESIS

Evidence for abnormal stem cells

The spectrum of clinical and hematologic features in MDS is a result of the gradual expansion of abnormal hematopoietic cells and an accompanying decrease in normal hematopoiesis. Cytogenetic, G6PD isoenzyme studies, and studies using molecular biologic techniques support the theory that the abnormal cells in MDS are clones derived from an abnormal stem cell.[4-8] Chromosome abnormalities are present at diagnosis in more than 50% of patients. These abnormalities, detected by standard karyotyping, are present in all hematopoietic cell lines except the lymphoid cell line, which is usually normal, indicating the abnormal clone arises from a stem cell that can differentiate into different cell lineages. Normal clones are found to coexist in the marrow with the abnormal clones. In those MDS that progress to acute leukemia, additional abnormalities in cell cultures and karyotypes can be demonstrated.

Isoenzyme studies in females who are heterozygous at the G6PD locus also indicate that the abnormal clone is derived from an abnormal stem cell. Because of random inactivation of one X chromosome, females heterozygous for enzymes determined by genes on this chromosome will normally demonstate random activity of one or the other isoenzyme within cells. All cells originating from the same stem cell, however, should have the same isoenzyme. The abnormal clones in MDS have been shown to contain the same G6PD isoenzyme, indicating a common progenitor cell. Conversely, both G6PD isoenzymes are found in normal skin and fibroblast cells in MDS patients.

The role of oncogenes

Control of cellular differentiation, maturation, and proliferation occurs through the interaction of hematopoietic growth factors with specific cellular receptors. This interaction causes activation of intracellular messengers and eventually DNA synthesis. The entire process is controlled by cellular proto-oncogenes. When these genes are mutated to oncogenes, they can disrupt the process and cause disordered control and neoplasia.[3] Studies using molecular techniques indicate that proto-oncogene mutations are present in all hematopoietic cell lineages in MDS, including lymphoid, suggesting the disorder originates in the pluripotent stem cell.[8]

It has been hypothesized that MDS is preceded by a phase in which genetic alterations of hematopoietic cells accumulate before hematologic change or chromosome aberrations occur.[4,9,10] The exact event that causes initial development of the abnormal clone is unknown but the process probably involves damage to the cell's genetic material. The damage could be produced by chemotheraputic or radiologic agents or by environmental or industrial toxins. For example, it has been shown that RAS and FMS proto-oncogene mutations to oncogenes occur in healthy individuals treated previously for lymphoma.

The significance of chromosomal changes in malignant cells is not fully understood, but there is mounting evidence that rearrangements of genetic material may be an important event in the activation of proto-oncogenes to oncogenes.[11,12] Tumor suppressor genes also may play a role in the development of MDS.[8] These are recessive oncogenes that serve to regulate growth and differentiation in a negative fashion, suppressing malignant growth. Chromosome deletions, often associated with MDS, may result in the loss of these tumor suppressor genes. Mutations of the P53 tumor-suppressor gene is the most common genetic mutation in human neoplasia.

The most frequent chromosome abnormalities in MDS involve chromosomes 5, 7, and 8, all of which carry proto-oncogenes. Chromosome 5 carries the FOS, RAS, and FMS proto-oncogenes; chromosome 7 carries the ERB-D proto-oncogene; and chromosome 8 carries the MYC proto-oncogene. Mutations of the RAS proto-oncogene have been reported in up to 50% of MDS patients[10] and FMS in up to 16% of MDS.[9] The RAS, MYC, and FOS proto-oncogenes have been implicated in growth factor-mediated signaling mechanisms. If these proto-oncogenes are activated, the abnormal clone in MDS may become immortalized by losing the normal control mechanisms that regulate growth. Some oncogene proteins may be responsible for inhibition of normal hematopoiesis. The role of oncogenes in myelodysplasia needs further exploration.

Maturation and proliferation abnormalities

Progression of MDS to acute leukemia is characterized by a gradual or sudden increase in the blast population with a block in maturation. It has been suggested that this progression to AML is compatible with multi-step transformation of the abnormal clone.[13] This is supported by the finding of additional chromosome karyotype abnormalities as progression occurs.

In vitro studies of hematopoietic cells from patients with MDS reveal both maturation and proliferation abnormalities. Many erythroblasts and myeloblasts are apparantly unable to mature.[13] The bone marrow morphologically reflects this maturation defect by exhibiting hypercellularity with an increase in blasts and other immature cells. With progressive impairment in maturation, the disease may evolve to an acute leukemia. In addition to abnormal maturation, proliferative activity of erythroid and myeloid cells is decreased in MDS as indicated by an increase in DNA synthesis time.[14] Other quantitative abnormalities in the myeloid and erythroid stem cells have been reported.[13-15] Evaluation of the stroma in myelodysplastic marrow reveals that its normal supportive hematopoietic function is preserved.[15]

Secondary MDS

Originally, all MDS were classified as idiopathic (primary myelodysplasia). Evidence now indicates that a portion of MDS, especially those occurring in patients younger than 50 years of age, are probably secondary to chemotherapy, radiation therapy (therapy-related myelodysplasia, t-MDS), or environmental mutagens.[16,17] In children, MDS may be associated with predisposing conditions such as constitutional chromosome disorders (Down's syndrome) and immunodeficiency disorders.[18]

INCIDENCE

MDS occurs primarily in individuals older than 50 years of age. There is a strong correlation between the proportion of elderly patients and frequency of MDS. Due to the lack of definition and classification of MDS before 1982, the actual incidence of these disorders has not been accurately assessed by large scale epidemiologic studies. Morbidity and mortality statistics also are lacking, partly because MDS is not included in the International Classification of Diseases (ICD). The difficulty in making correct diagnoses in the early stages of the disease also contribute to unreliable incidence figures. A recent study in Germany found that both the average annual crude incidence and age-specific incidence of MDS increased between 1976 to 1989.[19] MDS was more common than AML in patients between 50 and 70 years of age. This rise in incidence may be due to an increased awareness of MDS on the part of physicians and clinical laboratory scientists as well as an increased application of diagnostic procedures in these elderly individuals.

There is a paucity of reports of MDS in children. This may be due to lack of a widely accepted classification system and clear diagnostic criteria. It has been recommended that pediatricians accept and use the adult classification system. Dysplasia in children with MDS is less pronounced, there is a predominance of the more aggressive subtypes (RAEB, RAEB-t), and progression to acute leukemia is faster than in adults.[18,20] These problems in diagnosis may contribute to an underestimation of MDS in children. The incidence of MDS may be approximately the same as the incidence of AML in children. About 15% of acute leukemias in children are AML.[22] One retrospective study indicated that 17% of children with AML had a preleukemic phase (MDS).[21] The median age of children at presentation of MDS is about 6 years, except for CMML, in which the median age is 2.5 years. The male/female ratio is about 1.6.

CLINICAL FINDINGS

The most frequent presenting symptoms, fatigue and weakness, are related to an anemia that is refractory to treatment. Less commonly, hemorrhagic symptoms resulting from thrombocytopenia or infection resulting from neutropenia precede diagnosis. Infection is a common and life-threatening complication in patients with diagnosed MDS. Neutropenia ($<1 \times 10^9$/L) and the more aggressive subgroups (RAEB, RAEB-t) are associated risk factors for infectious complications.[23] Infection is the most common cause of death. Splenomegaly or hepatomegaly may be present, especially in CMML.

TABLE 16-1 *HEMATOLOGIC ABNORMALITIES IN MYELODYSPLASTIC SYNDROMES*

	Erythroid Series	*Myeloid Series*	*Thrombocyte Series*
Peripheral blood findings	anemia, macrocytes, oval macrocytes, dimorphism, basophilic stippling, nucleated RBC, Howell-Jolly bodies, sideroblasts, anisocytosis, poikilocytosis, reticulocytopenia	neutropenia, hypogranulation, abnormal granulation, shift-to-the-left, nuclear abnormalities including pseudo-Pelger-Huët and ring nuclei, monocytosis	thrombocytopenia, or thrombocytosis, giant forms, hypogranulation, micromegakaryocytes, functional abnormalities
Bone marrow findings	megaloblastoid erythropoiesis, nuclear fragmentation and budding, karyorrhexis, multiple nuclei, defective hemoglobinization, vacuolization, ringed sideroblasts	abnormal granules in promyelocytes, increase in Type I and Type II blasts, absence of secondary granules, nuclear abnormalities, decreased myeloperoxidase, Auer rods in blasts	micromegakaryocytes, megakaryocytes with multiple, separated nuclei, large mononuclear megakaryocytes, hypogranulation or large abnormal granules in megakaryocytes

● LABORATORY FINDINGS

The MDS present with a range of abnormal morphologic features that can be demonstrated on stained peripheral blood and bone marrow smears. FAB criteria for classification of MDS into subtypes based on the degree of dysplasia and cytopenia will be presented later in this chapter. Included here are the general hematologic features used to initially define the presence of a MDS (Table 16-1).

● Peripheral blood

Hematologic findings include anemia, neutropenia, and/or thrombocytopenia and occasionally monocytosis. Anemia is the most consistent finding, occurring as an isolated cytopenia in 35% of cases. Bicytopenia occurs in 30% of cases and pancytopenia in 19%.[24] Less commonly, an isolated neutropenia or thrombocytopenia is found. Dysplastic features of one or more cell lines is typical. Functional abnormalities of hematologic cells also is common.[25] Studies show that the higher the degree and number of cytopenias, the worse the prognosis.[26]

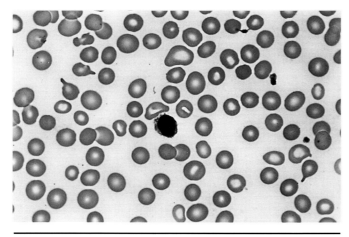

FIGURE 16-1. A peripheral blood film of a patient with MDS. Notice the macrocytic cells, anisocytosis, basophilic stippling and Howell-Jolly body. (250× original magnification)

ERYTHROCYTES

The degree of anemia is variable, but the hemoglobin is generally less than 10 g/dL. The erythrocytes are usually macrocytic (Fig. 16-1), and less often normocytic. Oval macrocytes, similar to those found in megaloblastic anemia, are frequently present. A dimorphic anemia with normochromic and microcytic hypochromic cells is a common initial finding in the RARS group. Reticulocytes show an absolute decrease but may appear normal if only the uncorrected relative number (percent) is reported. In addition to anemia, qualitative abnormalities indicative of dyserythropoiesis are present. These include anisocytosis, poikilocytosis, basophilic stippling, Howell-Jolly bodies, and nucleated erythrocytes. Often hemoglobin F is increased (5% to 6%) and distributed in a heterogeneous pattern. Acquired hemoglobin H also has been reported in MDS. Other erythrocyte changes include altered A, B, and I antigens, enzyme changes, and an acquired erythrocyte membrane change similar to, but not identical with, that found in paroxysmal nocturnal hemoglobinuria (PNH).

LEUKOCYTES

Neutropenia is the second most common cytopenia observed in MDS. Neutropenia may be accompanied by the finding of metamyelocytes and myelocytes on the blood smear. Blasts and progranulocytes also may be present. Morphologic abnormalities in granulocytes indicative of dysgranulopoiesis are a hallmark finding in MDS (Fig. 16-2). Dysgranulopoiesis is characterized by agranular or hypogranular neutrophils, persistent basophilia of the cytoplasm, abnormal appearing granules, hyposegmentation (pseudo-Pelger-Huët) (Figs. 16-3A and 16-3B), or hypersegmentation of the nucleus and donut- or ring-shaped nuclei. Care should be taken to distinguish hypogranular neutrophils with pseudo-Pelger-Huët anomaly from lymphocytes, and neutrophilic-band forms with hypogranulation from monocytes. Neutrophils also may demonstrate enzyme defects, such as decreased myeloperoxidase and decreased leukocyte alkaline phosphatase. In some cases, neutrophils exhibit severe functional impairment, including defective bactericidal, phagocytic, or chemotactic properties.

Absolute monocytosis is a common finding, even in leukopenic conditions.

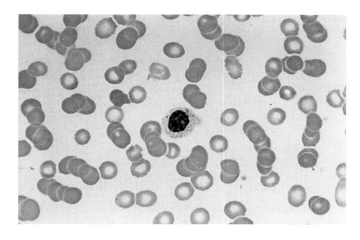

FIGURE 16-2. A peripheral blood film of a patient with MDS shows a neutrophil with the round pseudo-Pelger-Huët nucleus. The nuclear chromatin is condensed and the cell contains granules, making identification possible. In many cases, these types of neutrophils are agranular, which makes it difficult to differentiate them from lymphocytes. (250× original magnification).

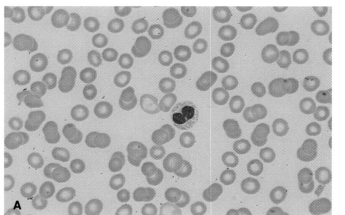

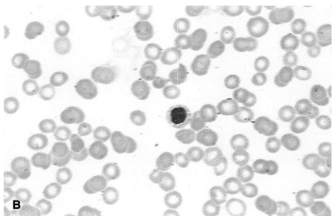

FIGURE 16-3. **A**, Bilobed segmented neutrophil (psuedo-Pelger-Huet) (PB; 250× original magnification; Wright Giemsa stain). **B**, Single lobed mature neutrophil in MDS (pseudo-Pelger-Huet; PB; 250× original magnification; Wright Giemsa stain).

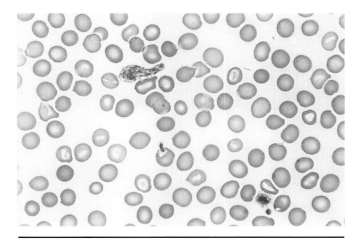

FIGURE 16-4. A peripheral blood film of a patient with MDS shows abnormally large platelets. Notice also the anisocytosis of erythrocytes. (250× original magnification.)

PLATELETS

Qualitative and quantitative platelet abnormalities are often present. The platelet count may be normal, increased, or decreased. The lowest platelet counts are associated with RAEB-T and CMML. Giant platelets, hypogranular platelets, and platelets with large fused granules may be seen in the peripheral blood (Figs. 16-4 and 16-5). Sometimes circulating micromegakaryocytes can be found. These may be difficult to define and are frequently overlooked, unless cytoplasmic blebs are present. Functional platelet abnormalities include abnormal adhesion and aggregation. As a result, the bleeding time may be prolonged, and other platelet function tests may give abnormal results.

● Bone marrow

Bone marrow examination is necessary to identify the dyshematopoietic element, to determine cellularity, and to establish a diagnosis. In most cases, the bone marrow is

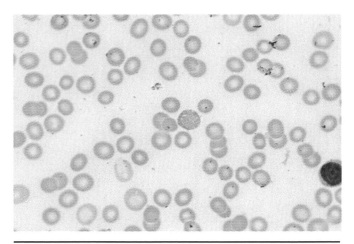

FIGURE 16-5. Large, agranular platelet (center) in the peripheral blood of a patient with myelodysplastic syndrome (MDS). (250× original magnification; Wright-Giemsa stain).

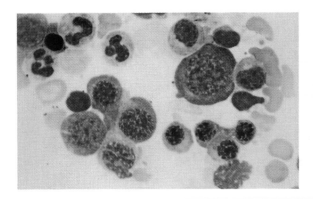

FIGURE 16-6. Megaloblastoid erythroblasts in the bone marrow of a patient with MDS. (RARS) (250× original magnification; Wright-Giemsa stain).

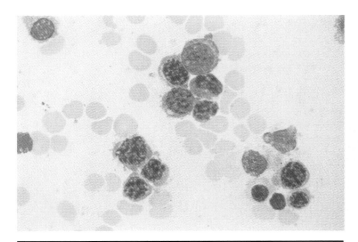

FIGURE 16-7. Bone marrow from a case of RAEB. The polychromatophilic erythroblasts have a megaloblastoid appearance. The cytoplasmic membrane is irregular in many of the erythroblasts. (250× original magnification; Wright-Giemsa stain).

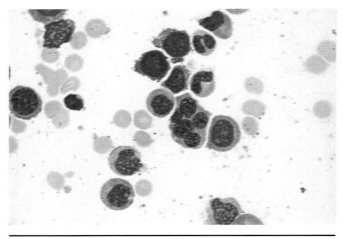

FIGURE 16-8. Multinucleated polychromatophilic erythroblast in the bone marrow of a patient with MDS. It is also megaloblastoid. (250× original magnification; Wright-Giemsa stain).

hypercellular with erythroid hyperplasia, although normocellular and hypocellular marrows also have been described. The cellularity of the marrow should be interpreted in relation to the patient's age because MDS is commonly found in the elderly. The number of myeloblasts can range from normal to 30% (promonocytes, erythroblasts, promyelocytes, and megakaryoblasts are not included in the blast count). Generally, all cell lines exhibit evidence of dyshematopoiesis.

Bone marrow trephine biopsy may be helpful in establishing the diagnosis of MDS in difficult cases.[27] Abnormal localization of immature myeloid precursors (ALIP) clustering centrally may be seen in biopsy before an increase in myeloblasts is detected in bone marrow smears.[28] ALIP has been shown to be an indicator of increased risk for transformation to leukemia and is associated with poor survival. In patients with less than 5% blasts, ALIP may indicate evolution to a more aggressive disease. A biopsy also gives an exact assessment of cellularity and an indication of the amount of reticulin fibers. Conversely, ringed sideroblasts, nuclear fragmentation and budding, Auer rods, irregular cytoplasmic basophilia, and abnormal staining of primary granules in promyelocytes are more easily identified in bone marrow aspirate smears. Thus, both aspirate smears and biopsy preparations are necessary for accurate diagnosis.

DYSERYTHROPOIESIS

The most common bone marrow finding in MDS is a megaloblastoid erythropoiesis (Fig. 16-6). However, the abnormal erythrocytic maturation is not responsive to vitamin B12 or folic acid therapy. Giant, multinucleated erythroid precursors can be found (Figs. 16-7 and 16-8). Other nuclear abnormalities include nuclear fragmentation, abnormal nuclear shape, nuclear budding, karyorrhexis, and irregular staining properties. The cytoplasm of normoblasts may show defective hemoglobinization, vacuoles, and basophilic stippling. The presence of ringed sideroblasts, reflecting the abnormal erythrocyte metabolism, is a common finding. Ringed sideroblasts are defined as normoblasts in which mitochondrial iron deposits encircle one third or more of the nucleus.

DYSGRANULOPOIESIS

Granulopoiesis is usually normal to increased, unless the overall marrow is hypocellular. Abnormal granulocyte maturation (dysgranulopoiesis), however, is almost always present. One of the major findings of dysgranulopoiesis in the bone marrow is abnormal staining of the primary granules in promyelocytes and myelocytes. Sometimes the granules are larger than normal, and in others the granules are absent. Secondary granules may be absent in myelocytes and other more mature neutrophils, giving rise to the hypogranular peripheral blood neutrophils. Irregular cytoplasmic basophilia with a dense rim of peripheral basophilia also is characteristic. Nuclear abnormalities, similar to those found in the peripheral blood granulocytes, may be present in bone marrow granulocytes.

DYSMEGAKARYOPOIESIS

Megakaryocytes may be decreased, normal, or increased. Abnormalities in maturation are reflected by the presence of micromegakaryocytes, megakaryocytes with small, multiple separated nuclei, and large mononuclear megakaryocytes (Figs. 16-9 and 16-10). The lack of granules or presence of giant abnormal granules also is characteristic.

● Other laboratory findings

Serum iron is normal or increased, and the TIBC is normal or decreased. Cobalamin (vitamin B12) and folic acid levels are normal to increased, a feature that helps to differentiate the megaloblastoid features of MDS from the typical megaloblastic features of megaloblastic anemias.

Immunologic analysis has revealed that MDS is associ-

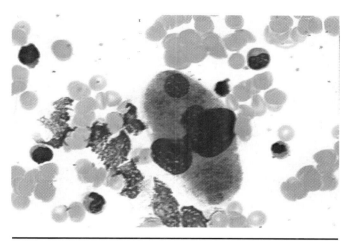

FIGURE 16-10. Abnormal megakaryocyte from a patient with MDS (BM). (250× original magnification; Wright-Giemsa stain).

ated with a significant decrease in the total number of T-lymphocytes together with a decrease in both CD4 and CD8 T-lymphocyte subsets.[29] The responses of T-lymphocytes to mitogens PHA and Con A may be significantly decreased. Although B-lymphocytes are quantitatively normal, serum immunoglobulins often are increased, and circulating immune complexes are frequently present.

Granulocytic oxidative metabolism as measured by the nitroblue tetrazolium reduction test may be abnormal and chemotaxis impaired.

● BLAST CELL CLASSIFICATION

● Morphologic identification of blasts

The blast count appears to be the most important prognostic indicator of survival and progression to acute leukemia in MDS. The maximum number of blasts compatible with a diagnosis of MDS is 30%. The minimum criteria for a diagnosis of acute leukemia includes more than 30% blasts.

The dysgranulopoiesis that affects primary azurophilic granules in neoplastic blasts changes the standard criteria for identification and classification of blast cells and promyelocytes. The standard criteria for a blast cell includes a cell with a central nucleus with fine nuclear chromatin, prominent nucleoli, a high nuclear cytoplasmic ratio, and deeply basophilic and agranular cytoplasm. It is now recognized that in MDS and acute leukemia there are some blast-like cells that contain primary azurophilic granules. These early azurophilic granules are not indicative of differentiation but rather of abnormal neoplastic cells.[30] Consequently, two types of blasts that occur in MDS and acute myeloid leukemia are recognized: Type I and Type II. More recently, it has been suggested that a third type of blast cell be recognized in MDS to improve predictions of progression to acute leukemia and survival.[30] These are called Type III blasts. Typical agranular blasts are included in the Type I category. Type II and Type III blasts have typical blast-like features except they contain pri-

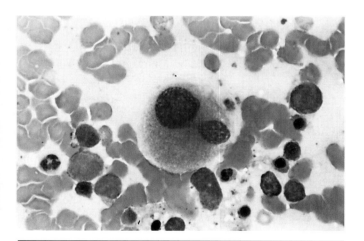

FIGURE 16-9. The bone marrow of a patient with MDS (RAEB) shows a megakaryocyte with the megaloblastoid nuclear feature. Notice that the nucleus is not lobular as is typical of a mature megakaryocyte but rather there are two, almost completely separate lobes. (250× original magnification).

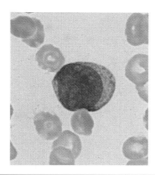

FIGURE 16-11. Myeloblast (PB). (250× original magnification; Wright-Giemsa stain).

mary azurophilic granules. The following morphologic criteria have been established for identifying Type I blasts, Type II blasts, Type III blasts, and promyelocytes in MDS and acute leukemia.[30]

TYPE I BLASTS (FIG. 16-11)

These cells include typical myeloblasts and unclassifiable cells. The nuclear chromatin is finely dispersed with prominent nucleoli. The nuclear cytoplasmic ratio is variable but is higher in the smaller blasts than the larger ones. The cytoplasm contains no granules.

TYPE II BLASTS (FIG. 16-12)

These cells resemble Type I blasts except that the cytoplasm contains primary granules (less than 20) and the nucleus is in a more central position. The nuclear cytoplasmic ratio tends to be lower (more cytoplasm) than that of Type I blasts.

TYPE III BLASTS

These cells are similar to Type II blasts except they contain more than 20 granules in the cytoplasm.

PROMYELOCYTES

The nucleus is eccentrically placed, and the chromatin pattern is more condensed. The Golgi apparatus is obviously seen as a clear area adjacent to the nucleus. The nuclear cytoplasmic ratio is low due to the increase in cytoplasm. There are many primary granules present. In some cases

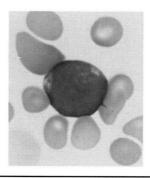

FIGURE 16-12. Type II myeloblast with a few primary granules (PB; 250× original magnification; Wright-Giemsa stain).

of MDS, the promyelocyte appears hypogranular or even agranular. In these cases, the abnormal cell can be identified as a promyelocyte by the other nuclear and cytoplasmic criteria. If the azurophilic granules are clumped and heterogeneous in size, the promyelocyte is classified as abnormal.

Using these criteria for distinguishing blasts and promyelocytes, the minimum criteria for a diagnosis of acute leukemia includes more than 30% Type I, Type II, and Type III blasts (exclusive of promyelocytes) in the bone marrow. The maximum number of blasts compatible with a diagnosis of MDS is 30% Type I, Type II, and Type III blasts. Often the blast count in the blood is greater than that in the marrow. It has been suggested that when the blast count exceeds 30% in the blood but the bone marrow concentration is less than 30%, the case be regarded as acute leukemia. The blasts in MDS, with the exception of RAEB-t and CMML, do not have Auer rods present.

● Cytochemical and immunological identification of blasts

Although the blast cells in MDS are primarily derived from granulocytic or monocytic precursors, a panel of cytochemical and immunocytochemical reactions should be performed and interpreted to enhance the accuracy of diagnosis.[31] Peroxidase and Sudan Black B identify blasts with a myeloid origin. However, in MDS, the blasts may have lower peroxidase activity than normal blasts. Iron stain may reveal abnormal iron metabolism in erythroblasts with the presence of increased iron stores and ringed sideroblasts. Abnormal carbohydrate metabolism is indicated by the presence of blocks of periodic acid–Schiff-positive material in erythrocyte precursors. Abnormal small megakaryoblasts can be difficult to distinguish from lymphoblasts or Type I myeloblasts. They can be readily identified, however, by immunochemistry with antibodies against platelet-specific glycoproteins IIB/IIIA (CD41), gpIIIA (CD61), or by antibody against Factor VIII in histiologic sections. Diaminobenzidine can be used to identify platelet peroxidase in electron micrographs.[31]

Only a few studies have been reported on the prognostic value of immunophenotyping in MDS. In general, there is no correlation between immunophenotypes and the FAB classification. It has been suggested that increased expression of CD33 and CD13 (found on immature myeloid cells) and decreased expression of NAT-9 (found on mature myeloid cells) may be an early indicator of transformation to acute leukemia.[32] Immunological phenotyping using monoclonal antibodies may be useful in identifying the lineage of blasts in those cases of acute leukemia derived from therapy-related MDS. Many of these cases show trilineage dysplasia and are difficult to define according to FAB subgrouping.[33] The specific cellular markers found on different cell lineages in acute leukemia are described in Chapter 18 with acute leukemia.

● DESCRIPTIONS OF SUBGROUPS OF MDS

The most widely recognized classification system for MDS is the revised FAB classification proposed in 1982.[2] Some

TABLE 16-2 *DIFFERENTIATING CHARACTERISTICS OF FAB SUB-TYPES OF MYELOCYSPLASTIC SYNDROMES*

Subtype	Bone Marrow		Peripheral Blood	
	Blasts (%)	Ringed Sid* (%)	Blasts (%)	Monocytes
RA†	<5	<15	<1	—
RARS	<5	≥15	<1	—
CMML	≤20	—	<5	>1 × 10^9/L
RAEB	5–20	—	<5	—
RAEB-t	>20–30 and/or Auer rods	—	≥5	—

* Ringed sideroblasts. The FAB group recommended that ringed sideroblasts be expressed as percent of total bone marrow cells. More commonly, they are expressed as percent of total erythroid precursors.

† RA, refractory anemia; RARS, RA with ringed sideroblasts; CMML, chronic myelomonocytic leukemia; RAEB, RA with excess blasts; RAEB-t, RAEB in transformation.

(From: Lee GR, et al: Wintrobe's Clinical Hematology, 9th ed. Philadelphia, Lea & Febiger, 1993.)

features of the five subgroups of MDS overlap, and some are exclusive to a particular group. The criteria used for classification include: percentage of bone marrow blasts, percentage of peripheral blood blasts, presence or absence of ringed sideroblasts, percentage of monocytes present, extent of cytopenias, and degree of dyspoiesis (Table 16-2).

Refractory anemia

Refractory anemia (RA) occurs with anemia as the primary clinical finding. The anemia is refractory to all conventional forms of therapy. Erythrocytes usually appear macrocytic, but occasionally they are microcytic or normocytic. The peripheral blood shows reticulocytopenia and signs of dyserythropoiesis, but leukocytes and platelets are usually quantitatively and qualitatively normal. Blast cells are usually absent in the peripheral blood but, if present, they constitute less than 1% of the nucleated cells.

The bone marrow is hypercellular with erythroid hyperplasia and signs of dyserythropoiesis. Megaloblastoid erythropoiesis that is unresponsive to folic acid or cobalamin is present. Ringed sideroblasts are absent or present in low numbers. Maturation of neutrophils and megakaryocytes is generally normal. Blast cells compose less than 5% of marrow cells.

For convenience, the rare isolated refractory thrombocytopenias and neutropenias are included in this category, even though anemia is absent. Some prefer to call these cases refractory cytopenia.

Refractory anemia with ringed sideroblasts or acquired idiopathic sideroblastic anemia

Refractory anemia with ringed sideroblasts (RARS) or acquired idiopathic sideroblastic anemia (AISA) is similar to RA, except that ringed sideroblasts account for more than 15% of the nucleated cells in the bone marrow. The anemia is usually macrocytic and less often normocytic. Sometimes there is evidence of a dual population of normochromic and hypochromic cells. The peripheral blood shows reticulocytopenia and often leukopenia. The occurrence of leukopenia in one study was 33%, with neutropenia occurring in 7%.[24] Another study found neutropenia in 48% of cases.[34] Occasionally, the platelet count is increased. A few cases exhibit granulocyte and platelet morphologic abnormalities.

The bone marrow is hypercellular with megaloblastoid dyserythropoiesis. If dysgranulopoiesis and dysmegakaryopoiesis are present, it is mild. There are fewer than 5% blast cells in the marrow.

Refractory anemia with excess blasts

In refractory anemia with excess blasts (RAEB), there is cytopenia in at least two cell lines and conspicuous qualitative abnormalities in all three cell lines. The anemia is normocytic or slightly macrocytic with reticulocytopenia. Evidence of dysgranulopoiesis is prominent and includes poorly granulated neutrophils, pseudo-Pelger-Huët anomaly, and, occasionally, decreased LAP and myeloperoxidase. There are fewer than 5% blasts in the peripheral blood. Monocytosis without leukocytosis may be present, but the absolute monocyte count does not exceed 1 × 10^9/L, and serum and urinary lysozyme levels are normal. Platelet abnormalities include giant forms, abnormal granularity, and functional aberrations. Sometimes circulating micromegakaryocytes can be found.

The bone marrow is hypercellular, less often normocellular, with varying degrees of granulocytic and erythrocytic hyperplasia. All three cell lines show signs of dyshematopoiesis. The percentage of blasts varies from 5% to 20%. Abnormal promyelocytes may be present.[35] These abnormal cells have blast-like nuclei with nucleoli, no chromatin condensation, and the cytoplasm contains large bizarre granules. There may be an increase in ringed sideroblasts, but the elevated blast count differentiates RAEB from RARS.

It has been shown that there is a difference in survival between patients having 5% to 10% blasts and those having 11% to 20% blasts. Those with more than 10% blasts have a poorer outcome. The separation of these two groups into RAEB-I (5% to 10% blasts) and RAEB-II (11% to 20% blasts) provides a more accurate prognostic classification.[30]

Refractory anemia with excess blasts in transformation

Refractory anemia with excess blasts in transformation (RAEB-t) includes those disorders that do not fit into any other MDS category due to an excess of blasts and/or the presence of Auer rods. They are also not typical of acute leukemia because the excess of blasts is insufficient to diagnose AML. In some cases, it is difficult to differentiate

RAEB-t from acute leukemia. Serial examinations are sometimes necessary to make an accurate diagnosis. This disorder generally has a shorter course than other types of MDS (10-month survival) and has a higher risk of evolving to acute leukemia. Rarely, have patients with RAEB-t had a previously established form of myelodysplasia.

RAEB-t is similar to RAEB except that any one of the following hematologic features may be found: 5% or more blasts in the peripheral blood, 20% to 30% Type I and Type II blasts in the bone marrow, or presence of unequivocal Auer rods in granulocyte precursor cells.

Chronic myelomonocytic leukemia

Chronic myelomonocytic leukemia (CMML) differs from the other subgroups in that it has a myeloproliferative element with a mature granulocytosis in the peripheral blood, and many patients have spenomegaly. Because it has features that straddle both myeloproliferative disorders and MDS, it is easily confused with chronic myelocytic leukemia (CML).

Synonyms for this disorder include subacute myelomonocytic leukemia and chronic erythromonocytic leukemia. Although other subgroups of MDS are not typically associated with organomegaly, between 30% and 54% of patients with CMML have splenomegaly and/or hepatomegaly. Lymphadenopathy is not present. There is usually no skin or gum involvement, as is commonly associated with acute myelomonocytic leukemia. The diagnosis is most often made when the patient is seen by a physician for symptoms of anemia, intercurrent infection, or hemorrhagic manifestations. These patients are found to have a predominantly monocytic cellular pattern in the peripheral blood and a myelocytic cellular pattern in the bone marrow. The average time lapse from onset of symptoms until diagnosis is 6 to 18 months. One study of 41 patients with CMML found that 24% had previously been diagnosed with another MDS subgroup or had peripheral cytopenia.[36] Two had agnogenic myeloid metaplasia. None, however, had been treated with cytotoxic drugs.

Although leukocytes are characteristically increased, erythrocytes and platelets are often decreased. Anemia is mild in CMML with an average hemoglobin of 11.7 g/dL. The erythrocytes are normocytic or slightly macrocytic. Thrombocytopenia is present in about 60% of cases.[37] Giant platelets and hypogranular forms are found. Circulating micromegakaryocytes are sometimes present. The leukocyte count is variable with many in the normal range, some increased and a few decreased. Regardless of the leukocyte count, there is an absolute monocytosis greater than 1×10^9/L and usually greater than 2×10^9/L. Monocytes frequently exhibit morphologic abnormalities. The nuclear pattern varies, but nucleoli are absent and the cells are easily distinguished from blasts. Neutrophils are often increased with or without dysgranulopoiesis. Immature granulocytes, monocytes, and nucleated erythrocytes may be identified on blood smears. Fewer than 5% blasts are found in the peripheral blood.

A constant and significant finding in CMML is the elevation of serum and urinary lysozyme levels. In addition, most patients have an increased uric acid level from increased cell turnover. Cobalamin and folic acid levels are normal or increased.

Protein electrophoresis reveals hypergammaglobulinemia in more than 50% of patients.[29,36] In most cases, it is polyclonal. Although it has been suggested that the abnormal monocytes may be responsible for this phenomenon, no relationship between degree of peripheral monocytosis and presence or absence of gammopathy has been established.

The bone marrow is hypercellular with a proliferation of immature and abnormal myelocytes. Some myelocytes have nuclei with nucleoli and an irregular chromatin pattern somewhere between that of blasts and myelocytes. Some myelocytes appear pyknotic or necrobiotic, whereas others have a monocytoid appearance. Even when myelocytes are increased, there is no apparent leukemic hiatus. Transitional forms in both directions are present. There are frequent reports describing an intermediate or abnormal cell, expressing staining and/or morphologic characteristics of both monocytoid and myeloid cells in the bone marrow. Promonocytes may be significantly increased, and up to 20% of the nucleated cells may be blasts. Auer rods may be present in some blasts, especially in progression of the disease. Erythrocyte precursors may be increased, particularly early in the disease. The morphology of erythroblasts often is abnormal, with megaloblastoid features and multiple nuclei. Megakaryocytes are usually quantitatively normal, but almost 50% show some degree of dysmegakaryopoiesis.[36]

The presence of a significant peripheral blood and bone marrow monocytosis, trilineage dysplasia, absence of the Philadelphia chromosome, and elevated serum and urine lysozyme levels help differentiate CMML from CML.

VARIANTS OF MDS

A number of patients have blood and/or marrow findings that cause problems in diagnosis and/or classification. Some of these findings occur often enough to consider them as variants of MDS.

Hypoplastic MDS

Although most cases of MDS are associated with hypercellular or normocellular bone marrows, about 10% have hypocellular marrows. In these cases, trephine biopsy is necessary to exclude a diagnosis of aplastic anemia or hypoplastic acute myeloid leukemia (AML). This distinction is important since the diagnosis will have an influence on treatment and prognosis.

Hypocellular MDS should be considered when the bone marrow cellularity is less than 30% or less than 20% in patients older than 60 years of age.[38] The criteria for MDS must be met in hypoplastic as well as hypercellular or normocellular cases. Dysplasia can be difficult to identify, and dyserythropoiesis has been described in aplastic anemia. Dysmegakaryopoiesis and dysgranulopoiesis, however, are most characteristic of MDS and may be a helpful finding. In addition, ALIP, indicating an abnormal bone marrow architecture, is typical of MDS. Chromosomal abnormalities, if present, help distinguish MDS from aplastic anemia.

The distinction of MDS from AML may be made by the blast count. A count over 30% is indicative of AML.

● MDS with fibrosis

Mild to moderate fibrosis has been described in up to 50% of patients with MDS. The incidence of fibrosis appears to be even greater in therapy-related MDS. If fibrosis is present, other diagnoses should be excluded, including myelofibrosis with myeloid metaplasia (MMM), chronic myelocytic leukemia, and acute megakaryocytic leukemia. Severe myelofibrosis in MDS is not common. In MDS patients with fibrosis, there is typically pancytopenia, hypocellular bone marrow with fibrosis, trilineage dysplasia, and small megakaryocytes with hypolobulated nuclei.[39]

● Unclassifiable MDS

In up to 10% of cases, the MDS does not fit the FAB subgrouping criteria. The most common reason is the presence of overlapping features of trilineage dysplasia and less than 5% blasts. Often the blast count favors the refractory anemia subgroup, but trilineage dysplasia favors the RAEB subgroup. Survival is poor, which favors RAEB. A new subgroup for these MDS cases has been proposed—refractory anemia with dysplasia.

To avoid overlap or contradiction in classifying MDS, a sequential approach has been suggested[40] (Fig. 16-13). Classification begins with the blast count and proceeds to the monocyte count and percentage ringed sideroblasts. In this system, the RA subgroup is a classification arrived at by exclusion of the other four.

● Therapy-related myelodysplasia

Myelodysplasia secondary to alkylating chemotherapy and/or radiotherapy for other malignant or nonmalignant diseases is frequently referred to as therapy-related or treatment-related MDS (t-MDS). It should be noted, however, that MDS may develop as a second primary disorder, unrelated to therapy, especially if MDS develops after a very short or a very long time after therapy. A study of 65 patients with t-MDS or acute leukemia suggests that panmyelosis related to therapy develops in three stages: (1) pancytopenia with myelodysplastic changes and less than 5% blasts; (2) frank MDS, which resembles RAEB or RAEB-t; (3) overt AML.[41] Not all stages are found in all patients, as some patients have overt AML while others die of infection, hemorrhage, or other disease before MDS or AML develops. Development of MDS or acute leukemia appears to be related to the duration, amount, and repetition of the therapy as well as the age of the patient.

The t-MDS are often difficult to classify according to the FAB criteria. In most cases, the qualitative changes are

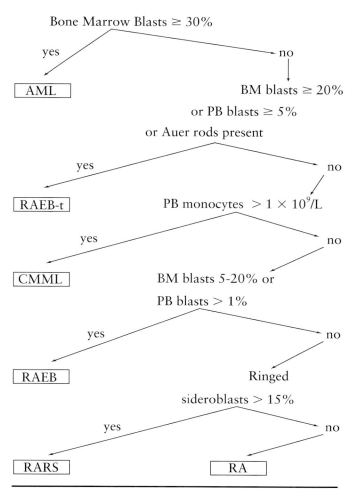

FIGURE 16-13. Sequential approach to classifying MDS according to the FAB criteria. Classification begins with the bone marrow blast count to differentiate MDS from acute leukemia. Abbreviations: BM, bone marrow; PB, peripheral blood; AML, acute myeloid leukemia.

marked with trilineage involvement, typical of RAEB or RAEB-t. The number of blasts, however, is usually less than 5%, typical of RA. Despite the low percentage of blasts, the clinical course of the disease reflects profound marrow failure, and the outcome is very unfavorable with a median survival of 4 to 6 months.[41] About 25% of patients have blast counts between 5% and 20%, which, together with the marked qualitative changes in all cell lines, qualifies for the RAEB classification. The bone marrow is most often hypercellular or normocellular. The finding of increased megakaryocytes is associated with increased fibrosis. Similar to primary MDS, about 30% of t-MDS evolve to acute leukemia. These leukemias are difficult to classify according to the FAB criteria for acute nonlymphocytic leukemia. In some cases, the proliferation of cells involve several or all cell lines bridging several classifications, while in others the problem is related to marked fibrosis and inadequate aspiration of marrow specimen.[41]

TABLE 16-3 *CYTOGENETIC FINDINGS IN PATIENTS WITH MDS*

Subtype	5q−	−5	−7	+8	del/t(11q)
RA	70	<5	5	15	<15
RARS	30	<5	<5	25	20
RAEB/RAEB-t	30	10	30	10	10
CMML	<5	<5	20	20	<5

* Data are expressed as percent of abnormal karyotypes in each group. RA, refractory anemia; RARS, RA with ringed sideroblasts; CMML, chronic myelomonocytic leukemia; RAEB, RA with excess blasts; RAEB-t, RAEB in transformation. (From Heim S, Mitelman F: Cancer Cytogenetics. New York, Alan R. Liss, 1987.)

CYTOGENETICS

Abnormal karyotypes can be demonstrated in up to 50% of individuals with MDS (Table 16-3). These are acquired clonal aberrations, similar to those seen in patient's with acute nonlymphoblastic leukemia.[32] The more frequent cytogenetic abnormalities involve structural or numeric abnormalities of chromosomes 5 and 7 and trisomy 8.

The best characterized and most common chromosome defect in MDS is the deletion of the long arm of chromosome 5, known as the 5q− syndrome. When present as the only genetic abnormality, it is associated with macrocytic anemia, dyserythropoiesis, hypolobulated megakaryocytes, and normal or increased platelet counts. The missing arm of chromosome 5 contains genes for five growth factors and for the M-CSF receptor. The significance of the deletion is not known but is probably related to the missing growth factor genes and receptor.

Another common abnormality is deletion of the long arm of chromosome 7 (7q-) or deletion of the whole chromosome (-7). The long arm contains the proto-oncogene ERB-B, which is the gene for the receptor of the epidermal growth factor (EGF). This abnormality is most common in pediatric MDS.[43]

Trisomy 8 (+8) is found in about 20% of the MDS abnormal karyotypes. Chromosome 8 contains the MYC proto-oncogene which codes for a nuclear transcription factor.

MDS patients with chromosome aberrations have a poorer prognosis than patients with a normal karyotype and show increased incidence of progression to acute leukemia and complications of marrow failure. The emergence of new abnormal clones is associated with transformation to a more aggressive subgroup or AML.

The t-MDS have more frequent and complex abnormalities than those found in primary MDS. Chromosome changes are almost always present in t-MDS and are usually multiple at diagnosis. The majority of karyotypic abnormalities include abnormalities of chromosomes 5 and/or 7 either singly or in combination with other abnormalities.[42] Additional abnormalities are listed in Table 16-4. In contrast to primary MDS, there may be extreme variability in karyotypic aberrations, with no two cells exhibiting the same abnormality.

TABLE 16-4 *CHROMOSOME CHANGES IN PATIENTS WITH THERAPY-RELATED MYELODYSPLASTIC SYNDROMES*

Single chromosome changes
  del(5q)
  del(7q)
  −5
  −7
  del(12p)
  t(1;7)(p11;p11)
Multiple chromosome changes
  Any of the above plus:
  +8
  +21
  3p(del or t)
  17q (del or t), 17p (del or t), −17
  6p (del or t)
  19p or q (t)
  Xq13 (t or dup)
  Xp11 (t)

(From: Third MIC Cooperative Study Group. Recommendations for a morphologic, immunologic, and cytogenetic (MIC) working classification of the primary and therapy-related myelodysplastic disorders. *Cancer Genet. Cytogenet.*, 32,1, 1988).

PROGNOSIS

The median survival for all types of MDS is less than 2 years; however, some patients may survive many years through transfusion dependency. The mortality rate varies from 58% to 72%. Leukemic transformation ranges in incidence from 10% to 40%.[44] The incidence of transformation appears to be less in RA and RARS. RA and RARS, however, may show progression to RAEB, RAEB-t, and, finally, acute leukemia. The most valuable prognostic factor appears to be the percentage of blasts in peripheral blood and bone marrow, with RAEB and RAEB-t having the lowest median survival[45] (Table 16-5).

Scoring systems, to be used in conjunction with the FAB

TABLE 16-5 *THE MEDIAN SURVIVAL AND LEUKEMIC PROGRESSION OF PATIENTS WITH PRIMARY MYELODYSPLASTIC SYNDROMES*

Subtype (%)	Median	Survival (months)	Leukemic Progression (%)
RA (28)	50	(18–64)	12
RA-S (24)	51	(14–76+)	8
RAEB (23)	11	(7–16)	44
CMMoL (16)	11	(9–60+)	14
RAEB-t (9)	5	(2.5–11)	60

RA–refractory anemia; RA-S–refractory anemia with ringed sideroblasts; RAEB–refractory anemia with excess blasts; CMMoL–chronic myelomonocytic leukemia; RAEB-t–refractory anemia with excess blasts in transformation.

(From: Third MIC Cooperative Study Group. Recommendations for a morphologic, immunologic, and cytogenetic (MIC) working classification of the primary and therapy-related myelodysplastic disorders. *Cancer Genet Cytogenet* 32,1, 1988).

TABLE 16-6 *A COMPARISON OF FOUR SCORING SYSTEMS USEFUL IN PROGNOSIS OF MDS. THE FOUR SYSTEMS USE A COMBINATION OF HEMOGLOBIN CONCENTRATION, NEUTROPHIL AND PLATELET COUNTS, BLAST COUNT AND DEGREE OF DYSHEMATOPOIESIS. AGE IS ALSO A FACTOR IN THE SANZ SYSTEM. IN ALL SYSTEMS, HIGHER SCORES ARE ASSOCIATED WITH A POORER PROGNOSIS*

Scoring System		Points	Range of Score	Good Prognosis	Intermediate Prognosis	Poor Prognosis
*Bournemouth			0–4	0–1	2–3	4
Hemoglobin <10 g/dL		1				
Neutrophils						
>16 × 10^9/L		1				
<2.5 × 10^9/L		1				
Platelets <100 × 10^9/L		1				
Blasts >5%		1				
**Dusseldorf			0–4	0	1–2	3–4
Hemoglobin <9 g/dL		1				
Lactate dyhydrogenase >200IU/L		1				
Platelets <100 × 10^9/L		1				
Blasts >5%		1				
***Varela			0–15	0–1	2–4	≥5
neutrophils or	platelets					
>3 × 10^9/L	>150 × 10^9/L	0				
1–3 × 10^9/L	100–150 × 10^9/L	1				
.5–1 × 10^9/L	50–99 × 10^9/L	2				
<.5 × 10^9/L	20–49 × 10^9/L	3				
	<20 × 10^9/L	4				
Megakaryocytes <1 per 1000 nucleated cells		2				
Dysgranulopoiesis						
Hypogranular (≥20%)		2				
Abnormal muclei (≥20%)		2				
Dysmegakaryopoiesis						
Micromegakaryocytes or						
Large mononuclear or						
Multiple small nuclei (≥30%)		2				
****Sanz			0–5	0–1	2–3	4–5
Platelets						
>100 × 10^9/L		0				
50–100 × 10^9/L		1				
<50 × 10^9/L		2				
Blasts						
<5%		0				
5–10%		1				
10–30%		2				
Age						
>60 years old		1				
<60 years old		0				

criteria, have been introduced to aid in prognosis (Table 16-6). The systems are similar, using easily obtained clinical and hematologic data.[46–49] Low scores correlate with prolonged survival. The use of scoring is recommended, especially in cases of t-MDS, to determine if those with a more favorable outcome can be identified at initial diagnosis.[31]

● THERAPY

In patients with pancytopenia, morbidity is associated with infection, bleeding, and anemia. The most common causes of death are hemorrhage and infection. Supportive care includes transfusions with leukocyte-depleted erythrocytes and platelets and prophylactic or curative antibi-

otic therapy. Patients with poor prognosis are treated more aggressively with AML-type chemotherapeutic regimens. Differentiation-inducing agents such as cytosine arabinoside (Ara-C) have shown limited success, with some patients achieving complete remission and others developing myelotoxicity or dying of treatment-related causes.[50,51] Bone marrow transplant is the only curative treatment available and is the treatment of choice for those younger than 50 years of age. In the last several years, investigators have studied hematopoietic growth factors as a possible treatment for MDS. Studies with GM-CSF, G-CSF, and IL-3 show that the growth factors improve the neutrophil count in most cases.[52] Erythropoietin is effective in some patients. Stimulation of megakaryopoiesis is least successful.[53] Further studies are needed using combinations of growth factors.

SUMMARY

The myelodysplastic syndromes are neoplastic pluripotential stem cell disorders characterized by one or more peripheral blood cytopenias and prominent cellular maturation abnormalities. The bone marrow is usually normocellular or hypercellular, indicating a high degree of ineffective hematopoiesis. Proto-oncogene mutations are commonly found in patients with MDS. Thus, oncogenes probably play a role in the pathogenesis of MDS.

Although anemia is the most common cytopenia, neutropenia and thrombocytopenia also occur. Erythrocytes are macrocytic or less frequently normocytic. Erythropoiesis in the bone marrow is abnormal, with megaloblastoid features commonly present. Neutrophils may show hypolobulation of the nucleus and hypogranulation. Megakaryocytes also show megaloblastoid features and hypolobulation of the nucleus. Platelets may be large and agranular.

The FAB group has classified the MDS into five subgroups dependent on the blast count, degree of dyspoiesis, and cytopenias and presence of ringed sideroblasts. These include refractory anemia (RA), refractory anemia with ringed sideroblasts (RARS), refractory anemia with excess blasts (RAEB), refractory anemia with excess blasts in transformation (RAEB-t). Those subgroups with higher blast counts and more involvement of cell lines in dyspoiesis are more aggressive disorders. The MDS frequently terminate in acute leukemia. There is no cure for MDS. Treatment is primarily supportive.

REVIEW QUESTIONS

A 65-year-old white man was seen in triage with complaints of fatigue, malaise, anorexia, and hemoptysis of recent onset. Laboratory tests revealed anemia and thrombocytopenia. Results of the CBC were:

Hb	5.8 gm/L
Hct	0.17 L/L
Erythrocyte count	1.60 x 10^{12}/L
Leukocyte count	10.5 x 10^9/L
Platelet count	38 x 10^9/L
Reticulocyte count	0.8%
Differential:	44% segmented neutrophils
	7% band neutrophils
	6% lymphocytes
	28% eosinophils
	1% metamyelocytes
	1% myelocytes
	9% promyelocytes
	4% blasts

The neutrophilic cells show marked hyposegmentation and hypogranulation.

A bone marrow was performed. The marrow showed a celluarity of about 75%. There was myeloid hyperplasia with 12% blasts, 26% promyelocytes, 18% myelocytes, 3% myelocytes, 4% bands and 37% eosinophils. The M:E ratio was 12:1. The myelocytes were hypogranular and some had two nuclei. The erythroid precursors showed megaloblastoid changes. Megakaryocytes were adequate in number but showed abnormal forms with nuclear separation and single nucleated forms. (Questions 1–5 relate to this case).

1. Which of the hematopoietic cell lines exhibit evidence of dyshematopoiesis?
   a. erythroid and myeloid
   b. erythroid, myeloid, and megakaryocytic
   c. erythroid only
   d. myeloid and megakaryocytic

2. How would you classify the bone cellularity?
   a. normocellular
   b. hypocellular
   c. hypercellular
   d. fibrotic

3. Which of the terms below best describes the M:E ratio?
   a. increased
   b. decreased
   c. normal
   d. reversed ratio

4. How would you classify the anemia morphologically?
   a. normocytic, normochromic
   b. microcytic, hypocyhromic
   c. normocytic, hypochromic
   d. macrocytic, normochromic

5. Given the laboratory results, what is the most likely subgroup of myelodysplasia?
   a. RA
   b. RARS
   c. RAEB
   d. RAEB-t

6. What is the minimum number of bone marrow blasts needed for a diagnosis of acute leukemia?
   a. 29%
   b. 50%
   c. 5%
   d. 30%

7. In addition to the number of blasts, what other criterion is essential for a diagnosis of RARS?
   a. More than 15% ringed sideroblasts
   b. More than 30% ringed sideroblasts
   c. Dyshematopoiesis in all three cell lineages
   d. Pancytopenia

8. CMML differs from the other subgroups of MDS because it has:
   a. a lymphocytosis in the peripheral blood
   b. a mature granulocytosis in the peripheral blood
   c. a hypocellular bone marrow
   d. a monocytopenia

9. The t-MDS differ from primary MDS in that t-MDS:
   a. is usually the less aggressive subgroup
   b. has more peripheral blood blasts

c. has fewer and less complex abnormal karyotypes

d. are more difficult to classify into a subgroup of MDS

10. Progression of MDS to acute leukemia is characterized by:

a. an increase in the blast population

b. decreased bone marrow cellularity

c. a decreased M : E ratio

d. splenomegaly

● REFERENCES

1. Coiffier, B., et al.: Dysmyelopoietic syndromes, a search for prognostic factors in 193 patients. Cancer, 52:83, 1983.
2. Bennett, M., et al.: Proposals for the classification of the myelodysplastic syndromes. Br. J. Haematol., 51:189, 1982.
3. Besa, E.C.: Myelodysplastic syndromes (Refractory Anemia): A perspective of the biologic, clinical, and therapeutic issues. Med. Clin. North. Am., 76:599, 1992.
4. Raskind, W.H., et al.: Evidence for a multistep pathogenesis of a myelodysplastic syndrome. Blood, 63:1318, 1984.
5. Musilova, J., Michalova, K.: Chromosome study of 85 patients with myelodysplastic syndrome. Cancer. Genet. Cytogenet., 33:39, 1988.
6. Okuda, T., et al.: Cytogenetic evidence for a clonal involvement of granulocyte-macrophage and erythroid lineages in a patient with refractory anaemia. Acta. Haemat., 80:110, 1988.
7. Prchal, J.T., et al.: A common progenitor for human myeloid and lymphoid cells. Nature, 274:590, 1978.
8. Weimar, I.S., Bourhis, J.H., DeGast, G.C., Gerritsen, W.R.: Clonality in myelodysplastic syndromes. Leuk. Lymph., 13:215, 1994.
9. Bartram, C.R.: Molecular genetic aspects of myelodysplastic syndromes. Hematol. Oncol. Clin. North. Am., 6:557, 1992.
10. Willemze, R., et al.: Biology and treatment of myelodysplastic syndromes—developments in the past decade. Ann. Hematol., 66:107, 1993.
11. Coll, D.C., List, A.F.: Myelodysplastic syndromes. West. J. Med., 151:161, 1989.
12. Hirai, H., et al.: Relationship between an activated N-ras oncogene and chromosomal abnormality during leukemic progression from myelodysplastic syndrome. Blood, 71:256, 1988.
13. Dormer, P.L., Hershko, C., Wilmanns, W.: Mechanisms and prognostic value of cell kinetics in the myelodysplastic syndromes. Br. J. Haemat., 67:147, 1987.
14. Dormer, P., Schalhorn, A., Wilmanns, W., Hershko, C.: Erythroid and myeloid maturation patterns related to progenitor assessment in the myelodysplastic syndromes. Br. J. Haemat., 67:61, 1987.
15. Coutinho, L.H.: Functional studies of bone marrow haemopoietic and stromal cells in the myelodysplastic syndrome (MDS). Br. J. Haemat., 75:16, 1990.
16. Degnan, T., Weiselberg, L., Schulman, P., Budman, D.R.: Dysmyelopoietic syndrome. Am. J. Med., 76:122, 1984.
17. Ciccone, G., et al.: Myeloid leukemias and myelodysplastic syndromes: Chemical exposure, histologic subtype and cytogenetics in a case-control study. Cancer Genet. Cytogenet., 68:135, 1993.
18. Gadner, H., Haas, O.A.: Experience in pediatric myelodysplastic syndromes. Hematol. Oncol. Clin. North. Am., 6:655, 1992.
19. Aul, C., Gattermann, Schneider, W.: Age-related incidence and other epidemiological aspects of myelodysplastic syndromes. Br. J. Haematol., 83:358, 1992.
20. Truncer, M.A., et al.: Primary myelodysplastic syndrome in children: The clinical experience in 33 cases. Br. J. Haematol., 82:347, 1992.
21. Blank, J., Lange, B.: Preleukemia in children. J. Pediatr., 98:565, 1981.
22. Hasle, H.: Myelodysplastic syndromes in childhood—classification, epidemiology, and treatment. Leuk. Lymph., 13:11, 1994.
23. Pomeroy, C., OKen, M.M., Rydell, R.E., Felice, G.A.: Infection in the myelodysplastic syndromes. Am. J. Med., 90:338, 1991.
24. Juneja, S.K., et al.: Haematological features of primary myelodysplastic syndromes (PMDS) at initial presentation: a study of 118 cases. J. Clin. Pathol., 36:1129, 1983.
25. Noel, P., Solberg, L.A.: Myelodysplastic syndromes: Pathogenesis, diagnosis and treatment. Crit. Rev. Oncol. Hematol., 12(3):193, 1992.
26. Sanz, G.F., Sanz, M.A.: Prognostic factors in myelodysplastic syndromes. Leuk. Res., 16:77, 1992.
27. Rios, A., et al.: Bone marrow biopsy in myelodysplastic syndromes: morphological characteristics and contribution to the study of prognostic factors. Br. J. Haemat., 75:26, 1990.
28. Yoshida, Y., Stephenson, J., Mufti, G.J.: Myelodysplastic syndromes: From morphology to molecular biology. Part K. Classification, natural history and cell biology of myelodysplasia. Int. J. Hematol., 57:87, 1993.
29. Colombat, P.H., Renoux, M., Lamagnere, J., Renous, G.: Immunologic indices in myelodysplastic syndromes. Cancer, 61:1075, 1988.
30. Goasguen, J.E., et al.: Prognostic implication and characterization of the blast cell population in the myelodysplastic syndrome. Leuk. Res., 15:1159, 1991.
31. Third MIC Cooperative Study Group: Recommendations for a morphologic, immunologic, and cytogenetic (MIC) working classification of the primary and therapy-related myelodysplastic disorders. Cancer Genet. Cytogenet., 32:1, 1988.
32. Kristensen, J.S.: Immunophenotyping in acute leukemia, myelodysplastic syndromes and hairy cell leukemia. Dan. Med. Bulle., 41:52, 1994.
33. Michels, S.D., McKenna, R.W., Arthur, D.C., Brunning, R.D.: Therapy related acute myeloid leukemia and myelodysplastic syndromes: a clinical and morphologic study of 65 cases. Blood, 65:1364, 1985.
34. Kushner, J.P., Lee, G.R., Wintrobe, M.M.: Idiopathic refractory sideroblastic anemia. Clinical and laboratory investigations of 17 patients and review of the literature. Medicine, 50:139, 1971.
35. Sultan, C., Imbert, M., Ricard, M.F., Marquet, M.: Myelodysplastic Syndromes. In Dyserythropoiesis. Edited by Lewis, S.M., Verwilgen, R.L., London: Academic Press, 1977.
36. Tefferi, A., Hoaglund, H.C., Therneau, T.M., Pierre, R.V.: Chronic myelomonocytic leukemia: natural history and prognostic determinants. Mayo. Clin. Proc., 64:1246, 1989.
37. Miescher, P.A., Farquet, J.J.: Chronic myelomonocytic leukemia in adults. Semin. Hematol., 11:129, 1974.
38. Dickstein, J.I., Vardiman, J.W.: Issues in the pathology and diagnosis of the chronic myeloproliferative disorders and the myelodysplastic syndromes. Am. J. Clin. Pathol., 99:513, 1993.
39. Kampmeier, P., Anastasi, J., Vardiman, J.W.: Issues in the pathology of the myelodysplastic syndromes. Hematol. Oncol. Clin. North. Am., 6:501, 1992.
40. Ho, P.J., Gibson, J., Vincent, P., Joshua, D.: The myelodysplastic syndromes: Diagnostic criteria and laboratory evaluation. Path., 25:297, 1993.
41. Michels, S.D., McKenna, R.W., Arthur, D.C., Brunning, R.D.: Therapy-related acute myeloid leukemia and myelodysplastic syndrome: A clinical and morphologic study of 65 cases. Blood, 65:1364, 1985.
42. Iurlo, A., et al.: Cytogenetic and clinical investigations in 76 cases with therapy-related leukemia and myelodysplastic syndrome. Cancer Genet. Cytogenet., 43:227, 1989.
43. Noel, P., Tefferi, A., Pierre, R.V., Jenkins, R.B., Dewald, G.W.: Karyotypic analysis in primary myelodysplastic syndromes. Blood Rev., 7:10, 1993.
44. Ganser, A., Hoelzer, D.: Clinical course of myelodysplastic syndromes. Hematol. Oncol. Clin. North. Am., 6:607, 1992.
45. Kirkhofs, H., Hermans, J., Haak, H.L., Leeksma, C.H.W.: Utility of the FAB classification for myelodysplastic syndromes: investigation of prognostic factors in 237 cases. Br. J. Haemat., 65:73, 1987.
46. Mufti, G.J., et al.: Myelodysplastic syndromes: a scoring system with prognostic significance. Br. J. Haemat., 59:425, 1985.
47. Varela, B.L., Chuang, C., Wall, J.E., Bennett, J.M.: Modifications in the classification of primary myelodysplastic syndromes: the addition of a scoring system. Hemat. Onc., 3:55, 1985.

48. Aul, C., Schneider, W.: Myelodysplastic syndromes. A prognostic factor analysis of 221 untreated patients. Blut., 57:234, 1988.

49. Sanz, G.F., et al.: Two regression models and a scoring system for predicting survival and planning treatment in myelodysplastic syndromes: A multivariate analysis of prognostic factors in 370 patients. Blood, 74:395, 1989.

50. Cheson, B.D.: The myelodysplastic syndromes: Current approaches to therapy. Ann. Intern. Med., 112:932, 1990.

51. Willemze, R., et al: Biology and treatment of myelodysplastic syndromes—developments in the past decade. Ann. Hematol., 66:107, 1993.

52. Ganser, A., Hoelzer, D.: Treatment of myelodysplastic syndromes with hematopoietic growth factors. Hematol. Oncol. Clin. North. Am., 6:633, 1992.

53. Arcenas, A.G., Vadhan-Raj, S.: Hematopoietic growth factor therapy of myelodysplastic syndromes. Leuk. Lymph., 11(suppl 2):65, 1993.

General aspects and classification of leukemia

17

KEY TERMS

leukemia
leukemic hiatus
oncogene
proto-oncogenes
anti-oncogene
tumor suppressor gene
epitope

INTRODUCTION TO THE CLASSIFICATION OF LEUKEMIAS

Leukemia is a progressive, neoplastic disease of the hematopoietic system characterized by unregulated proliferation of uncommitted or partially committed stem cells. It includes a heterogeneous group of neoplasms that differ with respect to aggressiveness, cell of origin, clinical features, and response to therapy.

The disease is classified into two broad groups, based on the aggressiveness of the illness: (1) acute, which if untreated causes rapid death, usually within months, and (2) chronic, a less aggressive form, which, if untreated, causes death in months to years. Both of these major groups are further classified into myeloid or lymphoid according to the origin of the leukemic stem cell clone. If myelocytic cells or other cells derived from the CFU-GEMM stem cell predominate, the disease is called myelogenous leukemia. If the lymphoid cells predominate, the disease is termed lymphocytic leukemia. Thus, using these two classification systems for aggressiveness of the disease and cell of origin, four types of leukemia are recognized: acute myelocytic leukemia (AML) (sometimes referred to as acute nonlymphocytic leukemia), chronic myelocytic leukemia (CML), acute lymphocytic leukemia (ALL), and chronic lymphocytic leukemia (CLL).

Further subtypes of each major classification can be identified based on morphologic, cytochemical, immunologic, and cytogenetic criteria of the malignant cells (Table 17-1). Acute leukemias involving the myelocytic monocytic, erythrocytic, or megakaryocytic cell lines are classified as subtypes of acute myelocytic leukemia (acute nonlymphocytic) since these cell types develop from the common stem cell, CFU-GEMM.

In addition to the above, three subtypes of acute leukemia are recognized: mixed lineage, undifferentiated, and myeloid/natural killer cell. Mixed lineage leukemia, as its name implies, is characterized by blasts with both lymphoid and myeloid features. Undifferentiated leukemia is characterized by blasts that cannot be identified as lymphoid or myeloid by currently available techniques.

TABLE 17-1 *CLASSIFICATION OF LEUKEMIAS*

	Myeloid	*Lymphoid*	*Other*
Acute Leukemia	myeloblastic promyelocytic monocytic myelomonocytic erythrocytic megakaryocytic	T-lymphocytic B-lymphocytic null cell (undifferentiated)	undifferentiated mixed lineage myeloid/natural killer cell
Chronic Leukemia	myelocytic myelomonocytic	lymphocytic plasmocytic (multiple myeloma) hairy cell prolymphocytic large granular cell lymphocytosis	

These leukemias will be discussed in more detail in the next chapter.

Acute leukemia

The acute leukemias are a heterogeneous group of diseases characterized by unregulated, progressive proliferation and accumulation of immature, malignant, hematopoietic precursors in the bone marrow. There is a gap in the normal maturation pyramid of cells, with many blasts and some mature forms but very few intermediate maturational stages. This gap in maturation is frequently referred to as the *leukemic hiatus*. Eventually, the immature neoplastic cells spill over into the peripheral blood, producing leukocytosis. In the laboratory, the diagnosis of acute leukemia is suggested when examination of the peripheral blood smear reveals the presence of many undifferentiated or minimally differentiated cells. If left untreated, the patient succumbs to complications of the disease within weeks to months of diagnosis. This short duration of the disease from diagnosis to death is what prompted hematologists to term the disease "acute." There has been remarkable progress in the treatment of ALL since 1970, with more than 50% of patients achieving remission of five years or longer. In these cases, the term "acute" is misleading.

Chronic leukemia

The chronic leukemias most often have an insidious onset. Diagnosis is frequently made during a routine physical examination for nonspecific patient complaints such as weight loss or weakness. The bone marrow typically exhibits an accumulation of differentiated lymphocytic (CLL) or myelocytic (CML) elements. These cells spill over into the peripheral blood, producing a leukocytosis. The differential count of the bone marrow and peripheral blood are similar with all stages of maturation present but with a predominance of the more mature forms. Chronic leukemias progress slowly. The course of the disease is measured in years rather than in months, as is typical for acute leukemias. In the past, chronic leukemias were commonly classified as a distinct group of hematopoietic disorders. More recently they have been grouped with other chronic neoplastic stem cell disorders. CML is now considered one of the four subgroups of chronic myeloproliferative disorders (Chapter 15). Chronic myelomonocytic leukemia is included as a subgroup of the myelodysplastic syndromes (Chapter 16). CLL is discussed in Chapter 19 with other chronic lymphoproliferative disorders. This chapter and the next will primarily include discussions of the acute leukemias.

HISTORY

In 1845, two individuals, John Bennet in Edinburgh and Rudolf Virchow in Berlin, independently published their observations of leukemia patients. They are generally credited with defining leukemia and recognizing its significance as a discrete disease entity.[1,2] Clinical histories of their patients were similar; both men described symptoms of increasing weakness, swelling of the abdomen, and serious nosebleeds in their patients. At autopsy, the two most remarkable findings were a greatly enlarged spleen and a peculiar appearance in the consistency and color of blood. Bennett thought the blood looked as though it was mixed with pus. Microscopically, he affirmed that the blood did contain many large corpuscles similar to those found in pus; however, Bennett remarked that there was no apparent sign of inflammation, a condition that was usually associated with the finding of pus. Virchow preferred the term "white blood" to describe the unusual pale whitish color of the blood, preferring to avoid the insinuation that the blood changes were associated with an inflammatory process. Two years later, the term "white blood" was translated into Greek, becoming "leukemia."[3]

As additional cases of leukemia were found, Virchow recognized that not all leukemias were associated with an increase in the same type of white cell. In some cases, white corpuscles were granular with divided or irregular nuclei, and the spleen was particularly enlarged. In other cases, the corpuscles were agranular with round nuclei, and the lymph nodes of the patient were enlarged. These observed distinctions were probably in reference to what we now classify as myeloid and lymphoid leukemias. The variety of cell types described by Virchow were verified by Ehrlich when he introduced his method of differential staining for blood cells.

An additional classification of leukemias was proposed by Ebstein in 1889.[4] One type appeared to have a grim prognosis and was unresponsive to treatment. He called this type acute leukemia. The second type was called chronic leukemia because the patient could be temporarily relieved of symptoms.

● EPIDEMIOLOGY

In the United States, leukemias and lymphomas account for 8% of all male cancers and 6% of all female cancers.[5] In 1993, there were about 12,600 new cases of leukemia in this country. Deaths from leukemia range from 3.8 per 100,000 for females to 6.3 per 100,000 for males.

Approximately 50% of all leukemias are diagnosed as acute. Although there is some difference in incidence of the acute leukemias between countries and regions of countries, the differences are not great. However, all leukemias are more prevalent in Jews of Russian, Polish, and Czeck ancestry than in non-Jews. Acute leukemia also is more common in whites than blacks. Whether these differences reflect the impact of environmental or genetic factors is unknown.

Of particular interest is the incidence and morphologic variation of acute leukemia among age groups. Although leukemia occurs at all ages, there is a peak incidence in the first decade, particularly from the ages of 2 to 5. This is followed by a decreasing incidence in the second and third decade. Thereafter, the incidence begins to increase, rising steeply after 50 years of age. The cellular type of

leukemia, occurring at these peak periods, differs significantly. Most childhood acute leukemias are of the lymphoid type, whereas those occurring in adults are typically myeloid in origin. Chronic leukemias are rare in children. Most chronic myeloid leukemias occur in young to middle-aged adults, while chronic lymphocytic leukemia is found primarily in older adults. In 1993, it was estimated that overall about 40% of all new cases of leukemia were lymphocytic and 42% were granulocytic.

ETIOLOGY

It has been known for some time that exposure to certain chemicals and irradiation can induce cancer in experimental animals. These agents also have been associated with cancer in humans. However, until recently, the actual pathogenic mechanisms of malignancy have remained obscure. The last several decades have seen enormous progress in our understanding of the pathogenesis of cancer.

● Oncogenes

In 1976, J. Michael Bishop and Harold Varmus of the University of California, San Francisco, discovered that normal cells contain genes that can cause cancer/tumors if they become altered or activated.[6] These altered cell genes that cause tumors are referred to as *oncogenes* (onco means tumor), while the normal unaltered cellular counterparts of oncogenes are known as *proto-oncogenes*. Proto-oncogenes may become activated to oncogenes as a consequence of gene mutation or gene rearrangement. This alters gene expression or activity/structure of its protein product.

Oncogenes are identified by a three-letter abbreviation derived from either a retrovirus or from the tissue specificity (e.g., SRC, ABL, SIS, ERB, RAS). [It has recently been recommended that the three letter proto-oncogene/oncogene abbreviation be capitalized. In some of the borrowed art for this book, the older lower case abbreviation is used.] The three-letter code is often preceded by a c- or v- to specify if it is a normal cellular gene or a viral derived form. To date, more than 60 proto-oncogenes have been identified.

The detection of proto-oncogenes in evolutionary diverse organisms suggests that these genes are highly conserved and play a key role in cell biology. In the normal cellular state, proto-oncogenes direct cellular growth, proliferation, and differentiation by encoding proteins that are involved at every level of growth regulation. When altered, however, these genes are capable of inducing and maintaining cell transformation.[7]

The normal growth of cells involves an intricately regulated cascade of events which can be organized into a first, second, third messenger concept. Each organ system has a set of molecules that regulate the proliferation and differentiation of its cells. These molecules include growth factors, growth factor receptors, cytoplasmic and nuclear proteins.

The growth factor/growth factor receptor complex composes the first messenger system. The growth factor receptor has an extracellular ligand-binding domain, a membrane spanning region and a cytoplasmic tail. The signal for cell proliferation and differentiation begins when growth factors bind to specific growth-factor receptors on the cell membrane. This transiently activates the receptor and triggers a cascade of intracellular biochemical reactions that regulate the expression and function of protein products. Only cells that have receptors for a specific factor are responsive to it. Some of the growth factors and their receptors are protein products of proto-oncogenes.

Activated receptors activate intracellular proteins of the second messenger system. These second messengers carry the message from the activated receptor to other cell sites, including the nucleus. In the nucleus are third messenger proteins that bind to the DNA and regulate transcription.

Signal transmission from the activated receptor to the nucleus via secondary messengers is not completely understood. The mechanism for signal transmission in tyrosine kinase receptors is activation of tyrosine kinase activity in the cytoplasmic portion of the receptor after growth factor binding. The tyrosine kinase phosphorylates appropriate substrates causing an increase in intracellular phosphorylated proteins. Transmission of the signal occurs through a further set of substrate reactions that connect the receptor-mediated signal to other pathways. Other growth factor receptors lack intrinsic catalytic activity but when activated interact with and activate cytosolic protein kinases. Still another type of receptor has tyrosine phosphatase activity when activated. Reversible phosphorylation of cellular proteins plays a key role in the regulation of many metabolic processes. Therefore it is not surprising that the kinases and phosphatases are involved in the second messenger system.

Another mechanism for signal transduction from a growth-factor receptor is coupled to guanine nucleotide binding proteins (G-proteins). The activity of this family of molecules is regulated by guanine nucleotide binding. The binding of the G-protein to an activated receptor and to GTP activates G-protein function. Conversely, binding GDP inhibits its function. The activated G-protein activates an enzyme that generates the second messenger.

Some of the known second messengers produced by activated growth factor receptors are listed in Table 17-2.

TABLE 17-2 *IMPORTANT SECOND MESSENGERS PRODUCED FROM THE INTERACTION OF ACTIVATED GROWTH FACTOR RECEPTORS AND CYTOSOLIC EFFECTOR PROTEINS*

Receptor associated effector protein	Second Messenger Produced
Calcium ion channel	Ca^{++}
Adenylate cyclase	cAMP
cGMP phosphodiesterase	cGMP
Phosphatidylinositol-specific phospholipase C	Diacylglycerol and inositol triphosphate (IP_3)

Notice that one of these mechanisms produces the second messenger diacylglycerol which activates protein kinase C and IP3 which stimulates release of intracellular calcium from intracellular storage sites. This leads to cell proliferation.

The second messengers activate third messengers which are the transcription factors located in the nucleus. Transcription of DNA is controlled by interaction of transcription factors with specific DNA sequences usually upstream of the gene to be transcribed. These transcription factors bind both DNA and an RNA polymerase. The DNA binding domain binds to an enhancer or promoter region of DNA and the activating domain binds to RNA polymerase. The transcription factor's receptor site for the RNA serves to provide an appropriate start site for transcription of DNA by the RNA polymerase. These transcription factors include those that control the expression of genes that are involved in cell proliferation and differentiation. The MYC oncogene and other oncogenes that are associated with neoplastic diseases of the leukocytes code for transcription factors.

This system of cell growth signaling has precise controls, growth-inhibitory signals, to prevent the proliferation from going on indefinitely and to initiate cell death signals.[8] RB and P53 are examples of tumor suppressor genes that serve to stop or slow cell division. Loss of or mutations in these genes may result in tumors.

Programmed cell death occurs through a process called apoptosis. In this nonpathologic form of cell death, the nucleus and cytoplasm condense and the nucleus fragments. The cell breaks up into membrane bound bodies which are phagocytosed or shed into a lumen. The process depends on endonuclease cleaving of DNA. These endonucleases are activated by an intracellular increase in Ca^{++} or protein kinase A. These same endonucleases are inhibited by protein kinase C. It is proposed therefore that growth activation and inhibition signals must be balanced for cell survival.

ONCOGENES AND CELL GROWTH

Oncogenes can disrupt the normal pathways of signal transduction and gene transcription. This causes an interruption of the regulation of cell proliferation and differentiation and production of a cell that has a growth advantage. This disruption results from a structural or quantitative change in the oncogene protein product that allows the protein to exceed its normal function.[8,10] The protein products encoded by oncogenes include growth factors, growth factor receptors, protein kinases and other proteins that are involved in the transduction of the signal from the activated cellular receptor to other cell sites, and transcriptional factors. It also is possible that some oncogenes may produce proteins that prolong cell survival by interfering with apoptosis.

The exact role of oncogene products in transforming normal cells to malignant cells is unknown but they may provide independence from normal cell signaling by causing abnormalities in the first, second or third messenger pathways.[11] (Table 17-3). First, the tumor cell oncogene may indirectly stimulate expression of a growth factor that acts on the tumor cell or encode the growth factor and cause excessive excretion of the factor. Either way the

TABLE 17-3 *POSSIBLE MECHANISMS IN WHICH ONCOGENES DISRUPT THE REGULATED FIRST, SECOND, THIRD MESSENGER CASCADE OF CELL PROLIFERATION AND DIFFERENTIATION*

Proliferation/ Differentiation Messenger	Abnormalities Associated With Oncogene Protein Product
First (extracellular and membrane receptor)	Excessive growth factor excretion; constitutively activated receptor
Second (cytoplasmic)	Abnormal cellular proteins involved in signal transduction that send out stimulatory signals without being activated by first messengers
Third (nuclear)	Transcription factor activated independently of secondary messenger

cell is stimulated in an autocrine fashion because the cell produces growth factor that stimulates the cell itself. Second, the growth factor receptor may be abnormal sending stimulatory signals to the cell even though a growth factor has not bound to the receptor. The receptor acts as though it is permanently activated (constitutively activated). The most common mode of permanent activation of a tyrosine kinase type receptor is deletion of the extracellular ligand binding domain of the receptor (Figure 17-1). Third, the

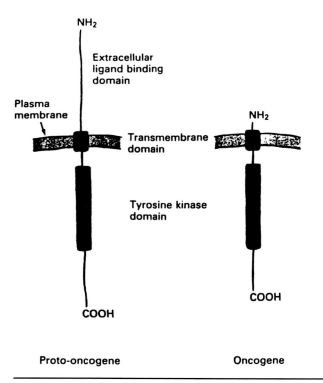

FIGURE 17-1. Comparison of a growth factor receptor product from a proto-oncogene and the mutated product from an oncogene. Notice that the extracellular ligand binding domain of the mutated receptor has been lost. This results in a receptor that is permanently activated (without growth factor binding). (From: Cooper, G.M.: Oncogenes. Boston: Jones and Bartlett, 1990).

intracellular protein that transduces signals from the receptor to other cell sites may send out stimulatory signals without activation from the growth factor receptor. Other downstream events that respond to the stimulatory signals also may be abnormal due to mutated gene products. Lastly, oncogenes coding for transcriptional proteins may produce abnormal proteins that are activated independently of activation by second messengers. This results in a cell that is constantly growing and dividing.

● Anti-oncogenes/tumor suppressor genes

Another recently recognized type of gene is the *anti-oncogene* or *tumor suppressor gene* (TSG). These TSGs function by suppressing cellular proliferation and, hence, neoplastic transformation. In most cases, it is believed that both alleles of a TSG must be deleted or mutated for neoplastic growth to occur. This is the reason these genes have been described as recessive oncogenes. The first well-described TSG is RB, located on chromosome 13 at 13q14. This gene is associated with a rare malignancy called retinoblastoma. In familial cases of retinoblastoma there is an inherited deletion or mutated allele of RB, present in all cells of the body. Then, a second event occurs after birth affecting the other RB allele, only in the retinal cells of the eye, causing development of an eye tumor, retinoblastoma. Another TSG, P53, is located at 17p13.1 and may be important in hematopoietic neoplasms, as a deletion of this area is frequently seen in cases of leukemia. The P53 gene appears to indirectly slow cell division.

It appears that neoplasia is a multistep process that involves a series of progressive changes. Both oncogenes and tumor suppressor genes play a role in this process. Activation of one oncogene or loss of one tumor suppressor gene is only one step in tumor development. It is probable that multiple oncogenes and tumor suppressor genes acting together may be necessary for development of a malignant neoplasm. This concept of multiple genetic mutations helps explain the high incidence of leukemia in nonhematopoietic disorders associated with hereditary genetic mutations such as Down's syndrome. In these conditions, the genetic mutation associated with the nonhematopoietic disorder may be one of the first of multiple steps leading to malignancy. Thus these individuals are at a higher risk of developing a neoplasm. Some neoplasms may progress to more malignant disorders as additional genetic mutations occur over the course of the disease. For instance, myelodysplasia and chronic leukemia often evolve to acute leukemia as progressive genetic abnormalities occur.

The role of oncogenes and tumor suppressor genes in the pathogenesis of leukemia is currently being investigated. Oncogenes have been identified at the breakpoints of chromosomal aberrations that are commonly present in specific types of leukemia. It appears that activation of these genes by viruses or other mutagens, or by chromosome breaks and translocations, results in the aberrant expression of proteins. These proteins seem to play a role in regulating hematopoietic cell growth and differentiation.

TABLE 17-4 *FACTORS PROPOSED TO PLAY A ROLE IN LEUKEMOGENESIS*

Factor	Example
Hereditary abnormalities	Down syndrome
	Fanconi anemia
	Kleinfelter syndrome
	Bloom syndrome
	Wiskott-Aldrich syndrome
	Blackfan-Diamond syndrome
Somatic mutation	Radiation
	Chemicals
	Drugs
Viral infection	Retroviruses—HTLV-I
Immunologic disorders	Wiskott-Aldrich syndrome
	Bruton's type X-linked agammaglobulinemia
	Ataxia telangiectasia
	Immunosuppressive therapy

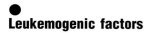

Leukemogenic factors

From studies on laboratory animals, four factors have been proposed as playing a role in causation of leukemia: (1) genetic susceptibility; (2) somatic mutation; (3) viral infection; and (4) immunologic dysfunction (Table 17-4).

GENETIC SUSCEPTIBILITY

There is strong evidence that hereditary factors and abnormal genetic material have important leukemogenic effects. A number of individuals who have congenital abnormalities associated with karyotypic abnormalities, including homogeneously staining extra chromosomes, translocations, inversions, and deletions, have a markedly increased risk of developing acute leukemia. Each of these genetic events may potentially activate proto-oncogenes. The best known of the genetic abnormalities associated with leukemia is Down syndrome. Various other congenital disorders also are associated with an increased risk for leukemia, including Fanconi anemia, Kleinfelter syndrome, Bloom syndrome, Wiskott-Aldrich syndrome, and Blackfan-Diamond syndrome.

Further evidence supporting the association of genetic factors with the occurrence of leukemia comes from family studies. An increased incidence of leukemia has been reported among monozygotic twins (more than what is expected by chance alone). The concordance rate in twins appears to be more prevalent in young children, and the onset of the disease tends to occur in very close succession. It should be remembered that the occurrence of leukemia in twins is extremely rare, making interpretation of concordance difficult. Some studies have reported an increase of leukemia in family groups. These studies have found an excess of leukemia in first-degree relatives of patients with CLL and acute leukemia (AL).[12–14]

SOMATIC MUTATION

Somatic cell mutation is an acquired change in the genetic material of cells other than those involved in reproduc-

tion. With the discovery of proto-oncogenes, it is likely that mutations in the chromosome near these proto-oncogenes could play a role in leukemogenesis. This helps explain the role of radiation and chemical toxins in acute leukemia. Radiation, some chemicals, and drugs can cause chromosome mutations. Ionizing radiation has long been recognized as capable of inducing leukemia, which is evident from observations of human exposure to radiation from nuclear reactions, therapeutic radiation, and occupational radiation. In Japan, following the 1945 nuclear explosions in Hiroshima and Nagasaki, there was a marked increase in the occurrence of leukemia among survivors. The peak incidence occurred 6 to 7 years after the explosion. All forms of leukemia were found to be increased, with the exception of CLL. The occurrence of leukemia was related directly to radiation exposure levels, with increased incidence occurring in those victims exposed to 100 rad or more. An increased incidence of leukemia also has been described in individuals receiving therapeutic radiation for ankylosing spondylitis, Hodgkin's disease, and polycythemia vera. For years before our knowledge of the hazards of radiation, the incidence of leukemia among radiologists was several times greater than that of the general population. With the advent of safety precautions, the mortality rate among radiologists has decreased considerably. These reports of leukemia in radiologists support the leukemogenic role of small doses of radiation over prolonged periods.

An increase in leukemia has been observed after treatment with alkylating agents and other chemotherapeutic drugs used in treatment of many kinds of malignancy. The only specific chemical implicated in causing leukemia, other than those used in medication, is benzene. Chronic exposure to benzene was an occupational hazard of shoemakers in Italy and Turkey in the 1960s. The incidence of leukemia among these individuals was about 13/100,000, well above the incidence in the general population. After benzene was replaced with another solvent the incidence returned to that of the general population.

More than 50% of patients with leukemia can be demonstrated to have acquired abnormal karyotypes. As the data accumulate from cytogenetic studies, specific, consistent mutations have been found in certain subgroups of leukemia. In particular, t(8;21)(q22;q22) is associated with AML-M2 type and t(15;17)(q22;q11) is virtually diagnostic of acute promyelocytic leukemia (AML-M3) (refer to Chapter 18). Research studies have shown that the 17q11 breakpoint involves the gene for retinoic acid receptor-alpha, and the 15q22 breakpoint involves a yet uncharacterized gene which is possibly a proto-oncogene. Initial treatment studies using transretinoic acid in patients with acute promyelocytic leukemia have shown that the leukemic cells can be induced to mature, and the patients may eventually enter remission. It is very likely that further research, similar to the story of the Philadelphia translocation (Chapter 15), will demonstrate a causal relationship of the specific chromosome aberrations and type of leukemic expression.

VIRAL INFECTION

Retroviruses are proven to be responsible for leukemia in laboratory animals, but definite evidence for a similar viral role in human leukemia is lacking. Retroviruses contain a reverse transcriptase that allows them to produce a DNA copy of the viral RNA core. The DNA can then be copied to produce more viral cores, or it can be incorporated into the nuclear DNA of the host cell. The strongest evidence for the existence of a leukemogenic virus in humans comes from the isolation of a human type-C retrovirus known as human T-cell leukemia/lymphoma virus (HTLV-I) from cell lines of patients with mature T-cell malignancies. This virus appears to be particularly prevalent in Japan and parts of the Caribbean region. Exactly how viruses induce leukemia is unclear, but it is suspected that the incorporation of the viral genome into host DNA may lead to activation of proto-oncogenes.

IMMUNOLOGIC

Increased incidence of lymphocytic leukemia has been observed in both congenital and acquired immunologic disorders. These disorders include the hereditary immunologic diseases Wiskott-Aldrich syndrome, Bruton's type X-linked agammaglobulinemia, and ataxia telangiectasia. An association between long-term treatment of patients with immunosuppressive drugs (e.g., renal transplant) and leukemia also has been observed. Possibly, a breakdown in the cell-mediated immunologic self-surveillance system and/or deficient production of antibodies against foreign antigens leads to the emergence and survival of neoplastic cells.

OTHER POSSIBILITIES

Certain hematologic diseases appear to pose a leukemogenic risk. The leukemia development sometimes appears to be related to the treatment used for the primary disease, whereas in others no such relationship can be found. The highest incidence of acute leukemia is found in individuals with chronic myeloproliferative or myelodysplastic diseases. This has prompted some hematologists to use the term "preleukemia" for these disorders. Acute leukemia occurs frequently in CML, with a terminal phase indistinguishable from acute leukemia developing in more than 70% of these patients. Other diseases with an increased incidence of leukemia include paroxysmal nocturnal hemoglobinuria (PNH), aplastic anemia, multiple myeloma, and lymphoma. It is interesting to note that all these hematologic disorders are considered stem cell disorders wherein the primary hematologic defect lies in the myeloid, lymphoid, or pluripotential stem cells.

More than likely, no single factor is responsible for leukemia, but, rather, the disease is produced by a variety of etiologic factors, including genetic factors and environmental exposures. The cause probably varies from patient to patient, and some individuals may be more susceptible than others to oncogene activation.

● DIFFERENTIATION OF LEUKEMIC CELLS

As mentioned, classifications of leukemias have been attempted since Virchow in the 1800s. Classifications are considered to be important for three reasons: (1) they allow clinicians and researchers a method of comparison of various therapeutic regimens; (2) they allow a system for identification and comparison of clinical features and laboratory findings; and (3) they permit meaningful associations of cytogenetic abnormalities with disease. Classification is based on identification of the leukemic cell lineage and its stage of cell differentiation.

Within the acute and chronic classifications, leukemias are subdivided into myeloid (nonlymphocytic) and lymphoid, depending on the predominant cell types present. The chronic myeloid and chronic lymphoid leukemias are relatively easy to identify because of the presence of easily recognizable differentiated cells. The acute myeloid and acute lymphoid leukemias are more difficult to identify solely by morphologic characteristics because of the undifferentiated cells. In many cases, it is impossible to morphologically differentiate lymphoblasts, myeloblasts, monoblasts, megakaryoblasts, or erythroblasts. However, the distinction of cell lineage is important for the physician to select the appropriate therapy. It must be recognized, however, that there is overlap between acute and chronic leukemias, complicating diagnosis in some cases. Cytogenetic studies suggest that CML occasionally may have a symptomless chronic phase, which may be undetected until the CML has transformed to the acute stage; this suspicion is supported by the presence of the Ph chromosome, a karyotypic abnormality strongly associated with CML, in patients with AML.

Differentiation of leukemic blasts allows classification of acute leukemia into various subtypes. Differentiation may be determined by morphology, immunologic marker analysis, cytochemical stains and/or chromosome analysis. Identification of leukemic blasts is sometimes complicated because the blast cells in leukemia are neoplastic and may not conform to the criteria used to differentiate normal blasts. None of the classification criteria is specific or diagnostic by itself.

In the late 1980s, a group of scientists from around the world met to investigate the subtyping of acute lymphoid and myeloid leukemias using morphologic, immunologic, and cytogenetic (MIC) criteria.[15,16] As a result of their work, the scientists recommended that physicians identify and code acute leukemias on the basis of combined MIC criteria of the blast cell population. The purpose was to simplify communication of results and findings, help identify subgroup commonalities, and help in classification of difficult cases that lack common markers. Most often, a combination of morphologic review of Romanowsky-stained bone marrow and blood smears, immunologic analysis of membrane markers, cytochemical analysis of cellular constituents, and chromosome analysis is used to differentiate leukemic blasts and arrive at a classification.

Although classification of leukemias according to predominant cell line is useful to the clinician, it is important to recognize that leukemia is not a limited disorder of one hematopoietic cell line; it is a stem cell disorder in which all cell progeny may be involved. This spectrum concept becomes evident when one type of leukemia transforms and terminates in another. Occasionally, definitive diag-

TABLE 17-5 *FAB CLASSIFICATION OF ACUTE LEUKEMIA*

1. Acute nonlymphocytic leukemias
   - M0   Acute myeloblastic leukemia without differentiation
   - M1   Acute myeloblastic leukemia with minimal differentiation
   - M2   Acute myeloblastic leukemia with maturation
   - M3   Promyelocytic leukemia, hypergranular
   - M3v   Promyelocytic leukemia, hypogranular (microgranular) variant
   - M4   Acute myelomonocytic leukemia
   - M4eo   Acute myelomonocytic leukemia with abnormal eosinophils
   - M5a   Acute monoblastic leukemia without differentiation
   - M5b   Acute monoblastic leukemia with differentiation
   - M6   Acute erythroleukemia
   - M7   Megakaryocytic leukemia
2. Acute lymphocytic leukemia
   - L1   Lymphoblastic leukemia with homogeneity
   - L2   Lymphoblastic leukemia with heterogeneity
   - L3   Burkitt's type lymphoblastic leukemia

nosis is delayed and can only be made by following the patient's disease over a period of time. Not infrequently with disease progression, it is difficult to determine which cell line is the most prominent.

Morphologic review

In 1976, in an effort to improve and standardize the classification of acute leukemias, a group of French, American, and British (FAB) physicians proposed a classification and nomenclature system based on the morphologic characteristics of blast cells on Romanowsky-stained smears and on the results of cytochemical stains.[17] This widely accepted system is known as the FAB classification and is only of value in untreated patients because cytotoxic therapy tends to distort both normal and malignant cells, making cell identification difficult. The FAB group also emphasizes that the criteria be applied only to those cases in which bone marrow fragments and trails are hyper- or normocellular. Caution should be used in diagnosing leukemia when the marrow is hypocellular.

In the FAB classification system the acute myeloid leukemias are subdivided into eight FAB groups, M0 to M7, depending on the predominant cell lineage (e.g., granulocytic, monocytic, erythrocytic, megakaryocytic) and the degree of cell differentiation (Table 17-5). The acute lymphoid leukemias are divided into three groups, L1 to L3 (Table 17-5). These three groups are defined by the individual cytologic features of blasts, and the degree of heterogeneity of these features within the leukemic cell population Tables 17-6 and 17-7).

Immunologic Analysis

DEVELOPMENT OF MONOCLONAL ANTIBODIES
Surface marker analysis began with identification and study of lymphocyte markers in the late 1960s and 1970s. Lymphocytes were divided into T- and B-lymphocytes depending on the presence or absence of specific markers. T-lymphocytes have a receptor for sheep erythrocytes. Thus, when sheep erythrocytes are incubated with T-lymphocytes, rosettes are formed, with the T-lymphocyte forming the center of the rosette and the sheep erythrocytes forming the petals. B-lymphocytes lack the sheep erythrocyte receptor but have receptors for complement and mouse erythrocytes. B-lymphocytes also synthesize immunoglobulin, which is incorporated into the membrane surface. These surface markers were the first to be used in studying lymphocytic leukemias, lymphomas, and immunodeficiency disease. Technical problems with these methods, however, limited the accuracy of the results.

Immunologic techniques with monoclonal antibodies, relatively new laboratory tools with increased accuracy, are now widely used to identify cell membrane antigens on a variety of cells. The development of a large number of monoclonal antibodies (produced commercially using hybridomas) to surface antigens on normal and leukemic cells together with technical advances in flow cytometry, have greatly enhanced the ability to define leukemic cell lineage, stage of cell development,[18] and clonality. The monoclonal antibody produced by the hybridoma is specific for an epitope of a particular membrane antigen (marker). The same epitope may be expressed on normal cells and on neoplastic cells or may be aberrantly lost from the original antigen on the normal cell when the cell becomes neoplastic.[19] If an antigen is expressed only on a single lineage, it is known as a "lineage-restricted" marker. If the antigen is present on more than one lineage, it is said to be "lineage-associated." Many monoclonal antibodies originally believed to be lineage-restricted are now found to have a much broader distribution. It is important to keep in mind that hypothetical maturation schemes of lymphoid and myeloid cells and their neoplastic counterparts are based on a less than perfect understanding of normal cell ontology and neoplastic cell transformation. In addition, not all cells of a particular lineage neoplasm always express the same antigens. Neoplastic cells may also express antigens of more than one cell lineage. For these reasons, reactivity of cells with a single monoclonal antibody should not be used as the sole evidence of cell lineage. Reactivity with a panel of monoclonal antibodies will give more complete information concerning a cell's lineage.

MONOCLONAL ANTIBODY NOMENCLATURE
There are several laboratories generating monoclonal antibodies and assigning them designations unique to their laboratory to identify the antibody's reactivity with cell antigens. These antibodies with unique designations frequently identify the same antigen. For example, Coulter's T11 monoclonal antibody and Becton-Dickinson's Leu5b monoclonal antibody both identify the same T-lymphocyte antigen. In an effort to organize this confusing situation, an international team designed a nomenclature system that identifies cell surface antigens, which appear on cells of certain lineages and during specific stages of differentiation. Antibodies from different laboratories are tested against standard cell lines. Those antibodies that have the same or very similar specificity define a cluster of differentiation (CD) on the cells. Each cluster is assigned a

TABLE 17-6 *MORPHOLOGIC (FAB) CLASSIFICATION OF ACUTE NONLYMPHOCYTIC LEUKEMIA*

	Subtype	Morphologic Features	Auer Rods	Cytochemical Features		
				Myeloperoxidase or Sudan Black B	Chloroacetate Esterase	Nonspecific Esterase
M0	Acute myeloblastic leukemia with no maturation	Myeloblasts without granules	−	−	−	−
M1	Acute myeloblastic leukemia with minimal maturation	Myeloblasts, with or without scant granules	± *	+	±	−
M2	Acute myeloblastic leukemia with maturation	Myeloblasts with granules, promyelocytes, few myelocytes	+	+	±	−
M3	Acute promyelocytic leukemia	Promyelocytes with prominent granules	+ +	+	+	−
M4	Acute myelomonocytic leukemia	Myeloblasts and promyelocytes >20% marrow cells; promonoblasts and monoblasts, >20%	±	+	+	+ †
M5a	Acute monoblastic leukemia without differentiation	Large monoblasts with lacy nuclear chromatin and abundant cytoplasm	−	−	−	+ ‡
M5b	Acute monoblastic leukemia with differentiation	Monoblasts, promonocytes, monocytes. Blood monocytosis	−	−	−	+ ‡
M6	Acute erythroleukemia	Megaloblastic erythroid precursors (>50%); myeloblasts (>30%)	+	+	−	±
M7	Megakaryocytic leukemia	Megakaryoblasts, "lymphoid" morphology (L1, L2, M1), cytoplasmic budding	−	−	±	± ‡

* +, usually present; + +, present in abundance; −, usually absent; ±, may or may not be present.
† Incompletely inhibited by sodium fluoride.
‡ Inhibited by sodium fluoride.
(From: Lee, GR: Wintrobe's Clinical Hematology, 9th ed. Philadelphia, Lea & Febiger, 1993.)

TABLE 17-7 *MORPHOLOGIC (FAB) CLASSIFICATION OF ACUTE LYMPHOCYTIC LEUKEMIA*

Morphologic Features	L1	L2	L3
Cell size	**Small**	Large	Large
Nuclear chromatin	Fine or clumped	Fine	Fine
Nuclear shape	Regular, may have cleft or indentation	Irregular, may have cleft or indentation	**Regular, oval to round**
Nucleoli	**Indistinct or not visible**	**One or more per cell; large, prominent**	One or more per cell; large, prominent
Amount of cytoplasm	**Scanty**	**Moderately abundant**	Moderately abundant
Cytoplasmic basophilia	Slight	Slight	**Prominent**
Cytoplasmic vacuoles	Variable	Variable	**Prominent**
Cytochemistry: Myeloperoxidase	Negative	Negative	Negative
Periodic Acid Schiff (PAS)	Negative or chunky positive	Negative or chunky positive	Negative or chunky positive

The most helpful features for differentiating subtypes are in bold type.

number. For example, T11 and Leu5b monoclonal antibodies react with T-lymphocytes, which have the sheep erythrocyte receptor (antigen). This antigen and these antibodies are represented by the CD2 cluster of differentiation. Thus, if a cell reacts with either T11 or Leu5b, the cell is said to be CD2-positive. The cluster of differentiation term was used because the exact epitopes identified by the various antibodies was not known. See Tables M and N in the Appendix for CD nomenclature for cell antigens and representative monoclonal antibodies used to identify these antigens.

MONOCLONAL ANTIBODY PROCEDURE

In the monoclonal antibody procedure, cell suspensions are incubated with monoclonal antibody and allowed to react. The cells are washed to remove excess antibody and exposed to fluorescein-conjugated anti-mouse immunoglobulin. Many monoclonal antibodies are directly conjugated with fluorochromes, making analysis easier and faster. The cells are analyzed by standard phase and fluorescent microscopy or by flow cytometry.

This technique has primarily been used to define and subgroup lymphoid leukemias (ALL). The use of immunologic markers to characterize AML subtypes and myeloid antigenic development has lagged behind the use of these markers in ALL. There are two possible explanations for this lag.[19] The first is that AML, unlike ALL, has two specific cytochemical markers—peroxidase and nonspecific esterase—which help in identifying the myeloid origin of the cells. The second is that to subtype AML, markers for myeloblasts, erythroblasts, monoblasts, and megakaryoblasts need to be identified. Recently, there has been an increasing repertoire of antibodies developed to myeloid antigens. These antibodies have helped not only in subtyping the myeloid luekemias, but also in identifying the lineage of leukemias that lack specific morphologic and cytochemical characteristics. These will be discussed in the next chapter.

● Cytochemical analysis

Cytochemistry in hematology refers to in vitro staining of cells that allows microscopic examination of the cells' chemical composition. Cell morphology is not significantly altered in the staining process. Most cellular cytochemical markers represent organelle-associated enzymes and other proteins. The cells are incubated with substrates that react with specific cellular constituents. If the specific constituent is present in the cell, its reaction with the substrate is confirmed by the formation of a colored product within the cell. The stained cells are examined and evaluated on blood smears with an ordinary light microscope, although, occasionally, electron microscopy is necessary to identify very weak reactions at the subcellular level. The results of these cellular reactions in normal and disease states are well established. Cytochemistry is particularly helpful in differentiating cell lineage of the blasts in acute leukemias, especially when morphologic identification on Romanowsky-stained smears is impossible (Table 17-6 and 17-7)

It is important to remember that the blast cells seen in leukemias are neoplastic cells and may therefore differ from normal blasts in both morphology and metabolic activity. Leukemic cells appear to develop with nuclear/cytoplasmic asynchrony, similar to that of megaloblastic cells. As a result, although the nucleus appears very immature, the cytoplasm of leukemic blasts may contain constituents normally present only in more mature cells. This is the basis for the revised definition of leukemic blasts to include three different types—I, II, and III. These will be discussed in the next chapter. In addition, there may be abnormal accumulation and distribution of cellular metabolites.

Some cellular constituents identified by cytochemical stains are sensitive to heat, light, storage, and processing technique. To demonstrate their presence, fresh smears must be used. Other constituents are more stable, and aged or processed specimens can be used.

The cytochemical staining reactions are of two types, enzymatic and nonenzymatic. The enzymatic group includes stains for myeloperoxidase, esterases, alkaline, and acid phosphatases. The nonenzymatic stains include Sudan black B for lipids, periodic acid–Schiff (PAS) for glycogen, and toluidine blue O for mucopolysaccharides.

A thorough discussion of these staining procedures and their expected reactions are included in the hematology procedure chapter of this book. A brief discussion is included here.

MYELOPEROXIDASE AND SUDAN BLACK B

The most helpful stain is the myeloperoxidase stain, which is used to differentiate the myeloblasts from lymphoblasts. The stain is positive in myeloid-derived cells and negative in lymphoid cells. The results of the Sudan black B stain closely parallel those of the myeloperoxidase stain. However, both stains should be used because sometimes leukemic blasts may stain positive with only myeloperoxidase or with only Sudan black B, but not with both. Sudan black B stains lipids.

ESTERASES

Another major stain is the one for nonspecific esterases. Alpha-naphthyl acetate or alpha-naphthyl butyrate esterase serve as substrates. The nonspecific esterase stain is used primarily to differentiate the granulocytic leukemias from those that have a monocytic origin. In monocytes, nonspecific esterase shows a strong positive reaction that is inhibited by sodium fluoride. A negative or weaker reaction that is not inhibited by sodium fluoride is typical of myeloblasts or other cells of the granulocyte series. Specific esterase using napthol AS-D chloroacetate as the substrate is found primarily in granulocytic cells.

PERIODIC ACID–SCHIFF

The PAS stain is used to identify glycogen deposits in lymphoblasts and erythroblasts. PAS also stains glycoproteins, mucoproteins, and high molecular weight carbohydrates. In some malignant hematologic disorders, the cells show intense, large granular deposits of activity. This is particularly evident in lymphoid cells of lymphoproliferative diseases and erythroblasts of M6 AML. This accumulation of activity is believed to be the result of disturbed glycogen metabolism and is the reaction of interest.

LEUKOCYTE ALKALINE PHOSPHATASE

The leukocyte alkaline phosphatase (LAP) stain is used in a semiquantitative method to help differentiate CML from a leukemoid reaction and polycythemia vera from secondary erythrocytosis. Activity is increased in leukemoid reactions and polycythemia vera, normal in secondary erythrocytosis, and decreased in CML. High values also are found in newborns and in normal pregnancy. Decreased values are associated with idiopathic thrombocytopenic purpura, paroxysmal nocturnal hemoglobinuria, and collagen disorders. The range of possible values is 0 to 400. A score greater than 160 is generally considered increased, and one less than 13 is considered decreased.

ACID PHOSPHATASE

Acid phosphatase is present in most human cells. It is a constituent of lysosomes. In blood cells, seven different isoenzymes exist: 0, 1, 2, 3, 3b, 4, 5. All but isoenzyme 5 are sensitive to tartrate inhibition. The staining reaction for acid phosphatase is primarily used to identify the hairy cells of hairy cell leukemia. These cells contain an increase in isoenzyme 5, often localized around the Golgi zone. Tartrate resistant acid phosphatase also is seen in Sezary cells, in prolymphocytes of prolymphocytic leukemia, in activated lymphocytes (especially T-lymphocytes), and in activated macrophages. Neoplastic T-lymphocytes will show a characteristic polarized positivity.

TOLUIDINE BLUE

Toluidine blue is a basic dye that reacts with acid mucopolysaccharides to form metachromatic granules. A positive reaction is specific for basophils and mast cells. However, a negative reaction should not rule out neoplasms of these cells, because the acid mucopolysaccharides may be scarce or negative in neoplastic disorders.

TERMINAL DEOXYNUCLEOTIDYL TRANSFERASE

Terminal deoxynucleotidyl transferase (TdT) is a DNA polymerase found in cell nuclei. It is present in lymphocytes in the thymus, in immature lymphocytes and in 1% to 3% of normal bone marrow cells. It is present in 90% of ALL cases but in only about 5% of AML cases. It is useful in defining leukemic cells in the spinal fluid in ALL, in differentiating ALL from AML blasts, in defining the blasts in CML blast crisis and in distinguishing lymphoblastic lymphoma (strong TdT activity). TdT can be measured by biochemical assays, immunoperoxidase, enzyme immunoassay (EIA) and by indirect or direct immunofluorescence using monoclonal antibodies.

RETICULIN STAIN

Reticulin stain is used to examine the reticulin fibers that form the major framework of the bone marrow. In hypercellular marrow, the reticulin becomes prominent, but its structural framework is preserved. In myelofibrosis, reticulin is markedly increased, but the structural framework is distorted.[20] A modified version of this stain, Gomori methenamine silver, often is used.

METHYL GREEN-PYRONINE

This stain identifies RNA (pyroninophilia) in the cytoplasm of plasma cells, immunoblasts and the B-cells of Burkitt's lymphoma. The blasts of ALL are usually negative or only weakly positive.

● Cytogenetic analysis

Advances in cytogenetics have allowed cytogeneticists to identify characteristic cytogenetic changes in the majority of the acute leukemias studied.[15,16] Some specific chromosome changes are consistently associated with particular FAB subgroups while others are not. In the lymphoid leukemias, nonrandom chromosome changes are often associated with either the B- or T-lymphocyte lineage. In addition to helping physicians evaluate their patients, cytogenetic studies help provide new insights into the pathogenesis of leukemia. Due to its importance, Chapter 20 has been devoted to cytogenetic analysis.

● Molecular analysis

Molecular genetic analysis, the process of using DNA technology to identify genetic defects, is increasingly being used as a diagnostic tool in neoplasms. Some abnormal cytogenetic chromosome karyotypes are commonly found in certain types of leukemia, such as the Philadelphia chromosome in CML. When present, this helps establish or confirm the diagnosis. In some cases, however, the Philadelphia chromosome is not detectable by cytogenetic analysis, even though the clinical features of CML are present. Molecular analysis in many of these atypical Philadelphia-negative cases has shown the identical genetic defect at the molecular level. This helps establish the diagnosis of CML.

Molecular analysis also is helpful in providing clues to the pathogenesis of leukemia. For example, the specific t(15;17) mutation found only in acute promyelocytic leukemia (M3 AML) produces an abnormal nuclear hormone receptor. The receptor in its normal form is important in transcription of certain target genes. This specific abnormality is likely involved in the maturation blockage of M3 cells. Chapter 21 discusses molecular genetic techniques and their application in diagnosis of hematopoietic diseases.

In summary, the most important initial classification of leukemias into acute lymphocytic or acute nonlymphocytic depends on identification of blast lineage (Table 17-8). A combination of cytochemistry, morphologic review, and immunologic marker analysis will assist the laboratory scientist in assigning cell lineage so that the physician can make an accurate diagnosis. Cytogenetic and molecular analysis give further clues to specific genetic mutations associated with particular FAB subgroups.

● PATHOPHYSIOLOGY

Leukemia occurs as the result of a somatic mutation of a single hematopoietic stem cell. Evidence for the clonal

TABLE 17-8 *CYTOCHEMICAL AND IMMUNOLOGIC FEATURES OF BLASTS IN ACUTE LEUKEMIA THAT HELP IN CLASSIFICATION (ACUTE LYMPHOCYTIC OR ACUTE NONLYMPHOCYTIC LEUKEMIA)*

Feature Observed	Lymphoblast	Myeloblast
Cytochemical stain:		
Peroxidase or Sudan Black B	negative	negative or positive at microscopic level (1000×) but positive (peroxidase) at ultrastructural level
PAS	negative or chunky positive	negative or diffusely positive
TdT	positive (90%)	usually negative
Immunological:		
CD13	negative	positive
CD33	negative	positive
CD2	positive (T-lineage)	usually negative
CD10	positive (B-lineage)	usually negative
CD19	positive (B-lineage)	usually negative
Morphological:		
Auer rods	not present	may be present
Abnormal granules	not present	may be present

evolution of acute leukemia (AL) cells come from cytogenetic studies. More than 50% of individuals with leukemia show an acquired abnormal karyotype in hematopoietic cells, whereas other somatic cells are normal. Using these specific cytogenetic markers, normal and malignant cells can be demonstrated to populate the marrow simultaneously. In untreated leukemias and during relapse, the leukemic cells dominate, whereas during remission usually only normal cells can be detected.

As mentioned previously, glucose-6-phosphate dehydrogenase (G6PD) is an enzyme determined by genes on the X chromosome. Several isoenzymes exist. In females, one of the two X-chromosomes in a cell is inactivated randomly in embryogenesis. All progeny of this cell will demonstrate the same X-chromosome inactivation. Females, heterozygous for G6PD isoenzymes, have inherited a different G6PD gene on each X chromosome. Because of random inactivation of one X chromosome, these individuals will demonstrate random activity of one or the other G6PD isoenzymes within cells. In G6PD heterozygote females with leukemia, the leukemic cells originating from a single stem cell should have either one isoenzyme or another; this is confirmed by analysis of G6PD isoenzymes in heterozygote females with acute leukemia. The leukemic cells contain a single type of isoenzyme, whereas other normal cells exhibit a normal heterogeneous distribution.

The cell in which the mutation occurs may be a committed lymphoid or myeloid stem cell or a more primitive cell that has the potential of differentiation into either lymphoid or myeloid cells, the pluripotential stem cell.[21] The mutation can often be identified as a chromosome alteration when cells in mitosis are studied. Occasionally, when chromosome studies are normal, aberrations in DNA at the molecular level can be found. The mutation leads to a neoplastic proliferation of the affected stem cell and/or its progeny, most probably through activation of a proto-oncogene. In acute leukemia, this unregulated proliferation is accompanied by an arrest in maturation at the primitive blast cell stage. It has been proposed that the neoplastic cell population reaches a tumor size of 1×10^{21} cells before overt leukemia can be diagnosed through bone marrow examination. As the neoplastic cell population increases, the concentration of normal cells decreases (Fig. 17-2). The most serious consequences of the disease are related to the inevitable cytopenias of normal blood

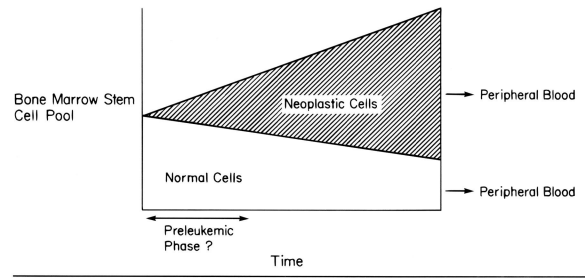

FIGURE 17-2. Clonal expansion of neoplastic cells in the bone marrow in leukemia over a period of time.

TABLE 17-9 *GROWTH PROPERTIES OF ACUTE LEUKEMIA PROGENITOR CELLS IDENTIFIED BY IN VITRO CULTURE ASSAYS*[22]

1. AL progenitor cells require growth factors for proliferation and survival but show limited maturation under the influence of these factors.
2. Regulatory factors other than growth factors (TNF, IFN-γ, TGF-β, IL-4) can synergize or antagonize proliferation of AL cells but do not directly stimulate proliferation.
3. Many AL progenitor cells have some spontaneous proliferative activity that is frequently mediated by autocrine growth stimulation.
4. Leukemic events may block programmed cell death (apoptosis) and extend cell survival. Growth factors may influence the expression of proteins that block or promote apoptosis.
5. Chromosome translocations in AL cells result in mutated genes (oncogenes) that may code for functionally abnormal growth factors or their cellular receptors or cause enhanced expression of these genes.

cells. The decrease in normal cell production was at one time believed to be caused by a crowding out by neoplastic cells together with competition for essential nutrients. Evidence, however, suggests that normal progenitor cells may be inhibited from proliferating either directly or indirectly through a humoral mediator from leukemic cells. Normal cells cultured in vitro with leukemia cells or leukemic cell extracts do not proliferate normally. Leukemic cells, on the other hand, appear to be resistant to the inhibitory substance, giving the leukemic cells a growth advantage.

In vitro cell culture studies have enlightened our understanding of the pathophysiology of acute leukemias (Table 17-9). The AL progenitor cells generally require hematopoietic growth factors (HCF) for survival and proliferation.[22] These leukemic cells, however, have mixed responses to HGFs, indicating that acute leukemias are a heterogeneous group of disorders. The growth factors IL-3, GM-CSF, and G-CSF stimulate colony growth or DNA synthesis in 80% of AML patients, while M-CSF stimulates growth in about 50% of cases. Stem cell factor (SCF, kit ligand [KL]) amplifies the response of AML cells to IL-3, GM-CSF, or G-CSF by 10- to 20-fold. Thus, the tissue concentration of SCF in vivo may affect the growth rate of AL cells. Other regulatory factors may synergize or antagonize the response of AL cells to HGFs but do not directly stimulate proliferation. These factors include tumor necrosis factor (TNF), interferon-gamma (IFN-γ), transforming growth factor-beta (TGF-β), and IL-4.

In vitro culture of AML-CFU has revealed that AL progenitor cells exhibit a certain level of spontaneous growth. This spontaneous growth may be mediated by autocrine growth stimulation. The AL blasts can produce HGFs as well as other cytokines such as TNF but not enough to maintain optimal growth. It appears that release of these cytokines is induced by IL-1 and TNF. It is questionable whether this autocrine growth plays a role in the pathophysiology of AL.

Although AL cells require HGF to proliferate, the cells show an inability to mature. Even when cell cultures are supplemented with growth factors known to induce maturation of normal cells, the AL cells do not mature. The inability of AL cells to mature toward terminally differentiated cells may interrupt apoptosis. Terminally differentiated normal myeloid cells lose proliferative potential and have a short lifespan. The maturation blockade of AL cells may result in expansion of the tumor clone by preventing cells from maturing into the nonproliferative mature cells with a limited lifespan.

An important area of research in AL is focused on the possibility that chromosome translocations may result in mutated genes that code for functionally abnormal HGFs and/or their receptors or cause overexpression of normal HGFs and/or their cellular receptors. Studies have found that AL cells have high-affinity receptors for some HGFs. This does not predict, however, that cells will proliferate in response to the bound HGF. The possibility exists that some function of the receptor is altered, resulting in abnormal activation. For example, a translocation commonly found in promyelocytic leukemia, t(15;17), causes formation of a new fusion gene composed of a portion of the retinoic acid receptor-alpha gene. This apparently causes altered function of the retinoic acid receptor, a nuclear receptor involved in transcription of certain genes. The AL cells can be stimulated to mature to granulocytes with all-transretinoic acid at concentrations above the physiologic level.

Further evidence for the role of abnormal proteins produced by mutated genes in the pathophysiology of leukemia is provided by molecular studies of the translocation found in 95% of CML patients. This translocation causes a genetic rearrangement of the oncogene ABL and the BCR gene. A new fusion gene is produced, BCR/ABL, which codes for a new protein, p210. This protein is a transmembrane signal transducer with abnormally high tyrosine kinase activity.

Another translocation, t(5;14), found in ALL is associated with overexpression of the IL-3 gene. In this translocation, the IL-3 gene on chromosome 5 is juxtaposed to the J region of the IgM gene on chromosome 14.

CLINICAL FINDINGS

Failure of normal hematopoiesis is the most serious consequence of leukemias. The most frequent symptoms are related to anemia, thrombocytopenia, or neutropenia. The major clinical problems are anemia, infection, and bleeding episodes, occurring as frank hemorrhages, petechiae, or ecchymoses. Bone pain due to marrow expansion and weight loss are common complaints. Physical examination shows hepatosplenomegaly and occasionally lymphadenopathy. Organomegaly is more common in chronic leukemias than in the acute forms.

Although the disease originates in the bone marrow, leukemic cells may infiltrate any tissue of the body, especially the spleen, liver, lymph nodes, central nervous system, and skin. The lesions produced vary from rashes to tumors. Skin infiltration is most commonly found in AML, especially those with a monocytic component. Central nervous system (CNS) involvement is especially common in ALL of childhood. Chloromas, green tumor masses of immature leukocytes, are associated with AML and CML. They are usually found in bone but can be found throughout the body. The green color, which fades to a dirty yellow after exposure to air, is responsible for the descriptive name given to this unique tumor. Presumably, the green color results from the myeloperoxidase content of malignant cells.

HEMATOLOGIC FINDINGS

A normocytic (occasionally macrocytic) normochromic anemia is present at diagnosis. (In the chronic leukemias, anemia may not be present initially, but it invariably develops during progression of the disease.) Sometimes a refractory anemia is present months before leukemia is evident. In addition to the leukemic inhibition of normal hematopoiesis already mentioned, ineffective erythropoiesis is partly responsible for the anemia as evidenced by the presence of megaloblastic features and ringed sideroblasts in erythrocyte precursors in the bone marrow.

Thrombocytopenia is usually present at diagnosis in acute leukemia. This finding, like that of anemia, usually occurs during progression of the disease in chronic leukemias. Platelet morphology and function also may be abnormal. Especially common are large hypogranular forms. Occasionally, micromegakaryocytes are present.

The leukocyte count may be normal, increased, or decreased. More than 50% of patients with AML do not have a significant leukocytosis at diagnosis. However, if left untreated, leukocytosis eventually develops. On the other hand, in the chronic leukemias, leukocytosis at diagnosis is a prominent finding. Regardless of the leukocyte count, in most cases, an increase in immature precursors is found. Blasts are especially prominent in the acute leukemias. Both absolute and relative monocytosis is a common feature in the acute myeloid leukemias.

It is not unusual to find bizarre morphologic abnormalities within leukemic cells. These findings of dysplasia reflect the abnormal maturation and differentiation characteristics of neoplastic cells. The abnormalities may include large irregular nuclei with prominent abnormal nucleoli, variation of chromatin condensation, the pseudo-Pelger-Huët anomaly, and abnormal granulation. Sometimes eosinophilic and basophilic granulation are found in the same cell.

Unique pink-staining granular inclusions called Auer rods can be found in the blast cells and promyelocytes of some acute myeloid leukemias. These abnormal granules are believed to be formed from fused primary granules. When AML is suspected, the finding of Auer rods can help establish the diagnosis because these inclusions are not found in ALL. Auer rods stain with myeloperoxidase, Sudan black B, and napthol AS-D-chloroacetate. Another type of giant pink-staining granule can be found in the malignant cells of acute leukemia. These giant granules stain positive with myeloperoxidase and Sudan black B. This morphologic granular aberration is termed pseudo-Chediak-Higashi anomaly. It has been described in AML, AMML, CML, and myelodysplastic syndromes.[23]

The bone marrow is hypercellular, although occasionally normocellularity or hypocellularity is found. Reticulin is increased, often worsening with progression of the disease. In acute leukemias, blasts constitute more than 30% of the nonerythroid marrow nucleated cells. In dysmyelopoietic syndromes and chronic leukemia, blasts compose less than 30% of marrow cells.

Maturation abnormalities are commonly present in all three cell lines. Megaloblastoid erythropoiesis may be prominent but proves to be unresponsive to vitamin B12 or folic acid treatment.

Because of the intense increase in cell turnover, other laboratory tests reflecting cell destruction may be abnormal. An increase in uric acid, a normal product of nucleic acid metabolism, is a consistent finding in all types of leukemia. The rate of excretion may increase to 50 times normal. Serum lactic dehydrogenase (LD) levels appear to correlate closely with the concentration of leukemic cells. Isoenzyme studies reveal that the LD is derived from immature leukocyte precursors. Muramidase (lysozyme) is a lysosomal enzyme present in monocytes and granulocytes. The serum and urine muramidase concentration in leukemia, although highly variable, is related to the cellular type. The highest concentrations are found in M4 and M5, the leukemias with a monocytic component.

PROGNOSIS AND TREATMENT

Prognosis

Before the 1960s, a patient diagnosed with acute leukemia could expect to die within a few months. With new treatment modalities (especially combined drug therapy), remission rates for both ALL and AML have improved dramatically. Remission is defined as a period of time in which there is no clinical or hematologic signs of the disease.

Approximately 50% of children with ALL can be expected to enter a prolonged remission with an indefinite period of survival. The prognosis of ALL in adults is not as good as in children. Two years is the median survival for adults after remission has been acheived. Only 10% to 25% have achieved a 5-year survival. Patients with poor prognostic factors in ALL include patients past puberty and infants, as well as those with extremely high blast counts, those presenting with the Philadelphia chromosome, and those with extensive mediastinal or CNS involvement.

The remission rate in AML is about 55% to 65%. Approximately 50% of these patients will remain in remission for 3 to 10 years. Patients who receive bone marrow transplants have a better prognosis, especially younger patients. Patients who had a previous myelodysplastic syndrome or chronic myeloproliferative disorder respond poorly to standard chemotherapy.

Accurate data for overall survival in CML is not available but appears to be in the range of 1 to 3 years. After onset of blast crisis, survival is only 1 to 2 months.

Survival in CLL depends on the severity of the disease at diagnosis and ranges from 30 to more than 120 months.

● Chemotherapy

Chemotherapy is the treatment of choice for leukemia. The goal of this type of therapy is to eradicate all malignant cells within the bone marrow, allowing repopulation with normal hematopoietic precursors. The problem with this type of therapy is that the drugs used in treatment are not specific for leukemic cells. Thus, during treatment, many normal cells also are killed. Most drugs used to treat leukemia can be included in three groups: antimetabolites, alkylating agents, and antibiotics.

The antimetabolites are purine or pyrimidine antagonists, which inhibit the synthesis of DNA. These drugs kill cells in cycle, affecting any rapidly dividing cell. In addition to leukemic cells, the antimetabolites also kill cells lining the gut, germinal epithelium of the hair follicles, and normal hematopoietic cells. This leads to complications of gastrointestinal disturbances, loss of hair, and life-threatening cytopenias.

The alkylating agents (chemical compounds containing alkyl groups) are not specific for cells in cycle but kill both resting and proliferating cells. The drug attaches to DNA molecules, interfering with DNA synthesis. The side effects of these compounds include myelosuppression, stomatitis, nausea, and vomiting.

Antibiotics bind to both DNA and RNA molecules, interfering with cell replication. Toxic effects of this therapy are similar to those of alkylating agents.

Since the 1970s, various drug combinations have been found to be more effective than single drug administration. The drugs commonly used and their mode of action are included in Table 17-10.

Therapy for ALL is divided into several phases. The induction phase is designed to reduce the disease into complete remission (i.e., eradicating the leukemic blast population). This is followed by the CNS prophylactic phase. CNS leukemia is the most common form of relapse in young children who have not undergone specific treatment to the brain and spinal column early in remission. The two modes of treatment in the CNS prophylactic phase are cranium irradiation and intrathecal chemotherapy. The third phase is maintenance chemotherapy, also called cytoreductive therapy or remission consolidation. The need for this type of therapy is controversial. Some studies have shown a slight increase in survival with its use, whereas others reveal no improvement. Before the institution of CNS prophylactic treatment, there was a high incidence of relapse. The maintenance therapy was designed to prevent this relapse and prolong remission. The purpose of maintenance therapy is to eradicate any remaining leukemic cells. Drug treatment usually continues for 2 to 3 years. The relapse rate after cessation of all therapy is about 25%.

The treatment regimen for AML is similar to that of ALL. The combination of antileukemic agents is different, but the purpose of chemotherapy is the same—to eradicate the leukemic blasts. CNS involvement is not a common complication of AML; therefore, CNS prophylactic treatment is not a part of the therapy regimen. The induction phase is followed by maintenance therapy, which increases the length of complete remission.

Chemotherapy, especially busulfan, irradiation and interferon are used to induce remission in CML. However, the only form of treatment that has provided long-term survival is a combination of chemoradiotherapy with bone marrow transplantation before blast crisis develops.

As in CML, permanent remission in CLL is rare. Treatment is conservative and usually reserved for patients with

TABLE 17-10 *CHEMOTHERAPEUTIC AGENTS USUALLY USED IN AL TREATMENT*

Drug	Class	Action
Cytosine arabinoside	Pyrimidine antimetabolite	Inhibits DNA synthesis
Daimpribocin	Anthrocycline antibiotic	Inhibits DNA and RNA synthesis
Doxorubicin	Anthracycline antibiotic	Inhibits DNA and RNA synthesis
5-Azacytidine	Pyrimidine antimetabolite	Inhibits DNA and RNA synthesis
6-Thioguanine	Purine antimetabolite	Inhibits purine synthesis
Methylglyoxal Bis (guanylhydrazone)	Unknown	Unknown
4'-(9-acridinylamino) methanasulfon-m-anisidide (AMSA)	Unknown	Binds to DNA
Prednisone	Synthetic glucocorticoid	Lyses lymphoblasts
Vincristine	Plant alkaloid	Inhibits RNA synthesis and assembly of mitotic spindles
Asparaginase	E. coli enzyme	Depletes endogenous asparagine
Daunorubicin	Anthracycline antibiotic	Inhibits DNA and RNA synthesis
Doxorubicin	Anthracycline antibiotic	Inhibits DNA and RNA synthesis
Methotrexate	Folic acid antimetabolite	Inhibits pyrimidine synthesis
6-Mercaptopurine	Purine antimetabolite	Inhibits pyrimidine synthesis
Cyclophosphamide	Synthetic alkylating agent	Cross-links DNA strands
Cytosine arabinoside	Pyrimidine antimetabolite	Inhibits DNA synthesis

more aggressive forms of the disease. Alkylating agents, chlorambucil and cyclophosphamide, are used. Radiotherapy, bone marrow transplantation and immunotherapy are also used to treat CLL.

Bone marrow transplant

Bone marrow transplants may provide new hope for a possible cure for leukemia; the highest rate of success in transplant patients has occurred with those younger than 40 years of age in a first remission with a closely matched donor. In this procedure, drugs and irradiation are used to bring about remission and eradicate any evidence of leukemic cells. Bone marrow from a suitable donor is then transplanted into the patient to supply a source of normal stem cells.

Autologous transplants have been used when a compatible donor cannot be found. In this procedure, some of the patient's marrow is removed while the patient is in complete remission. The marrow specimen is then treated in vitro with monoclonal antibodies or 4-hydroperoxycyclophosphamide to remove any residual leukemic cells (purged) and cryopreserved. After all traces of leukemia have been removed from the patient by chemotherapy and radiotherapy, the treated marrow is given back to the patient. Peripheral stem cells also have been used to re-establish hematopoiesis in the marrow after intensive chemo- or radiotherapy. In this procedure, apheresis is used to collect stem cells from peripheral blood over a period of several days. Autologous bone marrow transplantation is applied to patients in remission and to those in early relapse. Overall survival appears to be better in those transplanted during the first complete remission. Although bone marrow transplantation appears to be successful in some cases, the number of patients who have undergone this type of therapy is too small to attempt meaningful interpretation of data.

Hematopoietic growth factors

A variety of HGFs and cytokines are being investigated for their role in improving the treatment outcome of AL. In vitro studies indicate that GM-CSF stimulates proliferation of leukemic blasts but does not induce maturation.[24] Taking advantage of this observation, GM-CSF is being used to manipulate leukemic cell kinetics so that response to treatment with S-phase specific cytotoxic drugs is enhanced.[25] Growth factors also may be of benefit in stimulating normal hematopoietic cell proliferation and differentiation after chemo- or radiotherapy and bone marrow transplantation to decrease the period of neutropenia.

Complications of treatment

Treatment for leukemia can actually aggravate the clinical situation of the patient. Although uric acid levels are commonly elevated in leukemia from an increase in cell turnover, the concentration of this constituent can increase many fold during effective therapy because of the release of nucleic acids by lysed cells. Uric acid is a normal end product of nucleic acid degradation and is excreted mainly by the kidney. In excessive amounts, the uric acid precipitates in renal tubules, leading to renal failure (uric acid nephropathy). Renal damage can be prevented by maintenance of adequate urine flow and administration of an inhibitor of uric acid production. Lysed blast cells also can release procoagulants into the vascular system, precipitating disseminated intravascular coagulation. The resultant decrease in platelets and coagulation factors can lead to hemorrhage. This complication is especially prevalent in M3 promyelocytic leukemia. Evidently, the granules of the promyelocytes are potent activators of the coagulation factors. As already mentioned, the chemotherapeutics destroy normal as well as leukemic cells. The cytopenia that develops during aggressive chemotherapy can lead to death from infection, bleeding, or complications of anemia. To prevent these life-threatening episodes, the patient needs supportive treatment, including transfusions with blood components and antimicrobial therapy.

SUMMARY

Proliferation and differentiation of hematopoietic stem cells are normally highly regulated. HGFs play an important role in these processes. Leukemia is a progressive malignant disease of hematopoietic stem cells characterized by an inability of these cells to mature into functional peripheral blood cells. Leukemias may be classified as acute or chronic based on the aggressiveness of the disease. Acute leukemias are characterized by accumulation of immature cells and have a rapid progressive course. Chronic leukemias are characterized by an accumulation of more differentiated cells and have a slow progressive course. Further classification is based on the cell lineage of the malignant stem cell—lymphoid or myeloid (nonlymphocytic).

The role of oncogenes in the pathogenesis of leukemias is under intense investigation. Oncogenes are altered proto-oncogenes that are known to cause tumors. Many proto-oncogene protein products are involved in cell growth and include HGFs as well as their cellular receptors, protein kinases (secondary messengers), and transcription factors. Proto-oncogenes may be mutated to oncogenes by mutagens, viruses, or by chromosome breaks and translocations. Oncogenes may cause production of abnormal growth factors, abnormal amounts of growth factors, abnormal growth factor receptors, or other abnormalities in the regulatory mechanisms of proliferation and differentiation.

Differentiation and classification of acute leukemias depends on accurate identification of the blast cell population. Since the lineage of blast cells is difficult to differentiate using only morphologic characteristics, immunologic phenotyping using monoclonal antibodies and cytochemistry analysis are used routinely to help identify blast phenotypes and stage of cell differentiation. Chromosome analysis also is helpful since specific karyotypes are often associated with specific types of leukemias.

Hematologic findings include anemia, thrombocytopenia (in acute leukemia) and leukocytosis. A shift to the left is consistently found with a combination of blasts and mature cells in acute leukemia. In the chronic leukemias there is more of a continuum of cells from immature to mature. Morphologic abnormalities of leukemic cells is not unusual including pseudo-Pelger-Huët anomaly and abnormal granulation. Auer rods may be found in blasts of AML.

Leukemia is usually treated using a combination of cytotoxic drugs (chemotherapy). The goal is to induce remission by eradicating the leukemic cells. Approximately 50% of ALL cases in children and 55% to 65% of AML cases in adults can be induced into remission. A much smaller number have a long-term survival. Bone marrow transplants are being used increasingly in restoring the marrow after intense chemo- or radiotherapy. Treatment with HGFs is used in some cases to stimulate leukemic cells to proliferate, making these cells more susceptible to S-phase cytotoxic drugs. This therapy also has been used to decrease the neutropenic period after chemo- or radiotherapy. Molecular studies aimed at identifying the specific cell or HGF abnormality appears to be the best hope for finding a "cure" for this disease.

● REVIEW QUESTIONS

A 22-year-old woman was seen by her physician. Her major complaints were increased fatigue and easy bruising. Results of physical examination showed purpuric lesions on her legs and mild splenomegaly.

Initial laboratory data:
Erythrocyte count	$3.16 \times 10^{12}/L$
Hb	9.6 gm/dL
Hct	0.29 L/L
Platelet count	$85 \times 10^9/L$
Leukocyte count	$5.8 \times 10^9/L$

Differential:
Segmented neutrophils	10%
Lymphocytes	8%
Blasts	82%

Erythrocyte morphology: Erythrocytes are normochromic and normocytic.

1. Which cytochemical stain is most useful in the differentiation of a myeloblast from a lymphoblast?
   a. Periodic acid-Schiff reaction
   b. Acid phosphatase
   c. Myeloperoxidase
   d. α-naphthyl acetate esterase

2. A gap in the normal maturation of pyramid cells with many blasts and some mature forms is known as:
   a. Leukemic hiatus
   b. Chronic leukemia
   c. Mixed cell leukemia
   d. Lineage restricted

3. This patient's peripheral blood cell counts are most likely the result of:
   a. immunosuppression of the hematopoietic cells
   b. destruction of the hematopoietic cells
   c. leukemic infiltration of the hematopoietic tissue
   d. decreased hematopoietic growth factor stimulation

4. Immunologic phenotyping of the blast cells is important to:
   a. help determine cell lineage
   b. identify the etiology of the leukemia
   c. determine if cytogenetic analysis is necessary
   d. replace the need to do multiple cytochemical stains.

5. If these blasts stain positive with myeloperoxidase and negative with PAS, they are most likely:
   a. lymphoblasts
   b. CFU-GEMM
   c. BFU-E
   d. myeloblasts

6. The esterase cytochemical stains are useful to differentiate:
   a. granulocytic leukemias from monocytic leukemias
   b. lymphocytic leukemias from myelocytic leukemias
   c. monocytic leukemias from megakaryocytic leukemias
   d. lymphocytic leukemias from monocytic leukemias

7. The PAS cytochemical stain is utilized to identify:
   a. reticulin
   b. glycogen
   c. acid phosphatase
   d. lipids

8. Oncogenes may cause leukemia by:
   a. suppressing proliferation of normal cells
   b. activating retroviruses
   c. encoding for an aberrant growth protein
   d. encoding proteins that cause DNA damage

9. Auer rods are inclusions found in:
   a. myeloblasts
   b. lymphoblasts
   c. erythrocytes
   d. prolymphocytes

10. The FAB classification of a leukemia with large blasts that are myeloperoxidase and specific esterase negative but have strong positivity for nonspecific esterase inhibited by sodium flouride is:
    a. M1
    b. M4
    c. M5
    d. M7

11. A two-year-old child has 75% blasts in the peripheral blood. The blasts are myeloperoxidase negative, CD13 and CD33 negative, CD2 positive. The most likely disorder is:
    a. AML

b. CML

c. ALL

d. CLL

12. A chromosome translocation, t(15;17) that results in an abnormal retinoic acid receptor is found in this leukemia:

a. ALL

b. CLL

c. acute promyelocytic

d. CML

13. The highest levels of serum and urine muramidase are found in this leukemia:

a. M0 AML

b. M2 AML

c. CML

d. M5 AML

14. Genes that can cause tumors if activated are:

a. cancer genes

b. proto-oncogenes

c. preleukemia genes

d. tumor-suppressor genes

15. A 40-year-old man had a leukocyte count of $50 \times 10^9/L$. The differential showed 35% blasts, 55% neutrophils, and 10% lymphocytes. The blasts contained Auer rods and myeloperoxidase positive. Which of the following CD markers should be expected to be positive?

a. CD2

b. CD13

c. CD19

d. CD10

16. Which of the following factors have NOT been proposed as playing a role in the causation of leukemia?

a. benzene

b. therapeutic radiation for Hodgkin's disease

c. living at high altitudes

d. chromosome translocations

REFERENCES ●

1. Bennett, J.H.: Two cases of disease and enlargement of the spleen in which death took place from the presence of purulent matter in the blood. Edinburgh. Med. Surg. J., 64:413, 1845.

2. Virchow, R.: Weisses blut. Frariep's Notizen, 36:151, 1845.

3. Wintrobe, M.M.: Blood, Pure and Eloquent. New York: McGraw-Hill Book Co., 1980.

4. Ebstein, W.: Ueber die acute leukamie und pseudoleukamie. Dtsch. Arch. Klin. Med., 44:343, 1888-1889.

5. Boring, C.C., Squires, T.S., Tong, T.: Cancer Statistics, 1993. CA, 43(1):7, 1993.

6. Marx, J.L.: Cancer gene research wins medicine Nobel. Science, 246:326, 1989.

7. Slamon, D.J.: Proto-oncogenes and human cancers. N. Engl. J. Med., 117:955, 1987.

8. Druker, B.J., Mamon, H.J., Roberts, T.M.: Oncogenes, growth factors and signal transduction. N. Engl. J. Med., 321:1383, 1989.

9. Hall, E.J.: From chimney sweeps to oncogenes: the quest for the causes of cancer. Radiology, 179:297, 1991.

10. Sullivan, A.K.: Classification, pathogenesis, and etiology of neoplastic diseases of the hematopoietic system. In G.R. Lee, T.C. Bithell, J. Foerster, J.W. Athens, J.N. Lukens (eds). Wintrobe's Clinical Hematology. Philadelphia: Lea & Febiger, 1993.

11. Rosenberg, N., Krontiris, T.G.: The molecular basis of neoplasia. In: Hematology Basic Principles and Practice. Edited by R. Hoffman, et al. New York: Churchill Livingstone, 1995.

12. Barber, R., Spiers, P.: Oxford survey of childhood cancers: progress report ll. Monthly Bull Ministry of Health, 23:46, 1964.

13. Gunz, F.W., Veale, A.M.O.: Leukemia in close relatives—accident or predisposition? J. Natl. Cancer. Inst., 42:517, 1969.

14. Miller, R.W.: Relation between cancer and congenital defects: an epidemiological evaluation. J. Natl. Cancer. Inst., 40:1079, 1968.

15. First MIC Cooperative Study Group: Morphologic, immunologic, and cytogenetic (MIC) working classification of acute lymphoblastic leukemias. Cancer. Genet. Cytogenet., 23:189, 1986.

16. Second MIC Cooperative Study Group: Morphologic, immunologic and cytogenetic (MIC) working classification of the acute myeloid leukemias. Br. J. Haematol., 68:487, 1988.

17. Bennett, J.M., et al.: Proposals for the classification of the acute leukaemias. Br. J. Haematol., 33:451, 1976.

18. Kaplan, S.S., et al.: Immunophenotyping in the classification of acute leukemia in adults. Interpretation of multiple lineage reactivity. Cancer, 63:1520, 1989.

19. Keren, D.F.: Flow cytometry. Chicago, ASCP, 1989.

20. Li, C-Y., Uam, L.T.: Cytochemistry and immunochemistry in hematologic diagnoses. Hematol. Oncol. Clin. North. Am., 8:665, 1994.

21. Bain, B.J.: Leukaemia diagnosis. Philadelphia: J.B. Lippincott Co., 1990.

22. Lowenberg, B., Touw, I.P.: Hematopoietic growth factors and their receptors in acute leukemia. Blood, 81:281, 1993.

23. Gallardo, R., Kranwinkel, R.N.: Pseudo-Chediak-Higashi anomaly. Am. J. Clin. Pathol., 83:127, 1985.

24. Fanin, R., Baccarani, M.: Granulocyte-macrophage colony stimulating factor in acute non-lymphocytic leukaemia. J. Intern. Med., 236:487, 1994.

25. Mazanet, R., Griffin, J.D.: Hematopoietic growth factors. In: J.O. Armitage, K.H. Antman (eds). High-dose cancer therapy. Baltimore: Williams and Wilkins, 1992.

Acute leukemia

KEY TERMS

●

acute leukemia
fagot cells
mixed lineage acute leukemia
bilineage acute leukemia
biphenotypic acute leukemia

INTRODUCTION

The *acute leukemias* (ALs) are stem cell disorders characterized by a malignant neoplastic proliferation and accumulation of immature hematopoietic cells in the bone marrow. The cells are unable to differentiate into normal functional blood cells and appear by immunologic assays to be frozen in a specific maturational stage. These leukemic cells apparently escape programmed cell death (apoptosis). The net effect is expansion of the leukemic clone.[1]

There are two major categories of acute leukemias classified according to the cellular origin of the primary stem cell defect. If the defect affects primarily the myeloid stem cell, the leukemia is classified as acute myelocytic leukemia (AML) (nonlymphoid). If the defect affects primarily the lymphoid stem cell, the leukemia is classified as acute lymphocytic leukemia (ALL). Immunologic investigations reveal that both these types of acute leukemia are actually composed of heterogeneous subtypes even though the morphologic appearance of the blasts in the subtypes may be similar. It is not unusual for one subtype to evolve into another, especially when the primary lesion occurs in the CFU-GEMM stem cell. Often, it is difficult to determine which cell line is predominant, as several cell lines appear to proliferate abnormally at the same time. In these cases, diagnosis may become possible only with disease progression.

The most reliable parameters for defining the neoplastic cells and classifying the acute leukemias into major categories and subtypes are combinations of the FAB morphologic criteria, cytochemical reactions, immunologic probes of cell markers, cytogenetic and molecular genetic abnormalities.

ACUTE MYELOCYTIC LEUKEMIAS (AML) (NONLYMPHOCYTIC)

The acute myelocytic leukemias (AMLs) occur primarily in adults and in infants younger than 1 year. Acute myelocytic leukemia accounts for only 15% to 20% of the leukemias in children. There appears to be a sharp increase in incidence of AML in adults after 50 years of age. This also is the type of leukemia that is seen most frequently when myelodysplastic syndromes transform into leukemia.

Pathophysiology

For a discussion of the pathophysiology of leukemia, refer to the previous chapter. A brief review and insights into the molecular defect in acute promyelocytic leukemia will be given here. Leukemia is a clonal disorder, which means that leukemic cells originate from a single mutant progenitor cell. The mutant cell retains the ability to proliferate but has lost the capacity to differentiate and mature. The disease originates from hematopoietic tissue in the bone

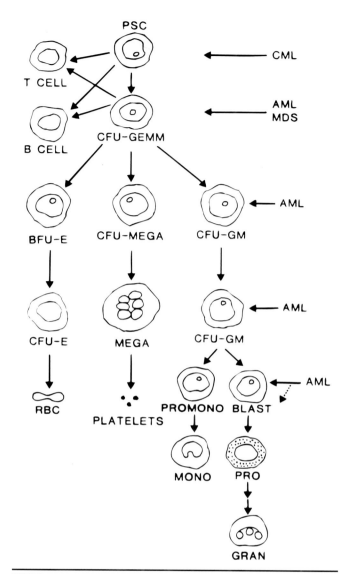

FIGURE 18-1. The cell of origin of AML. This is a schematic summary of data from surface marker and G6PD analysis indicating possible sites of origin of AML, chronic myeloid leukemia (CML), and myelodysplastic syndromes (MDS). [PSC, pluripotential stem cell; mega, megakaryocyte; CFU, colony-forming unit; GEMM, granulocytic, erythroid, monocytic, megakaryocytic; GM, granulocytic, monocytic; Promono, promonocyte; mono, monocyte; pro, promyelocyte; gran, granulocyte; BFU-E, burst-forming unit, erythroid, CFU-E, colony-forming unit, erythroid.] (From: Griffin, J.D., and Lowenberg, B. Clonogenic cells in acute myeloblastic leukemia. Blood, 68(6):1185, 1986).

marrow, but, with progression, malignant cells can be found to infiltrate multiple organs.

Investigations of clonogenic cells in AML have shown that the mutant neoplastic stem cell may arise at multiple points in the differentiation scheme of myeloid cells (Fig. 18-1). In some patients with AML, similar cytogenetic abnormalities are found in all progeny of the myeloid stem cell, including erythrocytes, granulocytes, monocytes, and megakaryocytes. This suggests the involvement of a neoplastic CFU-GEMM cell. This appears to be the target neoplastic cell in approximately one third of patients with AML.[2] In other patients, the cytogenetic abnormality is only present in granulocytes, suggesting the target neoplastic cell is a more mature precursor stem cell, perhaps the CFU-GM.

Evidence is mounting that the neoplastic clone develops from a stem cell with a genetic mutation(s) that affects the proliferation and differentiation of cells. The mutated gene is known as an oncogene, and its normal counterpart is a proto-oncogene. The oncogenes initiate a process that results in malignancy. The exact mechanism by which the oncogene causes malignancy has not been determined. In acute leukemia, research has focused on proto-oncogenes that code for hematopoietic growth factors and growth factor receptors.[3–6] Alterations in the growth factor/membrane receptor interactions, disruptions in the transduction of the message from the receptor to the nucleus, and defects in the transcription of genes have the potential to produce a cell that escapes normal regulatory mechanisms.

Many oncogenes have been identified at breakpoints associated with chromosome abnormalities in specific types of leukemia. The most common oncogenes in AML are mutated RAS family proto-oncogenes found in up to 30% of AML cases. RAS proto-oncogenes code for G-proteins, which bind and hydrolyze GTP and are important in modulating signal transduction from activated growth factor receptors. Thus, they are a part of the second messenger system (see Chapter 17). These G-proteins are located on the inner side of the plasma membrane and on other cytoplasmic organelle membranes. It has been shown that most RAS oncogenes produce increased active G-proteins. This suggests that signal transduction for cell proliferation and/or differentiation is increased.

One of the most intense areas of leukemia research is focused on the highly specific t(15;17) cytogenetic translocation of acute promyelocytic leukemia (APL). This translocation involves the retinoic acid receptor-alpha (RAR-α) gene on chromosome 17 and the PML gene on chromosome 15. This translocation is limited to neoplastic promyelocytes, has never been reported in other neoplastic diseases, and is present in virtually all APL cases.[7] Some APL cases have a cytogenetically normal karyotype, but molecular analysis has shown rearrangement of the PML and RAR-α genes. These findings suggest that the t(15; 17) translocation is involved in the pathogenesis of the disease. The gene rearrangement results in a fusion RAR-α/PML gene and a reciprocal PML/RAR-α gene. The PML/RAR-α mRNA has been identified in all APL patients, while the RAR-α/PML mRNA is found in about two thirds of APL patients.[8]

The RAR-α is a member of the superfamily of nuclear receptors. These receptors have two domains, one domain binds DNA and the other domain binds the retinoid hormones. Retinoids are regulators of cell proliferation, differentiation, and embryonal morphogenesis.[8] The RAR-α is activated by binding retinoid. The activated RAR-α then binds to specific sites in DNA where it functions in direct transcriptional control of specific target genes.

Thus, RAR-α is a part of the third messenger system in regulation of cell growth and differentiation. The role of the fusion gene products in APL has not been determined. It is proposed that the abnormal PML/RAR-α may not act as a normal retinoid receptor, thereby impairing or blocking differentiation.

Retinoic acid has proven to be an effective treatment for inducing complete remission in APL.[8] Molecular analysis has revealed that retinoic acid induces the neoplastic promyelocytes to differentiate to mature granulocytes, thus overcoming the maturation arrest.[9] It is possible that a high concentration of retinoic acid, as is given in induction therapy for APL, somehow overcomes the interference with receptor activation.

These findings in APL provide important insights into our understanding of leukemogenesis. Although the specific lesion is different in other leukemias, the pathogenic model may be similar.

● Clinical findings

As noted in the previous chapter, presenting signs and symptoms of the disease are related to the suppression of normal hematopoiesis. Pallor, fatigue, and weakness from the anemia are found in almost all patients. Bleeding, bruising, and petechial hemorrhages caused by thrombocytopenia also are constant features of the disease. Infection that fails to respond to appropriate therapy may be the first sign of leukemia. The infection is usually minor but, on occasion, may be more serious (pneumonia, meningitis). When fever is present, it is usually related to an underlying infection. Bone pain is not as common in AML as it is in ALL. Bone tenderness, however, is noted on physical examination in approximately two thirds of patients. Splenomegaly, hepatomegaly, and lymphodenopathy occur in approximately 50% of patients at the time of diagnosis.

The clinical findings of the M3 subgroup, acute promyelocytic leukemia, differ from other types of AML. A life-threatening coagulation disorder is a common presenting symptom. Patients are younger, have lower leukocyte counts, and organomegaly is uncommon.[10]

● Hematologic findings

PERIPHERAL BLOOD (TABLE 18-1)

A normocytic, normochromic anemia of variable severity is almost always present at the time of diagnosis. Occasionally, a macrocytic anemia with hypersegmented neutrophils is found, but the anemia does not respond to cobalamin or folic acid treatment, distinguishing it from megaloblastic anemia. Nucleated erythrocytes are often found on the blood smear. Anisocytosis and poikilocytosis may be present in variable degrees. The platelet count is usually moderately depressed. Thrombocytosis in AML is associated with abnormalities of chromosome 3, t(3;3) and inv(3). Hypogranular and giant platelet forms are commonly found. The leukocyte count is variable, ranging

TABLE 18-1 *LABORATORY FINDINGS CHARACTERISTIC OF AML*

PERIPHERAL BLOOD

Normochromic, normocytic anemia

Nucleated erythrocytes

Variable anisocytosis and poikilocytosis

Platelets usually decreased: hypogranular and giant forms present

Leukocyte count usually increased but may be normal or decreased

Blasts (15–95%), Auer rods may be present

Monocytosis

Neutropenia

Dysplastic neutrophils

Variable eosinophilia and basophilia

BONE MARROW

Hypercellular

Dysplastic

>30% blasts

from less than $1 \times 10^9/L$ to more than $100 \times 10^9/L$; more than 50% of the patients have a normal or decreased leukocyte count at the time of diagnosis but less than 20% have counts over $100 \times 10^9/L$. Regardless of the leukocyte concentration, diagnosis of AL is suggested by the presence of blasts on the blood smear. Blasts usually compose from 15% to 95% of all leukocytes. If AL is suspected by the physician but no blast cells can be detected on the blood smear, or if the leukocyte count is low (< 2 $\times 10^9/L$), a buffy coat smear should be prepared. This preparation will reveal the presence of blast cells even when present in very low concentrations if AL is present. The finding of blasts with azurophilic granules is helpful in identifying the myeloid nature of the leukemia. When Auer rods are present in blasts, they exclude a diagnosis of ALL. Auer rods can be found in myeloblasts, monoblasts, and occasionally in more differentiated monocytic or myelocytic cells.

Other abnormal findings on the blood smear often include monocytosis and neutropenia. The monocytosis frequently precedes overt leukemia. The few mature neutrophils present frequently demonstrate signs of myelodysplasia: pseudo Pelger-Huët anomaly, hypogranulation, and small nuclei with hypercondensed chromatin. This is especially common in M2 AML.[11,12] Eosinophils and basophils may be mildly to markedly increased. When present, basophilia may help to differentiate leukemia from a leukemoid reaction. Absolute basophilia is not present in a leukemoid reaction.

BONE MARROW

A bone marrow examination is always indicated when leukemia is suspected. Aspiration may yield a dry tap due to the packed marrow (hypercellular), however, biopsy will reveal sheets of blasts with a decrease in normal cells. In leukemia with severe peripheral leukopenia, blasts are difficult to find in the blood but are always present in abnormal amounts in the bone marrow. According to the FAB criteria for acute leukemia, blasts must compose more than 30% of the nonerythroid nucleated cells in the marrow to distinguish leukemia from the myelodysplastic syndromes. Frequently, the blast count is close to 100%. Auer rods bodies are present in bone marrow blasts in about half the cases of AML. Auer rods are considered to be abnormal primary granules and stain for myeloperoxidase and acid phosphatase. Phi bodies, considered a morphologic variant of Auer rods, are inclusion bodies found in AML that stain positive for hydroperoxidase.

When Auer rods are absent, blast morphology alone does not permit distinction of myeloblasts from lymphoblasts. Cytochemistry is necessary to define the myeloid nature of the blast cell population. As mentioned previously, myeloblasts are peroxidase and/or Sudan black B positive, whereas lymphoblasts are negative. At least 3% of the blasts should be positive for peroxidase or stain positive with Sudan black B to assign myeloid lineage to the blasts. To identify monocytic differentiation more than 20% of the blast cells should show diffuse positivity for nonspecific esterase. To identify megakaryoblasts, the blasts should show the presence of ultrastructural peroxidase.[13]

Rarely the bone marrow appears hypocellular, resembling aplastic anemia. Hypocellular AML is defined as a leukemia with a bone marrow cellularity of less than 30% and more than 30% blasts.[14] In these cases, distinction of AML from aplastic anemia may be made by staining the biopsy specimens for reticulin. An increase in fibroblasts is typical of AL but not aplastic anemia.

Dysplasia of leukocytes, erythrocytes, hypolobulation of megakaryocyte nuclei, abnormal granulation of granulocytes, and pseudo-Pelger-Huët anomaly may be present.

OTHER LABORATORY FINDINGS

Other laboratory findings may reflect the increased proliferation and turnover of cells. Hyperuricemia and an increase in lactate dehydrogenase are common findings resulting from the increase in cell turnover. Hypercalcemia, when present, is believed to be caused by increased bone resorption, associated with leukemic proliferation in the bone marrow. Increased serum and urine muramidase are typical findings in those leukemias with a monocytic component.

In the APL subtype (M3), prolonged prothrombin time and partial thromboplastin time, hypofibrinogenemia, and elevated fibrin degradation products are frequently found in association with ecchymoses and overt bleeding.[10]

● Classification

Since 1976, assignment to either major leukemia group (myeloid or lymphoid) and to subgroups within each major group has been based on morphologic and cytochemical characteristics established by the FAB classification system.[15] In the last decade, immunophenotyping of leukemic cells and cytogenetic analysis for chromosome aberrations also have been used to supplement morphological and cytochemical data. It is now widely accepted that the best approach to classifying acute leukemia uses a combination of morphologic, cytochemical, immunologic, and cytogenetic criteria.[14–18]

CYTOCHEMISTRY

As noted previously, initial classification of acute leukemias requires the distinction of AML from ALL. The cytochemical peroxidase stain is the most widely used parameter to make this distinction. In AML, at least 3% of the blasts are peroxidase and/or Sudan black B positive, whereas in ALL the blasts are negative. The finding of Auer rods or granules in blasts on Romanowsky-stained smears also will help identify blasts of the myeloid lineage.

Common cytochemical stains, if positive, contribute only negative evidence for ALL. If negative, they do not confirm ALL. Thus, further testing is suggested when blasts are negative with myeloperoxidase and Sudan black B.

IMMUNOPHENOTYPING

Immunofluoresence can be used to demonstrate terminal deoxynucleotidyl transferase (TdT) in individual cells. High levels are common in ALL. Although originally believed to be lymphoid-specific, TdT is now believed to be present on the more immature hematopoietic cells including those of early myeloid lineage.[19] It is consistently identified in up to 20% of AML cases.[20] Therefore, TdT should not be used alone in determining lymphoid lineage.

Immunophenotyping is a necessary component of AL classification, especially when the morphologic appearance and cytochemistry reactions do not clearly define cell lineage or when it is suspected that more than one neoplastic cell population is present. Some investigators have suggested that a specific sequence of testing with monoclonal antibodies be followed so that if insufficient cells are obtained for complete testing, the most useful information can be obtained.[14] The use of extensive panels also is costly and time-consuming. In most cases, lineage can be determined using a limited, representative panel of monoclonal antibodies.

The first panel of monoclonal antibodies should be those that can differentiate AML from ALL and T-ALL from B-ALL. About 90% to 99% of AML can be discriminated from ALL using the panel of antibodies in Table 18-2.[16,20] Immunophenotyping using monoclonal antibodies for differentiating AML from ALL should include typing for CD33, CD13, and CD65, which are present on mye-

loid cells, CD19, CD10, and CD24 present on B lymphoid cells, CD7 and CD2 present on T-lymphoid cells, HLA-DR present on myeloid and B-lymphoid cells (Table 18-2). Occasionally, myeloperoxidase may be identified in blasts at the ultrastructural level when negative by light microscopy. These blasts with myeloperoxidase identifiable only at the ultrastructural level are considered myeloid in nature if immunophenotyping reveals at least one lineage-specific myeloid antigen.[13]

When cytochemistry and immunophenotyping are used together, most cases of AL can be classified into lymphoid or myeloid. Rarely a population of malignant blasts is cytochemically negative by conventional and ultrastructural methods and nonreactive with both lymphoid and myeloid monoclonal antibodies. These leukemias are classified as undifferentiated. Another uncommon type of acute leukemia is characterized by a blast population with both myeloid and lymphoid markers on the same cell or with two separate populations of malignant blasts, one myeloid and the other lymphoid. These are considered to be mixed lineage leukemias. The definition and actual existance of mixed-lineage leukemia is controversial. Some believe that the presence of both myeloid and lymphoid markers on the same cell is an example of lineage infidelity of malignant cells.

The second panel of monoclonal antibodies should include antibodies to subtype the AML into granulocytic, monocytic, erythrocytic, and megakaryocytic lineages (Table 18-3). The M0, M1, M2, and M3 subtypes exhibit granulocytic differentiation, differing from each other in the degree of granulocyte maturation. The M4 exhibits both granulocytic and monocytic differentiation, whereas M5 shows predominantly monocytic differentiation, M6 shows erythrocytic differentiation, and M7 shows megakaryocytic differentiation.

The association of specific immunologic phenotypes with various FAB subgroups has not been established, although some associations have been made. The monoclonal antibodies that react with most cases of AML (subgroups M0–M5) include CD33, CD13, and CD65.[21] In addition, the monoclonal antibody that identifies myeloperoxidase, MAI, is helpful especially when cytochemistry for myeloperoxidase is negative. The CD34 marker and TdT are present on the least differentiated myeloid cells and are characteristically associated with M0 and M1. The CD34 marker also is found on the neoplastic megakaryoblasts of M7. The AMLs with monocytic differentiation generally have the CD14 and CD11b markers in addition to CD13 and CD33. The promyelocytic cells

TABLE 18-2 *DIFFERENTIATION OF ALL FROM AML USING IMMUNOPHENOTYPING WITH SELECTED MONOCLONAL ANTIBODIES*

Leukemia	HLA-DR	CD33	CD13	CD65	CD19	CD10	CD24	CD7	CD2
AML	+	+	+	+	−	−	−	−	−
B-Lymphocyte	+	−	−	−	+	+	+	−	−
T-Lymphocyte	−	−	−	−	−	−	−	+	+

TABLE 18-3 *THE PATTERN OF REACTIVITY WITH MONOCLONAL ANTIBODIES MOST COMMONLY OBSERVED IN THE FAB SUBTYPES OF AML.*

Subgroup	HLA-DR	CD34☆	CD13	CD33	CD11B	CD14	CD71 Glycophorin A	CD41, CD42*, CD61
M0	+	+	+	+ or −	usually −	usually −	−	−
M1	+	usually +	usually +	+	+ or −	usually −	−	−
M2	+	usually −	+	+	+ or −	usually −	−	−
M3	−	−	+	+	usually −	usually −	−	−
M4	−	−	+	+	+	+	−	−
M5	+	usually −	+ or −	+	+	+	−	−
M6	+ or −	−	+ or −	+ or −	−	−	+	−
M7	usually +	+	−	+ or −	−	−	−	+ *

TdT is usually used to identify early lymphoid precursors but may also be found in 10–20% of AML, particularly those of M0 and M1 subgroups.

* CD42 recognizes only more mature megakaryocytes

☆ recognizes stem cells

of M3 are usually negative for the immature myeloid markers HLA-DR and CD34, but positive for CD13 and CD33. Monoclonal antibodies that react with the transferrin receptor (CD71) are helpful in identifying the blasts of M6 as are the lineage specific markers for spectrin and glycophorin A. The blasts of M7 are positive for CD34 and CD33 in early cells. The presence of platelet peroxidase, glycoprotein IIIa (CD61), the glycoprotein IIb and IIb/IIIa complex (CD41) and glycoproteins IX and Ib (CD42a, CD42b) will help identify more mature megakaryoblasts. Cases not defined by either of these panels should be tested by antibodies that identify other subtypes of ALL.

CYTOGENETIC ANALYSIS OF AML

In acute leukemia, normal polyclonal cells are increasingly replaced by an abnormal clone of cells derived from a single neoplastic stem cell. In cytogenetic study, bone marrow cells are examined directly or after culture with mitogens. Chromosome abnormalities, if present, can be detected in cells in metaphase. In the majority of AML cases, consistent nonrandom chromosomal aberrations can be identified in the abnormal clone. The same abnormality is found in all progeny of the leukemic stem cell. Additional abnormalities may develop in subclones. A clone is present if two or more cells show identical structural chromosome change or additional chromosomes or if three cells show the same missing chromosome.[22]

It is estimated that approximately two thirds of those patients with AML have detectable cytogenetic abnormalities.[16] Of these, about 60% were found by the MIC Study Group to have specific, consistent aberrations. The most common cytogenetic abnormalities in AML are trisomy 8, monosomy 7, and deletion of the long arm of chromosome 7 (7q-), monosomy 5 and deletion of the long arm of chromosome 5 (5q-). The nonrandom chromosome abnormalities most commonly associated with the FAB subgroups are listed in Table 18-4 and will be discussed in the sections on FAB subgroups that follow.

BLAST COUNT

The FAB approach to diagnosing acute leukemia requires a minimal marrow leukocyte blast count of greater than 30%. Occasionally, blasts in the peripheral blood are greater than 30% but blasts in the bone marrow are less than 30%. To permit a diagnosis in this case, it has been proposed that the diagnosis of AML be made if the blast count in the bone marrow and/or peripheral blood is greater than 30%.[13] Recognizing that leukemic blasts are abnormal cells and frequently exhibit nuclear/cytoplasmic asynchrony with nuclear maturation lagging, it is recommended that when evaluating cells for the purpose of establishing a diagnosis of AML the following cells be included in the total blast count:[13]

TABLE 18-4 *NONRANDOM STRUCTURAL CHROMOSOMAL ABNORMALITIES IN ACUTE NONLYMPHOCYTIC LEUKEMIA*

Chromosomal Abnormality	Morphologic Association
Trisomy 8	Variable
Monosomy 7	M2,M4,M5
Monosomy 5, del(5q)	M1,M2
t(8;21)(q22;q22)	**M2**,*M4
t(15;17)(q22;q11-12)	**M3**
t(9;11)(p22;q23)	**M5**,M4,M2
del(11)(q22-23)	**M5**,M4,M2
inv(16)(p13;q22), del(16q)	**M4Eo**,M2,M5
t(6;9)(p23;q34)	M1,M2,M4; marrow basophilia
t(9;22)(q34;q11)	M1

* FAB subtypes in bold type identify strong associations with chromosomal abnormalities.

(From: Lee, GR, Bithell, TC, Foerster, J, Athens, JW, Luken JN.: Wintrobe's Clinical Hematology. 9th ed. Philadelphia, Lea & Febiger, 1993.)

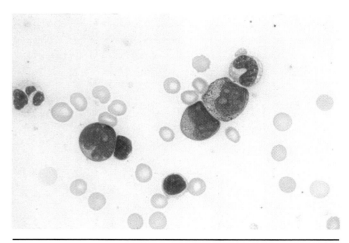

FIGURE 18-2. A type I blast on the left; type III blast in the center and a promyelocyte on the right. The nuclear chromatin pattern in the two blasts is similar but the type III blast has granules. (Bone marrow; 250 × original magnification; Wright-Giemsa stain)

1. Type I myeloblasts (Figure 18-2): typical myeloblasts with lacy open chromatin and prominent nucleoli, immature deep blue cytoplasm without granules.
2. Type II myeloblasts (Figure 18-3): blasts similar to Type I blasts except for the presence of up to 20 discrete azurophilic granules.
3. Type III myeloblasts (Figure 18-2): cells resembling the typical myeloblast except for the presence of numerous azurophilic granules. These cells are typically found in M2 with a t[8;21] chromosome abnormality, some cases of myelodysplasia and a rare form of M1.
4. Neoplastic promyelocytes associated with M3 AML.
5. Monoblasts and promonocytes of M5 AML.
6. Megakaryoblasts of M7 AML.

For a diagnosis of AML, there must be a minimum of 30% blasts present. It is recognized that the percentage of erythroblasts in the marrow influences the assessment

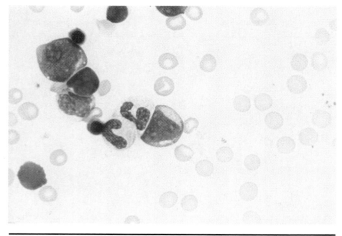

FIGURE 18-3. Type II blast (center) with only a few granules near the periphery of the cell. (Bone marrow; 250 × original magnification; Wright-Giemsa stain).

of the nonerythroid blast cells, if the differential count includes erythroblasts.[23] When a diagnosis of AML or myelodysplastic syndrome is suspected, the first step in bone marrow assessment is an estimation of the bone marrow cellularity, followed by an assessment of the percentage of erythroblasts. Further evaluation of the bone marrow depends on the number of erythroblasts present, greater than 50% or less than 50% of all the nucleated marrow cells.

If erythroblasts compose more than 50% of all nucleated bone marrow cells, the percentage of nonerythroid blast cells is determined by performing a differential count excluding the erythroid cells. This will help make a differential diagnosis between M6 AML and myelodysplastic syndrome. If 30% or more of all nonerythroid cells are blasts, the diagnosis is M6 AML, whereas if there are less than 30% blasts in the remaining nonerythroid population, the diagnosis is myelodysplastic syndrome.

If there are fewer than 50% erythroblasts in the bone marrow, it is not necessary to exclude the erythroblasts from the differential count to reach a diagnosis of acute leukemia or myelodysplastic syndrome. The diagnosis of AML (M0–M5) is made when 30% or more of all nucleated bone marrow cells are blasts. This method for counting blast cells when erythroblasts exceed 50% of all nucleated marrow cells, means that the criteria for a diagnosis of M6 AML are different from that of other AML subgroups because the marrow must reveal not only a minimum of 30% myeloblasts but also a minimum of 50% erythroblasts (Figure 18-4). For further assessment of the M0–M5 subtypes of AML, only the myeloid cells are evaluated, excluding lymphocytes, plasma cells, mast

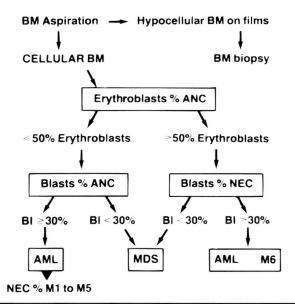

FIGURE 18-4. Suggested steps in the analysis of a bone marrow aspirate to reach a diagnosis. Suggested steps in the analysis of a bone marrow (BM) aspirate to reach a diagnosis of acute myeloid leukemia (AML, M0-M7) or myelodysplastic syndrome (MDS). B1 = blast cells; ANC = all nucleated bone marrow cells; NEC = nonerythroid cells. (From: Bennett, J.M., et al.: Proposed revised criteria for the classification of acute myeloid leukemia. Ann. Intern. Med., 103(4):620, 1985.)

TABLE 18-5 *BONE MARROW CRITERIA FOR CLASIFICATION OF AML*

	M1	M2	M3	M4	M5	M6
Blasts (as a % of all nonerythroid cells)	≥90%	30–89%	>30%	>30%	>80% of monocytic cells (5A) <80% of monocytic cells (5B)	>30%
Erythroblasts (as a % of all nucleated cells)	—	<50%	<50%	<50%	—	>50%
Granulocytic component (as a % of all nonerythroid cells)	<10%	>10%	>10%*	>20%†	<20%	variable
Monocytic component (as a % of all nonerythroid cells)	<10%	<20%	<20%	>20% to <80%‡	>80%‡	variable

* many promyelocytes with heavy granulation

† includes myeloblasts

‡ includes monoblasts

(Modified from Bennett, J. M., et al.: Proposed revised criteria for the classification of acute myeloid leukemia. Ann. Intern. Med. 103:620, 1985)

cells, macrophages, and nucleated erythrocytes (Table 18-5). Other criteria designed to distinguish between M1 and M2, between M2 and M4, and between M4 and M5 will be discussed within the description of each subtype in this section.

FAB SUBGROUPS OF AML

Although the subgroups of AML may originate from a common stem cell, CFU-GEMM or CFU-GM, the phenotype, clinical findings, cytogenetic abnormalities, and predominant neoplastic hematopoietic cell in the bone marrow and peripheral blood may differ among the subgroups (Table 18-6). This section will discuss these parameters in the eight AML subgroups.

M0 acute myeloid leukemia with minimal differentiation This AML shows minimal myeloid differentiation and may have formerly been classified as undifferentiated AML.[13,24] The blasts are negative with conventional cytochemical stains for myeloid cells, and morphologic differentiation is absent. In some cases, the blasts resemble ALL morphology, most often of the L2 subgroup. The blasts may show peroxidase activity by techniques designed to analyze cells at the ultrastructural level. If ultrastructural peroxidase is negative, the cells should show positivity with at least one monoclonal antibody of the myeloid lineage (CD13, CD33, CD11b, CD11c, CD14, CD15) to be classified as M0 AML.[25,26] Cells fulfilling these criteria that also show evidence of ultrastructural platelet peroxidase and platelet glycoproteins IIb/IIIa (CD 41) may repre-

TABLE 18-6 *CELLULAR CHARACTERISTICS OF ANLL SUBTYPES**

	AML	APL	AMMoL	AMoL	AEL	AMegL
Relative frequency						
Adults[11]	58%	7%	28%	6%	1%	—
Children[4]	52%	9%	21%	12%	3%	3%
Morphology						
FAB classification	M0,M1,M2	M3	M4	M5	M6	M7
Associated features						Cytoplasmic budding Myelofibrosis
Cytochemical features						
Myeloperoxidase	±†	+	+	±	−	−
Chlorocetate esterase	+	+	+	−	−	−
Nonspecific esterase	−	−	+	+	−	−
PAS	−	−	−	−	+	−
Platelet peroxidase	−	−	−	−	−	+
Cytogenetic abnormalities	t(8;21)	t(15;17)	del(16)(q22) inv(16)(p13q22)	t(11q) del(11q)		Abnormalities involving chromosomes 5,7,21

* ANLL, acute nonlymphocytic leukemia; AML, acute myelocytic leukemia; AMMoL, acute myelomonocytic leukemia; AMoL, acute monocytic leukemia; AEL, acute erythroleukemia; AMegL, acute megakaryocytic leukemia; APL, acute promyelocytic leukemia; PAS, periodic acid-Schiff.

† +, usually present or increased; −, usually absent or decreased; ±, may or may not be present.

(From: GR Lee, et al.: Wintrobe's Clinical Hematology. Philadelphia: Lea & Febiger, 1993)

TABLE 18-7 *DISTINGUISHING CHARACTERISTICS OF M1 AND M0 MYELOBLASTS FROM L2 LYMPHOBLASTS*

Characteristic	L2	M0	M1
Myeloperoxidase	negative	usually positive at ultrastructural level	>3% positive; may be seen at ultrastructural level
PAS	negative or chunky positive	negative	negative or diffusely positive
TdT	positive	usually negative	usually negative
CD2	helpful if positive	may be positive	usually negative
CD7	helpful if positive	may be positive	usually negative
CD13	negative	usually positive	usually positive
CD33	negative	usually positive	positive
TCR gene rearrangement	helpful if positive	negative	negative
Immunoglobulin gene rearrangement	helpful if positive	negative	negative

sent megakaryocytic lineage and are more appropriately classified as AML-M7.[13] Diagnosis of M0 AML cannot be made on morphology alone but requires immunophenotyping to exclude lymphoid lineage. Some M0 cases have been reported in which TdT, CD2, CD4, and CD7 (lymphoid markers) are present but MP0 at the ultrastructural level is present and T-cell receptor genes are not rearranged. It is recommended that these cases be considered M0 AML rather than biphenotypic AL.[27]

M1 myeloblastic leukemia without maturation (Figure 18-5)

This AML variant is most common in adults and in infants younger than 1 year. Leukocytosis is present in about 50% of patients at the time of initial diagnosis. The predominant cell in the peripheral blood is usually a poorly differentiated myeloblast with fine lacy chromatin and nucleoli. Occasionally, only a few blast cells are seen, but the bone marrow always reveals a sharp increase in blasts. Platelets are generally decreased.

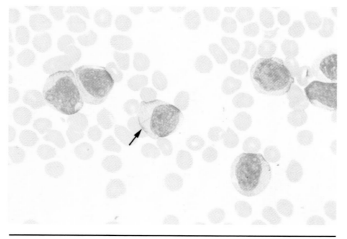

FIGURE 18-5. Myeloblasts in the peripheral blood from a case of M1 AML. Auer rod (arrow) is present in the center blast. Note the high nuclear to cytoplasmic ratio, the fine, lacy chromatin and prominent nucleoli. (250 X original magnification, Wright-Giemsa stain.)

The hypercellular bone marrow reveals that 90% or more of the nonerythroid cells are myeloblasts. The remaining cells are promyelocytes or more mature granulocytes and monocytes. Auer rods are rarely found in the blasts. A few blasts may have scant azurophilic granules. If no evidence of granules or Auer rods is present, the blasts may resemble L2 lymphoblasts. However, cytochemical stains and immunophenotyping will help differentiate the myeloblasts from lymphoblasts (Table 18-7).

The myeloblasts are large with a small to moderate amount of blue-gray cytoplasm. The nucleus is round, oval, or irregular with fine lacy chromatin and several distinct nucleoli. Vacuoles may be present. Dysmyelopoiesis is almost always present. Dyserythropoiesis and dysthrombopoiesis also may be found.

The myeloperoxidase or Sudan black B stain is positive in more than 3% of the blasts, indicating granulocyte differentiation. Naphthol AS-D chloroacetate (specific esterase) may be positive, but the nonspecific esterases, alpha-naphthyl butyrate and alpha-naphthyl acetate, are negative. Napthol AS-D acetate is weakly positive and insensitive to NaFl inhibition. Auer rods stain similar to reactions in myeloblasts (Table 18-8).

Approximately 50% of patients will have acquired clonal chromosome aberrations in the leukemic cells. If the karyotype is abnormal, the prognosis is significantly worse. Chromosome aberrations associated with this subgroup include trisomy 8(+8), t(9;22), t(6;9), del(5q-) and monosomy 5. Trisomy 8 is the most frequent chromo-

TABLE 18-8 *CYTOCHEMICAL REACTIONS FOR AUER RODS*

SBB	+
MPO	+
Napthol AS-D Chloroacetate Esterase	±
PAS	±
Romanowsky (occasionally only seen with MPO or SBB)	+ or −

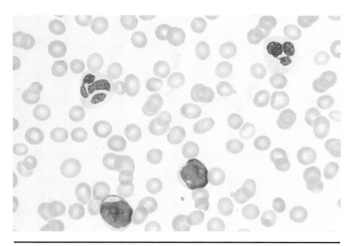

FIGURE 18-6. Myeloblasts and hypogranular segmented neutrophils from a case of M2 AML. (Peripheral blood; 250 × original magnification; Wright-Giemsa stain).

some abnormality in AML and although found most commonly in M1; it also may be found in M3, M4, and M5.

M2 myeloblastic leukemia with maturation (Figure 18-6)
The M2 variant of AML is most common in adults and accounts for about 30% of AML cases. As in the M1 variant, leukocytosis is present in approximately 50% of patients at initial diagnosis. The remaining 50% have normal counts or are leukopenic. Thrombocytopenia is almost always present. Myeloblasts can usually be found in the blood smears and may be the predominant cell type.

The bone marrow is hypercellular and myeloblasts make up from 30% to 89% of the nonerythroid nucleated cells. The myeloblasts are large with variable amounts of cytoplasm and azurophilic granules. Auer rods are a common finding. The nucleus may be round, oval, or reniform, resembling that seen in monocytic cells with fine lacy chromatin and nucleoli. The monocytic component is less than 20%, differentiating M2 from M4. The differentiation characteristic from M1 is that maturation of granulocytes from the promyelocyte stage and beyond is present in more than 10% of the nucleated nonerythroid cells.

Myelocytes and metamyelocytes often show abnormal morphologic characteristics, including nuclear/cytoplasmic maturation asynchrony, hypogranularity, or abnormal granules. Pseudo-Pelger-Huët anomaly in neutrophils and binucleated blasts, promyelocytes, myelocytes, and metamyelocytes can be found.

Eosinophils, basophils, and occasionally plasma cells may be increased. Although in most cases maturation occurs along the line to neutrophils, occasionally bone marrow eosinophilia or basophilia occurs, suggesting the neoplastic cells have entered alternate maturation pathways. These cases are sometimes designated M2E0 or M2 BASO.[24]

Peroxidase, and Sudan black B stains are more strongly positive and a larger percentage of cells show reactivity in M2 than in M1. The specific and nonspecific esterase reactions are usually negative.

Cases of M2 are strongly associated with a chromosome translocation involving chromosomes 8 and 21, t(8;21) (q22;q22).[28] The proto-oncogene, c-myc, is involved in this translocation. This abnormality also has been reported in M4. When the t(8;21) abnormality is present, additional chromosome changes such as loss of a sex chromosome and 9q-, are common. The presence of the t(8;21) is usually associated with a better prognosis, unless additional aberrations are present. There is a strong association between the t(6;9) chromosome abnormality in M2 and basophilia and/or a previous myelodysplastic syndrome.[29] Basophilia in M2 also is associated with deletion of the short arm of chromosome 12(12p-). The t(9; 22) abnormality also may be found but not as frequently as in M1.

M3 hypergranular promyelocytic leukemia
The M3 subgroup accounts for 5% to 10% of AML cases. It occurs in a younger age group than M1 or M2 and is more virulent than other AML variants. The median age at diagnosis is 39, and survival averages about 18 months. The most common clinical finding in initial diagnosis is bleeding. It is believed that the release of large numbers of promyelocytic granules that contain a procoagulant initiate disseminated intravascular clotting (DIC). This is the most serious complication of M3 AML. Effective therapy potentiates this complication when large numbers of granules are released from lysed promyelocytes. There may be a 50-fold increase in tissue factor from dying cells during cytotoxic therapy.[10] Tissue factor release into the blood can activate the clotting process. There also is evidence of fibrinolysis. Heparin therapy is usually administered with initiation of chemotherapy to prevent DIC, but the treatment is controversial. Other abnormalities of coagulation may be present. Two forms of M3 have been described: the typical hypergranular type and the hypogranular or microgranular variant (M3v).

HYPERGRANULAR M3 (FIGURE 18-7) Most patients with the hypergranular type are leukopenic or exhibit only slightly increased leukocyte counts. The count is rarely high. Blasts and promyelocytes with heavy granulation and multiple Auer rods are found on blood smears. In some cases, the typical hypergranularity of promyelocytes is less evident in the peripheral blood than in the bone marrow.[30] Anemia and thrombocytopenia are typical findings.

Most cells in the bone marrow are abnormal promyelocytes with heavy azurophilic granulation. Sometimes the granules are so densely packed that they obscure the nucleus. There also are some cells filled with fine dust-like granules. Cells with multiple Auer rods, sometimes occurring in bundles *(fagot cells)*, are characteristic (Figure 18-8). The cytoplasm of fagot cells is frequently clear and pale blue, but it may contain a few azurophilic granules or lakes of clear pink material. The nucleus varies in shape but is often folded or indented or sometimes bilobed. Often a high number of promyelocytes appear to be disrupted on the blood smear, with azurophilic granules and

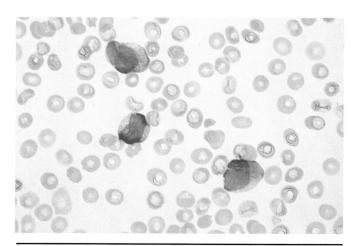

FIGURE 18-7. Abnormal promyelocytes from a case of hypergranular promyelocytic leukemia (M3). (Peripheral blood; 250 × original magnification; Wright-Giemsa stain).

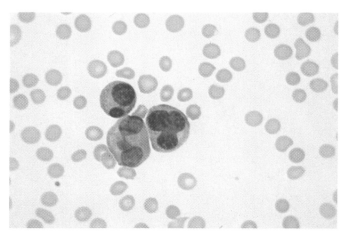

FIGURE 18-9. Abnormal promyelocytes from a case of hypogranular variant of promyelocytic leukemia (M3). (Peripheral blood; 250 × original magnification; Wright-Giemsa stain)

Auer rods lying over and between intact cells. It is important to distinguish M3 from M2, which also may have an increase in promyelocytes. In M2, the granulation is not as heavy and does not pack the cytoplasm as in M3.

MICROGRANULAR M3 VARIANT In contrast to typical hypergranular M3, the leukocyte count in microgranular M3 is usually markedly increased. The predominant cell in the peripheral blood is a promyelocyte with a bilobular, reniform, or multilobed nucleus (resembling that of a monocyte) and cytoplasm devoid of granules or with only a few fine azurophilic granules (Figure 18-9).

The nuclear chromatin is fine with nucleoli often visible. A small abnormal promyelocyte with a bilobed nucleus, deeply basophilic cytoplasm and sometimes cytoplasmic projections, is present as a minor population in most cases but occasionally may be the predominant cell. When cytoplasmic projections are present, the cells resemble megakaryoblasts. Fagot cells are scarce or absent but

single Auer rods may be found. The finding of a few cells with the typical cytoplasmic features of hypergranular M3 will help to distinguish this leukemia from a monocytic leukemia. In contrast to the hypogranular appearance of peripheral blood promyelocytes, the bone marrow promyelocytes are more typical of the cells found in the hypergranular form of M3 (Figure 18-10).

Peroxidase, Sudan black B, and naphthol AS-D chloroacetate esterase are strongly positive. Naphthol AS-D acetate esterase may be positive but is not inhibited by NaFl. The alpha-naphthyl butyrate and alpha-naphthyl acetate esterases for nonspecific esterases are negative. In some cases, cytochemistry results are confusing because the neoplastic cells stain for nonspecific esterase that is fluoride-sensitive or for both specific and fluoride-sensitive nonspecific esterases.

Recently, a form of M3 has been described in which some promyelocytes contain metachromatic granules

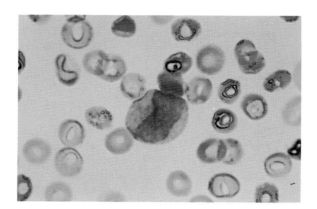

FIGURE 18-8. A fagot cell from promyelocytic leukemia. Notice the bundle of Auer rods. (Bone marrow; 250 × original magnification; Wright-Giemsa stain)

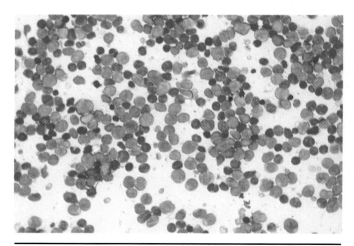

FIGURE 18-10. Bone marrow aspirate from the patient in Figure 18-9. The abnormal promyelocytes are the predominant cell. (100 × original magnification, Wright-Giemsa stain).

(when stained with toluidine blue).[31] Distinctive features include folded nuclei, hypergranular cytoplasm, and coarse metachromatic granules.

APL is associated with a diagnostic translocation involving chromosomes 15 and 17, t(15;17). This aberration has only been seen in APL. As described earlier, this translocation involves rearrangement of the retinoic acid receptor-alpha (RAR-α) gene and the PML gene.

Treatment with all-trans retinoic acid is the standard therapy used to induce remission. This induces the leukemic cells to differentiate into short-lived mature myeloid cells. The leukocyte count progressively increases, reaching a peak at 12 to 14 days. Abnormal promyelocytes gradually disappear. The duration of the remission is often brief. In some cases, retinoic acid therapy is followed by chemotherapy. Reverse-transcription polymerase chain reaction (RT-PCR) assay to detect the presence of the PML/RAR-α hybrid gene has been suggested to monitor therapy and predict relapse.[32] The presence of the mutated gene is correlated with relapse and its absence is associated with prolonged survival.

About 25% of patients given retinoic acid therapy become acutely ill. The mortality rate in these individuals is high. The illness is similar to capillary leak syndrome with fever, respiratory disease, renal impairment, and hemorrhage.[8] The management of the "retinoic acid syndrome" has not been defined.

M4 myelomonocytic leukemia (Naegeli type)   This variant of AML derives its name from the finding of both myelocytic and monocytic differentiation in the peripheral blood and bone marrow. It is distinguished from M1, M2, and M3 by an increased proportion of leukemic monocytic cells in the bone marrow or peripheral blood or both (Figure 18-11). It is one of the most common AML variants, ac-

counting for 20% to 30% of AML cases. Infiltrations of leukemic cells in extramedullary sites is more frequent than in the pure granulocytic variants. Gingival hyperplasia is present in about 10% of patients. Serum and urinary levels of muramidase are usually elevated because of the monocytic proliferation.

The leukocyte count is usually increased. Monocytic cells (monoblasts, promonocytes, monocytes) are increased to 5 × 10^9/L or more. Anemia and thrombocytopenia are present in almost all cases.

The bone marrow resembles M2, with blasts composing more than 30% of the nonerythroid component. However, the marrow differs from M1, M2, and M3 in that monocytic cells (monoblasts, promonocytes, monocytes) exceed 20% of the nonerythroid nucleated cells. The sum of the myelocytic cells, including myeloblasts, promyelocytes, and later granulocytes, is greater than 20% and less than 80% of the nonerythroid cells. This bone marrow picture together with a peripheral blood monocyte count of 5 × 10^9/L or more (including all stages of monocytic maturation) is compatible with a diagnosis of M4. The myeloblasts appear as described in M1 and M2. Monoblasts are usually large with abundant bluish-gray cytoplasm. The nucleus is round or convoluted with delicate chromatin and one or more nucleoli. The bone marrow may reveal erythrophagocytosis by monocytes.

There are two situations in which either the blood or bone marrow picture does not conform to the above criteria. In these cases, ancillary laboratory tests are used to confirm the presence of a significant monocytic component and establish a diagnosis of M4. The ancillary tests suggested are lysozyme levels or cytochemical methods (Table 18-9).

SITUATION 1   If the bone marrow findings are as described above but the peripheral blood monocyte count is less

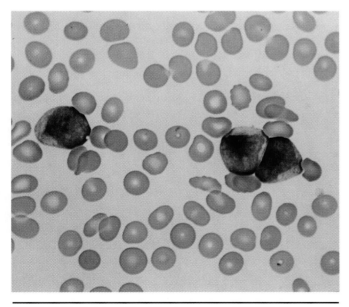

FIGURE 18-11. Peripheral blood film from a case of M4 AML. These nucleated cells are monoblasts. (250 × original magnification; Wright-Giemsa stain).

TABLE 18-9   *FAB CRITERIA FOR AN M4 DIAGNOSIS*

1) Peripheral blood ≥5 × 10^9/L monocytic cells
Bone marrow:
  Blasts ≥30% of nonerythroid cells
  Monocytic cells >20% to <80% nonerythroid cells
  Granulocytic component >20% to <80%

OR

2) Peripheral blood <5 × 10^9/L monocytic cells and bone marrow monocytic cells ≥20% to <80% of nonerythroid nucleated cells

and

  Ancillary tests:
    Serum or urinary lysozyme 3 times normal or
    Naphthol AS-D chloroacetate esterase and alpha-naphthyl acetate esterase or naphthol AS-D acetate esterase with and without NaFl reveal >20% monocytic cells in bone marrow

OR

3) Peripheral blood: ≥5 × 10^9/L monocytic cells
Bone marrow: Similar to M2 AML criteria
Ancillary tests: As shown in (2) above

than 5×10^9/L, a diagnosis of M4 can be made if serum or urinary lysozyme concentrations exceed three times the normal reference values. If cytochemical methods are used, a double esterase reaction with specific napthol AS-D chloroacetate esterase and nonspecific α-naphthyl esterase or naphthol AS-D acetate with and without NaFl should demonstrate that more than 20% of bone marrow cells are of the monocytoid lineage for a diagnosis of M4.

SITUATION 2 If the peripheral blood monocyte count is 5×10^9/L or more but the bone marrow resembles M2 rather than M4, either the lysozyme test or cytochemical methods described above should be used. If either of these tests reveals a significant monocytic component, a diagnosis of M4 can be made.

Cytochemical methods demonstrate two cell populations: myeloblasts and promyelocytes; monoblasts and promonocytes. Myeloblasts are positive for peroxidase, Sudan black B, and naphthol AS-D chloroacetate esterase. The nonspecific esterase, α-naphthyl acetate esterase, is negative. Monoblasts are negative or only slightly positive for peroxidase, and naphthol AS-D chloroacetate esterase and demonstrate a negative or fine granular Sudan black B positivity. The nonspecific esterases are positive and inhibited by sodium fluoride. Some blasts are impossible to distinguish as either myelocytic or monocytic because they have cytochemical reactions of both cell lines.[33] For example, in some cases, there is an overlap of blasts with peroxidase and nonspecific esterase positivity.

In some cases of M4 with eosinophilia, abnormal eosinophils account for 5% or more of the nonerythroid nucleated cells in the marrow. There are both eosinophilic and large, atypical basophilic granules within the same cell. The nucleus is often monocytoid. These cells stain positive with naphthol AS-D chloroacetate esterase and PAS, whereas normal eosinophils do not. The M2 AML variant (M2EO) also may have an increase in eosinophils, but these cells have normal granules and stain as typical eosinophils. The eosinophilic variant of M4 (M4EO) is strongly correlated with translocation, deletion or inversion of the long arm of chromosome 16, t(16;16), del(16q) and inv(16). Differentiation also may be along the basophilic pathway (M4BASO). Basophilia is associated with t(6;9). Trisomy 4 (+ 4) and a variety of deletions and translocations involving 11q23 are associated with M4.

M5 monocytic leukemia (Schilling type)

This subgroup accounts for 5% to 15% of AML cases. The most common clinical findings in the M5 variant are weakness, bleeding, and a diffuse erythematous skin rash. There is a high fre-

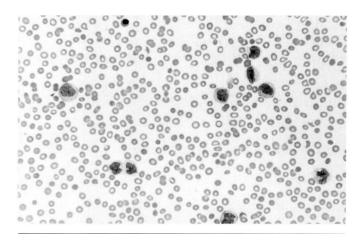

FIGURE 18-12. Peripheral blood film from a case of M5 AML. There is a predominance of monocytic cells with a monoblast on the left and many promonocytes. There is also a nucleated erythrocyte at the top. (100 × original magnification; Wright-Giemsa stain)

quency of extramedullary infiltrations of the lungs, colon, meninges, lymph nodes, bladder, and larynx. Serum and urinary muramidase levels are often extremely high.

The criterion for a diagnosis of M5 is that 80% or more of all nonerythroid cells in the BM are monocytic (including monoblasts, promonocytes, and monocytes) (Figure 18-12). There are two distinct forms, 5A and 5B, classified according to degree of differentiation (Table 18-10). The granulocytic component in the bone marrow usually accounts for less than 10% of the nucleated cells but may increase to 20%.

5A POORLY DIFFERENTIATED (FIGURE 18-13) This variant is the more frequent AML in children. Monoblasts account for 80% or more of all monocytic cells in the bone marrow. The remaining 20% of monocytic cells are monocytes with only rare promonocytes. Some monoblasts may be found in the peripheral blood. The monoblasts are large (up to 40 μm) with voluminous, variably basophilic cytoplasm. Pseudopods with transluscent cytoplasm are common. Azurophilic granules may be present. The nucleus is round or oval with delicate chromatin and one or more nucleoli but Auer rods are not found. Dyshematopoiesis is not conspicuous.

5B WELL DIFFERENTIATED (FIGURE 18-14) The well-differentiated form of M5 also reveals more than 80% monocytoid cells in the nonerythroid bone marrow but, in contrast to M5A, in M5B monoblasts account for less than 80% of the

TABLE 18-10 *CRITERIA FOR DIAGNOSIS OF M5 AML*

	Peripheral Blood	Bone Marrow Monocytic Component (nonerythroid)	Bone Marrow Monoblasts	Maturation Index
M5A	≥5 × 10⁹/L monocytic cells	≥80%	≥80% of all monocytic components	≤4%
M5B	≥5 × 10⁹/L monocytic cells	≥80%	<80% of all monocytic components	>4%

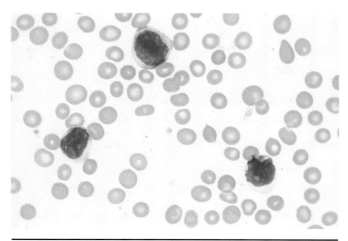

FIGURE 18-13. Monoblasts from a case of M5A AML. (Peripheral blood; 250 × original magnification; Wright-Giemsa stain).

monocytic component. More than 20% of the monocytic cells show evidence of maturation to the promonocyte or monocyte stage. In some cases, the percentage of blasts is less than 30%; however, if the total number of monocytes, promonocytes, and monoblasts is greater than 80% in the bone marrow, it still can be called acute leukemia. The promonocytes in the marrow are similar to monoblasts, except that they have a large cerebriform nucleus with delicate chromatin. Nucleoli may be present. The cytoplasm is less basophilic than that of the monoblast with a ground-glass appearance. Fine azurophilic granules are often present. Monocytes in the peripheral blood are increased and monoblasts are often present.

The diagnosis of M5A or M5B is usually confirmed from the results of cytochemical stains. The nonspecific esterase stains, alpha-naphthyl butyrate esterase or alpha-naphthyl acetate esterase, are positive. The specific esterase, naphthol AS-D chloroacetate esterase, is negative. Myeloperoxidase and Sudan black B show absent or weak diffuse activity in the monoblasts.

Abnormalities of the long arm of chromosome 11, with translocations or deletions, are characteristic although not diagnostic for monocytic leukemias. The t(8;16) abnormality is associated with significant phagocytosis. The expression of FOS proto-oncogene on chromosome 14 that has been linked to proliferation and differentiation of cells, appears to be enhanced in M4 and M5 leukemia cells.[34] There is a positive correlation between the amount of FOS transcripts and the percentage of cells expressing cell markers for monocyte maturation. This enhanced expression of FOS may be a molecular marker for monocytic cell differentiation in leukemia.

M6 erythroleukemia (DiGuglielmo's syndrome)   Erythroleukemia is a rare form of leukemia accounting for less than 5% of AML cases. It usually affects adults over 50 years of age. It is almost nonexistent in children. It primarily affects the erythroid cells. Clinical manifestations are similar to those observed in other subtypes of AML. The most frequent presenting symptoms are bleeding, or those related to anemia. As the disease progresses, myelocytic and megakaryocytic involvement in the leukemic process becomes more evident with gradual hyperplasia of these cell lines. Frequently, the disease evolves into M1 or M2 acute myeloblastic leukemia (Figure 18-15). Mean survival is about 11 months.

The most dominant changes in the peripheral blood are anemia with striking poikilocytosis and anisocytosis. Nucleated erythrocytes demonstrate abnormal nuclear configurations similar to those identified in myelodysplasia. The leukocyte alkaline phosphatase score is normal or increased. Leukocytes and platelets are usually decreased.

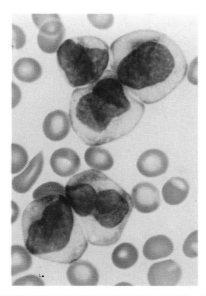

FIGURE 18-14. Monocytic cells, predominantly promonocytes, from acute monocytic leukemia (M5B). (Peripheral blood; 250 × original magnification; Wright-Giemsa stain).

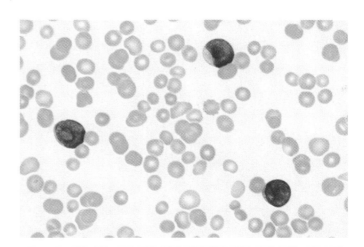

FIGURE 18-15. Blasts in the peripheral blood from a patient with M6 AML and in blast crisis. The blast morphology is typical of M1 AML. (250 × original magnification; Wright-Giemsa stain).

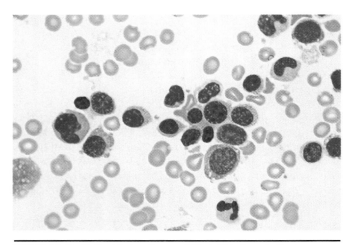

FIGURE 18-16. Erythroblasts with megaloblastoid features in the bone marrow from a case of M6 AML. (250 × original magnification; Wright-Giemsa stain).

The diagnosis of erythroleukemia can be made when more than 50% of all nucleated bone marrow cells are erythroid and 30% or more of all remaining nonerythroid cells are myeloblasts. A rare form of "true erythroid leukemia" occurs when the bone marrow is replaced by proliferating erythroblasts showing no maturation beyond basophilic normoblasts. In this entity, there is no myeloblast proliferation.

The bone marrow erythroblasts are distinctly abnormal, with bizarre morphologic features. The cells are megaloblastoid with distinct chromatin and parachromatin arranged in a "tortoise" pattern (Figure 18-16). Cobalamin and folic acid levels are normal or increased. Giant multilobular or multinucleated forms are common (Figure 18-17). Other features include nuclear budding and frag-

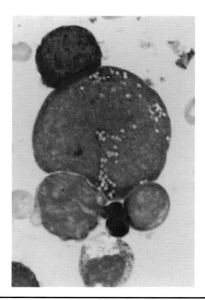

FIGURE 18-17. Multinucleated erythroid precursor from erythroleukemia (M6). (bone marrow) (Bone marrow; 250 × original magnification; Wright-Giemsa stain).

mentation, cytoplasmic vacuoles, Howell-Jolly bodies, and ringed sideroblasts. Erythrophagocytosis by the abnormal erythroblasts is a common finding. Auer rods may be found in the myeloblasts. Dysmegakaryopoiesis is common, with mononuclear forms or micromegakaryoblasts present. Neutrophils may exhibit hypogranularity and pseudo-Pelger-Huët anomaly.

Normal erythroblasts are PAS negative, however, in erythroleukemia, some erythroblasts, especially pronormoblasts, demonstrate coarse positivity superimposed on diffuse or granular positivity. PAS-positive erythroblasts also are found in MDS, other subgroups of AML, iron deficiency anemia, thalassemia, severe hemolytic anemia, and sometimes in megaloblastic anemia. The myeloblastic component of M6 shows reactions similar to those found in M1. Aneuploidy (abnormal number of chromosomes) and abnormalities of chromosomes 5 and 7 are associated with this subtype. The chromosome 5 and 7 abnormalities are often associated with secondary leukemia.

M7 acute megakaryoblastic leukemia This acute leukemia has been known by several different names: acute malignant myelosclerosis, acute myelodysplasia with myelofibrosis, and acute myelofibrosis. Because of the similarity of clinical and hematologic findings, all these disorders are believed to represent the same entity, acute megakaryoblastic leukemia. The disease is rare (3 to 12% of AML) and may occur de novo or as a leukemic transformation of CML and myelodysplastic syndromes. Various chemotherapy regimens have been used, but remission has not been achieved.

Patients usually present with pallor and weakness because of anemia and bleeding. Results of physical examination show no significant organomegaly.

Pancytopenia is characteristic at initial diagnosis, followed by a high peripheral blood blast count in the later stages of the disease. On careful examination of the blood smear, micromegakaryocytes and undifferentiated blasts may be found. The blasts are pleomorphic without any specific distinguishing characteristics and may resemble L2 lymphoblasts or M1 myeloblasts. However, the finding of cytoplasmic blebs is suggestive that these cells are megakaryoblasts. Megakaryocyte fragments may be present.

Bone marrow aspiration usually results in a dry tap. Biopsy reveals increased fibroblasts and/or increased reticulin and greater than 30% blasts. The fibrosis is believed to be secondary to the increase in megakaryocytes. It has been suggested that megakaryocytes secrete a platelet mitogenic factor that stimulates fibroblast proliferation.[2] The blasts may be identified as megakaryocytic by immunophenotyping, cytochemistry, and electron microscopy.[35] The blasts are highly variable ranging from small round cells with scant cytoplasm and dense heavy chromatin to cells with moderately abundant cytoplasm with or without granules and nuclei with lacy chromatin and prominent nucleoli. Some blasts may have cytoplasmic blebs. About 20% to 30% of the blasts are two to three times the size of lymphocytes. Occasionally megakaryocytes with shedding platelets are seen. Dysplasia of all cell lines is a common finding.

Peroxidase, Sudan black B, and naphthol AS-D chloroacetate esterase for specific esterase are negative, distinguishing the megakaryoblasts from myeloblasts. In more mature cells, the PAS is positive with distinct localized deposits. The acid phosphatase also shows localized positivity. The alpha-naphthyl butyrate esterase is negative but the alpha-naphthyl acetate esterase is positive, a reaction typical for megakaryoblasts. Undifferentiated blasts may be identified as megakaryoblasts by electron microscopy. These immature cells exhibit demarcation of the membrane system and a positive platelet peroxidase (PPO) reaction at the ultrastructural level. The PPO activity occurs in the perinuclear space and in the endoplasmic reticulum.

The monoclonal antibodies that react with platelet glycoproteins, Ib (CD42b), IIb/IIIa(CD41), and IIIa(CD61), have been used to identify cells of the megakaryocytic lineage. The antibodies against IIb/IIIa or IIIa recognize both the megakaryoblast and mature megakaryocyte, but the antibody against Ib recognizes only the more mature megakaryocytes.

Abnormalities of chromosomes 21 and 8 have been described in association with M7. Among patients with Down syndrome in whom acute megakaryoblastic leukemia developed, all had a translocation of chromosome 21. Abnormalities of chromosomes 5 and 7 are associated with secondary leukemia.

Maturation index

In an attempt to provide a sharper distinction between M1 and M2 and between M5a and M5b, it has been proposed that a maturation index (MI) be used in addition to the FAB criteria.[36] The original FAB criteria for M1 and M2 and for M5a and M5b are primarily based on the degree of maturation of leukemic cells. The maturation index is an attempt to objectively quantify this maturation. From a bone marrow or peripheral blood differential, the percentage of promyelocytes/promonocytes and blasts are determined and entered into the following formula:

$$MI = \frac{\text{promyelocytes (in myeloblastic)/promonocytes (in monoblastic)} \times 100}{\text{blasts} + \text{promyelocytes/promonocytes}}$$

The highest degree of maturation (either in peripheral blood or bone marrow) is used to determine the AML subtype. In most cases of the original study, higher maturation occurred more frequently in the bone marrow than in the peripheral blood. The dividing line between subtypes is 4% (M1 ≤ 4%, M2 > 4%, and M5a ≤ 4%, M5b > 4%). It has been suggested that distinction between these particular subtypes is important in prognosis since a smaller degree of maturation (M1 and M5A) is associated with a larger tumor mass and a shorter remission period.

ACUTE LYMPHOBLASTIC LEUKEMIA

Acute lymphoblastic leukemia (ALL) is primarily a disease of young children with a peak incidence between the ages of 2 and 5 years. It is characterized by a malignant proliferation of lymphoid stem cells. The malignant lymphocytes replace normal hematopoietic tissue in the bone marrow and infiltrate the lymph nodes, spleen, liver, and other organs. The predominant cell in the bone marrow and peripheral blood can be identified as a lymphoblast. Like AML, ALL is a heterogeneous disorder with a variety of morphologic and immunologic subtypes. Without treatment, survival is short, but with recently developed treatment regimens, most children enter a period of prolonged remission and many appear to be "cured."

Pathophysiology

The basic abnormality appears to be the mutation of a single lymphoid stem cell giving rise to a clone of malignant lymphocytes. These lymphoid cells retain the ability to proliferate in an unregulated manner but appear to be frozen in their maturation sequence. As discussed in the previous chapter, the trigger for the original leukemic genetic mutation is unknown but may be a combination of leukemogenetic factors. As in AML, the impairment of normal hematopoiesis is the primary cause of concern.

Clinical findings

The onset of the disease is usually abrupt and continues in a progressive manner. Symptoms are related to anemia, thrombocytopenia, and neutropenia. Common complaints include fatigue, pallor, fever, weight loss, irritability, and anorexia. Fever is often related to a concomitant infection. Petechiae and ecchymoses are present in more than half of patients; frank hemorrhage is less common. Bone pain is noted in about 80% of patients with tenderness, especially over the long bones. Often the child refuses to walk or stand. Occasionally children have symptoms related to CNS involvement, including headaches and vomiting. Splenomegaly, hepatomegaly, and lymphadenopathy are common findings.

Hematologic findings (table 18-11)

PERIPHERAL BLOOD

The leukocyte count may be increased, decreased, or normal. About 60% of the patients have leukocytosis due to

TABLE 18-11 *LABORATORY FINDINGS CHARACTERISTIC OF ALL*

PERIPHERAL BLOOD
Leukocyte count usually increased but may be normal or decreased
Neutropenia
Lymphoblasts
Normocytic, normochromic anemia
Thrombocytopenia

BONE MARROW
Hypercellular
>30% lymphoblasts

an abundance of immature lymphoid cells. Neutropenia is often marked even when the total leukocyte count is increased. Blast cells usually appear in the blood. The blasts are small with scant cytoplasm, indistinct chromatin, and absent or poorly defined nucleoli. The platelet count is usually decreased. Normocytic, normochromic anemia is almost always present and can be severe. Anisocytosis, poikilocytosis, and nucleated erythrocytes, however, are not usually present. Thrombocytopenia is present in over 90% of cases.

BONE MARROW

The hypercellular bone marrow reveals replacement of normal hematopoietic cells by lymphoid elements. By definition, there are 30% or more lymphoblasts but in reality most patients have more than 65% blasts present. The morphology of the blasts is variable and will be described with the FAB classification discussed below. Auer rods are not present in lymphoblasts. Intracytoplasmic inclusions have been described in the lymphoblasts of patients with ALL. The punctate staining and cytochemistry of these inclusions syggest they are probably lysosomal in origin.[37,38] Cytochemistry, enzyme analysis for TdT, and immunophenotyping help identify the lymphoid nature of these abnormal cells (Table 18-12).

In lymphoblasts, the peroxidase, Sudan black B, and napthal AS-D chloroacetate esterase are negative. The PAS reaction usually demonstrates a coarse granular or block-like positivity. Some myeloid leukemias also may demonstrate this type of reactivity. In AML, however, the granular pattern is superimposed on a diffusely positive back-ground, whereas in lymphoblasts there is no background positivity. Napthol AS-D acetate, alpha-naphthyl acetate, and alpha-naphthyl butyrate are negative or weakly positive in null cell ALL and B-ALL but show localized coarse positivity in T-ALL. Acid phosphatase shows an intense localized positive reaction in T-ALL. This reaction is not diagnostic of T-ALL, however, since it may be seen in M6 AML and M7 AML as well as in rare cases of B-ALL. In L3 ALL, the vacuoles stain with oil red O, indicating the presence of lipid.

FAB classification

The FAB group has defined three subtypes of ALL (L1, L2, L3) based on the morphology and heterogeneity of bone marrow lymphoblasts (Table 18-13).[15] Cytologic features used to evaluate blast morphology include:

1. cell size
2. nuclear chromatin
3. nuclear shape
4. nucleoli
5. amount of cytoplasm
6. amount of basophilia in cytoplasm
7. cytoplasmic vacuolation

Up to 10% of the cells may vary from each specific feature within the subgroup.

L1 ALL (FIGURE 18-18)

This is the most common ALL found in children. It appears to have the best prognosis. The key to this subtype

---

TABLE 18-12 *CHARACTERISTICS OF BLASTS IN ACUTE LYMPHOCYTIC LEUKEMIA SUBTYPES*

Characteristic	Early B Precursor	Common B (CALLA)	Pre-B Cell	B Cell	Early T-Precursor	T Cell
Gene rearrangement:						
Immunoglobulin	+	+	+	+	−	−
T-cell receptor (TCR)	−	−	−	−	+	+
Immunologic features:						
Cytoplasmic μ	−	−	+	−	−	−
Membrane Ig	−	−	−	+	−	−
CD19	+	+	+	+	−	−
CD24,CD10	−	+	+	+ (CD10 usually negative)	−	−
CD20	−	−	+	+	−	−
CD2,CD7	−	−	−	−	+ (CD2 may be negative)	+
Cytochemical stains:						
TdT	+	+	+	−	+	+
Acid phosphatase	−	−	−	−	+	+
Cytogenetic abnormalities	t(4;11), t(9;22)	6q-, t(12p), 12p-, t(9;22)	t(1;19), t(9;22)	t(8;14), t(2;8), t(8;22), 6q-	t(9p), 9p-	t(11;14), 6q-
FAB subgroup (most frequent)	L1, L2	L1, L2	L1	L3	L1, L2	L1, L2

+ usually present; − usually absent

(Adapted from: Lee, G. R. et al.: Wintrobe's Clinical Hematology. Philadelphia: Lea & Febiger, 1993)

TABLE 18-13   *FAB CRITERIA FOR THE SUBTYPES OF ALL*

Cytological Features	L1	L2	L3
Cell size	Small cells predominate	Large, heterogeneous in size	Large and homogeneous
Nuclear chromatin	Homogeneous in any one case	Variable-heterogeneous in any one case	Finely stippled and homogeneous
Nuclear shape	Regular, occasional clefting or indentation	Irregular; clefting and indentation common	Regular-oval to round
Nucleoli	Not visible, or small and inconspicuous	One or more present, often large	Prominent; one or more vesicular
Amount of cytoplasm	Scanty	Variable; often moderately abundant	Moderately abundant
Basophilia of cytoplasm	Slight or moderate, rarely intense	Variable; deep in some	Very deep
Cytoplasmic vacuolation	Variable	Variable	Often prominent

(From Bennett, J.M., et al., Proposals for the classification of the acute leukaemias. Br. J. Haematol., 33:451, 1976)

is homogeneity of lymphoblasts. Most cells within any one case are homogeneous in size but heterogeneity is compatible with L1 if all other features considered suggest L1. The lymphoblasts are predominantly small, up to twice the size of a small lymphocyte. The chromatin is usually finely dispersed but may appear more condensed in small cells. The chromatin pattern may vary from case to case but is homogeneous within cases. The nuclear shape is regular with occasional clefts or identations. Nucleoli are not prominent and may be absent. The cytoplasm is scant and only slightly or moderately basophilic.

L2 ALL (FIGURE 18-19)

This is the most frequent ALL found in adults. Occasionally, the cells have granular inclusions, making it difficult to distinguish L2 from M2 AML, if cytochemical stains are not performed. In contrast to granules in myeloid cells, the granules in lymphoblasts are peroxidase-negative and the cells are positive for TdT. In contrast to the blasts of L1, the blasts in L2 demonstrate a marked heterogeneity in any one case and between cases. There is a great deal of variability in cell size within each case, but the cells are generally two times the size of small lymphocytes. The nucleus is irregular with clefting and indentations. The chromatin pattern in any one case is heterogeneous, varying from finely reticular to condensed. Nucleoli are always present but vary in size and number. Often they appear very large. The cytoplasm is abundant with variable basophilia.

L3 ALL (BURKITT TYPE)(FIGURES 18-20 AND 18-21)

This is the rarest form of ALL. It occurs in both adults and children. The lymphoblasts are similar in appearance to those found in Burkitt's lymphoma. The blasts are homogeneous both within and between cases. The cells are large with abundant, intensely basophilic cytoplasm. There is prominent cytoplasmic vacuolization. Vacuoles also may be present in L1 and L2 lymphoblasts but it is much less intense than in L3. The nucleus is oval to round, with dense but finely stippled chromatin and one or more prominent nucleoli.

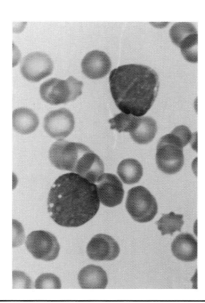

FIGURE 18-18. Lymphoblasts in peripheral blood from L1 acute lymphocytic leukemia. Notice the nuclear cleavage. (250 × original magnification; Wright-Giemsa stain).

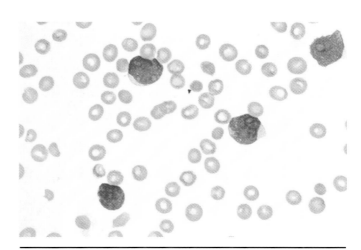

FIGURE 18-19. Lymphoblasts in peripheral blood from L2 acute lymphocytic leukemia. (250 × original magnification; Wright-Giemsa stain).

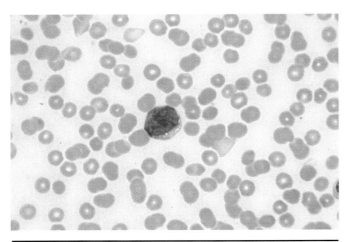

FIGURE 18-20. Lymphoblast in peripheral blood from L3 acute lymphocytic leukemia. Notice the vacuoles. (250 × original magnification; Wright-Giemsa stain).

SCORING SYSTEM FOR FAB CRITERIA IN ALL

Although the above criteria has served to help classify most cases of ALL, it was recognized that it is sometimes difficult to distinguish between L1 and L2. The cells in L3 are so unique that there is little difficulty in classifying this type of ALL. To improve the FAB classification, a scoring system for assessing both qualitative and quantitative morphologic features of the blasts has been proposed (Table 18-14).[39] The total score may range from −4 to +2. A score of 0 to +2 classifies the ALL as L1, whereas a score of −1 to −4 classsifies the ALL as L2. A positive, negative, or no score may be assigned to each criteria. The categories and criteria for scoring are:

1. Nuclear/cytoplasmic ratio (−1 to +1 score possible):
   Positive score—if 75% or more of cells have a high N:C ratio.
   Negative score—if 25% or more of cells have a low N:C ratio.

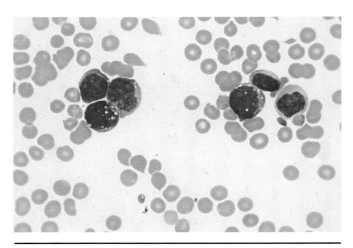

FIGURE 18-21. Lymphoblasts in the bone marrow from the patient in Figure 18-20. (250 × original magnification; Wright-Giemsa stain).

TABLE 18-14 *SCORING SYSTEM FOR L1 AND L2*

Criteria*	Score†
High N/C ratio ≥75% of cells	+
Low N/C ratio ≥25% of cells	−
Nucleoli: 0 to 1 (small) ≥ 75% of cells	+
Nucleoli: 1 or more (prominent) ≥25% of cells	−
Irregular nuclear membrane ≥25% of cells	−
Large cells ≥50% of cells	−

* The following are not scored: (1) intermediate or indeterminate criteria, (2) regular nuclear membrane in ≥75% of cells, and (3) <50% large cells, regardless of cell size heterogeneity.

† Positive (+) or negative (−).

(From Bennett, J.M., et al. The morphologic classification of acute lymphoblastic leukaemia: concordance among observers and clinical correlations. Br. J. Haematol., 47:553, 1981)

No score—if cells do not conform to either of the above criteria.
2. Nucleoli (−1 to +1 score possible):
   Positive score—if 75% or more of the cells have ill-defined small nucleoli.
   Negative score—if 25% or more of the cells have well-defined prominent nucleoli.
   No score—if cells do not conform to either of the above criteria.
3. Nuclear membrane (only a negative or no score possible):
   Negative score—if 25% or more of the cells have an irregular nuclear membrane.
   No score—if membranes are regular or possess irregularity in less than 25% of cells.
4. Cell size (only a negative or no score possible):
   Negative score—if 50% or more of the cells are large (at least two times the size of small lymphocytes).
   No score—if cells do not meet the above criteria.

● Immunologic phenotype of ALL

Research with surface markers and intracellular markers has shown that lymphoblasts in ALL vary considerably in immunologic maturation. In normal lymphoid cells, some antigenic determinants (surface markers) appear at a very early developmental stage and disappear with maturity, whereas others appear on more mature cells. Monoclonal antibodies have demonstrated that leukemic cells may have phenotypes of normal cells but appear to be frozen in a certain maturational stage. However, a significant number of acute leukemias express inappropriate combinations of antigens, making diagnosis challenging. Treatment protocols and prognosis are proving to be more effective and accurate when the leukemic cell is immunologically classified. In addition, evaluation of therapy response and detection of residual leukemic cells is possible using immunophenotyping, especially when the leukemic cell phenotype deviates from its normal cell counterpart.

The MIC classification of acute ALL recognizes four

TABLE 18-15 *CELLULAR MARKERS USEFUL IN DIAGNOSIS AND CLASSIFICATION OF B-ALL*

Subgroup P	TDT	HLA-DR	CD19	CD24	CD10	CD20	Rearrangment of Ig Genes	Cytoplasmic μ	Membrane Ig
Early B precursors	+	+	+	−	−	−	+	−	−
Common ALL (CALLA)	+	+	+	+	+	−	+	−	−
Pre-B-ALL	+	+	+	+	+	+	+	+	−
B-ALL	−	+	+	+	usually −	+	+	−	+

TABLE 18-16 *MONOCLONAL ANTIBODIES USEFUL IN THE DIAGNOSIS AND CLASSIFICATION OF T-ALL*

Subgroup	Tdt	CD7	CD2(E-receptor)
Early T-precursor ALL	+	+	−
T-ALL	+	+	+

immunologic subgroups of B-ALL and two immunologic subgroups of T-ALL.

B-ALL

The B-ALL subgroups include early B-precursor-ALL, common ALL (cALL), pre B-ALL, and B-ALL (Table 18-15).[14] Early B-precursor-ALL was formerly included in undifferentiated ALL (U-ALL). Recently, however, it was found that the characteristic cell in this ALL had the early B-cell marker, CD19, as well as rearranged immunoglobulin genes. As discussed in Chapter 4, the assembly of the D-J immunoglobulin genes is the first genetic event that identifies a B-cell progenitor. The next stage of B-cell maturation is identified by the presence of the common acute lymphocytic antigen, CALLA (CD10), and the early B-cell marker CD24. If the neoplastic cell has these markers, the ALL is known as common ALL. Common ALL is the most frequent ALL found in children in the western world. It seems to have the best prognosis of the immunologic subtypes. This is also the type of ALL found most frequently when chronic myelocytic leukemia (CML) transforms to an ALL. The next two subgroups of B-ALL, pre-B ALL and B-ALL, are identified by the B-lymphocyte surface antigens mentioned above plus the CD20 antigen that appears in the more differentiated B-cell. In addition, cytoplasmic or surface membrane immunoglobulin (CyIg, SmIg) are also identified at the pre-B and B-lymphocyte developmental stages. Malignancies of later stages of B-lymphocyte differentiation are included in chronic neoplastic lymphoproliferative disorders.

T-ALL

The two T-ALL subgroups, early T-precursor ALL and T-ALL, are differentiated using only two CD markers, CD7 (gp40 protein), CD2 (E-receptor), and TdT (Table 18-16). This classification does not recognize the antigenic heterogeneity of T-ALL but when used with the B-ALL

markers of CD19, CD10, TdT, HLA-DR, CyIg, and SmIg, 90% of ALL will be classifiable into one of the B-ALL or T-ALL subgroups.[14]

A wider panel of monoclonal antibodies can be used to further classify the ALL into subgroups that are believed to reflect normal maturation (Figures 18-22 and 18-23). Between 18% and 35% of ALLs in adults express myeloid antigens, while 10% to 20% of ALLs in children express these antigens.[36] This phenotype is probably a reflection of the abnormal maturation and differentiation of the neoplastic cell.

T-ALL occurs most often in males. A mediastinal mass is a common finding, and the total leukocyte count is usually higher than in other immunologic subtypes.

UNCLASSIFIED ALL (U-ALL)

Unclassified ALL (also known as null cell ALL, or non-B, non-T-ALL) is classified as such because the lymphoblasts lack any of the markers for the other subtypes. However, with the discovery of additional markers for B cells, it can be demonstrated that most of the null ALL lymphoblasts are actually B cells. Very few ALLs are now classified as U-ALL. In some cases, the cells are only positive for the HLA-DR and TdT. These two markers are common to less mature T- and B-lymphocytes, indicating that the common precursor of T- and B-lymphocytes probably also possesses these markers. Thus, it is possible that the blasts found in U-ALL may represent the committed lymphoid stem cell.

CORRELATION OF IMMUNOLOGIC AND FAB CLASSIFICATIONS

Although attempts have been made to correlate the FAB subtypes of ALL with the immunologic subtypes, there appears to be no clear distinctions with the exception of L3 which are all B-ALL.

Terminal deoxynucleotidyl transferase

In addition to identification of lymphocytes by immunophenotyping, certain intracellular enzymes are proving to be helpful in identifying cellular subtypes. The most important of these is terminal deoxynucleotidyl transferase (TdT), a DNA polymerase found in cell nuclei. Its presence

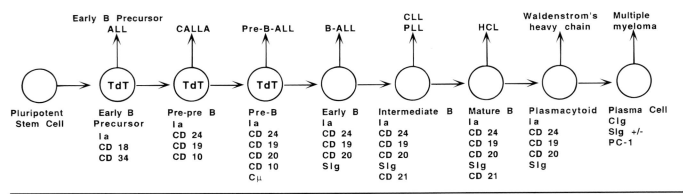

FIGURE 18-22. Normal B-lymphocyte maturation scheme with leukemic and other lymphoproliferative counterparts. (Adapted from Keren, D.F.: Flow cytometry in Clinical Diagnosis. Chicago, ASCP. 1989). (ALL = acute lymphocytic leukemic; CLL = Chronic lymphocytic leukemia; PLL = Prolymphocytic leukemia; HCL = hairy cell leukemia; CIg = cytoplasmic immunoglobulin; SIg = surface immunoglobulin.)

can be determined by direct enzyme assay, and indirect or direct immunofluorescence, using monoclonal antibodies. This enzyme is not present in normal mature lymphocytes but can be found in 65% of the total thymic population of lymphocytes. The TdT positive cells are localized in the cortex. It also can be found in very early B cells and blasts of early myeloid lineage. About 1% to 3% of normal bone marrow cells are TdT positive. Its value in ALL is to iden-

tify primitive lymphoblasts from more mature cells.[40] It also can be identified in M0 and M1 AML.

●
Cytogenetic abnormalities in ALL

Abnormal karyotypes can be demonstrated in 50% to 60% of the cases of ALL (Table 18-17). Abnormalities appear to be more common in B-ALL and common-ALL than in T-ALL. Both hyperdiploidy and hypodiploidy have been described. Patients who have chromosome counts greater than 50 have a better prognosis with long-

FIGURE 18-23. Normal T-lymphocyte maturation scheme with leukemic counterparts. (ALL = acute lymphocytic leukemia; CLL = Chronic lymphocytic leukemia).

TABLE 18-17 NONRANDOM STRUCTURAL CHROMOSOME ABBERATIONS IN ALL

Immunophenotype	Chromosomal Abnormality	Genes Involved
B-Lineage ALL	t(4;11)(q21;q23)	
	t(5;14)(q31;q32)	IL-3, IgH
Pre-B cell ALL	t(1;19)(q23;p13)	prl, E2A
B cell ALL	t(8;14)(q24;q32)	c-myc, IgH
	t(2;8)(p11;q24)	c-myc, Igκ
	t(8;22)(q24;q11)	c-myc, Igλ
T cell ALL	t(11;14)(p13;q11)	tcl-2, TCRα
	t(1;14)(p34;q11)	TCRα
	t(8;14)(q24;q11)	c-myc, TCRα
	t(10;14)(q24;q11)	Tcl-3, TCRα
	t(1;14)(p32;q11)	TCRα
	t(14;14)(q11;q32)	TCRα
	t(7;9)(q35−36;q34)	TCRβ
	t(7;14)(q35−36;q11)	TCRβ
	t(7;7)(p15;q11)	TCRγ
	t(7;14)(p15;q11)	TCRγ
	inv(14)(q11;q32)	TCRα
	inv(14)(q11;q32)	tcl-1, TCRα
Variable	t(9;22)(q34;q11)	c-abl, bcr
	del 9(p21−22)	If-α, if-β1

* IL-3, interleukin 3; IgH, κ,λ, immunoglobulin heavy, kappa and lambda light chains; TCRα,β,γ, T cell receptor α,β,γ-genes; bcr, breakpoint cluster region; If-α,β1, interferon α,β1-genes

(From: Lee, GR, et al.: Wintrobe's Clinical Hematology. 9th ed. Philadelphia, Lea & Febiger, 1993).

term remission. A normal karyotype is also associated with a better prognosis. Patients with numerical and/or structural abnormalities with modal counts less than 50 have a worse prognosis. About 10% to 15% of children with ALL have the Ph chromosome, which is associated with a poor prognosis. The FAB L3 subtype is characterized by a translocation of 8 to 14, t(8;14). In particular, the following aberrations are associated with a poor prognosis; t(9;22), t(8;14), t(4;11). A summary of the immunologic, morphologic, cytochemical, and cytogenetic characteristics of ALL subtypes is given in Table 18-9.

MIXED LINEAGE LEUKEMIA

The terminology concerning *mixed lineage acute leukemias* is confusing and controversial. The term *"bilineage"* is generally used to define those leukemias that have two separate populations of leukemic cells, one which phenotypes as lymphoid and the other as myeloid. The term *"biphenotypic"* describes acute leukemias that have myeloid and lymphoid markers on the same population of neoplastic cells. Lack of lineage specificity could be the result of genetic misprogramming or the leukemic clone could represent a bipotential cell that has retained both lymphoid and myeloid markers during development.[41,42]

Immunologic phenotyping is necessary to define mixed lineage leukemias because there are no definitive morphologic and cytochemical features for lymphoid cells.[21,43] Since lineage markers are generally "lineage associated" and not "lineage specific," a single inappropriate surface marker should not be used as sole evidence for biphenotypic leukemia. Cells should have at least two inappropriate markers to be considered biphenotypic.[44] Biphenotypic leukemia is suspected if the percentage of blasts having myeloid markers overlaps with the percentage having lymphoid markers. More specific diagnosis is possible if a double labeling technique using two immunologic markers or a combination of cytochemistry and immunologic markers is used. This procedure distinguishes between bilineage and biphenotypic acute leukemias because it can be determined if the same cell has two separate markers.

A more inclusive scheme for identifying mixed-lineage leukemia requires a combination of morphologic, cytochemical, immunologic, and cytogenetic evaluation and subsequent association of these features with one or the other lineage.[45] The importance of an inclusive scheme for classification of leukemia is emphasized by the finding of T-cell markers (CD7 and CD2) and a B-cell marker (CD19) in a significant number of cases of AML.[41,42] The blasts in these cases lack any other features of lymphoid lineage and many express abnormal karyotypes associated with AML rather than ALL. Based on these findings, it has been proposed that some cell markers may have a broader spectrum of reactivity than previously believed.[42] Alternatively, lineage infidelity may be a characteristic of some malignant cells.

Although mixed-lineage leukemias are uncommon, it is important to identify them to determine their actual occurrence, to identify appropriate therapy, and to correlate karyotypic abnormalities.[16]

ACUTE UNDIFFERENTIATED LEUKEMIA (AUL)

Occasionally, the blasts of acute leukemia may not stain with the standard cytochemical stains and surface markers. In these cases, the morphology of the blasts is nonspecific. Before a diagnosis of AUL is made, electron microscopic studies should be performed to detect ultrastructural evidence of primary granules and/or peroxidase. A positive finding with this technique indicates nonlymphocytic leukemia and is important for treatment decisions. A negative finding with electron microscopy together with the other negative findings indicates a diagnosis of acute undifferentiated leukemia. AUL is predominantly found in adults and only about one third of patients respond to the chemotherapy regimens of AML and ALL.

MYELOID/NATURAL KILLER (NK) CELL ACUTE LEUKEMIA

Investigators from the Southwest Oncology Group (SWOG) recently proposed a new group of acute leukemia, myeloid/natural killer cell acute leukemia.[46] These leukemic cells coexpress myeloid antigens (CD33, CD13, and/or CD15) and NK cell-associated antigens (CD56, CD11b), while they lack HLA-DR and T-lymphocyte associated antigens, CD3 and CD8. Most cases morphologically resemble M3v AML with invaginated nuclear membranes, scant to moderate amounts of cytoplasm, fine to moderately coarse azurophilic granules, and finely granular myeloperoxidase and Sudan black B positivity (weaker than in M3). No fagot cells are present. In contrast to M3 AML, however, the leukemic cells of this group demonstrate cell-mediated cytotoxicity characteristic of NK cells. The initial leukocyte count is usually high. The percentage of bone marrow blasts is high (47% to 99%).

In contrast to M3 AML, the leukemic cells of myeloid/NK cell acute leukemia do not show the t(15;17) abnormality or express the PML/RAR-α fusion transcript. Furthermore, patients do not respond to all-trans retinoic acid therapy. Other cytogenetic abnormalities are sometimes present.

Clinical findings overlap with other acute leukemias. Some patients have a bleeding diathesis consisting of petichial and/or mucosal hemorrhage or disseminated intravascular coagulation. Most do not have splenomegaly or hepatomegaly. The median survival is 30 months.

It is suggested that myeloid/NK cell acute leukemia is a distinct disorder and should not be considered a subgroup of M3 AML or NK-large granular lymphocyte (LGL) leukemia, a lymphoproliferative disorder. Rather the myeloid/NK cell acute leukemia is believed to be derived from a transformation of a stem cell common to myeloid and NK lineages.

SUMMARY

The acute leukemias (AL) are a heterogeneous group of neoplastic stem cell disorders characterized by unregulated proliferation and blocked maturation. The two major groups of AL are acute myelocytic leukemia (AML) and acute lymphocytic leukemia (ALL). These two major groups are further classified into subtypes based on FAB morphologic criteria, cytochemical stains, immunologic analysis, cytogenetic and molecular abnormalities. The FAB classification describes eight subtypes for AML and three for ALL. The AML subgroups are defined based on the degree of cellular differentiation and lineage of blasts. The subgroups include myeloid (M0–M3), monocytic (M4–M5), erythrocytic (M6), and megakaryocytic (M7). The FAB ALL subgroups are based on morphology of blasts and include L1, L2, and L3. Immunophenotyping in ALL helps subtype the blasts into B-ALL or T-ALL. There is no clear-cut association between FAB subgroups of ALL and immunologic phenotype except that all L3 ALLs are B-ALLs.

The peroxidase and/or Sudan back B cytochemical stains help differentiate AML (peroxidase positive) from ALL (peroxidase negative). Subgrouping the AMLs further requires additional cytochemical stains.

Also helpful in differentiating ALs is cytogenetic analysis. The most specific abnormality associated with FAB subgroups is the t(15;17) found only in M3. This abnormality has been shown at the molecular level to involve the retinoic acid receptor (RAR) gene and the PML gene. Other cytogenetic abnormalities are not specific for a particular subgroup but some are associated with particular subgroups.

Mixed lineage leukemia is used to describe ALs that have two separate populations present (myeloid and lymphoid) or have blasts that possess myeloid and lymphoid markers on the same cell. This lack of specific lineage may be due to genetic misprogramming of the leukemic cell or the leukemic clone could represent a bipotential stem cell that has retained markers of both cell lineages.

The onset of AL is usually abrupt and, without treatment, progresses. Symptoms are related to anemia, thrombocytopenia, and/or neutropenia. Splenomegaly, hepatomegaly, and lymphadenopathy are common findings. Hematologic findings include a normocytic, normochromic anemia, thrombocytopenia and usually an increased leukocyte count. Blasts are almost always found in the peripheral blood. A bone marrow examination is always indicated if leukemia is suspected. The bone marrow reveals more than 30% blasts.

Treatment of leukemia is discussed in Chapter 17.

REVIEW QUESTIONS

A 34-year-old Latin American male had been in excellent health until two weeks before admission when he noticed a mild sore throat, and was seen at a neighborhood clinic where penicillin was prescribed. He was able to return to work and felt better until four days prior to admission when he noticed some fever and easy bruising. He noticed no other bleeding symptoms, no epistaxis, gingival bleeding, or petechiae. He reported to the emergency room where an abnormal blood count was noted and he was admitted for further evaluation.

Admission laboratory data:

Erythrocyte count	3.2×10^{12}/L
Hb	9.7 gm/dL
Hct	0.31 L/L
Platelet count	31×10^9/L
Leukocyte count	26.2×10^9/L
Differential:	
Promyelocytes	79%
Myelocytes	9%
Lymphocytes	12%

Erythrocyte morphology: Erythrocytes are normochromic and normocytic.

A bone marrow aspirate and biopsy was performed to aid in diagnosis. The bone marrow biopsy revealed a hypercellular marrow. The bone marrow aspirate revealed an M:E ratio of 7.8:1. The predominant cell was an atypical immature cell with an indented or lobulated nuclear configuation. Heavy cytoplasmic granulation was present and multiple Auer rods were seen in several cells.

Cytochemical stains showed that these cells were Sudan Black B positive, specific esterase positive, and non-specific esterase positive with only slight fluoride inhibition present. (Use this data for questions 1-4.)

1. Based on the morphology and cytochemical stains of these cells, what is the most likely diagnosis?
   a. acute myelogenous leukemia with maturation (AML-M2)
   b. acute promyelocytic leukemia (AML-M3)
   c. acute myelomonocytic leukemia (AML-M4)
   d. acute monocytic leukemia (AML-M5)

2. What is the major complication associated with this leukemia:
   a. central nervous system involvement
   b. severe leukopenia
   c. bone marrow failure
   d. disseminated intravascular coagulation (DIC)

3. What chromosome abnormality is associated with this leukemia?
   a. t(15;17)
   b. inv(16)
   c. t(8;21)
   d. t(9;11)

4. If this patient was treated with all-trans retinoic acid and two weeks later the blood count was repeated, what would you expect to find?
   a. a decreased leukocyte count
   b. pancytopenia
   c. an increased leukocyte count
   d. erythrocytosis

5. In attempting to subtype a case of acute leukemia, the clinical laboratory scientists noted that the blasts were negative with myeloperoxidase, Sudan black B, naphthol AS-D chloracetate esterase, alpha-naphthyl acetate. Peroxidase was positive at the ultrastructural level. These blasts should show positivity with the following monoclonal antibodies:
   a. CD24
   b. CD7
   c. glycophorin A
   d. CD41, CD42, CD61

6. In a case of ALL, the lymphoblasts showed strong localized positivity with acid phosphatase and were positive for CD7 and CD2, negative for CD19, CD24, CD20. These blasts are most likely:
   a. T-lymphoblasts
   b. B-lymphoblasts
   c. lymphoid stem cells
   d. biphenotypic blasts

7. Acute leukemia blasts that have myeloid and lymphoid markers on the same cells most likely define what subgroup of leukemia?
   a. bilineage
   b. Myeloid/NK
   c. biphenotypic
   d. Undifferentiated

8. The FAB classification of AML is based on:
   a. cytogenetic abnormalities
   b. morphology and cytochemistry of blasts
   c. immunophenotyping of blasts
   d. molecular genetic abnormalities

9. An acute leukemia that is characterized by the presence of morphologically undifferentiated blasts that are negative with conventional cytochemical stains should be:
   a. classified as undifferentiated acute leukemia
   b. classified as myeloid/NK leukemia
   c. immunophenotyped before classifying
   d. classified as undifferentiated acute lymphocytic leukemia

10. When Auer rods (bodies) are found in blasts of a case of acute leukemia, the leukemia is most probably:
   a. undifferentiated leukemia
   b. B-lymphocytic leukemia
   c. T-lymphocytic leukemia
   d. myelocytic leukemia

● REFERENCES

1. Lowenberg, B., Touw, I.P.: Hematopoietic growth factors and their receptors in acute leukemia. Blood, 81:281, 1993.
2. Griffin, J.D., et al.: Use of surface marker analysis to predict outcome of adult acute myeloblastic leukemia. Blood, 68:1232, 1986.
3. Delwel, R., et al.: Growth regulation of human acute myeloid leukemia: effects of five recombinant hematopoietic factors in a serum free culture system. Blood, 72:1944, 1988.
4. Delwel, R., et al.: Human recombinant multilineage colony stimulating factor (interleukin-3): stimulator of acute myelocytic leukemia progenitor cells in vitro. Blood, 70:333, 1987.
5. Vellenga, E., Ostapavicz, D., O'Rourke, B., Griffin, J.D.: Effects of clonogenic cells in short term and long term cultures. Leukemia, 1: 584, 1987.
6. Miyauchi, J., et al.: The effects of three recombinant growth factors, IL-3, GM-CSF and G-CSF on the blast cells of acute myeloblastic leukemia maintained in short term suspension culture. Blood, 70: 657, 1987.
7. Grignani, F., et al: Acute promyelocytic leukemia: From genetics to treatment. Blood, 83:10, 1994.
8. Warrell, R.P. Jr., DeThe', H., Wang, Z-Y., Degas, L.: Acute promyelocytic leukemia. N. Engl. J. Med., 329:177, 1993.
9. LoCoco, F., Pelicci, P.G., Biondi, A.: Clinical relevance of the PML/RAR-α gene rearrangement in acute promyelocytic leukaemia. Leuk. Lymph., 12:327, 1994.
10. Frankel, S.R.: Acute promyelocytic leukemia. Hematol. Oncol. Clin. North. Am., 7:109, 1993.
11. Xue, Y., et al.: Translocation (8;21) in oligoblastic leukemia: Is this a true myelodysplastic syndrome? Leuk. Res., 18:761, 1994.
12. Hamblin, T.J.: Pseudo-myelodysplastic syndrome with (8;21). Leuk. Res., 18:767, 1994.
13. Cheson, B.D., et al.: Report of the National Cancer Institute-sponsored workshop on definitions of diagnosis and response in acute myeloid leukemia. J. Clin. Oncol., 8:813, 1990.
14. First MIC Cooperative Study Group: Morphologic, immunologic, and cytogenetic (MIC) working classification of acute lymphoblastic leukemias. Cancer Genet. Cytogenet., 23:189, 1986.
15. Bennett, J.M.: Proposals for the classification of the acute leukemias. Br. J. Haematol., 33:451, 1976.
16. Second MIC Cooperative Study Group: Morphologic, immunologic, and cytogenetic (MIC) working classification of the acute myeloid leukaemias. Br. J. Haematol., 68:487, 1988.
17. delCanizo, M.C., et al.: Discrepancies between morphologic, cytochemical, and immunologic characteristics in acute myeloblastic leukemia. Am. J. Clin. Pathol., 88:38, 1987.
18. Neame, P.B., et al.: Classifying acute leukemia by immunophenotyping: a combined FAB-immunologic classification of AML. Blood, 68:1355, 1986.
19. Kaplan, S.S., et al.: Simultaneous evaluation of terminal deoxynucleotidyl transferase and myeloperoxidase in acute leukemias using an immunocytochemical method. Am. J. Clin. Pathol., 87: 732, 1987.
20. Bradstock, K.F.: The diagnostic and prognostic value of immunophenotyping in acute leukemia. Pathology, 25:367, 1993.
21. Huh, Y.O., Andreeff, M.: Flow cytometry. Hematol. Oncol. Clin. North. Am., 8:703, 1994.
22. Standing Committee on Human Cytogenetic Nomenclature: An international system for human cytogenetic nomenclature. Cytogenet. Cell Genet., 21:309, 1978.
23. Bennett, J.M., et al.: Proposed revised criteria for the classification of acute myeloid leukemia. Ann. Intern. Med., 103:626, 1985.
24. Bain, B.J.: Leukaemia diagnosis. A guide to the FAB classification. Philadelphia, J.B. Lippincott Co., 1990.
25. Parreira, A., et al.: Terminal deoxynucleotidyl transferase positive acute myeloid leukemia: an association with immature myeloblastic leukemia. Fr. J. Haematol., 69:219, 1988.
26. Imamura, N., Kuramoto, A.: Acute unclassifiable leukaemia in adults, demonstrating myeloid antigens and myeloperoxidase proteins. Br. J. Haematol., 69:427, 1988.
27. Bennett J.M., et al: Proposal for the recognition of minimally differentiated acute myeloid leukemia (AML-M0), Br. J. Hematol., 78: 325, 1991.
28. Davey, D.D., et al.: 8;21 Translocation in acute nonlymphocytic leukemia. Am. J. Clin. Pathol., 92:172, 1989.
29. Lillington, D.M., MacCallum, P.K., Lister, T.A., Gibbons, B.: Translocation t(6;9)(p23;93) in acute myeloid leukemia without myelocysplasia or basophilia: Two cases and a review of the literature. Leukemia, 7:527, 1993.
30. Bennett, J.M., et al.: A variant form of hypergranular promyelocytic leukaemia (M3). Br. J. Haematol., 44:169, 1980.
31. Castoldi, G.L., Liso, V., Specchia, G., Tomas, P.: Acute promyelocytic leukemia: Morphological aspects. Leukemia, 8:1441, 1994.

32. Diverio, D., et al.: Monitoring of treatment outcome in acute promyelocytic leukemia by RT-PCR. Leukemia, 8:1105, 1994.

33. Huhn, D.: Morphology, cytochemistry and ultrastructure of leukemia cells with regard to the classification of leukemias. Recent Results Cancer Res., 93:51, 1984.

34. Mavilio, F., et al.: Selective expression of fos proto-oncogene in human acute myelomonocytic and monocytic leukemias: A molecular marker of terminal differentiation. Blood, 69:160, 1987.

35. Bennett, J.M., et al.: Criteria for the diagnosis of acute leukemia of megakaryocyte lineage (M7). Ann. Intern. Med., 103:460, 1985.

36. van Rhenen, D.J., Verhulst, J.C., Huijgens, P.C., Langenhuijsen, M.M.A.C.: Maturation Index: A contribution to quantification in the FAB classification of acute leukemia. Br. J. Haematol., 46:581, 1980.

37. Weinberg, J.B., Hammer, S.P.: Blast cell leukemia with IgM monoclonal gammopathy and intracytoplasmic vacuoles and Auer-body-like inclusions. Am. J. Clin. Pathol., 71:151, 1979.

38. Yanagihara, E.T., et al.: Acute lymphoblastic leukemia with giant intra-cytoplasmic inclusions. Am. J. Clin. Pathol., 74:345, 1980.

39. Bennett, J.M.: The morphological classification of acute lymphoblastic leukemia: Concordance among observers and clinical correlations. Br. J. Haematol., 47:553, 1981.

40. Miettinen, M., Schwarting, R., Hyun, B.H.: Immunohistochemical evaluation of hematologic malignancies. Hematol. Oncol. Clin. North. Am., 8:683, 1994.

41. Ball, E.D., et al.: Prognostic value of lymphocyte surface markers in acute myeloid leukemia. Blood, 77:224, 1991.

42. LoCoco, F., et al.: CD7 positive acute myeloid leukaemia: A subtype associated with cell immaturity. Br. J. Haematol., 73:480, 1989.

43. Kaplan, S.S., et al.: Immunophenotyping in the classification of acute leukemia in adults. Interpretation of multiple lineage reactivity. Cancer, 63:1520, 1989.

44. del Vecchio, L., et al.: Immunodiagnosis of acute leukemia displaying ectopic antigens: proposal for a classification of promiscuous phenotypes. Am. J. Haematol., 31:173, 1989.

45. Mirro, J., Kitchingman, G.R.: The morphology, cytochemistry, molecular characteristics and clinical significance of acute mixed-lineage leukemia. In Leukaemia Cytochemistry: Principles and Practice. Edited by C.S. Scott. Chichester: Ellis Horwood Limited, 1989.

46. Scott, A.A., et al.: HLA-DR-, CD33-, CD56-, CD16-myeloid/natural killer cell acute leukemia: A previously unrecognized form of acute leukemia potentially misdiagnosed as French-American-British acute myeloid leukemia—M3. Blood, 84:244, 1994.

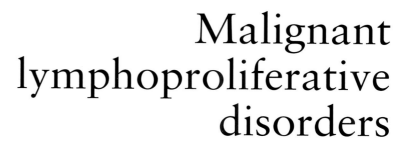

Malignant lymphoproliferative disorders

KEY TERMS

erythrophagocytosis
Hodgkin's disease
lymphadenopathy
lymphoma
lymphoproliferative disorders
lymphosarcoma
splenomegaly

INTRODUCTION

Malignant *lymphoproliferative disorders* may occur in the hematopoietic system (bone marrow and peripheral blood), in the lymphoreticular system (lymph nodes and spleen), or in other organ systems such as the gastrointestinal tract, central nervous system, and so forth. When the neoplastic cells are found predominantly in the hematopoietic system, the disorder is referred to as lymphocytic leukemia. If the neoplastic cells are predominantly in the lymphoreticular and other organs, the term *lymphoma* is used. There can be considerable overlap between leukemia and lymphoma. A primary leukemic disorder may also involve the lymph nodes and other tissue, and a primary lymphoma may show bone marrow and peripheral blood involvement.

The study and diagnosis of lymphoproliferative disorders has been one of the most confusing areas of hematology because of the multiple classification systems and differing terminology. Originally, the diagnosis of the lymphoproliferative disorders was based solely on morphologic findings. In recent years, however, morphologic findings alone have become insufficient; immunocytologic studies have also been found to be important for accurate classification into B-cell, T-cell, or undifferentiated (U)-cell origin and subsets (see Chapter 18). Cytogenetic analysis has recently been used to add important information concerning the origin of malignant lymphocytes. The newest method used in lymphoma diagnosis is molecular DNA testing to detect rearrangements of B-immunoglobulin genes, T-cell antigen receptor genes, BCL2 gene, and so forth. It is hoped that the application of new techniques to the study of lymphocytic malignancies will help to unify theories and terminology and simplify diagnosis. One form of malignant lymphoproliferative disorder, acute lymphocytic leukemia, has been discussed in Chapter 18 with the other acute leukemias. This chapter will include the lymphomas and other lymphoproliferative disorders. Lymphoma is basically divided into two major categories: Hodgkin's disease and non-Hodgkin's lymphoma. The clinical, morphologic, and treatment parameters differ among these basic types. Different responses to treatment have made accurate diagnosis important.

HODGKIN'S DISEASE

Hodgkin's disease was first described by Thomas Hodgkin in 1832.[1] He reported the terminal course of seven patients who had marked *lymphadenopathy* and some of whom also had *splenomegaly*. When first described, controversy existed as to whether this disorder was an unusual infectious entity or a true neoplasm. Although the exact cell of origin is still unknown, investigators now agree that Hodgkin's disease is indeed a true malignant neoplasm.

Hodgkin's lymphoma may occur at any age; however, there is a bimodal distribution occurring with a peak in the 20- to 30-year age group and a second peak in patients older than 50 years of age. Hodgkin's disease is the most common malignancy of young adults in the United States and Europe. Patients may have adenopathy and no symptoms, or they may experience fever, night sweats, weight loss, malaise, and unusual complaints such as pain in enlarged nodes after alcohol consumption. Most frequent sites involved are the cervical and supraclavicular lymph nodes with later spreading to contiguous nodal regions, spleen, liver, and bone marrow. The occurrence of primary extranodal Hodgkin's disease, although possible, is uncommon.

The diagnosis of Hodgkin's disease depends on the demonstration of the classic Reed-Sternberg (RS) cell (Fig. 19-1A). This cell has a lobated nucleus that may appear as two separate nuclei. Each nuclear lobe has a prominent eosinophilic (inclusion-like) nucleolus with chromatin clumping around the nuclear membrane, making a halo effect around the nucleolus. The nuclear membrane is thickened, and there is a moderate amount of eosinophilic cytoplasm that sometimes is artifactually clear-staining. There are four RS cell variants referred to as the single and multinucleated variants, lacunar cells, and lymphocytic-histiocytic (LH) cells (Figs. 19-1B to 19-1E). The single nucleated (Hodgkin's cell) and multinucleated variants have the same chromatin, nucleolus, and cytoplasm as the described RS cell, except the variants have either one nucleus or more than two nuclei. The multinucleated variants may actually have a single large multilobated nucleus. Lacunar cells, when seen in formalin fixed tissue, have an artifactually clear cytoplasm with a centrally placed nucleus, giving a "lacunar" appearance. The nucleus is single to multilobated and has small basophilic nucleoli with irregularly clumped chromatin. The LH cell is a relatively large cell with a single indented or lobated nucleus, thin nuclear membrane, and small nucleoli. The lacunar cell is seen predominantly in nodular sclerosing type, whereas the LH cell is seen in lymphocyte-predominant Hodgkin's disease. The RS cell and variants are the malignant cells of Hodgkin's disease. Regardless of the type of RS variant cells identified in any given case, the classic RS cell also must be present to establish the diagnosis. The typical RS cell and Hodgkin's cell will have positive staining for CD15 and CD30. The exception to this is lymphocyte predominant Hodgkin's disease, as described below.

Hodgkin's disease has been subclassified into four different types, based on the histopathology of involved lymph nodes[2,3] (Table 19-1).

Lymphocyte predominance

This type usually occurs in males of younger ages and is frequently confined to a single lymph node or node group. Histopathologic examination reveals a nodular or diffuse pattern. Either pattern will show a predominance of small mature lymphocytes with clusters of epithelioid histiocytes. RS cells are rare and difficult to find while the LH variant cells are more prevalent. The nodules of the nodular variant also are composed predominantly of small lymphocytes, and in some cases the nodular pattern may be

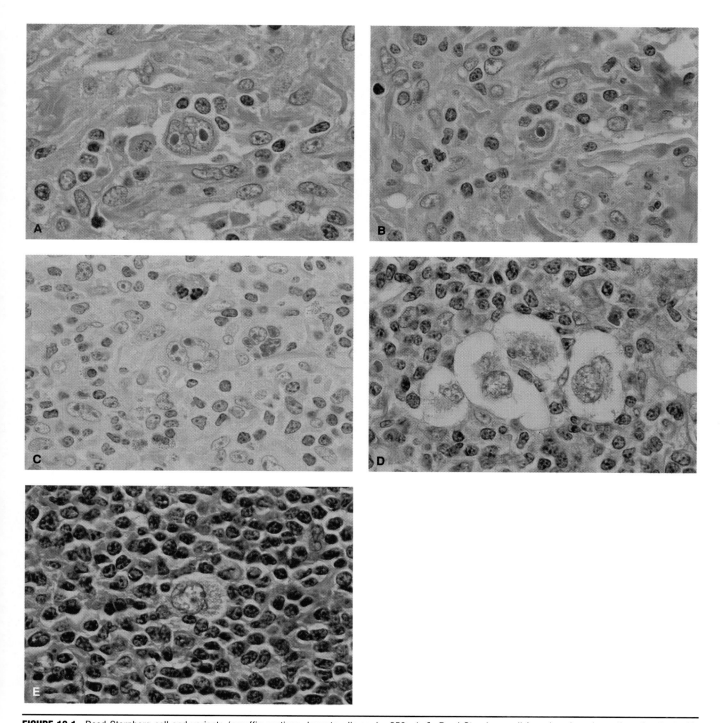

FIGURE 19-1. Reed-Sternberg cell and variants (paraffin sections, hematoxylin-eosin, 250×). **A,** Reed-Sternberg cell from lymph node section of patient with Hodgkin's disease showing two mirror image nuclei each with a prominent nucleolus; cytoplasm is abundant and eosinophilic. **B,** Single nucleated RS variant—"Hodgkin" cells. **C,** Multinucleated RS variant. **D,** Lacunar cells as seen in nodular sclerosing Hodgkin's disease. **E,** LH, cell as seen in lymphocyte predominant Hodgkin's disease.

TABLE 19-1 *MORPHOLOGIC SUBTYPES OF HODGKIN'S DISEASE*

Subtype	Typical Features
Lymphocyte predominance	Small round lymphocytes, LH cells, Hodgkin's cells, and rare RS cells
Nodular sclerosing	Bands of collagen defining nodules; lacunar cells, Hodgkin's cells, RS cells
Mixed cellularity	Heterogeneous cell population, Hodgkin's cells, RS cells
Lymphocyte depleted	Many RS cells and Hodgkin's cells; diffuse fibrosis

subtle. The malignant cells of the nodular variant have a distinctive phenotype, different from all other types of Hodgkin's disease. These cells are positive for the B-cell antigen CD20 and negative for CD15.[4] This variant form also has the potential to transform to a large B-cell lymphoma. Hence, nodular lymphocyte predominant Hodgkin's disease may represent an unusual neoplasm of follicular center cells.

● Nodular sclerosing

A diagnosis of nodular sclerosing (Fig. 19-2) depends on the presence of bands of collagen that extend down from the capsule into the node, causing compartmentalization of the more cellular areas. Also, lacunar cells must be present, and RS cells must be seen for the diagnosis of Hodgkin's disease. The background cellularity consists of a varying number of lymphocytes, histiocytes, plasma cells, and eosinophils. Nodular sclerosing type typically occurs in females, with limited spread, and frequently involves the mediastinum.

● Mixed cellularity

In mixed cellularity Hodgkin's disease, there is replacement of the normal architecture with a proliferation of lymphocytes, histiocytes, plasma cells, and eosinophils. Granuloma-like areas may be seen. RS cells are moderate in number with single and multinucleated variants. Mixed cellularity type usually occurs in the 20- to 30-year age group with Stage II or III disease at the time of diagnosis.

● Lymphocyte depleted

Few lymphocytes are seen in lymphocyte-depleted Hodgkin's disease, and there is a predominance of RS cells with single and multinucleated variants. Some cases may show diffuse fibrosis of the lymph node. This type of Hodgkin's disease is usually seen in males of an older age group, and patients frequently present with multiple-site involvement.

Extranodal occurrence of Hodgkin's disease has been reported in various organs, including spleen, liver, skin, lungs, and bone marrow. The histologic appearance is identical to that described in the lymph node setting; however, characteristic features of the subtypes may be missing. Hodgkin's disease in the bone marrow is usually not aspirable, as there is a dense background fibrosis with a mixture of lymphocytes, eosinophils, plasma cells, and histiocytes. Single-nucleated Hodgkin's cells may be sparse, and diagnostic RS cells may not be present (Fig. 19-3). When seen on the Wright-stained bone marrow aspirate slide, the Hodgkin's cells are large, approximately the size of megakaryocytes, and the nuclei are irregular with a prominent nucleolus. Occasionally, Hodgkin's disease may be found in body fluids, such as pleural or peritoneal fluid. The malignant cells seen on cytocentrifuged, Wright-stained preparations are large cells with large, irregular nuclei and prominent nucleoli. Circulating Hodgkin's cells in peripheral blood have been reported in rare cases.

The prognosis of Hodgkin's disease is related to the morphologic subtype and extent of organ involvement. Generally, prognosis is better when the morphology shows a higher number of lymphocytes and fewer numbers of RS cells. More importantly, however, prognosis

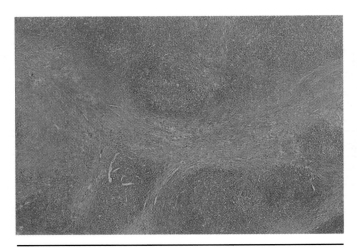

FIGURE 19-2. Lymph node section from a patient with nodular sclerosing type Hodgkin's disease with thick bands of collagen surrounding nodules of tumor (paraffin section, hematoxylin-eosin, 25×).

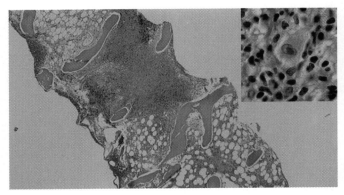

FIGURE 19-3. Bone marrow containing Hodgkin's disease shows focal disruption of architecture, distinct from surrounding normal marrow, with dense background fibrosis, heterogeneous cell infiltrate, and occasional Hodgkin's cells (inset) (paraffin sections, hematoxylin-eosin, 25×).

TABLE 19-2 *CLINICAL STAGES OF HODGKIN'S DISEASE*

Stage	Characteristics
I	Tumor in one anatomic region or two contiguous anatomic regions on the same side of the diaphragm
II	Tumor in more than two anatomic regions or two noncontiguous regions on the same side of the diaphragm
III	Tumor on both sides of the diaphragm not extending beyond lymph nodes, spleen, or Waldeyer's ring
IV	Tumor in bone marrow, lung, etc.—any organ site outside of the lymph nodes, spleen, or Waldeyer's ring

varies with the clinical stage (Table 19-2). The initial histologic type of Hodgkin's disease in a given case may progress to a more aggressive form.

Depending on the histologic type and clinical stage, Hodgkin's disease may be treated with either combined chemotherapy or radiation therapy.

● NON-HODGKIN'S LYMPHOCYTIC LYMPHOMA

The existence of malignant neoplasms arising primarily from the lymphatic system was first proposed by Virchow in 1863. This concept lay dormant for nearly 30 years until redescribed in more detail. *Lymphosarcoma* was then observed microscopically to be a heterogeneous group of tumors. This realization led to the use of different terms in the literature, such as lymphosarcoma, nodular lymphoma (Brill-Symmers disease), and reticulum cell sarcoma. In 1966, Rappaport presented a formalized classification that is still used by some institutions (Table 19-3).[5] The Rappaport terminology is popular because of its simplicity and clinical correlation. The explosion of immunologic research that began in the 1960s inevitably led to new theories concerning cell origin, based on functional characteristics of T- and B-cells and their subsets (see Chapter 4). Subsequently, the Lukes-Collins[6] classification emerged as an alternative to the purely morphologic scheme of Rappaport (Table 19-4). Several other classifications have been reported; however, for various reasons, these have not been as widely accepted. The International Working Formulation was proposed as a grouping of lymphomas correlating tumor aggressiveness to histologic ap-

TABLE 19-3 *RAPPAPORT CLASSIFICATION OF NON-HODGKIN'S LYMPHOMA*

Diffuse
  Well differentiated lymphocytic
Nodular or diffuse
  Poorly differentiated lymphocytic
  Mixed (lymphocytic-histiocytic)
  Histiocytic
  Undifferentiated

TABLE 19-4 *LUKES-COLLINS CLASSIFICATION OF NON-HODGKIN'S LYMPHOMA*

U-Cell
T-Cell
  Small lymphocyte
  Convoluted lymphocyte
  Sezary cell-mycosis fungoides
  Immunoblastic sarcoma
  Lennert's lymphoma
B-Cell
  Small lymphocyte
  Plasmacytoid lymphocyte
  Follicular center cell
    small cleaved
    large cleaved
    small non-cleaved
    large non-cleaved
  Immunoblastic
  Hairy cell
Histiocytic

pearance (Table 19-5).[7] The most recent classification is the Revised European-American Classification of Lymphoid Neoplasms (REAL).[8] This classification includes all of the more recently described types of lymphoma and uses different terms for the follicular center cell lymphomas (Table 19-6).

Generally, lymphomas can be grouped morphologically into small, intermediate, or large size cells with a diffuse or follicular (nodular) pattern of growth, and functionally into B-cell, T-cell, and U-cell (undifferentiated cell) disorders. The clinical setting varies with the type of lymphoma and the prognosis generally worsens with increasing cell size and mitotic activity.

Demonstration of surface and/or intracytoplasmic markers of lymphocytes is extremely valuable in the classification of the lymphomas. In most cases, the marker studies can determine the T- or B-cell nature of the cells and will sometimes demonstrate an abnormal phenotype distinguishing benign versus malignant cells.[9] The marker studies can be performed using either flow cytometry, immunoperoxidase techniques on frozen sections, or immu-

TABLE 19-5 *INTERNATIONAL WORKING FORMULATION OF LYMPHOMA*

Low Grade
  Small lymphocytes
  Follicular, small cleaved cell
  Follicular, mixed, small cleaved, and large cell
Intermediate Grade
  Follicular, large cell
  Diffuse, small cleaved
  Diffuse, mixed, small, and large cell
  Diffuse, large cell
High Grade
  Diffuse, large cell, immunoblastic
  Lymphoblastic
  Small noncleaved cell

TABLE 19-6 *REVISED EUROPEAN-AMERICAN LYMPHOMA CLASSIFICATION[8]*

B-cell Neoplasms
Peripheral B-cell neoplasms
    Precursor B-lymphoblastic leukemia/lymphoma
      Small lymphocytic lymphoma/CLL/prolymphocytic
      Lymphoplasmacytoid/immunocytoma
      Mantle cell
      Follicular center lymphoma, grades I, II, and III
      Marginal zone: MALT and monocytoid B-cell
      Splenic marginal zone (provisional)
      Hairy cell leukemia
      Plasmacytoma/multiple myeloma
      Diffuse large B-cell lymphoma
      Burkitt's lymphoma
      High grade, Burkitt-like
T-cell
    Precursor T-lymphoblastic lymphoma/leukemia
    Peripheral T-cell
      T-chronic lymphocytic leukemia/prolymphocytic
      Large granular lymphocyte leukemia (LGL)
      Mycosis fungoides/Sezary syndrome
      Peripheral T-cell lymphomas
      Angioimmunoblastic T-cell
      Angiocentric
      Intestinal T-cell
      Adult T-lymphoma/leukemia
      Anaplastic large cell lymphoma

TABLE 19-7 *LEUKOCYTE DIFFERENTIATION ANTIGENS COMMONLY USED*

Cluster Designation	Antibody	Antigen
CD1	T6	Thymocyte
CD2	T11, 35.1, Leu5	Sheep RBC Receptor
CD3	T3, UCHT1, Leu4	T-Cell Receptor
CD4	T4, Leu3	Class II MHC, "Helper"
CD5	T1, Leu1	Pan T
CD6	T12	Pan T
CD7	3A1, G3, 7, Leu9	Pan T
CD8	T8, Leu2	Class I MHC, "Suppressor"
CD9	BA-2, J2	B Leukemia Assoc.
CD10	BA-3, J5	CALLA
CD11C	LeuM5	Granulocyte
CD13	My7	Granulocyte/Monocyte
CD14	LeuM3	Histiocytic
CD15	LeuM1, Myl	Granulocyte, Monocyte
CD16	Leu11	NK cells
CD19	B4, Leu 12	B Lineage Assoc.
CD20	B1, Leu 16	B Lineage Specific
CD21	Ba-5, B2	EBV virus/C3d Receptor
CD22	Leu 14, B3	B Lineage Assoc.
CD23	B6	B Lineage
CD24	BA-1	B Lineage Assoc.
CD25	TAC	Il-2 Receptor
CD30	Ki-1, Ber-H2	Reed-Sternberg
CD33	My9, LeuM9	Granulocyte
CD34	My10	Progenitor cell
CD41	gly. IIb IIIa	Megakaryocytes
CD42	Glycophorin	RBC precursors
CD43	Leu22	T-cell
CD45	CLA	Leukocytes
CD45RO	UCHL-1	Post-thymic T-cell
CD56	Leu19	NK cells
CD57	Leu7	Natural killer cell
CD68	KP-1	Monocyte

noperoxidase techniques on air-dried smears or paraffin sections. In general, mature cells, such as the small cell lymphomas, have only surface antigens and are best studied by flow cytometry or frozen sections and smears. The large cell lymphomas tend to have intracytoplasmic and surface antigens and can be studied using paraffin sections. Table 19-7 is a list of the monoclonal antibodies commonly used in the diagnosis of lymphocytic disorders, and Table 19-8 lists these antigens by cell type. Table 19-9 is a list of monoclonal antibodies used for tissue sections. Commonly observed results of marker studies are listed in Table 19-10. It should be remembered, however, that any individual case may have a different or unusual pattern of antigen markers. These results must be correlated with standard morphology to determine the best diagnosis.

Cytogenetic studies in lymphoproliferative disorders have been invaluable as a research tool and more recently as an aide in clinical diagnosis and prognosis. A discussion of chromosome aberrations in lymphoma will be found in Chapter 20.

● B-cell lymphomas—small cell types

SMALL LYMPHOCYTIC LYMPHOMA

Small lymphocytic lymphoma (SLL) (Figs. 19-4A and 19-4B), (previously known as well-differentiated lymphocytic lymphoma [WDLL]) occurs almost entirely in middle age and elderly persons. Patients often have asymptomatic lymphadenopathy and hepatosplenomegaly. The pattern of growth in lymph nodes is always diffuse because the cell of origin is not derived from germinal centers. The cells of SLL are small lymphocytes (6 to 9 μ diameter) with round nuclei, having a block-type chromatin clumping and small amount of light blue cytoplasm. Only rare mitotic figures are seen. Focal collections of larger lymphocytes, paraimmunoblasts, may be seen. These are called proliferation centers and should not be mistaken for a follicular lymphoma or for transformation to an aggressive cell type. The majority of cases are of B-cell lineage and show faint monoclonal surface immunoglobulin as well as marking with CD5. SLL may involve the bone marrow in a focal or diffuse pattern. When circulating lymphoma cells are present in the peripheral blood, the

TABLE 19-8 *LIST OF COMMONLY USED CD BY CELL TYPE*

TABLE 19-8 *LIST OF COMMONLY USED CD BY CELL TYPE*

Lymphoid-T-cell
  CD1, 2, 3, 4, 5, 7, 8, 25, 45RO

Lymphoid-B-cell
  CD10, 19, 20, 21, 22, 23, 24

NK cells
  CD16, 56, 57

Myelomonocytic
  CD13, 14, 15, 33, 11c, 68

Platelet-Megakaryocyte
  CD41

Erythrocyte- and Erythrocyte Precursors
  CD42

Others
  CD34-Progenitor cell
  HLA-DR B lymphocyte, monocyte, activated T-cell

picture may be identical to chronic lymphocytic leukemia (CLL). Differentiation between these two diagnoses is not important because SLL and CLL have the same prognosis and are treated identically. Some cases may show progression to a large cell, high grade lymphoma, known as Richter's syndrome. Studies have shown that Richter's syndrome represents transformation of the original cell line, not development of a new primary malignancy, as was originally speculated. If the cell infiltrate also consists of plasmacytoid lymphocytes and plasma cells, the term lymphoplasmacytoid cell lymphoma is used. This variant of SLL has the same prognosis as the standard SLL. Patients with SLL have a long term survival; treatment is only instituted when symptoms or complications develop.

Terminology is as follows:

Rappaport:	Well-differentiated lymphocytic lymphoma
Lukes-Collins:	(B-cell) small lymphocyte
Working Formulation:	Low grade, small lymphocytic
REAL:	B-cell, small lymphocytic

TABLE 19-9 *COMMON MONOCLONAL ANTIBODIES USED FOR IMMUNOPEROXIDASE STAINING OF FROZEN SECTIONS AND/OR FIXED TISSUE*

Lymphoid-T-cell
  UCHL-1 (CD45RO), Leu22 (CD43), Leu4 (CD3), Leu3a&b (CD4), Leu2A (CD8), Leu5 (CD2), Leu1 (CD5), Leu7 (CD57)

Lymphoid-B-cell
  Leu14 (CD22), L26 (CD20), kappa, lambda

Myelomonocytic
  LeuM1 (CD15)

Histiocytic
  KP-1 (CD68), Mac387, HAM56, LeuM3 (CD14)

Others
  CLA (CD45)
    EMA (epithelial membrane antigen)
    Factor VIII—megakaryocytes

SMALL-CLEAVED CELL LYMPHOMA

Small-cleaved cell lymphoma (SCCL) (Figs. 19-5A and 19-5B) was originally termed poorly differentiated lymphocytic lymphoma (PDLL) by Rappaport because, as the name implies, the cells are not round, easily identifiable lymphocytes. Cells of SCCL are small- to moderate-sized lymphocytes (6 to 12 μ) with irregular, angulated, and elongated nuclei. The chromatin is partially clumped, nucleoli are indistinct, and mitotic figures are only occasionally seen.[10,11] Lukes-Collins used the term "cleaved" for the irregular nuclear shape; the deep indentations or cleaves are more readily identified in whole cell preparations. The cleaved lymphocyte is derived from the germinal center of the lymph node, and, therefore, the histologic pattern of growth is most often follicular, simulating a germinal center. The follicular SCCL is the most common lymphocytic lymphoma of adults in the United States and is only seen rarely in patients younger than 20 years of age. Patients usually have widespread disease, showing lymphadenopathy of multiple sites and possible spleen, liver, bone marrow, and peripheral blood involvement. When cells of SCCL are seen in the peripheral blood, they are moderately enlarged with partially clumped chromatin and occasional or frequent cleaved nuclei, also known as "butt" cells (Fig. 19-5C). The leukocyte count may be moderately to markedly elevated at greater than 100 $\times$ 10^9/L. When patients present with a leukemic phase, the differential diagnosis includes chronic lymphocytic leukemia, acute lymphocytic leukemia, and lymphoma. In chronic lymphocytic leukemia, cells have rounded nuclei with block-type chromatin clumping and only rare cleaved nuclei. Blasts of acute lymphocytic leukemia are small to moderately enlarged cells with a diffuse, nonclumped chromatin and minimal cytoplasm; nuclei may be round, oval, or folded. In addition, patients with acute lymphocytic leukemia will frequently show anemia and thrombocytopenia, whereas the leukemic phase of SCCL will more often have erythrocyte cell and platelet counts.

Follicular SCCL has a relatively good prognosis, with 70% of patients having a 5-year survival, although usually not disease-free. Diffuse SCCL shows the same clinical and morphologic features; however, prognosis is worse, with 28% 5-year survival. The cells of follicular and diffuse SCCL are of B-cell origin, demonstrate strong surface monoclonal immunoglobulin, and are frequently positive for CD10. Marrow involvement may be focal or diffuse, frequently showing a paratrabecular distribution (aggregates of lymphoma cells lining bone trabeculae), a location that is believed to be a homing site of B-lymphocytes. SCCL may progress to a more aggressive large cell type of lymphoma.

Terminology:

Rappaport:	Poorly differentiated lymphocytic lymphoma, nodular or diffuse
Luke-Collins:	B-cell follicular center cell lymphoma, small cleaved cell type
Working Formulation:	Low grade—follicular, small cleaved cell type; Intermediate grade—diffuse, small cleaved cell type
REAL:	Folluclar center cell lymphoma, grade I

TABLE 19-10. RESULTS OF CELL ANTIGEN MARKERS THAT ARE FREQUENTLY USED TO DISTINGUISH DIFFERENT TYPES OF LYMPHOMAS. THESE REPRESENT THE COMMONLY OBSERVED RESULTS; HOWEVER, INDIVIDUAL CASES MAY VARY

I. Surface Marker Studies Performed by Flow Cytometry

	T-cell Markers, CD no.	B-cell Markers, CD no.	CALLA CD10	Granulocytic Markers CD no.	SIg (monoclonal)	TdT
CLL/WDLL	5	19, 20, 23, ±22	−		weak Ig	−
SCCL	−	19, 20, 22 ± 23	+		+ Ig, M > D > G	−
Mantle/IL	5	19, 20, 22	−		+ Ig, D > M	−
Hairy Cell	25, ±5	19, 20, 22	−	11c	+ Ig, M > G	−
LGL—T cell	2, 3, 8, 16, ±57	−	−		−	−
LGL—NK cell	2, 16, ±8, 56, 57					
T-CLL	2, 3, 4, 5, 7	−	−		−	−
Sezary	2, 3, 4, 5	−	−		−	−
SNCL	−	19, 20, 22, 24	+		+ Ig	−
T-Lymphoblastic	3, 7, ±2, 5, 4, 8	−	−		−	+
pre-B Lymphoblastic	−	19, 20	+		−	+
pre-preB Lymphoblastic	−	19	+		−	+

II. Surface and Cytoplasmic Marker Studies Performed by Immunoperoxidase Staining of Parafin Sections

	Positive	Negative
Hodgkin/RS cells mc, ns, ld	CD15, 30	20, 45, EMA
NLPHD	CD20, 30, 45, EMA	15
ALCL	CD30, 45, EMA	15

SIg - surface immunoglobulin; TdT - terminal deoxynucleotidal transferase; CLL - chronic lymphocytic leukemia; WDLL - well differentiated lymphocytic lymphoma; SCCL - small cleaved-cell lymphoma; IL - intermediate lymphoma; LGL - large granular cell lymphocytosis; SNCL - small non-cleaved cell lymphoma; ALL - acute lymphocytic leukemia; RS - Reed-Sternberg; mc - mixed cellularity; ns - nodular sclerosing; ld - lymphocyte depleted; NLPHD - nodular lymphocyte predominant Hodgkin's disease; ALCL - anaplastic large cell lymphoma; EMA - epithelial membrane antigen.

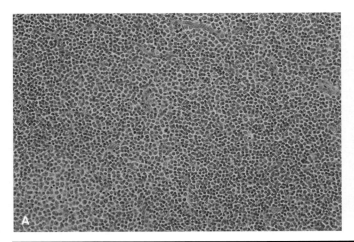 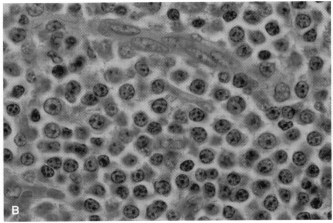

FIGURE 19-4. Small lymphocytic lymphoma with **A,** diffuse pattern (25×) and **B,** predominantly small lymphocytes showing round nuclei with dense chromatin clumping (250×). An occasional large lymphocyte is seen with open chromatin (paraffin section, hematoxylin-eosin).

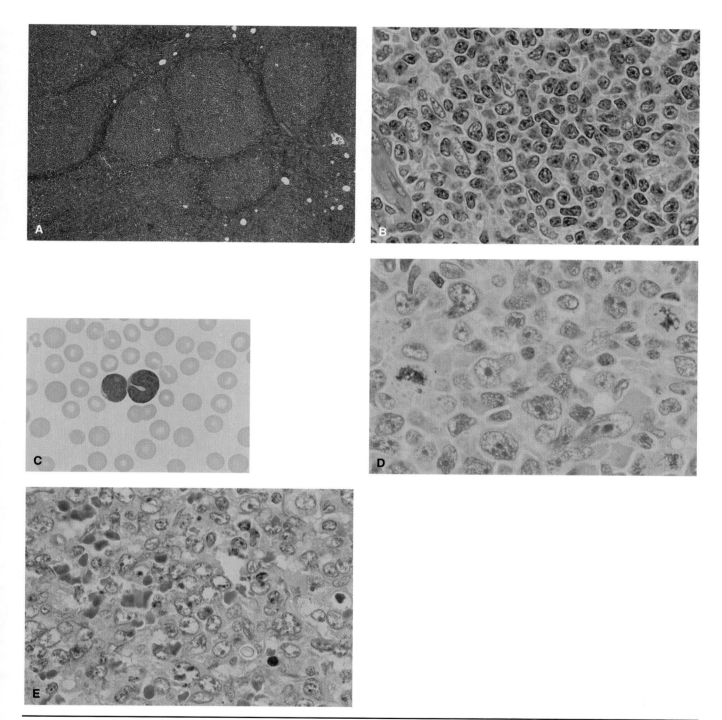

FIGURE 19-5. Follicular center cell lymphomas (paraffin sections, hematoxylin-eosin) **A,** Section of lymph nodes showing effacement of normal architecture caused by nodular pattern of lymphoma (25×). **B,** Small cleaved cell lymphoma with a predominance of small lymphocytes with irregular, angulated and elongated nulcei and clumped chromatin. A few larger lymphocytes are also present (250×). **C,** Circulating lymphoma cell of small cleaved cell lymphoma showing typical "butt" cell appearance (Wright-Giemsa stain, 250×). **D,** Large cleaved cell lymphoma showing a predominance of large lymphocytes with open chromatin, irregular nuclei and occasional nucleoli (250×). **E,** Large noncleaved cell lymphoma with large lymphocytes showing round, oval or slightly irregular nuclei with open chromatin and one to several nucleoli (250×).

MANTLE CELL/INTERMEDIATE CELL LYMPHOMA

This lymphoma is most often seen in older adults (median age, 60 years) and is predominant in males. The lymphoma is frequently advanced at the time of presentation, and bone marrow and peripheral blood involvement can be seen.

As the name implies, this neoplasm derives from the mantle zone, the small lymphocytes that normally surround the germinal centers.[8] These lymphocytes have morphology "intermediate" between the small lymphocyte of SLL and the cleaved cell of SCCL. Therefore, some of the cells will have round nuclei with dense chromatin, and some will have irregular, cleaved nuclei with partially clumped chromatin. In the early stages of the disease, the lymph node sections will show large, expanded mantle zones surrounding small, crowded out germinal centers. As the disease progresses, the expanding mantle zones become confluent, and the lymph node shows a diffuse pattern. If the diagnosis is made at the diffuse stage, the term intermediate cell lymphoma is used.

Although not listed in the original Working Formulation, the nodular pattern-mantle cell lymphoma corresponds with a low grade classification and the diffuse pattern-intermediate cell lymphoma has a more aggressive course corresponding with an intermediate grade lymphoma. Surface marker studies will show the cells from both types of patterns to be positive with CD19, CD20, CD22, CD24, CD5, and HLA-DR.

● B-cell lymphomas—large cell type

The large cell lymphomas were originally believed not to be of lymphocytic origin because of their typically large size and nuclear characteristics. Therefore, they were grouped under the term "histiocytic" by Rappaport. Lukes-Collins have split this category into the following four types, based on functional and morphologic features: large cleaved cell (Fig. 19-5D), large noncleaved cell (Fig. 19-5E), immunoblastic B-cell (Fig. 19-6), and true histio-

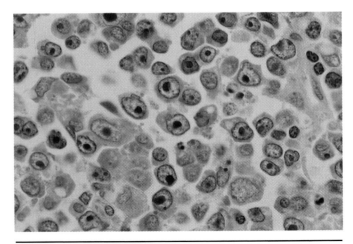

FIGURE 19-6. B-cell immunoblastic lymphoma. Large B immunoblasts have round nuclei, open chromatin and one to two prominent nucleoli. The immunoblasts show a moderate amount of cytoplasm. (Paraffin section, hematoxylin-eosin, 250×).

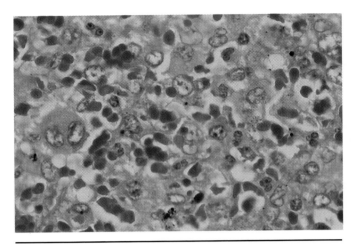

FIGURE 19-7. True histiocytic malignancy. Large malignant histiocytes can be seen with irregular nuclei, open chromatin and abundant cytoplasm. Tumor cells have phagocytosed red blood cells (paraffin section, hematoxylin-eosin, 250×).

cytic lymphoma (Fig. 19-7). The large cleaved and large noncleaved lymphomas are of follicular center cell origin, and, therefore, they may show a follicular pattern. However, usually the pattern is diffuse. The large cell lymphomas (as opposed to small cell types) usually present as limited disease with single node replacement; however, they act aggressively and progress to dissemination. Likewise, bone marrow infiltration is usually not seen early and circulating malignant cells in the peripheral blood are rarely reported. The cells are large (20 to 40 μ) and have an open and vesicular chromatin pattern with one to several prominent nucleoli. The nuclear shape may be round or ovoid (large noncleaved cell, immunoblastic) or irregular and cleaved (large cleaved cell). Immunologic studies show surface and cytoplasmic monoclonal immunoglobulin, except for the true histiocytic malignancies. Large cleaved and noncleaved lymphocytic lymphoma have a fairly homogeneous population of cells with greater than 80% of cells being large cleaved or large noncleaved lymphocytes. The immunoblastic B-cell type differs in that some cases will show a mixture of plasma cells, plasmacytoid lymphocytes, and B-immunoblasts,[3] while other cases consist almost entirely of B-immunoblasts. The B-immunoblast is a large cell with a moderate amount of cytoplasm showing peripheral basophilia because of increased amounts of RNA (pyroninophilia). The nucleus is round with open, irregularly distributed chromatin, and a single prominent nucleolus.

True histiocytic malignances (Fig. 19-7) are rare and may present with predominantly lymph node replacement (true histiocytic lymphoma) or splenomegaly (histiocytic medullary reticulosis). A key feature for the diagnosis of histiocytic malignancy is to find erythrophagocytosis by the tumor cells.

Terminology:

Rappaport:	Histiocytic lymphoma
Lukes-Collins:	B-cell, follicular center, large cleaved cell
	B-cell, follicular center, large non-cleaved cell
	B-cell immunoblastic
	True histiocytic lymphoma
Working Formulation:	Intermediate grade—diffuse, large cell (cleaved or noncleaved)
	High grade—diffuse, immunoblastic
REAL:	Follicular center cell lymphoma, grade III
	Diffuse large B-cell lymphoma

● B-cell lymphomas—other types

MIXED CELL LYMPHOMA

Mixed cell lymphoma is a B-cell lymphoma of follicular center cell origin where the predominant cell is a small cleaved cell, with at least 20% but not more than 50% of the large cleaved/noncleaved cell type present. These may have a follicular or diffuse pattern, and the cell morphology is identical to that described for SCCL and large cleaved and noncleaved cells. The REAL classification[8] uses the term follicular center cell lymphoma and subtypes grade I (small cleaved cell), grade II (mixed cell) and grade III (large cell cleaved and/or noncleaved). This lymphoma occurs mainly in adult ages and may be widespread at presentation. Bone marrow or other extranodal involvement may show only the large cell or only the small cell component.

Terminology:

Rappaport:	Mixed (lymphocytic-histiocytic) nodular or diffuse
Working Formulation:	Low grade—follicular mixed, small and large cell
	Intermediate grade—diffuse mixed, small and large cell
REAL:	Follicular: center cell lymphoma, grade II

BURKITT'S LYMPHOMA

Burkitt's lymphoma (Figs. 19-8A and 19-8B) also known as small noncleaved cell (SNC), is more often seen in the pediatric population.[12] The endemic type occurs in Africa and usually presents with maxillary and mandibular tumors. The tumor cells are moderate in size (15 to 20 μ) with finely dispersed chromatin and distinct nucleoli seen along the nuclear membrane. The nuclear membrane is round without indentations or folds. There is a moderate amount of pyroninophilic cytoplasm. Mitoses are frequent and tissue sections show a prominent "starry sky" pattern because of the presence of large macrophages.[10]

This is one of the first lymphomas described to have a characteristic cytogenetic aberration.[13] Most cases will have a translocation involving chromosomes 8 and 14, t(8;14)(q24;q32). In this translocation, the break in chromosome 8 occurs just proximal to the MYC oncogene locus, transposing it to the gene region in chromosome 14, which is responsible for immunoglobulin heavy chain production. This translocation has been seen in other B-cell malignancies and two variants have been described, t(2;8) and t(8;22).[14] In the latter two examples, the break in chromosome 8 is just distal to the MYC region and either the gene for kappa light chain (chromosome 2) or lambda light chain (chromosome 22) is transposed to this area. This is an example of a chromosome translocation with rearrangement of oncogenes and gene regions pertaining to the functional expression of the malignant cell line.

The tumor cells of Burkitt's lymphoma are of follicular center cell origin and have demonstrable surface and cytoplasmic immunoglobulin. This tumor may show an initial response to chemotherapy; however, it frequently recurs. Wright-stained cells with bone marrow and peripheral blood involvement are large with a moderate amount of vacuolated basophilic cytoplasm and large nuclei. The vacuoles stain prominently with oil red O. This morphology is identical to the L3 type of acute lymphocytic leukemia (Chapter 18).

Terminology:

Rappaport:	Undifferentiated cell or histiocytic lymphoma
Lukes-Collins:	B-cell, follicular center cell, small non-cleaved cell
Working Formulation:	High grade—small non-cleaved cell
REAL:	Burkitt's lymphoma

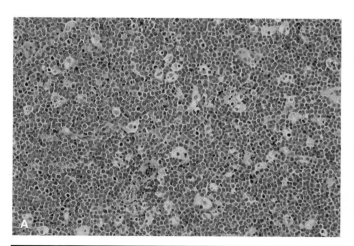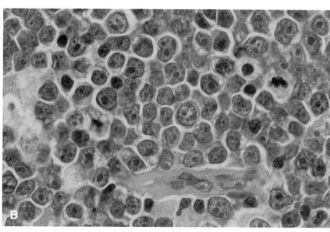

FIGURE 19-8. A, Small noncleaved lymphoma, Burkitt type with "starry sky" appearance caused by benign macrophages interspersed among the tumor cells (25×). **B,** Small noncleaved cell lymphoma, Burkitt type with intermediate size cells showing round to slightly irregular nuclei, reticular chromatin and prominent nucleoli. (250×).

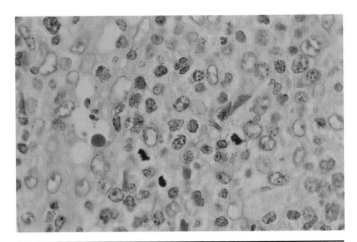

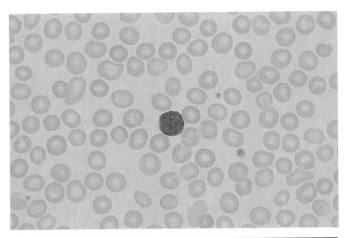

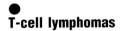

FIGURE 19-9. T-cell lymphoma with eosinophils/large lymphocytes with open chromatin and small irregular, convoluted lymphocytes (250×) (paraffin section, hematoxylin-eosin).

FIGURE 19-10. Sezary cell. Small lymphocytes with a convoluted nucleus and partially clumped chromatin. Nuclear membrane fold lines can be seen throughout the nucleus (Wright-Giemsa stain, 250×).

T-cell lymphomas

T-cell lymphomas have long been recognized in Japan where they are the most common form of lymphocytic malignancy; however, this type of lymphoma also is seen in the United States.[3] The use of monoclonal antibodies for T-cell subsets caused an explosion of information concerning diagnosis of T-cell disorders, thus causing currently used classifications to become insufficient. T-cell lymphomas tend to show general features which aid in their recognition.[10] Because T-cells are predominantly in paracortical areas as opposed to germinal centers, the pattern of involvement in the node is always diffuse. There is frequently a heterogeneous population of eosinophils, plasma cells, histiocytes, and small and large lymphocytes (Fig. 19-9). The nuclei of the lymphocytes may be tightly convoluted. The T-cell lymphomas also may be composed of a homogeneous population of small-, large-, or intermediate-sized lymphocytes. There is frequently widespread disease commonly with skin involvement. Bone marrow and peripheral blood involvement also can be seen. A few T-cell disorders will be discussed here.

T-CELL LYMPHOMA—SMALL LYMPHOCYTE

T-cell lymphoma, small lymphocyte is almost identical, morphologically, to small lymphocytic lymphoma and chronic lymphocytic leukemia. The distinction between T- and B-cell type is important, as the T-cell type has a poor prognosis. This distinction can only reliably be made by surface marker studies. Richter syndrome has been known to occur with the T-cell type lymphoma.

MYCOSIS FUNGOIDES

Mycosis fungoides is a primary T-cell malignancy of skin. It usually occurs in adults, ages 40 to 60 years. Skin lesions are usually scaly plaques that progress to a tumor stage. Skin biopsies show an infiltrate of small and/or large cells. The small lymphocyte is 8 to 10 μ with minimal cytoplasm

and highly convoluted (cerebriform) nuclear shape. The large cell is approximately 15 to 20 μ with convoluted and hyperchromatic nuclei and prominent nucleoli. Although the primary tumor site is skin, spreading to the lymph nodes, lungs, spleen, liver, and bone marrow can occur. Peripheral blood involvement with the small cerebriform cell is known as Sezary syndrome (Fig. 19-10). Most cases with the surface marker studies tag the T-cells as helper cells.

ADULT T-CELL LEUKEMIA/LYMPHOMA

Patients with adult T-cell leukemia/lymphoma frequently present with widespread disease including bone marrow and peripheral blood involvement. There is frequently hypercalcemia, with or without lytic bone lesions. This lymphoma is known to be linked with the human T-cell lymphotropic virus (HTLV virus). Although this lymphoma is endemic in certain regions of Japan as well as the southeastern United States and Caribbean, sporadic cases have been reported from many other locations.

Histologically, the lymph node architecture is diffusely replaced by the lymphoma cell infiltrate, which may be comprised of small-, intermediate-, and/or large-sized lymphocytes. Regardless of the predominant cell size, the nuclei display marked folds of the nuclear membrane, resulting in convoluted and cerebriform shapes. The mitotic activity is increased. There also may be associated an infiltrate of eosinophils and plasma cells. In the peripheral blood, the nuclear shapes also show the multiple folds and may appear "clover-leaf" shaped. This is classified as a high-grade lymphoma.

T-LYMPHOBLASTIC LYMPHOMA/LEUKEMIA

T-lymphoblastic lymphoma/leukemia (Fig. 19-11) is reported most often in adolescent males; however, it may be seen in either sex at any age. Presentation is usually with lymphadenopathy, mediastinal mass, bone marrow, and peripheral blood circulating blasts. The blast cells also

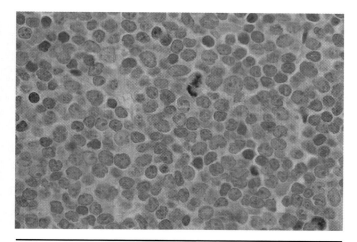

FIGURE 19-11. Lymphoblastic lymphoma with intermediate size cells showing round to irregular nuclei, homogeneous fine chromatin and small inapparent nucleoli. Mitotic figures can also be seen (250×) (paraffin section, hematoxylin-eosin).

may be present in spinal fluid. The malignant cells are frequently convoluted; however, this is not specific for T-cells. Acid phosphatase staining shows a characteristic polarized positivity in the cytoplasm. Most cases of lymphoblastic lymphoma are of T-cell type (80%); however, some cases are pre-B and pre-pre-B similar to acute lymphocytic leukemia. The morphology in tissue sections of the B-cell type is similar to T-cell lymphoblastic lymphoma, except the nucleus is not as folded or convoluted. It is very important to differentiate lymphoblastic lymphoma from Burkitt's lymphoma (small non-cleaved cell) as treatment differs. This can be done in most cases by immunophenotyping and TdT nuclear stain (see Table 19-10). The cells of pre-B and pre-pre-B lymphoblastic lymphoma will not show punctate staining with acid phosphatase.

ANAPLASTIC LARGE CELL LYMPHOMA

Anaplastic large cell lymphoma (ALCL) is composed of very large cells with large nuclei of varying shapes, some appearing like Reed-Sternberg cells. The chromatin is irregularly clumped and open, and the nucleoli are prominent. There is abundant cytoplasm. The pattern of growth is variable and many times the neoplastic cells will be growing in cohesive appearing clusters. This pattern can be difficult to distinguish from metastatic carcinoma.

The tumor cells stain positive for CD30 and CD45, but negative for CD15, which helps to distinguish this lymphoma from Hodgkin's disease.[4] Some cases also will be positive for epithelial membrane antigen (EMA) and some will have T-cell markers, although very few will have B-cell markers. Most cases will not have T- or B-cell antigens expressed. Because of the positive staining for Ki-1 (CD30), which is sometimes referred to as "Ki-1 positive anaplastic large cell lymphoma."

ALCL was not listed in the original Working Formulation, but corresponds with a high-grade classification. Recently, a chromosome translocation, t(2;5)(p23;q35), has been described in ALCL and may become helpful for the diagnosis. Refer to Chapter 20.

● OTHER LYMPHOCYTIC MALIGNANCIES

● Chronic lymphocytic leukemia

Chronic lymphocytic leukemia (CLL) (Fig. 19-12a) is almost exclusively a disease of adults, rarely occurring in patients younger than 40 years of age. The diagnosis is frequently made incidentally when a complete blood count is ordered for routine physical examination or other disease workup. The diagnosis can be made from peripheral blood by finding an absolute lymphocytosis (usually between 10 to 150 × 10⁹/L) with lymphocytes that are monotonous in appearance having round nuclei, block-

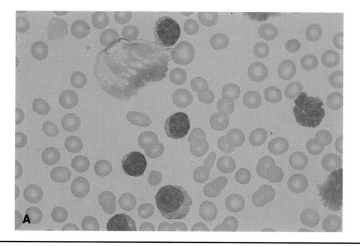

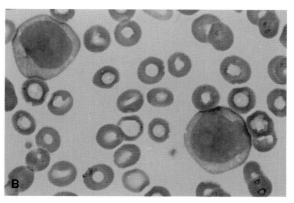

FIGURE 19-12. A, Chronic lymphocytic leukemia showing small round lymphocytes with dense chromatin clumping; a larger prolymphocyte is noted (Wright-Giemsa stain, 250×). **B,** Prolymphocytic transformation of CLL (Wright stain, 250×).

type chromatin clumping, and a small amount of light blue cytoplasm. Varying numbers of "smudge" cells are seen as the lymphocytes are fragile and tend to rupture when the peripheral smear is made. Occasional large lymphocytes are present with less clumped chromatin and single nucleoli; these are referred to as prolymphocytes. A normocytic normochromic anemia, neutropenia, and thrombocytopenia develop with disease progression as the lymphocytes in the bone marrow replace normal hematopoietic cells. Approximately 10% of patients may acquire an autoimmune hemolytic anemia.

The bone marrow is focally or diffusely infiltrated by lymphocytes of the same morphology as seen in the peripheral blood. More than 90% of cases are of B-cell origin, and the morphologic character of T-cells versus B-cells may be indistinguishable. The type of cell markers present on B-lymphocytes in CLL is identical to those of lymphocytes in the lymph node in patients with small lymphocytic lymphoma. The cells have a uniform distribution of surface immunoglobulin, but the density is less than that of normal lymphocytes. The heavy chain is usually associated with a monoclonal light chain. B-CLL cells usually mark with CD19, CD20, CD24, and the T-cell marker CD5. This helps distinguish CLL from peripheralized cells of SCCL, but not from mantle cell/intermediate cell lymphoma.

Serum immunoglobulins may be normal early in the disease, but as the disease progresses hypogammaglobulinemia develops. About 5% of the patients develop Ig monoclonal spikes.

CLL may transform to a prolymphocytic leukemia, showing a predominance of prolymphocytes (Fig. 19-12b), or it may transform to a large cell lymphoma known as Richter's syndrome. The clinical course is usually prolonged and treatment is initiated only when patients become symptomatic.

Differential diagnosis is most often not a problem in CLL because few other diseases produce a sustained increase in small mature appearing lymphocytes. Usually, lymphocytosis caused by infectious disorders are easily distinguished from CLL because of the presence of heterogeneous populations of reactive lymphocytes and because of the distinctive clinical features of the patient. Infectious lymphocytosis, a self-limiting disease that primarily affects children, is associated with an absolute lymphocytosis that subsides in 4 to 6 weeks. The lymphocytes, normal appearing, type as T cells. Pertussis (whooping cough) is also associated with a reactive proliferation of small mature lymphocytes. As mentioned previously, SLL may present a blood picture identical to CLL when circulating lymphoma cells are present; differentiation is not important because both diseases have the same prognosis and are treated identically.

Hairy cell leukemia

Hairy cell leukemia (HCL) (Fig. 19-13), originally referred to as leukemic reticuloendotheliosis, also is a disorder seen predominantly in adults with a male:female ratio of approximately 7:1. A patient with hairy cell leukemia typi-

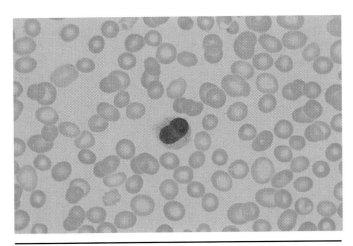

FIGURE 19-13. Hairy cell leukemia. Large lymphocyte with indented nucleus, diffusely distributed chromatin, small nucleolus and abundant pale staining cytoplasm with peripheral projections or "hairs" (Wright-Giemsa stain, 250×).

cally has pancytopenia and prominent splenomegaly. HCL cells on a peripheral smear are large lymphocytes with a moderately large nucleus. The nucleus has a diffuse homogeneous chromatin distribution and may have a single nucleolus. The cytoplasm is a pale light-blue, sometimes vacuolated, and frequently shows projections or "hairs." The "hairy" projections may be easier to demonstrate with wet preparations using phase microscopy. The nuclei may be round, indented, or folded.

The cellular origin of hairy cells is a B-lymphocyte that also shows features of phagocytosis. Bone marrow involvement may be focal or diffuse, and on tissue sections the cytoplasm is clear. There is a dense production of reticulum by the tumor cells, frequently causing a "dry tap" with marrow aspiration attempts. The spleen also shows a characteristic appearance with diffuse red pulp infiltration and pseudosinuses lined with leukemic cells and filled with red blood cells (referred to as "blood lakes").

The leukemic cells stain show tartrate resistant acid phosphatase (TRAP) staining. TRAP staining, although characteristic, is not diagnostic of hairy cell leukemia and has been reported in other hematopoietic malignancies. Typical surface marker studies in hairy cell will show positive staining with CD19, CD20, CD22, CD24, CD25, and CD11c, as well as surface monoclonal immunoglobulins.[15] Some cases also will have CD5.

With appropriate chemotherapy, patients frequently do well for long periods of time.

Large granular lymphocytic leukemia

This disorder has several synonyms—large granular cell lymphocytosis, natural-killer cell leukemia, and T-gamma lymphocytosis.[16]

This is a chronic lymphoproliferative disorder characterized by a proliferation in bone marrow and peripheral blood of lymphocytes that have a moderate to abundant amount of cytoplasm with sometimes prominent granules. The morphology is not different from benign, reactive granular lymphocytes, so the key is to recognize the homogeneity of the lymphocytic population; most of the circulating lymphocytes will have this same morphology. There is usually an associated cytopenia, either anemia, neutropenia or thrombocytopenia or any combination. The bone marrow may have pure red blood cell aplasia when anemia is a prominent feature. However, in patients with neutropenia or thrombocytopenia the myeloid precursors and megakaryocytes usually show adequate marrow maturation. Patients frequently have a history of rheumatoid arthritis and splenomegaly is a common physical finding. The diagnosis is best established by finding the lymphocytic proliferation in the bone marrow and by surface marker studies of the peripheral blood and/or bone marrow lymphocytes. The cell phenotype shows two main patterns, a T-cell type with positive CD2, CD3, CD8, CD16, and $\pm$CD57, and a natural-killer cell (NK) with positive CD2, CD16 and $\pm$CD8, CD56, and CD57.

Most cases have a long disease course with symptoms and complications related to the degree of peripheral cytopenias, and some have been reported to show a transformation to large cell lymphoma.

● Multiple myeloma (plasma cell myeloma)

Multiple myeloma (Figs. 19-14A and 19-14B) is usually seen in older adults; nevertheless, cases have been reported in young adults and, rarely, in childhood. The usual presentation includes multiple osteolytic bone lesions, bone marrow infiltration, monoclonal gammopathy, and generalized hypoagammaglobulinemia with Bence Jones proteinuria. The marrow infiltration shows a varying number of mature and immature plasma cells that may be seen diffusely or in proliferating sheets. These malignant plasma cells are sometimes referred to as myeloma cells.

The plasma cells frequently are enlarged with less chromatin clumping than is seen in benign plasma cells. Multi-nucleated plasma cells can be found. The more atypical appearing neoplastic cells also show centrally placed nuclei, a high nuclear to cytoplasmic ratio, and prominent nucleoli. When sheets of plasma cells and plasma cells with atypical features are seen in the bone marrow, the diagnosis of a plasma cell neoplasm can be made with confidence. If, however, the plasma cell more closely resembles normal plasma cells and no aggregates are seen, the diagnosis must be established by combining the clinical, laboratory, and bone marrow findings.

In contrast to the normal individual who synthesizes all five classes of immunoglobulin, in multiple myeloma a single immunoglobulin is produced in excess (M-component). Thus, the patient is said to have a monoclonal gammopathy. In addition, the synthesis of normal immunoglobulins is suppressed. The most common immunoglobulin secretion is IgG, then IgA, and IgD. The production of immunoglobulins is abnormal, and overproduction of light chains results in the presence of light chains in urine, a condition called Bence Jones proteinuria. A small percent of cases will secrete only light chains. The light chains are rapidly cleared by the kidneys and may only be seen in the urine and not in serum. A common complication of this disease is renal impairment from an obstruction of renal tubules by proteinaceous casts. Approximately 1% of cases do not secrete any immunoglobulin; however, the presence of immunoglobulin can be demonstrated in the cytoplasm of the malignant plasma cells with immunoperoxidase techniques. With dense bone marrow infiltration, patients may be anemic and have a myelophthisic blood picture. Rouleaux and rapid erythrocyte sedimentation caused by hyperglobulinemia are hallmark features of the disease.

Wright's stained blood smears will frequently show a blue background because of the excess of plasma protein. Occasional circulating plasmacytoid lymphocytes or plasma cells are seen. Rarely, plasma cell leukemia may occur with many circulating myeloma cells (usually greater than 2×10^9/L).

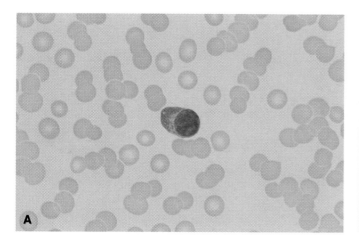
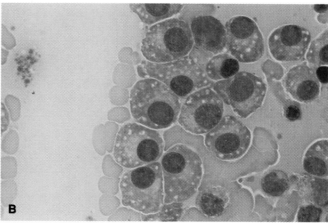

FIGURE 19-14. Multiple myeloma. (Wright-Giemsa stain) **A,** Peripheral smear with circulating myeloma cell and rouleaux formation of the red cells (250×). **B,** Bone marrow smear with cluster of atypical, large plasma cells (250×).

Asymptomatic patients are followed but usually not treated. Symptomatic patients are treated with alkylating agents, radiotherapy, and prednisone. Infection is the most common cause of death.

Waldenstrom's macroglobulinemia

Waldenstrom's macroglobulinemia is a plasma cell dyscrasia that secretes monoclonal IgM. This entity differs from multiple myeloma in that instead of osteolytic bone lesions there is soft tissue involvement.[9] The bone marrow infiltration shows lymphocytes, plasmacytoid lymphocytes, and plasma cells. The malignant cell in this disease is believed to be at a stage of development between the mature B-lymphocyte and the most differentiated B cell, the plasma cell. This cell, called the plasmacytoid lymphocyte, has surface immunoglobulin and CD20 antigen, but it lacks the CD21 antigen of mature B lymphocytes and the PC-1 antigen of the plasma cell. The major complications of Waldenstrom's macroglobulinemia relate to hyperviscosity syndrome because of the presence of large amounts of IgM. Bleeding problems may arise because of interference in the complex formation between coagulation factors and platelets by the IgM macroglobulins.

Heavy chain disease

Heavy chain disease is a lymphoproliferative disease characterized by the overproduction of abnormal heavy chains of the immunoglobulin molecule. The malignant cell is most probably the plasmacytoid lymphocyte. Diagnosis is based upon the demonstration of these heavy chains in the serum or urine by immunochemical methods. To date, four types of heavy chain disease have been found: τ, α, δ, and μ. The clinical manifestations are similar to those of malignant lymphoma, including lymph node enlargement, hepatosplenomegaly, fever, and malaise.

SUMMARY

Malignant neoplasms of lymphocytes may either arise in the peripheral blood and bone marrow (leukemia) or in tissue (lymphoma). Lymphomas can arise in virtually any organ site, but most often lymphoma begins in lymph nodes. For treatment purposes, lymphoma is initially classified as Hodgkin's disease versus non-Hodgkin's lymphoma. The hallmark for diagnosis of Hodgkin's disease is the presence of Reed-Sternberg cells, Reed-Sternberg cell variants, and a background of benign lymphocytes, plasma cells, and histiocytes.

Non-Hodgkin's lymphomas are classified as B- or T-cell and as low grade, intermediate grade, or high grade. Classification of lymphoma is necessary for each individual case to determine prognosis and appropriate treatment. Accurate diagnosis and classification requires not only tissue preparation for morphology, but also immunophenotyping by flow cytometry or immunoperoxidase stains. Cytogenetic analysis is also helpful in some cases.

REVIEW QUESTIONS

Patient L.M. is a 62-year-old male who presented with weakness and fatigue. The patient has been in good health until the last three months when he noted becoming increasingly tired after a routine workday, and not being able to maintain his usual exercise schedule. Physical exam reveals an enlarged spleen, but no lymphadenopathy. CBC shows the following:

Hgb.—	8.1 g/dL
Hct.—	.25 L/L
MCV—	88 fL
WBC—	2.5 × 10⁹/L
Platelet count—	85 × 10⁹/L

Examination of the peripheral smear shows 80% lymphocytes that have an abnormal morphology with a large, immature nucleus, single prominent nucleolus and abundant pale staining cytoplasm. Flow cytometry for surface markers show the cells to be marking with CD19, CD20, CD22, CD24, CD25, and CD11c, as well as IgG-lambda.

1. The most likely diagnosis is:
   a. chronic lymphocytic leukemia.
   b. acute lymphocytic leukemia.
   c. hairy cell leukemia.
   d. reactive lymphocytosis.
   e. peripheralized lymphoma.

2. The most appropriate special stain to perform on a peripheral blood smear would be:
   a. acid phosphatase, with and without tartrate.
   b. alkaline phosphatase.
   c. Sudan black.
   d. myeloperoxidase.
   e. chloroacetate esterase.

3. The bone marrow would most likely show:
   a. aspirable marrow with focal lymphocytic infiltrate.
   b. aspirable marrow with diffuse lymphocytic infiltrate.
   c. nonaspirable marrow with 10% cellularity.
   d. nonaspirable marrow with diffuse lymphocytic infiltrite.
   e. aspirable marrow with 10% cellurarity.

REFERENCES

1. Hodgkin, T.: On some morbid appearances of the absorbent glands and spleen. Trans. Med. Chir. Soc., London, 17:68, 1832.
2. Lukes, R.S., et al.: Report of the nomenclature committee. Cancer Res., 26:1311, 1966.
3. Jaffe, E.S.: Surgical Pathology of the Lymph Nodes and Related Organs. Philadelphia: W.B. Saunders, 2nd ed., 1995.
4. Knowles, D.M., ed. Neoplastic Hematopathology. Baltimore: Williams & Wilkins, 1992.
5. Rappaport, H.: Tumors of the Hematopoietic System. Atlas of Tumor Pathology. Armed Forces Institute of Pathology, 3:8, 1966.
6. Lukes, R.J., Collins, R.D.: Immunological characterization of human malignant lymphoma. Cancer, 34:1488, 1974.
7. Rosenberg, S.A., et al.: National Cancer Institute sponsored study

of classification on non-Hodgkin's lymphomas. Summary and description of a working formulation for clinical usage. Cancer, 49: 2112, 1982.

8. Harris, N.L., Jaffe, E.S., Stein, H., et al.: A revised European-American classification of lymphoid neoplasms: a proposal from the International Lymphoma Study Group. Blood 84:1361-1392,1994.

9. Keren, D.F., Hauson, C.A., Hurtibise, P.W.: Flow Cytometry and Clinical Diagnosis. Chicago: ASCP Press, 2nd ed., 1994.

10. Iochim, H.L.: Lymph Node Biopsy. Philadelphia: J.B. Lippincott, 1993.

11. Swerdlow, S.H.: Biopsy Interpretation of Lymph Nodes. New York: Raven Press, 1992.

12. Kjeldsberg, C.R., Wilson, J.R., Bernard, C.W.: Non-Hodgkin's lymphoma in children. Hum. Pathol., 14:612, 1983.

13. Manalov, G., Manalova, Y.: Marker band in one chromosome 14 from Burkitt's lymphoma. Nature, 237:33, 1972.

14. Croce, L., Tsujimoto, Y., Erikson, J., Nowell, P.: Biology of diseases; chromosome translocations and B cell neoplasia. Lab. Invest., 51: 258, 1984

15. Sun, T.: Color Atlas/Text of Flow Cytometric Analysis of Hematologic Neoplasms. New York: Igaku-Shoin, 1993.

16. Schumacher, H.R., Cotelingam, J.D.: Chronic Leukemia Approach to Diagnosis. New York: Igaku-Shoin, 1993.

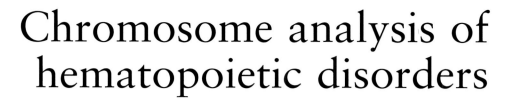

Chromosome analysis of hematopoietic disorders

20

KEY TERMS

acquired aberration
acrocentric
allogeneic
aneuploid
anti-oncogene
autosome
centriole
centromere
chiasmata
chimerism
chromatid
chromosome
congenital aberration
cytogenetics
diploid
euchromatin
G-band
haploid
heterochromatin
hyperdiploid
hypodiploid
metacentric
nondisjunction
polyploid
pseudodiploid
Q-band
satellite
submetacentric
synaptonemal complex
tumor suppressor gene

INTRODUCTION

Cytogenetics is the study of chromosome morphology particularly as it relates to a normal or abnormal state. In 1956, the normal number of chromosomes per human cell was established at 46 and since that time, many chromosome abnormality syndromes have been reported. The use of cytogenetics has markedly improved patient diagnosis and family counseling in the field of congenital aberrations and prenatal diagnosis. Cytogenetic studies also are responsible for major advances in the field of hematopoietic malignancies and solid tumors. Chromosome analysis of many of the malignant disorders has become a critical factor for diagnosis, prognosis, and for research studies as well. This chapter will cover the basic techniques of human chromosome analysis and standard nomenclature and will discuss the practical uses of cytogenetics in patients with hematopoietic disorders.

CHROMOSOME STRUCTURE AND MORPHOLOGY

Nuclear chromatin of human cells is composed of nucleic acid and protein and is organized into 46 chromosomes. The nucleic acids, deoxyribonucleic acid (DNA) and ribonucleic acid (RNA), also are called polynucleotides. A single nucleotide consists of a phosphate, a sugar (deoxyribose for DNA and ribose for RNA), and a base. The base may be a purine (A = adenine, G = guanine) or a pyrimidine (C = cytosine, T = thymine, or U = uracil for RNA). The bases are aligned on the polynucleotide strand in a triplet code so that three bases code for a single amino acid; the succession of bases in this triplet code determines the genes that will be transcribed and translated by messenger RNA and transfer RNA into the resultant protein products. There are approximately 100,000 genes in human cells, each located at a specific site on a specific chromosome (gene loci). The different possible expressions of a gene are known as alleles. For example, the gene for the ABO blood group has three alleles: A, B, and O.

The DNA exists as a double-stranded helix, with the two polynucleotide strands held together by hydrogen bonds between complimentary bases so that G will bind only with C and A only with T (or U for RNA). The bonding of A-T and G-C are called *base pairs*. This double helix has a diameter of approximately 20 A° and is of variable length. For example, the amount of DNA that is contained in the smallest chromosome, no. 21, is composed of approximately 50 million base pairs, while the largest chromosome, no. 1, has approximately 250 million base pairs. The double helix initially coils around histone proteins resulting in a structure called a *nucleosome* (Fig. 20-1). This nucleosome forms a superhelix with the histone proteins, calcium and magnesium forming a *chromatin fiber* (also called solenoid) with a diameter of 250 A°. The chromatin fiber continues to coil with nonhistone proteins and forms a *chromomere*. The chromomere coils to form an identifiable *chromatid* with a diameter of 0.2 to 0.5 μm. After DNA synthesis, identical sister chroma-

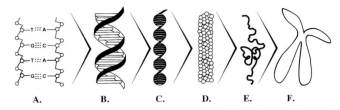

FIGURE 20-1. Chromosome morphology and ultrastructure. **A,** Molecular structure of DNA with two polynucleotide chains held together by hydrogen bonding of base pairs (T = thymine, C = cytosine, A = adenine, G = guanine). **B,** Double helical structure of DNA. **C,** Coiling of double helix strand around histone proteins to produce nucleosome. **D,** Superhelix of nucleosome producing chromatin fiber. **E,** Coiling of chromatin fiber to produce chromomere. **F,** Final structure of chromosome consisting of two identical sister chromatids (condensed chromomere) held together at the centromere.

tids are connected at the *centromere* giving the final structure of a chromosome.

The centromere connects sister chromatids and divides them into short "p" and long "q" arms (Fig. 20-2). If the centromere is in the center of the chromosome so that the length of p = q, it is referred to as a *metacentric* chromosome (chromosomes 1, 3, 16, 19, and 20). If the centromere is off-center so that p < q, the chromosome is called submetacentric (chromosomes 2, 4, 5, 6 to 12, 17, 18, X, and Y), and when the centromere is located close to the end of the chromosome so that p is very short, the chromosome is called *acrocentric* (chromosomes 13 to 15, 21, and 22). The terminal portion of the p arm on the acrocentric chromosomes is tightly coiled into chromatin masses called *satellites* that are attached to the rest of the p arm by less tightly coiled *chromatin stalks* (Fig. 20-2). *Heterochromatin* refers to the chromatin that stains dark, is composed of highly repetitive DNA sequences, and is genetically inactive; *euchromatin* refers to the areas that stain light and are genetically active during interphase.

A normal human cell has 46 chromosomes consisting of 23 pairs. Chromosome pairs 1 to 22 are autosomes and the X and Y chromosomes are sex chromosomes. Before

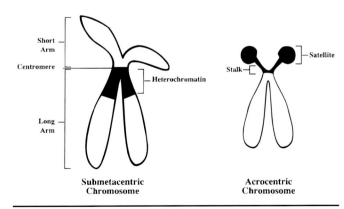

FIGURE 20-2. Chromosome structure of a typical submetacentric chromosome and an acrocentric chromosome.

banding, the chromosome numbers were assigned by total length of the chromosome beginning with no. 1 as the longest and no. 22 as the shortest. With banded analysis, it was discovered that chromosome 21 is actually shorter than 22, but the designations were not changed. A *homologous* chromosome pair consists of two morphologically identical chromosomes that have identical gene loci, but may have different gene alleles as one member of a homologous pair is of maternal origin and the other is of paternal origin. For example, a homologous pair consisting of both chromosomes no. 9 have the gene locus for the ABO blood group on the long arm. An individual may inherit the allele for blood group A on the maternal no. 9 chromosome and the allele for blood group B on the paternal no. 9 chromosome. A *heterologous* pair consists of morphologically non-identical chromosomes that have different gene loci.

● MITOSIS, MEIOSIS

The life of a cell is called the *cell cycle*, which consists of four major phases (Fig. 20-3). Beginning with phase G1, the cell is performing its designated function. During this time, the nuclear chromatin is dispersed and is not recognizable as individual chromatids. The next phase, S, is the time of DNA synthesis when the DNA is replicated and identical sister chromatids are then attached at the centromere. This is followed by a short resting phase, G2, after which the cell enters mitosis. The length of time that a cell spends in each phase is quite variable. For example, the mature cell such as a segmented neutrophil will remain in G1 for the remainder of its life and will not progress through DNA synthesis. The average time that a cell spends in mitosis is estimated to be 45 minutes.

To study human chromosomes, cells must be mitotically active. *Mitosis* is the process of division of somatic cells so that each daughter cell has the same genetic composition as the parent cell. A cell that is not dividing, but is performing its designated function is in *interphase*. Interphase begins at phase G1 of the cell cycle and continues until the end of phase G2. During this time, the nuclear chromatin is dispersed and chromosome morphology is not identifiable. *Prophase* is the first stage of mitosis (Fig. 20-4) during which the DNA begins to coil, chromosome morphology becomes recognizable, and a pair of cytoplasmic organelles known as *centrioles* migrate to opposite poles of the cell. In *metaphase*, the DNA is tightly coiled and the chromosomes align in the center of the cell *(equatorial plate, metaphase plate)* while the contractile fibers *(spindle apparatus)* extend from the centrioles and attach to the chromosome centromere. *Anaphase* begins with the contraction of the spindle fibers pulling apart the sister chromatids so that one sister chromatid migrates to one pole of the cell and the other sister chromatid migrates to the opposite pole of the cell. *Telophase* occurs with a simple division of the cytoplasmic membrane, and the two daughter cells then enter G1 phase of the cell cycle. Each resultant daughter cell has the identical genetic composition of the parent cell.

Meiosis is the specialized division of diploid primary gametocytes that results in each gamete, oocyte, and sperm, having a haploid (n = 23) number of chromosomes. Normal gametes must have one chromosome of each homologous pair so that all gene loci are present. The first stage of meiosis (meiosis I) is the reduction division and the second stage (meiosis II) is a simple mitotic division (Fig. 20-5). Meiosis I begins with prophase I in which the DNA coils and the chromosomes become shorter and thicker. Prophase I has several successive stages (leptotene, zygotene, pachytene, diplotene, and diakinesis) during which there is an exact gene-for-gene pairing of the homologous chromosomes; the X and Y chromosome align end-to-end. This very close association of the homologous pairs is referred to as the *synaptonemal complex*. A crossing over of the chromatids of the homologous pairs may occur, forming *chiasmata*, a point where there may be breakage and rejoining to the opposite chromosome with crossing over of gene alleles. In metaphase I, the spindle fibers from the centrioles connect to the centromeres of the chromosomes. During anaphase I, the spindle fibers contract, and the intact chromosomes are pulled to opposite poles so that the chromosomes of each homologous pair migrate to opposite poles of the cell. By the end of telophase I, the resultant two cells have a haploid number of chromosomes with each gene loci being represented. These two cells (secondary gametocytes) then enter directly into metaphase of a simple mitotic division where the spindle apparatus connects to the centromeres, contracts, and the sister chromatids migrate to opposite poles. The cytoplasmic membrane then splits and the mature gametes are formed.

After puberty in the male, spermatogenesis occurs continuously, and four mature sperm result from meiosis of a single primary spermatocyte. In oogenesis in the female, the primary oogonium begins meiosis I during embryogenesis and will not complete it until years later when ovulation occurs. At that time, the primary oogonia divides resulting in one polar body (a nondividing cell) and the secondary oogonia. The secondary oogonia will then pro-

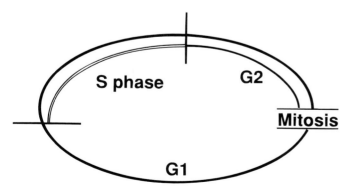

FIGURE 20-3. Diagram of the cell cycle beginning with G1, the stage that the cell is performing its designated duties. The DNA is uncoiled and exists as 46 single chromatids. S phase is the time of DNA synthesis, after which the DNA is still uncoiled and consists of 46 chromosomes (sister chromatids joined at the centromere). G2 is a resting phase followed by mitosis.

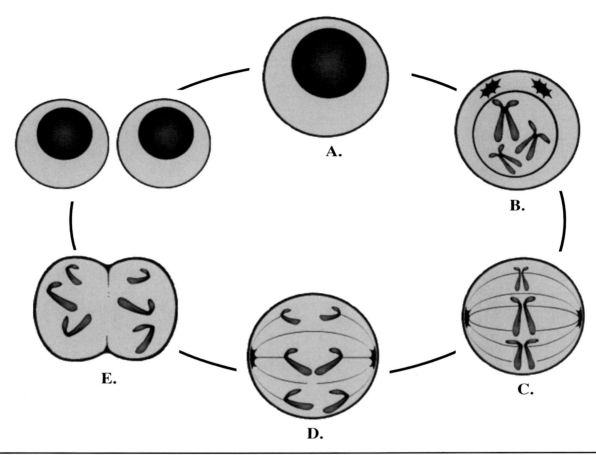

FIGURE 20-4. Mitosis. **A,** Interphase. Chromatin is dispersed. **B,** Prophase. Chromosome structure is discernible and centrioles begin to migrate. **C,** Metaphase. Chromosomes are lined up in the center, spindle fibers from the centrioles connect to the centromeres, and the nuclear membrane is not visible. **D,** Anaphase. Spindle fibers contract and sister chromatids migrate to opposite poles of the cell. **E,** Telophase. Chromatid migration is complete and the cytoplasmic membrane forms down the center, completing the cell division.

ceed directly into metaphase of meiosis II, completing this only if fertilization occurs.

CYTOGENETIC PROCEDURES

Specimen preparation

Specimens used for cytogenetic analysis must have viable cells capable of undergoing mitotic activity; the choice of appropriate specimens depends upon the clinical situation of the patient (Table 20-1). For the evaluation of possible *congenital aberrations,* peripheral blood is the most appropriate sample as circulating lymphocytes can be easily manipulated to undergo mitosis by the use of various mitogens, most commonly phytohemagglutinin (PHA) that stimulates predominantly the T lymphocytes. However, if the patient has a lymphocytopenia or if the case requires work-up for mosaicism, a punch-biopsy of skin may be cultured for growth of fibroblasts. When the clinical situation involves a spontaneous abortion (miscarriage), stillbirth, or death shortly after birth, the appropriate sample would be fetal tissue (products of conception) or autopsy acquired organ samples (lung, liver, kidney, diaphragm). A *prenatal evaluation* requires culturing either amniotic fluid cells or chorionic villous biopsy processed by direct harvest and tissue culture. These various cultures are harvested at the time of maximal mitotic activity, usually 72 to 96 hours for peripheral blood and 7 to 21 days for amniotic fluid and fibroblast cultures.

Evaluation of *malignant processes* such as leukemia, lymphoma or other tumors requires that the neoplastic cells be sampled directly, either by peripheral blood, bone marrow, or solid tumor biopsies. These samples are harvested immediately (direct harvest) or by short-term unstimulated cultures to obtain mitoses of the neoplastic cells and not the associated nontumor cells.

The first step of the cytogenetic procedure is to have cells active in mitosis. Once this has been accomplished by any of the above methods, the cells are "harvested."

Harvest procedure and banding

Mitotically active cells from any of the above methods are stopped in metaphase by incubation with agents that

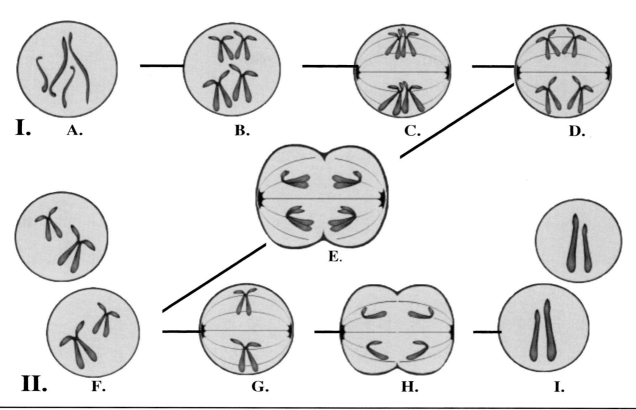

FIGURE 20-5. Meiosis I and II. **A,** Prophase I. Primary gametocyte begins meiosis I with DNA coiling. **B,** Homologous chromosomes pair to form synaptonemal complex. **C,** Metaphase I. Homologous pairs line up in the center of the cell and the spindle fibers connect to the centromeres. **D,** Anaphase I. Spindle fibers contract and homologous chromosomes begin to migrate to opposite poles. **E,** Telophase I. Migration is complete and homologous chromosomes have segregated to opposite poles. **F,** Secondary gametocytes are formed with 23 chromosomes. **G,** Metaphase II. Chromosomes are lined up in the center of the cell and the spindle fibers connect to the centromeres. **H,** Anaphase-Telophase II. Spindle fibers contract, chromatids migrate to opposite poles and cytoplasmic membrane splits. **I,** Mature gametes are formed.

disrupt the spindle apparatus, most commonly colchicine or colcemid.[1] The cells are then incubated with a hypotonic solution (frequently 0.075 M KCL) that will totally hemolyze erythrocytes and partially swell the nucleated cells. Fixation and washing of the cells is then accomplished with Carnoy's fixative, 3:1 methanol:glacial acetic acid. After washing the cells 3 to 4 times, a trial slide is prepared by dropping 3 to 4 drops of the final cell suspension onto a clean glass slide. The slide is dried on a slide warmer and examined by phase microscopy for appropriate spreading and number of mitotic figures. If the first slide does not show optimal quality, the suspension may be concentrated or diluted, or other manipulations may be tried to obtain improved chromosome morphology. The remainder of the slides are then prepared and "aged" for banding; this often involves heating the slides in a 60° C oven for 1 to 2 days.

Chromosome banding is obtained by various staining

TABLE 20-1   *APPROPRIATE SPECIMENS FOR CYTOGENETIC ANALYSIS*

Clinical Situation	Appropriate Specimen	Type of Processing
Congenital Aberrations	Peripheral blood	Mitogen stimulation of lymphocytes with phytohemagglutinin
	Skin biopsy	Tissue culture
	Autopsy organ samples	Tissue culture
	Products of conception	Tissue culture
Prenatal Diagnosis	Amniotic fluid	Tissue culture
	Chorionic villus biopsy	Direct harvest, tissue culture
Acquired Aberrations of Neoplastic Cells	Peripheral blood/Bone marrow	Direct harvest, unstimulated culture
	Lymph node/spleen	Direct harvest, unstimulated culture of cell suspension
	Solid tumor biopsy	Short-term tissue culture

TABLE 20-2 *CYTOGENETIC BANDING TECHNIQUES AND SPECIAL PROCEDURES*

Type of Banding/Procedure		Result
Q banding	quinacrine fluorescence A-T rich areas = bright G-C rich areas = dull	distinct bright and dull band patterns of homologous chromosomes
G banding	Giemsa stain after enzyme pretreatment A-T rich areas = dark G-C rich areas = pale	distinct dark and pale band patterns of homologous chromosomes identical to Q bands
R banding	A-T rich areas = pale G-C rich areas = dark	distinct pale and dark band patterns of homologous chromosomes reverse of Q and G bands
C banding	Giemsa stain after acid-alkali denaturation	stains heterochromatic pericentric regions of chromosomes 1, 9, 16 and long arm of Y chromosome
NOR Staining	silver stain of nucleolar organizing region	stains stalk region of acrocentric chromosomes 13, 14, 15, 21 and 22
FISH	fluorescent labeled DNA probes	depending on probe used, will stain specific chromosome centromere, region, arm, or whole chromosome
Synchronization	synchronization of cells in cell cycle with cold or with blocking agent (methotrexate)	increases number of cells in mitosis
High-resolution banding	cells are synchronized and are stopped in late prophase or early metaphase	chromosomes are less condensed than in metaphase and are banded at the 500–850 band stage
Fragile site	cells are cultured with folate/thymidine deprivation	reveals areas of chromosome gaps, most useful for fra(X).
SCE	sister chromatid exchange is detected by incubation through 2 cell cycles in BrdU and stained with fluorescent Hoechst-33258	sister chromatids will stain dark or light showing areas of exchange, indicating mutagenicity

procedures that result in a specific pattern of dark-, medium-, and light-stained bands for each homologous chromosome pair. The first chromosome banding was reported in 1970[2] with the use of quinacrine, a fluorescent stain that reveals a pattern of bright and dull bands (Q-bands).[2] Q-banding techniques are relatively simple, however, the banding fades when examined microscopically with ultraviolet illumination, and the resolution of bands is not as detailed as with G-bands. Most laboratories routinely analyze G-bands using Giemsa stain and some form of enzyme pretreatment, usually trypsin.[3] These techniques result in a high quality banding pattern that does not fade with microscopic examination. The pattern of bright or dull Q-bands and dark or pale-staining G-bands is essentially the same. Reverse banding (R-bands) yields a band pattern opposite to that of Q- and G-bands so that a pale G-band will be dark staining with R-banding.

The most recent advance in cytogenetic procedures has been the development of fluorescent-labeled cloned DNA probes for specific chromosome centromeres, whole arms or whole chromosomes (fluorescent in situ hybridization, FISH).[4] This allows specific identification of chromosomes involved in structural aberrations and allows partial analysis of interphase cells for the X and Y chromosome and for numerical chromosome abnormalities. Other banding techniques or special harvest procedures may be helpful for evaluation in certain clinical situations (Table 20-2).

● Chromosome analysis

Analysis of chromosomes is best performed microscopically. The adequacy of analysis depends on the mitotic rate of the cells and on banded chromosome morphology. An optimal preparation will have mitotic spreads with moderately long chromosomes, few chromosome overlaps, and good quality banding (Fig. 20-6). Photomicrographs are taken of representative cells using black and white film that enhances contrast between bands. The

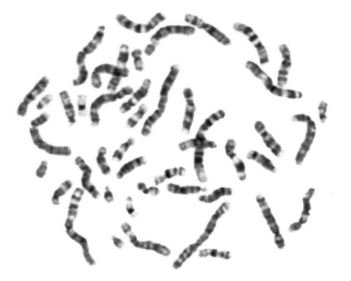

FIGURE 20-6. Metaphase spread of chromosomes belonging to a single cell, obtained by direct harvest of bone marrow aspirate (G-banded, original magnification, 100×).

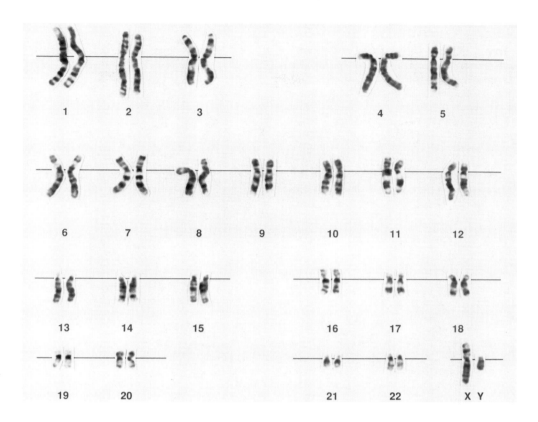

FIGURE 20-7. Karyotype of normal human male cell, G-banded.

karyotype is prepared from the photographs or by a video-computer linked analysis system. To prepare a karyotype, the chromosomes are grouped initially by size and centromere position, then by the specific pattern of dark, intermediate, and light staining bands (Fig. 20-7). The number of cells analyzed per case will vary according to the clinical situation. Preliminary standardized guidelines for cytogenetic analysis have been published and are being used as minimal guidelines by most laboratories.[5] Accrediting agencies, such as the College of American Pathologists (CAP) also have standards for laboratory inspection.

CHROMOSOME ABNORMALITIES

Chromosome abnormalities may either be numerical or structural and may involve the autosomes (1 to 22) and/or the X and Y sex chromosomes. *Congenital* abnormalities are present at the time of birth. These abnormalities will be present in all cells if they are inherited from a parent carrier or if they occurred during gametogenesis. Congenital aberrations may also occur in the embryo shortly after fertilization resulting in a *mosaic*, so that some cells will have the aberration and some will be normal. If the aberrations occur at some time after birth they are *acquired*, and this usually is seen in a single cell line identifying a neoplastic clone.

Numerical aberrations

A normal human cell with 46 chromosomes is called *diploid*. *Aneuploid* refers to a chromosome count other than 46, which is not a multiple of n (n = 23). If a cell has greater than 46 chromosomes the term *hyperdiploid* is used and if a cell has less than 46 chromosomes it is called *hypodiploid*. Most numerical aberrations are felt to be caused by a process of *nondisjunction*. Nondisjunction occurs during meiotic or mitotic cell division when a spindle fiber from the centriole does not connect to the chromosome centromere, or the spindle fiber connects but does not contract (Fig. 20-8). This results in one daughter cell with an extra chromosome *(trisomy)* and one daughter cell with a chromosome loss *(monosomy)*. In most cases, the cell with the chromosome loss does not survive the next cell cycle. Another process, termed *anaphase lag*, results when one chromatid does not completely migrate to the opposite pole but "lags behind" and gets caught outside of the nuclear membrane (Fig. 20-9), yielding one daughter cell with a chromosome loss and one daughter cell that is normal.

The term *polyploid* refers to cells that have a chromosome count that is a multiple of the n number. Hence, a tetraploid cell is polyploid and has a chromosome count of 4n = 92. *Endomitosis* is the process that results in polyploid cells when there are multiple mitotic divisions without dissolution of the nuclear membrane. The megakaryocyte is an example of a normal polyploid cell. The term *pseudodiploid* is used when the chromosome count is 46 and there are numerical and/or structural aberrations. For example, 46,XX,+8,−21 is an abnormal cell but has a chromosome count of 46, and therefore is pseudodiploid.

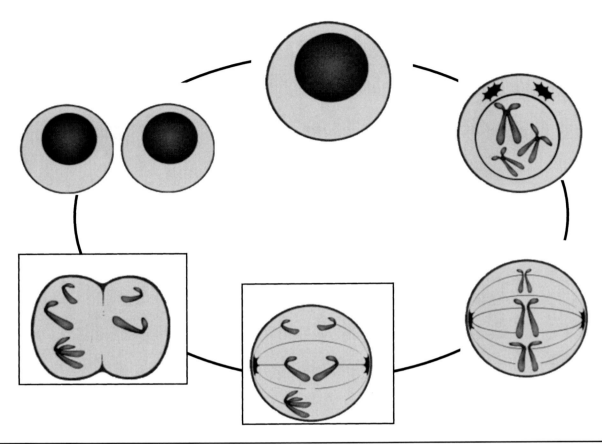

FIGURE 20-8. Nondisjunction. During anaphase the sister chromatids of a chromosome do not disjoin, resulting in one daughter cell with an extra chromosome (trisomy) and the other with a chromosome loss (monosomy).

Structural aberrations

Structural chromosome aberrations occur when there is chromosome breakage and the repair process results in structural loss or in abnormal recombinations. Table 20-3 lists structural aberrations with a short description, example nomenclature, and illustration. Any of these may be seen as congenital or acquired, with the exception of homogeneously staining regions and double minutes that have only been seen in neoplastic cells.

Polymorphic variation

Morphologic variations are known to occur in certain chromosomes. These variations have no clinical significance, but if present, will be inherited consistently through each generation. *Polymorphic variants* are easily demonstrated with various banding techniques and can be used to identify maternal vs. paternal origin of homologous chromosomes. This has become particularly useful for following same-sex allogeneic bone marrow transplant recipients. Some of the more commonly seen polymorphic variants include a pericentric inversion of chromosome 9, variable amounts of pericentric heterochromatin on chromosomes 1, 9, 16 and a variable amount of heterochromatin on the long arm of the Y chromosome. Also, there can be variable amounts of satellite material on the short arms of the acrocentric chromosomes.

CYTOGENETIC NOMENCLATURE

The designation of chromosome number, region, band, and karyotype nomenclature has been established by an international committee whose goal is to have one usable system. The International System for Human Cytogenetic Nomenclature (ISCN)[6] has published guidelines for use by clinical and research laboratories, and, in 1991, the ISCN published specific rules for cancer cytogenetics.[7] The short and long arms of each chromosome are divided into regions by major landmark bands (Fig. 20-10). Each region is further divided into the individual pale-, intermediate-, and dark-staining bands. The numbering of regions and bands always begins at the centromere and proceeds distally to the terminal portions, *pter* and *qter*. The num-

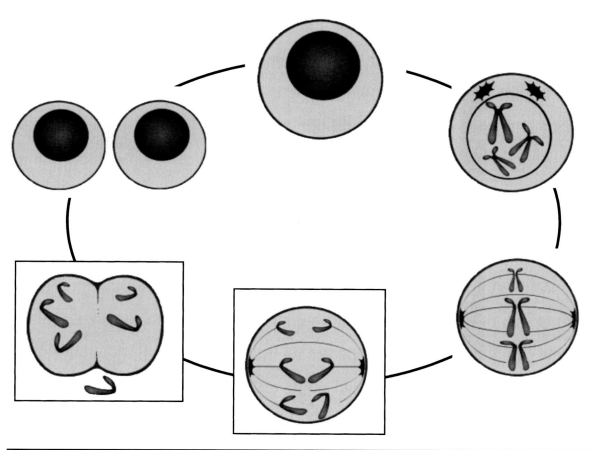

FIGURE 20-9. Anaphase lag. Chromatid does not complete migration resulting in one daughter cell with a normal chromosome count and the other with a chromosome loss.

bering of bands begins with the number 1 for each region. To designate a specific band of a chromosome, the order is written as chromosome number, arm, region, band. For example, in Figure 20-10, the band designated at the arrow on chromosome 7 would be 7q32.

The karyotype of a cell is designated first by the total number of chromosomes followed by the sex chromosomes. If aberrations are present, sex chromosome abnormalities are listed first, followed by abnormalities of autosomes listed in numerical order of the chromosomes involved. Numerical abnormalities are designated by a " + " or " − " in front of the chromosome number. Structural abnormalities are listed by the appropriate abbreviation, followed by the chromosomes involved in parenthesis, followed by the break-point band designation in parentheses. Therefore, normal female and normal male karyotypes, respectively, would be listed: 46,XX and 46,XY. A male cell with trisomy for chromosomes 8 and 21 would be listed as: 48,XY, + 8, + 21. A female cell with trisomy for chromosomes 3, 8, and 15, and a translocation involving chromosome 9 and 22 would be listed as: 49,XX, + 3, + 8,t(9;22)(q34;q11), + 15. See Table 20-3 for other examples of nomenclature.

● CYTOGENETIC ANALYSIS OF HEMATOPOIETIC DISORDERS

In the past 5 to 10 years, the field of cytogenetics related to the study of neoplasms has literally exploded. Certain chromosome aberrations have been found to be characteristic and sometimes diagnostic of particular hematopoietic disorders, lymphoproliferative disorders, or solid tumors. These findings have contributed greatly to the clinical services giving valuable information for diagnosis and prognosis. In addition, some of these findings have led researchers to significant discoveries of gene loci and theories of tumorigenesis including protooncogene activation and tumor suppressor genes. Chromosome aberrations that are found in neoplastic cells are referred to as *acquired, clonal* aberrations. An acquired aberration is one that occurs at some time after birth and is present only in the neoplastic cells. A clone exists if numerical and/or structural aberrations are identical in at least 2 cells, unless the abnormality is a single chromosome loss (monosomy), then 3 cells must have the same chromosome loss. Identification of an abnormal clone by cytogenetics indicates the presence of a neoplastic cell line. Table 20-4

TABLE 20-3 *STRUCTURAL CHROMOSOME ABERRATIONS WITH DIAGRAMS, EXPLANATIONS AND EXAMPLE NOMENCLATURE*

Structural Aberration and Nomenclature	Explanation	Structural Aberration and Nomenclature	Explanation
Chromosome/ Chromatid Breaks	Break occurs in chromosome/ chromatid and is usually repaired. Increased random breaks may be seen with toxins, radiation, and virus exposure.	**Inversion, Paracentric** ex: inv(7)(q21q32)	Two breaks occur and the material between the breaks inverts, then is repaired. When the inversion does not involve the centromere = paracentric.
Terminal Deletion ex: del(7)(q32)	Break occurs and acentric fragment is lost during mitosis/meiosis.	**Ring Chromosome** ex: r(7)(p21q35)	Breaks occur in the short and long arm and the broken ends are repaired together; the acentric fragments are lost.
Interstitial Deletion ex: del(7)(q31q32)	Two breaks occur in one arm and material between breaks is lost; ends are repaired together.	**Isochromosome** ex: i(7p) or i(7q)	Centromere splits horizontally and results in chromosome with only short or long arm material. The remaining arm of the chromosome is usually lost
Translocation, balanced ex: t(7;8)(q32;q23)	Breaks occur in two different chromosomes with fragments repaired to the opposite chromosome; no loss of DNA occurs.	**Dicentric** ex: dic(7;8)(q32;q23)	Breaks occur in two chromosomes and the chromosomes – including centromeres- are repaired together; the acentric fragments are lost.
Translocation,Robertsonian ex: t(14q21q)	Breaks occur at centromeres of two acrocentric chromosomes; the centromeric regions fuse and the short arm/ satellite material is lost.	**Duplication** ex: dup(7)(q31→q32)	Region of a chromosome is duplicated; may be direct or inverted.
Translocation, unbalanced (derivative chromosome) ex: der(7)t(7;8)(q32;q23)	The first chromosome listed as der( ) is the one that retains the centromere. In this example, der(7) results in a partial trisomy for 8q and partial monosomy for 7q.	**Homogeneously Staining Region** ex: hsr(7)(q31)	Region of chromosome that is amplified and stains homogeneous, light or dark.
Inversion, Pericentric ex: inv(7)(p15q21)	Two breaks occur and the material between the breaks inverts, then is repaired. When the inversion involves the centromere = pericentric.	**Double Minutes** dmin	Small acentric pieces of DNA, usually paired, representing amplified genes.

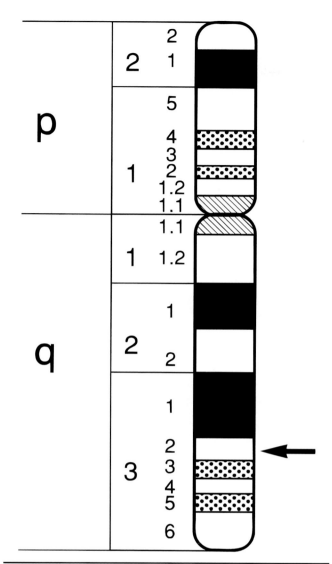

FIGURE 20-10. Diagram of chromosome 7 with arm, region, and band designations. The band located at the arrow is designated 7q32.

TABLE 20-4 *PRESENT APPLICATIONS OF CYTOGENETICS IN HEMATOPOIETIC DISORDERS*

- confirm or establish the diagnosis of chronic myelocytic leukemia (CML)
- confirm or predict blast crisis of CML
- aid in diagnosis and prognosis of acute leukemia
- confirm or establish remission and relapse of acute leukemia
- aid in the diagnosis and prognosis of myelodysplastic states
- evaluation of bone marrow transplant for donor vs. recipient cells and possible recurrence of original neoplasm
- aid in the diagnosis and prognosis of lymphoproliferative disorders

neoplastic clone and will only have congenital aberrations if present.

Processing of specimens

The best sample for cytogenetic analysis of hematopoietic disorders, excluding lymphomas, is bone marrow aspirate; even when blast cells are present in the peripheral blood, a greater mitotic rate is usually achieved from the bone marrow sample. These cells are processed by direct harvest and/or unstimulated cultures. The overall cellularity of the marrow aspirate or peripheral blood sample can vary greatly and will affect the mitotic yield and chromosome morphology. Therefore, it is best for the cytogenetic laboratory to prepare a smear of the sample received and harvest an amount appropriate for the specimen cellularity. The smear can be easily stained with a Wright-Giemsa-type stain, and this smear also may be useful if the patient diagnosis is not known or if unsuspected results are found. The best specimen for study of lymphoma is an involved lymph node. In general, the morphology of chromosomes from a peripheral blood or bone marrow/lymph node specimen is not as good as that from a phytohemagglutinin stimulated study; this may reflect an inherent feature of the malignant cells. In fact, cells with particularly poor morphology may represent the abnormal clone whereas the cells with better morphology may be the remaining normal population. Therefore, when working in cancer cytogenetics, a technologist must be careful to analyze each mitotic spread and not skip the poorly banded cells. Some laboratories have been successful in improving chromosome morphology and/or mitotic yield of malignant-type specimens by using synchronization and/or media supplements.

There also may be differences in the mitotic rate of neoplastic versus normal cells, which will lead to misinterpretation. For example, it has been well documented that specimens from patients with acute promyelocytic leukemia (AML-M3) may demonstrate the diagnostic t(15;17) only after unstimulated culture as opposed to direct harvest which may yield only a normal karyotype or a markedly reduced number of cells with the t(15;17). Occasionally, another type of leukemia may have a demonstrable clonal aberration from directly harvested cells and only a normal karyotype after unstimulated culture.

gives a list of the most practical uses of cytogenetic analysis in the hematopoietic disorders.

Occasionally, congenital chromosome aberrations are coincidentally found when analyzing neoplastic cells. This is most often true for congenital aberrations that may not be associated with clinical findings. For example, a female patient with acute leukemia and a 47,XXX karyotype may have the +X as an acquired aberration indicative of the malignant cells or the +X may represent a congenital finding and be present in all the patient's cells. However, if the karyotype is 47,XX,+8, this most certainly is acquired as trisomy 8 is not compatible with life. The presence of congenital aberrations must be accurately interpreted and distinguished from acquired clonal aberrations. This is most often accomplished by stimulated peripheral lymphocyte analysis or occasionally by skin biopsy fibroblast culture, as these cells are not part of the

TABLE 20-5 *APPROPRIATE SPECIMENS AND TYPE OF PROCESSING FOR CYTOGENETIC ANALYSIS OF NEOPLASTIC CELLS*

Possible Diagnosis	Specimen	Processing
Acute Leukemia Myeloproliferative Disorders Myelodysplastic States	Bone Marrow Peripheral Blood	Direct harvest, 24-48-72 hour unstimulated culture
Acute Promyelocytic Leukemia	Bone Marrow Peripheral Blood	Unstimulated culture
Lymphoproliferative Disorder	Lymph Node, Spleen, Bone Marrow, Peripheral Blood	Direct harvest, unstimulated culture; T-Cell: phytohemagglutinin stimulation; B-Cell: pokeweed, lipopolysaccharide, or EBV stimulation
Solid Tumor	Tumor Tissue Effusion (pleural, peritoneal, etc.)	Direct harvest (if adequate cell suspension), short-term tissue culture Direct harvest, unstimulated culture

The processing of cells from lymphoma may include incubation with mitogens in addition to the unstimulated cultures. The neoplastic cells from B-cell lymphomas will sometimes respond to pokeweed, lipopolysaccharide, or EBV antigen and neoplastic cells from T-cell lymphomas will occasionally respond to phytohemagglutinin stimulation. A summary of specimen processing is given in Table 20-5.

● Chronic myelocytic leukemia

The first chromosome abnormality reported to be associated with a malignancy was described in 1960 as an abnormally small chromosome seen in patients with chronic myelocytic leukemia (CML).[8] This was designated the Philadelphia or Ph[1] (now designated as Ph) chromosome and was believed to be a deletion of the long arm of chromosome 22. With the advent of banding techniques, it was found to actually be a balanced translocation involving chromosomes 9 and 22, t(9;22)(q34;q11).[9] This translocation is seen in at least 90% of patients with CML. Approximately 5% to 10% of these patients will have a variant translocation involving chromosome 22 and a chromosome in addition to or instead of chromosome 9. In fact, every chromosome except the Y chromosome has been reported in variant Ph translocations and some complex rearrangements may involve three or more chromosomes. Patients with variant translocations have the same clinical features and prognosis as those with the typical 9;22 translocation (see Chapter 15).

The t(9;22) is present in myeloid precursors, erythroid precursors, megakaryocytes, and some lymphocytes. This is used as evidence that the malignant change occurs at the level of the pluripotent stem cell affecting all marrow cells. The Ph is found in nearly 100% of the bone marrow cells analyzed. Patients who are treated and have achieved an apparent remission with normal peripheral white blood cell counts still have the t(9;22) in bone marrow cells. One exception involves interferon therapy where some patients have shown a significant reduction in the percent of cells with the t(9;22).[10] It is not yet known if this will relate to an improved prognosis. Most cases of CML terminate in a blast crisis, and the majority of these patients will have a change in the karyotype with chromosome aberrations in addition to the t(9;22). The most frequently observed additional aberrations are a duplication of the Ph, +der(22)t(9;22), a duplication of chromosome 8, +8, and an isochromosome for the long arm of chromosome 17, i(17q). This cytogenetic transformation may be detected days or weeks before the actual morphologic transformation to blast crisis is seen in the marrow or peripheral blood. The prognosis of the blast crisis may be relatively better if no change in the karyotype occurs.

Investigators have attempted for some time to decipher why a specific chromosome translocation should be so closely associated with a single morphologic type of leukemia. It is now known that the proto-oncogene ABL (Abelson murine leukemia virus) is normally located at 9q34 and is translocated to 22q11 in the Philadelphia translocation.[11] The site of breakage in chromosome 22 is clustered within a 5-6 kilobase (kb = sequence of 1000 base pairs) region, termed breakpoint cluster region, BCR. This translocation then results in a new chimeric gene consisting of a portion of the ABL and a portion of the BCR. The ABL is activated to a functioning oncogene and a 210 kD polypeptide product of BCR-ABL is present in the leukemic cells. It is not yet known if this new abnormal polypeptide is at least partially responsible for the neoplastic proliferation of the myeloid cells. Molecular studies and fluorescent in situ hybridization have shown that in some of the cases of Philadelphia chromosome negative CML, the molecular rearrangement of BCR-ABL has still occurred while cytogenetically the chromosomes appear normal.[12] These molecular level rearrangements may have occurred by a process of insertion of the ABL gene into the region of the BCR on chromosome 22 or by an initial 9;22 translocation followed by a second translocation, resulting in a cytogenetically normal chromosome 9 and 22, with a gene level rearrangement of the BCR-ABL. Similar studies have shown that variant Ph translocations have the molecular level BCR-ABL even in cases where the chromosome 9 appears cytogenetically uninvolved. The t(9;22) also is seen in approximately 15% of cases of acute lymphocytic leukemia (ALL), particularly in adult ages, and <5% of cases of acute nonlymphocytic leukemia (ANLL). Although the translocation appears cytogenetically the same as that seen in CML, there is in fact a difference in the site of breakage through the BCR locus, resulting in a 190 kD protein. Perhaps this molecular level difference is responsible for the morphologic expression as ALL. The cases of Ph-positive ALL and ANLL must be distinguished from a patient presenting in blast crisis of CML, as the prognosis in the latter is relatively worse. In most cases of Ph-positive ALL and ANLL, the number of the cells with the Ph is significantly less than 100%, while in blast crisis of CML it is almost always seen in 100% of the cells. If complete remission is achieved in ALL or ANLL, the karyotype will be normal; in apparent remission of blast crisis of CML, the Ph will still be present.

Myeloproliferative disorders other than CML

The other myeloproliferative disorders, polycythemia rubra vera (PRV), myelofibrosis with myeloid metaplasia (MMM), and essential thrombocythemia (ET), have clonal acquired chromosome aberrations in approximately 50% to 60% of cases. The prognosis does not seem to be worse if clonal aberrations are present. No specific chromosome aberrations have been reported, but some correlation has been found with abnormalities of chromosome 20, particularly del(20q), in PRV. Frequently seen aberrations in the myeloproliferative disorders include abnormalities of 1q, −7, +8, +9, del(13q), and del(20q). Demonstration of a clonal aberration can be very helpful in cases where the diagnosis of a myeloproliferative disorder is difficult to distinguish from a non-neoplastic reactive proliferation.

Acute nonlymphocytic leukemia

Approximately 70% of patients with primary acute nonlymphocytic leukemia (ANLL) have clonal acquired chromosome aberrations in the leukemic cells. These aberrations are present only in the leukemic blasts and not in the other hematopoietic precursors. Therefore, primary ANLL appears to be a malignancy of the committed stem cell. The chromosome abnormalities found may be single, numerical or structural, or may be multiple karyotypic aberrations. Some aberrations such as trisomy 8 occur frequently in ANLL, but are not diagnostic for a specific type of leukemia. Chromosome aberrations when present in the original leukemic cells can be valuable in following the progression or regression of the leukemia. If the original leukemic cells have a clonal aberration, such as +8, a complete remission sample should have only a normal karyotype. In subsequent samples the presence of even one cell with +8 would indicate an early relapse, which may not be detectable morphologically. Some patients may have additional aberrations at the time of relapse indicating cytogenetic transformation to a more aggressive and resistant disease. If the original leukemic cells have a normal karyotype, it will usually remain normal during relapse; however, a few of these cases may show newly acquired aberrations in relapse indicative of transformation. Initially, prognosis was related to whether 100% of the

TABLE 20-6 *CORRELATION OF NONRANDOM CHROMOSOME ABERRATIONS AND FAB CLASSIFICATION OF ANLL*

FAB Classification	Chromosome Aberration
M0	Various clonal, numerical and/or structural
M1	Various clonal, numerical and/or structural
M2	t(8;21)(q22;q22), & as above
M3	t(15;17)(q22;q11)
M4	abn. 11q; eos-abn.16q
M5	abn. 11q, t(9;11)(p22;q23)
M6	Various clonal, numerical and structural
M7	abn. 3q; t(1;22)
Secondary leukemia	−5, del(5q), −7, del(7q)

cells have a chromosome aberration (AA), 100% have a normal karyotype (NN) or if the cells show a combination of normal and abnormal karyotypes (AN). Patients with AA have a significantly worse prognosis than patients with NN. Patients with AN have a prognosis intermediate between AA and NN. Emphasis is now also placed on the actual chromosome aberration found. The abnormalities that are associated with a relatively better prognosis with shorter time to complete remission include t(8;21), t(15;17), and 16q abnormalities. A relatively worse prognosis has been seen with −5/del(5q), −7/del(7q), +8, t(9;22), t(8;16), rings, and double minutes (dmin). Table 20-6 shows the chromosome aberrations reported in different types of ANLL listed by FAB classification. Other abnormalities that have been frequently reported include +4, t(6;9)(p23;q34), +9, del(9q), +11, +12, del(12p), del(13q), del(20q), +21, and markers. Figure 20-11 shows some examples of the structural aberrations.

Most interesting of the chromosome aberrations in acute leukemia is the t(15;17). This aberration is virtually diagnostic of acute promyelocytic leukemia (M3). It has not been reported in other types of malignancy and is seen in more than 80% to 90% of cases of M3. The translocation is seen in the hypergranular form as well as microgranular variant of M3. It has recently been shown that the translocation breakpoint on chromosome 17 lies within the gene locus for retinoic acid receptor alpha (RARα) and a more recently described PML gene locus on chromosome 15.[13,14] Incubation of cells in vitro with retinoic acid has been shown to result in maturation and differentiation of the leukemic cells to segmented neutrophils; treatment trials have now been initiated with trans-retinoic acid.[15] It is likely that further research will show this type of causal relationship between the other chromosome rearrangements, type of leukemic expression and possibly treatment response.

Cytogenetic studies of pediatric age patients with ANLL have shown similar findings to those of adults, however, with a higher incidence of the 16q abnormalities and of t(8;21).

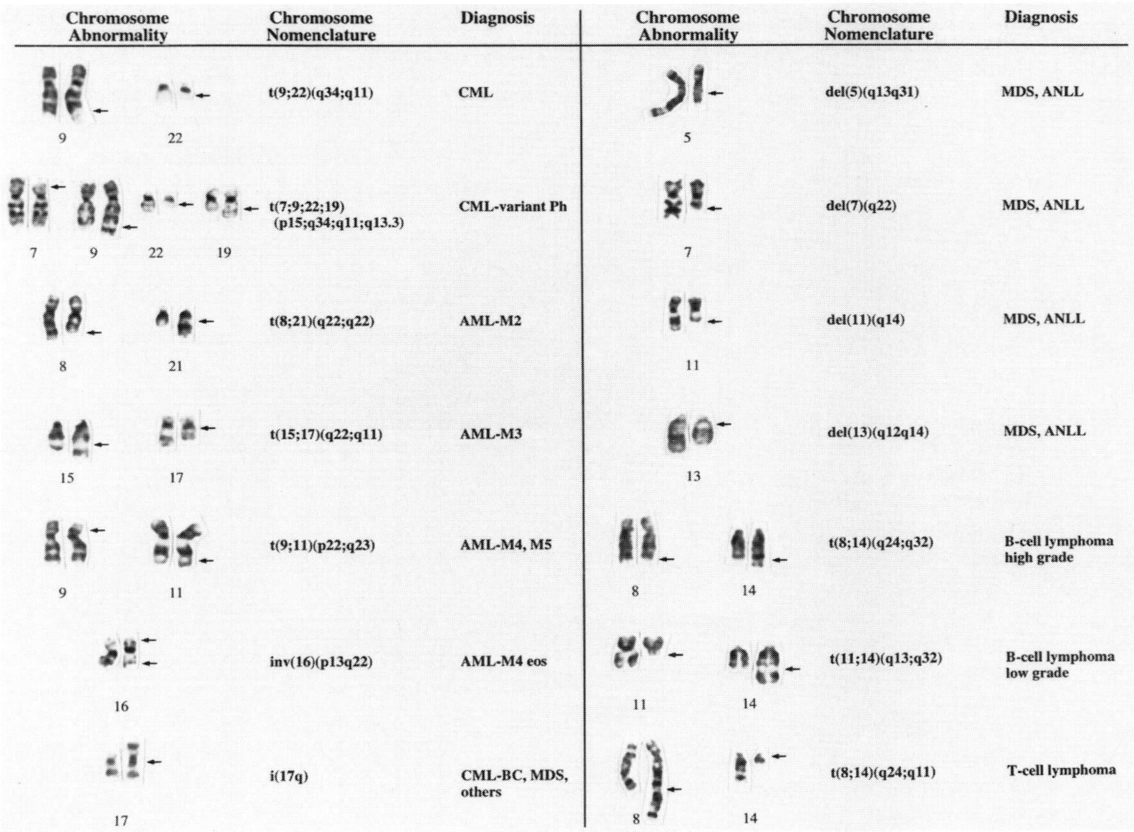

Chromosome Abnormality	Chromosome Nomenclature	Diagnosis	Chromosome Abnormality	Chromosome Nomenclature	Diagnosis
9 22	t(9;22)(q34;q11)	CML	5	del(5)(q13q31)	MDS, ANLL
7 9 22 19	t(7;9;22;19) (p15;q34;q11;q13.3)	CML-variant Ph	7	del(7)(q22)	MDS, ANLL
8 21	t(8;21)(q22;q22)	AML-M2	11	del(11)(q14)	MDS, ANLL
15 17	t(15;17)(q22;q11)	AML-M3	13	del(13)(q12q14)	MDS, ANLL
9 11	t(9;11)(p22;q23)	AML-M4, M5	8 14	t(8;14)(q24;q32)	B-cell lymphoma high grade
16	inv(16)(p13q22)	AML-M4 eos	11 14	t(11;14)(q13;q32)	B-cell lymphoma low grade
17	i(17q)	CML-BC, MDS, others	8 14	t(8;14)(q24;q11)	T-cell lymphoma

FIGURE 20-11. Partial karyotypes of structural chromosome aberrations in hematopoietic malignancies. The abnormal chromosome is on the right of each chromosome pair with an arrow at the site of rearrangement. Refer to text for explanations.

Myelodysplastic states

Chromosome analysis of the myelodysplastic states (MDS) has shown clonal acquired aberrations in 50% to 70% of patients studied. These aberrations are similar to those found in ANLL except for the more specific t(15; 17) and t(8;21), which are not seen in MDS. Cytogenetics has become very valuable in the diagnosis and prognosis of patients with MDS.[16] Some cases of MDS are difficult to diagnose as the peripheral blood and bone marrow findings may be subtle. In these cases, the demonstration of a clonal, acquired chromosome aberration establishes the diagnosis of a hematopoietic neoplasm. In general, patients with MDS that have clonal acquired aberrations have a worse prognosis than those with a normal karyotype. When categorized by type of myelodysplastic state, clonal chromosome aberrations are more often seen in refractory anemia with excess blasts and refractory anemia with excess blasts in transformation, as opposed to refractory anemia and refractory anemia with ringed sideroblasts. The chromosome aberrations are present in all three cell lines, myeloid, erythroid, and megakaryocytic, indicating that the neoplastic proliferation begins at the pluripotent stem cell as was seen in the myeloproliferative disorders. Clonal chromosome aberrations have also been reported in chronic myelomonocytic leukemia; however, no specific aberration has been found. Some of the more commonly seen aberrations in the MDS include: t(1; 3)(p36;q11), der(1)t(1;7)(p11;p11), −5, del(5q), −7, del(7q), +8, +9, i(17q), +19, del(20q), +21, abnormalities of Xq.

Secondary leukemia

Acute leukemia is known to occur with increased incidence in patients who have previously received chemotherapy, radiation therapy, or have had exposure to other toxins. These cases are called secondary or iatrogenic leukemia and many times these patients initially present with a myelodysplastic state. The majority of cases of secondary leukemia are found to be nonlymphocytic and usually occur 18 months to 2 years after exposure. The patients who seem to be at greatest risk are those who received radiation and chemotherapy; chemotherapy alone is an intermediate risk and radiation alone is the lowest risk. The type of chemotherapeutic agent used also makes a difference in the leukemic risk. Alkylating agents such as melphalan have a significantly higher leukemogenic potential than nonalkylating agents. In contrast to patients with primary ANLL, more than 90% of patients with secondary acute leukemia/MDS will have clonal, acquired chromosome aberrations in the leukemic cells.[17] Abnormalities frequently seen are a loss of chromosome 5 and/or 7, or long arm deletions of chromosome 5 and/or 7, or der(1)t(1;7). The modal chromosome number is often hypodiploid and the prognosis is generally poor.

● Acute lymphocytic leukemia

Approximately 60% to 75% of patients with acute lymphocytic leukemia (ALL) will have clonal acquired aberrations of the malignant cells. Cytogenetic findings are a crucial part of the leukemia workup for pediatric cases and the results are directly related to prognosis.[18,19] Patients who have the best overall prognosis are those who have hyperdiploid karyotypes of the leukemic blasts with a chromosome count greater than 50, usually ranging from 51 to 65. Chromosomes frequently duplicated are 4, 6, 10, 14, 17, 18, 20, 21, and X. Some cases with hyperdiploidy will also have structural aberrations; it is not known if this changes the prognostic category. Most cases with hyperdiploidy of greater than 50 also have clinically favorable findings such as 3 to 7 years of age, total white cell count less than 10,000, FAB classification type L1, and pre-B CALLA positive phenotype. The next best prognostic group of ALL is in individuals with a normal karyotype. The remaining cases, when grouped by cytogenetics, have an intermediate to poor prognosis. Hyperdiploidy with a chromosome count of 47 to 50 is associated with an intermediate prognosis and no clinically distinguishing features.[20] Chromosomes most often increased are 8, 13, and 21. Pseudodiploidy is seen with variable structural and/or numerical aberrations. In general, cases with pseudodiploid karyotypes have an intermediate to poor prognosis depending upon the specific structural aberrations. Hypodiploidy is a more unusual finding and is most often due to a single chromosome loss, resulting in a chromosome count of 45. Rarely seen is severe hypodiploidy with a near haploid chromosome count. These cases have a relatively poor prognosis. Some of the more commonly seen structural aberrations in ALL are listed in Table 20-7.

● Lymphoma and lymphoproliferative disorders

Chromosome analysis of the lymphomas and other lymphoproliferative disorders has lagged behind that of the acute leukemias due to the difficulty of obtaining tumor cells for cytogenetic procedures. In recent years, chromosome analysis in these disorders has added greatly to the understanding of the importance of the gene loci involved in chromosome aberrations seen with specific types of lymphoma. These results have also led to the development of molecular gene probes and their use in the clinical laboratory. Most cases of lymphoma are not particularly difficult to diagnose by routine histology; cytogenetics is only practically helpful in cases that have difficult morphology, or to confirm the presence of small numbers of tumor cells.

TABLE 20-7 *CORRELATION OF CHROMOSOME ABERRATIONS SEEN IN ALL WITH IMMUNOPHENOTYPE AND PROGNOSIS*

ALL Phenotype	Chromosome Aberration	Known Gene Loci	Prognosis
Early B cell CALLA +	Hyperdiploid >50		good
	Hyperdiploid 47–50		intermediate
	Hypodiploid		poor
	del(6q)		intermediate
	del/t 9p	IFNA/IFNB	intermediate
	del/t 12p		intermediate
	t(9;22)(q34;q11)	ABL/BCR	poor
eosinophilia	t(5;14)(q31;q32)	IL3/IGH	intermediate
CIg +	t(1;19)(q23;p13)	PBL1/E2A	poor
Biphenotypic & CALLA-	t(4;11)(q21;q23)		poor
B cell SIg +	t(8;14)(q24;q32)	MYC/IGH	poor
	t(2;8)(p12;q24)	IGK/MYC	poor
	t(8;22)(q24;q11)	MYC/IGL	poor
T cell	t(11;14)(p13;q11)	TCL2/TCRα-δ	poor
	t(8;14)(q24;q11)	C-MYC/TCRα	poor
	inv(14)(q11q32)	TCRα/IGH/TCL1	poor
	t(v;14)(v;q11)	TCRα	poor
	t(7;v)(q34–36;v)	TCRβ	poor
	t(7;v)(p15;v)	TCRγ	poor

Some of the cases with poor prognosis listed may change to intermediate with aggressive therapy; IFNA = interferon alpha; IFNB = interferon beta; IL3 = interleukin 3; IGH = immunoglobulin heavy chain; E2A = IG enhancer; IGK = kappa chain; IGL = lambda chain; MYC&ABL = oncogenes; BCR = breakpoint cluster region; PBL1 = leukemia genes; TCL1&2 = putative proto-oncogene; TCRα,β,δ,γ = T cell receptor genes; v = variable chromosome involved.

(Adapted from LeBeau, M.: The role of cytogenetics in the diagnosis and classification of hematopoietic neoplasms. In: Knowles, D., ed. Neoplastic Hematopathology. Williams and Wilkins, Baltimore, 1992, Table 9.4, pg. 309).

The first abnormality described in the lymphomas was the 14q+[21] seen in Burkitt's lymphoma (see Chapter 19). This was later characterized as t(8;14)(q24;q32) and is seen in approximately 75% of cases of Burkitt's lymphoma. Two variant translocations, t(2;8)(p12;q24) and t(8;22)(q24;q11), have been reported in 10% to 15% of Burkitt's lymphoma. The 14q32 is the site of the gene for the heavy chain of immunoglobulin and the break at 8q24 is just proximal to the site of the proto-oncogene MYC. Therefore, the MYC gene is translocated to the heavy chain locus at 14q32.[22] This was the first demonstration of a protooncogene that was translocated to a location known to be active in B-cell lymphoma and resulting in the activation of the oncogene. The t(2;8) results in the juxtaposition of a gene for kappa light chain to MYC and the t(8;22) results in the juxtaposition of a gene for lamda light chain to MYC. In cases of Burkitt's lymphoma that have the two variant translocations, the tumor cells are found to mark with surface kappa chain when the t(2;8) is found and to mark with lamda chain when the t(8;22) is found.

Information regarding prognosis of lymphoproliferative disorders related to the cytogenetic findings is currently emerging.[23] There does seem to be a correlation of prognosis with karyotype in chronic lymphocytic leuke-

TABLE 20-8 *CORRELATION OF CHROMOSOME ABERRATIONS SEEN IN NON-HODGKIN'S LYMPHOMA WITH GENE LOCI IDENTIFIED*

Chromosome Aberration	Lymphoproliferative Disorder	Known Gene Loci
+12, 11q− t(11;14)(q13;q32)	CLL, small lymphocytic and multiple myeloma	BCL1/IGH
t(14;18)(q32;q21)	follicular center cell - small cleaved cell	IGH/BCL2
t(14;18), +8, 2q-	follicular mixed	
t(14;18), +7, +12, + others	follicular/diffuse large cell	
t(8;14)(q24;q32) t(2;8)(p11;q24) t(8;22)(q24;q11)	small noncleaved cell and other B cell high grade tumors	MYC/IGH IGK/MYC MYC/IGL
inv(14)(q11q32) t(14;v)(q11;v) t(7;v)(q34;v) t(7;v)(p15;v) t(2;5)(p23;q35)	T cell neoplasms T cell neoplasms T cell T cell Ki-1 + anaplastic large cell	TCRα/IGH TCRα,δ TCRβ TCRγ

BCL1 = B cell leukemia/lymphoma 1; IGH = immunoglobulin heavy chain; BCL2 = B cell leukemia/lymphoma 2; C-MYC = protooncogene; IGK = kappa light chain; IGL = lamda light chain; TCR = T cell receptor genes, alpha, beta, delta, and gamma.

(Adapted from LeBeau, M.: The role of cytogenetics in the diagnosis and classification of hematopoietic neoplasms. In: Knowles, D., ed. Neoplastic Hematopathology. Williams and Wilkins, Baltimore, 1992, Table 9.4, pg. 309).

mia and in multiple myeloma. Further studies are necessary in these areas.

Interestingly, the chromosome rearrangements that have been found in T-cell lymphomas have now been shown to involve gene loci for T-cell receptor genes alpha, beta, delta, and gamma. Table 20-8 lists the characteristic chromosome aberration with the lymphoproliferative disorder and gene loci known to be involved in these rearrangements.

Bone marrow transplantation

Some of the hematopoietic disorders presented in this chapter are treated by allogeneic bone marrow transplantation, depending on the clinical situation and availability of donors. Cytogenetics is a valuable tool in following the engraftment and progression of donor versus recipient cells. If the recipient marrow cells have an initial chromosome aberration, such as t(9;22), or if the donor and recipient are of opposite sex, it is helpful to follow the engrafting marrow cells with cytogenetic analysis to detect the possible presence of recipient cells. Occasionally, the donor or recipient may have a polymorphic chromosome variant such as inv(9) that can be used to follow the cell line if the donor and recipient are of the same sex. Following a successful allogeneic transplant only donor cells should be present. Occasionally, 1% or 2% of recipient cells may be detectable shortly after transplant, but will then diminish. If recipient cells recur with a normal karyo-

type a *chimerism* develops. For example, a female recipient after a male donated transplant may show 60% 46,XY and 40% 46,XX. This would suggest a likely relapse of the original disease; however, in some cases the chimeric state may last for months or longer without leukemic relapse.[24–26] If the recipient cells recur with an abnormal karyotype, for example 60% 46,XY and 40% 46,XX,t(9; 22), then relapse has occurred. Rarely, patients have developed leukemic transformation of the donor cells.[27] In some of these cases, the donor remained normal and in other cases the donor also had developed leukemia. There is a somewhat greater risk for the latter when donor and recipient are identical twins, as the overall risk of leukemia occurrence in one twin is approximately 15 times higher than the normal population once leukemia has occurred in the first twin.

Autologous bone marrow transplant is performed mainly on patients with lymphoma or solid tumor, but occasionally in cases of leukemia. In these situations cytogenetics may be useful to follow possible disease recurrence only if the patient originally showed an abnormal karyotype of the malignant cells.

Solid tumors

Chromosome analysis of solid tumors has been hampered in the past by the difficulty in obtaining cell suspensions and in successful short-term tissue culture growth. There have been great improvements in recent years; however, some tumors remain too difficult to study. Many of these findings will be more helpful on a research level than on a practical clinical level. Some of the tumors that have been studied, benign and malignant, have shown interesting associations with specific chromosome aberrations[28,29] (Table 20-9). The cytogenetic work performed with retinoblastoma has added a new dimension to our understanding of tumorigenesis.[30] The occurrence of retinoblastoma is related to the loss of a specific type of gene now termed *tumor suppressor gene* or *"anti-oncogene."* These genes are normally responsible for suppressing cell dedifferentiation and tumor growth. If both gene alleles are mutated certain types of neoplasms occur. The tumor suppressor gene associated with retinoblastoma is designated RB1 and is located at 13q14.[31] Some patients inherit a chromosome 13 that has a molecular level mutation of RB1 or more rarely an identifiable chromosome deletion, del(13), that involves q14. A second event occurs in a single retinal cell that results in a loss or mutation of the remaining normal RB1 locus, leading to tumor development. Noninheritable cases of retinoblastoma (sporadic) represent about 60% of patients and mutation of both RB1 loci occurs only in the retinal cells. This same process is known to occur in Wilms' tumor with the affected tumor suppressor gene at 11p13 or 15.[32] No doubt many more tumor suppressor genes will be found associated with specific neoplasms.

Some of the pediatric tumors known as "small round blue cell tumors" can present with bone marrow metastasis and cause difficulty in diagnoses as the morphology

TABLE 20-9 *NON-RANDOM CHROMOSOME ABERRATIONS THAT HAVE BEEN IDENTIFIED IN VARIOUS NEOPLASMS*

Neoplasm	Chromosome Aberration
Alveolar rhabdomyosarcoma	t(2;13)
Bladder carcinoma	struct. abn. no. 1 & 11 i(5p) +7 −9
Breast carcinoma	struct. abn. no. 1, 16q
Ewing's/Askin Tumor/Neuroepithelioma	t(11;22)(q24;q12)
Glioma	double minutes
Renal carcinoma	t(5;14)(q13;q22) t or del 3p11−21
Colon carcinoma	struct. abn. no. 1 & 17 +7, +12, −18
Lipoma	t(12)(q13−14)
Melanoma	t or del 1p12−22 t(1;19)(q12;p13) t or del 6q +7
Meningioma	−22
Myxoid Liposarcoma	t(12;16)(q13;p11)
Neuroblastoma	del(1)(p31−32) HSR/dmin
Ovarian carcinoma	struct. abn. no. 1 t(6;14)(q21;q24)
Pleomorphic adenoma	t(13)(p21) t or del (8)(q12) t or del (12)(q13−15)
Prostatic carcinoma	del(7)(q22) del(10)(q24)
Retinoblastoma	struct. abn. no. 1 i(6p), −13 del(13)(q14)
Small Cell Ca-lung	del(3)(p14p23)
Synovial Sarcoma	t(X;18)(p11;q11)
Testicular teratoma/sarcoma	i(12p)
Wilms'	struct. abn. no. 1 t or del (11)(p13)

(Adapted from Heim, S., Mitleman, F.: Cancer Cytogenetics. Alan R. Liss, Inc., New York, 1987, Table 1, Chapter 11, pg. 229.)

of tumor cells can mimic leukemia and lymphoma. Cytogenetic analyses will at times be very helpful in the evaluation of these malignancies.[33] Ewing's sarcoma, Askin tumor, and neuroepithelioma fall in the above category and all three have a characteristic chromosome abnormality, t(11;22)(q24;q12).

Molecular genetics

New techniques are now available that allow evaluation of not just the gross chromosome morphology, but of the individual gene composition. This field is rapidly advancing in knowledge and improvement of techniques, so that

the list of disorders that can be diagnosed or detected is increasing. The reader is referred to Chapter 21 for a thorough discussion of the techniques and clinical application.

The neoplastic states that can be diagnosed with molecular DNA studies are the following:

BCR gene rearrangement in CML
IG gene rearrangement in B-cell neoplasms
T-receptor gene rearrangement in T-cell neoplasms
BCL2 gene rearrangement in follicular center cell lymphoma
RARα gene rearrangement in acute promyelocytic leukemia.

The advantage of these techniques over cytogenetic studies is that molecular DNA techniques do not require viable cells capable of mitotic activity. A sample of tumor cells including nonmitosing peripheral blood cells and paraffin embedded tissue can be used. The disadvantage of molecular DNA studies is that it only gives information about a single gene mutation as opposed to other chromosome aberrations that might be present. In addition, molecular DNA studies are not quantitative, so it is not possible to tell in a given sample the percent of cells with the abnormality. The following scenario illustrates the use of the two different techniques. A 25-year-old man is known to have CML and has received an allogeneic transplant from his sister. The first post-transplant specimen did not have cells sufficient for cytogenetics, so a sample also was sent for molecular DNA studies. Southern blot analysis revealed the presence of the BCR gene rearrangement, indicating persistence of leukemic cells. A second sample obtained 3 months later was sufficient for cytogenetics and yielded the following results:

80%—46,XX—pBMT
10%—46,XY,t(9;22)(q34;q11)
10%—47,XY,+8,t(9;22)(q34;q11)

In the first sample, molecular studies were critical to show persistence of the leukemia. Cytogenetics performed on the second sample was critical to show the percent of leukemia cells, and in addition, demonstrated a cytogenetic transformation towards blast crisis with the +8.

The use of cytogenetics and/or molecular DNA studies in neoplastic disorders must be well coordinated so that there is minimal duplication of work and billing to the patient.

SUMMARY

Clinical laboratory specialists in the hematology laboratory are frequently asked when cytogenic studies are indicated and what specimens are appropriate to submit. For these reasons, it is important to have a basic understanding of the specimen requirements, processing, and clinical indications for chromosome analysis. Acquired, clonal chromosome aberrations may be seen in most of the hematopoietic disorders, including acute leukemias, myelodysplastic states, and myeloproliferative disorders. These results are used for diagnosis and prognosis in many cases. In addition, cytogenetics can be used to follow the progression or regression of a malignant cell line if the original pretreatment sample revealed a clonal aberration.

The chromosome aberrations found in hematopoietic disorders are present only in the malignant cell line. Some aberrations have been found to be specific for a particular diagnosis. For example, the t(15;17) is diagnostic for AML-M3. Identification of these specific aberrations has been instrumental in leading researchers to gene loci that are critical in neoplastic transformation of cells. In the future, this information will hopefully result in more effective treatment.

REVIEW QUESTIONS

The patient A.S. is a 35-year-old male who presented with a severe nose bleed. The patient has been previously healthy; however, in the last three weeks he has noticed easy bruising and on the day of admission to the hospital he had a nose bleed that he couldn't stop. Initial CBC revealed:

Hgb.- 10 g/dL
Hct.- 0.30 L/L
MCV- 85 fL
WBC- 50×10^9/L
Plt. ct.- 20×10^9/L

The peripheral smear showed the majority of cells to have "butterfly" shaped nuclei, immature chromatin, and pale cytoplasm. Preliminary cytogenetic analysis performed on bone aspirate revealed 75% of cells to have t(15;17)(q22;q11); 25% of cells have a normal male karyotype.

1. The most likely diagnosis is:
   a. AML-M2.
   b. AML-M3, microgranular variant.
   c. ALL-L1.
   d. AML-M7.
   e. ALL-L3.

2. The breakpoint on chromosome 17 involves which gene?
   a. C-ABL
   b. C-MYC
   c. BCR
   d. RARA
   e. MLL

3. The identification of this cytogenetic aberration has led to treatment of these patients with which of the following?
   a. Interferon
   b. Interleukin
   c. Retinoic acid
   d. Vitamin K
   e. Vitamin B_{12}

REFERENCES

1. Barch, M., ed.: The ACT Cytogenetics Laboratory Manual, 2nd ed. New York: Raven Press, 1991.

2. Caspersson, T., Lomakka, G., Zach, L.: The fluorescence patterns of the human metaphase chromosomes—distinguishing characters and variability. Hereditas, 1971; 67:89–102.

3. Seabright, M.: A rapid banding technique for human chromosomes. Lancet, 1971; 2:971–972.

4. Schad, C., Kraker, W., Talal, S., et al.: Use of fluorescent in situ hybridization for marker chromosome identification in congenital and neoplastic disorders. Am. J. Clin. Path., 1991; 96:203–210.

5. Knutsen, T., Bixenman, H., Lawce, H., Martin, P.: Association of cytogenetic technologists task force: Chromosome analysis guidelines preliminary. Karyogram, 1989; 6:131–135.

6. Harden, D.G., Klinger, H.P., eds.: ISCN 1985: An International System for Human Cytogenetic Nomenclature. New York: Karger, 1985.

7. Mitelman, F., ed.: ISCN 1991: Guidelines for Cancer Cytogenetics. New York: Karger, 1991.

8. Nowell, P.C., Hungerford, D.A.: A minute chromosome in human chronic granulocytic leukemia. Science, 1960; 132:1497.

9. Rowley, J.D.: A new consistent chromosomal abnormality in chronic granulocytic leukemia. Nature, 1973; 243:290–293.

10. Claxton, D., Deissorth, A., Spitzer, G., et al.: Polyclonal hematopoiesis in interferon-induced cytogenetic remissions of chronic myelogenous leukemia. Blood, 1992; 79:997–1002.

11. Bartram, C.R., deKlein, A., Groffen, J., et al.: Translocation of c-abl oncogene correlates with the presence of a Philadelphia chromosome in chronic myelocytic leukemia. Nature, 1983; 306:239–242.

12. Morric, C.M., Heisterkamp, N., Kennedy, M.A., Groffen, J., et al.: Ph-negative chronic myeloid leukemia: Molecular analysis of Abl insertion into M-bcr on chromosome 22. Blood, 1990; 76:1812–1818.

13. detheh, Chomienne, C., Lanotk, M., Deja, A., et al.: The t(15;17) translocation of acute promyelocytic leukemia fuses the retinoic acid receptor alpha gene to a novel transcribed locus. Nature, 1990; 247:558–561.

14. Grignani, F., Fagioli, M., Pelicci, P.G., et al.: Acute promyelocytic leukemia: From genetics to treatment. Blood, 1994; 1:10–25.

15. Wu, X., Wang, X., Yao, H., et al.: Four years experience with the treatment of all-trans-retinoic acid in acute promyelocytic leukemia. Am. J. Haematol., 1993; 43:183–189.

16. Morel, P., Hebba, M., Fenaux, P., et al.: Cytogenetic analysis has strong independent prognostic value in de novo myelodysplastic syndromes and can be incorporated in a new scoring system: A report on 408 cases. Leukemia, 1993; 7:1315–1323.

17. Carbone, P., Santoro, A., Giglio, M.C., Barbata, G., et al.: Cytogenetic findings in secondary acute nonlymphocytic leukemia. Cancer Genet. Cytogenet., 1992; 58:18–23.

18. Rubin, C., LeBeau M.: Cytogenetic abnormalities in childhood acute lymphoblastic leukemias. Am. J. Pedi. Hematol. Oncol., 1991; 13:202–216.

19. LeBeau, M.: The role of cytogenetics in the diagnosis and classification of hematopoietic neoplasms. In: Knowles, D., ed. Neoplastic Hematopathology. Baltimore: Williams and Wilkins, 1992.

20. Raimondi, S.C., Roberson, P.K., Pui, C.H., et al.: Hyperdiploid (47-50) acute lymphoblastic leukemia in children. Blood, 1992; 79:3245–3252.

21. Menolov, G., Manolaova, Y.: Marker band in one chromosome 14 from Burkitt lymphoma. Nature, 1972; 237:33.

22. Dalla Favera, R., Bregui, M., Erickson, J., Patterson, D., Gallo, R., Croce, C.: Human c-myc onc gene is located in the region of chromosome 8 that is translocated in Burkitt lymphoma cells. Proc. Natl. Acad. Sci. USA., 1982; 79:7824–7827.

23. Offit, K., Chagenti, R.S.: Chromosomal aberrations in non-Hodgkin's lymphoma. Biologic and clinical correlations. Hematol. Oncol. Clin. North. Am., 1991; 5:853–869.

24. Van den Berg, H., Beverstock, G., Westerhof, J.P., Vossen, J.M.: Chromosomal studies after bone marrow transplantation for leukemia in children. Bone Marrow Transplant, 1991; 7:335–342.

25. Arthur, C.K., Apperley, J.F., Guo, A.P., Rassol, F., Gao, L.M., Goldman, J.M.: Cytogenetic events after bone marrow transplantation for chronic myeloid leukemia in chronic phase. Blood, 1988; 5:1179–1186.

26. Offit, K., Burns, J.P., Cunningham, I., Jhawar, S.C., Black, P., Kunan, N.A., O'Reilly, R.J., Chaganti, R.S.: Cytogenetic analysis of

chimerism and leukemia relapse in chromic myelogenous leukemia patients after T-cell depleted bone marrow transplantation. Blood, 1990; 75:1346–1355.

27. Browne, P.V., Lawler, M., Humphries, P., McCann, S.R.: Donor-cell leukemia after bone marrow transplantation for severe aplastic anemia. N. Engl. J. Med., 1991; 325:710–713.
28. Heim, S., Mitleman, F.: Cancer Cytogenetics. New York: Alan R. Liss, 1987.
29. Mitleman, F.: Catalog of Chromosome Aberrations in Cancer. 4th ed. New York: John Wiley, 1991.

30. Cavener, W.K., Koufos, A., Hansen, M.F.: Recessive mutant genes predisposing to human cancer. Mutat. Res., 1986; 168:3–14.
31. Yunis, J.J., Ramsay, N.: Retinoblastoma and subband deletion of chromosome 13. Am. J. Dis. Child., 1978; 32:161–163.
32. Benedict, W.F.: Recessive human cancer susceptibility genes (retinoblastoma and Wilms' loci). In: Advances in Viral Oncology, Vol. 7. New York: Raven Press, 1987; pp. 19–34.
33. Sainati, L., Stella, M., Montaldi, A., et al.: Value of cytogenetics in the differential diagnosis of the small round cell tumors of childhood. Med. Pediatr. Oncol., 1992; 20:130–135.

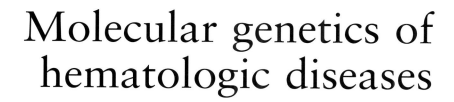

Molecular genetics of hematologic diseases

21

KEY TERMS

allele
base pair
cDNA (complementary DNA)
DNA (deoxyribonucleic acid)
gene
genotype
gene rearrangement
genome
hybridization
in situ hybridization
linkage analysis
locus
mutation
nucleotide
oncogene
polymerase chain reaction
  (PCR)
probe
replication
restriction endonuclease
RNA (ribonucleic acid)
Southern blot
transcription
translation
translocation

INTRODUCTION

Molecular genetics is the process of analyzing molecules of deoxyribonucleic acid (DNA). In the past few years, tremendous advances have been made in applying DNA technology to the practice of laboratory medicine. Nowhere have these applications impacted as strongly as in the field of hematology where new and improved tests have been implemented to diagnose a wide variety of hematologic diseases. It appears that this revolutionary progress will continue in the coming years as technology improves and as new discoveries are brought from the basic science level to their practical realization in clinical laboratories.

The types of diseases that are amenable to DNA technology include inherited diseases which by definition have a genetic basis, and infectious diseases where the identification of foreign DNA signals the presence of a particular pathogen. In addition, it appears that virtually all cancers result from genetic defects, and the laboratory detection of these defects will undoubtedly play a role in improved diagnosis and treatment of patients with leukemia and lymphoma.

To understand how DNA technology is implemented in diagnostic laboratories, first we must review the basic structure of human DNA. The terminology used in describing DNA structure may be new to some readers of this chapter. If so, please be aware that most of the terms mentioned in this chapter are defined in the Glossary section of this textbook.

DNA is the blueprint that cells use to catalog, express, and propagate information. Each nucleated cell of a person's body contains a complete set of DNA inherited from the person's parents and constituting the person's *genome*. The DNA of the human genome is composed of 3 billion *base pairs* of *nucleotides* divided among 46 chromosomes and encoding approximately 100,000 different genes. *Genes* are the functional units of DNA that serve as templates for RNA *transcription* and ultimately protein *translation*. The sequence of nucleotides in each gene determines the structure of the encoded protein.

One person's genome differs from another person's by about 0.2%, or by one of every 500 nucleotide pairs.[1] Interestingly, the human genome differs from the chimpanzee genome by only about 1%. Some gene sequences are so critical to basic cell function that they are nearly the same across all species including bacteria, yeast, and humans. In contrast, other parts of the genome are highly variable and are exploited in forensic tests[1] and parentage assays[2] to distinguish persons from one another. For example, genes of the HLA complex are highly variable among persons, while genes involved in the repair of damaged DNA are virtually identical from person to person.

DNA is composed of two complementary strands of nucleotides (Fig. 21-1). In living cells, these complementary strands are bound together by hydrogen bonds except in very short segments that are being actively transcribed or *replicated*. In the laboratory, however, the two strands of DNA can be fully dissociated by simply heating to 95° C or by placing the DNA in a solution of high pH. Once the strands are separated, a particular nucleotide sequence of interest can be identified using a DNA *probe*. A probe is simply a single stranded segment of DNA whose nucleotide sequence is complementary to the target sequence. The probe binds to the target DNA in a process called *hybridization*. This process forms the basis for all of the laboratory tests that have been developed to analyze specific portions of the human genome (Fig. 21-2).

Following is a list of the most commonly used laboratory tests and a brief overview of the procedures involved. These tests are described in greater detail in the remainder of this chapter, and potential medical applications of these tests are illustrated.

LABORATORY METHODS IN MOLECULAR DIAGNOSTICS

Southern blot analysis

DNA is isolated, cleaved with restriction endonucleases that cut DNA at specific nucleotide sequences, separated by size using gel electrophoresis, transferred to a membrane, and detected with probes complementary to the nucleotide sequence of interest. (Tissue requirements: fresh or frozen tissue, fresh body fluid or frozen cell pellet, blood, or marrow.)

Polymerase chain reaction (PCR)

DNA is isolated, and a specific segment of the DNA is copied a billion-fold so that it can be more easily detected

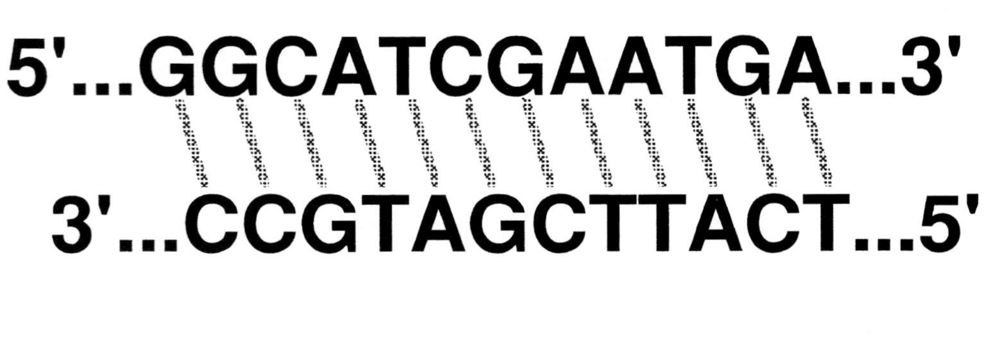

5'...GGCATCGAATGA...3'
3'...CCGTAGCTTACT...5'

FIGURE 21-1. The structure of DNA. DNA is composed of a strand of nucleotides that is bound by hydrogen bonds (shown as diagonal bridges) to a strand of complementary nucleotides. This forms a double-stranded DNA molecule where the nucleotide adenine (A) is complementary to thymine (T), and guanine (G) is complementary to cytosine (C).

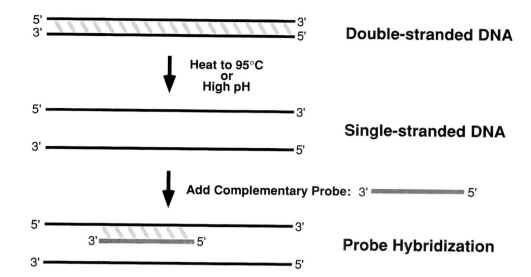

FIGURE 21-2. The two strands of DNA may be dissociated *in vitro* by treating them with heat or a solution of high pH. Once separated, the strands can bind to a DNA probe of complementary nucleotide sequence by a process known as hybridization.

and, in some cases, further analyzed for structural defects. (Tissue requirements: fresh, frozen, or paraffin-embedded tissue, blood, or body fluid.)

In situ hybridization

DNA or *RNA* (ribonucleic acid) in tissue sections on glass slides is identified by complementary probes. The architecture and cytology of the tissue is preserved to permit localization of the target sequence by microscopy. (Tissue requirements: frozen or paraffin-embedded tissue.)

Fluorescence *in situ* hybridization (FISH)

Whole chromosomes (metaphase or interphase) are hybridized to complementary probes and visualized by microscopy. (Tissue requirements: fresh cells for metaphase analysis, fixed cells or tissue sections for interphase analysis.)

INHERITED DISEASES

In the past few years, molecular biologists have identified specific genetic defects underlying many common inherited diseases. When a disease-associated genetic defect is identified, the abnormal DNA can be excised and used as a probe to study other patient DNA samples for the presence of the defect. Table 21-1 lists some of the inherited hematologic diseases for which specific genetic defects have been identified.

In inherited diseases, the genetic defect responsible for the disease is present in every nucleated cell of the patient's body, even if gene expression or clinical manifestation is restricted to only one organ or stage of development. Because the defect is present in all cells, it can be identified in samples that are easily collected such as blood or scrapings of oral mucosa. Furthermore, the defect can be identified before the onset of clinical disease, and even in

prenatal samples of amniotic fluid. For example, hemoglobinopathies involving the β-globin gene can be identified in a fetus even though it is not yet expressing the β-globin gene product or any clinical evidence of disease.[3,4]

Sickle cell anemia

Sickle cell anemia is an autosomal recessive disease that affects 1/260 African Americans and almost always shortens their lifespan. The biologic basis of sickle cell anemia is known to be a defect in the β-globin protein of hemoglobin. At the DNA level, the mutation always involves the substitution of a single nucleotide (thymine instead of adenine in the sixth codon), but that small change results in a dramatic alteration of hemoglobin molecules such that

TABLE 21-1 *INHERITED OR CONGENITAL HEMATOLOGIC DISORDERS AMENABLE TO MOLECULAR GENETIC ANALYSIS*

Chronic granulomatous disease

Gaucher disease

Hemoglobinopathies, including sickle cell anemia, alpha and beta thalassemias, and hereditary persistence of fetal hemoglobin

Hemolytic anemias such as glucose-6-phosphate dehydrogenase deficiency and McLeod syndrome

Bleeding and thrombotic disorders, including deficiency of coagulation factors V, VII, VIII, IX, XI, XII, and XIII, protein C, protein S, plasmin, plasminogen, and antithrombin, Bernard-Soulier syndrome, platelet storage pool deficiency, and von Willebrand's disease

Immunodeficiencies including adenosine deaminase, purine nucleoside phosphorylase, and leukocyte adhesion deficiencies, DiGeorge and Wiskott-Aldrich syndromes, and X-linked lymphoproliferative disorder

Myeloperoxidase deficiency

Porphyrias

Red cell membrane defects including hereditary spherocytosis and elliptocytosis, and paroxysmal nocturnal hemoglobinuria

they tend to polymerize under conditions of dehydration or low oxygen concentration. Hemoglobin polymerization diminishes erythrocyte deformability, thus impairing blood flow through small capillaries. Affected individuals suffer from chronic anemia and recurrent pain as a consequence of small vessel occlusion and ischemia.

Traditionally, laboratory diagnosis of sickle cell anemia has relied on examination of the blood smear combined with hemoglobin electrophoresis. When these procedures are inconclusive, or when prenatal diagnosis is requested, DNA technology is a useful means of detecting the genetic defect.

SOUTHERN BLOT ANALYSIS OF THE SICKLE MUTATION

To detect the sickle mutation by the *Southern blot* technique, DNA is first extracted from the patient specimen by (1) detergent solubilization of lipids in cell membranes, (2) protease digestion of proteins, and (3) separation of DNA from the remaining material. The purified DNA is then cleaved with a *restriction endonuclease* that reproducibly cuts the strands at specific nucleotide sequences to produce smaller fragments of DNA. The resultant DNA fragments are size-fractionated by gel electrophoresis, and transferred to a nylon membrane where they are hybridized to a radiolabeled probe targeting the gene of interest, in this case the β-globin gene. The pattern of probe hybridization determines whether the sickle mutation is present or absent (Fig. 21-3).

The Southern blot assay may be adapted to detect many other disease-associated alterations besides the sickle mutation. A key step in the Southern blot procedure is the step in which DNA is cleaved at specific nucleotide sequences by the action of restriction endonucleases. If a patient's DNA sequence is altered by *mutation, translocation,* or any other structural defect, then the number and/or size of the resulting restriction fragments is altered accordingly. The restriction fragment(s) containing the gene of interest are identified by probe hybridization. Radiolabeling of the probe permits its subsequent detection by autoradiography. Alternatively, the probe may be labeled with biotin or digoxigenin and detected using colorimetric procedures analogous to what is done in immunohistochemical assays of antigen-antibody complexes.

DETECTION OF THE SICKLE MUTATION BY POLYMERASE CHAIN REACTION

An alternate method of detecting the sickle mutation is by DNA amplification, a procedure in which a particular segment of DNA is copied a billionfold. DNA amplification techniques are revolutionizing our ability to analyze DNA in the clinical laboratory because we now have the capacity to examine an otherwise virtually undetectable sequence of DNA from a small tissue specimen or even a single cell. While several new amplification methods have been recently introduced,[5] the first and most commonly used method is *polymerase chain reaction* (PCR).[6] PCR

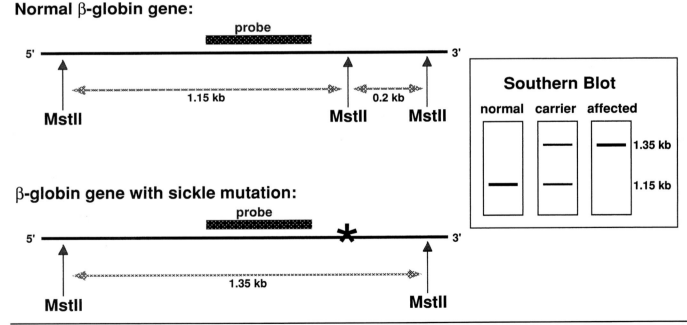

FIGURE 21-3. Southern blot analysis of the sickle cell mutation is accomplished by first isolating patient DNA and cutting it with MstII restriction endonuclease that cleaves DNA at a specific nucleotide sequence (shown by arrows). Since that specific sequence is present many times in the human genome, MstII cuts genomic DNA into many small fragments. The resultant DNA fragments are separated by size using gel electrophoresis, and then transferred to a nylon membrane by a blotting procedure. The membrane is soaked in a radiolabeled DNA probe (shown as a bar) that hybridizes to a complementary segment of the β-globin gene. The pattern of bands recognized by the probe reflects the size of the corresponding restriction fragments, measured in kilobases (kb). A β-globin gene harboring the sickle mutation (shown as a star) fails to cut with MstII at the mutation site, thus altering the band pattern. In this way, a person affected by sickle cell anemia can be distinguished from a carrier (sickle trait) and from a person of normal genotype.

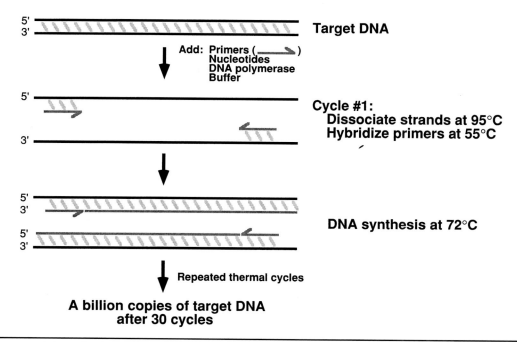

5' ///////////////////////////////// **Target DNA**
3' /////////////////////////////////

Add: Primers (————➤)
     Nucleotides
     DNA polymerase
     Buffer

5' ————————————————————————— **Cycle #1:**
                                        Dissociate strands at 95°C
3' —————————————————————————   **Hybridize primers at 55°C**

5' ///////////////////////////////// **DNA synthesis at 72°C**
3'

5'
3' /////////////////////////////////

Repeated thermal cycles

**A billion copies of target DNA
after 30 cycles**

FIGURE 21-4. Polymerase chain reaction is a method of enzymatically amplifying a particular segment of DNA through a process of repeated cycles of heating, cooling, and DNA synthesis. First, patient DNA is mixed with the chemicals needed for DNA synthesis. Included in these chemicals are two short DNA probes called primers (shown as half-arrows) that are designed to span the particular segment of DNA that needs to be amplified. A thermocycler instrument is programmed to sequentially heat and cool the sample. In cycle #1, the sample is heated to 95° C to dissociate complementary strands of DNA, then cooled to 55° C to permit binding of the short DNA probes that serve as primers for enzymatic DNA replication at 72° C. This replication generates new complementary strands that represent an exact copy of the original target DNA. In subsequent cycles, the products of previous cycles can serve as templates for DNA replication, allowing an exponential accumulation of DNA copies. After 30 cycles, which takes only a couple of hours, approximately a billion copies of the target DNA have been produced.

works by enzymatically replicating one particular segment of DNA (up to about 5000 nucleotides in length) from amid the entire 3 billion base pair human genome. This permits rapid, sensitive, and specific identification of a segment of DNA that can then be further tested for a disease-specific genetic defect (Fig. 21-4).

Diagnosis of the sickle cell genotype can be accomplished by PCR amplification of a segment of the β-globin gene harboring the sickle mutation site.[7] The amplified DNA can then be cleaved with the MstII restriction enzyme and electrophoresed in an agarose gel. Since MstII differentially cleaves normal DNA but leaves sickle DNA intact, the pattern of bands in the agarose gel depends on whether the sickle mutation is present.

Alternatively, short DNA probes that serve as PCR primers have been designed to preferentially amplify either the normal β-globin sequence or the defective sickle β-globin sequence depending on the specific primer used. This preferential amplification is based on the premise that mutations interfering with primer hybridization result in inhibition of amplification reactions (Fig. 21-5).

A major advantage of PCR over Southern blot analysis is that PCR is more sensitive and can therefore be performed on a much smaller volume of patient blood or tissue. Other advantages of PCR are its rapidity (approximately 1 to 2 days compared with more than 4 days for Southern blot analysis), relatively low cost, and the capa-

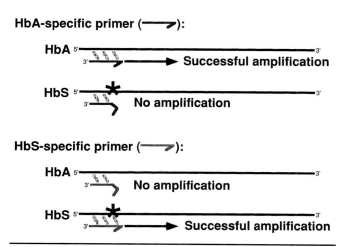

HbA-specific primer (————➤):

HbA 5' ——————————————————— 3'
     3' ————➤ **Successful amplification**

HbS 5' ——————*——————————— 3'
     3' ——➤ **No amplification**

HbS-specific primer (————➤):

HbA 5' ——————————————————— 3'
     3' ——➤ **No amplification**

HbS 5' ——————*——————————— 3'
     3' ————➤ **Successful amplification**

FIGURE 21-5. One way that polymerase chain reaction can be used to facilitate detection of the sickle mutation is to design primers (shown as half-arrows) that preferentially bind to either normal β-globin or sickle β-globin sequences. If a primer does not match its target sequence perfectly, particularly at the 5' end of the primer where the DNA polymerase initiates replication, then amplification is inhibited. If the primer matches its target, then abundant PCR products are generated. By comparing the yield of PCR reactions, it is possible to determine if the sickle mutation is present.

bility of using formalin-fixed paraffin-embedded tissues. However, a drawback of PCR is the meticulous attention to detail that must be used to prevent carryover or contamination of laboratory samples by extraneous DNA.

The sickle cell genotype is relatively easy to diagnose because the specific genetic mutation is identical among all affected individuals. Nearly all other inherited diseases described to date are much more complex in that diverse genetic defects can result in the same clinical syndrome. For example, only about half of patients with hemophilia A have an identifiable mutation or deletion of the factor VIII gene, while the remaining patients presumably have a genetic defect that somehow inhibits expression of the factor VIII protein. In families where the precise genetic defect is known, laboratory tests can be designed to identify the particular defect. Even if the defect is not known, a process called *linkage analysis* often can be used to follow inheritance patterns among family members to predict whether the disease is likely to affect a given individual. This is accomplished by analyzing "marker" DNA that lies on the same chromosome as the inherited defect.[8]

● Cancer

DNA technology provides a powerful new tool for assisting in the diagnosis of cancer. Unlike inherited disease in which every nucleated cell in the body contains defective DNA, cancer results when one cell acquires genetic defects that stimulate uncontrolled cell division and tumor formation. It is believed that virtually all cancers harbor genetic defects. The specific genes that are altered in tumors and are thereby responsible for tumor formation are called *oncogenes*. The unaltered counterpart of an oncogene generally functions to regulate cell growth or differentiation, whereas in tumor cells its function has gone awry as a result of abnormal expression or structural alteration. Each time a malignant cell divides, the genetic defect is passed on to its progeny. Therefore, all of the cells within a particular tumor contain the same defective DNA that gave rise to the tumor, a concept known as tumor clonality. Because cancers harbor clonal genetic defects, cancer cells may be distinguished from normal cells by DNA probe analysis of the defective gene sequences. Certain oncogene defects are highly characteristic of particular types of cancer and can be used to assist in the diagnosis of that cancer.

CHRONIC MYELOGENOUS LEUKEMIA

Traditional cytogenetics demonstrates that hematopoietic neoplasms frequently harbor characteristic chromosomal translocations. This is exemplified by chronic myelogenous leukemia (CML) where the characteristic Philadelphia chromosome (Ph) represents a shortened chromosome 22 resulting from a reciprocal translocation between the abl gene on chromosome 9 and the bcr gene on chromosome 22. This translocation produces a new fusion gene called bcr/abl that encodes hybrid RNA and protein containing elements of both genes. The abnormal juxtaposition of BCR enhances the potency of the abl gene prod-

uct (a tyrosine kinase enzyme), which results in altered myeloid cell proliferation. Using a single DNA probe, the molecular equivalent of the t(9;22) translocation can now be detected in virtually all cases of CML by Southern blot analysis.[9]

Approximately 90% of all patients who have clinical and laboratory features of CML have an identifiable Ph by karyotyping. An additional 5% apparently have an occult translocation that is detectable only by molecular analysis of bcr/abl. Regardless of karyotype, all patients with molecular evidence of bcr/abl gene rearrangement should be considered to have CML since they share a similar natural history and predisposition to blast crisis.[10] In blast crisis of CML, the bcr/abl defect is retained while additional genetic defects seem to account for the more aggressive cytologic appearance and clinical behavior of the tumor. The remaining 5% of tumors suspected of being CML but lacking bcr/abl do not behave in the same fashion as CML, and these tumors are believed to represent other myeloproliferative diseases or myelodysplastic syndromes masquerading as CML.

While DNA technology is slightly more sensitive than karyotyping in detecting the CML-associated genetic defect, karyotyping has the advantage of revealing other chromosomal abnormalities besides t(9;22). Therefore, a cost-effective approach to the laboratory work-up of suspected CML might be to first perform karyotyping and only proceed to a molecular assay if the karyotype is nondiagnostic.

In monitoring tumor burden during therapy, karyotyping is just about as sensitive as Southern blot analysis in detecting minimal numbers of leukemic cells. By either assay, tumors comprising over 5% of sample cellularity are generally detectable. One advantage of molecular technology is the capability to analyze cells that are resistant to entering cell cycle and are therefore difficult to karyotype. For example, blood neutrophils are fully amenable to DNA analysis whereas they are not amenable to karyotyping because they are not capable of dividing.

AMPLIFICATION OF THE BCR/ABL JUNCTION

An alternative method of detecting bcr/abl translocation is called reverse transcription PCR (rtPCR). In this procedure, RNA is extracted from tissues and then converted to *complementary DNA* (cDNA) using an enzyme called reverse transcriptase. The cDNA is then subjected to PCR amplification using primers spanning the translocation breakpoint, and the product is detected by electrophoresis (Fig. 21-6).[11]

rtPCR is a 1000-fold more sensitive than Southern blot analysis or karyotyping in detecting minimal numbers of affected cells, so rtPCR test results are beneficial in predicting relapse of CML following therapy.[12] Another unique benefit of rtPCR is the ability to distinguish bcr/abl breakpoints that are characteristic of CML (called p210) from those of de novo acute leukemia (called p190).[13] While these alternate breakpoints appear identical by karyotyping, they are distinct at the molecular level and from a clinical standpoint. They separate patients with de novo acute leukemia from those presenting in blast crisis

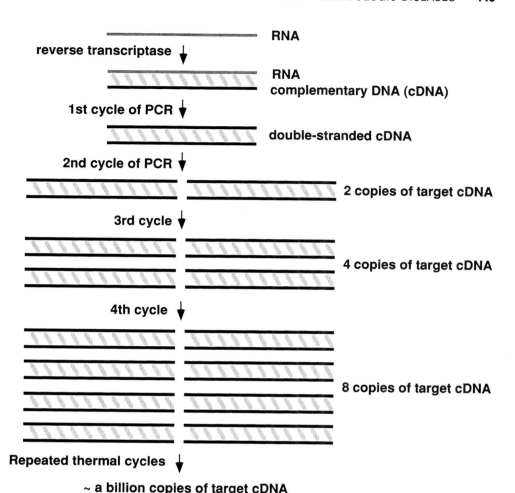

RNA

reverse transcriptase ↓

RNA
complementary DNA (cDNA)

1st cycle of PCR ↓

double-stranded cDNA

2nd cycle of PCR ↓

2 copies of target cDNA

3rd cycle ↓

4 copies of target cDNA

4th cycle ↓

8 copies of target cDNA

Repeated thermal cycles ↓

~ a billion copies of target cDNA

FIGURE 21-6. The rtPCR procedure is a means of determining whether a particular RNA transcript is present in a tissue sample. RNA is extracted from the sample followed by conversion to complementary DNA (cDNA) using the enzyme reverse transcriptase. This cDNA serves as a template for DNA amplification by the polymerase chain reaction, as described in Figure 21-4. After 30 cycles, about 1 billion copies of the target cDNA sequence have been produced. These abundant copies can then be readily detected or further analyzed in a way that provides important information on the type of RNA in the patient sample.

of CML. Furthermore, detection of bcr/abl p190 identifies a subset of acute lymphoblastic leukemia patients who are less responsive to standard chemotherapy regimens.[14]

ACUTE PROMYELOCYTIC LEUKEMIA (ANLL-M3)

Table 21-2 displays the characteristic chromosomal defects of myeloid leukemias. Perhaps the most interesting of these from a diagnostic standpoint is acute promyelocytic leukemia (ANLL-M3). Its characteristic t(15;17) involves the PML gene on chromosome 15 and the retinoic acid receptor alpha (RARα) gene on chromosome 17. Amazingly, leukemias harboring this genetic defect respond to treatment with retinoic acid derivatives, providing one of the first examples where cancer therapy specifically targets a gene product thought to be involved in tumorigenesis. Unfortunately, retinoic acid therapy alone is not sufficient for cure since the cells harboring the basic genetic defect eventually become resistant to the effects of retinoic acid.[15]

Molecular tests have been developed to detect the underlying PML/RARα translocation. These tests are used to assist in the diagnosis and classification of acute leukemia and to predict which patients will respond to retinoic acid therapy. More importantly, a sensitive test is now

TABLE 21-2 *RECURRENT TRANSLOCATIONS IN MYELOID LEUKEMIAS*

Leukemia	Karyotype	Genes	Clinical Significance
CML	t(9;22)	ABL/BCR	predisposed to blast crisis
ANLL-M1 or M2	t(8;21)	ETO/AML1	good response to high dose ARA-C
ANLL-M3	t(15;17)	PML/RARα	responds to retinoic acid therapy
ANLL-M4eo	inv(16)	MYH11/CBFβ	good response to high dose ARA-C
ANLL	t(6;9)	DEK/CAN	marrow basophilia is seen
ANLL	t(16;21)	FUS/ERG	
CMML	t(5;12)	PDGFRβ/TEL	

CML = chronic myelogenous leukemia; ANLL = acute non-lymphocytic leukemia; CMML = chronic myelomonocytic leukemia; t = translocation; inv = inversion.

available to monitor tumor burden during remission, and the results of this test appear to predict which tumors will relapse.[16]

The molecular test that is most sensitive for detecting PML/RARα is rtPCR. In this assay, RNA from the patient's tumor is converted to cDNA, and then primers spanning the breakpoint between the PML and RARα genes are used to specifically detect the translocation. In patients who have been induced into clinical remission, positive results in the rtPCR assay appear to be predictive of tumor relapse. In contrast, patients having consistently negative assays for PML/RARα enjoy prolonged survival.[16]

Southern blot analysis also can be used to detect PML/RARα, but because the translocation breakpoints vary widely from patient to patient, multiple probes are needed to detect all possible translocations. In contrast, mRNA encoded from the translocation breakpoint is remarkably homogeneous and therefore can be more easily analyzed, notwithstanding the fact that RNA is much less stable than DNA and must be handled carefully to avoid degradation.

GENE TRANSLOCATIONS IN LYMPHOID LEUKEMIAS AND LYMPHOMAS

Lymphomas and lymphoid leukemias commonly contain chromosomal translocations that involve the antigen receptor genes, namely the immunoglobulin (Ig) genes expressed in B cells, or the T cell receptor (TCR) genes expressed in T cells. Translocations involving these genes are believed to represent errors occurring during physiologic gene rearrangement (to be described in the next section). Genes located at or near the reciprocal translocation breakpoint are considered to be putative oncogenes. Expression of these oncogenes is frequently dysregulated by juxtaposition of an antigen receptor gene.

Table 21-3 lists the most common recurrent translocations of lymphoid neoplasms. In most cases, either Ig or TCR genes are translocated with genes that function in regulating cell growth. For example, the myc oncogene of Burkitt's lymphoma and the putative bcl1 oncogene (also called CCND1 or PRAD1) of mantle cell lymphoma encode proteins that promote cell division. In follicular lymphomas, the protein product of the bcl2 oncogene inhibits cell death. In either case, inappropriate overexpression of these oncogenes appears to be responsible for the development of lymphoid tumors.

Clonal genetic defects often can be detected by Southern blot analysis of the affected oncogene, or by amplification of the translocation breakpoint by PCR.[17-20] These types of assays, in conjunction with traditional morphologic examination and other laboratory studies, can be used to diagnose and classify tumors. Although the Southern blot assay is too insensitive to detect minimal residual disease, PCR assays of IgH/bcl2 translocation have been successful in predicting which patients are likely to relapse with follicular lymphoma.[21]

In theory, the best treatment for a tumor would be to eliminate the genetic defect(s) that are responsible for its uncontrolled growth. Alternatively, if we understood the

TABLE 21-3 *RECURRENT TRANSLOCATIONS IN LYMPHOMAS AND LYMPHOID LEUKEMIAS*

Lymphoid neoplasm	Karyotype	Genes*
B CELL LYMPHOMAS		
Burkitt's lymphoma	t(8;14, 2 or 22)	myc/IgH, Igκ, or Igλ
mantle cell lymphoma	t(11;14)	bcl1/IgH
follicular lymphoma	t(14;18)	IgH/bcl2
diffuse large cell lymphoma	t(3;14)	bcl6/IgH
diffuse large cell lymphoma	t(3;14)	bcl6/IgH
lymphoma	t(11;14)	RCK/IgH
lymphoma	t(10;14)	LYT-10/IgH
B CELL LEUKEMIAS		
acute lymphoblastic leukemia	t(9;22)	ABL/BCR
pre-B ALL	t(1;19)	PBX1/E2A
pre-B ALL	t(17;19)	HLF/E2A
pre-B ALL	t(5;14)	IL3/IgH
mixed lineage acute leukemia	t(various;11)	various/MLL
chronic lymphocytic leukemia	t(14;19)	IgH/bcl3
T CELL LEUKEMIAS/LYMPHOMAS		
	t(8;14)	myc/TCR$\alpha\delta$
	t(1;7 or 14)	TAL1/TCR$\alpha\delta$ or β
	t(7;9)	TCRβ/TAL2
	t(7;19)	TCRβ/LYL1
	t(7;14)	TCRβ/tcl1
	t(7;9)	TCRβ/TAN1
	t(1;7)	LCK/TCRβ
	inv(7)	TCRβ/TCRγ
	t(11;14)	TTG1/TCR$\alpha\delta$
	t(11;7 or 14)	TTG2/TCR$\alpha\delta$ or β
	t(10;7 or 14)	HOX11/TCR$\alpha\delta$ or β
anaplastic large cell lymphoma	t(2;5)	NPM/ALK

* In each case, the order of the genes corresponds to the order of the karyotype.

consequences of a particular genetic defect, we may be able to intervene in a biochemical pathway that would thwart tumor growth or trigger tumor cell death. As further progress is made in tailoring therapy to specific genetic defects, there will be increasing demands on clinical laboratories to detect these genetic defects in patient samples.

IMMUNOGLOBULIN AND T-CELL RECEPTOR GENE REARRANGEMENT

In addition to any translocation that a lymphoid neoplasm may have, B cell tumors have an additional clonal marker in their rearranged Ig genes that code for antibody specificity (Fig. 21-7). B cell tumors are believed to arise from a single transformed B cell harboring a particular Ig *gene rearrangement*, and that particular rearrangement is inherited by all tumor cell progeny. Therefore, clonal gene rearrangement serves as a marker to distinguish tumor cells from normal cells.[22,23] Tumor-associated gene rearrangement can be detected by Southern blot analysis using probes to the Ig genes (Fig. 21-8). Ig gene rearrangement

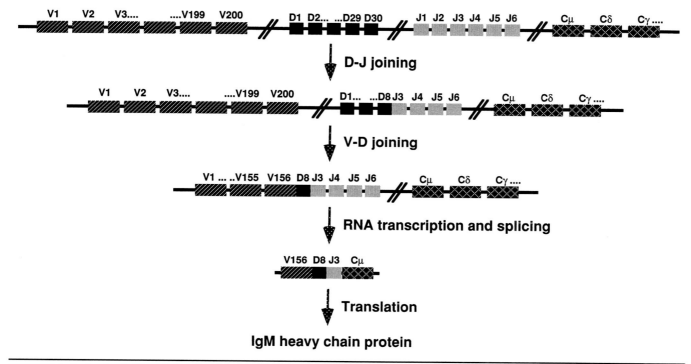

FIGURE 21-7. During B cell differentiation, the immunoglobulin heavy chain gene rearranges to produce a unique coding sequence that determines antibody specificity. This occurs through a process of splicing and deletion whereby one of 30 diversity (D) regions is juxtaposed with one of 6 joining (J) regions, and then with one of 200 variable (V) regions. Finally, constant (C) region splicing determines antibody isotype (IgM, IgD, IgG, IgA, or IgE). In the example depicted here, V, D, J, and Cμ segments are sequentially spliced together to generate a nucleic acid sequence that encodes IgM heavy chain proteins. These heavy chain proteins complex with kappa or lambda light chain proteins (that are also encoded by rearranged genes) to produce a functional antibody molecule.

also serves as a marker of commitment to the B cell lineage. Information on clonality and lineage is helpful in distinguishing a B-cell neoplasm from benign lymphoid hyperplasia or from a non-B cell tumor.

Just as B cells rearrange their Ig genes, T lymphocytes rearrange their TCR genes to encode a unique antigen receptor expressed on the surface of T cells. Therefore, Southern blot analysis of gene rearrangement can serve as a clonal marker for T cell tumors analogous to what was described above for B cell tumors. In the case of T cells, there are four different TCR genes that are capable of rearranging (called TCRα, β, γ, and δ). Any particular T cell tumor may exhibit rearrangements of one, two, three, or all four of these TCR genes. DNA probes targeting the TCRβ gene are the most useful in distinguishing monoclonal T cell neoplasms from polyclonal reactive processes.

Cossman et al.[24] have published guidelines for laboratory implementation of gene rearrangement testing by the Southern blot method. As with all clinical laboratory tests, appropriate quality control and proficiency testing are essential.

CLINICAL UTILITY OF GENE REARRANGEMENT STUDIES

The most valuable aspect of laboratory analysis of gene rearrangement is in distinguishing malignant from benign lymphoproliferations. In general, malignant lymphoid tumors exhibit clonal antigen receptor gene rearrangement, while benign reactive lymphoid hyperplasias do not.[25]

The converse principle is not always true, as exemplified by a few hematopoietic disorders where clonality does not necessarily imply malignancy. These include large granular lymphocytosis and lymphomatoid papulosis, both of which frequently demonstrate clonal gene rearrangements even though they may regress without therapy. Because clonality is not always synonymous with malignancy, it is important that DNA probe results be interpreted in the context of clinical information and in correlation with morphologic examination of the tissue to obtain accurate diagnostic and prognostic information.

A second benefit of gene rearrangement testing is in determining the lineage (B versus T cell) of a lymphoid proliferation. Table 21-4 reveals that B cell tumors usually have clonal rearrangements of the Ig heavy chain and kappa light chain genes, while T cell tumors usually have clonal rearrangement of the TCRβ gene.[22,25] Acute lymphoblastic leukemias sometimes harbor simultaneous Ig and TCR gene rearrangements even though flow cytometric immunophenotyping suggests that they are not biphenotypic. Likewise, lymphoid gene rearrangements have been reported in occasional cases of acute myeloid leukemia (but not in nonhematopoietic tumors), implying that gene rearrangement does not necessarily indicate lymphoid origin. Therefore, immunophenotypic methods

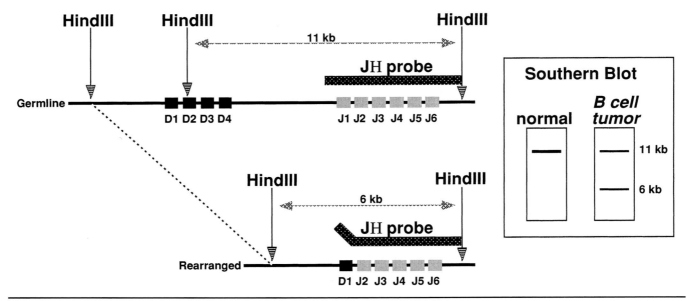

FIGURE 21-8. Rearrangement of the immunoglobulin heavy chain gene involves random splicing of D and J segments to produce a new coding sequence. This process alters the size of DNA fragments produced by the cleaving action of the HindIII restriction endonuclease (shown by arrows). In a B cell tumor, all tumor cells contain exactly the same rearrangement that was present in the original transformed B cell from which the tumor arose. This tumor-related clonal rearrangement is identified as an extra band on a Southern blot hybridized to a JH probe (shown as a bar). In the normal sample, an 11kb band corresponds to the size of the unrearranged (germline) DNA fragment. Although some B cells may be present in the normal sample, their corresponding gene rearrangements are not visible on the Southern blot because the rearrangements are polyclonal and they lie below the threshold of assay sensitivity. In the tumor, an extra band is identified that represents the tumor-specific clonal immunoglobulin gene rearrangement. Residual germline DNA is also present in the tumor, and it is generated from two potential sources: 1) the unrearranged allele of the immunoglobulin gene in tumor cells, or 2) the unrearranged genes present in nontumor cells of the specimen.

are more reliable than gene rearrangement analysis in assigning the lineage of immature hematopoietic neoplasms. In contrast, mature lymphoid tumors may be confidently classified as B or T cell type based on their pattern of gene rearrangements.

In morphologically equivocal hematopathology specimens, immunophenotyping is generally recommended as the first-line ancillary laboratory test, with gene probe studies reserved as a secondary option.[26] In cases where diagnostic uncertainty remains after morphologic and im-

munophenotypic examination, gene rearrangement studies were shown to be helpful in 72% of cases (confirmatory in 41%; essential to the diagnosis in 31%).[27]

In recent years, PCR has been explored as an alternate method of detecting clonal gene rearrangements.[28,29] Current protocols successfully identify clonal Ig rearrangement in about 80% of B cell neoplasms. Even though about 20% of B cell neoplasms are missed, amplification techniques still hold promise as laboratory tools because they are fast and they are applicable to paraffin-embedded tissue. Furthermore, the particular rearranged sequences that characterize each lymphoid tumor might be exploited as tumor-specific markers to assist in staging the extent of tumor spread and in monitoring response to therapy.[30]

● INFECTIOUS DISEASE

DNA technology has provided new methods of detecting micro-organisms based on the unique genetic code of each species. Amplification strategies are promising because they are sensitive, specific, and rapid in detecting pathogen-specific nucleic acid sequences. While DNA technology is only beginning to be applied in diagnostic laboratories, it will undoubtedly be quite useful in detecting those pathogens that are difficult to identify by conventional culture or serology. Table 21-5 lists hematology-related pathogens for which molecular strategies have already been reported.

TABLE 21-4 *CLONAL GENE REARRANGEMENT BY DIAGNOSIS*

	Immunoglobulin		T Cell Receptor
	IgH	kappa	TCRβ
B-acute lymphoblastic leukemia	100%	40%	30%
CLL, B cell lymphoma	100	100	<10
Hairy cell leukemia	100	100	0
Myeloma	100	100	5
T-acute lymphoblastic leukemia	10–20	0	95
Peripheral T cell lymphoma	0	<1	80
mycosis fungioides, ATLL	<1	<1	100

CLL = chronic lymphocytic leukemia (B cell type), ATLL = acute T cell leukemia/lymphoma.

TABLE 21-5 *PATHOGENS OF HEMATOLOGIC SIGNIFICANCE DETECTABLE BY MOLECULAR TECHNIQUES*

Epstein-Barr virus (EBV)

Cytomegalovirus (CMV)

Human herpesvirus 6 (HHV6)

Human herpesvirus 8 (HHV8)

Human immunodeficiency virus (HIV)

Human T-lymphotropic virus type 1 (HTLV1)

Malaria

Mycobacteria

Mycoplasma

Parvovirus B19

Toxoplasma

Lymphoma-associated viruses

Two viruses have been consistently linked to lymphoid neoplasms, human T lymphotropic virus type 1 (HTLV1) and Epstein-Barr virus (EBV). HTLV1 infects T-helper lymphocytes and causes them to proliferate by stimulating expression of interleukin 2 and its receptor. Asymptomatic HTLV1 infection is found in 15% of the population in Japan, the Caribbean Islands, and the southeastern United States. About 0.1% of infected individuals eventually develop adult T-cell leukemia/lymphoma characterized by hypercalcemia and a proliferation of peculiar multilobated helper T lymphocytes harboring the virus. Integration of viral cDNA into host chromosomal DNA can be detected in the malignant lymphocytes by Southern blot analysis or by PCR.[31]

EBV infects oropharyngeal epithelial cells and lymphocytes. Virtually all persons are infected before adulthood, and once infected they periodically shed infectious virus in their saliva for the remainder of their lives. EBV is known to cause infectious mononucleosis, and it is suspected of playing a role in the development of certain lymphomas. EBV DNA is found in the majority of immunodeficiency-related lymphomas, in 40% of all Hodgkin's disease tissues, and in 20% of sporadic Burkitt's lymphomas.

Both Southern blot analysis and PCR have been used to detect EBV in clinical specimens, but the best method for confirming tumor-associated EBV is *in situ hybridization* to EBV encoded RNA (EBER).[32] In this procedure, probes are hybridized to viral RNA transcripts in paraffin tissue sections on glass slides. Microscopic visualization localizes the virus to particular cells in the lesion (Fig. 21-9).

SUMMARY

In summary, DNA technology provides a powerful new tool for laboratory diagnosis of a wide variety of hematopoietic diseases including inherited diseases, infectious diseases, and malignancies. On the horizon are many new implementations of DNA technology based on discoveries of the genetic defects underlying certain diseases. At the same time, improvements in the technology itself will facilitate adoption of these new tests in clinical laboratories.

ACKNOWLEDGMENT

The author thanks Dennis W. Ross, MD, PhD, for sharing his knowledge and enthusiasm for hematopathology and

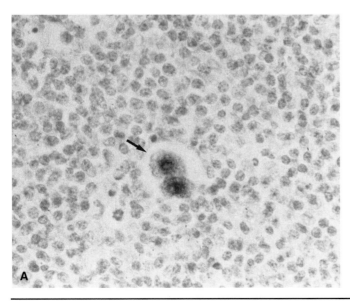
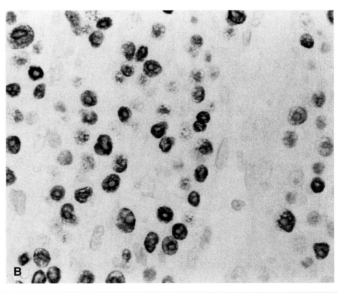

FIGURE 21-9. *In situ* hybridization to Epstein-Barr virus EBER transcripts reveals the localization of virus to (A) a Reed-Sternberg cell of Hodgkin's disease (arrow), and (B) the malignant cells of a diffuse large cell lymphoma, immunoblastic subtype, arising in an immunocompromised patient. The nuclei of the virus-infected cells are darkly stained as a consequence of probe binding, while uninfected cells are seen as pale cell ghosts.

molecular diagnostics. Polymerase chain reaction patents are owned and licensed by Hoffmann-LaRoche Molecular Systems, Inc.

REVIEW QUESTIONS

Case 21-A:

A 38-year-old woman complained of dizziness, fatigue and abdominal pain. On physical examination she appeared pale and her spleen was enlarged. Laboratory studies revealed anemia and an elevated white blood cell count of 69×10^9/L. A complete spectrum of granulocytic cells from myeloblasts to neutrophils was present in the blood, and basophils were increased. The neutrophil alkaline phosphatase score was low. The bone marrow was inaspirable, but a biopsy revealed that the marrow was packed with myeloid elements. Cytogenetics could not be performed due to the inability to induce division of blood cells and the lack of an adequate marrow aspirate. Blood is submitted for molecular diagnostic testing.

1. For Case 21-A, the most appropriate molecular test to assist in diagnosis of the patient's hematologic disorder is:
   a. Polymerase chain reaction to detect adenovirus infection.
   b. Flourescence in situ hybridization to detect t(15; 17) PML/RARα translocation.
   c. Southern blot analysis to detect clonal bcr gene rearrangement.
   d. In situ hybridization to detect the β-globin gene.

2. The test you chose in the question above was performed, and the result was positive. If further molecular testing reveals clonal rearrangement of the immunoglobulin heavy chain gene, it most likely indicates that the patient:
   a. Does not have leukemia.
   b. Has multiple chromosomal translocations.
   c. Is progressing to blast crisis.
   d. Has a hemoglobinopathy with superimposed B cell lymphoma.

3. Is there any reason to do molecular testing at a later date on the patient described in Case 21-A?
   a. No. The positive test results are definitive, and nothing more can be accomplished.
   b. Yes. The patient can be monitored to detect residual disease following therapy.
   c. Yes. If bone marrow transplantation is indicated, molecular testing of the patient and her family members for human leukocyte antigen (HLA) profiles could help identify a marrow donor.
   d. B and C.

4. All molecular tests that analyze specific portions of the human genome rely on the principle that:
   a. DNA is different in every cell of a particular individual.
   b. Probes bind to their complementary target sequence through a process called hybridization.

   c. DNA can be analyzed only after it has been cut with restriction endonucleases.
   d. DNA strands are bound together by hydrogen bonds that can never be broken.

5. Which of the following assays would be most appropriate for detecting a genetic defect that is present in only 0.1% of the cells in a patient sample?
   a. Polymerase chain reaction.
   b. Southern blot analysis.
   c. Restriction endonuclease digestion.
   d. Cytogenetics.

6. Polymerase chain reaction (PCR) differs from reverse transcription PCR (rtPCR) in the following way(s):
   a. PCR only works on human-derived samples since humans are the only species having a DNA genome, whereas rtPCR only works on samples containing foreign organisms (such as retroviruses) that have RNA genomes.
   b. Following amplification, PCR generates a DNA product, whereas rtPCR generates an RNA product.
   c. Prior to PCR amplification you usually extract DNA from the patient sample, whereas rtPCR requires extraction of RNA.
   d. All of the above.

7. Immunoglobulin and T cell receptor gene rearrangement studies can be used to:
   a. Distinguish B cell leukemia from B cell lymphoma.
   b. Determine whether a lymphoid clone is present in a tissue specimen.
   c. Prove that a tissue sample is benign.
   d. Detect Epstein-Barr virus in a tissue specimen.

8. Which of the following is true about the molecular genetics of cancer?
   a. Virtually all cancers are thought to harbor genetic defects.
   b. DNA probe analysis can be helpful in diagnosing cancer.
   c. The genes responsible for tumor formation are called oncogenes.
   d. All of the above.

9. Which of the following is true about the Southern blot procedure?
   a. Before electrophoresis, the DNA is cut into fragments using proteinase enzymes.
   b. The electrophoresis step is critical because it permits mutations to accumulate.
   c. The probe binds to its target during the hybridization step, and therefore the probe does not need to be labeled (ie. tagged with a marker).
   d. Interpretation of results relies on visualization of the band pattern.

10. Inherited diseases are characterized by:
    a. Defective DNA that does not affect gene structure, transcription, or function.
    b. Acquisition of mutations in DNA that are detected only in the diseased organs.

c. The inability to predict inheritance patterns among family members unless you know the precise genetic defect that underlies the disease.

d. A genetic defect that is generally present in all tissues of the patient's body.

● REFERENCES

1. Weedn, V.W., Roby, R.K.: Forensic DNA testing. Arch. Pathol. Lab. Med., 117:486–491, 1993.
2. Walker, R.H.: Molecular biology in paternity testing. Lab. Med., 23:752–757, 1992.
3. Anonymous: Guidelines for the fetal diagnosis of globin gene disorders. J. Clin. Pathol., 47: 199–204, 1994.
4. Camaschella, C., Saglio, G.: Recent advances in diagnosis of hemoglobinopathies. Crit. Rev. Oncol. Hematol., 14:89, 1993.
5. Wiedbrauk, D.L.: Molecular methods for virus detection. Lab. Med., 23:737–742, 1992.
6. Faloona, F.A.: Specific synthesis of DNA in vitro via a polymerase catalyzed chain reaction. Methods in Enzymol., 155:335, 1987.
7. Saiki, R.K., et al.: Enzymatic amplification of β globin genomic sequences and restriction site analysis for diagnosis of sickle cell anaemia. Science, 230:1350, 1985.
8. Sommer, S.S., Sobell, J.L.: Application of DNA-based diagnosis to patient care: The example of hemophilia A. Mayo Clin. Proc., 62: 387–404, 1987.
9. Blennerhassett, G.T., et al.: Clinical evaluation of a DNA probe assay for the Philadelphia (Ph') translocation in chronic myelogenous leukemia. Leukemia, 2:648–657, 1988.
10. Kurzrock, R., Gutterman, J.U., Talpaz, M.: The molecular genetics of Philadelphia chromosome-positive leukemias. N. Engl. J. Med., 319:990–998, 1988.
11. Kawasaki, E.S., et al.: Diagnosis of chronic myeloid and acute lymphocytic leukemias by detection of leukemia-specific mRNA sequences amplified in vitro. Proc. Natl. Acad. Sci. USA., 85: 5698–5702, 1988.
12. McClure, J.S., Litz, C.E.: Chronic myelogenous leukemia: molecular diagnostic considerations. Hum. Pathol., 25:594–597, 1994.
13. Kantarjian, H., et al.: What is the contribution of molecular studies to the diagnosis of bcr-abl-positive disease in adult acute leukemia? Am. J. Med., 96:133–138, 1994.
14. Westbrook, C.A., et al.: Clinical significance of the bcr-abl fusion gene in adult acute lymphoblastic leukemia: A Cancer and Leukemia Group B study (8762). Blood, 80:2983–2990, 1992.
15. Grignani, F., et al.: Acute promylocytic leukemia: From genetics to treatment. Blood, 83:10–25, 1994.
16. Miller, W.H., et al.: Detection of minimal residual disease in acute promyelocytic leukemia by a reverse transcription polymerase chain reaction assay for the PML/RAR-a fusion mRNA. Blood, 82: 1689–1694, 1993.
17. Williams, M., Meeker, T., Swerdlow, S.: Rearrangement of the chromosome 11 bcl-1 locus in centrocytic lymphoma: Analysis with multiple breakpoint probes. Blood, 78:493–498, 1991.
18. Rimokh, R., et al.: Detection of the chromosomal translocation t (11;14) by polymerase chain reaction in mantle cell lymphomas. Blood, 83:1871–1875, 1994.
19. Crisan, D., Anstett, M.: Bcl-2 gene rearrangements in follicular lymphomas. Lab. Med., 24:579–588, 1993.
20. Shiramizu, B., Magrath, I.: Localization of breakpoints by polymerase chain reaction in Burkitt's lymphoma with 8;14 translocation. Blood, 75:1848–1852, 1990.
21. Gribben, J.G., et al.: Detection by polymerase chain reaction of residual cells with the bcl-2 translocation is associated with increased risk of relapse after autologous bone marrow transplantation for B-cell lymphoma. Blood, 81:3449–3457, 1993.
22. Cossman, J., et al.: Molecular genetics and the diagnosis of lymphoma. Arch. Pathol. Lab. Med., 112:117–127, 1988.
23. Gill, J.I., Gulley, M.L.: Immunoglobulin and T-cell receptor gene rearrangement. Hematol. Oncol. Clin. North Am., 8:751–770, 1994.
24. Cossman, J., et al.: Gene rearrangements in the diagnosis of lymphoma/leukemia: Guidelines for use based on a multiinstitutional study. Am. J. Clin. Pathol., 95:347–354, 1991.
25. Greisser, H., Tkachuk, D., Reis, M.D., Mak, T.: Gene rearrangements and translocations in lymphoproliferative disease. Blood, 73: 1402–1415, 1989.
26. Kamat, D., et al.: The diagnostic utility of immunophenotyping and immunogenotyping in the pathologic evaluation of lymphoid proliferations. Mod. Pathol., 3:105–112, 1990.
27. Davis, R.E., Warnke, R.A., Dorfman, R.F., Cleary, M.L.: Utility of molecular genetic analysis for the diagnosis of neoplasia in morphologically and immunophenotypically equivocal hematolymphoid lesions. Cancer, 67:2890–2899, 1991.
28. Medeiros, L., Weiss, L.: The utility of the polymerase chain reaction as a screening method for the detection of antigen receptor gene rearrangements. Hum. Pathol., 25:1261–1263, 1994.
29. Trainor, K.J., et al.: Gene rearrangement in B and T-lymphoproliferative disease detected by the polymerase chain reaction. Blood, 78: 192, 1991.
30. Yamada, M., et al.: Minimal residual disease in childhood B-lineage lymphoblastic leukemia: Persistence of leukemic cells during the first 18 months of treatment. N. Engl. J. Med., 323:448, 1990.
31. Takemoto, S., Matsuoka, M., Yamaguchi, K., Takatsuki, K.: A novel diagnostic method of adult T-cell leukemia: Monoclonal integration of human T-cell lymphotropic virus type I provirus DNA detected by inverse polymerase chain reaction. Blood, 84: 3080–3085, 1994.
32. Gulley, M.L., Raab-Traub, N.: Detection of Epstein-Barr virus in human tissues by molecular genetic techniques. Arch. Pathol. Lab. Med., 117:1115–1120, 1993.

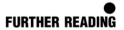

FURTHER READING

Ross, D.W.: Introduction to Molecular Medicine. 2nd ed. New York, Springer-Verlag, 1996.
Bernstam, V.A.: Handbook of Gene Level Diagnostics in Clinical Practice. Ann Arbor MI, CRC Press, 1992.

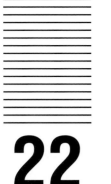

Morphologic analysis of body fluids in the hematology laboratory

22

CHAPTER OUTLINE

●

KEY TERMS

●

arachnoid mater
ascitic fluid
birefringence
cardiac tamponade
central nervous system
cerebrospinal fluid
chylous
cytocentrifuge
dura mater
effusion
exudate
meninges
pericardial cavity
peircardium
peritoneal cavity
peritoneum
pleura
pleural cavity
pia mater
pseudochylous
synovium
transudate

453

INTRODUCTION

In the past few years, the hematology laboratory has played an increasingly important role in the morphologic evaluation of body fluids. This is primarily due to the use of the cytocentrifuge, which markedly improves morphology over the previously used direct smear technique. The Wright-stained, cytocentrifuge-prepared slide is made in the hematology laboratory for the purpose of performing a differential white blood cell count. However, this slide also is valuable in making many important diagnoses, both benign and malignant. Most malignant cells can be recognized, including hematopoietic malignancies, carcinomas, and sarcomas. The hematopoietic malignancies are generally easier to diagnose from the Wright-stained slide as opposed to the routine cytology preparation, performed by alcohol fixation of cells and Papanicolaou stain. Another advantage of the slides made in the hematology laboratory is that these slides are prepared within an hour of receiving the specimen, whereas cytology preparations are more time-consuming. Important non-malignant findings that may be diagnostic on Wright stain, such as intracellular bacteria, fungi, and so forth, are frequently not seen on cytology slides. Hematologic slides, however, should not replace cytology preparations. Cytologic preparations have better retention of nuclear detail and are superior to hematologic slides when attempting to determine the specific type of carcinoma or sarcoma present. Both techniques are necessary and aid in arriving at the most accurate diagnosis.

This chapter is presented in atlas format, as this is believed to be the most helpful way to discuss morphology of body fluid cells. Other studies, such as those performed in the chemistry and microbiology laboratories, will not be discussed in this chapter.

TYPES OF BODY FLUIDS

The body fluids discussed in this chapter that are most commonly sampled are derived from the pleural, pericardial, and peritoneal cavities and from the *central nervous system* and joint spaces (Table 22-1). The pleural, pericar-

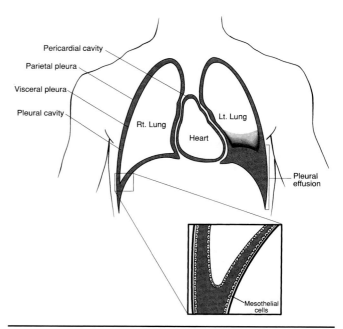

FIGURE 22-1. Diagram of right lung illustrating the pleural cavity and inset showing mesothelial cells of the parietal and visceral pleura. Illustration of heart shows the pericardial cavity. Diagram of left lung shows the abnormal accumulation of fluid (effusion) in the pleural cavity compressing the lower left lung.

dial, and peritoneal cavities are actually potential spaces and do not contain any appreciable amount of fluid in the normal setting. The central nervous system, however, normally contains a specific amount of fluid for protection of the brain and spinal cord. The joint spaces also have a consistent amount of fluid present for the continual lubrication of the bone surfaces and delivery of nutrients. The pleural cavities (left and right) consist of the space between the lung and the inside portion of the chest wall. This area is lined by a continuous single layer of cells called the pleura (Fig. 22-1). The pleural lining that covers the lung is the *visceral pleura,* and the lining that covers the inside of the chest wall is the *parietal pleura.* The lining cells are mesothelial cells that are derived from embryonic mesoderm. The purpose of the pleural lining is to provide a moist surface to minimize friction between the lung and chest wall as respiration occurs. In disease states, the mesothelial cells multiply, the lining thickens and fluid collects in the cavity. The contents of the fluid will depend on the pathologic process causing the fluid accumulation.

The peritoneal cavity consists of the space between the inside of the abdominal wall and the outside of the stomach, small and large intestine, liver, and superior aspect of the urinary bladder and uterus. The kidneys are positioned posterior to the peritoneal lining and are referred to as *retroperitoneal.* Other organs that are retroperitoneal in location are the pancreas, duodenum, some lymph nodes, abdominal aorta, etc. The peritoneal lining is identical to the pleural lining consisting of one layer of mesothelial cells. The lining covering the inside of the abdominal wall is the *parietal peritoneum* and the lining covering the

TABLE 22-1   *LIST OF SITE OF ORIGIN OF BODY FLUIDS WITH TERMINOLOGY OF PROCEDURE TO OBTAIN FLUID AND TYPE OF FLUID*

Anatomic Site	Procedure	Fluid Obtained
pleural cavity	thoracentesis	pleural fluid
peritoneal cavity	paracentesis	peritoneal fluid (ascitic fluid)
pericardial cavity	pericardial aspiration	pericardial fluid
joint space	joint aspiration (arthrocentesis)	synovial fluid
spinal cord	spinal tap, lumbar puncture	cerebrospinal fluid

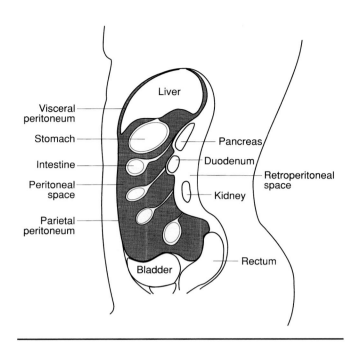

FIGURE 22-2. Abdominal cavity illustrating the peritoneal space between the inside of the abdominal wall and the outside of the liver, stomach, intestines, and dome of the bladder.

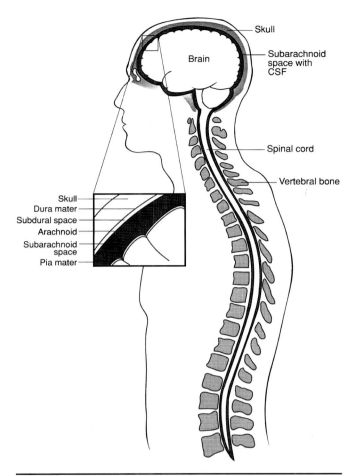

FIGURE 22-3. Central nervous system showing the subarachnoid space containing cerebral spinal fluid (CSF) covering the brain and spinal cord. Inset illustrates the meninges—dura mater, arachnoid mater, and pia mater.

organ surfaces is the *visceral peritoneum* (Fig. 22-2). In disease states the cell layers will thicken and fluid may accumulate, referred to as *ascitic fluid* or *ascites*.

The heart is enclosed in a sac-like structure called the pericardial sac, which also is lined by mesothelial cells. The lining covering the outside of the heart is the *visceral pericardium,* and the lining covering the inside of the pericardial sac is the *parietal pericardium* (Fig. 22-1). During certain pathologic events, fluid may accumulate in the pericardial sac. If the fluid accumulates rapidly (a minimum of 250 mL), or if a relatively large amount (1000 mL) accumulates over a longer period of time, there may be a serious restriction to the normal heart beat, creating a life-threatening event. This is called *cardiac tamponade.* In this situation, fluid must be removed quickly, either by pericardial aspiration or surgery, to save the life of the patient.

The CNS, consisting of the brain and spinal cord, is normally lined by special membranes referred to as meningeal membranes or meninges. The meninges consist of a relatively thick *dura mater,* the outermost membrane, a thinner *arachnoid mater,* the middle membrane, and an innermost *pia mater* that lies directly on the surface of the brain and spinal cord. The *cerebrospinal fluid* (CSF) occupies the subarachnoid space between the arachnoid mater and pia mater (Fig. 22-3). The CSF is produced by the choroid plexus cells and ependymal lining cells found in the ventricles. This fluid circulates through the ventricular system in the cerebrum, cerebellum, and brain stem and completely covers the surface of the brain and spinal cord. The CSF is a product of ultrafiltration and active secretion and is produced at a rate of approximately 21

mL/hour.[1] The CSF is reabsorbed by the *arachnoid cells.* The total volume of CSF in adults is 90 to 150 ml. Neonates have a CSF volume of 10 to 60 ml. In certain disease states, the content of the CSF will change.

Some bony joints of the body are lined by special membranes called the *synovium* that normally consists of a single layer of synovial cells (Fig. 22-4). The joint space contains synovial fluid that acts as a lubricant and a transport medium for nutrients to get to the bone surfaces of the joint. The synovial fluid is produced in part by the synovial cells and is an ultrafiltrate of plasma. Synovial fluid also contains a mucopolysaccharide called hyaluronate, which sometimes makes the fluid so thick that it hampers laboratory studies.

● COMMON CELL TYPES SEEN IN BODY FLUIDS

Segmented neutrophils (segs) are frequently seen in the pleural, pericardial, and peritoneal fluids in varying numbers. The neutrophils have the same appearance as in peripheral blood smears. Sometimes, however, cytocentri-

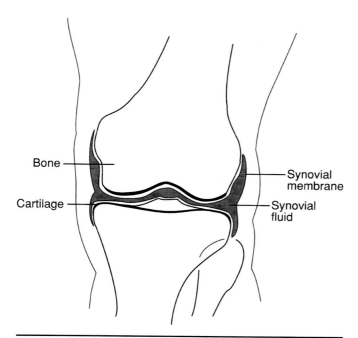

FIGURE 22-4. Knee joint illustrating synovial membrane lining and synovial fluid.

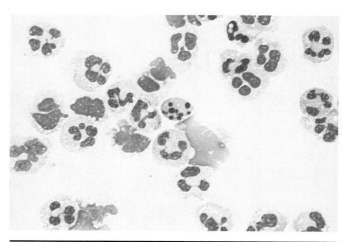

FIGURE 22-6. Degenerating neutrophil with separation of nuclear lobes and dense staining of the chromatin.

fuge artifactual changes can be seen with nuclear segments being thrown to the periphery of the cytoplasm creating a "hypersegmented" appearance (Fig. 22-5). Degeneration of neutrophils is seen more frequently in body fluid samples than in peripheral blood smears. The dying cells show cytoplasmic vacuolization and separation of nuclear segments with dense staining chromatin (Fig. 22-6). These cells may be mistaken for nucleated red blood cells or even for yeast organisms. Neutrophilic precursors, such as promyelocytes, myelocytes, and metamyelocytes are not commonly seen but if present may represent a chronic inflammatory process or true marrow disorder such as myeloproliferative disorders and myelodysplastic states. Myeloblasts are usually only seen in the latter two.

Lymphocytes are frequently present in all types of fluids in variable numbers. The lymphocytes vary in morphology from small to large and transformed (reactive). In cytocentrifuge preparations, the lymphocyte nucleoli are artifactually more prominent than in peripheral blood smears, the nuclear shape may be irregular and the cytoplasm may have artifactual projections[2] (Figs. 22-7 and 22-8). If the lymphocytes are neoplastic (leukemias, lymphomas) the morphology will depend on the type of neoplasm, and the cells will be homogeneous in appearance. Flow cytometry or immunoperoxidase techniques may be helpful in distinguishing benign versus malignant lymphocytes.

Monocytes in body fluids may have an appearance similar to that seen in peripheral blood smears or may be larger with abundant, vacuolated cytoplasm (histiocyte), or may have actual phagocytosed material (macrophage,

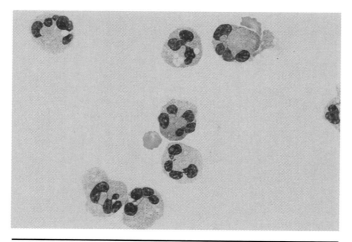

FIGURE 22-5. Artifactual change in neutrophils showing nuclear lobes thrown to the periphery of the cytoplasm. Slides in this chapter are all cytocentrifuge prepared, Wright stained. Original magnification 250×, unless otherwise noted.

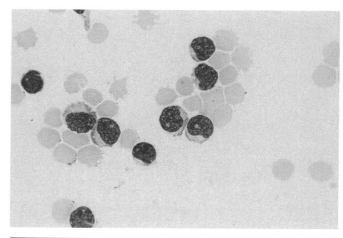

FIGURE 22-7. Artifactual change in lymphocytes with overly prominent nucleoli.

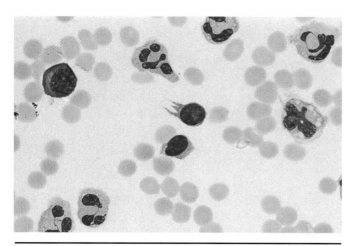

FIGURE 22-8. Artifactual change in lymphocytes with cytoplasmic projections.

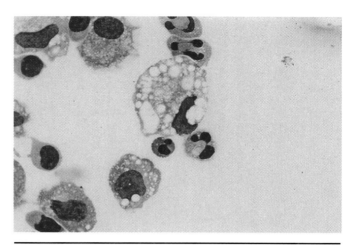

FIGURE 22-10. Histiocyte in pleural fluid.

phagocyte) (Figs. 22-9, 22-10, and 22-11). The distinction among the three morphologic types (monocytes, histiocytes, and macrophages) is not clinically important; however, in some cases the phagocytosed cells or organisms may be of diagnostic importance. When large vacuoles fuse, a "signet ring" appearance occurs with the nucleus flattened against the cell membrane (Fig. 22-12). Only a few monocytes are present in CSF and histiocytes/macrophages are usually only seen in pathologic states in the CSF.

Plasma cells are not seen in normal fluids and are usually present only in chronic inflammatory disorders (Fig. 22-13).

Eosinophils, basophils, and *mast cells* may be present in small numbers in pleural, pericardial, peritoneal, or joint fluids. Increased numbers of these cell types are seen in various disorders and may or may not correlate with peripheral eosinophilia or basophilia.[3] Mast cells can be distinguished from basophils, as mast cells have a round—not segmented—nucleus, and mast cells have a

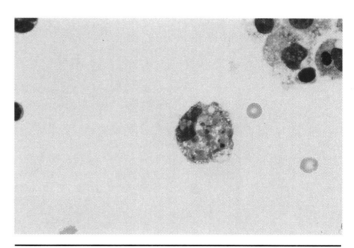

FIGURE 22-11. Macrophage in pleural fluid.

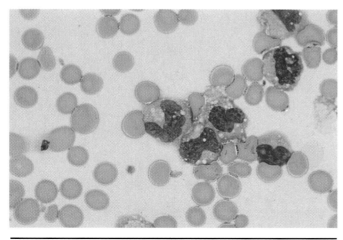

FIGURE 22-9. Monocytes in pleural fluid.

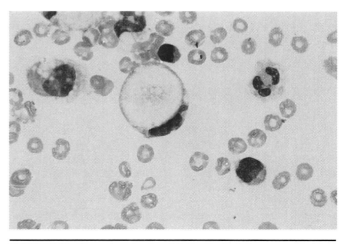

FIGURE 22-12. Macrophage in pleural fluid with single large vacuole giving a "signet ring" appearance.

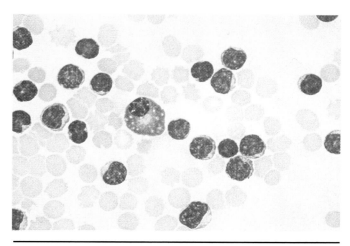

FIGURE 22-13. Plasma cell in pleural fluid.

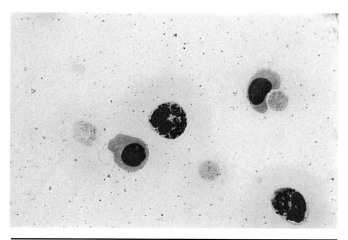

FIGURE 22-14. Basophil in pleural fluid.

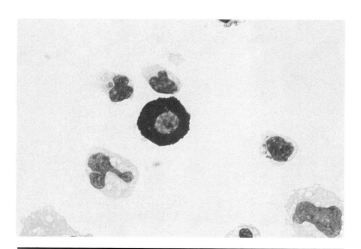

FIGURE 22-15. Mast cell in pleural fluid.

TABLE 22-2   *NORMAL EXISTING TISSUE CELLS FOUND IN THE VARIOUS BODY FLUIDS*

Fluid Type	Normal Tissue Cells
CSF	ependymal, choroid plexus cells, arachnoid cells
pleural, pericardial, peritoneal	mesothelial cells
joint	synovial cells

higher number of cytoplasmic granules than basophils. The granules in mast cells are smaller than those seen in basophils (Figs. 22-14 and 22-15). An increase in the number of basophils may correlate with myeloproliferative disorders involving body fluids.

Benign *tissue cells* can be seen in any of the body fluids (Table 22-2) and must be differentiated from malignant cells. Benign mesothelial cells can be seen in the pleural, pericardial, and peritoneal fluids. These are large cells that have a moderate to abundant amount of cytoplasm. The cytoplasm may be light or dark blue and occasionally may contain granules or phagocytosed debris. The nucleus is eccentric with a homogeneous chromatin pattern. Nucleoli may or may not be seen, and if present, are blue and will have a smooth membrane (Fig. 22-16). The tissue cells present in joint fluids are synovial cells that have a similar appearance to mesothelial cells with a somewhat denser cytoplasm (Fig. 22-17). The tissue cells that may be seen in CSF tend to be in clusters and may have cytoplasmic granules and slightly irregular nuclei. These are the ependymal cells, choroid plexus cells, and arachnoid cells (Fig. 22-18). The arachnoid cells are frequently seen as a syncytium with a mass of cytoplasm containing several nuclei (Fig. 22-19). Benign tissue cells are usually seen only in CSF from infants or from adults that have had recent neurosurgery or a reservoir in place.

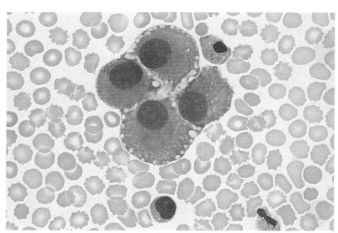

FIGURE 22-16. Benign mesothelial cells in pleural fluid.

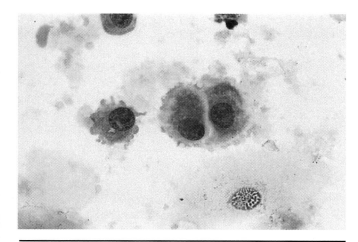

FIGURE 22-17. Synovial cells in joint fluid.

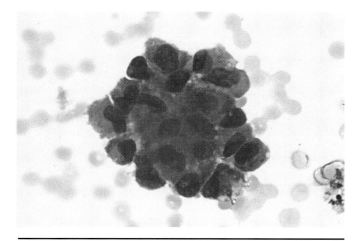

FIGURE 22-18. Choroid plexus cells in CSF.

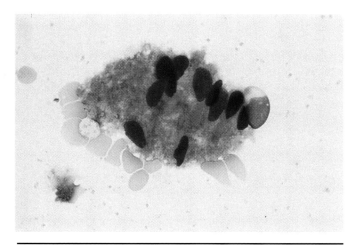

FIGURE 22-19. Arachnoid cell syncytium in CSF.

TABLE 22-3 *ARTIFACTS THAT CAN BE SEEN WITH WRIGHT STAINED CYTOCENTRIFUGE PREPARED SLIDES AND THE FINDINGS THAT CAN BE MISTAKENLY DIAGNOSED*

Artifact	Mistaken Interpretation
1. Peripheral localization of nuclear lobes in neutrophils	hypersegmented neutrophils
2. Degenerating neutrophil	yeast organisms nucleated red blood cell
3. Overprominence of nucleoli in lymphocytes	blast cells
4. Cytoplasmic projections of lymphocytes	hairy cell leukemia
5. Single large vacuole in histiocyte	signet ring carcinoma
6. Talc particles	yeast organisms
7. Stain precipitate	bacterial organisms
8. Degenerating tissue cells	malignant cells

● MORPHOLOGIC FINDINGS DUE TO ARTIFACT

Some artifactual findings have already been mentioned, such as peripheral displacement of the nucleus in neutrophils, cytoplasmic extensions of lymphocytes, and overly prominent nucleoli of lymphocytes (Table 22-3). Other artifactual changes may resemble actual pathologic findings and interpretation must be made cautiously. Talc powder particles may be an in vitro contaminant in any type of body fluid. This powder is on sterilized surgical gloves used by the physician obtaining fluid from the patient. *Talc* particles can look like yeast organisms, even budding yeasts if there are two particles closely associated. Usually the talc particle will have a refractile center that is not a feature of yeast and the talc particles are birefringent, showing up as bright Maltese cross-like figures with polarized light (Fig. 22-20). *Stain precipitate* may look like bacterial organisms. If the precipitate appears to be intracellular, changing the fine focus will usually show the precipitate to be in a different plane of focus from the cell. True intracellular bacteria will be in the same plane of focus as the cell. Stain precipitate is darker in color than bacteria, variable in size, and will be seen extracellularly, sometimes in distant areas of the slide (Fig. 22-21). In difficult cases, an extra slide should be prepared for a gram stain. *Early cellular degeneration* is exaggerated by the cytocentrifuge and shows irregular nuclear margins and separating chromatin. This can be mistaken for malignant cells (Fig. 22-22).

● PLEURAL, PERICARDIAL, AND PERITONEAL FLUIDS

Fluids obtained from the pleural, pericardial, and peritoneal cavities have similar findings in various pathologic states and will be discussed together. The pleural, pericardial and peritoneal spaces normally contain a minimal

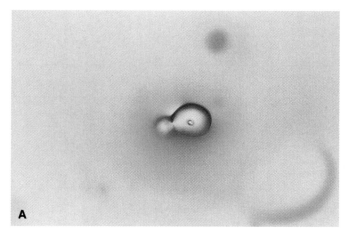

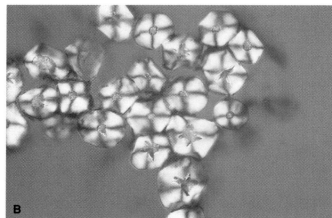

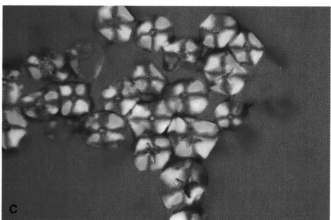

FIGURE 22-20. A, Talc particle with plain light resembling yeast. **B,** Talc particles as seen with polarized light appearing as a "Maltese cross" shape. **C,** Talc particles with polarized light and quartz compensator.

amount of fluid (less than 25 mL in the pleural cavity), only enough to keep the lining membranes moist. The fluid is produced by the parietal lining and absorbed by the visceral lining. Fluid is produced by plasma filtration through capillary endothelial cells and is dependent on four factors: capillary hydrostatic pressure, plasma osmotic pressure, lymphatic resorption, and capillary permeability.[2] Any pathologic state affecting one or several of these four factors may result in abnormal fluid collection, or *effusion* in the pleural, pericardial, and peritoneal spaces. In the pleural spaces, accumulation of at least 300 mL is necessary to be detected on chest x-ray and in the

peritoneal cavity accumulation of at least 500 mL is necessary to be detected by abdominal x-ray.[2]

An effusion may accumulate due to a systemic disease state *(transudate)* or as a result of a primary pathologic state of the area *(exudate)*. Transudates are frequently a result of increased capillary hydrostatic pressure such as seen with congestive heart failure or decreased plasma oncotic pressure such as seen with hypoproteinemia due to nephrotic syndrome or liver failure. A transudate will most often have a specific gravity of 1.015 or less, a total protein of 3.0 g/dL or lower, a ratio of effusion total protein/serum total protein of less than 0.5, and a ratio of

TABLE 22-4 *COMPARISON OF MORPHOLOGY OF PATHOLOGIC YEAST AS SEEN WITH WRIGHT STAIN*

Histoplasma	*Cryptococcus*	*Candida Albicans*	*Candida Tropicalis*
usually small, often intracellular, distinct non-staining cell wall, partially staining interior	wide variation in size, usually extra-cellular, capsule not visible on air dried preparations, either solidly stained with "wrinkled" appearance, or partial internal staining	can be extracellular and intracellular, moderate size, stains solid; rarely may see pseudohyphae formation	can be extracellular and intracellular, moderate size, dark blue with red internal staining

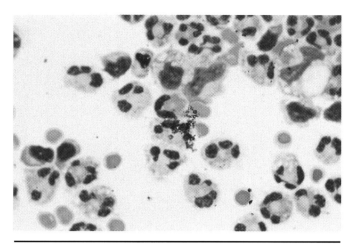

FIGURE 22-21. Stain precipitate on top of cell, with precipitate in focus and cells slightly out of focus.

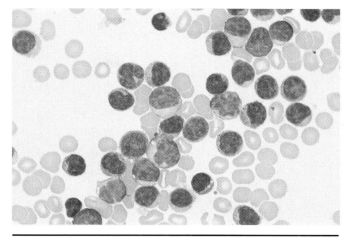

FIGURE 22-23. Reactive lymphocytes in pleural fluid.

effusion lactate dehydrogenase (LD) to serum LD of less than 0.6.[1,2]

An exudate is formed by increased capillary permeability and/or decreased lymphatic resorption. An exudative effusion can be caused by many different pathologic processes including bacterial infections, viral infections, neoplasms, collagen vascular diseases, etc.

A *chylous* effusion has a characteristic milky, opaque appearance which remains in the supernatant after centrifugation. Chylous effusions result from leakage of lymphatic vessels. In the pleural cavity (chylothorax) this is due to leakage of the major thoracic duct. In the peritoneal cavity chylous effusions result from blockage of the lymphatic vessels. In both the pleural and peritoneal cavities, this most often results from malignancy such as lymphoma or carcinoma, or trauma. This type of fluid is rich in chylomicrons. A pseudochylous effusion is also milky and results from a chronic, long standing effusion due to tuberculosis, rheumatoid pleuritis, etc.[2] Pseudochylous effusions do not contain chylomicrons.

●
Nonspecific reactive changes

In various pathologic states, certain types of white blood cells may be present in increased numbers. Bacterial infections will have a predominance of segmented neutrophils while viral, fungal, and mycobacterial infections may have a predominance of lymphocytes or show a mixed inflammatory response. As in peripheral blood, neutrophils may have toxic granulation, Döhle bodies and cytoplasmic vacuoles.

Lymphocytes are frequently reactive and transformed, simulating lymphoma cells. The most helpful feature in distinguishing reactive lymphocytes from lymphoma cells is that reactive lymphocytes consist of a heterogeneous population of cells with varying nuclear shape, amount of cytoplasm and degree of cytoplasmic basophilia (Figs. 22-23 and 22-24). Lymphoma cells will be homogeneous with the same nuclear and cytoplasmic features. The morphology of the lymphoma cells will depend on the particular type of lymphoma.

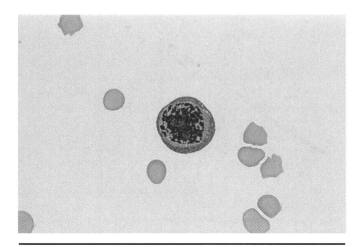

FIGURE 22-22. Early cell degeneration.

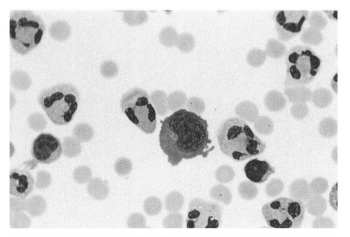

FIGURE 22-24. Reactive lymphocytes in pleural fluid.

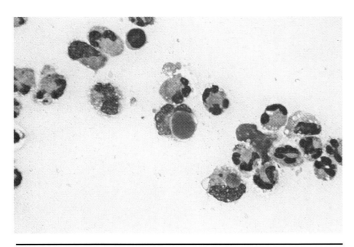

FIGURE 22-25. Spontaneous LE cell formation in pleural fluid.

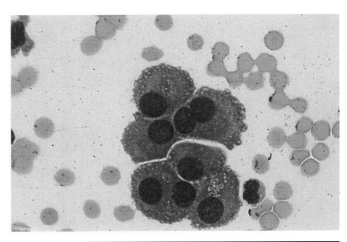

FIGURE 22-28. Reactive mesothelial cells in pleural fluid.

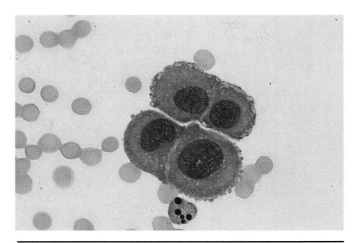

FIGURE 22-26. Reactive mesothelial cells in pleural fluid.

In rare cases, spontaneous formation of lupus erythematosus (LE) cells is apparent. An LE cell is a macrophage, either neutrophil or monocyte, that has phagocytosed a nucleus showing a homogeneous, smooth chromatin pattern (Fig. 22-25). The finding of these cells is suspicious but not diagnostic for systemic lupus erythematosus (SLE). Other autoimmune type disorders may also show the LE cell phenomenon. Nevertheless, identification of these cells can be extremely helpful in arriving at a difficult diagnosis. The LE cell should not be mistaken for simple phagocytosis of cells by macrophages, which is frequently seen. The chromatin of the usual phagocytosed cell is not smooth and homogeneous.

Mesothelial cells may show nonspecific reactive changes, which include multinuclearity, presence of nucleoli, mitotic activity and sometimes an increase in cell size (Figs. 22-26 and 22-27). Occasionally, there also may be an increased nuclear-cytoplasmic ratio and nuclear folding simulating carcinoma. Reactive mesothelial cells also may tend to cluster and appear cohesive; however, nuclear molding is not seen (Fig. 22-28). In cases where it is very difficult to distinguish reactive mesothelial cells versus malignant cells, cytology preparations will usually be definitive as alcohol fixation and Papanicolaou stain yield better nuclear detail.

● Micro-organisms

Most types of pathogenic bacterial and fungal organisms will stain with Wright stain and are detectable on a routine cytocentrifuge preparation. Bacteria will stain blue regardless of the gram-stain features. It is important to demonstrate the organisms intracellularly as this is an indication of true pathogenicity versus in vitro contamination (Figs. 22-29 and 22-30). Once bacteria are recognized with Wright stain, it is helpful to prepare a second cytocentrifuge slide for a gram stain to confirm the presence of bacteria and to be able to give additional information to the physician while cultures are pending.

Most pathogenic yeasts are found in CSF, as opposed to

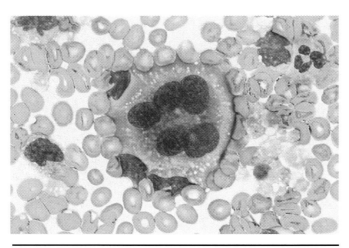

FIGURE 22-27. Multinucleated reactive mesothelial cells in pleural fluid.

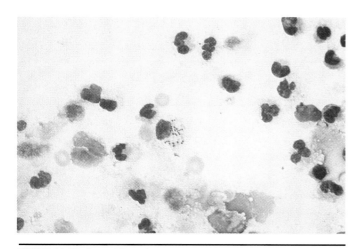

FIGURE 22-29. Bacterial cocci, intracellular, joint fluid.

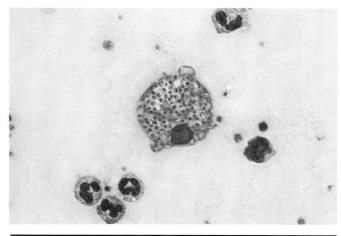

FIGURE 22-32. Histoplasma, multiple organisms in histiocyte; buffy coat, peripheral blood.

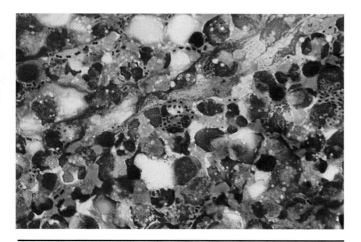

FIGURE 22-30. Intracellular and extracellular bacteria, bacilli, peritoneal fluid.

pleural, pericardial, or peritoneal fluids. These organisms may or may not be found intracellularly. The different types of pathogenic yeast show some distinguishing features on Wright stain. This morphologic variance can be used as a clue for an initial impression of the specific type of yeast, but cultures must be obtained for definitive identification. The most frequently seen fungal organisms in fluids are *Cryptococcus, Histoplasm, Candida albicans,* and *Candida tropicalis* (Figs. 22-31, 22-32, 22-33, and 22-34). Refer to Table 22-4 for a comparison of morphology.

● Malignant cells in fluids

The pleural, pericardial or peritoneal fluids may contain malignant cells and their identification is critical for accurate diagnosis.[4,5] In some patients, a diagnosis of malignancy may already have been established by other tissue sampling (biopsy or excision) and finding the malignant cells in fluid establishes a condition of tumor metastasis.

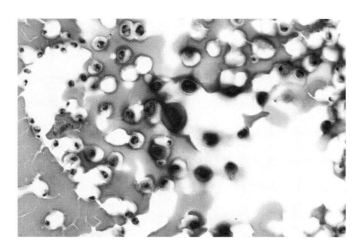

FIGURE 22-31. *Cryptococcus,* CSF.

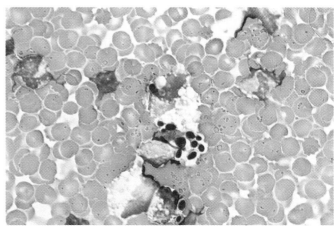

FIGURE 22-33. *Candida albicans,* CSF.

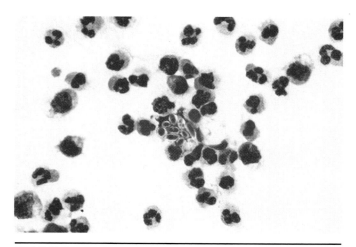

FIGURE 22-34. *Candida tropicalis,* peritoneal fluid.

TABLE 22-5 *COMPARISON OF MORPHOLOGIC FEATURES OF REACTIVE MESOTHELIAL CELLS VERSUS MALIGNANT CELLS*

Cell Features	Reactive Mesothelial Cells	Malignant Cells
nuclear membrane	smooth	irregular, jagged
chromatin	evenly distributed	unevenly distributed
nucleoli	absent or present with smooth membrane	prominent, frequently multiple, irregular membrane
nuclear molding	none	present in non-hematopoietic malignancies

For other patients, the finding of malignant cells in fluid may be the initial diagnosis of a malignancy and if a sample is not also sent to cytology, the recognition of malignancy on the hematology laboratory preparation is critical in establishing an early diagnosis. Malignant cells in fluids can usually be distinguished as *hematopoietic* in origin (leukemia, lymphoma) versus *nonhematopoietic* (carcinoma, sarcoma) and in some cases further specification of cell type is also possible. It is important to look at the entire cellular area of the slide with a low power objective (10×) to detect suspicious clusters of cells. In any one sample, there may be only few malignant cells present that are difficult to find.

General features that can be seen in almost any type of malignant cell include an irregular nuclear membrane, unevenly distributed chromatin, and nucleoli that also have irregular membranes (Table 22-5).[5] The nuclear/cytoplasmic ratio will vary, with small cell carcinoma cells having minimal cytoplasm and adenocarcinoma cells having as much or more cytoplasm as a benign mesothelial cell. The nuclear membrane irregularity may be jagged or may show multiple folds. When nucleoli are present they are frequently prominent and irregular in shape (Fig. 22-35). Mitotic activity by itself is not a reliable sign of malignancy as reactive mesothelial cells may undergo mitosis. Cytoplasmic vacuoles are also not a reliable finding for malignancy as this may be seen as a part of early degeneration in many cells.

None of the features described can be used alone to diagnose malignancy. All the features must be looked for and evaluated together. For example, one type of malignancy may show smooth nuclear membranes, but with unevenly distributed chromatin and irregular nucleoli (Table 22-6).

The most common nonhematopoietic malignancies seen in body fluids are *small cell carcinoma* (oat cell) and *adenocarcinoma*. Small cell carcinoma cells have the same general morphologic findings of malignant cells, but can be distinguished from other types of carcinoma cells because of the characteristic high nuclear-cytoplasmic ratio,

blast-like chromatin, absence of nucleoli or nonprominent nucleoli, and frequent nuclear molding (Fig. 22-36). Nuclear molding is the process of the nucleus of one cell molding around the shape of an adjacent cell. Nuclear molding occurs with cohesive growth requiring the presence of desmosomes and tight junctions. Therefore, this may be seen in any type of carcinoma, but is most often seen with small cell carcinoma. Some cells also may have a paranuclear "blue body," which is an inclusion that has not yet been characterized and may represent early cell degeneration or phagocytosed material. Depending on the orientation of the cell, the blue body may appear to be intranuclear. The blue body has only been described in small cell carcinoma and rarely in sarcoma.[6] The blue body is seen only with air dried, Wright stained preparations (Fig. 22-37). If the malignant cells are noncohesive, small cell carcinoma could be mistaken for a hematopoietic malignancy, and the finding of a blue body would be a good clue for the diagnosis of small cell carcinoma.

Adenocarcinoma differs from small cell carcinoma in that the overall size of an adenocarcinoma cell is larger than a small cell carcinoma cell with a moderate to abundant amount of cytoplasm (Fig. 22-38). The nuclear chromatin is partially clumped and heterogeneous and there are prominent nucleoli. The presence of cytoplasmic vacuoles is not specific and may represent early cell degeneration.

Other types of carcinoma and sarcoma can be found in body fluids (Figs. 22-39, 22-40, 22-41, and 22-42). The features seen with Wright stain are not as specific as from a cytology preparation and the latter is necessary to specifically identify the type of malignancy. For example, squamous cell carcinoma can look like adenocarcinoma with Wright stain; however, in most cases these are readily distinguishable on cytology preparations (Fig. 22-43). Certain types of malignant cells may contain clues for the cellular origin. Melanoma cells may have melanin pigment that will be demonstrable with Wright stain and hepatocellular carcinoma may have bile pigment (Figs. 22-44 and 22-45). The presence of these pigments can be suspected with Wright stain but must be confirmed with more specific staining techniques.

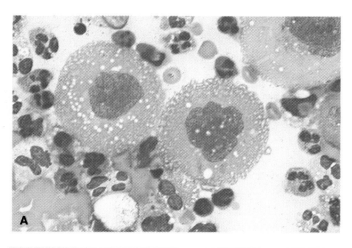
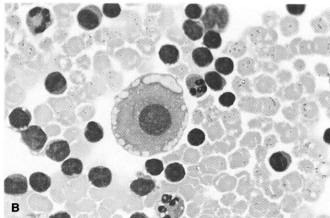
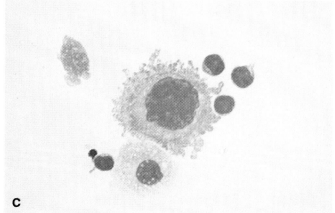

FIGURE 22-35. A, Malignant cells, pleural fluid. **B,** Benign mesothelial cell to contrast features with malignant cells. **C,** Single malignant cell, pleural fluid.

TABLE 22-6 *GENERAL MORPHOLOGIC FINDINGS OF BENIGN MESOTHELIAL CELLS AND MALIGNANT CELLS. ANY GIVEN CELL MAY SHOW VARIABLE FEATURES SO THAT ALL MUST BE EVALUATED BEFORE DECIDING IF A BODY FLUID SAMPLE IS BENIGN OR MALIGNANT. NO SINGLE FEATURE CAN BE USED TO DIAGNOSE MALIGNANCY*

	Mesothelial Cell	*Adenocarcinoma*	*Small Cell Carcinoma*	*Large Cell Lymphoma*	*Leukemic Blasts*
Cell size	large—15–30 μ	large to giant	moderate to large	moderate to large	small to moderate
Chromatin	loose, homogeneous	partially clumped heterogeneous	slightly course, homogeneous	partially clumped, heterogeneous	smooth, lace like homogeneous
Nucleoli	none to small and regular	prominent, multiple, irregular	none to small and not prominent	small to prominent, irregular	variable
Nuclear membrane	smooth	irregular, jagged	irregular, jagged, folded	irregular, jagged, folded	smooth or irregular, folded
N:C ratio	low, 1:3–5	low, 1:3 or less	high, 1:1.25	high to moderate 1:1.25–1:2	high to moderate 1:1.25–1:1.75
Intercell relationship	individual or clumped, no nuclear molding	usually clumped, ± nuclear molding	clumped with nuclear molding; occasionally individual	individual, no clumping, no nuclear molding	individual, no clumping, no nuclear molding

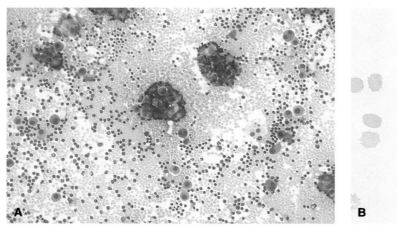

FIGURE 22-36. A, Small cell carcinoma, pleural fluid, showing tight cell clusters (original magnification, 25×). **B,** Small cell carcinoma.

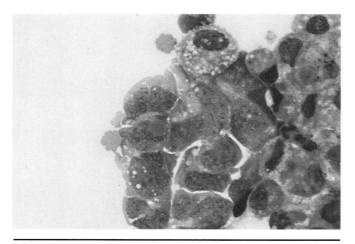

FIGURE 22-37. Small cell carcinoma, paranuclear "blue body" in malignant cell.

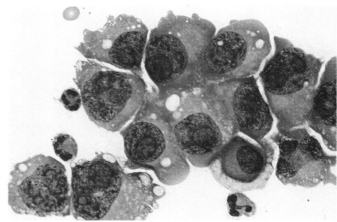

FIGURE 22-39. Pancreatic carcinoma in peritoneal fluid.

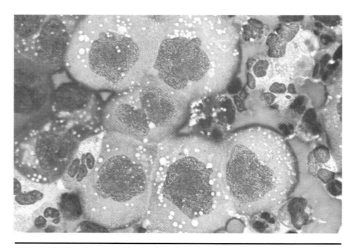

FIGURE 22-38. Adenocarcinoma in pleural fluid.

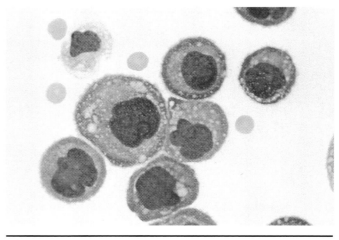

FIGURE 22-40. Gastric adenocarcinoma in pleural fluid.

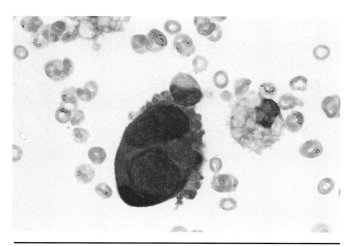

FIGURE 22-41. Liposarcoma in pleural fluid.

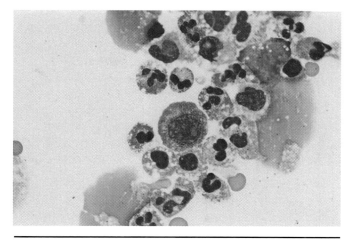

FIGURE 22-44. Malignant melanoma in pleural fluid with melanin pigment in malignant cell.

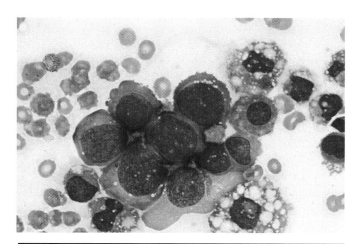

FIGURE 22-42. Germ cell tumor (spermatocytic seminoma) in pleural fluid.

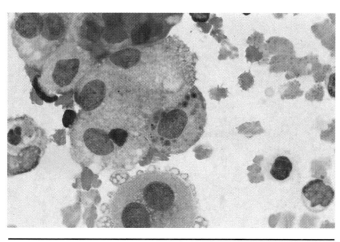

FIGURE 22-45. Bile pigment in macrophage in peritoneal fluid that also has cells of cholangiocarcinoma.

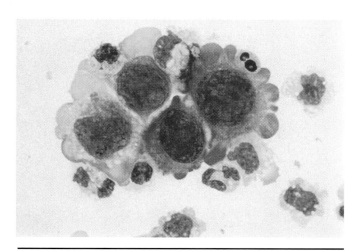

FIGURE 22-43. Squamous cell carcinoma in pleural fluid.

Practically any type of hematopoietic malignancy can be found in body fluids, including lymphocytic and non-lymphocytic leukemias, lymphomas, Hodgkin's disease, and plasma cell[7] neoplasms. Generally, the abnormal cells found in the body fluids in these disorders will have the same morphologic features as are seen in peripheral blood and bone marrow. The acute leukemias will only occasionally involve the pleural, pericardial, or peritoneal cavities and more often will be seen in the CSF. Blasts appear larger on cytocentrifuge preparations than on peripheral blood smears and the nuclear membrane may be surprisingly irregular. Auer rods can be seen and if necessary unstained slides can be prepared for cytochemistry stains and terminal deoxynucleotidyl transferase (TdT) to differentiate the blasts. Lymphoblasts will have a very high nuclear/cytoplasmic ratio and the nucleus may be folded or convoluted.

The morphology of non-Hodgkin's lymphoma in the body fluids will depend on the particular type of lym-

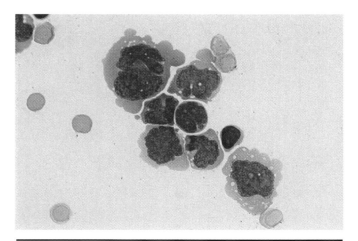

FIGURE 22-46. Large cell lymphoma in pleural fluid.

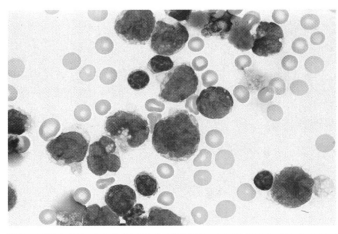

FIGURE 22-48. Lymphoblastic lymphoma, T-cell type, in pleural fluid.

phoma. Again, the nuclear membrane may be surprisingly irregular. Large cell lymphoma will have cells that are moderate to large in size with irregular nuclei, partially clumped chromatin and sometimes prominent nucleoli (Fig. 22-46). The cytoplasm is small to moderate in amount and basophilic. The cells are discohesive, but if the fluid is very cellular, the cells may be thrown together and have the appearance of carcinoma cell clusters; nuclear molding will not be seen. Small noncleaved lymphoma (Burkitt's or non-Burkitt's) will have intermediate size cells with more than one nucleoli and an immature blast-like chromatin (Fig. 22-47). Frequently, prominent cytoplasmic vacuoles are apparent. Small cell lymphoma is the most difficult to diagnose and may look like a benign lymphocytic infiltrate. In these cases, flow cytometry is valuable in demonstrating a clonal population of cells. T-cell lymphoma may show markedly irregular, convoluted nuclei; however, marker studies are necessary to confirm T- or B-cell origin of the neoplastic cells (Figs. 22-48 and

22-49). This may be accomplished by flow cytometry or by immunoperoxidase techniques on cytocentrifuge prepared slides.

Hodgkin's lymphoma can occasionally be seen to involve pleural fluid (Figs. 22-50 and 22-51). The malignant Hodgkin cell is large with a moderate to abundant amount of cytoplasm, large nuclei, and prominent nucleoli. If the nucleus is bilobated or if the cell has two nuclei, it may be a Reed-Sternberg cell. The other cells present consist of varying numbers, small lymphocytes, eosinophils, histiocytes, and plasma cells. If a patient has a diagnosis of Hodgkin's disease already established by other tissue biopsy, the malignant cells (either Hodgkin cell, Reed-Sternberg cell, or multinucleated variants) must still be identified in the effusion sample to diagnose involvement of the fluid.

●
CEREBROSPINAL FLUID

Cerebrospinal fluid (CSF) is different from the pleural, pericardial, and peritoneal fluids in that it exists in the

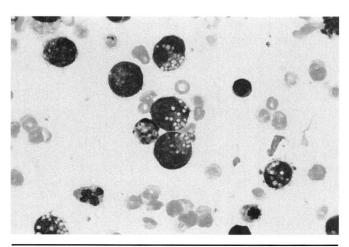

FIGURE 22-47. Small noncleaved cell (Burkitt) lymphoma in pleural fluid.

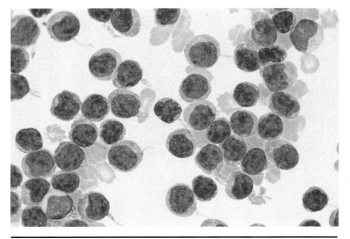

FIGURE 22-49. Small lymphocytic lymphoma, T-cell type, in pleural fluid.

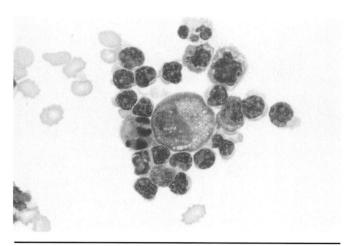

FIGURE 22-50. Hodgkin's disease, pleural fluid.

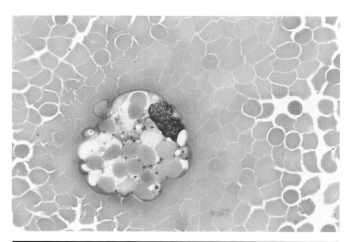

FIGURE 22-52. Erythrophagocytosis in CSF.

normal state. However, CSF is normally acellular so that the presence of any cells even at a low count is suggestive of a pathologic state. A common problem when evaluating CSF is to distinguish a true CNS hemorrhage versus a spinal tap procedure that causes hemorrhage (traumatic tap). Both of these will present as grossly bloody fluids. If the total erythrocyte count (red blood cell, RBC, count) in the first tube collected is significantly higher than in the last tube collected, it is in favor of a traumatic tap. *Xanthochromia* is a pink to orange color of the fluid supernatant produced by the breakdown products of hemoglobin and is usually thought to indicate true CNS hemorrhage. Xanthochromia will occur, however, if a grossly bloody fluid from a traumatic tap sits for some time before it is centrifuged. A definitive sign of CNS hemorrhage is phagocytosis of erythrocytes by histiocytes *(erythrophagocytosis)* (Fig. 22-52). It takes approximately 18 hours for histiocytes to mobilize and phagocytose erythrocytes after a hemorrhage. If the hemorrhage is older, hematoidin crystals may be seen intra- or extracellularly (Fig. 22-53).

● Nonspecific reactive changes

The normal leukocyte counts (white blood cell, WBC, count) of CSF have been difficult to determine but are reported to be 0 to $5/\mu L$ for adults and 0 to $30/\mu L$ for infants younger than 1 year of age, 0 to $20/\mu L$ for children 1 to 4 years of age, and 0 to $10/\mu L$ for children aged 5 years to puberty.[1,2] The normal ranges listed above for pediatric ages are somewhat controversial as they have a high upper limit. Most important for interpretation is to consider the types of white blood cells present and to correlate that with clinical findings.

The total WBC count cannot be interpreted without the total RBC count. When a specimen is obtained as a traumatic tap, the WBC and RBC will reflect the same WBC/RBC ratio as the peripheral blood of the same patient. A general rule is to expect 1 to 2 WBC for every 1000 RBC in the CSF. For example, if the total WBC in a CSF specimen is $10/\mu L$ and the RBC is $10,000/\mu L$, then

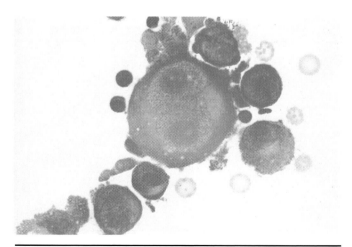

FIGURE 22-51. Hodgkin's disease with Reed-Sternberg cell, pleural fluid.

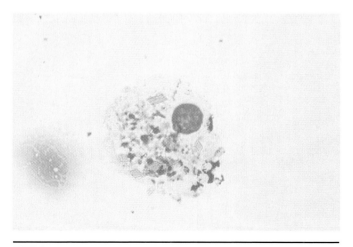

FIGURE 22-53. Hematoidin crystals in macrophage in CSF.

TABLE 22-7 *CAUSES OF INCREASED NEUTROPHILS IN CSF**

Meningitis
  bacterial meningitis
  early viral meningoencephalitis
  early tuberculous meningitis
  early fungal meningitis
  aseptic meningitis

Other Infections
  cerebral abscess
  subdural empyema

Other
  CNS trauma
  cerebral infarct
  tumor necrosis
  spinal anesthesia
  intrathecal drug injection
  previous lumbar puncture

* Adapted from Kjeldsberg C, Knight J. Body Fluids. ASCP Press, Chicago, 1993, p. 78.

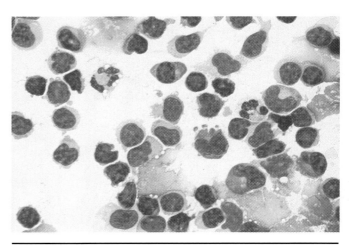

FIGURE 22-54. Reactive lymphocytes—CSF.

there is no significant increase of WBC (pleocytosis). If, however, the total RBC is $100/\mu L$ with a WBC of $10/\mu L$, then there is a significant WBC indicative of a pathologic state.[8] When a patient has an elevated or decreased peripheral blood WBC or RBC, then it is best to use the following calculation to determine if the CSF WBC is significant:[1,2]

$$\text{corrected CSF WBC} = \text{total WBC of fluid}$$
$$- \frac{\text{WBC of blood} \times \text{RBC of fluid}}{\text{RBC of blood}}$$

If the predominant cell is a segmented neutrophil, bacterial meningitis is a strong possibility. Early viral meningitis, however, may have increased neutrophils as well (Table 22-7).[9] A lymphocytic pleocytosis may be seen with viral (aseptic) meningitis, fungal meningitis, tuberculous meningitis, and so forth (Table 22-8). As with the pleural, pericardial, and peritoneal fluids, reactive lymphocytes must be distinguished from lymphoma cells (Fig. 22-54).

Rarely, eosinophils may be the predominant cell type. Eosinophilic pleocytosis is nonspecific and sometimes associated with drug reactions and parasitic infections (Table 22-9). Monocytes are usually seen in a mixed-cell inflammatory reaction and not as a pure monocytic pleocytosis (Table 22-10).

Hematopoietic precursors including megakaryocytes are present if the spinal tap needle penetrated the vertebral bone drawing back a portion of bone marrow. This is more often seen in infants, but may occur in adults with osteoarthritis.[10]

Mesothelial cells are not present in CSF but other tissue cells such as arachnoid cells and choroid plexus cells can be seen. These are most often present in CSF from infants or from adults that have had some type of manipulation such as surgery, shunt, or reservoir. It is very unusual to see these cells from a simple spinal tap procedure in an adult.

● Micro-organisms

The same type of micro-organisms described in pleural, pericardial, and peritoneal fluids may be present in CSF

TABLE 22-8 *CAUSES OF INCREASED LYMPHOCYTES IN CSF**

Meningitis
  viral meningoencephalitis
  aseptic meningitis
  tuberculous meningitis
  syphilitic meningoencephalitis
  leptospiral meningitis
  fungal meningitis
  parasitic disease

Degenerative Disorders
  Multiple Sclerosis
  Guillain-Barré syndrome

Other Inflammatory States
  polyneuritis
  sarcoidosis
  drug therapy

* Adapted from Kjeldsberg C, Knight J. Body Fluids. ASCP Press, Chicago, 1993, p. 77.

TABLE 22-9 *CAUSES OF INCREASED EOSINOPHILS IN CSF**

Common Causes
  parasitic infection
  fungal infection
  idiopathic eosinophilic meningitis
  foreign material reaction
  acute polyneuritis

Rare Causes
  hypereosinophilic syndrome
  tuberculous meningoencephalitis
  viral meningitis
  rickettsial infection
  hematopoietic malignancy
  primary CNS tumor
  sarcoidosis

* Adapted from Kjeldsberg C, Knight J. Body Fluids. ASCP Press, Chicago, 1993, p. 79.

TABLE 22-10   *CAUSES OF INCREASED MONOCYTES IN CSF. MONOCYTIC PLEOCYTOSIS FREQUENTLY IS SEEN WITH OTHER CELL TYPES PRESENT (MIXED INFLAMMATORY RESPONSE)**

Meningitis
  tuberculous meningitis
  chronic meningitis
  partially treated bacterial meningitis
  syphilitic meningoencephalitis
  viral meningoencephalitis
  fungal meningitis
  leptospiral meningitis
  toxoplasma meningitis
  amebic encephalomyelitis
  ruptured brain abscess
Other
  CNS hemorrhage
  cerebral infarct
  multiple sclerosis
  foreign material reaction
  CNS malignancy

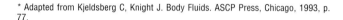

* Adapted from Kjeldsberg C, Knight J. Body Fluids. ASCP Press, Chicago, 1993, p. 77.

samples. As mentioned earlier, it is critical to distinguish intracellular bacteria from stain precipitate. A gram stain is most helpful in this situation. The most common yeast organism seen in CSF is cryptococcus (Fig. 22-31). Once cryptococcus is suspected from the cytocentrifuge prepared slide, an India ink preparation should be performed by the microbiology laboratory to confirm the presence of the characteristic large capsule of cryptococcus. If only very few organisms are present, however, the India ink preparation may be negative as unconcentrated CSF is used for the India ink. Cultures must be obtained to confirm the type of organism present.

● Malignant cells

Much of the description of malignant cells in pleural, pericardial, and peritoneal fluids holds true for spinal fluid examination as well.[11] Carcinoma cells tend to be less cohesive in spinal fluid than in other fluids and may simulate hematopoietic malignancies. Since mesothelial cells do not exist in the CSF, the presence of any large tissue cells should be considered suspicious for malignancy (Figs. 22-55, 22-56, and 22-57). Malignant cells, however, must be differentiated from the benign choroid plexus cells, ependymal cells, and arachnoid cells. This is done by evaluating the cells for standard features of malignancy as described earlier. Cytology preparations will usually be definitive.

Rarely, cells from primary CNS neoplasms may be found in the CSF. Medulloblastoma is a malignant tumor usually occurring in the cerebellum and has a morphologic appearance similar to small cell carcinoma (Fig. 22-58). Patient history from the physician would be necessary to distinguish the origin of the tumor.

Acute lymphocytic leukemia more often involves the CNS than acute nonlymphocytic leukemia (Figs. 22-59,

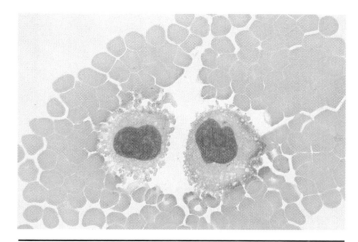

FIGURE 22-55. Adenocarcinoma, CSF.

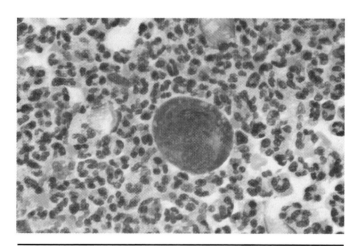

FIGURE 22-56. Large cell undifferentiated carcinoma with intense chemical acute meningitis, CSF.

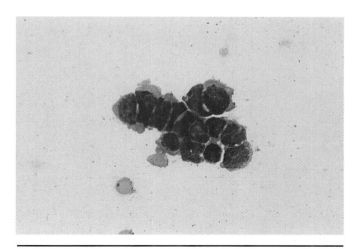

FIGURE 22-57. Small cell carcinoma, CSF.

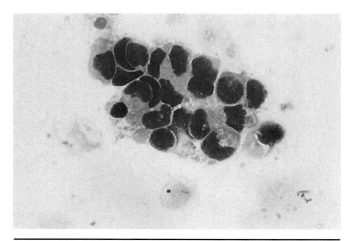

FIGURE 22-58. Medulloblastoma, CSF.

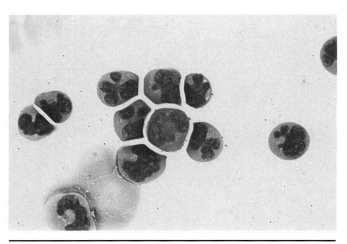

FIGURE 22-60. Acute myelomonocytic leukemia, CSF.

22-60, and 22-61). When erythrocytes are present, care must be taken not to overinterpret the presence of blasts that simply represent peripheral blood contamination. If no erythrocytes are present, even a low number of blasts (1% to 2%) may be indicative of CNS involvement.[12] Special studies such as cytochemistry stains, TdT, and surface markers by immunoperoxidase stains or flow cytometry may be helpful.[13]

Any type of lymphoma may involve the CNS, but more often seen are the high grade lymphomas such as lymphoblastic, immunoblastic, and small noncleaved cell. Primary CNS lymphoma is seen more often in recent years because of the relatively high incidence of this malignancy in patients that are HIV-positive. The lymphoma in a HIV-positive patient is high grade and frequently corresponds to small noncleaved cell, pleomorphic type, or B-immunoblastic (Fig. 22-62).

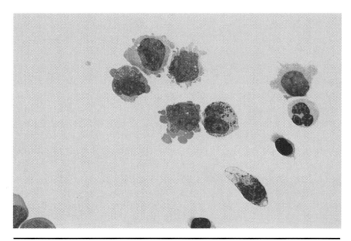

FIGURE 22-61. Blast crisis of chronic myelocytic leukemia with myeloblasts in CSF.

● JOINT FLUID

Synovial fluids tend to be thick and viscus due to the presence of hyaluronate, a mucopolysaccharide substance se-

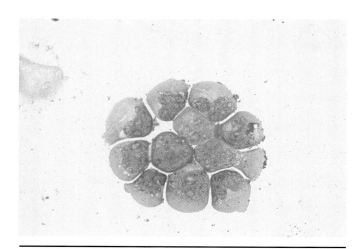

FIGURE 22-59. Acute lymphocytic leukemia, L3, CSF.

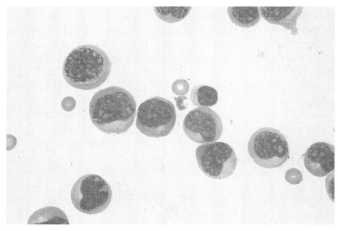

FIGURE 22-62. High grade lymphoma, small noncleaved cell type, in CSF.

TABLE 22-11 *GENERAL GROUPING OF DIAGNOSIS BY TOTAL WBC AND PERCENT NEUTROPHILS IN SYNOVIAL FLUID ANALYSIS; THERE IS SOME OVERLAP OF DIAGNOSTIC GROUPS AND OTHER STUDIES ARE NECESSARY TO REACH AN ACCURATE DIAGNOSIS*

Total WBC 0–5,000/µL <30% neutrophils
osteoarthritis, traumatic arthritis, neuropathic arthropathy, pigmented villonodular synovitis

Total WBC 2,000–200,000/µL >50% neutrophils
rheumatoid arthritis, Lupus erythematosus, Reiter's syndrome, rheumatic fever, ankylosing spondylitis

Total WBC 50,000–200,000/µL >90% neutrophils
Infectious—bacterial, mycobacterial, fungal

Total WBC 500–200,000/µL <90% neutrophils
Crystal induced—gout, pseudogout, apatite arthropathy

Total WBC 50–10,000/µL <50% neutrophils RBC present
Hemorrhagic—trauma, hemophilia, anticoagulant, pigmented villonodular synovitis, neuropathic arthropathy, hemangioma

creted by the lining synovial cells. If the fluid is too thick to proceed with cell counts, hyaluronidase may be added to loosen the fluid. Joint fluid is most often aspirated to distinguish crystal-inducing diseases (gout, pseudogout) from septic joints. Other disease states can induce an inflammatory response; however, it is usually not possible to diagnose these by joint fluid examination alone. Certain diagnoses can be suspected when comparing the total WBC count with percent segmented neutrophils present, however, there is great overlap and morphologic examination by cytocentrifuge preparations can be extremely helpful (Table 22-11).[14,15]

Joint fluids that have a total WBC of 50,000 to 200,000/µL are suggestive of an infectious or crystal-induced etiology. If the differential count shows 90% or more segmented neutrophils, then an infectious agent is most likely and cultures must be obtained. Micro-organisms can be seen in joint fluid if present in sufficient numbers and will have the same morphology as previously described. Bacterial organisms are more common and pathogenic yeasts are only rarely seen.

When the total WBC is in the range of 2000 to 200,000/µL with greater than 50% neutrophils in the differential count, entities such as rheumatoid arthritis (RA), systemic lupus erythematosus (SLE), Reiter's syndrome, and so forth should be considered. Rarely, spontaneous LE cell

formation may occur. The LE cell is suggestive of SLE; however it is not diagnostic and also may be seen in RA. The so-called RA cell is a neutrophil containing granules of immune complexes. These cells are not specific for a diagnosis of RA. The Reiter's cell is a macrophage with vacuoles containing debris of phagocytosed neutrophils. The debris may also be unrecognizable blue material. These cells are also nonspecific and not diagnostic for Reiter's disease.

Synovial cells can become proliferative in a reactive setting similar to mesothelial cells. Reactive synovial cells may also be multinucleated, may occur in clusters and nuclei may have small, regular nucleoli. Theoretically, malignant cells may be seen in synovial fluid; however, this is extremely rare.[16]

● Examination for crystals

The three most common types of crystals present in joint fluid are *monosodium urate crystals* seen in gout, *calcium pyrophosphate crystals* seen in pseudogout, and *cholesterol crystals* present in different types of chronic arthritides such as RA. Examination for crystals on a cytocentrifuge-prepared slide is superior to a standard wet preparation as the cytocentrifuge concentrates the specimen. Samples that may be negative with wet preparation may actually show crystals on the concentrated cytocentrifuge slide. Using cytocentrifuge prepared slides also decreases the chance of contamination when handling wet preparations. If sufficient numbers of crystals are present they can be seen with plain light microscopy on a Wright-stained cytocentrifuge slide. However, polarized light must be used to confirm *birefringence*. If fewer crystals are present, polarization is necessary to initially see them. Every joint fluid sent to the hematology laboratory for cell counts should have a crystal examination. Some Wright stain techniques result in dissolution of the monosodium urate crystals. Therefore, it is best to prepare two cytocentrifuge slides, one for Wright stain and one left unstained. Both slides should be examined for crystals on multiple specimens to determine if a particular stain technique dissolves the monosodium urate crystals (Table 22-12).

Monosodium urate (MSU) crystals should be reported as intracellular and/or extracellular. MSU crystals are typically long, thin and needle-like with pointed ends (Fig. 22-63A). They may be seen singly or in bundles. MSU crystals are strongly birefringent and are brilliant with po-

TABLE 22-12 *MORPHOLOGIC COMPARISONS OF COMMONLY SEEN BIREFRINGENT CRYSTALS AND PARTICLES*

Crystal	Birefringence	Color Parallel to Quartz Compensator	Morphology
monosodium urate	strong	yellow	long, thin, needle-like, intra- and extra-cellular
calcium pyrophosphate	weak	blue	short, rectangular, intra- and extra-cellular
cholesterol	strong	variable	large plate-like, notched, extracellular
steroids	strong	variable	amorphous, intra- and extracellular
talc particles	strong	yellow and blue	maltese cross shape, extracellular

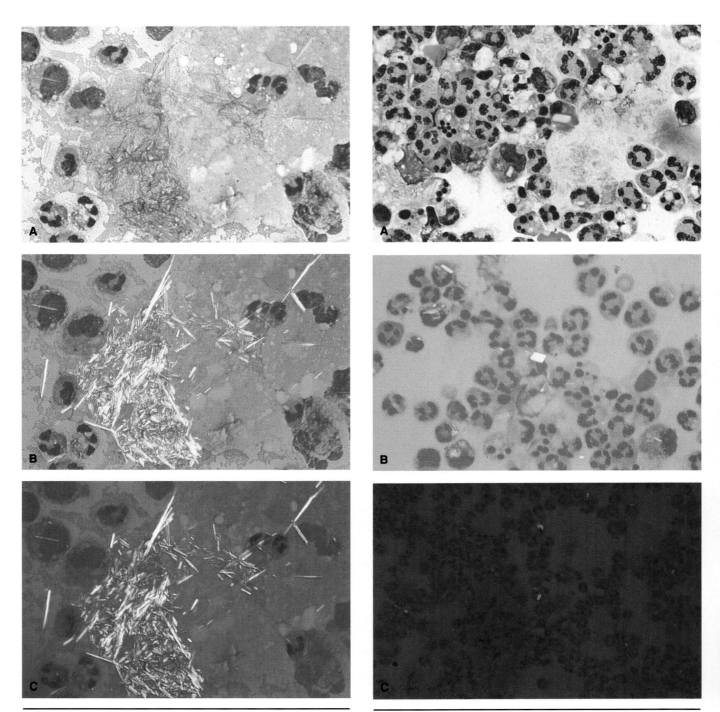

FIGURE 22-63. MSU crystal with **A,** plain light, **B,** polarized light, and **C,** quartz compensator with crystal showing yellow color parallel to quartz line and crystal with blue color perpendicular to quartz line.

FIGURE 22-64. CPP crystal with **A,** plain light, **B,** polarized light showing weak birefringence, and **C,** quartz compensator; yellow crystal is perpendicular to quartz line and blue crystal is parallel to quartz line.

larized light (Fig. 22-63B). A quartz compensator must be used to determine positive or negative birefringence. MSU are negatively birefringent and when aligned parallel to the compensator will show a yellow color and when turned perpendicular to the compensator the color changes to blue (Fig. 22-63C).[1,2]

Calcium pyrophosphate crystals (CPP) may also be seen intra- and/or extracellularly. CPP crystals are typically short, rectangular in shape and weakly birefringent so that they may be difficult to see with polarized light (Figs. 22-64A and 22-64B). When aligned parallel to a quartz compensator, the CPP crystals are blue and the color changes to yellow when crystals are perpendicular to the compensator (Fig. 22-64C).[1,2] Occasionally, a joint

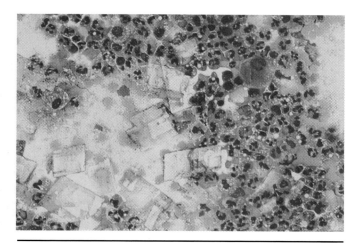

FIGURE 22-65. Cholesterol crystals in joint fluid.

fluid may have MSU and CPP crystals; the presence of one does not exclude the other.

Cholesterol crystals have a characteristic notched-plate shape and are birefringent (Fig. 22-65). These crystals are present in chronically inflamed joints such as seen in rheumatoid arthritis.

Talc particles are distinguished from pathogenic crystals by a characteristic Maltese-cross shape with polarized light. If a joint has been injected with steroids, the steroid particles can be seen intra- and extracellularly. Steroid particles do not have a crystal shape and are amorphous but birefringent.

SUMMARY

Examination of cellular morphology in body fluids is a critically important procedure for hematology laboratories. Not only is this performed for a differential leukocyte count, but for the possible demonstration of diagnostic findings such as microorganisms, malignant cells, etc. The cytocentrifuge prepared Wright stained slide yields excellent morphology of cells and can significantly aid in timely diagnosis of patients with effusions of unknown etiology. The hematology laboratory must take an active role in correlating morphologic findings with additional studies that may be necessary such as cultures, special stains, cytology, etc.

REVIEW QUESTIONS

The patient T.C. is a 55-year-old male who was brought to the emergency room in a comatose state. He was found at home by his son and appears to have fallen from a ladder. After physical exam, a spinal tap was performed and revealed the following:

color-	red
appearance-	bloody
RBC-	100×10^9/L
WBC-	0.100×10^9/L

differential white cell count reveals:

80% segmented neutrophils
15% lymphocytes
5% monocytes

1. Which of the following would be the most specific finding for a true CNS hemorrhage vs. traumatic spinal tap?
   a. Crenated red blood cells seen on the cytocentrifuge slide
   b. Xanthochromia of the supernatant after centrifugatioin of the fluid
   c. Erythrophagocytosis by histiocytes, seen on the cytocentrifuge slide
   d. WBC of 0.200×10^9/L in the spinal fluid
   e. 15% monocytes in the differential count

2. What is the significance of the white cell count of 0.100×10^9/L?
   a. This is diagnostic for acute meningitis.
   b. This is diagnostic for early viral meningitis.
   c. This white cell count is expected for the amount of hemorrhage and does not indicate infection.
   d. This is diagnostic for fungal meningitis.

REFERENCES

1. Kreig, A.F., Kjeldsberg, C.R.: Cerebrospinal fluid and other body fluids. In: Henry SB, ed. Clinical Diagnosis and Management by Laboratory Methods. Philadelphia: W. B. Saunders, 1991.
2. Kjeldsberg, C., Knight, J.: Body Fluids, 3rd ed. Chicago: ASCP Press, 1993.
3. Lau, M.S., Pien, F.D.: Eosinophilic pleural effusions. Hawaii Med. J., 1990; 49:206–207.
4. Ultmann, J.: Malignant effusions. CA-Cancer, 1991; 41:166–179.
5. Clare, N., Rone, R.: Detection of malignancy in body fluids. Lab. Med., 1986; 17:147–150.
6. Wittchow, R., Laszewski, M., Walker, W., Dick, F.: Paranuclear blue inclusions in metastatic undifferentiated small cell carcinoma in the bone marrow. Mod. Pathol., 1992; 5:555–558.
7. Mitchell, M.A., Horneffer, M.D., Standiford, T.J.: Multiple myeloma complicated by restrictive cardiomyopathy and cardiac tamponade. Chest, 1993; 103:946–947.
8. Bonadio, W.A., Smith, D.S., Goddard, S., Burroughs, J., Khaja, G.: Distinguishing cerebrospinal fluid abnormalities in children with bacterial meningitis and traumatic lumbar puncture. J. Infect. Dis., 1990; 162:251–254.
9. Greenlee, J.E.: Approach to diagnosis of meningitis. Cerebrospinal fluid evaluation. Infect. Dis. Clin. North. Am., 1990; 4:583–598.
10. Craver, R.D., Carson, T.H.: Hematopoietic elements in cerebrospinal fluid in children. Am. J. Clin. Pathol., 1991; 95:532–535.
11. Bigner, S.H.: Cerebrospinal fluid (CSF) cytology: Current status and diagnostic applications. J. Neuropathol. Exp. Neurol., 1992; 51:235–245.
12. Odom, L., Wilson, H., Jamieson, B., et al.: Significance of blasts in low cell count cerebrospinal fluid specimens from children with acute lymphoblastic leukemia. Cancer, 1990; 66:1748–1754.
13. Homans, A.C., Barker, B.E., Forman, E.N., Cornell, C.J. Jr., Dickerman, J.D., Truman, J.T.: Immunophenotypic characteristics of cerebrospinal fluid cells in children with acute lymphoblastic leukemia at diagnosis. Blood, 1990; 76:1807–1811.
14. Shmerling, R.H., Delbanco, T.L., Tosteson, A., Trentham, D.: Synovial fluid tests what should be ordered? JAMA, 1990; 264:1009–1014.
15. Freemont, A.J., Denton, J., Chuck, A., Holt, P.J., Davies, M.: Diagnostic value of synovial fluid microscopy: A reassessment and rationalisation. Ann. Rheum. Dis., 1991; 50:101–107.
16. Li, C.Y., Yam, L.T.: Blast transformation in chronic myeloid leukemia with synovial involvement. Acta. Cytol., 1991; 35:543–545.

Primary hemostasis

CHAPTER OUTLINE
●

KEY TERMS
●

● INTRODUCTION

Blood normally circulates within a closed system of vessels. A traumatic injury, such as a cut to the finger, severs blood vessels and results in bleeding.

To minimize blood loss, normally inert platelets and dissolved proteins in the plasma mobilize to form an insoluble mass or structural barrier that occludes the injured vessels. The barrier is limited to the injury site so that normal circulation is maintained in vessels elsewhere in the body. The same elements provide a continuous surveillance system that prevents leakage of plasma and cells into the tissues in normal circumstances.

The process of forming the barrier to blood loss and limiting it to the injured site is *hemostasis*. Hemostasis is from the Greek words "heme" meaning blood and "stasis" meaning to halt. The barrier mass is known as the *hemostatic plug*, *blood clot*, or *thrombus*. It is formed by the process of *blood coagulation*.

Hemostasis occurs in stages called *primary hemostasis*, *secondary hemostasis*, and *fibrinolysis*. During primary hemostasis, the platelets interact with the injured vessels and with each other. A clump of platelets results from this interaction, and at this point the hemostatic plug is known as the *primary hemostatic plug*. The primary plug temporarily arrests bleeding but it is fragile and easily dislodged from the vessel wall. Subsequently, insoluble strands of fibrin become deposited on the primary platelet plug to make it strong and stable and to allow healing of the wound without further blood loss. Generation of fibrin constitutes the stage of secondary hemostasis. Fibrin is formed by a series of complex biochemical reactions from soluble plasma proteins called coagulation factors as they associate with the injured blood vessels and with the platelet plug. The plug, or clot, is then termed the *secondary hemostatic plug* (Fig. 23-1). After the wound has healed, additional components of the hemostatic system break down and remove the clot in the fibrinolysis stage. All of the phases and components of the hemostatic system are controlled by physiologic and biochemical inhibitors.

Injury also can occur to intact, unsevered blood vessels. In this case, blood clot formation occurs on an interior surface of the damaged vessel wall and results in an abnormal condition called *thrombosis*.

This chapter will focus on primary hemostasis. The structure and functions of the blood vessels (vascular system) and the platelets as they form the primary hemostatic plug will be described. Secondary hemostasis and fibrinolysis will be discussed in Chapter 24 and the disorders of all components of hemostasis in Chapters 25 and 26.

● ROLE OF THE VASCULAR SYSTEM

The vascular system (vasculature) consists of three types of blood vessels: arteries, veins, and capillaries. The arteries carry blood from the heart to the capillaries. The veins return blood from the capillaries to the heart. The vessels

Stages of Hemostasis with Vascular Injury

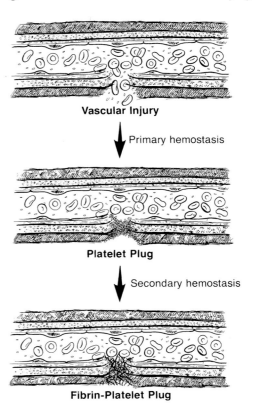

FIGURE 23-1. Bleeding occurs after an injury to a blood vessel. The hemostatic system is activated to prevent excessive blood loss. Hemostasis occurs in two stages. During primary hemostasis the platelets aggregate at the site of the injury and form the platelet plug (primary hemostatic plug). During secondary hemostasis, fibrin forms around the platelet plug to form the fibrin-platelet plug (secondary hemostatic plug).

in which hemostasis occurs are the smallest arteries (arterioles) and the smallest veins (venules).

● Structure of blood vessels

The structure of all blood vessels is similar (Figs. 23-2A and 23-2B). It consists of a central cavity, the lumen, through which the blood flows. The lumen is lined with a continuous single layer of flattened cells called *endothelial cells*. The endothelial cells separate the blood from the underlying tissues. They provide a protective environment for the cellular elements of the blood and the dissolved constituents of the plasma. The individual endothelial cells are usually interconnected by overlapping portions of their cytoplasm. However, in some tissues the cytoplasmic connections are cemented together in tight junctions and in other tissues there are small gaps between the cells. The lumenal surface of the endothelial cells has a thin coating of complex protein and carbohydrate substances (mucopolysaccharides) called the *glycocalyx*. The ablumenal surface (the surface on the tissue side of the cell) is attached

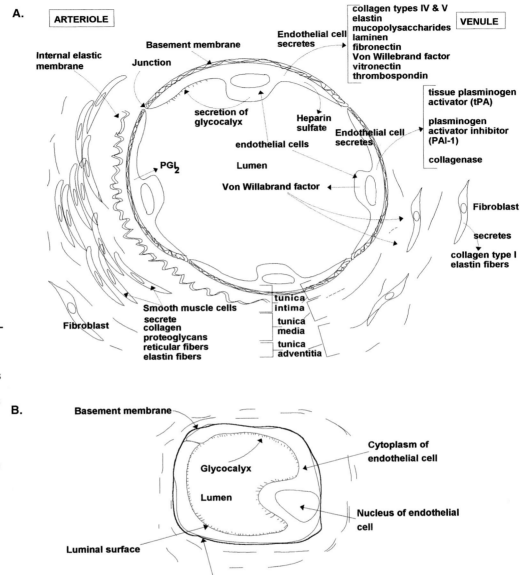

A.

ARTERIOLE

VENULE

Internal elastic membrane

Basement membrane

Junction

Endothelial cell secretes

collagen types IV & V
elastin
mucopolysaccharides
laminen
fibronectin
Von Willebrand factor
vitronectin
thrombospondin

secretion of glycocalyx

Heparin sulfate

endothelial cells

Endothelial cell secretes

tissue plasminogen activator (tPA)

plasminogen activator inhibitor (PAI-1)

collagenase

PGI₂

Lumen

Von Willabrand factor

Fibroblast

secretes

collagen type I
elastin fibers

tunica intima

tunica media

tunica adventitia

Smooth muscle cells secrete collagen proteoglycans reticular fibers elastin fibers

Fibroblast

B.

Basement membrane

Cytoplasm of endothelial cell

Glycocalyx

Lumen

Nucleus of endothelial cell

Luminal surface

Abluminal surface

FIGURE 23-2. Structure and functions of the blood vessel wall, comparison among arterioles, venules, and capillaries. **A,** Arterioles and venules. Endothelial cells, smooth muscle cells, and fibroblasts synthesize and secrete the components of the subendothelial matrix of connective tissue and the basement membrane proteins. The wall of arterioles is primarily smooth muscle cells and contains elastin in contrast to the venule which has only sparse smooth muscle cells. The media layer of arterioles is the most prominent while the adventitia layer is the largest in venules. **B,** A capillary has very little connective tissue in the vessel wall. It is primarily composed of endothelial cells and basement membrane.

to a basement membrane that consists of a unique form of collagen, type IV, embedded in a protein matrix. Layers of tissue beneath the basement membrane vary in thickness and composition depending on the size and type of vessel. These layers under the ablumenal surface of the endothelial cells are the *subendothelium.*

Histologically on cross section, the layers of veins and arteries appear distinct (Fig. 23-2A). The innermost layer, tunica intima, consists of the endothelial cell monolayer, the basement membrane, connective tissue which holds them together and, in arteries, an organized internal elastic membrane. The middle layer, tunica media, is thicker in arteries than in veins. In arteries smooth muscle cells predominate and are surrounded by loose connective tissue primarily consisting of elastin fibers, collagen fibers,

reticular fibers, and proteoglycans. In veins there are only a few smooth muscle cells, less elastin fibers and a similar matrix of connective tissue. The tunica adventitia, the outer coat, is thicker in veins than arteries. In this layer there are a few fibroblasts embedded in the collagen and other connective tissue. The fibroblasts synthesize and secrete the fibers and other components of the matrix.

CAPILLARIES

The *capillaries* (Fig. 23-2B) compose, by far, the largest surface area of all types of blood vessels, although they are, individually, the smallest. They are approximately 5 to 10 μm in diameter, just large enough for single blood cells to traverse. The lumen of a capillary is formed from single endothelial cells with their cytoplasm wrapped

TABLE 23-1 *STRUCTURE AND FUNCTIONS OF BLOOD VESSELS*

Blood Vessel	Structural Characteristics	Functions
Capillaries	5 to 10 μm diameter Single endothelial cell lumen Basement membrane No smooth muscle cells No collagen fibers No elastic fibers	No hemostatic function except those of endothelial cells Exchange nutrients, oxygen and waste products
Venules	20 to 200 μm diameter Basement membrane Few smooth muscle cells Few fibroblasts Primary component is thin layer of collagen and extracellular matrix No elastic fibers	Major site of hemostatic activity following traumatic injury Exchange nutrients, oxygen and waste products Regulate vascular permeability Endothelial cell hemostatic functions
Arterioles	20 to 200 μm diameter Basement membrane Primary component is smooth muscle cells Fibroblasts Thicker wall of collagen and extracellular matrix Few elastic fibers	Site of hemostatic activity following traumatic injury Regulate blood pressure by change in diameter Endothelial cell hemostatic functions

around in circular form. Tissue beneath the basement membrane of a capillary is sparse and contains no smooth muscle cells (Table 23-1).

VEINS

Blood vessels approaching or leaving the capillaries become progressively larger in diameter as they near the heart. Veins immediately leaving the capillaries are the *venules* (Fig. 23-2A). Venules are approximately 20 to 200 μm in diameter and are a major site of hemostatic activity after traumatic injury. Venules are composed of endothelium and basement membrane surrounded by a layer of extracellular connective tissue (Table 23-1) with a few fibroblasts and smooth muscle cells embedded in it. The connective tissue contains type I collagen fibers. In larger veins there are a few scattered fibers of elastin but they are not organized into a membrane. Mast cells are present in some layers (see Chapter 4).[1]

Blood flow in the veins is slow compared with that in the arteries, but valves in medium and large veins prevent backflow and keep the blood flowing toward the heart.

ARTERIES

Blood is pumped from the heart to the tissues through arteries. The lumena of the arteries become progressively smaller, forming the precapillary vessels referred to as *arterioles* (Fig. 23-2A). Arterioles, also a major site of hemostasis, are similar in structure to the veins except that a definite membrane of elastic tissue surrounds the basement membrane. The underlying tissues are composed primarily of smooth muscle cells with some fibroblasts in an extracellular connective tissue matrix (Table 23-1). Larger arteries contain progressively more elastic tissue that is condensed into one or more distinct layers.

● Functions of blood vessels

After injury, the damaged vessels initiate hemostasis. The first response of the vessels to the injury is constriction or narrowing of the lumen of the arterioles to minimize the flow of blood to the wounded area and the escape of blood from the wound site. *Vasoconstriction* occurs immediately and lasts a short period of time. The mechanism is not known entirely. It is, in part, caused by neurogenic factors and, in part, by several regulatory molecules that interact with receptors on the surface of cells of the blood vessel wall. The molecules include serotonin and thromboxane A_2, both products of platelet activation, and endothelin which is produced by the endothelial cells. These substances may aid in prolonging vasoconstriction. In contrast, the endothelial cells synthesize and secrete a prostaglandin, PGI_2, also called prostacyclin. PGI_2 counteracts constriction by causing vasodilation of the arterioles. Vasodilation increases the blood flow in the injured area and causes redness of the skin. As a result, a mechanism of checks and balances is present that prevents either process from becoming too powerful.

Also after injury, the endothelial cells of the venules contract producing gaps between them. Fluid from the plasma leaks into the tissues and causes swelling (edema). This is called increased vascular permeability.

The endothelial cells lining the lumen of blood vessels are the principle element regulating many vascular functions. Some of the functions modulated by the endothelial cells are hemostatic and, as such, aid the body in either forming (thrombogenic) or preventing the blood clots (non-thrombogenic). Some of the functions are nonhemostatic in nature (Table 23-2).

Hemostatic functions that inhibit clot formation include the provision of a nonreactive environment for the components of the hemostatic system. These components are inert in the presence of normal endothelium. Both physiologic and biochemical interactions provide the nonreactive environment. Physiologically, the surface of the endothelial cells is negatively charged and repels circulating proteins and platelets, which also are negatively

TABLE 23-2 *FUNCTIONS OF ENDOTHELIAL CELLS*

Function	Consequence
HEMOSTATIC Functions	
Non-thrombogenic	
Negatively charged surface	Repels platelets and hemostatic proteins
Heparin sulfate	Inhibits fibrin formation
Thrombomodulin	Inhibits fibrin formation
PGI$_2$ (Prostacyclin)	Vasodilation
	Inhibits platelet aggregation
Tissue plasminogen activator (tPA)	Activates fibrinolytic system
Plasminogen activator inhibitor (PAI-1)	Inhibits activation of fibrinolytic system
Endothelin	Vasoconstriction
Thrombogenic	
Produce and process von Willebrand factor	Carrier of Factor VIII in fibrin formation
Tissue thromboplastin	Platelet adhesion
	Initiate fibrin formation
NON-HEMOSTATIC Functions	
Selective blood/tissue barrier	Keep cells and macromolecules in vessels
	Allow nutrient and gas exchange
Process blood-borne antigens	Cellular immunity
Synthesize and secrete connective tissue	
Basement membrane collagen	Back-up protection for endothelial cells
Collagen of the matrix	Platelet adhesion
Elastin	Vasodilation and vasoconstriction
Fibronectin	Bind cells to one another. Platelet adhesion after tissue injury
Lamenin	Bind cells to one another. ? platelet adhesion
Vitronectin	Bind cells to one another. ? platelet adhesion
Thrombospondin	Bind cells to one another. ? platelet adhesion

charged. Biochemically, a wide variety of the substances that are synthesized and secreted by the endothelial cells contribute to the nonreactive environment. Examples are heparan sulfate, a mucopolysaccharide of the glycocalyx, and thrombomodulin, a protein of the endothelial cell surface, both of which inhibit thrombin formation. PGI$_2$, in addition to causing vasodilation of blood vessels, inhibits activation of platelets. Additionally, endothelial cells synthesize tissue plasminogen activator (tPA) and an inhibitor of tPA called plasminogen activator inhibitor (PAI-1). These proteins are involved in the control of fibrinolysis.

Thrombogenic functions of the endothelial cells include the production and processing of von Willebrand factor (vWf) (see Chapter 26). vWf is made by the endothelial cells and stored in structures called Weible-Palade bodies. It is secreted both into the plasma from the luminal side and into the subendothelium from the ablumenal side of the cells. The vWf in the subendothelium binds to collagen fibers in the extracellular matrix[2] and supports the binding of platelets in the initial stage of clot formation. The endothelial cells also contain tissue thromboplastin, which is released during injury and initiates the formation of fibrin for secondary hemostasis (see Chapter 24).

Nonhemostatic functions of the endothelial cells are, first, that as a barrier between the blood and underlying tissues, they selectively prevent erythrocytes and macromolecules from leaving the lumen. Several types of openings called pores or vesicles on the flat surfaces allow for transport of nutrient molecules from the plasma to the tissues and of waste products from the tissues into the blood. Second, they process blood-borne antigens for cellular immunity. Third, they synthesize and secrete the connective tissue of the wall of the vessels: basement membrane collagen, collagen fibers of the deeper layers, and elastin. Fibronectin, a glycoprotein that coats several cell types, as well as thrombospondin, lamenin and vitronectin are also synthesized and secreted to become part of the extracellular matrix.[1] These proteins are "glue" that allow cells to adhere to one another, to the extracellular connective tissue and to platelets.

When endothelial injury occurs, platelets and coagulation proteins in the plasma are exposed to subendothelial tissues. Interaction between the vessel wall components and the plasma components leads to the formation of the hemostatic plug.

The amount of blood lost from a vessel depends on its size and type as well as on the efficiency of the hemostatic mechanism. Hemostasis is most effective in smaller vessels and in capillaries. When larger vessels are severed, plug formation takes longer and may not be sufficient to stop bleeding. The pressure is much higher in arteries and the flow may be so rapid that clots cannot form.

● PLATELETS IN HEMOSTASIS

The second major component of the hemostatic system is the blood platelets. The role of platelets in hemostasis was first established by Bizzozero in 1882.[3] He noted their

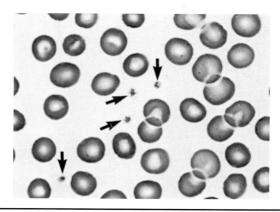

FIGURE 23-3. Peripheral blood smear. The arrows point to platelets (Wright-Giemsa stain: 250×).

adhesion and participation in formation of a thrombus in the mesenteric vessels of rabbits and guinea pigs.

Platelets are seen on a Romanowsky stained peripheral blood smear as small bluish, granular structures (Fig. 23-3). They circulate as discoid-shaped, anuclear cells, approximately 2 to 3 μm in diameter. The normal concentration of platelets in the blood is 150 to 440 × 10^9/L.

The following section of this chapter will discuss the production of platelets in the bone marrow, their ultrastructure, and their various roles in hemostasis.

Platelet production

PROGENITOR CELL COMPARTMENT

Platelets are produced in the bone marrow from the same stem cell (CFU-GEMM) as the erythroid and myeloid series. Under hormonal influence, this stem cell differentiates into megakaryocyte progenitor cells (see Chapter 2, Fig. 2-8). At least two stages of progenitor cell maturation have been identified: the immature megakaryocyte progenitor cell (BFU-Meg) and the committed megakaryocyte progenitor cell (CFU-Meg). Morphologically, these cells appear as small indistinguishable lymphoid-like cells.[4]

An adequate concentration of platelets in peripheral blood is maintained by a regulatory process. Production can be increased or decreased in response to a stimulus, which is probably the platelet mass and/or the megakaryocyte mass. As the stimulus decreases or increases, there is a corresponding inverse increase or decrease in the level of regulating factors.

Two types of regulating factors have been described. Some act on stem and progenitor cells, while others influence the more mature recognizable cells of the megakaryocyte series (see Chapter 2, Fig. 2-11). Interleukin-3 (IL-3) and GM-CSF are early acting growth factors that synergistically cause stem cells to differentiate into megakaryocyte progenitor cells and also induce them to proliferate.[5] They, therefore, influence the number of megakaryocytes being formed.

The second type of regulating factor is called *thrombopoietin*. Thrombopoietin primarily influences the matura-

tion stages of the megakaryocytes. This includes the eventual size of the cells, and, therefore, the number of platelets produced. It may also affect the rate of release of platelets to the peripheral blood. Thrombopoietin may be more than one substance. It has not yet been isolated and characterized molecularly.

STAGES OF MEGAKARYOCYTE DEVELOPMENT

Stimulation of stem cell receptors by the early-acting factors, IL-3 and GM-CSF, results in the formation of a megakaryoblast. The blast cell undergoes a maturation sequence that is different from that of other marrow cells in that nuclear maturation takes place first and is largely complete before cytoplasmic maturation begins. The unique nuclear maturation process consists of a series of *endomitoses*. With each endomitosis, the DNA content of the cell is doubled but cell division does not take place. The DNA content, or ploidy level, of the cells may become 4N to 32N, or potentially larger. The 8N stage is the first recognizable stage on a bone marrow smear and is the most common ploidy class found.

Cytoplasmic maturation may begin at ploidy levels of 8N or greater, but the stage at which maturation occurs varies from cell to cell. The reason for variability in cytoplasmic maturation at different ploidy levels is not known. Clinical conditions associated with the presence of large platelets are noted to have megakaryocytes with ploidy shifted left (lower ploidy). Lower ploidy megakaryocytes also appear to produce platelets that are more dense and

TABLE 23-3 *CHARACTERISTICS OF DEVELOPMENTAL STAGES OF MEGAKARYOCYTES*

Stage	Name	Characteristics
Stage I	Megakaryoblast	6 to 24 μm diameter Scant basophilic cytoplasm No visible granules Round nucleus Visible nucleoli
Stage II	Promegakaryocyte	14 to 30 μm diameter More cytoplasm, primarily blue in color Few visible granules Nucleus lobulated or indented Beginning demarcation membrane system seen on electron microscopy
Stage III	Megakaryocyte	16 to 56 μm diameter More granules in cytoplasm Abundant cytoplasm with pinkish color developing Multilobulated nucleus No nucleoli visible
Stage IV	Mature megakaryocyte	20 to 60 μm diameter Abundant pinkish very granular cytoplasm Demarcation zones indistinctly present Multilobulated nucleus No nucleoli visible

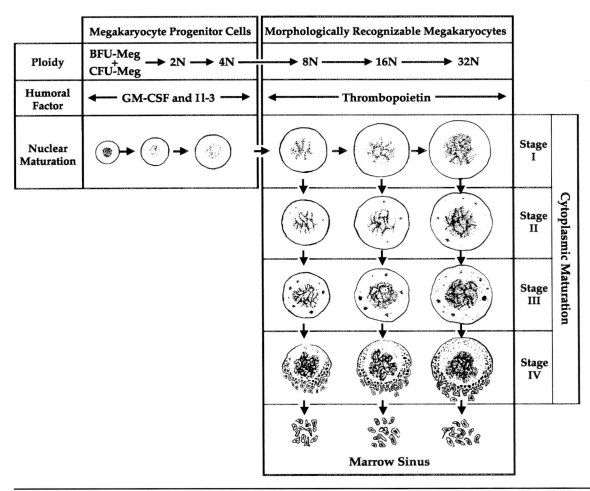

	Megakaryocyte Progenitor Cells		Morphologically Recognizable Megakaryocytes		
Ploidy	BFU-Meg + CFU-Meg → 2N → 4N		8N	16N	32N
Humoral Factor	← GM-CSF and Il-3 →		← Thrombopoietin →		
Nuclear Maturation			Stage I / Stage II / Stage III / Stage IV		

Marrow Sinus

FIGURE 23-4. The maturation sequence of megakaryocytes. The committed stem cell (CFU-Meg) under the influence of humoral factors (GM-CSF and IL-3) differentiates to a 2N megakaryoblast. Nuclear maturation proceeds through a series of endomitoses. Cytoplasmic maturation, influenced by thrombopoietin, occurs in cells at ploidy levels of 8N or higher. Morphologic features of each stage of cytoplasmic maturation are described in the text. Platelets are first released through the endothelial cells that line the marrow sinuses as proplatelets, which then break apart into mature platelets.

more functionally active. Increased ploidy of the nucleus might result in more cytoplasm and thus more platelets from an individual megakaryocyte.

Four stages of megakaryocyte development have been described according to their morphologic appearance on Romanowsky stained smears (Fig. 23-4 and Table 23-3). The differentiating characteristics are the nuclear morphology, cytoplasmic appearance, and relative size of the cell as determined by the ploidy class. It should be pointed out that, in the practical day-to-day evaluation of bone marrow specimens, it is not necessary to distinguish the maturation stages of megakaryocytes. It is, however, important to recognize a cell as being of the megakaryocyte cell line.

Stage I megakaryocytes (megakaryoblasts)(Fig. 23-5) have scant basophilic cytoplasm. No granules are visible by light microscopy. The nucleus is usually round and nucleoli may be visible. Megakaryoblasts are 6 to 24 μm in diameter.

The cytoplasm of *Stage II* cells (promegakaryocytes)

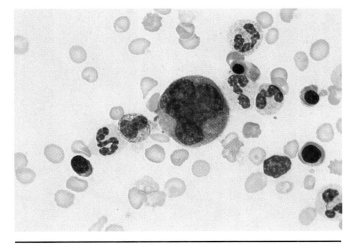

FIGURE 23-5. Megakaryoblast (BM).

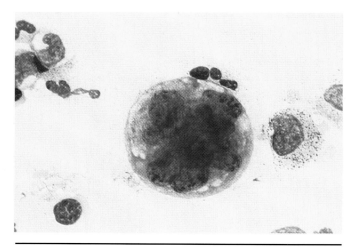

FIGURE 23-6. Promegakaryocyte (BM).

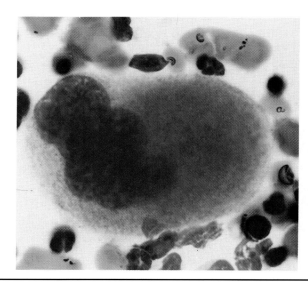

FIGURE 23-8. Megakaryocyte (BM).

(Fig. 23-6) contains visible azurophilic granules. The granules first appear in the perinuclear or Golgi region. The nucleus is lobulated and may appear indented or horseshoe-shaped. Nucleoli have disappeared. Promegakaryocytes measure 14 to 30 μm in diameter. A cytoplasmic membrane system termed the demarcation membrane system (DMS) begins to develop at this stage but it can only be seen with electron microscopy. The origin of the DMS is controversial. It is believed by some to be formed by invagination of the megakaryocyte cell membrane and by others to be produced by the Golgi apparatus. As it forms, small areas of megakaryocyte cytoplasm are separated. These areas will eventually become the platelets.[5]

Stage III megakaryocytes (granular megakaryocyte) (Fig. 23-7) are characterized by their larger size (16 to 56 μm) and increasing numbers of granules and demarcation membranes. The nucleus has multiple lobes and the amount of cytoplasm is greatly increased. It has developed a pinkish color with only a little blue remaining.

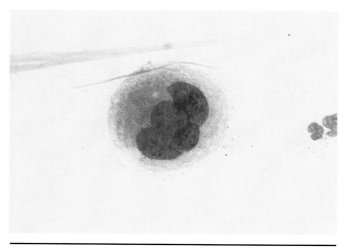

FIGURE 23-7. Early granular megakaryocyte (BM).

In *Stage IV* megakaryocytes (Fig. 23-8), the nucleus is compacted but lobulated. The cytoplasm is abundant and more pink in color. The granules are organized within zones that are separated by the demarcation membrane. Stage IV cells are 20 to 60 μm in diameter and are termed mature megakaryocytes.

RELEASE OF PLATELETS

Mature megakaryocytes, situated less than 1 μm from a bone marrow sinus, shed platelets directly into the sinuses. The mechanism is not yet fully understood. Platelets appear to be released from megakaryocytes in groups called proplatelets. Each megakaryocyte produces seven to eight proplatelets which are extruded through the cytoplasm of endothelial cells and into the marrow sinuses. It is thought that the proplatelets then break up into platelets, although the process has not yet been observed. Alternatively, the megakaryocyte cytoplasm could randomly break up into platelets within the marrow space.

The nucleus of the megakaryocyte remains in the marrow and is thought to degenerate and to be removed by the macrophage system. Whole intact megakaryocytes are occasionally released from the marrow, circulate in the peripheral blood, and migrate to lung tissue. These cells also may release platelets to the peripheral blood.[6]

Approximately 5 days are required for a megakaryoblast to develop into platelets. Two-thirds of the platelets that are released into the peripheral blood circulate in the bloodstream. The other third are sequestered in the spleen and are at equilibrium with those platelets in the blood. The average lifespan of platelets in the peripheral blood is approximately 9.5 days.

●
Micromegakaryocytes

Megakaryocytes may be present in the peripheral blood of normal persons, although it is exceedingly rare to observe

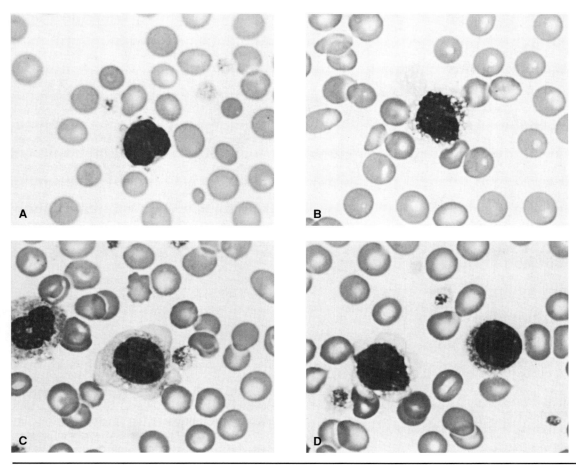

FIGURE 23-9. Micromegakaryocytes in peripheral blood smear of a patient in megakaryocytic blast crisis of CML. These photographs show several morphologic variations of these cells. Note the dense chromatin structure and the resemblance to lymphocytes. (A) A small micromegakaryocyte is shown with cytoplasmic tags of platelets. (B) This cell shows vacuolization and granulation of the cytoplasm. (C) In this cell the chromatin is less dense with a large amount of a granular cytoplasm. (D) The cell on the left is similar to Fig. 20–4C showing agranular and vacuolated cytoplasm. In contrast, the cell on the left has a small amount of densely granular cytoplasm (Wright-Giemsa Stain; ×1000).

them on a smear. In persons with myeloproliferative or myelodysplastic syndromes megakaryocytes may be seen in greater numbers and with abnormal morphology. One of these abnormal morphologic forms is the micromegakaryocyte, "dwarf" megakaryocyte, or megakaryocyte fragment. Micromegakaryocytes are believed to represent abnormal megakaryocytes that have lost their ability to undergo endomitosis. Most of these cells have a single-lobed nucleus and are the size of a lymphocyte. Morphologically, they may be confused with lymphocytes but can be distinguished by tags of one or more platelets attached to a nucleus (Fig. 23-9). Some may have pale blue, foamy or vacuolated cytoplasm that resembles a nongranular platelet. The nuclear structure is variable but many cells have very densely clumped chromatin and stain a brown-black color with Wright's stain. Others may have a finer, looser chromatin.

● Platelet structure

Circulating inert platelets are disc-shaped cells with smooth surfaces. Unlike the exterior surfaces of erythro-cytes and leukocytes, platelets have several openings resembling holes in a sponge. The openings are membranous channels which extend deep into the interior of the cell.

After an injury, many changes affecting the platelet morphology and biochemistry take place. The changes cause the platelets to become "activated." After they are activated platelets are then able to make a primary hemostatic plug. To understand the activation process, the normal platelet ultrastructure will be described next.

The platelet ultrastructure is divided into four arbitrary regions or zones: the peripheral zone, the structural zone, the organelle zone, and the membrane systems[7] (Fig. 23-10 and Table 23-4). The components of each region have specific functions in activated platelets and are discussed below.

PERIPHERAL ZONE
The peripheral zone of the platelet consists of a cytoplasmic membrane covered on the exterior by a fluffy surface coat and on the interior by a thin submembranous region between the peripheral zone and the next layer.

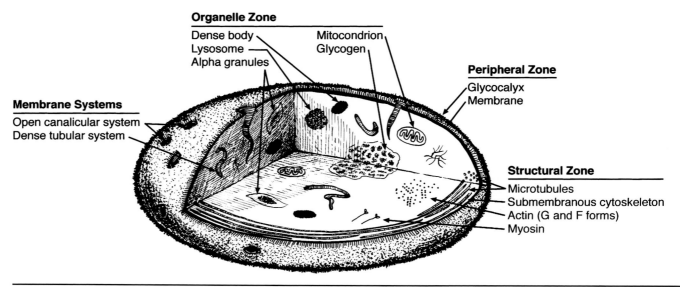

FIGURE 23-10. Diagram of the primary ultrastructural features of the resting platelet. The components of each of the four zones are shown. (Modified from Thompson, A.R., Harker, L.A.: Manual of Hemostasis and Thrombosis. 3rd Ed. Philadelphia: F.A. Davis, Co., 1982.)

TABLE 23-4   *PLATELET STRUCTURE*

1. Peripheral zone—Functions are adhesion and aggregation
    SURFACE COAT
      Glycocalyx—glycoproteins, proteins and mucopolysaccharides
    PHOSPHOLIPID BILAYER
      Phospholipids—asymmetric arrangement and source of arachidonic
        acid
    INTEGRAL PROTEINS
      Glycoproteins, especially Ib, IIb, IIIa, IX
      Enzymes

2. Structural zone—Functions are structure and support
    MICROTUBULES
    CYTOSKELETAL NETWORK
      Actin
      Actin binding protein
    CYTOPLASMIC MESHWORK
      Actin
      Myosin

3. Organelle zone—Functions are secretion and storage
    GRANULES
      Dense bodies
        Non-protein functional mediators
      Alpha granules
        Proteins
      Lysosomes
        Enzymes
    MITOCHONDRIA
    GLYCOGEN

4. Membrane systems—Functions are secretion and storage
    SURFACE CONNECTED OPEN CANNICULAR SYSTEM (OCS)
    DENSE TUBULAR SYSTEM
    FUSED SYSTEMS

This region has a few microfilaments, the nature of which are described below.

The surface coat, also called the *glycocalyx*, consists of several glycoproteins, proteins, and mucopolysaccharides that are most probably adsorbed from the plasma. Included are the coagulation factors V, VIII, and fibrinogen. The glycocalyx also is found on the surface membrane of the interior channels. Some of the surface proteins may be receptors for substances that cause platelet activation. The glycocalyx of platelets is thicker than that of other cells.

The cytoplasmic membrane has a typical trilaminar structure of a bilayer of phospholipid and embedded integral proteins. The membrane is the former demarcation membrane of the parent megakaryocyte.

An asymmetric arrangement of the phospholipids is an important factor in the function of activated platelets. Phosphatidylcholine and phosphatidylethanolamine are concentrated on the outer half, while phosphatidylserine, phosphatidylinositol, and sphingomyelin predominate on the inner half of the bilayer.[8]

The integral proteins may serve as receptors for stimuli involved in platelet function. Approximately 30 have been identified as glycoproteins. A nomenclature system has been developed for the major platelet glycoproteins. They may be abbreviated "gp" and are numbered with Roman numerals from I to IX according to electrophoretic migration by decreasing molecular weight. The function and structure of glycoprotein Ib and a complex of IIb and IIIa have been studied most extensively.

Glycoprotein Ib (Fig. 23-11A) is a receptor for von Willebrand factor. It is complexed with gp IX in the membrane, but the function of gp IX is unknown. Glycoprotein Ib has two chains called α and β. The gp Ibα chain is larger and contains the binding sites for vWf, thrombin,

A.

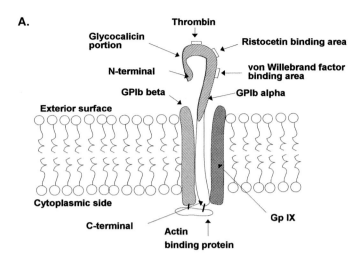

B.

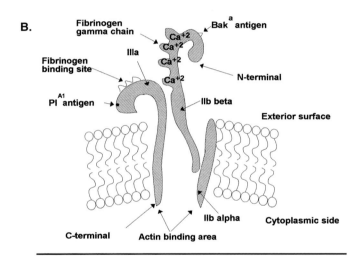

FIGURE 23-11. Structure of platelet membrane glycoproteins. **A,** Glycoprotein Ib is composed of an alpha and a beta chain. Both span the phospholipid bilayer. The alpha chain is larger and contains the binding sites for thrombin, ristocetin, and vWf. It is associated with glycoprotein IX. The cytoplasmic side has binding sites for actin. **B,** Glycoproteins IIb and IIIa associate in a complex after platelet activation. Binding sites for fibrinogen as well as platelet-specific antigens are present. The cytoplasmic portions of each component have binding areas for actin.

ristocetin (used in the platelet aggregation test), and auto-antibodies produced in individuals who are sensitive to quinidine.[9] The binding sites are located on the major portion of glycoprotein Ibα called *glycocalicin*. The glycocalicin portion is located on the surface of the platelet and can be removed by proteolytic enzymes. The remainder of the molecule is associated with the gp Ibβ chain spanning the phospholipid bilayer. On the cytoplasmic side both the α and β portions are associated with actin binding protein (see below). Each platelet contains approximately 25,000 glycoprotein Ib molecules.[10] Glycoprotein Ib functions in the platelet adhesion process described below.

The *glycoprotein IIb/IIIa complex* (Fig. 23-11B) is a receptor for fibrinogen. It also binds other circulating adhesive proteins such as von Willebrand factor, thrombospondin, vitronectin, and fibronectin. There are approximately 50,000 copies per platelet. Glycoprotein IIb, the larger of the two, is a two-chain protein. The α chain is embedded in the phospholipid bilayer, and the β chain protrudes from the platelet surface. Part of the β chain is the Bak^a antigen. Glycoprotein IIIa is a single chain and is associated with the gp IIb portion that lies within the phospholipid bilayer. The small surface portion of gp IIIa contains the Pl^{A1} antigen. The cytoplasmic sides of the two proteins are associated with actin in the platelet cytoskeleton. The glycoprotein IIb/IIIa complex is "hidden" in resting platelets and "appears" when platelets are activated.[9,10] It is required for platelet aggregation as described below.

Arachidonic acid, an unsaturated fatty acid, is a major component of the phospholipid portion of the membrane. It is a precursor of very potent stimulators that cause platelet aggregation and vessel constriction.

The submembranous region consists of filaments similar to those in the structural layer described next.

STRUCTURAL ZONE

The structural zone consists of *microtubules* and a network of proteins. The functions of the structural zone are to support the plasma membrane, maintain the resting discoid shape of the platelet and to provide a means of change in the shape when the platelet is activated. This layer was formerly called *thrombosthenin*.

Microtubules are composed of the protein tubulin. They are a bundle of 8 to 24 tubules, which are located beneath the submembranous region of filaments and completely surround the circumference of the platelet. They are important in maintaining the platelet's discoid shape.

The protein network consists of actin, actin binding protein and several other structural proteins and it forms a cytoskeleton that supports the plasma membrane (Fig. 23-12). Actin is the most abundant protein in platelets accounting for 15% to 20% of the total protein. It has two forms, G or globular and F or filamentous. The F form consists of several polymerized G molecules. Approximately 40% to 50% of the actin in a resting platelet is in the F form with the remainder in the G form. Actin binding protein is attached to the cytoplasmic side of the glycoprotein Ib/IX complex and anchors actin to the membrane.[6]

Actin also is part of a network of structural support throughout the cytoplasm. In the cytoplasm it is associated with myosin along with several other contractile proteins similar to those of smooth muscle. Unlike smooth muscle, in which the ratio of actin to myosin is about 7:1, the platelet ratio is 100:1. This network supports the resting discoid shape and when the platelet becomes activated significant biochemical and structural changes occur.

ORGANELLE ZONE

The organelle zone is beneath the microtubule layer and consists of mitochondria, glycogen particles, and at least

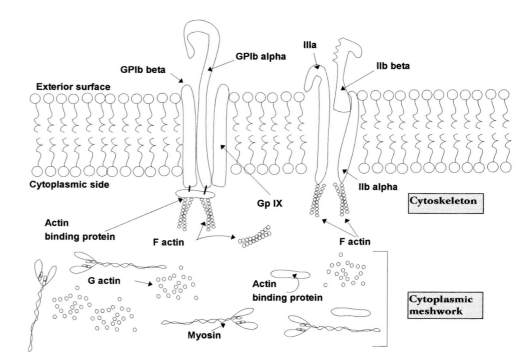

FIGURE 23-12. Cytoskeleton and cytoplasmic meshwork in the resting platelet. The cytoskeleton is composed of F-actin and actin-binding protein associated with the glycoproteins that span the phospholipid bilayer. The cytoplasmic meshwork consists primarily of F and G actin, actin-binding protein, myosin that are randomly distributed throughout the cytoplasmic interior of the platelet.

three types of granules dispersed within the cytoplasm: *dense bodies*, *alpha granules*, and *lysosomal granules*. The granules serve as storage sites for several proteins and other substances essential for platelet function. The *dense bodies* are named because they appear more dense in electron microscope preparations than the other types of granules. These bodies contain mediators of platelet function and hemostasis that are not proteins: ADP, ATP, and other nucleotides as well as phosphate compounds, calcium ions, and serotonin (Table 23-5). The ADP in the dense bodies is known as the nonmetabolic or storage pool of ADP to distinguish it from the metabolic ADP found in the cytoplasm. The metabolic pool provides energy for normal platelet metabolism, whereas the storage pool is important in the platelet aggregation reactions.

Alpha granules are the most numerous of the three types of granules. Alpha granules contain two major groups of proteins (Table 23-6). One group consists of proteins that are similar to hemostatic proteins found in

the plasma. Some, such as von Willebrand factor and factor V, are synthesized in the megakaryocyte when the platelets develop.[11] Others, such as fibrinogen, are absorbed from the plasma and packaged in the alpha granules. The second group includes proteins with a variety of functions. Some are found exclusively in platelets and are not found in other cells. Platelet factor 4, which combines with and neutralizes heparin, and β-thromboglobulin are examples.[12] Some proteins are growth factors

TABLE 23-6 *PROTEINS IN PLATELET ALPHA GRANULES*

Protein	Functions
Group I—Hemostatic Proteins	
Fibrinogen	Platelet aggregation and conversion to fibrin
Factor V	Helps in fibrin formation
von Willebrand factor	Platelet adhesion
Plasminogen activator inhibitor (PAI-1)	Inhibits fibrinolysis
α_2-antiplasmin	Inhibits fibrinolysis
Plasminogen	Converted to plasmin for fibrinolysis
Group II—Non-hemostatic Proteins	
Platelet-specific	
B-thromboglobulin	Chemotactic for fibroblasts in tissue repair
Platelet factor 4	Promotes platelet aggregation
Platelet derived growth factor	Promotes repair of smooth muscle cells
Not platelet-specific	
Albumin	?
Thrombospondin	Promotes platelet aggregation
Fibronectin	Cohesion of cells

TABLE 23-5 *COMPOSITION AND FUNCTIONS OF PLATELET DENSE BODY CONTENTS*

ADP (nonmetabolic)	Agonist for platelets. Recruits and activates new platelets for platelet aggregation
ATP (nonmetabolic)	Agonist for cells other than platelets
Other nucleotides	Unknown
Inorganic phosphates	Unknown
Calcium	Probable source of adequate extracellular calcium for variety of hemostatic reactions
Serotonin	Vasoconstriction

that affect the growth and gene expression of cells in the blood vessel wall. An example of this is platelet derived growth factor. Plasminogen activator inhibitor (PAI-1) also is synthesized in the megakaryocyte and stored in the alpha granules. When platelets are activated, PAI-1 is released and appears to protect newly formed clots from lysis.

Lysosomal granules contain several hydrolytic enzymes and are similar to the lysosomes found in other cells.

Platelets contain all the necessary enzymes for the glycolytic and tricarboxylic acid cycles and for glycogen synthesis and degradation. About 50% of the platelet's energy (ATP) is derived from the glycolytic pathway and about 50% is derived from the tricarboxylic acid cycle.

MEMBRANE SYSTEMS

The fourth structural zone of the platelet is a system of membranes. One type of membrane called the surface-connected open canalicular system (OCS) is the membrane that surrounds the twisted channels leading from the platelet surface to the interior of the platelet. This membrane is the remnant of the demarcation membrane system of the parent megakaryocyte.

A second type of membrane is the dense tubular system (DTS), which originates from the rough endoplasmic reticulum of the megakaryocyte. It is one of the storage sites for calcium ions. The channels of the dense tubular systems do not connect with the surface of the platelet.

The two membrane systems, OCS and DTS, fuse in various areas of the platelet cytoplasm to form membrane complexes.[7] The membrane complexes appear to be important regulators of the intracellular calcium concentration. The concentration of calcium ions within the platelet cytoplasm is important in regulating platelet metabolism and activation.

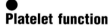

Platelet function

PLATELET ROLES IN HEMOSTASIS

Platelets are involved in several aspects of hemostasis (Table 23-7). One role appears to be that of passive surveillance of the blood vessel endothelial lining for gaps and breaks. Although the exact nature of this role is somewhat controversial, it has been shown that platelets maintain the continuity or integrity of the vessels by filling in the small gaps caused by the separation of endothelial cells. They attach to the underlying exposed collagen fibers of the subendothelium and prevent blood from escaping. A

TABLE 23-7 *PLATELET ROLES IN HEMOSTASIS*

1. Surveillance of blood vessel continuity
2. Formation of primary hemostatic plug
3. Formation of secondary hemostatic plug
4. Healing of injured tissue

decrease in the number of platelets in the peripheral blood results in leaking of blood through these gaps into the tissues.

When injury occurs and there is an actual break in the continuity of the lining of the vessels, the platelets react by forming the aggregate known as the *primary hemostatic platelet plug*. The bleeding stops because the openings in the vessels are mechanically filled in by the mass of platelets.

Following this plug formation, membrane phospholipids of the aggregated platelets provide a reaction surface for the formation of fibrin. Fibrin stabilizes the initial platelet plug and the entire mass of fibrin and platelets is the *secondary hemostatic plug*.

As a fourth role, secretions from the platelets help to heal the injured tissues. Platelet derived growth factor, a mitogen stored in alpha granules, stimulates smooth muscle cells and possibly fibroblasts to multiply and replace the cells that were damaged by the injury.

The steps and mechanisms which result in primary and secondary hemostatic plug formation are described below.

FORMATION OF THE PRIMARY HEMOSTATIC PLUG

Platelets are disc-shaped and inert in the environment of normal endothelium. Injury to the blood vessels causes a change in the normal environment. The platelets respond to the change by becoming activated. The primary hemostatic plug is the result of the transformation of the platelets from inactive to active. The plug forms in a specific sequence of steps that are called adhesion, activation, aggregation and secretion (Fig. 23-13).

Platelet adhesion   Platelet adhesion, the first step in primary hemostatic plug formation, is attachment of platelets to something besides other platelets. When endothelium is injured and bleeding occurs, platelets escape from the blood vessel and flow into the subendothelial tissues. They immediately stick to components of the subendothelium, the most important element of which is collagen fibers. The subendothelial surfaces are components to which platelets are not normally exposed. Platelet adhesion to collagen will only occur with the help of von Willebrand factor (vWf) and glycoprotein Ib of the platelet membrane.

vWf, which is synthesized by endothelial cells, is both stored within them and secreted into the subendothelial areas and into the plasma (see Chapter 25). In the subendothelium, it is adsorbed onto collagen fibers (Fig. 23-14). Some vWf, as we have seen above, also is found in platelet alpha granules. vWf molecules consist of a series of anywhere from 2 to 50 identical subunits. Each subunit has receptors by which it can bind to both collagen and to gpIb.[13] When platelet adhesion occurs, vWf binds to both collagen and to glycoprotein Ib on the platelet surface and becomes a "bridge" connecting the platelet to the collagen fiber (Fig. 23-14). As the binding continues the platelet "zippers" by attachment of its receptors to several adhesive proteins of the connective tissue matrix and eventually "spreads" itself over the surface of the collagen. Many platelets spread in a similar manner until a monolayer of platelets covers the surface of the collagen.

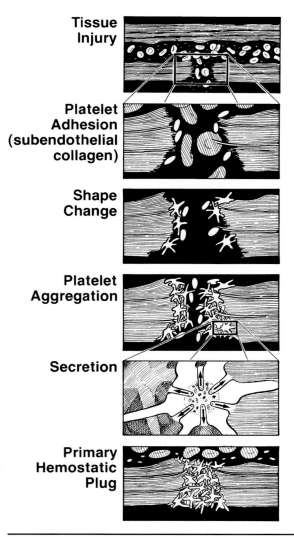

Tissue Injury

Platelet Adhesion (subendothelial collagen)

Shape Change

Platelet Aggregation

Secretion

Primary Hemostatic Plug

FIGURE 23-13. Diagram of platelets forming the primary hemostatic plug. Tissue injury causes platelets to adhere to subendothelial collagen. They undergo shape change, aggregate, and secrete granule contents. Additional platelets become activated by the secreted substances and clump together, eventually forming a mechanical barrier that halts the flow of blood from the wound.

Much of what is known about this phase of platelet function has been shown by studying patients with two diseases in which platelets fail to adhere properly: Bernard-Soulier disease and von Willebrand disease. Bernard-Soulier disease is characterized by lack of glycoprotein Ib on the platelet membrane. Patients with von Willebrand disease lack von Willebrand factor (vWf).

Activation Adhesion of platelets to collagen fibers via vWf triggers a series of morphologic and functional changes known as *activation*. Activation is a complicated process that is not totally understood. The most well-studied of the changes will be described below. They include changes in (1) metabolic biochemistry, (2) shape, (3) surface receptors, and (4) membrane phospholipid orienta-

tion. Only activated platelets are able to proceed with the subsequent steps in the formation of the primary hemostatic plug. Once activated, the platelet response becomes self-perpetuating.

Changes in metabolic biochemistry will be described first. A number of substances have been shown to stimulate platelets and cause the metabolic changes. Some substances are generated by the platelets themselves and some by other cells in the injured tissue. Some are normally present within cells but released when the cells are injured. Some have been tested experimentally in in vitro tests, but their in vivo actions are unknown. An agent that induces platelet activation is called an *agonist*. Each agonist binds to a specific platelet receptor and causes a series of reactions on the inside of the platelet. The result of binding by all agonists is similar to that described below.

The biochemical changes begin when vWf and collagen contact the receptor, glycoprotein Ib, on the surface of the platelet. Enzymes in the membrane become activated and cleave specific membrane phospholipids. The resulting products are "second messengers," which enter the platelet cytoplasm and transfer the signal to interior parts of the cells. Many sets of reactions are subsequently stimulated by the second messengers.

The pathways and second messenger products of three membrane enzymes, phospholipase C, phospholipase A_2, and adenyl cyclase, will be described. Products of all three cause rapid movement of intracellular calcium ions from storage sites in the dense tubular system as well as transport from the outside, through the membrane, and into the cytoplasm.[13] Resting platelets have very low levels of ionic calcium in the cytoplasm. Many cellular systems that are idle in resting platelets become activated by the presence of calcium ions. There is a direct relationship between the amount of cytoplasmic calcium and the extent of stimulation.

The substrate of *phospholipase C* is a derivative of phosphatidylinositol (PI). PI is one of the phospholipids found in greater quantity on the inner leaf of the bilayer. Several derivatives of PI are also present in the membrane. One or two phosphate groups may be enzymatically added to PI via ATP at positions 4 and 5 of inositol to form phosphoinositol-4-monophosphate or phosphoinositol-4,5-biphosphate (PIP_2), also called diphosphatidylinositol and triphosphatidylinositol, respectively (Fig. 23-15). Phospholipase C splits PIP_2. Two compounds are formed from the PIP_2, each of which cause a separate set of internal pathways. The first, inositol-1,4,5-triphosphate (IP_3), stimulates a series of reactions which result in the release of calcium ions from the dense tubular system. The second compound from PIP_2 cleavage is diacylglycerol (DG), which activates another enzyme called protein kinase C. Protein kinase C phosphorylates other proteins. Phosphorylation is a common regulatory process in all cells and results in activation of some proteins and inactivation of others. In the platelet, it is believed to lead to subsequent steps such as secretion from the granules and appearance of the fibrinogen receptor, glycoprotein IIb/IIIa.[6]

Phospholipase A_2 is stimulated by the increase in cytoplasmic calcium described above. Phospholipase A_2 hy-

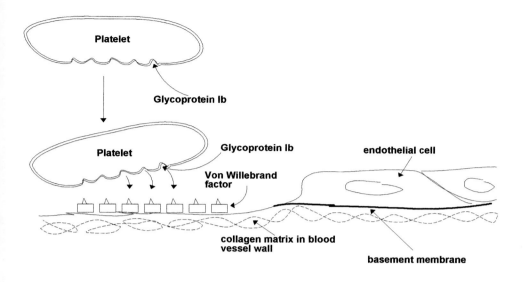

FIGURE 23-14. Platelets adhere to von Willebrand factor in the subendothelium after an injury. They then spread onto the subendothelial surfaces by attaching to other adhesive proteins that compose the matrix. Glycoprotein Ib is involved in the attachment of platelets to the subendothelium.

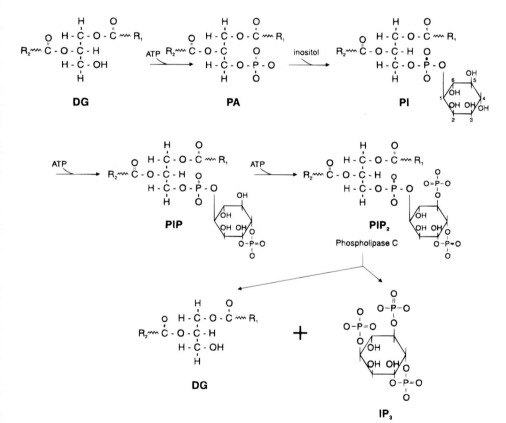

FIGURE 23-15. A second messenger system is mobilized when platelets become stimulated by agonists. When platelets are stimulated by injury, a message is transferred from the surface to the interior of the cell. When the message is received on the inside, changes occur in the platelet biochemistry and metabolism and the platelet becomes activated. Two second messengers are diacylglycerol (DG) and inositol-1,4,5-triphosphate (IP3). They are formed by cleavage of phosphatidyl inositol 4,5-bisphosphate (PIP2) by activated phospholipase C. PIP2 is formed by the addition of phosphate groups from DG with the help of ATP and the addition of inositol. The precursors of PIP2 by this pathway are phosphotidic acid (PA), phosphotidylinositol (PI), and phosphoinositol-4-monophosphate (PIP).

drolyzes arachidonic acid (AA) from the second carbon of the glycerol backbone of phosphatidylinositol and phosphatidylcholine.[13] Arachidonic acid is an unsaturated fatty acid and a precursor of a variety of regulatory substances. In the platelet, thromboxane A_2 is synthesized from AA by the enzymes *cyclo-oxygenase* and thromboxane synthase (Fig. 23-16). Within the platelet, thromboxane A_2 stimulates secretion from the platelet granules. Normal secretion will not occur if thromboxane A_2 synthesis is blocked and subsequent steps in platelet function will be seriously impaired. Ingestion of aspirin inhibits cyclo-oxygenase and prevents affected platelets from synthesizing thromboxane A_2. The consequences of aspirin ingestion will be discussed in Chapter 25. Thromboxane A_2 also can diffuse out of the cell and enhance vasoconstriction.[13] Thromboxane A_2 is a labile compound. It is spontaneously converted into an inert form, thromboxane B_2, a short time after its synthesis.

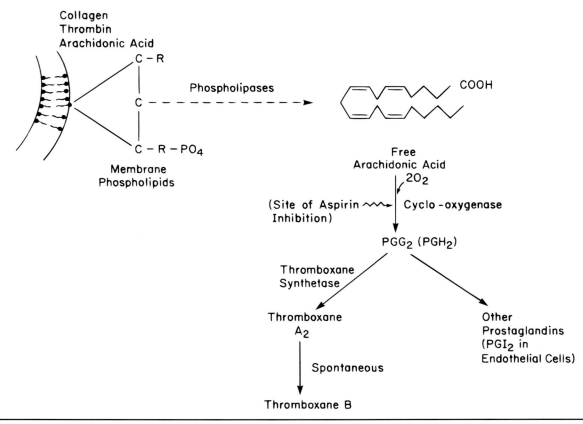

FIGURE 23-16. *Biochemical pathways of Thromboxane A2 formation in the platelet. Stimulation of platelet membranes (both intracellular granule and cytoplasmic membranes) by agonists such as collagen, thrombin, and arachidonic acid results in liberation of arachidonic acid from membrane phospholipids. The enzyme cyclo-oxygenase incorporates two molecules of oxygen forming the prostaglandin PGG2, which in its reduced form is PGH2. Thromboxane synthase in platelets converts PGG2 into the unstable but active Thromboxane A2. Thromboxane A2 is spontaneously converted into inactive Thromboxane B. Alternatively PGG2 can also be converted to other prostaglandins and in endothelial cells to PGI2 or prostacyclin, a powerful platelet inhibitor.*

The third membrane enzyme to be discussed, adenyl cyclase, is stimulated by agents that inhibit platelet aggregation and blocked by many agonists that promote platelet aggregation. Internal calcium levels are increased by its action but the mechanism by which it does this is unclear.[13]

Activation continues with a change in shape of the platelet when the internal calcium level reaches a threshhold. *Shape change* is the transformation from disc-shaped cells to spheres with spiny projections called *pseudopods* from the surface (Fig. 23-17). It involves the proteins in the structural zone including the membrane cytoskeleton proteins, actin and myosin of the cytoplasmic lattice, and the microtubules. During shape change, the microtubules dissolve. When pseudopods form, microtubules reappear within them.[14] At the same time, G actin polymerizes so that 70% to 80% of it is converted to filaments of F actin. The polymerized actin associates with actin binding protein and other proteins of the membrane skeleton to form a lattice network of structural support in the cytoplasmic membranes of the pseudopods. Through actin binding protein, this network attaches to the glycoprotein Ib/IX complex in the plasma membrane. Additionally, other F actin filaments associate with myosin forming

a meshwork of *actomyosin* throughout the cytoplasm of the pseudopods. Myosin becomes activated by phosphorylation by protein kinase C, myosin light chain kinase, and other enzymes as it associates with the F actin. Actomyosin provides a system of contractile units that is compared to that of smooth muscle. Contraction is the mechanical force that drives all of the succeeding platelet responses.[6,14]

Simultaneously, a band of actomyosin microfilaments replaces the microtubule layer surrounding the circumference of the resting platelet. This band contracts, bringing the granules and organelles into closer contact within a small area in the center of the sphere.[14]

The result of the shape change is that each platelet has a larger membrane surface area for biochemical reactions and a greater chance of contact with other platelets. Platelets adhering to collagen spread over the surface by filling in the space between the pseudopods over a period of time. The platelets thus fit together in a "jigsaw puzzle effect."

Shape change will lead to succeeding responses if the stimulus is strong enough and the intracellular calcium level becomes high enough. Without these, the platelet will return to its original discoid shape.

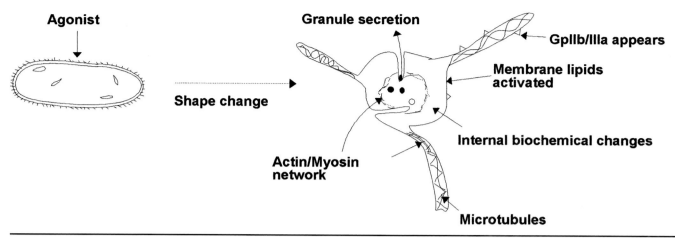

FIGURE 23-17. Platelet shape change after stimulation by an agonist. Pseudopods develop on the platelet surface and contain a network of actin and myosin, membrane phospholipids are activated, glycoprotein IIb/IIIa receptors appear, internal biochemical changes occur, and granule secretion follows.

The third element of activation results in the appearance of the glycoprotein IIb/IIIa receptor to which fibrinogen binds. This receptor is hidden in resting platelets but appears very soon after activation with any agonist. Platelets are able to bind fibrinogen only after the glycoprotein IIb/IIIa receptor appears.[10] Calcium is required for fibrinogen attachment.

The mechanism by which the fibrinogen receptor appears is not known. In the resting platelet glycoprotein IIb and glycoprotein IIIa are separate entities. Some authors describe the nature of the appearance of the glycoprotein IIb/IIIa receptor as a merging of the two after stimulation by an agonist (Fig. 23-18).

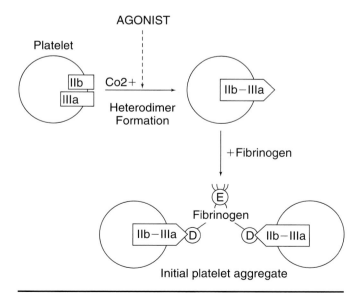

FIGURE 23-18. The initial steps in platelet aggregation. After stimulation by an agonist, glycoprotein IIb/IIIa receptors appear on the platelet surface. Fibrinogen becomes a "bridge" between two platelets by binding to the receptors.

The fourth aspect of activation is a change in the membrane surface which allows fibrin-forming proteins (coagulation factors) to bind to it (Fig. 23-19). This function is known as the platelet *procoagulant* activity. The proteins are bound in complexes that allow the correct orientation of enzymes and substrate molecules as fibrin is formed (see Chapter 24).

Activation is summarized schematically in Figure 23-19 and in Table 23-8.

Aggregation   After adherent platelets are activated, primary hemostatic plug formation continues with a phase known as aggregation. *Platelet aggregation* is the attachment of platelets to one another. New platelets flowing into the bleeding tissue become activated by contact with agonists such as ADP that are released by the damaged tissue and endothelial cells. With activation the new platelets undergo shape change, and their glycoprotein IIb/IIIa sites are exposed. The new platelets then stick to those that are adhering to collagen.

Aggregation occurs in two phases called primary and secondary. During *primary aggregation* platelets adhere loosely to one another. If the stimulus by agonists is weak, primary aggregation is reversible. *Secondary aggregation* takes a longer period of time and begins as the platelets start to release their own ADP and other granule contents and to synthesize thromboxane A_2 as described below. Presumably, the released substances become agonists, which continue the stimulation process. If platelets are unable to release ADP and/or to synthesize thromboxane A_2, secondary aggregation will not occur, and they will disaggregate. The result might be that bleeding from a wound would take a longer time to stop.

Fibrinogen and extracellular calcium are needed for aggregation to occur.[14] Both are plasma constituents. Both also are released by the platelets from internal storage granules to provide high concentrations in the injured area. The role of calcium in platelet aggregation is not known. The role of fibrinogen is that of a "bridge" linking

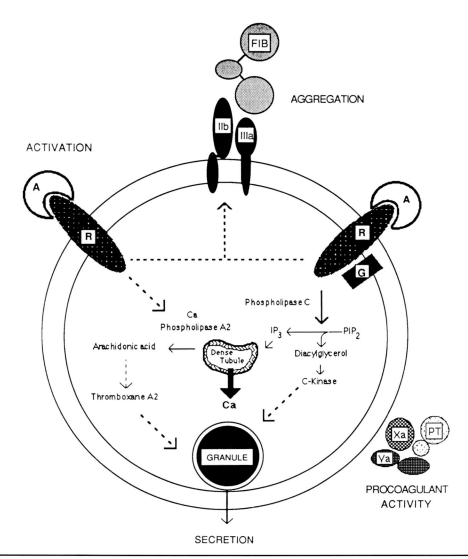

FIGURE 23-19. Schematic diagram showing platelet biochemical changes after activation. A-agonist; R-receptor; FIB-fibrinogen; Xa, Va, PT-coagulation proteins (factors); G-G actin form.

TABLE 23-8 *CHARACTERISTICS OF RESTING VS ACTIVATED PLATELETS*

Platelet Characteristic	Resting Platelet	Agonist Activated Platelet
Shape	Disc	Sphere with pseudopods
Actin	Mostly G form	Mostly F form
	Attached to gplb	Becomes actomyosin
		Lattice in pseudopods with actin-binding protein
Microtubules	Circumference	In pseudopods
Phospholipids	Intact	Thromboxane A_2 synthesized from arachidonic acid
Phospholipase A_2	Inactive	Activated—cleaves arachidonic acid from phospholipids
Phospholipase C	Inactive	Activated—cleaves phosphotidylinositol to become "second messengers"
Adenyl cyclase	Inactive	Activated—leads to phosphorylization of proteins
Cytoplasmic calcium	Low	High
Glycoproteins IIb and IIIa	Hidden	Appear as fibrinogen receptor

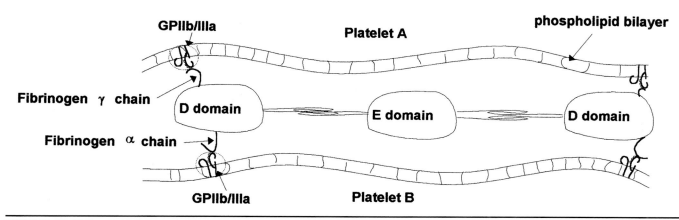

FIGURE 23-20. Fibrinogen binding to two platelets is horizontally. Peptides from the alpha and gamma chains of both D domains bind to glycoprotein IIb/IIIa receptors.

two adjacent platelets. Fibrinogen is able to link the two platelets because of its molecular structure. This structure is described in detail in Chapter 24. Briefly, fibrinogen is composed of two pair of three polypeptide chains, alpha, beta, and gamma. One set of the three peptide chains forms a D domain on each end of the molecule. All 6 chains meet in the center of the molecule in the E domain. One fibrinogen molecule may attach to the glycoprotein IIb/IIIa receptors on two different platelets by binding sites in the alpha and gamma chains of its D domains (Fig. 23-20). The extreme carboxy terminal end of the gamma chain and two sites on the alpha chain of fibrinogen bind to specific and complementary short amino acid sequences in the receptor. Approximately 16 to 80,000 molecules of fibrinogen are bound to each activated platelet.[11] Fibrinogen binding is reversible for a time but after about 10 to 30 minutes becomes irreversible.[10]

The need for calcium in platelet aggregation can be appreciated by observing platelets on a blood smear. Platelets are found in clumps of various sizes on smears prepared from needletip or capillary blood. On smears prepared from blood that has been anticoagulated by a calcium sequestering agent such as EDTA, platelets are singly dispersed, and platelet clumps are seen only rarely.[14]

The need for glycoprotein IIb/IIIa receptors in platelet aggregation was found by studying patients with a rare disorder called Glanzmann's thrombasthenia. Persons with this disease lack the gp IIb/IIIa receptors and platelets do not aggregate in response to various agonists in the platelet aggregation test described below. Patients who have decreased levels of fibrinogen also have abnormal platelet aggregation (see Chapter 25).

Other adhesive proteins such as vWf, thrombospondin, and fibronectin also bind to the gp IIb/IIIa receptor[13] but their functions in this are not clear.

Secretion (release) Following adhesion, shape change, and primary aggregation, platelets begin to discharge granule contents into the surrounding area. The process is known as *secretion* or *release*. Secretion is energy-depen-

dent and requires ATP. It occurs gradually over a period of time and before or concurrently with secondary aggregation.

Secretion occurs in two ways. By one mechanism, the open cannicular system fuses with membranes of granules that have been centralized deep within the interior of the platelet. The contents are then extruded through the OCS to the outside. Alternatively, the membranes of some granules fuse with each other and then with the plasma membrane. The contents are, again, emptied to the outside of the platelet.[10,14]

Secretion is self-supporting. Some of the released substances are agonists that stimulate additional membrane receptors. Stimulation of the receptors causes the internal calcium level to rise and then more release occurs. The platelets eventually become degranulated.

ROLES OF THE GRANULE CONTENTS The contents of the three types of granules were previously described. Each type of granule requires a threshold level of calcium in the cytoplasm before it begins to secrete. The order from lowest to highest calcium level is dense granules, alpha granules, and then the lysosomes.

The substances released from the dense bodies and the alpha granules have various functions, some of which are defined and most of which are unknown. They promote platelet plug formation by stimulating additional platelets to adhere, secrete, and aggregate. Examples of the functions of some of them are described below. The contents of the lysosomes will not be further considered here.

The dense bodies contain ADP, ATP, serotonin, and calcium. The release of ADP from the dense bodies into the surrounding tissue is considered to be of primary importance in the continued stimulation and recruitment of new platelets to the aggregate. After an injury, the first source of extracellular ADP may be the damaged tissue and endothelial cells. Extracellular ADP binds to a specific platelet membrane receptor that is coupled to the enzyme adenyl cyclase. One effect of this binding is to cause the intracellular calcium stores to move from storage sites to the cytoplasm. The increased cytoplasmic calcium causes the platelets to release their own ADP from the dense bodies to the outside. Another effect of the binding of ADP to its receptor is to cause fibrinogen receptors (gp IIb/IIIa) to appear on the platelet surface.[13] As the release continues, the amount of extracellular ADP increases and more platelet receptors are stimulated resulting in higher internal and external levels of calcium. While most investigators consider ADP release to be a prime factor in platelet stimulation, others have proposed that this role of ADP may be an artifact of the experimental process.[13]

The dense body pool of calcium is released extracellularly with the ADP. This calcium is nonmetabolic and is not involved in the internal stimulation processes. The purpose of the extruded calcium is believed to be to provide a high concentration outside the platelets for fibrinogen attachment and for other reactions that take place on the platelet exterior surface.

The roles of serotonin and ATP of the dense granules will not be discussed here because they are not associated with any diseases and they are either very complicated or as yet controversial.

The alpha granules contain a wide variety of proteins, some of which are specific for the platelet and others, such as fibrinogen, that are similar to hemostatic proteins found in the plasma. A partial list of the substances released from the alpha granules is found in Table 23-6.

The platelet-specific proteins are platelet factor 4 (PF4), β-thromboglobulin (βTG), and platelet derived growth factor (PDGF). PF4 is called the heparin neutralizing factor. Heparin is an anticoagulant used in the treatment of patients who clot excessively (thrombosis) (see Chapter 25). PF4 has the ability to neutralize the activity of heparin. It also has many other actions such as chemotactic activity for neutrophils, monocytes, and fibroblasts.[14] The role of βTG is uncertain, but it is believed to attract fibroblasts chemotactically and may, therefore, promote healing of the wound. PDGF is a mitogen and also may contribute to healing.

Thrombospondin is another protein released from the alpha granules but it is not platelet specific. It is synthesized by many other cells, including endothelial cells, and is found in the extracellular connective tissue. It may function in platelet adhesion and aggregation.

vWf, factor V, and fibrinogen are examples of proteins in the alpha granules that are similar to hemostatic proteins of the plasma. Factor V may function as a receptor on the platelet surface for hemostatic proteins and is a cofactor in the process of fibrin formation. The functions of vWf and fibrinogen have been discussed previously.

Primary hemostatic plug Eventually the platelets form a barrier that seals the injury and prevents further loss of blood. The barrier is called the *primary hemostatic plug*. The platelet plug is responsible for the initial cessation of bleeding from a cut. The time for bleeding to cease depends on the depth of the injury and the size of the blood vessel. Superficial wounds, in which only capillaries and small vessels are affected, usually stop bleeding within 10 minutes.

PLATELETS AND SECONDARY HEMOSTASIS

The primary platelet plug is relatively unstable and is easily dislodged. As an illustration, one can probably recall accidentally causing trauma to a fresh cut and having the bleeding begin again. The primary platelet plug is stabilized and anchored firmly to the vessel wall by the process of *secondary hemostasis*. Secondary hemostasis begins with fibrin formation around the aggregated platelets. The entire platelet-fibrin mass then contracts to a firmer, more cohesive clot. The contraction is called *clot retraction*. Platelets participate in both fibrin formation and clot retraction.

Platelet procoagulant activity Activation of platelets results in the exposure of binding sites for coagulation proteins involved in the formation of fibrin on the platelet surface. The biochemical mechanisms underlying this relationship are not known. Some believe that the more negatively charged phospholipids usually found on the inner leaflet of the bilayer "flip flop" to the outer leaflet and become the binding sites.

The binding of coagulation factors to specific platelet receptors provides proper orientation of the protein molecules for enzymatic reactions to occur and for eventual thrombin formation. The capacity of stimulated platelets to catalyze the coagulation process by providing phospholipid surfaces is known as *platelet factor 3* or *platelet procoagulant activity*. The fibrin stabilized platelet plug is termed the *secondary hemostatic plug*. This phase of hemostasis is discussed in Chapter 24.

Clot retraction Following fibrin formation, a final step in the coagulation process is contraction of the clot. As the clot retracts, serum is expressed. This can be observed in a test tube of blood when no anticoagulant is added. A few minutes after unanticoagulated blood is placed into the test tube it begins to gel. The gel is the fibrin with the blood cells caught in it. The mass of fibrin and trapped erythrocytes shrinks over a period of 2 to 24 hours as the serum is squeezed from the fibrin mass.

Clot retraction is believed to occur by the association of adjacent platelet pseudopods with each other and with the fibrin strands. Actin and other contractile proteins within the pseudopods cause the platelets to contract. In vivo, the result of clot retraction is a cohesive mass of platelets and fibrin that seals the wounded vessel and prevents further blood loss. Contraction also permits the return of a more normal blood flow through the vessel. The stabilized platelet-fibrin mass will remain in place until fibroblast repair of the wound results in permanent healing.

● LABORATORY INVESTIGATION OF PRIMARY HEMOSTASIS

Laboratory tests for platelets include the platelet count and evaluation of platelet function. A variety of platelet counting methods are used in clinical laboratories. The platelet function tests that will be described below are the bleeding time, the platelet aggregation test, and the clot retraction test.

Platelet count

Platelets may be counted by manual or automated methods.[16] Manual methods are performed by diluting a sample of whole blood, counting the platelets in an aliquot, and calculating the number per liter. Two commonly described procedures are the Rees and Ecker and the Brecker-Cronkite methods.

The Rees and Ecker method employs a diluting fluid containing brilliant cresyl blue. The stain helps to make the platelets more visible. Counting is done using a light microscope. The diluting fluid for the Brecker-Cronkite method is 1% ammonium oxalate, which is sold commercially in Unopettes (Becton-Dickson Co., Rutherford, NJ). A phase microscope and a special flat hemacytometer are suggested for accurate counting. A light microscope and regular hemacytometer may also be used.

Reliable automated or semiautomated instruments for platelet counting are available, and their use is preferred over manual methods because they are more accurate and can be controlled more easily. Some instruments use whole anticoagulated blood and others require centrifugation of the blood to obtain platelet rich plasma.

Whether manual or automated methods are used, it is necessary to correlate the count with the platelet concentration on a well-prepared peripheral blood smear. Normally, 8 to 20 platelets will be seen per field at $1000\times$ magnification.

The number of platelets can be estimated by multiplying the average number counted in five to ten fields (at $1000\times$ magnification) by 20,000 if the smear was made from the needle tip or from capillary blood. A factor of 15,000 should be used if the blood was anticoagulated. The estimated count should agree reasonably with the direct chamber count, the limits of which should be established by each laboratory. Correlation between the estimate and the direct count decreases with high platelet concentration. Morphology of the platelets also should be observed and notation made of the presence of large forms, agranular forms, or other abnormal platelets.[17]

Bleeding time

The bleeding time is an in vivo measurement of primary hemostasis. In this procedure, an incision is made in the skin and the length of time for the bleeding to stop is measured by a stopwatch. Three methods for performing this test are described. They differ primarily in the site and manner of making the incision.

The Duke method, first described in 1910, is the least reproducible method and has been abandoned by most laboratories. The ear lobe is punctured with a sterile disposable lancet and the time for bleeding to stop is recorded.

The Ivy method, which was introduced in 1941, is performed by placing a pressure cuff on the patient's arm at 40 mmHg. Two or three incisions 1 mm wide and 3 mm deep on the volar surface of the forearm are made with a sterile disposable lancet. The bleeding time of the cuts is averaged. Although use of the pressure cuff produces a longer bleeding time, it is more reproducible because the influence of the capillaries is decreased. Severed capillaries tend to collapse as blood leaves them which shortens the bleeding time in a manner that is not dependent upon platelet function. Venostasis produced by the pressure cuff causes the vessels to remain filled with blood. Therefore, the bleeding stops because the platelets aggregate and form the primary hemostatic plug.[18] With the Ivy method, however, the size of the cut is still variable and influences the reproducibility of the test.

In 1969, Mielke introduced the template bleeding time (a modified Ivy method) that produces a cut of standardized length and depth in addition to the stasis produced by the pressure cuff.[19] The template bleeding time has been found to be highly reproducible and is the method of choice today. Commercially available templates (The Template Bleeding Time, Hemakit, Inc., Malden, MA; Simplate Bleeding Time, General Diagnostics, Morris Plains, NJ; Surgicutt, ITC Commercial Group, Edison, NJ) produce cuts 9 mm or 5 mm wide and 1 mm deep. The depth of the cuts is superficial so that only the small vessels are severed. The normal bleeding time by the template method is 1 to 9 minutes. The direction of incision on the forearm has an effect on the result. Slightly longer times are recorded when the incision is horizontal than when it is vertical.[20]

Determination of the bleeding time by the template method measures the ability of the platelets to form a primary hemostatic plug. A defect in platelet function will cause a prolonged bleeding time. Thus, defects in the ability of the platelets to adhere, aggregate, or release will influence the bleeding time. Thrombocytopenia also causes a prolonged template bleeding time. There is a linear inverse relationship between the platelet count and the bleeding time when the platelet count is between $10 \times 10^9/L$ and $100 \times 10^9/L$. The bleeding time may be altered to some extent in certain diseases involving blood vessels and in von Willebrand disease.

The bleeding time should not be performed on patients who have ingested aspirin or aspirin containing products within 7 days. Aspirin causes a slight increase in the bleeding time in almost all normal individuals. It begins to correct within 48 hours after a dose is taken. The extent of prolongation, however, is usually not beyond the normal range except in patients who also have a functional platelet defect.[18] Patients should be aware that, occasionally, an abnormally prominent scar may form.[20]

Platelet aggregation test

The platelet aggregation test is an in vitro test of the ability of the platelets to aggregate with certain agonists. This test may be indicated in patients who have prolonged bleeding times in the presence of normal platelet counts, and may aid in pinpointing the cause of abnormal platelet function. Aggregation is measured spectrophotometrically and recorded by a platelet aggregometer. Measurement is based on the decrease in optical density that occurs in a solution as platelets aggregate. The required specimen depends on the type of instrument. Some use platelet rich plasma and others whole blood. Sodium citrate is the anticoagulant.

To perform the test, the specimen is placed in a cuvet, warmed to 37° C and maintained at that temperature throughout the procedure. The specimen is constantly agitated with a stirring bar to keep the platelets in an even suspension and to allow them to collide with one another. Aggregation will not occur if they are not stirred. Each agonist is added and tested individually with a separate aliquot of the specimen. A recording device monitors the aggregation obtained with each agonist for a period of about 15 minutes. Aggregation is measured as a decrease in optical density (absorbance) of the platelet suspension. Initially the suspension is cloudy. As the platelets aggregate the suspension becomes clearer and the optical density decreases. Alternatively, aggregation may be expressed as percentage of light transmittance, which is the negative log of the optical density. The decrease in optical density is recorded as graphs similar to Figure 23-21.

Aggregating reagents that are most often used clinically are ADP, epinephrine, collagen, and ristocetin, an antibiotic known to cause thrombocytopenia. At times, thrombin and arachidonic acid are used.

Typical normal curves obtained with each of the four common reagents are shown in Figure 23-21. ADP in an optimal concentration (Fig. 23-21A) and epinephrine (Fig. 23-21B) produce biphasic curves. In Figure 23-21A, the point "a" represents the baseline before the agonist is added. At "b" there is an initial increase in absorbance immediately after addition of the reagent due to shape change of the platelets. The curve at "c" represents a primary wave of aggregation in response to the agonist in the test tube. As ADP begins to be released from the platelets and thromboxane A_2 synthesized internally, a second wave of aggregation "d" is generated.

The curve obtained with ADP is dependent on the concentration of the reagent. If the concentration is too low, a primary wave will be obtained but the platelets will disaggregate. The primary wave will be seen on the graph but it will fall back toward the baseline rather than produce the secondary wave. If the concentration of ADP is too high, a single, monophasic wave will be seen.

Normal Platelet Aggregation Curves

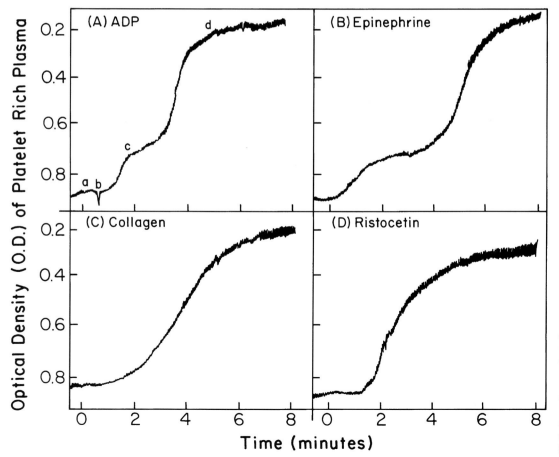

FIGURE 23-21. Platelet aggregation curves in response to the commonly used agonists, ADP, epinephrine, collagen and ristocetin. An explanation of the various parts of the curve in response to ADP is found in the text.

The curve with epinephrine is seen in Figure 23-21B. Epinephrine binds to α_2-adrenergic receptors and causes an opening in the membrane that allows extracellular calcium to move into the cell.[14] Epinephrine is unique in that it does not cause shape change but is still involved in platelet aggregation.[10] It, like ADP, requires the synthesis of thromboxane A_2 to stimulate secondary aggregation and secretion. The significance of epinephrine in vivo is unknown. It is useful, however, in vitro as part of the platelet aggregation test and helps to explain abnormal platelet function in some conditions.

The collagen curve (Fig. 23-21C) is a single wave of aggregation. Collagen does not cause a primary wave of aggregation. It does, however, induce platelets to secrete and to form thromboxane A_2. The single wave represents the aggregation resulting from the released substances. The lag seen before the aggregation wave represents the time during which the secretions are being generated.

Normal platelet aggregation with the above agonists also depends on adequate amounts of gp IIb/IIIa receptors on the surface of the platelet and of fibrinogen. Abnormal aggregation patterns can reflect abnormalities of the primary wave, the secondary wave, or both. With ADP and epinephrine, defects of primary aggregation, for instance, absence of gp IIb/IIIa or fibrinogen will result in lower height of the primary wave and no secondary wave. Defects in release of ADP or the formation of thromboxane A_2 will result in primary aggregation that will disaggregate and return to the baseline. Abnormal aggregation with collagen reflects the inability to release ADP and/or to form thromboxane A_2.

The mechanism of response with ristocetin is to produce agglutination of the platelets (Fig. 23-21D). vWf and glycoprotein Ib are required. The release reaction is not measured. The curve may show one or two waves.

Abnormal platelet aggregation in response to one or more agonists is seen in several disorders of platelet function (see Chapter 25). It is particularly useful as an aid in the diagnosis of von Willebrand disease, Bernard-Soulier disease, and Glanzmann's thrombasthenia. The test may be abnormal after administration of several drugs including aspirin. As with the bleeding time, the patient should be aspirin-free for 1 week before the test. Return to normal of the platelet aggregation test takes longer than the bleeding time after aspirin ingestion.

Clot retraction test

The clot retraction test is no longer a useful clinical procedure. The test consists of observing the retraction of a clot in a test tube 24 hours after drawing the blood. A semiquantitative method has been devised using platelet-rich plasma. Clot retraction is dependent on an adequate number of functionally normal platelets. The test is abnormal in thrombocytopenia and in Glanzmann's thrombasthenia.

SUMMARY

Blood clots after an injury by a series of complex biochemical reactions called hemostasis. The purpose of hemostasis is to temporarily reconstruct continuity of injured blood vessels so that external loss of blood is minimized. The components of hemostasis are found in the plasma and in the tissues that comprise the blood vessel walls. All of the components are inert until activated by the injury.

Hemostasis occurs in phases called primary hemostasis, secondary hemostasis, and fibrinolysis. This chapter discussed the primary hemostasis phase. During primary hemostasis, the blood vessels and the platelets cooperatively form an aggregate of the platelets that mechanically fills the openings in the injured blood vessels and stops bleeding from the wound. The injured blood vessels contribute by constricting and secreting a variety of biochemical mediators that affect all of the subsequent steps of hemostasis. The roles of the platelets are to adhere to the injured areas of the blood vessel walls, aggregate by attaching to one another and also by secreting substances that are stored in their granules. The secreted substances help to attract and activate new platelets that are added to the aggregate and that help the growth of new tissue that permanently heals the wound. The surface of the aggregated platelet is required for the reactions of secondary hemostasis.

REVIEW QUESTIONS

1. The cells that line the central cavity of all blood vessels and related tissues are called:
   a. Epithelial cells
   b. Endothelial cells
   c. Capillaries
   d. Smooth muscle cells

2. The normal lifespan of the platelets in the peripheral blood is:
   a. 8 hours
   b. 1 day
   c. 10 days
   d. 100 days

3. Platelet dense granules are storage organelles for _____, which are released after activation.
   a. calcium, ADP, and serotonin
   b. fibrinogen, glycoprotein Ib, and von Willebrand factor
   c. ADP, thromboxane A_2, and fibrinogen
   d. lysosomal granules, ATP, and factor V

4. Which of the following is needed for platelets to aggregate?
   a. thrombin
   b. actin
   c. von Willebrand factor
   d. fibrinogen

5. Platelet glycoprotein IIb/IIIa complex is:
   a. a membrane receptor for fibrinogen
   b. secreted from the dense bodies
   c. secreted by endothelial cells
   d. also called actin

6. The formation of thromboxane A$_2$ in the activated platelet:
   a. is needed for platelets to adhere to collagen
   b. is caused by the alpha granule proteins
   c. requires the enzyme cyclooxygenase
   d. occurs via a pathway involving von Willebrand factor

7. A humoral factor which regulates platelet production by speeding up the maturation time of the megakaryocyte is called:
   a. thrombocyte
   b. thrombopoietin
   c. interleukin-3
   d. prostaglandin

8. The function of microtubules in the resting platelet is:
   a. to keep a high level of calcium in the cytoplasm
   b. to store and sequester calcium
   c. to provide a negative charge on the platelet surface
   d. to keep the disc shape

9. Contents of the platelet granules are released from the platelet:
   a. through the open membrane system after fusion with the granules
   b. through the microtubules after fusion with the granules
   c. by disintegration of the platelet plasma membrane
   d. by the mitochondria

10. Which of the following is true about the relationship between ADP and platelets?
    a. ADP is necessary for platelet adhesion
    b. ADP released from the granules is required for platelet aggregation
    c. ADP is synthesized in the platelet from arachidonic acid
    d. ADP is released from the alpha granules of the platelets

REFERENCES

1. Kefalides, N.A.: Biochemical aspects of the vessel wall. In Hemostasis and Thrombosis: Basic Principles and Clinical Practice. 2nd Ed. Edited by R.W. Coleman, J. Hirsch, V.J. Marder, and E.W. Salzman. Philadelphia: J.B. Lippincott Co., 1987.

2. Jaffe, E.A.: Vascular function in hemostasis. In Hematology. 4th Ed. Edited by W.J. Williams, E. Beutler, A.J. Erslev, and M.A. Lichtman. New York: McGraw-Hill, Inc., 1990.

3. Bizzozero, J.: Uber einen neuen Formbe standtheil des Blutes und die rolle bei der thrombose und der Blutgerinnung. Virchows Arch. Pathol. Anat., 90:261, 1882.

4. Gerwirtz, A.M.: Human megakaryocytopoiesis. Semin. Hematol., 23:27, 1986.

5. Isenberg, W.M., Bainton, D.F.: Megakaryocyte and platelet structure. In Hematology: Basic Principles and Practice. 2nd Ed. Edited by R. Hoffman, E.J. Benz, Jr., S.J. Shattil, B. Furie, H.J. Cohen, and L.E. Silberstein. New York: Churchill Livingstone, 1995.

6. Brass, L.F.: Molecular basis for platelet activation. In Hematology: Basic Principles and Practice. 2nd Ed. Edited by R. Hoffman, E.J. Benz, Jr., S.J. Shattil, B. Furie, H.J. Cohen, and L.E. Silberstein. New York: Churchill Livingstone, 1995.

7. White, J.G.: Anatomy and structural organization of the platelet. In Hemostasis and Thrombosis: Basic Principles and Clinical Practice. 2nd Ed. Edited by R.W. Colman, J. Hirsh, V.J. Marder, E.W. Salzman. Philadelphia: J.B. Lippincott Co., 1987.

8. Phillips, D.R.: Platelet membranes and receptor function. In Hemostasis and Thrombosis: Basic Principles and Clinical Practice. Edited by R.W. Colman, J. Hirsh, V.J. Marder, and E.W. Salzman. Philadelphia: J.B. Lippincott Co., 1982.

9. Bithell, T.C.: Platelets and megakaryocytes. In Wintrobe's Clinical Hematology. 9th Ed. Edited by G.R. Lee, T.C. Bithell, J. Foerster, J.W. Athens, and J.N. Lukens. Philadelphia: Lea & Febiger, 1993.

10. Bennett, J.S., Shattil, S.J.: Platelet function. In Hematology. 4th Ed. Edited by W.J. Williams, E. Beutler, A.J. Erslev, and M.A. Lichtman. New York: McGraw-Hill, Inc., 1990.

11. Plow, E.F., Ginsberg, M.H.: Molecular basis of platelet function. In Hematology: Basic Principles and Practice. 2nd Ed. Edited by R. Hoffman, E.J. Benz, Jr., S.J. Shattil, B. Furie, H.J. Cohen, and L.E. Silberstein. New York: Churchill Livingstone, 1995.

12. Holt, J.C., Niewiarowski, S.: Biochemistry of α-granule proteins. Semin. Hematol., 22:151, 1985.

13. Bithell, T.C.: The physiology of primary hemostasis. In Wintrobe's Clinical Hematology. 9th Ed. Edited by G.R. Lee, T.C. Bithell, J. Foerster, J.W. Athens, and J.N. Lukens. Philadelphia: Lea & Febiger, 1993.

14. Brace, L.D.: Platelet physiology. In Hemostasis and Thrombosis in the Clinical Laboratory. Edited by D.M. Corriveau and G.A. Fritsma. Philadelphia: J.B. Lippincott, Co., 1988.

15. Nurden, A.T., Caen, J.P.: Specific roles for platelet surface glycoproteins in platelet function. Nature, 255:720, 1975.

16. Weisbrot, I.M., Hollenberg, C.M.: Platelet counting methods. Lab. Med., 11:307, 1980.

17. Evans, V.J.: Platelet morphology and the blood smear. J. Med. Tech., 1:689, 1984.

18. Mielke, C.H., Jr.: Aspirin prolongation of the template bleeding time: Influences of venostasis and direction of incision. Blood, 60:1139, 1982.

19. Mielke, C.H., Jr., Kaneshiro, M.M., Maher, I.A., Weiner, J.M., et al: The standardized normal Ivy bleeding time and its prolongation by aspirin. Blood, 34:204, 1969.

20. Mielke, C.J., Jr.: Measurement of the bleeding time. Thromb. Haemost., 52:210, 1984.

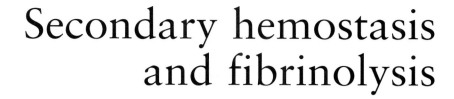

Secondary hemostasis and fibrinolysis

24

KEY TERMS

coagulation factors
zymogens
intrinsic pathway
extrinsic pathway
common pathway
prothrombin group
vitamin-K dependent factors
PIVKA
fibrinogen group
contact group
tissue factor
prothrombinase complex
fibrin monomer
fibrin polymer
thrombomodulin
plasmin
plasminogen
tissue plasminogen activator
  (t-PA)
urokinase-like tissue
  plasminogen activators
  (u-PA)
plasminogen activator
  inhibitor-1
plasminogen activator
  inhibitor-2
fragment X
fragment Y
fragment E
fragment D
primary fibrinolysis

INTRODUCTION

Secondary hemostasis occurs when soluble plasma proteins, called *coagulation factors,* interact in a series of complex enzymatic reactions to convert the soluble protein fibrinogen to insoluble fibrin. The reactions occur in a cascade- or waterfall-like fashion, whereby the circulating inactive coagulation factors *(zymogens)* are sequentially activated to enzymes. Each zymogen serves first as a substrate and then as an enzyme (Fig. 24-1). The final substrate in the cascade is fibrinogen and when acted upon by the final enzyme, thrombin, fibrinogen is converted to fibrin. Activation of the cascade begins when the zymogens are exposed to the subendothelial layers of the vessels. All enzymatic reactions except the last (the formation of fibrin from fibrinogen) require a phospholipid surface provided by the membranes of activated platelets and injured vessels. The requirement of a surface is important because it limits the site of reactions and fibrin formation to the site of injury.

All the enzymes in the cascade, except factor XIII (a transamidase), are serine proteases that act as cleaving enzymes with protease activity at the site of a serine residue (Table 24-1). The original reactions are amplified many times by means of the nonenzyme coagulation factors (cofactors) and positive feedback activation.

Schematic Representation of Factor Activation in Coagulation Cascade

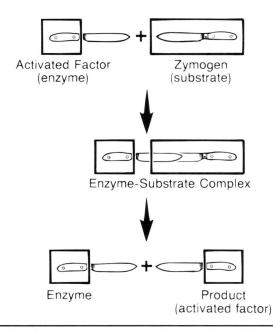

FIGURE 24-1. Schematic representation of factor activation in the coagulation cascade. The factors circulate as inert proteins (zymogens) until activated to an enzyme by proteolytic cleavage.

TABLE 24-1 *HEMOSTATIC FUNCTION OF COAGULATION FACTORS*

Serine Proteases	Cofactors	Transamidase	Substrate
XIIa	HMWK	XIII	Fibrinogen (I)
XIa	VIII		
IXa	V		
VIIa	Tissue Factor (III)		
Xa			
Thrombin (IIa)			
Kallikrein			

HMWK: High molecular weight kininogen.

INTERACTIONS AND CONTROLS OF HEMOSTASIS

Fibrin forms a meshwork in and around the primary hemostatic platelet plug like a spider web, producing a stable physical barrier to escaping blood. The barrier, sometimes referred to as a clot, is temporary, serving a purpose only until the vessel's endothelial wall is repaired. It is imperative to keep in mind that both primary hemostasis and secondary hemostasis are necessary for normal clot formation. The importance of both systems is supported by the finding that individuals with a deficiency in one system usually show clinical manifestations of a bleeding disorder, even though the other system is normal. Deficiencies in primary hemostasis usually produce small pinpoint hemorrhages beneath the skin called petechiae and bleeding from mucous membranes, whereas deficiencies in secondary hemostasis produce ecchymosis (large bruises) and more serious deep hemorrhages into joints and body cavities.

The process of fibrin formation is a well-balanced, controlled process, whereby clot formation is limited to the ruptured vessel, preventing widespread coagulation activation. The proteolytic activity of the activated clotting factors is limited by natural inhibitors or regulators. The process of fibrin formation is also controlled by negative feedback; large quantities of thrombin, the last enzyme formed in the cascade, destroy the coagulation cascade cofactors in the rate-limiting steps of its own production.

Once the fibrin clot has served its purpose of plugging the injured vessel and the vessel begins to repair itself, the fibrin is digested by plasmin, an enzyme of the fibrinolytic system. Plasmin, normally circulates as an inert protein, plasminogen, and is activated by the serine proteases of the coagulation cascade and by a factor released from the injured endothelium of the blood vessel.

Thus, it can be seen that the mechanisms of hemostasis are intricately regulated; coagulation factors, natural inhibitors, and fibrinolytic proteins activate and inhibit one another. These regulatory mechanisms serve to limit the coagulation process to the site of injury and to destroy the fibrin clot after it has served its purpose (Fig. 24-2).

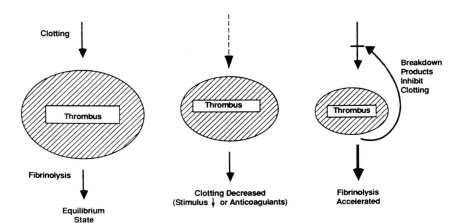

FIGURE 24-2. Activation of coagulation factors promotes the formation of a clot (clotting) while fibrinolysis breaks down the clot. Immediately after injury, the process of clotting predominates and the clot grows in size. When clotting and fibrinolysis are in equilibrium, the clot neither enlarges or decreases in size. If clotting is inhibited and/or if fibrinolysis is accelerated; however, the clot decreases in size. This occurs normally during the healing process. In the fibrinolytic process, the products released from the clot as it breaks down, serve to inhibit clotting. (With permission from: Sherry, S.: Fibrinolysis, Thrombosis and Hemostasis. Philadelphia: Lea & Febiger, 1992.)

COAGULATION FACTORS

The coagulation factors have been designated by Roman numerals, I through XIII, according to the order of their discovery, not their reaction sequence. Each factor also has one or more common names or synonyms (Table 24-2). Factor VI is no longer included in the coagulation sequence as this "factor" is now considered to be the activated form of factor V. When a factor becomes activated, it has enzymatic activity and the letter "a" accompanies the Roman numeral designation (e.g., activated factor XII is factor XIIa). There are several exceptions to this terminology. Factor II (prothrombin) in its activated form is preferentially known as thrombin rather than factor IIa, and when fibrinogen (factor I) is cleaved by thrombin it is preferentially called fibrin. Fibrin, the end product of the cascade, has no enzymatic properties. Tissue thromboplastin and calcium do not have an activated form.

The coagulation factors were discovered when patients with life-long histories of bleeding problems were seen by physicians. Studies of the affected patient's blood revealed that certain proteins were functionally deficient. Most of these proteins have now been isolated and characterized as to their composition and biochemical function (Table 24-3). In addition, the coagulation proteins have been sequenced and the chromosomal location of their genes identified (Table 24-4).

Sources of coagulation factors

The coagulation factors are synthesized in the liver. Plasminogen, from the fibrinolytic system, and the protease

TABLE 24-2 *NOMENCLATURE AND SYNONYMS FOR COAGULATION FACTORS*

Roman Numeral	Preferred Descriptive Name	Synonyms
I	Fibrinogen	
II	Prothrombin	
III	Tissue factor	Thromboplastin
IV	Calcium ions	
V	Proaccelerin	Labile factor, accelerator globulin (AcG), thrombogen
VII	Proconvertin	Stable factor, serum prothrombin conversion accelerator (SPCA)
VIII	Antihemophilic factor (AHF)	Antihemophilic globulin (AHG), antihemophilic factor A, platelet cofactor 1, thromboplastinogen
IX	Plasma thromboplastin component (PTC)	Christmas factor, antihemophilic factor B, autoprothrombin II, platelet cofactor 2
X	Stuart factor	Power factor, autoprothrombin III, thrombokinase
XI	Plasma thromboplastin antecedent (PTA)	Antihemophilic factor C
XII	Hageman factor	Glass factor, contact factor
XIII	Fibrin stabilizing factor (FSF)	Laki-Lorand factor (LLF), fibrinase, plasma transglutaminase, fibrinoligase
—	Prekallikrein	Fletcher factor
—	HMW kininogen	High molecular weight kininogen, contact activation cofactor, Fitzgerald factor, Williams factor, Flaujeac factor, Reid factor, Washington factor

(From: Lee, G.R., et al: Wintrobe's Clinical Hematology. Philadelphia: Lea & Febiger, 1993.)

TABLE 24-3 *SOME PROPERTIES OF THE COAGULATION FACTORS*

Factor* (1)	Biochemistry (2)	Biosynthesis (3)	Biologic Half-Life† (Hours) (4)	Activity in Serum (5)	Activity in Adsorbed Plasma (6)	Function (7)	Plasma Concentration (mg/L)
Fibrinogen	Multimeric glycoprotein; 3 paired peptide chains; MW 340,000	Liver	72–120‡	Absent	Unchanged	Precursor of fibrin; common pathway	2,500–3,000
Prothrombin	Monomeric glycoprotein; MW 69,000	Liver; vitamin K-dependent	67–106‡	Absent	Absent	Proenzyme; precursor of thrombin; common pathway	70–150
Factor V	Multimeric glycoprotein; MW 200,000–400,000	Liver	?12–36	Absent	Unchanged	Cofactor; common pathway	4–14
Factor VII	Monomeric glycoprotein; MW 63,000	Liver; vitamin K-dependent	4–6	Increased	Absent	Proenzyme; extrinsic pathway	0.5
Factor VIII-vWF complex	Multimeric glycoprotein; MW ~1,200,000; functionally heterogeneous subunits			Absent	Unchanged	Cofactor; intrinsic pathway; platelet adhesion	7
Factor VIIIc	Monomeric glycoprotein; MW 267,000	?	10–14	Absent	Unchanged	Cofactor, intrinsic pathway; "carrier" molecule for VIIIc	0.1
vW factor	Multimeric glycoprotein; MW ~1,200,000	Endothelium; megakaryocytes	22–40	Present	Unchanged	Platelet adhesion	—
Factor IX	Monomeric glycoprotein; MW 55,000	Liver; vitamin K-dependent	18–40	Increased	Absent	Proenzyme; intrinsic pathway	4
Factor X	Two-chain glycoprotein; MW 55,000	Liver; vitamin K-dependent	?24–60	Unchanged	Absent	Proenzyme, common pathway	10
Factor XI	Two-chain glycoprotein; MW 160,000	Liver	?48–84	Unchanged	Slightly decreased§	Proenzyme, intrinsic pathway	2–7
Factor XII	Monomeric glycoprotein; MW 80,000	?	52–60	Unchanged	Unchanged	Proenzyme; intrinsic pathway	27–45
Prekallikrein	Monomeric γ-globulin; MW 88,000	?Liver	?	Unchanged		Proenzyme; kinin system; intrinsic pathway	50
HMW kininogen	Monomeric α-globulin; MW 110,000	?Liver	?	Unchanged		?Cofactor; kinin system; intrinsic pathway	70–90
Factor XIII	Multimeric glycoprotein; two paired peptide chains; MW 320,000	Megakaryocytes, liver	?72–168	Decreased	Unchanged	Proenzyme; common pathway	1

* All data pertain to coagulation factors of human origin. Data concerning bovine material often are more complete, and are discussed in the text. MW, molecular weight. ?, insufficient data or significant disagreement between published figures.

† Biologic half-life, as distinguished from overall in vivo half-life or half disappearance time.

‡ Data obtained by using isotropic methods. Figures in column 4 not so indicated are based on studies in patients with hereditary deficiencies.

§ Variable, depending on concentration of adsorbent.

(Adapted from: Lee, G.R. et al.: Wintrobe's Clinical Hematology. Philadelphia: Lea & Febiger, 1993).

TABLE 24-4 *CHROMOSOMAL LOCATION CONTAINING COAGULATION FACTOR INFORMATION*

Factor	Inheritance	Chromosome	Region
I	Autosomal dominant	4	q26-31
II	Autosomal dominant	11	p11-q12
V	Autosomal recessive	1	q21-25
VII	Autosomal recessive	13	q34
VIII:C	Sex-linked recessive	X	q28
vWF	Autosomal dominant	12	p12-13
IX	Sex-linked recessive	X	q27
X	Autosomal recessive	13	q34
XI	Autosomal recessive	4	q35
XII	Autosomal recessive	5	q33
XIII	Autosomal dominant	6	p24-25
Antithrombin III	Autosomal dominant	1	p23
Protein C	Autosomal dominant	2	q13-14
Protein S	Autosomal dominant	3	p21
Plasminogen	Autosomal dominant	6	q26-27
TPA	Autosomal dominant	8	p12
TPA-I-1	Autosomal dominant	7	q21-22
TPA-I-2	Autosomal dominant	18	q21-22
Antiplasmin	Autosomal recessive	18	?
Prekallikrein	Autosomal recessive	?	?
HMWK	Autosomal recessive	?	?
Heparin cofactor II	Autosomal dominant	22	?

(From: Bick R.L.: Disorders of Thrombosis and Hemostasis. Chicago: ASCP, 1992).

inhibitors also are synthesized in the liver. In severe liver disease, these proteins can be markedly depressed, leading to bleeding diathesis.

Factor VIII is a large macromolecular complex composed of two distinct proteins: a small portion with procoagulant activity (VIII:C) and a larger multimeric portion that serves to bind platelets to collagen (the von Willebrand factor, vWf). Kupfer's cells in the liver appear to be the site of Factor VIII:C synthesis. vWf protein is believed to be synthesized by the endothelial cells throughout the body and by megakaryocytes.

●
Properties of coagulation factors

The coagulation process has traditionally been divided into three pathways based on the mode and sequence of coagulation protein activation in vitro: the intrinsic, extrinsic, and common pathways. Each of the 13 coagulation factors is assigned to one of these pathways (Table 24-5). The *intrinsic pathway* is activated by contact of coagulation proteins with negatively charged surfaces, whereas the *extrinsic pathway* is activated by contact of factor VII with tissue factor. The intrinsic and extrinsic pathways converge in the *common pathway*. These pathways and their reactions will be discussed later.

TABLE 24-5 *COAGULATION FACTORS IN INTRINSIC, EXTRINSIC AND COMMON PATHWAY*

Intrinsic Pathway	Extrinsic Pathway	Common Pathway
Prekallikrien	VII	X
HMWK	Tissue Factor (TF; III)	V
XII		II
XI		I
IX		
VIII		

In addition to being divided into three pathways based on their sequential roles in hemostasis, the coagulation factors can be divided into three groups dependent on their physical properties: prothrombin group, fibrinogen group, and contact group (Table 24-6).

PROTHROMBIN GROUP

The *prothrombin group* includes Factors II, VII, IX, and X. These factors have a molecular mass ranging from 50,000 to 100,000 Daltons and migrate on electrophoresis with the α- or β-globulins. Calcium ions are necessary for binding prothrombin factors to an acidic phospholipid surface where activation to the enzyme form occurs.

Vitamin K has a very important role in the synthesis of the functional factors in this group. Therefore, the prothrombin group factors also are known as the *vitamin K-dependent factors*. Vitamin K is found in some vegetable oils and leafy plants. It also is synthesized in the gut by various bacteria. This fat-soluble vitamin is only absorbed from the gastrointestinal tract in the presence of bile salts. Studies have revealed that vitamin K is needed for the attachment of an extra COOH (carboxyl) group to the γ-carbon of glutamic acid residues (γ-carboxylation) at the N-terminal end of the polypeptide chain (Fig. 24-3). This postribosomal modification provides the critical calcium

TABLE 24-6 *COAGULATION FACTOR GROUPS BASED ON PHYSICAL CHARACTERISTICS*

Contact Group	Prothrombin Group	Fibrinogen Group
Characteristic: require contact with a surface for activation	Characteristics: require vitamin K for synthesis; need Ca++ to bind to a phospholipid surface; adsorbed from plasma by BaSO₄.	Characteristics: large molecules; absent from serum (consumable).
XII	II	I
XI	VII	V
Prekallikrein	IX	VIII
HMWK	X	XIII

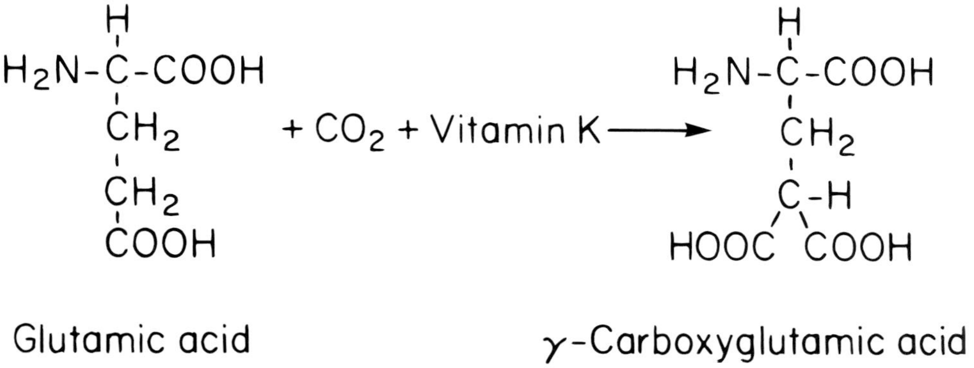

$$H_2N-\overset{\overset{\displaystyle H}{|}}{\underset{\underset{\underset{COOH}{|}}{\underset{CH_2}{|}}}{C}}-COOH \quad + CO_2 + \text{Vitamin K} \longrightarrow \quad H_2N-\overset{\overset{\displaystyle H}{|}}{\underset{\underset{\underset{HOOC \quad COOH}{}}{\underset{C-H}{|}}}{C}}-COOH$$

Glutamic acid γ-Carboxyglutamic acid

FIGURE 24-3. The vitamin K-dependent γ-carboxylation of glutamic acid. The coagulation factors in the prothrombin group must undergo this post-ribosomal carboxylation of glutamic residues in order to become functional. In factor activation, calcium binds to the carboxyl groups of the protein and to the phospholipid surface of the platelet.

receptor that is essential for binding the factor to phospholipid surfaces. Thus, in the absence of vitamin K, the factors are synthesized in the liver and can be found in plasma, but they are totally nonfunctional because they lack the COOH groups necessary for binding to phospholipid surfaces. These factors, without the COOH modification, are sometimes referred to as *PIVKA* (protein induced by vitamin K absence or antagonist). The nonfunctional and functional factor forms are identical with respect to antigenic determinants and amino acid composition.

FIBRINOGEN GROUP

The *fibrinogen group* includes factors I, V, VIII, and XIII. This group of factors also is referred to as the consumable group because they are consumed during the formation of fibrin and therefore absent from serum. Factors I, V, and XIII have molecular masses from 300,000 to 340,000 Daltons. Factor VIII is a macromolecular complex with a molecular weight of about 1,200,000 Daltons. The fibrinogen group migrates with the α or β globulins on electrophoresis.

CONTACT GROUP

The *contact group* includes Factors XI and XII as well as the plasma proteins, prekallikrein, and high molecular weight kininogens (HMWK). These factors are involved with the initial activation of the intrinsic coagulation pathway and require contact with a negatively charged surface for their activity. Except for factor XI, the contact factors do not appear to play an essential role in hemostasis in vivo.[1] This group of factors is integrally related to other biological systems, including the fibrinolytic, kinin, and complement systems. The activated forms of the contact group coagulation factors can activate these biological systems as well as the coagulation system. Factor XI and Factor XII have molecular weights of about 80,000 and 165,000, respectively, and migrate as α or β globulins on electrophoresis.

COAGULATION CASCADE

The coagulation cascade (Fig. 24-4) may be divided into three interacting pathways: the intrinsic, extrinsic, and common pathways. Each pathway includes reactions between a specific group of coagulation factors as indicated in Figure 24-5.

The activation of factor X, the first factor in the common pathway, may be accomplished by two separate pathways: the intrinsic and the extrinsic pathways. Factor X activation by the intrinsic and extrinsic pathways converges the cascade and is followed by a common course to thrombin and fibrin formation. Thus, the formation of Factor Xa, thrombin, and fibrin compose the common pathway.

The conceptualization of intrinsic, extrinsic, and common pathways has evolved from reactions occurring in vitro in test tubes and has contributed to our understanding of coagulation in vivo. It is important to realize that the pathways are not mutually exclusive of one another. Enzymes from one pathway may activate substrates in another. Additionally, some enzymes in the cascade are important as positive feedback activators, that is, they activate substrates that are necessary for their own production. These cross-reactions between intrinsic, extrinsic, and common pathways and feedback activation are important in amplifying the coagulation cascade to form adequate amounts of fibrin. Figure 24-6 shows the cross-reactions and feedback activation. The diagram of the cascade (Fig. 24-4) shows the primary physiologic reactions. Other reactions that may be physiologically important will be discussed in the text.

Overview of the coagulation cascade reactions

Blood coagulation occurs on cell-surface phospholipid membranes provided by subendothelial tissue that is exposed when the vessel endothelium is injured and by activated platelets. Clotting factors bind to the phospholipid

The Coagulation Cascade

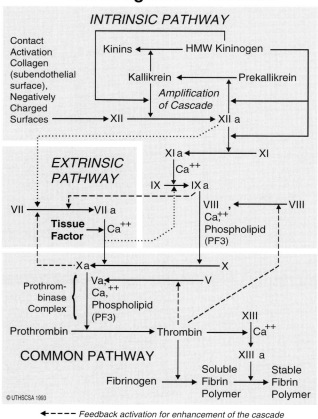

FIGURE 24-4. The coagulation cascade may be divided into three pathways: intrinsic, extrinsic, and common. The intrinsic pathway is physiologically activated by the binding of factor XII to collagen. The extrinsic system is activated by the release of tissue thromboplastin (tissue factor, TF) into the blood. The extrinsic pathway complex of factor VIIa/TF can also activate factor IX from the intrinsic pathway. Activated factors from both the extrinsic and intrinsic pathways activate factor X from the common pathway. Factor Xa and IXa feedback to activate factor VII. Thrombin also provides feedback activation to factor VIII and factor V to amplify the cascade.

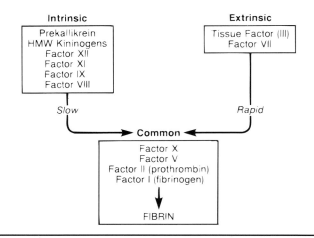

FIGURE 24-5. Coagulation factors in the intrinsic, extrinsic, and common pathways.

membrane surface and rearrange until a complex of enzyme, substrate, and cofactor is formed.[2] The membrane serves to decrease the Km of the reaction between enzyme and substrate and localizes the reaction to the site of injury.[3] Platelets must be activated to participate in coagulation. Platelets activated by collagen or thrombin undergo a transbilayer lipid movement that moves the procoagulant phosphatidylserine from the inside to the outside of the cell. These activated platelets also express receptors for factor VIIIa and Va.

The two ways to initiate blood coagulation are exposure of blood to a negatively charged surface such as collagen or to *tissue factor* (TF), an integral membrane protein of extravascular plasma membranes. Blood is exposed to both negatively charged surfaces and TF when the blood

vessel endothelium is interrupted and subendothelial tissue is exposed. Negatively charged surfaces initiate coagulation through activation of the contact factors in the intrinsic pathway and TF provides the receptor for factor VII, initiating activation of the extrinsic pathway.

Three enzyme complexes must form on the cell membrane for blood coagulation to occur: the factor VIIa/TF complex; factor IXa/factor VIIIa, Ca^{++} platelet phospholipid (platelet factor 3, PF3) complex; factor Xa/factor Va, Ca^{++}, PF3 complex.[4]

In vivo hemostasis is initiated at the wound site through the extrinsic pathway by exposure of blood to TF from the subendothelial tissue.[5] The integral membrane protein, TF, is tightly associated with membrane phospholipid. If stimulated, the endothelial cells can increase production of TF by 10- to 40-fold.[6] Agonists also can stimulate TF expression on monocytes, macrophages, and endothelial cells. The location of TF on extravascular plasma membranes permits initiation and localization of coagulation to the site of injury. The extracellular domain of TF is the receptor for factor VII.

Factor VII in the blood binds to TF generating the complex, factor VIIa/TF, which then activates factor X from the common pathway. Factor VIIa/TF also activates Factor IX from the intrinsic pathway. Factor IXa forms a complex with factor VIII, PF3 and Ca++ to activate additional factor X. Both factor IXa and Xa activate factor VII in positive feedback reactions.[7–9]

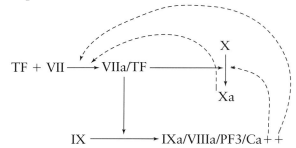

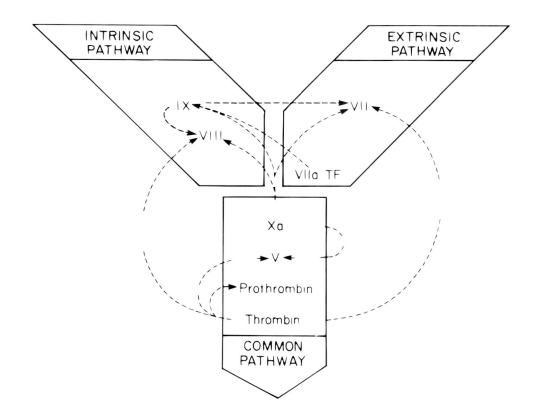

FIGURE 24-6. Although the coagulation cascade is usually illustrated as a one-way series of reactions, positive feedback from activated factors serve to accelerate and enhance the cascade. Activated factor X and thrombin play key roles in this feedback. In addition, activated factor IX from the intrinsic pathway can activate factor VII from the extrinsic pathway and factor VIIa-TF can, in turn, activate factor IX. This reciprocal activation process links the intrinsic and extrinsic pathways. (From: Lee, G.R., et al: Wintrobe's Clinical Hematology. Philadelphia: Lea & Febiger, 1993.)

Evidence indicates that initial activation of factor X is through the extrinsic pathway (VIIa/TF), but sustained and amplified coagulation is primarily via the intrinsic system (Factor IXa/VIIIa, Ca + +, PF3 activation).

Since the factor VIIa/TF complex from the extrinsic pathway can activate the intrinsic pathway via factor IX, contact factor activation of the intrinsic pathway may be an ancillary mode of activating factor IX. This is supported clinically by the observation that individuals deficient in the contact factors do not bleed. On the other hand, hemophiliacs (deficiency of factor VIII or IX) who cannot form the factor IXa, VIIIa, Ca + +, PF3 complex have severe bleeding problems attesting to the importance of these factors in normal hemostasis.

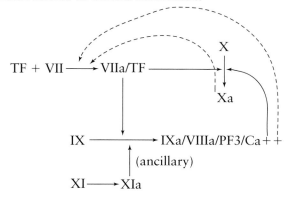

The factor Xa/Va, PF3, Ca + + complex proteolytically cleaves factor II (prothrombin) to form thrombin. Thrombin cleaves fibrinogen to form fibrin.

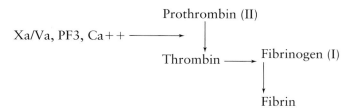

Thrombin is the central regulatory molecule in hemostasis. It serves as a positive feedback molecule by activating cofactors VIII and V and platelets; it serves as a negative feedback molecule by activating the thrombin inhibitor, Protein C.

The next sections will detail the reactions of the intrinsic, extrinsic, and common pathways. The functions and characteristics of the coagulation factors included in each pathway will be discussed.

●
Intrinsic pathway

The components of the intrinsic pathway are all contained within the blood stream, hence the name "intrinsic." The intrinsic pathway clotting factors include factors XII, XI, IX, VIII, high molecular weight kininogen (HMWK), and prekallikrein.

As stated previously, factor X may be activated by either the intrinsic or extrinsic pathway. Although initial activation of factor X is through factor VIIa/TF from the extrinsic pathway, the principal mechanism of continued, more efficient factor X activation is by the factor IXa/VIIIa, Ca + +, PF3 complex from the intrinsic pathway.[8,9]

Activation of Factor IX by the TF/VIIa complex is complemented and enhanced by factor XIa. Factor XIa may be activated by factor XIIa and cofactor HMWK.

CONTACT FACTORS

The intrinsic pathway is initiated by exposure of the contact factors to vessel structures beneath the endothelium (collagen, basement membrane). The four contact factors include the zymogens factor XII, factor XI, prekallikrein, and a cofactor, high molecular weight kininogen (HMWK). As subendothelial tissue surfaces with a net negative charge are exposed, the contact factors bind to them. Calcium ions are not required for this binding. The contact factors also may be adsorbed in vitro by negatively charged surfaces such as glass, kaolin, celite, and ellagic acid. Pathologically, the lipopolysaccharides of bacteria may serve as the site for adsorption of the contact factors. Adsorption of the contact factors to vessel substructure initiates the interaction and activation of the contact system.

Since patients deficient in the contact factors, factor XII, prekallikrien, and HMWK, do not bleed abnormally, it is unlikely that these factors play a significant role in in vivo hemostasis. On the other hand, at least 50% of patients with factor XI deficiency have bleeding abnormalities. This suggests factor XI may be an important accessory to blood coagulation but it is probably not essential.[8,9] The reactions of the contact phase are mutually reinforcing.

Factor XII and prekallikren The first factors adsorbed to the injured vessel are factor XII and prekallikrein. These two proteins are involved in reciprocal activation of each other using HMWK as a cofactor.

$$XII \longrightarrow XIIa$$
$$HMWK \Big| \qquad \Big\backslash HMWK$$
$$kallikrein \longleftarrow prekallikrein$$

Binding of factor XII to the exposed subendothelial surface of the vessel appears to be dependent on interaction of postively charged groups on factor XII with the negative charge of the vessel subendothelial surface. This binding results in a conformational change (but not cleaving) of the factor XII molecule that partially exposes its enzymatically active site. Surface bound factor XII then proteolytically cleaves prekallikrein to the protease kallikrein. Prekallikrein circulates as a complex with HMWK and binds to the same surface as factor XII. Kallikrein with HMWK as a cofactor will then, by a reciprocal reaction, proteolytically cleave surface bound factor XII to XIIa (Fig. 24-7). This generation of factor XIIa and kallikrein by reciprocal activation serves to amplify the initial reactions. Factor XIIa can be further cleaved by kallikrein, plasmin, and trypsin, yielding smaller factor XII fragments. These smaller fragments apparently increase the activation of prekallikrein to kallikrein but decrease the procoagulant activity of factor XII.

There may be another undetermined factor, in addition to kallikrein, that can activate surface bound factor XII. This possibility is suggested by the laboratory findings in those individuals with hereditary deficiencies of prekallikrein. Prekallikrein deficient plasma gives a prolonged activated partial thromboplastin time, but the test becomes normal if the plasma is exposed to clot promoting surfaces such as kaolin, for prolonged periods before the addition of calcium. Thus, factor XII is probably cleaved to factor XIIa by an alternate proteolytic enzyme(s). Prekallikrein deficiency does not result in abnormal bleeding.

In addition to activating prekallikrein to kallikrein, factor XIIa has at least two other enzymatic functions: it converts factor XI to its active form, XIa, in the presence of cofactor HMWK, and it activates the fibrinolytic system by its interaction with a plasminogen proactivator, probably kallikrein (generating plasmin from plasminogen). Thus, the products generated by factor XIIa include: kallikrein, factor XIa, and plasmin. It appears that factor

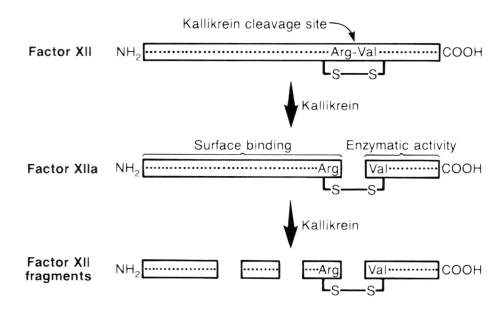

FIGURE 24-7. Factor XII, a single polypeptide chain, is cleaved by kallikrein into a two chain disulfide bonded molecule. This enzymatically active form can be further cleaved by kallikrein into factor XII fragments. The conversion of factor XIIa to fragments enhances its prekallikrein to kallikrein activity but decreases its procoagulant activity. Factor XII adsorbed to collagen undergoes a conformational change exposing its enzymatically active site but is not cleaved until acted upon by kallikrein. (From Schiffman, S.: Factor XII. In: CRC Handbook series in Clinical Factor Science. Edited by D. Seligson. Section I: Hematology Vol. III. Edited by R.M. Schmidt, Boca Raton: CRC Press, Inc. 1980.)

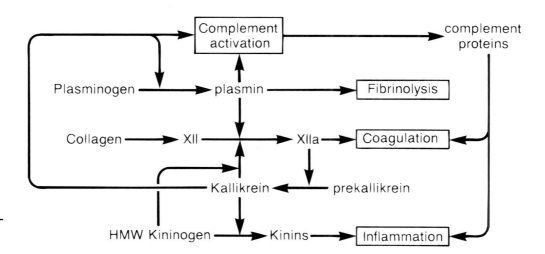

FIGURE 24-8. Role of contact factors in physiologic systems.

XIIa also activates factor VII, the first component of the extrinsic pathway, providing another link between the intrinsic and extrinsic systems.

Kallikrein may be released from its surface binding site, enter the plasma, and activate three other biologic systems, the kinin system, the fibrinolytic system, and the complement system. Kallikrein cleaves HMWK into smaller biologically active fragments called kinins. Kallikrein activates plasminogen to plasmin, a potent proteolytic enzyme that degrades fibrin, and plasmin, in turn, can activate the first and third components of the complement cascade (Fig. 24-8). Kallikrein also serves as a chemotactant for neutrophils and monocytes.

High molecular weight kininogen High molecular weight kininogen serves as a cofactor in activation of contact factors.

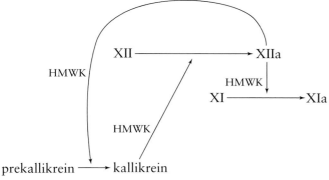

There are two forms of kininogen in plasma: a high molecular weight kininogen (HMWK) and a low molecular weight kininogen (LMWK). HMWK circulates in plasma in 1:1 noncovalently bonded complexes with both factor XI and prekallikrein. It appears that HMWK serves to localize these two substrates for interaction with factor XIIa by bringing them into close contact and optimal position at the site of vessel injury.

HMWK, the preferred substrate for kallikrein, is a single chain glycoprotein that can be cleaved by kallikrein into a two-chain disulphide bonded molecule with the re-

lease of a small fragment, bradykinin. The released kinin causes contraction of smooth muscles, increased vascular permeability, increased secretion from mucous glands, and pain. The larger two chain molecule of cleaved HMWK acts as a regulatory cofactor, similar to factor V and factor VIII, accelerating the conversion of factor XII to XIIa, prekallikrein to kallikrein, and factor XI to XIa.

Factor XI Factor XI is composed of two identical polypeptide chains joined by disulfide bonds. It circulates as a complex with HMWK. It is activated to a serine protease by factor XIIa and cofactor HMWK (Fig. 24-9).

$$XI \xrightarrow{\text{XIIa, HMWK}} XIa$$

Although patients with deficiencies of other contact factors (factor XII, prekallikrein, and HMWK) do not have bleeding problems, about 50% of patients with a factor XI deficiency have bleeding problems after surgery or injury. Whether bleeding occurs is not determined exclusively by factor XI levels since levels are similar in those who experience bleeding and those who do not.

It has been determined that both thrombin and factor XIa can activate factor XI in a positive feedback reaction.[1,10] The substrate for factor XIa is factor IX.

OTHER FACTORS IN THE INTRINSIC PATHWAY
Activation of the contact factors is followed by activation of factor IX, which forms a complex with factor VIII to activate factor X in the common pathway.

Factor IX Factor IX is a single polypeptide chain that is activated by factor XIa in the presence of Ca++ (Fig. 24-10).

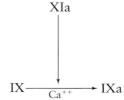

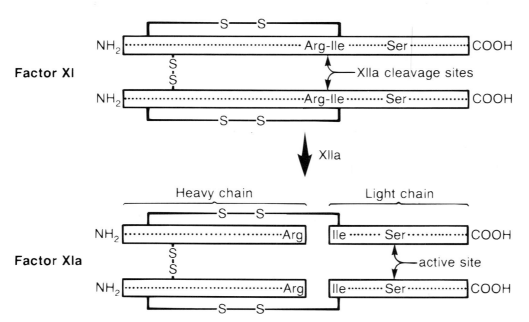

FIGURE 24-9. Factor XI activation: Factor XI contains two identical disulfide bonded chains. Activation by factor XIIa occurs by cleavage of each chain into two disulfide bonded fragments. The smaller fragments contain the active enzyme sites. (From Griffin, J.H., Bouma, B.N.: Blood coagulation Factor XI. In: CRC Handbook series in Clinical Laboratory Science. Edited by D. Seligson. Section I: Hematology Vol. III. Edited by R.M. Schmidt, Boca Raton: CRC Press, Inc. 1980.)

This is the first reaction in the intrinsic pathway that requires Ca++. Calcium is required to bind factor IX to a phospholipid surface but does not affect the activity of the activating protease, factor XIa.

After activation, factor IXa forms a complex with the cofactor, factor VIII, and Ca++ on the platelet phospholipid surface to activate factor X (Fig. 24-11).

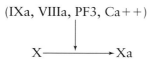

The extrinsic pathway complex, VIIa/TF, also can activate factor IX. This extrinsic pathway for factor IX activa-

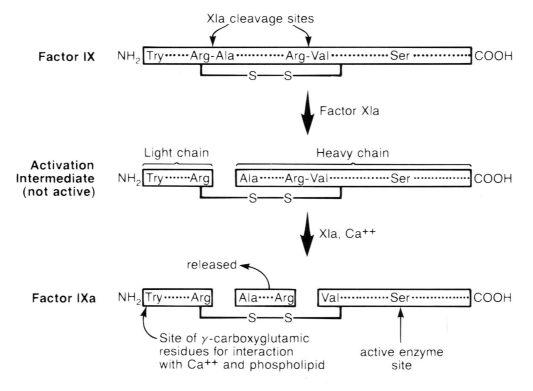

FIGURE 24-10. Factor IX is a single polypeptide chain. Activation occurs in a two step process. The first step involves a cleavage of the chain into a disulfide bonded light and heavy chain. The second step cleaves and releases an activation peptide. Apparently the intermediate form (IXα) has no enzymatic activity but may be the rate limiting step in factor IX activation. (From Malar, R.A.: Factor IX: Activation and Function. In: Prothrombin and Other Vitamin K Proteins. Vol I. Edited by W.H. Seegers, D.A. Walsy. Boca Raton: CRC Press, Inc. 1986.)

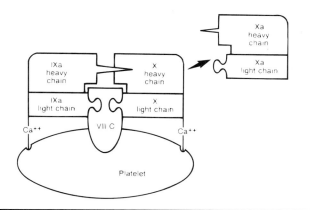

FIGURE 24-11. The complex formed by the sequential activation of the intrinsic pathway (factors IXa, VIII, Ca + +) activates factor X. The cofactor, factor VIII C, binds to the platelet phospholipids (PF3) and serves to orient factors IXa and X to enhance activation of factor X. Factors IX and X are bound to the platelet via Ca + + bridges.

tion bypasses the contact activation system and is another link between the intrinsic and extrinsic systems.

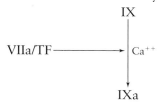

You will recall that the factor VIIa/TF complex also activates factor X.

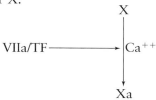

Evidence indicates that when both factor IX and factor X are presented together as substrates for VIIa/TF, the preferred substrate is factor IX. This occurs because factor Xa assists in the activation of factor IX by converting factor IX to the inactive intermediate form, factor IXα, a good substrate for VIIa/TF. The factor IXα is then rapidly cleaved to the activated form, IXβ (IXa), by the factor VIIa/TF complex.[8]

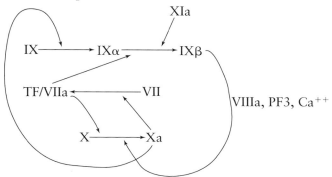

The activation of factor X by the factor IXa/VIIIa, PF3, Ca + + complex is accelerated 50-fold over activation of factor X by VIIa/TF.[8] Thus, factor IXa/VIIIa amplifies generation of factor Xa. The factor IXa/VIIIa complex is probably necessary for providing adequate quantities of factor Xa for in vivo hemostasis. This helps explain why patients deficient in factors IX and VIII bleed abnormally.

Although activation of the contact factors takes place on the subendothelial surface of the vessel, the activation of factor IX and subsequent cascade reactions take place on the phospholipid surface of the platelets in the primary hemostatic plug.

Factor VIII Factor VIII is composed of two distinct, noncovalently bonded subunits: factor VIII with procoagulant activity (VIII:C) and the portion that carries the von Willebrand factor activity (VIII:vWf). Each portion has distinct functions, biologic and immunologic properties. The coagulant portion is also known as the antihemophiliac factor and serves as the cofactor in factor X activation by factor IX. Its precise function in this reaction is not understood, but it is known to bind to the phospholipid platelet surface and it appears to govern the specificity between substrate (factor X) and enzyme (factor IXa). This cofactor function of factor VIII can be markedly enhanced by small amounts of thrombin. Thrombin activates factor VIII by proteolytic cleavage, which dissociates factor VIII:C from the vonWillebrand complex. This dissociation makes a factor VIII:C phospholipid binding site available. Larger amounts of thrombin, however, destroy the procoagulant function of factor VIII.

● Extrinsic pathway

Factor X also can be activated by the extrinsic pathway. The extrinsic activation involves factor VII and a cofactor, tissue factor (factor III, TF). TF also is referred to as tissue thromboplastin. The pathway gets its name "extrinsic" from the fact that this activation pathway requires a factor that does not circulate in the blood, TF. TF is an integral cell membrane protein found in subendothelial tissue.

When the subendothelium of a vessel is exposed to blood, factor VIIa forms a complex with TF and the complex binds by Ca + + bridges to the subendothelial phospholipid surface. This activation complex serves to activate surface bound factor X. As described previously, this extrinsic activation complex also is capable of activating the intrinsic pathway factor IX, thus providing a bypass of the need for contact activation of the intrinsic pathway.

$$\begin{array}{ccc}
 & & IX \\
VIIa + TF & \longrightarrow & |Ca^{++} \\
Ca^{++} & \searrow & IXa \\
 & & |VIIIa, PF3, Ca^{++} \\
X & \longrightarrow & Xa
\end{array}$$

FACTOR VII

Factor VII is a single chain glycoprotein. The chain is structurally similar to the peptide chains of other factors in the prothrombin group and requires a cofactor for activity. Factor VII has a shorter half-life (3 to 5 hours) than other vitamin K-dependent clotting factors but in its activated form is more stable than other activated factors. The activated form remains in circulation nearly as long as the zymogen.[11]

Current concepts in the conversion of factor VII to VIIa suggest that factor Xa is the principal physiologic activator. Factor VII complexed with TF, as opposed to factor VII in solution, is preferentially cleaved to VIIa by factor Xa.[11] Thrombin, factor XIIa and IXa also are capable of significantly enhancing factor VII activity. It is not known for certain if factor VII must be cleaved to become active, but it probably has some proteolytic activity in the single chain form.

FACTOR X ACTIVATION

Activation of factor X by factor VIIa requires the presence of TF. The TF does not require activation but rather serves in a cofactor capacity. Tissue factor is not normally found within the blood vessels. It is present on subvascular cells and made accessible for factor VII complex formation when the vessel endothelium is ruptured. Tissue factor is widely distributed in many tissues but is especially rich in brain, lungs, and placenta. Pathologic activation of the extrinsic pathway may occur with extensive tissue damage when large amounts of tissue factor are available for complex formation with factor VII. Blood monocytes and endothelial cells, which are in contact with plasma, can be stimulated to produce TF by endotoxin, complement component 5a, immune complexes, interleukin-1, or tumor necrosis factor.[11] The bilipid erythrocyte membranes are very rich in the protein-phospholipid complex. Thus, intravascular hemolysis exposes circulating coagulation factors to tissue factor and also may precipitate coagulation.

Tissue factor pathway inhibitor (TFPI) can alter the function of factor VIIa-TF complex and impede factor X activation via the extrinsic pathway.[12] TFPI binds to factor Xa, which then binds to factor VIIa/TF complex and prevents further factor X activation via VIIa/TF. This negative feedback of factor X activation is discussed under the next section of biochemical inhibitors.

● Common pathway

The common pathway includes three reactions each representing a key rate limiting step in the cascade:

(1) the activation of factor X by the products of the intrinsic and extrinsic pathways:

Intrinsic: IXa, VIIIa, PF3, Ca++

$$X \longrightarrow Xa$$

Extrinsic: VIIa, TF, Ca++

(2) conversion of prothrombin to thrombin by activated factor X:

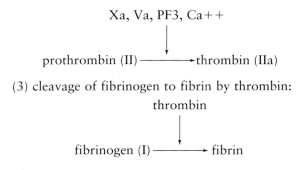

Xa, Va, PF3, Ca++

prothrombin (II) $\longrightarrow$ thrombin (IIa)

(3) cleavage of fibrinogen to fibrin by thrombin:

thrombin

fibrinogen (I) $\longrightarrow$ fibrin

FACTOR X

Factor X is a double chain glycoprotein held together by disulfide bonds. It can be activated in two ways: by the complex derived from the intrinsic pathway, factor IXa, factor VIIIa, Ca++; or by the complex derived from the extrinsic pathway, factor VIIa, TF, and Ca++ (Fig. 24-12). The activation of factor X takes place only if the factor has been bound to a phospholipid surface via a calcium bridge.

Factor Xa forms a complex with cofactor factor V, phospholipid, and Ca++ for optimal activation of prothrombin (Fig. 24-13). This complex is the first activation complex in the common pathway. The factor Xa, factor Va Ca++, and phospholipid complex is sometimes referred to as the *prothrombinase complex* and is remarkably similar to the factor IXa, factor VIIIa, Ca++, and phospholipid complex. In both complexes, the activity of cofactors, factors VIII and V, are markedly enhanced by thrombin, and the enzymatic portions of the complexes, factors IXa and Xa, are similar in structure being a part of the prothrombin group.

Russell's viper venom, obtained from the East Indian viper, contains a protease similar to factor VIIa that can selectively and directly activate factor X. Although now replaced by other laboratory assays, this venom was used in the laboratory to perform the Stypven time test. This test was used primarily to differentiate factor VII deficiency from factor X deficiency.

FACTOR V

Factor V is a single chain glycoprotein. Platelet granules contain about 25% of the factor V found in the blood. The cofactor activity of factor V is increased 13,000 times by thrombin. Since factor Va is needed for initial formation of thrombin, small amounts of factor V zyymogen may be activated by a proactivator other than thrombin or factor V may have some activity as a zymogen. The exact mechanism of the factor V enhancement of thrombin formation is unknown, but it is probably important in the formation of the substrate-enzyme complex by serving as a receptor on platelets for both factor Xa and prothrombin (Fig. 24-13).

PROTHROMBIN (FACTOR II)

Prothrombin is a single chain glycoprotein. As with the other vitamin K dependent proteins, the γ-carboxyglutamic acid residues at the amino end of the molecule are

Factor X Activation

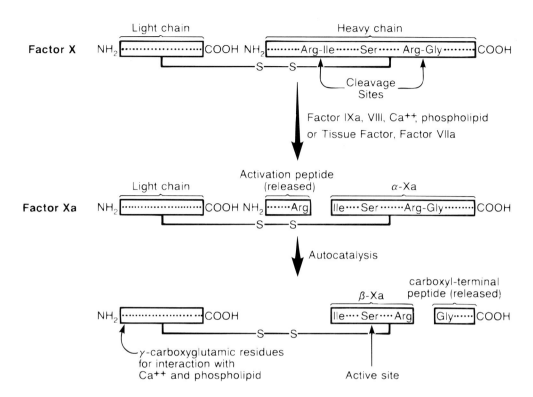

FIGURE 24-12. Factor X is composed of two polypeptide chains linked by a disulfide bond. The heavy chain contains the enzymatic site and the light chain contains the γ-carboxyglutamic acid residues that are responsible for binding the factor to phospholipid via Ca + +. This schematic diagram shows the widely studied pathways of bovine factor X activation. The first cleavage of the heavy chain releases an activation peptide and gives rise to the α-form of the enzyme. In the presence of phospholipid a second autocatalytic cleavage occurs forming the β-form of the enzyme. The two forms appear to have identical procoagulant activity. (From Marciniak, E.: Factor X: Activation and molecular forms. In: Prothrombin and Other Vitamin K Proteins. Vol. I. Edited by W.H. Seegers, D.A. Walz, Boca Raton: CRC Press, 1986.)

responsible for the interaction of prothrombin with phospholipid surfaces via calcium bridges. The molecule may be divided into two structural parts, the "pro" portion (fragment 1.2) and the thrombin portion, also called prethrombin 2. Fragment 1.2 is responsible for binding the prothrombin molecule to phospholipid via calcium and for its interaction with factor Va. Factor Xa cleaves the prothrombin molecule between the fragment 1.2 and prethrombin portions releasing fragment 1.2 and the potent enzyme portion, thrombin (Fig. 24-14). Thrombin then cleaves the substrate fibrinogen to form fibrin.

Elevated levels of fragment 1.2 are associated with a thrombotic tendency and may be a useful marker for identifying those at risk of thrombosis. A laboratory test for fragment 1.2 is now available for clinical use.

FIBRINOGEN (FACTOR I)

Fibrinogen is an elongated trinodular molecule with two identical halves (Fig. 24-15). Each half is composed of three pairs of chains Aα, Bβ, and γ, held together by three disulfide bonds, one between the α-chains and two between the γ chains. The letters A and B prefixing the α- and β-chains designate fibrinopeptides that are cleaved by thrombin in the formation of fibrin. Thus, fibrin includes α, β, and γ chains (minus the A and B peptides).

The two halves of fibrinogen are joined at the amino terminal ends of the Aα, Bβ, and γ chains, forming a central nodule called the central domain or *E domain*. The carboxy terminals of the β and γ chains plus a short se-

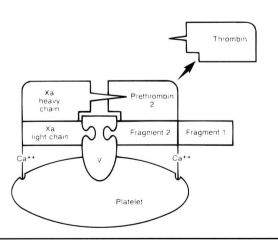

FIGURE 24-13. The prothrombinase complex (factors Xa, Va, Ca + +, PF3) activates prothrombin to thrombin. Factor V binds to the platelet phospholipid surface (PF3) and serves to orient factor Xa and prothrombin to enhance the formation of thrombin. Factor X and prothrombin are bound to the platelet surface via Ca + + bridges. This complex is very similar to the complex formed by the intrinsic pathway (factors IXa, VIIIa, Ca + +, PF3).

Prothrombin Conversion to Thrombin

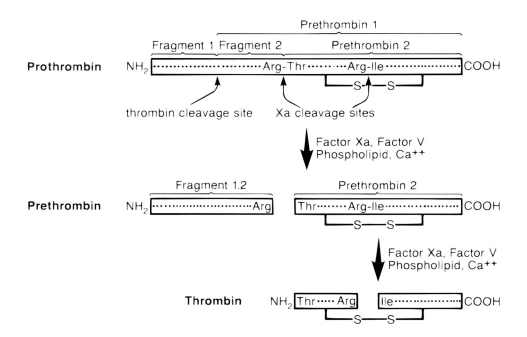

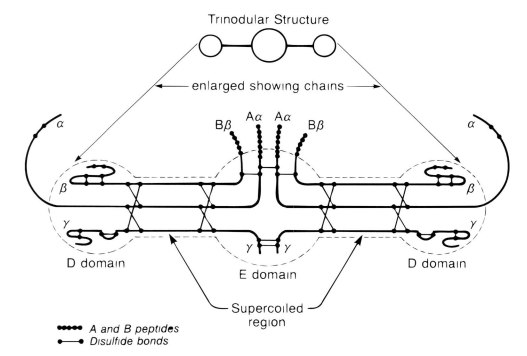

FIGURE 24-14. The prothrombin molecule is a single chain glycoprotein that can be divided into the "pro" portion (fragment 1 and fragment 2 or fragment 1.2) and the thrombin portion (prethrombin 2). Factor Xa proteolytically cleaves the molecule between the pro and prethrombin portions releasing fragment 1.2 and prethrombin. Prethrombin is further cleaved into two disulfide bonded chains forming the potent enzyme thrombin.

Fibrinogen Structure

FIGURE 24-15. Fibrinogen is a trinodular structure composed of three pairs (Aα, Bβ, γ) of disulfide bonded polypeptide chains. The central nodule is known as the E domain. Thrombin cleaves small peptides, A and B, from the α and β chains in this region to form fibrin. The central nodule is joined by supercoiled α-helices to the terminal nodules also known as the D domains.

quence of the α chain form the two terminal nodules, one on each end of the molecule. These terminal nodules are also referred to as the terminal domains or *D domains*. The three nodules are joined by elongated supercoiled α-helices. The Aα-chain has a long polar appendage at the carboxy terminal end. This exposed portion of the molecule is readily cleaved by proteolytic enzymes. In fact, this appendage is the first part of the molecule cleaved by plasmin digestion.

The insoluble fibrin clot is formed from fibrinogen in three distinct steps:

1. hydrolytic cleavage of arginine-glycine bonds by thrombin releasing A and B fibrinopeptides from the α and β chains, forming fibrin monomer.

2. spontaneous formation of fibrin polymers from fibrin monomers.

3. stabilization of the fibrin polymers by factor XIIIa.

Thrombin proteolytically cleaves the A and B fibrinopeptides from the α- and β-chains of fibrinogen. The resulting structure is very similar to that of fibrinogen with a decrease in molecular weight of only 3%. This thrombin cleaved molecule is referred to as *fibrin monomer.*

With thrombin cleavage, the negative charges around the central domain that normally cause the individual fibrinogen molecules to repulse each other are eliminated. As a result, the net charge of the central domain changes from a negative eight to a positive five. The terminal domains, however, retain their net negative charges.

These changes in electrostatic forces may play a role in the second step in fibrin formation, fibrin polymerization. Each nodule of the trinodular structure contains a polymerization site, which permits the longitudinal and lateral growth of fibrin polymers into a fibrin clot. The negatively charged terminal domain of one monomer spontaneously assembles with the positively charged central domain of another monomer molecule giving a polymer structure (Fig. 24-16).

Although these charge attractions are sufficient to account for polymerization, there also are structural features of complementary knobs and holes in the nodules that contribute to the linkage between monomers. These polymerization sites are initially bonded by hydrogen bonds that are readily dissociated (solubilized) by 5 M urea or monochloroacetic acid.

FACTOR XIII

The final reaction in fibrin formation is the stabilization of the fibrin polymer catalyzed by factor XIII. Factor XIII is activated by thrombin cleavage. Factor XIIIa is a calcium-dependent transamidase that is responsible for catalyzing the formation of covalent bonds between glutamine and lysine residues of the *fibrin polymer.* These bonds are formed between the terminal domains of γ-chains and between polar appendages of α-chains of neighboring monomers.

The expression of factor XIIIa activity requires its interaction with calcium ions. Calcium binds to the catalytic subunit (A2) of factor XIII causing a conformational change that exposes its active center.

The covalently cross-linked fibrin network produces a

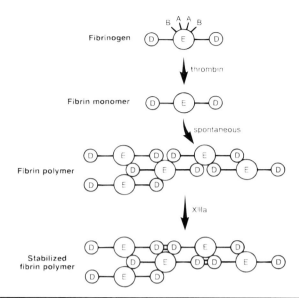

Formation of Fibrin Polymer

FIGURE 24-16. Thrombin cleaves the A and B peptides from the E domain of fibrinogen to form fibrin monomer. The cleavage apparently changes the negative charge of the domain to a positive charge. This permits the spontaneous growth of fibrin polymers as the positively charged E domain assembles with the negatively charged D domains of other fibrin monomers. The polymer is initially joined by hydrogen bonds. Factor XIIIa in the presence of Ca + + is responsible for catalyzing the formation of covalent bonds between glutamine and lysine residues of adjacent monomers, thus stabilizing the lattice formation.

fibrin clot with increased mechanical strength and increased resistance to proteolytic digestion by plasmin. The presence of these unique bonds is responsible for the liberation of specific fibrin degradation products when plasmin digests the clot. In contrast to the hydrogen bonded monomers, the factor XIIIa-stabilized fibrin polymer is not soluble in 5M urea or monochloroacetic acid.

Factor XIII is found evenly distributed between plasma and platelets. There is strong evidence that plasma factor XIII is synthesized in the liver. Platelet factor XIII is synthesized by the megakaryocyte and is present in the soluble nongranular fraction of the platelet. In plasma, factor XIII is composed of two nonidentical polypeptide chains, A and B, that are joined by noncovalent bonds in a tetrameric structure, A_2B_2. In the platelet, only the A chains are present in a dimeric form. The catalytic activity of the protein resides in the A chains. Factor XIII is trapped in the fibrin clot during clot formation or is provided by the platelets. The zymogen is activated by thrombin and calcium in a proteolytic cleavage of the A chains. The B chains dissociate in the activation process.

Factor XIIIa also is responsible for the cross-linking of another protein, fibronectin, to the α-chain of fibrin and to collagen. Fibronectin, a cold insoluble protein synthesized by endothelial cells, is found in plasma, in the granules of platelets, and is associated with cell surfaces. It has a number of interactions and roles, including the adherence of cells to surfaces. Thus, it may be important in promoting the adherence of the fibrin clot to the cell surface of the vessel structure. It also may be involved in wound healing and tissue repair by supporting new cell growth.

AMPLIFICATION OF THE CASCADE

The sequential activation of coagulation factors in a cascade-like fashion together with positive feedback activation by some of the activation products including kallikrein (activating factor XII), thrombin (activating cofactors V and VIII), and factor Xa (activating factors IX and VII) as well as enhancement of enzyme activity by cofactors, leads to a multifold amplification of the coagulation system. Evidence for the occurrence of amplification includes the difference in normal plasma between concentrations of factors involved in the early phases of activation and those involved in latter phases of the cascade (concentration gradient).[2] The plasma concentration of factors involved in the early reactions of the intrinsic system are much lower than that of the final substrate, fibrinogen. It has been estimated that on the basis of this mass difference alone, the amplication from contact activation to clot formation is about 500-fold.[13] The actual amplication, however, is more probably near 1,000,000-fold.

This amplification process necessitates that coagulation be confined to the site of injury and regulated to the formation of a fibrin clot just large enough to control bleeding. Without some form of regulation, the coagulation process could disseminate throughout the body. These regulatory mechanisms will be discussed in the next section.

PHYSIOLOGIC CONTROL OF HEMOSTASIS

The dynamic process of fibrin generation by activated clotting factors is normally limited to the site of vascular injury. Even with intense stimulation of coagulation, such as occurs in massive trauma, circulation remains fluid in uninvolved vessels. The physiologic mechanisms that are responsible for controlling coagulation include: blood flow, liver clearance of activated factors, feedback inhibition, biochemical inhibitors (naturally occurring anticoagulants), and fibrinolytic dissolution of fibrin.

Blood flow

Clots do not form in a vessel unless two events occur: vasoconstriction and activation of clotting factors. Initially, clot formation is enhanced by vessel constriction that temporarily slows the blood flow through the injured vessel. The constriction serves to force platelets and coagulation factors into contact with the injured vessel. This promotes activation of both primary and secondary hemostasis. Return of the normal flow of blood through the area of injury serves to limit coagulation by continually

diluting the area of activated factors and washing them away. Although stasis promotes the formation of clots, it alone will not produce thrombosis. Likewise, serine proteases (activated coagulation factors) will not promote clot formation if blood continues to flow freely. This is why initial vasoconstriction to slow down the blood flow at the site of injury is important for adequate fibrin formation.

Liver clearance

As the blood brings the activated coagulation factors to the liver, they are selectively removed by the hepatocytes. Plasmin from the fibrinolytic system and degraded fibrin complexes also are removed by the liver. Liver disease can lead to either systemic fibrinolysis or thrombosis, thus attesting to the importance of this organ in control of coagulation.

Feedback inhibition

Some of the activated factors have the potential to destroy other factors in the coagulation cascade. Thrombin has the ability to temporarily activate factors V and VIII, but as the concentration of thrombin increases, these factors undergo proteolytic destruction by the same enzyme. Factor Xa first enhances the activity of factor VII and then, through reaction with tissue factor pathway inhibitor, prevents further activation of factor X by the factor VIIa/TF complexes. By this process of feedback inhibition, these enzymes limit their own production. Clotting also is controlled indirectly by the end product, fibrin. Fibrin has a strong affinity for thrombin. Once adsorbed onto the fibrin complex, thrombin is very slowly released, limiting the amount of thrombin available to cleave additional fibrinogen to fibrin, a process that could be interpreted as an antithrombin mechanism. In addition, fibrin degradation products produced by plasmin digestion function as inhibitors of fibrin formation by interfering with the conversion of fibrinogen to fibrin and the polymerization of fibrin monomers.

Biochemical inhibitors

The biochemical inhibitors are soluble plasma proteins that regulate the enzymatic reactions of serine proteases, preventing the initiation or amplication of the clotting cascade (Table 24-7) (Fig. 24-17). These protease inhibitors include: (1) antithrombin III; (2) heparin cofactor II; (3) tissue factor pathway inhibitor; (4) protein C; (5) protein S; (3) α_2-macroglobulin; (4) α_1-antitrypsin; and (5) C1 inactivator.

In addition to these natural inhibitors, individuals sometimes develop antibodies that are capable of neutralizing the procoagulant properties of specific coagulation factors. These acquired inhibitors may cause bleeding or may be found in asymptomatic individuals. The antibodies usually occur after transfusion or treatment with factor replacement for coagulation factor deficiencies.

TABLE 24-7 *EFFECTS OF PHYSIOLOGIC INHIBITORS ON COAGULATION PROTEASES*

Factor	ATIII	Heparin Cofactor II	TFPI	Proteins C and S	alpha2-macroglobulin	alpha1-antitrypsin	C1 Inactivator	alpha2-antiplasmin	PAI
XIIa	+	−	−	−	−	−	+	+	−
XIa	+	−	−	−	−	+	+	+	−
IXa	+	−	−	−	−	−	−	−	−
Xa	+	−	+	−	−	−	−	+	−
VIII	−	−	−	+	−	−	−	−	−
V	−	−	−	+	−	−	−	−	−
VII	−	−	+*	−	−	−	−	−	−
Thrombin	+	+	−	−	+	+	−	+	−
Kallikrein	+	−	−	−	+	+	+	+	−
Plasmin	+	−	+	−	+	+	+	+	−
t-PA	+	−	−	−	+	+	−	+	+

* inhibits when complexed with TF; TFPI: tissue factor pathway inhibitor; t-PA: tissue plasminogen activator; PAI: plasminogen activator inhibitor; +, inhibition; −, no inhibition.

They also may occur spontaneously. These acquired inhibitors will be discussed in Chapter 26.

ANTITHROMBIN III

Antithrombin III, ATIII (recently renamed as antithrombin, AT), is a single chain glycoprotein with a molecular weight of 56,000 Daltons, produced in the liver, endothelial cells, and possibly the megakaryocytes. It is by far the most important inhibitor of coagulation. Antithrombin III is an antiserine protease that serves to inactivate all serine proteases in the coagulation cascade (XIIa, XIa, IXa, Xa, and IIa as well as plasmin and kallikrien) (Fig. 24-17). Its most significant function is inhibition of thrombin (IIa). Since thrombin plays a major role in coagulation, its inhibition provides a significant regulation of clot formation.

The ATIII molecule forms a 1:1 stoichiometric complex with thrombin. An arginine residue in ATIII interacts with the active serine residue of thrombin. This binding between inhibitor and enzyme causes a loss of thrombin's enzymatic activity.

Factor VIIa is relatively resistant to inactivation by ATIII. Perhaps the interaction of Factor VIIa with tissue factor protects this protease from forming complexes with ATIII.

Heparin, a glycosaminoglycan found endogenously in mast cells and many organ systems, and other heparin-like molecules appear to interact with ATIII (heparin cofactor) in the inhibition of coagulation. Heparin binds to ATIII and causes a conformational change. This change makes the reactive arginine site in ATIII more accessible to the serine site of thrombin, enhancing the rate of thrombin/ATIII complex formation by a factor of 1000 times[14] (Fig. 24-18). After interaction of the enzyme and ATIII, the heparin detaches from the complex and is free to cycle again. Inhibition of thrombin not only prevents formation of fibrin from fibrinogen but also inhibits activation of factor VIII and factor V by thrombin.

Decreased levels of ATIII may be hereditary or acquired and are associated with venous thrombosis. Hereditary ATIII deficiency is found in 2% to 3% of individuals with venous thromboembolisms. Acquired deficiencies of ATIII have been associated with oral contraceptives, surgery, septicemia, and liver disease. When the ATIII level is less than 60% of normal, patients are unresponsive to antithrombotic therapy with heparin.

HEPARIN COFACTOR II

Heparin cofactor II, a second anticoagulant protein with heparin cofactor activity, is a single chain glycoprotein with a molecular weight of 65,000. This anticoagulant inhibits thrombin but is inactive with other coagulation or fibrinolytic proteases.[15] Because the affinity of heparin cofactor II for heparin is less than that of ATIII, a higher concentration of heparin is necessary to accelerate thrombin inhibition by this cofactor. It has been suggested that heparin cofactor II may function as a second-line inhibitor of thrombin.

TISSUE FACTOR PATHWAY INHIBITOR (TFPI)

This inhibitor has only recently been identified and characterized. It was formerly known as extrinsic pathway inhibitor (EPI), lipoprotein-associated coagulation inhibitor (LACI), and anti-convertin. It is a Kunitz-type serine protease inhibitor. Kunitz-type inhibitors appear to act by feigning to be a good substrate for the enzyme, but, once it binds, the enzyme activity slows or ceases altogether. TFPI is produced by several cell lines including liver, lung, bladder, and endothelial tissue cells. Platelets also secrete TFPI after stimulation with thrombin or calcium. It is unknown as to which cell type is responsible for maintenance of plasma TFPI concentration. Heparin infusion increases plasma levels of TFPI, which appears to be related to the release of the protein from intra- or extra-cellular stores.

TFPI possesses three inhibitor domains, and, although unusual, this is consistent with its multiple inhibitory specificities. The first domain inhibits the factor VIIa/TF com-

Inhibitors of Coagulation

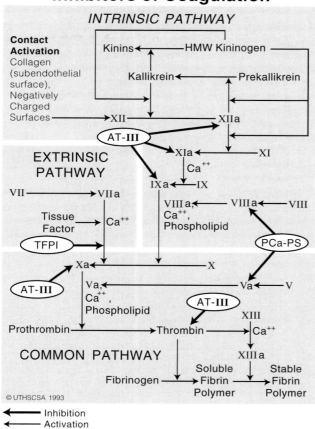

FIGURE 24-17. The most important inhibitors of coagulation are antithrombin III (ATIII) and activated protein C (PCa) and protein S (PS). ATIII accounts for about 80% of the inhibition. ATIII is an antiserine protease that primarily inactivates thrombin but also may inactivate all other serine protease coagulation factors. Protein C is activated by thrombin and a cofactor, thrombomodulin. PCa, together with PS, destroys factors Va and VIIIa. An important inhibitor of the extrinsic pathway is tissue factor pathway inhibitor (TFPI). Other less significant inhibitors are discusssed in the text.

plex and the second directly inhibits factor Xa. The inhibitory function of the third domain is not known.[11]

Plasma levels of TFPI are relatively stable, increasing moderately with age, but the range of normal is quite broad. The mean concentration in plasma is 100 ng/mL with a normal range of about 70 to 150 ng/mL.[16]

There are three pools of TFPI within the blood vessels (Table 24-8).[7,17] A major pool is bound to the endothelial surface, a smaller pool circulates in the plasma, and a third pool (<10% of the plasma pool) is found in platelets. The majority of the plasma pool is complexed with very low density lipoproteins (VDRL), low density lipoproteins (LDL), and high density lipoproteins (HDL) (LDL < HDL < VLDL). Only 5% to 10% of TFPI circulates carrier-free, but evidence suggests that this is the most biologically active form.[17] Heparin and streptokinase cause a rapid increase of TFPI activity in the plasma, suggesting this

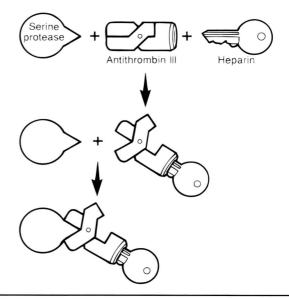

FIGURE 24-18. A schematic drawing depicting the possible mode of heparin catalyzed inactivation of serine proteases by ATIII. The heparin apparently causes a conformational change in the ATIII molecule that makes its active site more accessible to the protease.

treatment causes release of the TFPI bound to the vascular endothelium. The platelet pool of TFPI may play an important role in in vivo inhibition since its release from activated aggregated platelets may accumulate increased amounts at the site of vascular injury.[17]

The TFPI is a potent inhibitor of factor Xa, the factor VIIa/TF complex, and a modest inhibitor of plasmin.[11] The inhibitor inactivates factor Xa by binding to the factor's serine active site or close to the site in a 1:1 stoichiometry. This binding is not calcium-dependent. Heparin enhances this TFPI inhibition of factor Xa by 40-fold.[18] The inhibition of factor VIIa/TF by TFPI involves the formation of a complex of VIIa-TF-Xa-TFPI (Fig. 24-19). This quaternary complex apparently forms as a result of several binding steps. The TFPI first binds with factor Xa in a calcium-independent reaction followed by the binding of this TFPI/Xa complex to the VIIa/TF complex in a calcium-dependent reaction.[17] This TFPI-induced feedback inhibition of the extrinsic pathway emphasizes the need for both the intrinsic and extrinsic pathways. Once factor Xa is produced, TFPI inhibits further activation of factor X by the factor VIIa/TF complex as well as activation of factor IX by both factor Xa and factor VIIa/TF. Further factor Xa must be produced through the intrinsic activa-

TABLE 24-8 *LOCATIONS OF TISSUE FACTOR PATHWAY INHIBITOR (TFPI) WITHIN BLOOD VESSELS*

1. blood vessel endothelial cell surface
2. plasma: 90–95% bound to lipoproteins, 5–10% carrier-free (most biologically active form)
3. platelets

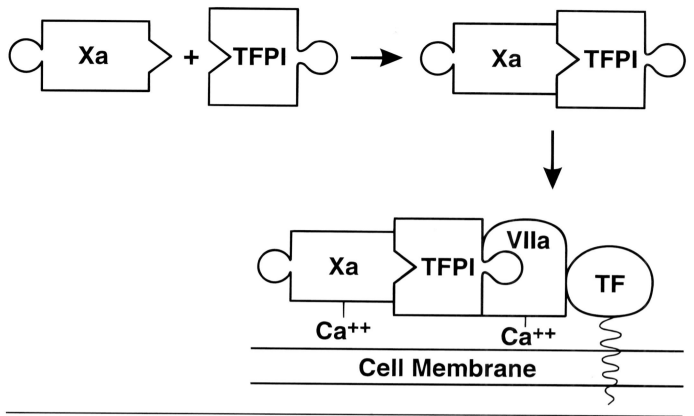

FIGURE 24-19. The inhibition of factor VIIa/TF by tissue factor pathway inhibitor (TFPI) occurs as the result of a multistep process. First, TFPI binds to factor Xa. This results in a conformational change of TFPI that promotes binding of the Xa/TFPI complex with the factor VIIa/TF complex in a calcium dependent reaction.

tion pathway. Thus, initial production of factor Xa occurs via the factor VIIa/TF pathway, but sustained hemostasis requires activation by factor IXa (produced via the intrinsic pathway).[18]

PROTEIN C AND PROTEIN S

Protein C is a vitamin K-dependent anticoagulant. In 1976, it was isolated and its properties described.[19] Later, it was recognized that Protein C was actually a protein that had been described several years before as a competitive inhibitor of factor Xa. It had been called autoprothrombin II-A.[20] Upon activation, protein C inhibits the activity of cofactors Va and VIIIa. Deficiencies of this protein are associated with venous thrombosis.

Protein C is activated to a serine protease by thrombin (Fig. 24-20). As with activation of other vitamin K-dependent coagulation proteins, the optimal activation of protein C requires a cofactor and calcium. The cofactor, *thrombomodulin* (named for its ability to change or modulate the specificity of thrombin from a procoagulant to an anticoagulant), is an intrinsic membrane glycoprotein present on endothelial cells. It dramatically enhances thrombin activation of protein C. Thombomodulin has a high affinity for thrombin, forming a 1:1 complex. When bound by thrombomodulin, thrombin cannot cleave fibrinogen but rather becomes a potent initiator of antico-

agulation by serving to activate protein C.[21] Activated protein C rapidly destroys factors Va and VIIIa, providing a mechanism for the regulation of thrombin formation. Activated protein C also contributes to fibrinolysis by inactivating plasminogen activator inhibitor-type I (PAI-1).[22]

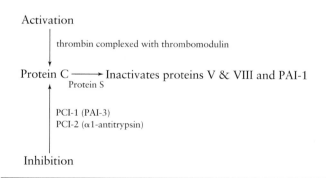

FIGURE 24-20. Protein C, an important inhibitor of coagulation, requires a cofactor, thrombomodulin, and calcium for optimal activation. Thrombomodulin binds thrombin in its cofactor activity, inhibiting the clot-promoting activity of this potent enzyme. Protein S enhances the activity of activated protein C presumably by promoting the binding of this protein to phospholipid surfaces.

The inhibitor activity of activated protein C is enhanced by another vitamin K-dependent protein, protein S. Only unbound Protein S (40%) is active in hemostasis. The remainder is bound to complement C4b. Protein S, which has a high affinity for phospholipid surfaces, promotes the binding of protein C to the phospholipid surface of platelets and to endothelial cells and accelerates the inactivation of factors Va and VIIIa.[21] This protein may be decreased in women taking oral contraceptives. Deficiencies of protein S are associated with thrombosis.

Activated protein C is inhibited by a specific serine protease inhibitor, protein C inhibitor-1 (PCI-1). This inhibitor has been found to be identical to plasminogen activator inhibitor-3 (PAI-3). The inhibitor forms a complex with protein C in a reaction similar to that between antithrombin and thrombin. The complex formation is enhanced in the presence of heparin. A second protein C inhibitor (PCI-2) has been identified and subsequently found to be identical to α1-antitrypsin. This inhibitor is heparin-dependent.

Individuals with protein C or protein S deficiency are at risk for development of thromboembolisms.[23] Resistance to activated protein C (APC resistance) also has been described in individuals predisposed to venous thrombosis.[24] A number of mechanisms for this resistance are possible, including functional protein S deficiency, mutated forms of factors VIII and V making them resistant to APC, and auto-antibodies against protein C.

α₂-MACROGLOBULIN

The glycoprotein α₂-macroglobulin is widely distributed in the body. Its concentration changes with age with highest levels in infants and children. It also may appear elevated in pregnancy, in women taking oral contraceptives, and in a number of other disorders. The α₂-macroglobulin is capable of forming complexes with proteases, including thrombin, plasmin, and kallikrein. Its binding to thrombin is slow and results in a proteolytic cleaving of α₂-macroglobulin followed by a decrease in the activity of thrombin. Thrombin bound to α₂-macroglobulin, however, can continue to slowly cleave fibrinogen to fibrin, suggesting α₂-macroglobulin may function primarily as a clearance mechanism for serine proteases since the thrombin/α₂-macroglobulin complexes are rapidly cleared from plasma, rather than as an inhibitor of enzymatic activity. On the other hand, α₂-macroglobulin is an important inhibitor of kallikrein accounting for binding of about 50% of plasma kallikrein.

α₁-ANTITRYPSIN

The glycoprotein, α₁-antitrypsin, identical to PCI-2 has the capacity to inhibit a number of proteases but its role in control of coagulation is probably secondary. Its activity is thought to be more important at the tissue level.

C1 INACTIVATOR

The C1 inactivator is a neuraminoglycoprotein that was first recognized as an inhibitor of the esterase activity of C1 from the complement cascade. Its role in the coagulation system is primarily as an inhibitor of the contact factors in the intrinsic pathway.

● THE FIBRINOLYTIC SYSTEM

The fibrinolytic system is activated in response to initiation of the coagulation cascade (activation of contact factors). Activation of fibrinolysis produces a proteolytic enzyme, *plasmin*, that is capable of digesting (by proteolysis) either fibrin or fibrinogen, as well as other factors in the cascade (Fig. 24-21). In addition, plasmin digestion of fibrin produces fragments called fibrin degradation products, which interfere with the thrombin catalyzed formation of fibrin. Plasmin is derived from its zymogen precursor, plasminogen, by plasminogen activators (Fig. 24-22).

The key components in the fibrinolytic system are: (1) plasminogen; (2) plasminogen activators; (3) plasmin; (4) fibrin; (5) fibrin/fibrinogen degradation products; and (6) inhibitors of plasminogen activators and plasmin.[25]

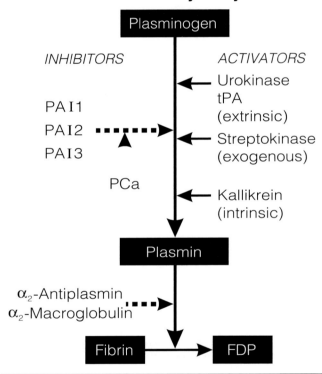

The Fibrinolytic System

FIGURE 24-21. The fibrinolytic system can be activated by the extrinsic activators, tissue plasminogen activator (tPA) derived from endothelial cells, and urokinase or the intrinsic activator, kallikrein. Exogenous activator, streptokinase, may also activate the system. Plasmin, the product of activation, controls coagulation by digesting fibrin to fibrin degradation products (FDP) and by degrading factors V, VIII, and XII. The inhibitors of plasminogen activation, plaminogen activator inhibitor-1 (PAI-1), plasminogen activator inhibitor-2 (PAI-2), plasminogen activator inhibitor-3 (PAI-3), and the inhibitors of plasmin (α₂-antiplasmin and α₂-macroglobulin) serve to control the fibrinolytic system. Activated protein C (PCa) inhibits PAI-1 and may enhance release of tPA, thus enhancing fibrinolysis. The fibrinolytic system, like the clotting system, is intricately regulated by these activators and inhibitors.

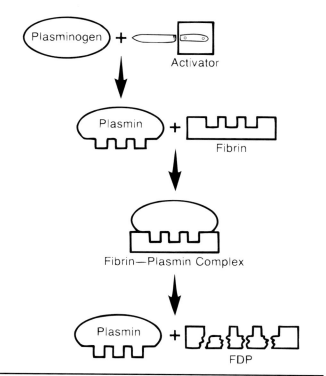

FIGURE 24-22. A schematic drawing of the steps in fibrinolysis. Plasminogen must be activated to plasmin, which then proteolytically degrades fibrin into fibrin degradation products (FDP).

● Plasminogen and plasmin

Plasminogen, a β-globulin with a molecular mass of about 80,000 Daltons, is a single chain glycoprotein that circulates in the blood as a zymogen. Like the coagulation factors, it is synthesized by the liver. Large amounts of plasminogen are adsorbed within the fibrin mass during clot formation.

Plasmin, an enzyme with trypsin-like specificity, is formed from plasminogen by various activators that cleave plasminogen into a serine protease. Plasmin can digest factors V and VIII, as well as fibrin and fibrinogen. Plasmin digestion of factor XII gives rise to successively smaller molecules that decrease in coagulant activity but increase in prekallikrien activating activity. If free in the plasma, plasmin can cause proteolytic degradation of many coagulation proteins, as well as components of the kinin and complement systems. This potentially dangerous proteolytic process is controlled by the rapid formation of plasmin/α2-antiplasmin complexes when free plasmin is present in the circulation.

Activators of plasminogen can be found in blood (intrinsic) and in most tissues (extrinsic). In addition, some substances not normally present in the blood during the coagulation and fibrinolytic processes (exogenous) can gain access to the circulation in pathologic states and activate plasminogen. The exogenous activators also include the commercially available therapeutic agents that are used in treatment of thrombotic disorders.

INTRINSIC ACTIVATORS

Plasminogen activators in the blood are referred to as intrinsic activators. These activators are involved in the contact phase of the intrinsic coagulation cascade. Factor XIIa activation of plasminogen is an indirect activation pathway and involves the interaction of factor XIIa with a plasminogen proactivator. This results in the conversion of the proactivator to an activator that subsequently cleaves plasminogen to form the enzyme plasmin. Evidence suggests that the plasminogen proactivator is prekallikrein and the activator is kallikrein, but the mechanism of activation by contact factors is not well understood.

EXTRINSIC ACTIVATORS

Tissue plasminogen activators (t-PA), derived primarily from the endothelium of the vasculature, and secreted plasminogen activators known as *urokinase-like plasminogen activators* (u-PA) compose the extrinsic activator route.

Tissue plasminogen activator, a serine protease, is a more rapid activator of plasminogen than the intrinsic activators. It has an affinity for fibrin with which it forms a bimolecular t-PA/fibrin complex. The catalytic efficiency of t-PA for activation of plasminogen is increased over a 1000-fold in the presence of fibrin. Contrastingly, nonbound t-PA in circulating plasma has a low affinity for plasminogen and, thus, is not efficient in activating this protein to plasmin.

Increased t-PA levels cause excessive fibrinolysis and may be associated with a bleeding tendency. A number of coagulation proteins enhance the release of t-PA, including factor Xa, thrombin, platelet activating factor, bradykinin, and protein C. The endothelium also can be stimulated to release t-PA into the vasculature by exercise, hypotensive shock, pharmacologic stimulators, and venous stasis. Tissue plasminogen activator can be found in the heart, kidney, and other organs. Theorectically, with extensive organ damage, t-PA is released into the circulation where it can cause extensive systemic fibrinogenolysis. This type of injury, however, is always associated with disseminated intravascular coagulation due to rapid activation of the extrinsic pathway by the simultaneous release of tissue thromboplastin.

Plasmin formed on the fibrin clot is only slowly inactivated by α2-antiplasmin because fibrin-bound plasmin has both its lysine-binding site and active site occupied by interaction with fibrin. The high-affinity lysine-binding site of plasmin must be available for the fast interaction with α2-antiplasmin. Plasmin in circulation, however, is rapidly inactivated because the lysine-binding site is available for interaction with α2-antiplasmin. Thus, the fibrinolytic process appears to be both triggered and limited by fibrin.[26]

Urokinase-type plasminogen activator (u-PA), as its name suggests, was originally believed to be present only in urine but later it was also found in many cell types as well as in plasma. Urokinase-type plasminogen activator exists in two forms: single-chain type glycoprotein (scu-PA) and two-chain type glycoprotein (tcu-PA). The scu-

PA has significant fibrin specificity, but in vitro studies reveal it is not effective in activating plasminogen.[25] Single-chain type glycoprotein is converted to tcu-PA by plasmin hydrolysis. Although tcu-PA has no specific affinity for fibrin, tcu-PA activation of plasminogen is increased 10-fold in the presence of fibrin. In plasma, tcu-PA activates fibrin-bound plasminogen and circulating plasminogen indiscriminately.

The proposed mechanism of action of u-PA is: first scu-PA directly activates a small amount of plasminogen to plasmin. Then plasmin hydrolyzes scu-PA to tcu-PA. More effective plasminogen activation then occurs by the action of tcu-PA. Thus, the conversion of scu-PA to tcu-PA during fibrinolysis is a positive feedback mechanism.

The urokinase-like plasminogen activator receptor (u-PAR) is present on a variety of cells. The receptor binds scu-PA and localizes it on the cell surface. This makes the scu-PA more readily accessible to plasmin cleavage producing tcu-PA. Binding increases the activation of plasminogen six-fold. The u-PAR is a glycosyl phosphatidyl-inositol (GPI) anchored protein. This protein is deficient in paroxysmal nocturnal hemoglobinuria.

Plasminogen activator inhibitor-1 (PAI-1) and *plasminogen activator inhibitor-2* (PAI-2) are rapid and specific inhibitors of the extrinsic plasminogen activators.

Lipoprotein(a), Lp(a), has been shown to inhibit the activation of plasminogen by t-PA and u-PA.[27] Lp(a) also competes with plasmin to bind to fibrin. This displaces plasmin into the blood where it is rapidly inactivated by α2-antiplasmin. These effects of Lp(a) are antifibrinolytic. Lp(a) also blocks inhibition of t-PA by PAI-1 in the presence of fibrinogen or heparin. This is a profibrinloytic effect. The overall effect of Lp(a) on fibrinolysis depends largely on the concentrations of PAI-1, t-PA, and Lp(a).

EXOGENOUS ACTIVATOR

Streptokinase, an enzyme derived from β-hemolytic streptococci also can activate plasminogen. This enzyme is not a serine protease but assumes enzyme activity when complexed stoichiometrically with plasminogen. Streptokinase is used primarily as a therapeutic agent to dissolve clots.

● Fibrin digestion

Plasmin is responsible for the asymmetrical, progressive degradation of fibrin (or fibrinogen), forming distinct protein fragments referred to as fibrin degradation (split) products (FDP or FSP). These fragments are rapidly cleared from circulation by the liver. Detection of the fragments in the plasma is of diagnostic value for some hemostatic disorders.

Plasmin digestion of fibrinogen has been widely studied and has been used as the model to explain the digestion of fibrin. The products formed include fragments X, Y, D, and E (Fig. 24-23). The first fragment formed is *fragment X* plus small peptides. Plasmin cleaves a few small peptides from the exposed polar appendages in the C-terminal region of the Aα-chains. The large remaining

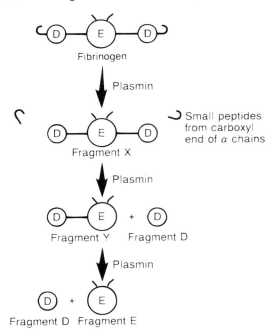

Plasmin Degradation of Fibrinogen

FIGURE 24-23. The degradation of fibrinogen by plasmin occurs in well-defined sequential steps. First, small peptides are cleaved from the carboxyl ends of α-chains producing fragment X. The E domain retains the A & B peptides. The Fragment X is still capable of reacting with thrombin to form fibrin. Next, one of the D domains is cleaved from the fragment X producing a fragment Y (DE) and a fragment D. Further cleavage of the fragment Y produces D and E fragments.

molecule is fragment X. The next step in plasmin digestion involves a single cleavage in the coiled region, midway between the D-terminal domain and the E-central domain, producing a uninodular *fragment D*, and a binodular fragment E,D. The larger binodular E,D fragment is referred to as *fragment Y*. Next, plasmin cleaves fragment Y in the coiled region between the E and D domains, producing *fragment E* and fragment D. Thus, with plasmin digestion, each fibrinogen molecule is degraded into two D fragments, one E fragment, and a few small peptides. These are the key cleavage sites. Many other cleavage sites exist, but their derivatives are not relevant for clinical assays.

Plasmin degradation of fibrin monomer and noncross-linked fibrin polymer is essentially identical to that of fibrinogen. Plasmin degradation of cross-linked fibrin, however, is slower, and structural derivatives are different because of the intermolecular bonds induced by factor XIIIa. The sites of proteolytic attack are the same but because of the cross-linking of the fibrin polymer the sites may not be as accessible to plasmin. Some of the cross-linked fibrin degradation products are combinations of X, Y, D, and E fragment complexes from two or more cross-linked fibrin monomers (e.g., DD/E, YD/DY, YY/DXD) (Fig. 24-24).

The fibrin fragments, if present in significant concentration, can exert an anticoagulant effect on the clotting

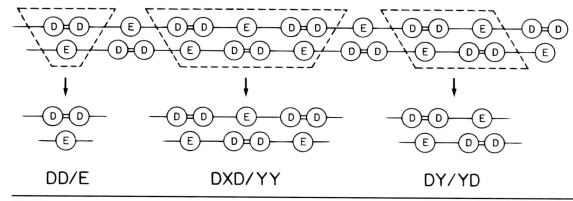

DD/E   **DXD/YY**   **DY/YD**

FIGURE 24-24. Fibrin digestion by plasmin occurs at cleavage sites identical to those of fibrinogen. However, because of the covalent bonds of the Factor XIIIa stabilized polymer, digestion is slower. Derivatives also are different as some sites are not as accessible in the lattice formation. In this schematic drawing, some of the derivatives of plasmin digestion of fibrin are depicted. (Adapted from: Marder, V.J., Francis, C.W., Doolittle, R.F.: Fibrinogen structure and physiology. In: Hemostasis and Thrombosis. Edited by R.W. Colman, J. Hirsh, V.F. Marder, E.W. Salzman. Philadelphia: J.B. Lippincott, 1982.)

system. Fragment X can still react with thrombin but very slowly. This slow reaction with fragment X results in competition for thrombin, preventing thrombin from reacting with fibrinogen. Fragment Y and fragment D inhibit the polymerization of fibrin monomers, and fragment E inhibits thrombin. These fragments can also interfere with primary hemostasis by inhibiting platelet aggregation.

Assays are available for the detection of fibrin(ogen) degradation products. The assays are based on the reaction of monoclonal antibodies with specific fibrin(ogen) derivatives. If an antiserum to fibrinogen fragments D and E is used, a positive result may be obtained with fibrinogen degradation products as well as fibrin degradation products (FDP). If, however, the antiserum is highly specific to an antigen on D-dimers (two linked D fragments), the test will be positive only if fibrin degradation has occurred (D-dimer test). Thus, the D-dimer test is a specific marker for plasmin degradation of fibrin.

●
Interaction of coagulation with fibrinolysis

From the discussion above, it can be seen that the fibrinolytic and coagulation systems are intricately related. Plasminogen proactivator is activated by the first factor in the intrinsic coagulation pathway, factor XIIa. Plasmin in turn will activate more factor XII. At the same time, however, plasmin degrades the coagulation cofactors, factor V, VIII, and the end product, fibrin. This plasmin degradation is normally limited to the site of injury because both plasminogen and plasminogen activators must be bound to the fibrin clot for optimal activation of plasminogen to plasmin. Rarely, pathologic activation of the fibrinolytic system may occur without activation of the coagulation system *(primary fibrinolysis)*. When this occurs, there is widespread degradation of fibrinogen and other clotting factors precipitating severe bleeding.

●
Physiologic control of fibrinolysis

As in the coagulation system, there are soluble protein inhibitors of the fibrinolytic system (Table 24-9). Plasmin

and t-PA are serine proteases whose action must be limited to the site of injury. The major protease inhibitors of these enzymes are α_2-antiplasmin, α_2-macroglobulin, PAI-1, and PAI-2. α_2-macroglobulin also is an inhibitor of the serine proteases involved in the coagulation cascade.

α_2-ANTIPLASMIN
The α_2-antiplasmin is a single chain glycoprotein that migrates with the α_2-globulins on electrophoresis. It is probably synthesized in the liver. Antiplasmin forms a 1:1 stoichiometric complex with plasmin or plasminogen. This complex formation appears to block free plasminogen's lysine binding sites, preventing its adsorption to fibrin. The enzymatic active site of free plasmin also is blocked. The α_2-antiplasmin inhibition of plasmin bound to fibrin is only slowly inactivated since its binding and active sites are occupied. The α_2-antiplasmin inhibits other serine proteases including the contact factors, factor Xa, and thrombin.

α_2-MACROGLOBULIN
The α_2-macroglobulin combines slowly with plasmin and is believed to neutralize excess plasmin once α_2-antiplasmin is saturated. The binding of this inhibitor appears

TABLE 24-9 *ACTIVATORS AND INHIBITORS OF FIBRINOLYSIS*

Activators	Inhibitors
Tissue plasminogen activator (tPA)	Plasminogen activator inhibitor-1 (PAI-1)
Urokinase-like plasminogen activator (uPA)	Plasminogen activator inhibitor-2 (PAI-2)
	Plasminogen activator inhibitor-3 (PAI-3)
Kallikrein	α2-antiplasmin
Streptokinase	α1-antitrypsin
	α2-macroglobulin
	Antithrombin III (ATIII)
	C1 inactivator

to occur as plasmin initiates a proteolytic attack on α2-macroglobulin. The plasmin becomes trapped within the inhibitor, preventing the enzyme from reaching fibrin.

PAI-1, PAI-2, AND PAI-3

Although t-PA is inhibited by α2-macroglobulin, α1-antitrypsin, ATIII, α2-antiplasmin, and plasminogen activator inhibitor-3 (identical to activated protein C inhibitor), more rapid, specific inhibition occurs with PAI-1 and PAI-2.[26]

PAI-1 is the primary inhibitor of t-PA and tcu-PA in plasma. It also activates protein C. Platelet PAI-1 accounts for most of the PAI-1 in blood but the PAI-1 in the plasma is the most active. PAI-1 is released from platelet α-granules during platelet activation. It also has been found in conditioned media of human endothelial cells, fibrosarcoma cells, hepatocytes, and in the placenta. Production and/or release is regulated by stimuli such as thrombin, endotoxin, interleukin-1, transforming growth factor-β, and tumor necrosis factor.

PAI-2 also inhibits t-PA and tcu-PA but less efficiently than PAI-1. It has been identified in human placenta and in the plasma of pregnant women. Secretion of PAI-2 is stimulated by endotoxin and phorbal esters. Neither PAI-1 or PAI-2 react with scu-PA.[25]

PAI-3 is an inhibitor of tcu-PA. Its interaction with activated protein C, however, is greater than its interaction with tcu-PA. Its activity is increased by heparin.

Deficient synthesis or release of t-PA or increased levels of PAI-1 impairs fibrinolysis and is associated with thrombosis. The levels of PAI have been found to be increased and fibrinolytic activity to be depressed in coronary artery disease and myocardial infarction. Recent reports indicate that high levels of PAI-1 are also associated with an increased incidence of recurrent cardiac thrombotic events in survivors of acute myocardial infarctions.

OTHER INHIBITORS

Other inhibitors that play a minor role in plasmin inactivation include ATIII, α1-antitrypsin and C1 inactivator.

The α1-antitrypsin slowly binds the active site of serine proteases. The C1 inactivator serves as a competitive substrate for plasmin, but it is of little importance in circulation because plasmin has a higher affinity for fibrin. This inhibitor is of primary importance in inhibition of complement and factors in the contact activation of the coagulation system.

● RELATIONSHIP OF THE HEMOSTATIC MECHANISM TO THE COMPLEMENT SYSTEM

The hemostatic mechanism, the complement system, and the kinin system are all involved in bodily defense to injury or invasion by foreign antigens. The relationship of the hemostatic mechanism and kinin system has already been mentioned in the discussion of activation of the contact factors in the intrinsic coagulation system. The complement system also has interrelationships with the hemostatic mechanisms at three levels: the platelets, secondary hemostasis, and fibrinolysis.

● Platelet level

Platelets appear to have some complement components bound to their surface membrane including C1. It also has been demonstrated that platelets can be induced to aggregate and secrete in the presence of antigen/antibody/complement complexes.

● Secondary hemostasis level

The coagulation and complement systems are similar in their activation reactions, and it is not surprising that the two may have crossover reactions. Both systems react in a cascade-like fashion, whereby protease zymogens are sequentially activated together with cofactors. Both systems also have two pathways for activation to take place. In the coagulation system, activation may occur through

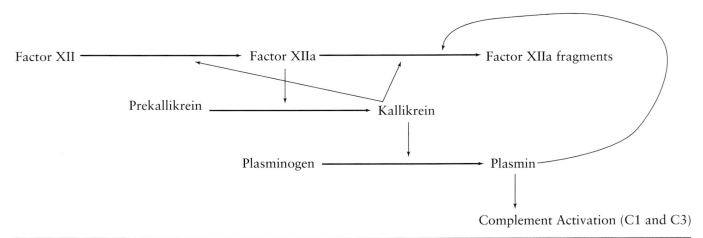

FIGURE 24-25. Complement activation in hemostasis. Factor XII indirectly activates complement through its activation of fibrinolysis. Plasmin can activate C1 and C3.

the intrinsic or extrinsic pathways, while in the complement system, activation occurs through either the classic or alternate pathways.

Factor XII from the intrinsic coagulation pathway can indirectly mediate complement activation through its activation of prekallikrein to kallikrein. Kallikrien activates plasminogen to plasmin and plasmin can activate complement (Fig. 24-25). Conversely, complement components also play a role in the coagulation system. Complement component C3b can markedly enhance tissue thromboplastin activity by monocytes. Additionally, fragment Bb from factor B in the alternate complement pathway is capable of cleaving prothrombin to form thrombin in the absence of factor X. The activity of C1 inhibitor, a major inhibitor of complement, also is an important inhibitor of the contact factors in the intrinsic pathway of coagulation.

Fibrinolysis level

Plasmin can initiate the classical pathway of complement activation by activating C1. In addition, the formation of bradykinin generates a kininogen fragment that is capable of augmenting the activity of C1 esterase. Conversely, C1 inhibitor also is an inhibitor of plasminogen activation.

LABORATORY INVESTIGATION OF SECONDARY HEMOSTASIS AND FIBRINOLYSIS

The clotting of blood and subsequent dissolution of the clot through fibrinolysis is an intricately regulated process. The process is kept in balance by the interaction of activators and inhibitors (Fig. 24-26). If this balance is upset by a deficiency of or an inappropriate activation of activators or inhibitors, thrombosis or bleeding may occur. Laboratory investigation is then initiated to identify the specific abnormality.

Abnormalities in secondary hemostasis often lead to serious bleeding disorders. Careful questioning of the patient by the physician to obtain an accurate medical history of the patient, as well as a thorough clinical evaluation and family studies are absolutely essential to establishing an accurate diagnosis of bleeding disorders.

Clinical evaluation includes laboratory tests that are designed to identify the specific cause of the bleeding. Laboratory tests of secondary hemostasis can be divided into two groups: screening tests and special tests. The screening tests are designed to test the overall integrity of the intrinsic, extrinsic, and common pathways. The most common screening tests include the prothrombin time (PT), the activated partial thromboplastin time (APTT), and thrombin time. Some laboratories prefer to add a number of other tests to their screening profiles before advancing to confirmatory tests. If the screening tests are abnormal, special tests are performed to identify the specific abnormality. The special tests include the mixing/substitution PT and APTT tests and/or factor assays. Occasionally, clinical findings suggest abnormal fibrinolysis and laboratory tests must be performed to evaluate the fibrinolytic system. A brief description of these commonly used tests follows. More details of the procedures can be found in Chapter 28.

Blood collection and preparation

Blood for coagulation testing may be drawn with either sodium citrate or sodium oxalate as the anticoagulant. Both anticoagulants prevent clotting by chelating calcium.

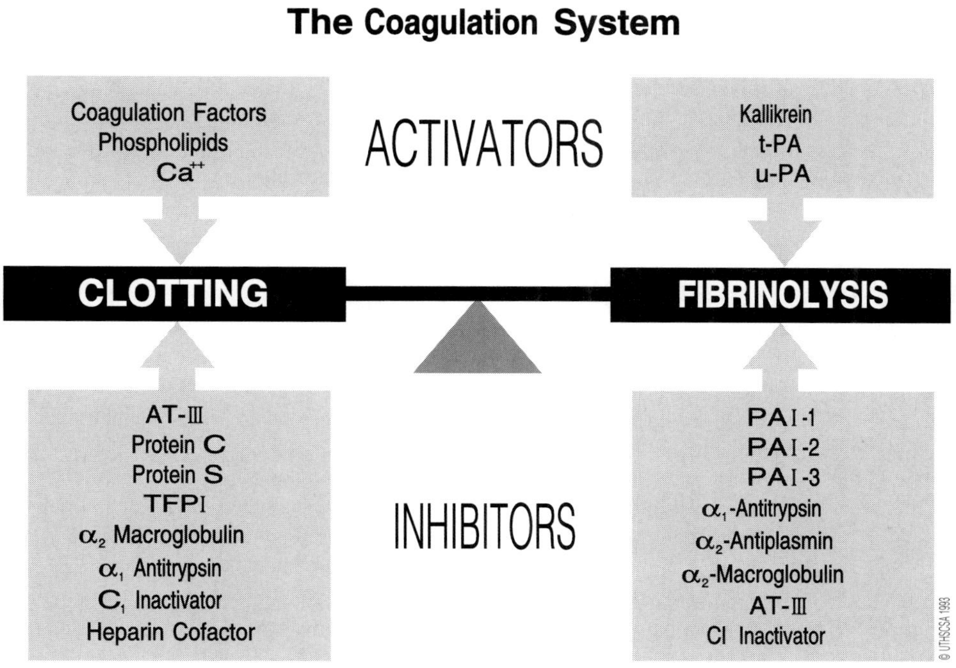

The Coagulation System

FIGURE 24-26. The coagulation system is kept in balance by activators and inhibitors of clotting and fibrinolysis. Clotting occurs when the blood vessels are damaged and activators of coagulation factors are released. Clotting is kept in control because fibrinolysis is initiated in response to clotting activation. Inhibitors of both clotting and fibrinolysis serve to bring the system back into balance. An upset in the activation or inhibition of either clotting or fibrinolysis will cause thrombosis or bleeding.

ACTIVATORS

| Coagulation Factors Phospholipids Ca++ | Kallikrein t-PA u-PA |

CLOTTING — FIBRINOLYSIS

INHIBITORS

| AT-III Protein C Protein S TFPI α₂ Macroglobulin α₁ Antitrypsin C₁ Inactivator Heparin Cofactor | PAI-1 PAI-2 PAI-3 α₁-Antitrypsin α₂-Antiplasmin α₂-Macroglobulin AT-III CI Inactivator |

Citrate, however, is the recommended anticoagulant since it is a better preservative of factor V and factor VIII. In addition, sodium oxalate may interfere with photooptical endpoints in automated coagulation instruments since precipitates of the calcium complexes are formed. Blood is drawn into tubes containing 3.8% sodium citrate with a final ratio of 9 parts blood to 1 part anticoagulant. If the hematocrit is over 55% or less than 20%, the amount of sodium citrate should be adjusted accordingly (see Chapter 28) as the ratio of calcium in the plasma to citrate is important for accurate results. An excess of citrate in the plasma may give a prolonged clotting time with the activated partial thromboplastin time and prothrombin time tests while an excess of calcium may promote clotting and give a shortened clotting time with these tests.

The use of a lower concentration of citrate, 3.2%, in the same blood to anticoagulant ratio (9:1) has been adopted by the International Committee for Standardization in Hematology and appears to overcome the problems in testing associated with high hematocrit samples.

Once blood is drawn for testing, the tests should be completed within a time frame of 30 minutes to 2 hours, because changes begin to take place as soon as the blood is drawn. In shed blood, the contact factors become activated as they come into contact with the surface of the tube. Thus, specimens that are deficient in the contact factors may show improved coagulability when testing is delayed, especially if the plasma is stored in glass tubes. Some glass tubes for coagulation testing are siliconized to minimize activation of these factors. Additionally, factor V and factor VIII are labile and may begin to decrease on prolonged storage.

Testing for screening of the integrity of the coagulation system requires platelet poor plasma (PPP). Platelet poor plasma should have a residual platelet count of less than 15×10^9/L. This plasma is prepared by centrifuging blood at a minimum RCF of 1000 xg for 10 to 15 minutes. The plasma is immediately removed from the cells and placed in stoppered plastic or siliconized tubes in the refrigerator at 4° C. The changes that occur in the sample within 2 hours are minimal. If freezing of the plasma is necessary, it should be rapidly frozen at $-70°$ C to prevent denaturation of the coagulation proteins. When testing commences, the plasma should be rapidly thawed at 37° C.

In addition to careful preparation of the blood specimen, accurate coagulation test results also depend on trauma-free venipuncture techniques. In traumatic punctures, tissue thromboplastin can enter the specimen and activate the extrinsic pathway of the coagulation cascade causing erroneous test results on preactivated plasma. To prevent contamination of the specimen with tissue thromboplastin some laboratories routinely draw two tubes of blood, discarding the first and using the second for coagulation testing.

●
Tests for secondary hemostasis

In most cases, the integrity of secondary hemostasis is evaluated in vitro by timing clot formation after calcium, thromboplastin, and/or an activator has been added to citrated plasma. The fibrin endpoint is detected by one of three means: visually, electromechanically (semiautomated), or spectrophotometrically (automated). The (manual) visual method involves tilting a tube containing plasma and reagents back and forth until visible fibrin strands appear.

The semiautomated method uses a fibrometer, which detects clots by electromechanical means (wire electrodes). Two electrodes are immersed in the plasma-reagent mixture, one a stationary electrode and the other a moving electrode. The moving electrode sweeps through the plasma and is lifted above the plasma level every half-second. When a clot forms, an electronic circuit is formed between the stationary and moving electrodes via fibrin as the moving electrode is lifted out of the plasma. This completed circuit stops a timer.

The automated coagulation systems use the principle of spectrophotometry, where clot formation causes a change in the optical density of the plasma. Other automated instruments that measure not only the fibrin endpoint but the kinetics of the reaction are helpful in detecting modest decreases in the coagulation factors in which the overall clotting time is normal.

SCREENING TESTS

After history and and physical examination of patients with suspected abnormalities of the hemostatic mechanism have been completed, laboratory screening tests of primary and secondary hemostasis are performed. The first procedure performed is usually the bleeding time for evaluation of primary hemostasis. This is followed by screening tests that evaluate the adequacy of the intrinsic, extrinsic, and common pathways of secondary hemostasis (Table 24-10). It is important to keep in mind that these

TABLE 24-10 *FACTORS EVALUATED IN SCREENING COAGULATION TESTS*

Factor	Bleeding Time	PT	APTT	TT	Urea Solubility
XII	−	−	+	−	−
XI	−	−	+	−	−
IX	−	−	+	−	−
Kallikrein	−	−	+	−	−
HMWK	−	−	+	−	−
VIII	−	−	+	−	−
X	−	+	+	−	−
V	−	+	+	−	−
VII	−	+	−	−	−
II	−	+	+	−	−
I	−	+	+	+	−
XIII	−	−	−	−	+
Platelets	+	−	−	−	−

+ evaluated

− not evaluated

screening tests are nonspecific as they measure the end-point of a series of reactions within the coagulation cascade. Thus, an abnormal test may signify an abnormality in any one of a group of factors. Special tests are required to identify the specific abnormality. Additionally, it is recognized that the screening tests lack sensitivity. Coagulation factors may be moderately to severely decreased before an abnormal clotting time is detected by screening tests. Thus, normal screening tests do not necessarily rule out coagulation factor deficiencies.

The two most common tests for coagulation screening are the APTT and the PT. The APTT tests for the integrity of the intrinsic pathway and the PT tests for the integrity of the extrinsic pathway. Both the APTT and PT include measurement of the common pathway. The time it takes for conversion of prothrombin to thrombin and fibrinogen to fibrin is relatively short when compared with the time for the reactions in the intrinsic and extrinsic systems. Therefore, the time involved in the reactions of the common pathway will affect the overall time of clot formation less than factors in the intrinsic or extrinsic pathways.

Prothrombin time

The PT is the best screening test for abnormalities in the extrinsic pathway. It measures the activation of factor X by the factor VIIa/TF complex, as well as the remaining reactions in the common pathway. Thus, the test measures factors I, II, V, VII, and X. In this test an optimal concentration of tissue thromboplastin (available commercially) is added to plasma, providing the tissue factor necessary to activate the extrinsic pathway. After a brief incubation, calcium is added to the mixture and the time required for a clot to form is measured. The normal time is about 11 to 15 seconds, depending on the tissue thromboplastin used. Automated procedures usually give shorter times than the manual tilt tube procedure.

In congenital heterozygous deficiencies of factors V, VII, and X, where the factor concentration is about 20% to 65% of normal, the PT is only prolonged by 1 to 3 seconds. The sensitivity of the PT to deficiencies of factors I and II also is limited. The PT may only be prolonged if factor II is less than 10% of normal and fibrinogen is less than 100 mg/dL. Dysfibrinogenemia also may prolong the PT test.

Abnormalities in the PT are seen in conditions other than congenital factor deficiencies. The PT is prolonged in liver disease and obstructive jaundice. Oral anticoagulants depress the vitamin K-dependent synthesis of the prothrombin group factors (II, VII, IX, X). Factor VII has the shortest half-life of these four factors, and within 24 hours after a large dose of coumarin this factor is deficient enough to prolong the PT. For this reason, the PT test is the test of choice for monitoring coumarin treatment of thrombotic conditions. The PT is also prolonged in heparin administration, in the presence of circulating anticoagulants, in 75% of patients with disseminated intravascular coagulation,[28] and in dysproteinemias.

Activated partial thromboplastin time

The APTT is the test of choice for screening abnormalities in the intrinsic pathway. The test measures all factors except factors VII and XIII. In this test, an activator substance, such as kaolin, celite, or ellagic acid, is incubated with plasma to activate the contact factors. Contact factor activation is followed by addition of a phospholipid substitute for platelets and calcium. The time for a clot to form is generally 32 to 46 seconds after addition of the phospholipid and calcium, but differs with the reagent system used. An abnormal APTT suggests an abnormality in the intrinsic or common pathways. Like the PT, the APTT is not sensitive to mild factor deficiencies. For example, factor VIII abnormalities are usually not detected unless the factor is less than 35% of normal.

Interpretation of PT and APTT results

The clinical laboratory scientist must be knowledgeable of the theory of the APTT and PT tests to interpret abnormal results and to subsequently choose appropriate, cost-effective, confirmatory testing.

PT ABNORMAL AND APTT NORMAL The only factor measured by the PT and not by the APTT is factor VII. Therefore, when the PT is abnormal but the APTT is normal, the most likely deficiency is factor VII. This can be verified by performing a factor VII assay.

PT ABNORMAL AND APTT ABNORMAL When both the PT and APTT tests are abnormal, the possibility of heparin contamination should be considered. This could be determined by performing a thrombin time and a reptilase time. Heparin will prolong the thrombin time but the reptilase time is unaffected. Heparin contamination also can be ruled out by performing a heparin neutralization step (with protamine sulfate) and repeating the test on neutralized plasma.

If these tests rule out heparin contamination, mixing studies to test for circulating inhibitors is necessary. Normal plasma and patient plasma are mixed in a 1:1 ratio. The PT and APTT are then repeated using aliquots of this mixture. In a factor deficiency, the normal plasma will provide enough of the deficient factor to significantly shorten the clotting time. If the clotting times are still prolonged after addition of normal plasma, the problem is probably a circulating inhibitor because the inhibitor affects the factors in normal plasma as well as in patient plasma. If normal plasma corrects both the PT and APTT, then the problem is most likely a deficiency in a factor of the common pathway: factors X, V, II, I. The plasma should be tested with the substitution APTT and PT tests or factor assay to identify the most likely abnormality.

PT NORMAL AND APTT ABNORMAL When only the APTT test is abnormal, a deficiency in a factor of the intrinsic pathway may be suggested: factors XII, XI, IX, VIII, prekallikrein, and HMWK. A lupus anticoagulant (LA) also can cause a normal PT and abnormal APTT. Although there are a variety of tests available for detection of LA, the APTT is a sensitive, screening assay depending on the sensitivity of the thromboplastin reagent used.[29]

The first step in determining the cause of a prolonged APTT is to repeat the APTT using a prolonged incubation with activator. If the APTT is corrected with prolonged incubation of plasma and kaolin, prekallikrein deficiency is suggested. If ellagic acid is used as the activator, prekallikrein deficient plasma gives a normal clotting time without prolonged incubation. The substitution APTT test and/or factor assay will help identify other specific factor deficiencies.

If a factor VIII inhibitor is suspected as the cause of a abnormal APTT, mixing studies for inhibitors has been suggested, using a 1:4 mixture of normal plasma and patient plasma. This is also helpful for detecting lupus anticoagulant. If this suspension is incubated at 37° C for 2 hours, all temperature-enhanced inhibitors can be detected, even the weak but clinically significant ones by performing an APTT to detect loss of factor activity in normal plasma. Sometimes in the presence of weak inhibitors, the 1:1 mixture of normal plasma and patient will show correction of the APTT.

Thrombin time   The TT test measures only the conversion of fibrinogen to fibrin. In this test, thrombin is added to citrated plasma and the time for a clot to form is measured. A prolonged TT indicates a deficiency in fibrinogen, dysfibrinogenemia, or the presence of circulating inhibitors such as heparin, plasmin, and FDPs. The TT may not be prolonged, however, unless the fibrinogen concentration is less than 100 mg/dL. The TT can be used to monitor heparin therapy or detect heparin contamination since heparin acts as an anticoagulant by inhibiting thrombin.

CONFIRMATORY TESTS FOR FACTOR ABNORMALITIES

Abnormalities in the screening tests should be followed by more specific diagnostic tests including the substitution APTT, and PT tests and/or factor assays. Since factor XIII is not included in any of the screening tests, if a deficiency of this factor is suspected, the urea solubility test is performed.

Substitution APTT and PT tests   The substitution APTT and PT tests involve mixing abnormal plasma from a patient

TABLE 24-11   *FACTOR CONTENT OF BLOOD COMPONENTS AND PRODUCTS USED IN MIXING/SUBSTITUTION PT AND APTT TESTS FOR DETERMINATION OF INHIBITORS AND FACTOR DEFICIENCIES*

Component or Product	Factors Present	Factors Absent
Normal Plasma	All	None
Aged Normal Plasma	I, II, VII, IX, X, XI, XII	V, VIII
Normal Serum	VII, IX, X, XI, XII	I, II,* V, VIII, XIII*
BaSO$_4$ or Al (OH)$_3$ Adsorbed Plasma	I, V, VIII, XI, XII, XIII	II, VII, IX, X

* May be present but significantly decreased.

and various blood components of known factor content, performing the PT and APTT on an aliquot of this patient plasma and blood component mixture, and observing whether the clotting time is corrected. The most commonly used components include: normal plasma, serum, barium sulfate-adsorbed plasma, and aged plasma (Table 24-11). If the abnormal test is corrected by the mixture of a patient's plasma and a blood component, the blood component can be assumed to have replaced the factor deficient in patient's plasma (Table 24-12). Specific confirmatory tests for suspected deficient factors are often performed, directly bypassing these time-consuming substitution tests.

NORMAL PLASMA   Normal plasma contains all coagulation factors and is mixed with patient plasma primarily to detect the presence of circulating inhibitors in the patient's plasma. If a factor deficiency is responsible for the abnormal clotting time, addition of normal plasma should provide the deficient factor and correct the APTT or PT time. However, if the abnormal clotting time is caused by a circulating inhibitor in the patient's plasma, the clotting time will remain prolonged even when normal plasma is

TABLE 24-12   *CORRECTION OF ABNORMAL PT AND APTT TESTS WITH MIXTURES OF PATIENT PLASMA AND VARIOUS BLOOD COMPONENTS AND PRODUCTS*

Factor Deficiency	PT	APTT	Test(s) Corrected With Aged Plasma	Test(s) Corrected With Serum	Test(s) Corrected With BaSO$_4$ Adsorbed Plasma
X	Abn	Abn	Yes	Yes	No
V	Abn	Abn	No	No	Yes
II	Abn	Abn	Yes	No	No
I	Abn	Abn	Yes	No	Yes
VII	Abn	N	Yes	Yes	No
XII	N	Abn	Yes	Yes	Yes
XI	N	Abn	Yes	Yes	Yes
IX	N	Abn	Yes	Yes	No
VIII	N	Abn	No	No	Yes

Key: Abn = Abnormal; N = Normal

added. The inhibitor inhibits factors in the normal plasma as well as in the patient's plasma.

SERUM Serum is lacking the consumable factors: factors I, V, VIII, XIII, and II. Thus, if normal serum is mixed with patient plasma and the clotting time is corrected, the factor deficiency involved one of the factors present in serum: factors VII, IX, X, XI, XII (XIII is not tested for in the PT or APTT test).

AGED PLASMA Aged plasma contains all factors except the labile factors, factors V and VIII. If aged plasma is mixed with patient plasma and the clotting time is corrected, the factor deficiency involved a factor present in aged plasma: factor I, II, VII, IX, X, XI, XII.

PLASMA ADSORBED Plasma adsorbed with the soluble salts, barium sulfate, or aluminum hydroxide will lack factors II, VII, IX, and X (the prothrombin group). If adsorbed plasma is added to patient's plasma and the clotting time is corrected, the factor deficiency involved a factor present in adsorbed plasma: factor I, V, VIII, XI, XII.

Factor assays Final proof of a factor deficiency requires measuring the activity of the suspected deficient factor in the patient's plasma. This is done by first performing an APTT or PT on various mixtures of a normal reference plasma and a factor deficient plasma and plotting an activity curve. As the concentration of normal plasma increases the clotting time becomes more normal. To test the patient's plasma, the APTT or PT is performed using mixtures of the patient's plasma (in place of the normal reference plasma) and the factor deficient plasma. The degree of correction of the clotting time of the factor deficient plasma by the patient's plasma is compared with the results plotted on the activity curve. The factor content in patient's plasma is then expressed as a percentage of normal. Substrates of factor deficient plasmas are available commercially and some can be easily prepared artificially. In this system, it is recommended to test more than one dilution of the patient's plasma to verify the validity of the test and to detect the possible presence of an LA. An LA can give abnormal assay results with undiluted patient plasma but corrects in serial dilutions.

Synthetic substrates One of the difficulties with coagulation tests based on fibrin endpoint reading is the lack of specificity for a particular proteolytic reaction. The fibrin endpoint of the APTT and PT tests measures the cascade reactions of the intrinsic or extrinsic and common pathways as a cumulative product, fibrin.

It is well established that the activated coagulation factors act as enzymes proteolytically cleaving substrates at specific sites within an amino acid sequence. With this knowledge has come the development of synthetic substrates that simulate the amino acid sequence near the cleavage site of natural substrates. These synthetic substrates have a chromophore or fluorophore indicator group attached to the C-terminal carboxyl group or the C-terminal amino acid of the peptide. The chromophore

product is released by enzymatic hydrolysis of the substrate, and its concentration is measured by either spectrophotometric or fluorometric methods. The rate of release of the indicator group is directly proportional to the amount of the enzyme present.

Fibrinogen assay A quantitative measurement of fibrinogen can be done using a modification of the thrombin time. A normal standard curve is made using dilutions of a fibrinogen reference plasma. The TT test is performed on each standard dilution and a graph is made, with TT in seconds plotted on the abscissa and fibrinogen concentration in mg/dL on the ordinate. A TT test is then performed on the patient plasma, noting the clotting time. The result is compared with the clotting times of the reference plasma on the graph. If calcium is added to the test system, a rough estimate of factor XIII activity can be made. The factor XIIIa crosslinks fibrin polymers, producing a stable, firm fibrin clot. A poor clot with the thrombin-calcium mixture suggests an abnormality of factor XIII.

Factor XIII screening test None of the routine screening tests measure factor XIII (except for the modified TT test). If factor XIII deficiency is suspected, the urea solubility test is performed. The urea solubility test is a simple test that is specific for factor XIII deficiency, based on the finding that factor XIII stabilized clots are not soluble in 5M urea (or 1% monochloracetic acid). The test is only sensitive to gross abnormalities of factor XIII (less than 2%).

TESTS FOR FIBRINOLYSIS

The overall fibrinolytic activity of blood is measured by clot lysis tests. Most commonly, tests for fibrinolysis are performed when excessive fibrinolytic activity caused by disseminated intravascular clotting (secondary fibrinolysis) is suspected. In this case, the excessive fibrinolysis is a normal response to disseminated activation of the coagulation factors. When hemorrhages occur in these cases, they are caused by consumption of clotting factors and the presence of fibrin degradation products that interfere with normal fibrin polymer formation. On the other hand, certain rare clinical situations are associated with the release of excessive quantities of plasminogen activators into the blood in the absence of fibrin clot formation (primary fibrinolysis). In these cases, the excess plasmin can degrade fibrinogen and the clotting factors, leading to a potentially dangerous hemorrhagic condition. Often, it is difficult to differentiate secondary fibrinolysis from primary fibrinolysis. However, it may be important for the physician to make an accurate diagnosis, since the treatment for individual cases may be different. Diagnosis is aided by the interpretation of a series of coagulation tests, including tests of the fibrinolytic system, scrutiny of a blood smear for the presence of schistocytes (noted in secondary fibrinolysis), and platelet counts (usually low in secondary fibrinolysis).

Normally, the rate at which fibrinolysis takes place is slow because of the presence of plasmin inhibitors.

Plasmin is inactivated more readily in blood that is collected in glass tubes. The sensitivity of tests for abnormal clot lysis is increased, if citrated plasma is clotted with thrombin in the absence of calcium. Calcium is needed for factor XIII activation, and this activated factor strengthens the clot. It also is important that tests for fibrinolysis are performed only if fibrinogen is present in normal concentrations. If fibrinogen is decreased, additional fibrinogen should be added to the test system.

Fibrinolysis is evaluated by testing for the presence of fibrin/fibrinogen degradation products (FDP) in plasma. The FDP are formed in vivo when procoagulant material gains entrance to the circulation causing activation of coagulation and/or fibrinolysis. Normally less than 5 μg/mL FDP are found in circulation, but in pathologic conditions such as disseminated intravascular coagulation, primary fibrinolysis, or in liver disease when the hepatocytes cannot clear the FDP, the concentration of these degradation products may increase significantly. The most common test to detect FDP is the latex agglutination test. The presence of FDPs are diagnostic of plasmin degradation of fibrin or fibrinogen.

Latex agglutination test Blood for the latex agglutination test is drawn in special tubes containing thrombin or reptilase to rapidly clot the blood and a trypsin inhibitor to prevent in vitro fibrinolysis. This test uses latex beads coated with antiserum to the small FDP fragments D and E.

A drop of serum is added to the beads and mixed. Agglutination is considered a positive test and indicates the presence of D and E fragments. A positive test is followed by repeats using diluted serum to obtain a semiquantitative measurement of FDP. This test does not differentiate between fibrin degradation products and fibrinogen degradation products.

D-dimer test The D-dimer assay is a newer assay that is specific for fibrin degradation products. D-dimers are only formed from plasmin digestion of cross-linked fibrin. The test is useful in the diagnosis of DIC. The principle of the test is identical to that for the latex agglutination test except that the antiserum is a highly specific monoclonal antibody to D-dimers.

ENZYME-LINKED IMMUNOSORBENT ASSAY (ELISA)

ELISA uses antibody (or antigen) bound enzymes to measure the concentration of antigens (or antibodies). The specificity of the assay is enhanced with the use of monoclonal antibodies. This method is also sensitive, detecting plasma concentrations in the nanogram per milliliter range.

In these assays, plasma is reacted with specific antibody immobilized on a solid surface like the wells of a microtiter plate. After incubation the test system is washed. Next, the antibody/antigen complexes in the wells are incubated with excess enzyme-labeled antibody that binds to the antibody-bound antigen. After washing, an enzyme substrate that can be detected by photometric, fluorescent, or luminescent endpoint is added. The enzyme product concentration is directly proportional to the concentration of the analyte in the sample.

The use of ELISA in the hemostasis laboratory has been adopted to measure a variety of inhibitors, coagulation activation products, and other coagulation proteins.[30]

SUMMARY

Blood coagulation is a system designed to arrest the bleeding that occurs when a vessel is injured. The proteins (factors) involved in this system circulate as inert forms until activated by exposure to negatively charged surfaces (intrinsic pathway) or to TF (extrinsic pathway). These surfaces and TF are normally subendothelial and extrinsic to the blood. When vessels are injured, however, the blood coagulation proteins are exposed to subendothelial tissue and activated platelets. This begins the activation of coagulation proteins. The sequence of activation is sequential in a cascade formation. The sequence begins with the least concentrated factors in the blood and proceeds to the most concentrated factor, fibrinogen. The activation sequence amplifies the proteolytic activity as the reactions occur.

The vitamin K-dependent factors (II, VII, IX, X) are zymogens and when activated become proteases. These proteases form complexes on a phospholipid surface with a cofactor (TF, V or VIII) and substrate.

Although the process of coagulation was originally divided into the intrinsic, extrinsic, and common pathways, there is now ample evidence that there is significant interaction and feedback between proteins of these pathways. The extrinsic pathway appears to be most important in initiation of the cascade but the intrinsic system is probably responsible for amplifying and sustaining coagulation. In the first step of the extrinsic pathway, TF binds factor VII forming the TF/factor VIIa complex that activates both factor X of the common pathway and factor IX of the intrinsic pathway. Factor IXa forms a complex with factor VIII to activate factor X. Factor Xa activates factor VII and IX in a positive feedback reaction. With the exception of factor XI, the contact factors (XII, HMWK, and prekallikrien) do not appear necessary for hemostasis in vivo.

In the common pathway, factor Xa forms a complex with factor Va and phospholipid. This complex cleaves prothrombin (factor II) to thrombin. Thrombin cleaves fibrinogen to form fibrin and in a positive feedback reaction activates factor V and factor VIII. Thrombin is the central regulatory molecule in hemostasis.

The entire coagulation process is regulated by positive and negative feedback loops. Thrombin is inhibited by ATIII. Factor Xa, TF/VIIa are inhibited by tissue factor pathway inhibitor (TFPI). Thrombin activates protein C, which in turn destroys the cofactors Va and VIIIa. The fibrinolytic system is activated by the activated contact factors of the coagulation system. This system ultimately destroys the fibrin clot. Fibrinolysis is also regulated by the presence of natural inhibitors. Thus, coagulation is a highly regulated process. Defects in these regulatory processes may result in thrombosis or bleeding.

The two primary laboratory screening tests for defects in secondary coagulation are the PT and APTT. The PT detects defects in the extrinsic and common pathways while the APTT detects defects in the intrinsic and common pathways. If a defect is suggested by abnormalities in these tests, further laboratory investigation is suggested.

REVIEW QUESTIONS

1. A patient had a prolonged PT but a normal APTT. What is the most likely factor deficiency?
   a. factor VII
   b. factor X
   c. factor IX
   d. TF

2. The D-dimer test is a specific test for:
   a. plasminogen activation
   b. plasmin degradation of fibrinogen
   c. plasmin degradation of fibrin
   d. factor XIII

3. The first step in determining the cause of a prolonged APTT is to:
   a. redraw the patient and repeat the test
   b. perform a mixing study for the presence of inhibitors
   c. perform a substitution test to determine the deficient factor
   d. repeat the APTT using a prolonged incubation with activator

4. Coagulation in vivo is most probably initiated by:
   a. activation of the contact factors
   b. TF/VIIa
   c. factor IXa
   d. complement activation

5. Which of the following cleaves prothrombin to thrombin?
   a. Xa, Va, PF3, Ca++
   b. IXa, VIIa, PF3, Ca++
   c. VIIa/TF
   d. XIa

6. Which of the following is **not** a PIVKA protein?
   a. II
   b. VII
   c. VIII
   d. IX

7. Which of the following factors is **not** present in BaSO4 adsorbed plasma?
   a. VIII
   b. II
   c. XII
   d. V

8. The most important inhibitor of coagulation is:
   a. heparin cofactor II
   b. protein S
   c. α1-antitypsin
   d. AT III

9. An important inhibitor of factor Xa and factor VIIa/TF complex is:
   a. AT III
   b. TFPI
   c. PAI-1
   d. tcu-PA

10. Activated protein C together with its cofactor, protein S is an inhibitor of:
    a. factors VIIIa and Va
    b. plasmin
    c. thrombin
    d. plasminogen activators

11. The integrity of the intrinsic coagulation system is evaluated by the:
    a. thrombin time test
    b. PT
    c. APTT
    d. bleeding time

12. If a patient has a prolonged PT and prolonged APTT but both are corrected by aged plasma and serum but not corrected with adsorbed plasma, the most likely deficiency is factor:
    a. X
    b. V
    c. II
    d. I

13. The urea solubility test is specific for detecting deficiencies of factor:
    a. X
    b. XII
    c. XIII
    d. IX

14. Factors involved with initial activation of the coagulation system and that require contact with a negatively charged surface for their activity belong to the following group of factors:
    a. prothrombin group
    b. fibrinogen group
    c. fibrinolytic
    d. contact group

15. The enzymatically active coagulation factors that promote coagulation are:
    a. cofactors
    b. serine proteases
    c. zymogens
    d. inhibitors

16. Which of the following is considered a profibrinolytic protein?
    a. PAI-1
    b. thrombin
    c. α2-antiplasmin
    d. t-PA

17. Deficiencies of the following protein(s) is (are) associated with thrombosis:
    a. protein C and protein S
    b. coagulation factors
    c. PAI-1
    d. PAI-2

18. Factor X can be activated by:
    a. factor XIa
    b. factor IXa, VIIIa, PF3, Ca + +
    c. factor XIIa
    d. factors Va and VIIa

19. The most concentrated coagulation factor in the blood is:
    a. XII
    b. IX
    c. X
    d. fibrinogen

20. An abnormal thrombin time is associated with:
    a. factor X deficiency
    b. fibrinogen deficiency
    c. excess plasminogen
    d. protein C deficiency

● REFERENCES

1. Rapaport, S.I.: Blood coagulation and its alterations in hemorrhagic and thrombotic disorders. West. J. Med., 158:153, 1993.
2. Scully, M.F.: The biochemistry of blood clotting: the digestion of a liquid to form a solid. Essays. Biochem., 27:17, 1992.
3. Hemker, H.C., Kessels, H.: Feedback mechanisms in coagulation. Haemost., 21:189, 1991.
4. Rapaport, S.I.: The extrinsic pathway inhibitor: a regulator of tissue factor-dependent blood coagulation. Thromb. Haemost., 66:6, 1991.
5. Flier, J.S., Underhill, L.H.: Molecular and cellular biology of blood coagulation. N. Engl. J. Med., 326:800, 1992.
6. Davies, G., Hagen, P.O.: The vascular endothelium. Ann. Surg., 218:593, 1993.
7. Rapaport, S.I.: Regulation of the tissue factor pathway. Ann. N.Y. Acad. Sci., 614:51, 1991.
8. Mann, K.G.: The coagulation explosion. Ann. N.Y. Acad. Sci., 714:265, 1994.
9. Mann, K.G., Bovill, E.G., Krishnaswamy, S.: Surface-dependent reactions in the propagation of blood coagulation. Ann. N.Y. Acad. Sci., 614:63, 1991.
10. Walsh, P.H.: Factor XI: A renaissance. Semin. Hematol., 29:189, 1992.
11. Broze, G.J., Girard, T.J., Novotny, W.F.: The lipoprotein-associated coagulation inhibitor. Prog. Hemost. Thromb., 10:243, 1991.
12. Jensen, R., Ens, G.E.: Characterization and function of tissue factor. Clin. Hemost. Rev., 6: 1, 1992.
13. Colman, R.W., Hirsch, J., Marder, V.J., Salzman, E.W.: Hemostasis and Thrombosis. Philadelphia: J.B. Lippincott Co., 1982.
14. Baxter Health Care Corporation: The interaction of antithrombin III and heparin in controlling coagulation. Clin. Hemost. Rev., 9: 10, 1995.
15. Tollefsen, D.M.: Heparin: Basic and clinical pharmacology. In Hematology: Basic Principles and Practice. Edited by R. Hoffman, E.J. Benz, S.S. Shattel, B. Furie, H.J. Cohen. New York: Churchill Livingstone, 1995.
16. Rapaport, S.I.: Inhibition of factor VIIa/tissue factor-induced blood coagulation: With particular emphasis upon a factor Xa-dependent inhibitory mechanism. Blood, 73:359, 1989.
17. Sandset, P.M., Abildgaard, U. Extrinsic pathway inhibitor—the key to feedback control of blood coagulation initiated by tissuethromboplastin. Haemost., 21:219, 1991.
18. Jensen, R., Ens, G.E.: Tissue factor pathway inhibitor. Clin. Hemost. Rev., 6:1, 1992.
19. Stenflo, J.: A new vitamin K-dependent protein. Purification from bovine plasma and preliminary characterization. J. Biol. Chem., 251:355, 1976.
20. Seegers, W.H., Novoa, E., Henry, R.L., Hassouna, H.I.: Relationship of 'new' vitamin K dependent protein C and 'old' autoprothrombin II-A. Thromb. Res., 8:543, 1976.
21. Walker, F.J., Fay, P.J.: Regulation of blood coagulation by the protein C system. FASEF. J., 6:2561, 1992.
22. Jensen, R.: Replacement therapy for protein C, protein S and antithrombin. Clin. Hemost. Rev., 9:1, 1995.
23. Pabinger, I., et al.: The risk of thromboembolism in asymptomatic patients with protein C and protein S deficiency: A prospective cohort study. Thromb. Haemost., 71:441, 1994.
24. Dahlbeck, B.: Physiological anticoagulation. J. Clin. Invest., 94:923, 1994.
25. Lijnen, H.R., et al.: Mechanisms of plasminogen activation. J. Intern. Med., 236:415, 1994.
26. Collen, D., Lijnen, H.R.: Molecular and cellular basis of fibrinolysis. In: Hematology: Basic Principles and Practice. Edited by R. Hoffman, E.J. Benz, S.S. Shattel, B. Furie, H.J. Cohen. New York: Churchill Livingstone, 1995.
27. Edeberg, J., Pizzo, S.V.: Lipoprotein (a) regulates plasmin generation and inhibition. Chem. Phys. Lipids., 67/68:363, 1994.
28. Bick, R.L., Scates, S.M.: Disseminated Intravascular coagulation. Lab. Med., 23:161, 1992.
29. Forastiero, R.R., Cerrato, B.S., Carreras, L.O.: Evaluation of recently described tests for detection of the lupus anticoagulant. Thromb. Haemost., 72:728, 1994.
30. Jensen, R., Ens, G.E.: ELISA application in hemostasis. Clin. Hemost. Rev., 7:1, 1993.

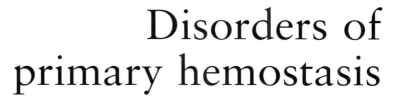

Disorders of primary hemostasis

25

KEY TERMS

petechiae
ecchymoses
easy bruisability
purpura
hematoma
excess bleeding
vasculitis
ischemia
necrosis
thrombocytopenia
thrombocytosis
idiopathic thrombocytopenic
  purpura (ITP)
acute ITP
chronic ITP
intermittent ITP
transplacental
  thrombocytopenia
neonatal thrombocytopenia
cardiopulmonary bypass
  surgery
Bernard-Soulier disease
von Willebrand disease
Glanzmann thrombasthenia
storage pool disease
cyclo-oxygenase
Gray platelet syndrome

INTRODUCTION

The functions of the hemostatic system are to prevent blood loss from intact blood vessels and to minimize the amount lost in the event of a disruptive injury. Equally important are factors that prevent inappropriate clot formation and allow the system to become active only when and where it is needed. Abnormalities of one or more components in the process of clot formation can lead to excessive bleeding or hemorrhage. Failure in the regulation of excessive clot formation leads to thrombosis.

This chapter is the first of two that will describe the disorders associated with abnormalities of the hemostatic system. It begins with a discussion of general clinical and laboratory aspects of the conditions that result in excess bleeding. Following these general topics, there is a discussion of the disorders of the vascular system and then of the platelets. These two hemostatic components are responsible for primary hemostasis. For each defect, the pathophysiologic basis and the clinical manifestations will be presented. A major emphasis will be placed on the laboratory involvement in diagnosis of the condition.

DIAGNOSIS OF BLEEDING DISORDERS

Clinical manifestations of bleeding disorders

A patient with a clinically significant bleeding disorder will present to the physician with some form of hemorrhagic symptoms. Manifestations are varied and their severity is generally in proportion to the severity of the defect. The type of bleeding may indicate the defective portion of the hemostatic mechanism.

Bleeding from subcutaneous blood vessels into intact skin may be seen as petechiae or ecchymoses (Figs. 25-1A and 25-1B). *Petechiae* are small red to purple spots less than 3 mm in diameter. They result from blood leaking through the intact endothelial lining of capillaries. Petechiae usually occur on the extremities because of the high venous pressure. When they arise spontaneously without trauma, they are painless. The lesions characteristically accompany abnormalities of platelets and blood vessels (Table 25-1).

Ecchymoses are bruises that are larger than 3 mm in diameter and also are caused by blood escaping through

TABLE 25-1 *BLEEDING SYMPTOMS AND ASSOCIATED DISORDERS OF HEMOSTASIS*

Symptom	Vascular Disorders	Platelet Disorders	Coagulation Factor Disorders
Petechiae	X	X	
Excessive bleeding from superficial wounds		X	
Retinal bleeding		X	
Ecchymoses		X	X
Gastrointestinal bleeding		X	X
Hematuria		X	X
Hypermenorrhea		X	X
Epistaxis		X	X
Gingival bleeding		X	X
Increased bleeding after tooth extraction		X	X
Intercranial bleeding		X	X
Deep muscular bleeding			X
Delayed bleeding			X
Spontaneous joint bleeding			X

intact endothelium and into subcutaneous tissue. They are red or purple in color when first formed and become yellowish green with age. Ecchymoses may appear spontaneously or with trauma and may be painful and tender. When ecchymoses are found in greater than normal numbers and with less than usual trauma, the condition is termed *easy bruisability*. They may occur in abnormalities of blood vessels, platelets, or coagulation factors.

The term *purpura*, meaning purple, is used to describe both petechiae and ecchymoses. Purpura is also used as part of the name of diseases in which these typical symptoms occur.

A bruise is called a *hematoma* (Fig. 25-1C) when blood leaks from an opening in a vessel and collects beneath intact skin. It is blue or purple in color and slightly raised. Hematomas can occur in any organ or tissue and may be in the form of a clot.

Another term used often in describing clinical manifestations of bleeding disorders is *excess bleeding*. Excess bleeding from superficial cuts and scratches occurs when platelets fail to form a primary hemostatic plug. Excess bleeding means that the bleeding occurs for a longer period of time and more profusely than is normal for the patient or compared with a "normal" person.

The bleeding symptoms seen in patients with coagulation factor deficiencies (see Chapter 26) contrasts with those of patients with platelet disorders. Rather than petechiae and superficial bleeds, the bleeding is into deeper tissues. When the coagulation factor deficiency is severe, patients may have large hematomas, spontaneous bleeding into deep muscles, hemarthroses (bleeding into joints), and delayed bleeding (Table 25-1).

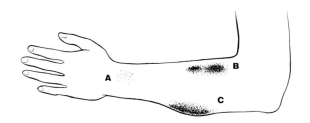

FIGURE 25-1. Schematic drawing of bleeding manifestations in intact skin. **A,** Petechiae. **B,** Ecchymosis. **C,** Hematoma.

Delayed bleeding occurs in these patients because they usually have normal platelet function. Therefore, a normal primary hemostatic plug is usually formed. With a superficial cut the blood flow may be arrested by formation of the primary plug. However, in the absence of stabilization with fibrin formation, the plug dislodges and the cut begins to bleed again. The second bleed may occur a day or more later and will continue for a long period of time.

Blood may escape into any body cavity or from any body orifice. Possible bleeding sites are listed in Table 25-1. Frank bleeding from visceral organs or mucous membranes is characteristic of both platelet and coagulation abnormalities.

● Clinical evaluation of abnormal bleeding

Excessive bleeding may be caused by a local situation such as a bleeding ulcer or by a generalized failure of the hemostatic mechanism. In some cases both may be present, and then the local problem is compounded. It is the physician's responsibility to determine the cause of the bleeding and prescribe proper treatment. This is done by obtaining an accurate medical history, performing a thorough physical examination, and ordering proper laboratory tests.

Questions in several categories are included in the patient's history. The answers should enable the physician to decide if a bleeding disorder exists, to determine if the abnormality is inherited or acquired, and help define the affected portion of the hemostatic mechanism.

The first category concerns the age at which symptoms first began. Occurrence at or shortly after birth indicates an inherited disorder, although onset later in life does not rule this out. Bleeding from the umbilical cord and circumcision suggest coagulation factor defects.

A second category concerns the persistence and severity of the symptoms, which may be revealed by inquiring if the symptoms have continued throughout life, occurred as a single incident, or have been intermittent. Bleeding in excess of that expected from a tonsillectomy, tooth extraction, trauma, injury, surgery, or childbirth may provide clues.

A third category of questions involves the family history, which is helpful to determine if other family members have similar symptoms. A pedigree analysis may determine the type of inheritance. Patients with inherited abnormalities do not always have a positive family history, however.

A fourth category involves excluding the presence of associated disease such as malignancy, aplastic anemia, leukemia, uremia, liver disease, or infections. These conditions are associated with coagulation defects and/or platelet disorders.

A fifth category involves history of drug therapy. Many drugs are known to affect the hemostatic mechanism. Different portions of the mechanism are affected by different drugs. Aspirin, chemotherapeutic drugs for malignancies, and coumarin anticoagulants are examples, but there are many others. The reader is referred to other texts that provide extensive lists of specific drugs that have been implicated.[1-3]

A final category that should be investigated is past or present exposure to toxic chemicals such as benzene, insect sprays, or hair dyes.

On physical examination, the type and sites of bleeding will be noted. The presence of petechiae or hemarthosis, for example, will provide a clue as to the affected portion of the hemostatic system. Whether the bleeding is from single or multiple sites and whether it is spontaneous or the result of trauma also is important.

Using the information from the history and physical examination, the physician will order appropriate laboratory tests to confirm and classify the presence of abnormal hemostasis.

● Laboratory evaluation of abnormal bleeding

No individual laboratory test can fully evaluate defective hemostasis. Initially, a battery of screening tests is usually ordered. Based on the results of these tests, the physician can determine if a detectable abnormality does exist and order the confirmatory tests necessary to define the disorder (see Chapters 23 and 24).

A minimal screening battery consists of a platelet count, and the determination of both the prothrombin time and activated partial thromboplastin time. Some also include a fibrinogen level and thrombin clotting time, and when the history indicates, tests for fibrin split products and/or antithrombin III levels. The significance of the results of these screening procedures and the definitive procedures which follow them will be discussed with each disease process.

In some patients with mild disease, the screening tests will not be sensitive enough to detect an abnormality. In such cases, a knowledgable physician in the field of bleeding disorders is needed to direct the clinical investigation using the information of the clinical history and physical examination.

● DISORDERS OF THE VASCULAR SYSTEM

The blood vessels are actively involved in the hemostatic system in a variety of ways (see Chapter 23). A structural abnormality or damage to either the endothelial lining of blood vessels or to the subendothelial structures may result in a variety of clinical manifestations and disease conditions. The symptoms are, for the most part, of the superficial type: easy bruising, petechiae, and excess or spontaneous bleeding from mucous membranes.

The platelet count and screening tests for coagulation factors are usually normal in blood vessel disorders (Table 25-2). A template bleeding time is usually normal but may be prolonged in some disease states.

An outdated and infrequently performed test for primary hemostasis is the tourniquet test, also called the Rumple-Leede test or the capillary fragility test. This test consists of applying a pressure cuff to the upper arm at 80 to 100 mmHg for 5 minutes. After a resting period of 10 to 15 minutes, an area about $1\frac{1}{2}$ inches in diameter

TABLE 25-2 *SIGNIFICANT LABORATORY TESTS IN THE DIAGNOSIS OF DEFECTS OF THE VASCULAR SYSTEM*

Screening Test	Result
Platelet count	Normal
Prothrombin time	Normal
Activated partial thromboplastin time	Normal

Additional Tests	Result
Template bleeding time	Normal or abnormal
Tourniquet test	Normal or abnormal

TABLE 25-4 *CLASSIFICATION OF ACQUIRED DISORDERS OF THE VASCULAR SYSTEM*

Purpura due to decreased connective tissue
  Senile purpura
  Cushing syndrome
  Corticosteroid therapy
  Scurvy
Purpura associated with paraproteins
  Paraproteinemias
  Amyloidosis
Purpura due to vasculitis
  Allergic purpura (Henoch Schoenlein)
  Infections
  Drugs
Mechanical purpura
  Increased venous pressure
  Self abuse
  Abuse by others
  Suction purpura
Purpura simplex

on the volar surface of the forearm is examined for the presence of petechiae. An increased number of the petechiae indicates increased permeability of the vessels, which allows blood to escape from the lumen. This can occur when blood vessels have certain diseases, when the number of platelets is decreased or when the platelets have abnormal function. The test does not contribute anything that the clinical history and physical examination does not reveal. In addition, the tourniquet test can cause diffuse hemorrhagic rash in patients with compromised hemostasis.

The diagnosis of blood vessel disorders is most often made by exclusion. That is, by finding no positive evidence for a disorder of platelets or coagulation factors in a patient who has bleeding symptoms.

Blood vessel disorders can be either inherited or acquired secondary to another condition (Tables 25-3 and 25-4). The hereditary diseases are caused by abnormal synthesis of subendothelial connective tissue structures. The disorders that will be discussed are hereditary telangiectasia, Ehlers-Danlos syndromes, Marfan syndrome, osteogenesis imperfecta, and pseudoxanthoma elasticum.

Of the acquired types, some are caused by abnormal subendothelium and others by altered endothelial cells. These diseases are commonly called nonthrombocytopenic purpuras because the platelet count is normal in the presence of bruising.

● Hereditary disorders of the vascular system

HEREDITARY TELANGIECTASIA

Hereditary hemorrhagic telangiectasia, also called Osler-Weber-Rendu disease, is inherited as an autosomal dominant trait. The disease was first described in 1864 by Sutton and further reviewed by Osler, Weber, and Rendu and named by Hanes.[4]

Characteristics of the disease include a family history of hemorrhage and the presence of flat, red, or purple lesions on mucous membranes. The lesions occur on the lips, the tongue, the entire gastrointestinal tract, respiratory tract, and on the palms and soles of the feet (Fig. 25-2). At autopsy, they can be found in any organ. The spots may be up to 3 mm in diameter and sometimes coalesce to become layered and spider-like and they blanch with pressure. The cause of the lesions is unknown but a lack of elastic fibers in the vessel wall is often demonstrated. They are composed of dilated capillaries and small venules. The walls of the vessels are thin and lack perivascular

TABLE 25-3 *CHARACTERISTICS OF INHERITED DISORDERS OF THE VASCULAR SYSTEM*

Disorder	Probable Cause	Significant Laboratory Findings
Hereditary telangiectasia	Unknown: possibly lack of elastic fibers	Usually normal
Ehlers-Danlos syndromes	Variable mutations of genes of collagen synthesis	Prolonged template bleeding time Platelet dysfunction
Marfan syndrome	Possible defective crosslinking of collagen	Prolonged template bleeding time
Osteogenesis imperfecta	Patchy, defective bone matrix and Abnormal type I procollagen	Prolonged template bleeding time and Abnormal platelet aggregation
Pseudoxanthoma	Abnormal elastic tissue, especially of arteries and skin	Prolonged template bleeding time

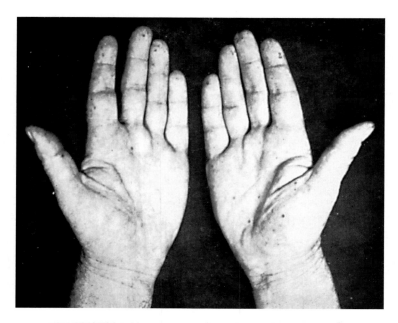

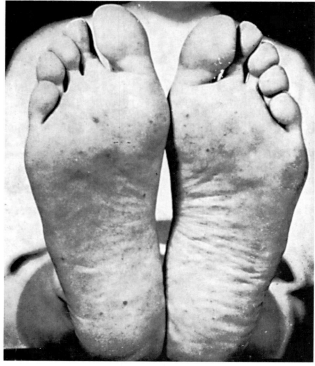

FIGURE 25-2. Hands and feet of a 55-year-old man with hereditary hemorrhagic telangiectasia. (With permission from: Wintrobe, M., et al: Clinical Hematology, 8th Ed. Philadelphia: Lea & Febiger, 1981.)

support because of abnormal connective tissue. The endothelial junctions also are defective.

The telangiectases begin to develop in childhood and become more numerous with age. Symptoms may begin early in adult life to middle age. Epistaxis is the most common manifestation. Slow bleeding from lesions in the gastrointestinal tract can lead to a hypochromic anemia. Disseminated intravascular coagulation (described later) has been reported. In the homozygous state, the disease is fatal.

Laboratory screening tests are normal. Treatment for hereditary telangiectasia is supporting and symptomatic only.

EHLERS-DANLOS SYNDROMES

The Ehlers-Danlos syndromes are a group of disorders in which there is abnormal and decreased synthesis of subendothelial connective tissue, particularly collagen and possibly elastin. Synthesis of collagen is very complex. Twenty genes are known to code for the primary amino acid sequences and several enzymes are involved in posttranslational modification of the proteins. From these, at least 10 distinct types of collagen are produced. An abnormality in any one gene can result in decreased synthesis of one of the collagen types or in the production of one type of collagen with a variant amino acid sequence. The result is the phenotype recognized as Ehlers-Danlos syndrome. At least 10 syndromes are included in the Ehlers-Danlos group based on clinical characteristics and inheritance pattern.

Most of the Ehlers-Danlos syndromes are inherited with an autosomal dominant pattern. Autosomal recessive and x-linked inheritance are represented as well.

Clinical characteristics are heterogeneous and vary from patient to patient. Bleeding manifestations occur because extreme fragility of the vessels allows blood to leave the lumen and enter the tissues. Easy bruising, spontaneous bruising, rupture of large vessels, petechiae, gastrointestinal, gingival, and dental bleeding are common. Other clinical features include extraordinary stretchability of the skin, fragility of the skin producing large wounds with trauma, difficulty in surgical closures of wounds, and hyperextensible joints.

The bleeding time may be abnormal. Platelet function abnormalities have been reported in some patients. Therapy is supportive.

MARFAN SYNDROME

Marfan syndrome demonstrates autosomal dominant inheritance. Characteristic defects are long extremities, spidery fingers, aortic aneurysm (dissecting and ascending), dislocation of the lens, hyperextensible joints, and easy bruising. The bruising may be caused by obscure abnormalities of platelet function or of the vessels. Laboratory features may include a prolonged template bleeding time and variable abnormalities of the platelet aggregation.

OSTEOGENESIS IMPERFECTA

Osteogenesis imperfecta also is transmitted in an autosomal dominant manner. It is a group of disorders of the genes for type I procollagens which cause a patchy, defective bone matrix. The result is extremely brittle bones that fracture easily. The phenotype ranges from the probability of death in utero or at birth because of collapse of the cranial bones to fractures with trauma only. Bleeding symptoms include intracranial hemorrhage, easy and spontaneous bruising, epistaxis, and hemoptysis. Laboratory tests show an abnormal template bleeding time and abnormal platelet aggregation studies.

PSEUDOXANTHOMA ELASTICUM

This rare disorder, inherited in an autosomal recessive manner, is the result of abnormal elastic tissue in the skin and all arteries. The molecular basis is as yet unclear. Symptoms may not appear until the second or third decade of life and then may involve hemorrhage in any organ, particularly the gastrointestinal tract, eyes, kidney, and skin. Easy bruising, petechiae, and purpura are commonly found. Some patients may have a tendency to develop

thrombosis and acute myocardial infarction.[5] The template bleeding time may be prolonged.

● Acquired disorders of the vascular system

Acquired disorders of the vascular system are seen quite often. Bruising and petechiae may occur with acquired defects of either the vessel wall or the endothelial cells themselves. A classification scheme is seen in Table 25-4.

Acquired disorders of the vascular system that primarily involve subendothelial structures are senile purpura, Cushing syndrome, administration of high doses of corticosteroids, and scurvy. In these conditions, the subendothelial supporting connective tissue is diminished, leading to easy bruising and the presence of ecchymoses.

Abnormal proteins in paraprotein disorders and amyloidosis cause bleeding. Allergic purpura, purpura due to infection and purpura due to drugs are caused by vasculitis. In addition, bruises can be inflicted by a variety of mechanical means. An idiopathic type of purpura characterized by the appearance of small ecchymoses or petechiae, either spontaneously, or after minor trauma, is called purpura simplex. Bleeding in congenital disorders is usually external, resulting from tears in the skin. Bleeding in the acquired disorders is usually from breaks in the vessels into intact skin.

SENILE PURPURA

Senile purpura is seen in older individuals. Ecchymoses appear spontaneously or with slight pressure, particularly in body areas that have been exposed to sunlight. Degeneration of supportive collagen fibrils develops with age and exposure to actinic radiation. Lack of support causes small blood vessels to burst and form bruises.

CUSHING SYNDROME

The origin of bruising in Cushing syndrome is similar to that of senile purpura. The mechanism leading to bruising is unknown but may be related to altered connective tissue support of the blood vessel wall, or to abnormalities of mucopolysaccharides in the supporting tissues.[5]

CORTICOSTEROID THERAPY

Therapy with high doses of corticosteroids causes bruising similar to that seen with Cushing syndrome.

SCURVY

Scurvy is a disease caused by a deficiency of vitamin C. This vitamin is needed for collagen synthesis. In its absence, collagen is insufficient or abnormal and bleeding occurs because of lack of subendothelial support for the vessels. Bleeding gums and bleeding around hair follicles on arms and thighs are characteristic. Also seen are ecchymoses and intramuscular hemorrhages. The bleeding time is normal. Treatment is oral vitamin C.

PARAPROTEIN DISORDERS

Paraproteins are monoclonal immunoglobulins produced by a single clone of identical abnormal plasma cells. They occur in a variety of malignant conditions such as multiple myeloma and lymphoproliferative disorders.

Symptoms related to hemostasis include purpura, bleeding, and thrombosis. The mechanisms leading to the symptoms are varied and speculative. They include qualitative platelet defects, acquired inhibitors and deficiencies of coagulation factors, binding of calcium by paraprotein leading to interference with coagulation, and deposition of the protein in the vascular wall. Thrombocytopenia may be present because of the underlying disease and contribute to the bleeding.

Hyperviscosity due to the abnormal protein leads to stasis in the vessels, which results in ischemia and acidosis and then to increased vascular permeability. Bleeding symptoms resulting from this include epistaxis, which is seen in 25% of patients with paraproteinemias, petechiae, purpura, and hemorrhage into other organs, particularly the retina.[5] The IgM and IgG paraproteins may fix complement and lead to release of histamine from mast cells, chemotaxis of leukocytes and aggregation of platelets with release of granule contents. These all cause an increase of the vascular permeability and may result in thrombosis of the small vessels.[5]

AMYLOIDOSIS

Amyloidosis occurs as a primary disorder as well as secondary to paraproteinemias such as multiple myeloma. It is a condition in which deposits of amyloid form in the skin, perivascular tissue, and vessel walls. It leads to fragility of the vessels and to bruising. Bleeding into visceral organs can also occur and thrombosis is common.

ALLERGIC PURPURA

Allergic purpura are a group of related disorders in which characteristic petechial and purpuric lesions are associated with various other generalized symptoms. Anaphylactoid purpura and Henoch-Schonlein purpura are synonyms.

The disease usually occurs in children older than 2 years of age and is believed to be immunologic in nature, perhaps due to antibody directed specifically against the endothelium.[5] Evidence for this is scant, except that a previous infection is noted in about half of patients.

There is a sudden onset of variable symptoms such as rash, malaise, headache, fever, gastrointestinal disorder, or joint pain. The skin lesions begin as urticaria, change to pink, then to red, and become hemorrhagic. Single lesions may fuse and become large patches. In addition, petechiae may be present. Henoch's description of the disease concentrated on the gastrointestinal symptoms accompanying the lesions. Schonlein reported the joint complications. The disease is self-limited.

Laboratory tests are negative, with the exception of the tourniquet test which may be positive.[6]

INFECTIONS

Purpura may be caused by infections with many kinds of organisms. Meningococci and other bacteria, viruses, and their toxins have been reported.

Purpura associated with infections is most often related to thrombocytopenia. When platelets are normal in num-ber, the purpura is considered to be caused by damage to the blood vessels (nonthrombocytopenic purpura). Nonthrombocytopenic purpura is related to nonspecific immune complexes formed by the antigenic agent and its corresponding antibody. The complexes attach to either the endothelial cells or to the underlying subendothelial structures.[5] The result is inflammation and destruction of the blood vessels (vasculitis) (Fig. 25-3). In vasculitis, the deposition of the immune complexes results in activation of complement and formation of complement fragments. The complement fragments initiate several processes: (1) Neutrophils migrate to the area by chemotaxis and phagocytize the immune complexes. Enzymes, free oxygen radicals, and other substances are then released from the neutrophils. The released substances cause damage to the vascular tissue. (2) Complement components C3a and C5a cause increased vascular permeability resulting in vasodilation and edema. (3) The lytic complement cascade can be completed resulting in damage to the vascular cell membranes.

The antigen-antibody complexes also cause aggregation of platelets and activation of factor XII (see Chapter 24), which both contribute to the formation of thrombosis. Thrombi may occlude blood vessels (*ischemia*) and could result in destruction of tissue supplied by the vessel (*necrosis*). Activated factor XII results in release of kinins from prekallikrein, which contributes to the vasodilation and edema of the inflammation. The damaged vessels may rupture and produce localized purpura.

DRUG INDUCED

Several drugs are known to cause vasculitis with the appearance of ecchymoses in the absence of thrombocytopenia. Aspirin, quinine, and warfarins (see below) are a few of those reported.[2] A variety of immune mechanisms result in pathology similar to that seen with infections as described above.

PURPURA SIMPLEX

A benign condition known as purpura simplex or "easy bruising" syndrome commonly occurs in young women. Spontaneous small ecchymoses appear on the skin of the thighs or upper arms and are sometimes called "devil's pinches."[2] In some patients, all laboratory tests are negative and in others various phases of the platelet aggregation test are abnormal. The cause of the condition is unknown although it is believed that some may have mild disorders of platelet dysfunction or unknown drug sensitivities that cannot be detected by present laboratory methods. Approximately 30% to 40% of individuals have increased numbers of large platelets and antiplatelet antibodies indicating an immune platelet process.

MECHANICAL PURPURA

Petechial hemorrhages in the skin may be caused by increased pressure within the lumen of capillaries after intense exercise, coughing spasms, or epileptic seizures.

ARTIFICIALLY INDUCED PURPURA

Artificially induced bruises may be self-inflicted or result from abuse by others. The cause is difficult to distinguish

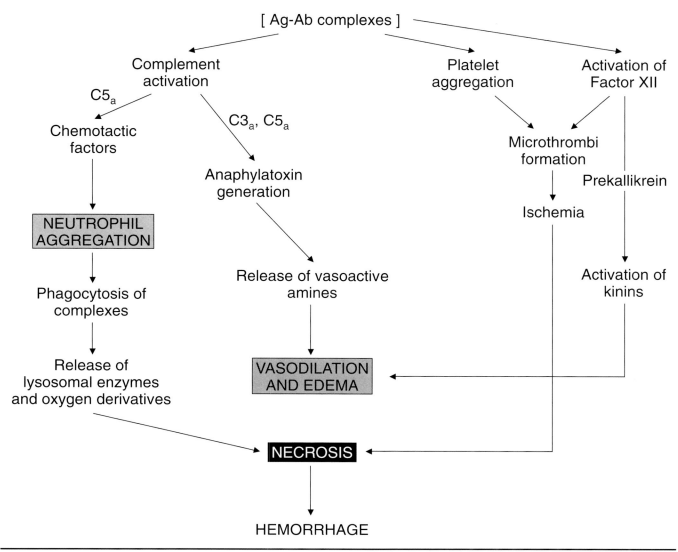

FIGURE 25-3. Vascular damage (vasculitis) caused by immune complexes leads to the activation of the complement cascade, platelet aggregation, and activation of factor XII. As a result, tissue necrosis and hemorrhage accompanied by dilation of blood vessels and edema develop. The hemorrhage results in nonthrombogenic purpura. See text for explanation.

from a true pathologic process. Another artificially induced cause of purpura and bleeding is the unnecessary, secretive overuse of anticoagulant drugs such as heparin and coumadin. This type of abuse may be suspected in health professionals who are aware of the consequences of anticoagulant drugs and have knowledge of ways of obtaining them. Often they have psychological problems that lead to the abuse of the drugs.

Petechial purpura may be induced by placing negative pressure on the skin for a prolonged period as, for instance, sucking the air from a glass held to the mouth. Petechiometer devices are based on this principle.

Autoerythrocyte and DNA sensitivities

Painful, single ecchymoses develop spontaneously in patients with anomalies called autoerythrocyte sensitivity and DNA sensitivity. The cause of the lesions is unclear but can be reproduced by intradermal injection of various erythrocyte fractions or DNA, respectively.

Other symptoms such as nausea and vomiting and bleeding from other sites may occur at the time of development of the bruises. Patients are almost always middle-aged women who also have emotional or psychological disturbances. No effective treatment has been found.

PLATELET DISORDERS

The function of platelets in hemostasis is to form the primary hemostatic plug. Platelet plugs are a response to injury to blood vessels and minimize blood loss. Platelets also aid in subsequent fibrin formation and clot retraction which comprise the secondary hemostatic plug.

TABLE 25-5 *CLASSIFICATION OF NUMERICAL PLATELET ABNORMALITIES*

THROMBOCYTOPENIA

Increased destruction
    Immune
    Nonimmune

Decreased production
    Megakaryocyte hypoplasia
    Replacement of normal marrow
    Ineffective thrombopoiesis
    Inherited disorders

Increased splenic sequestration

Dilution

Multifactorial causes

THROMBOCYTOSIS

Primary

Secondary

Platelet disorders are classified as quantitative or qualitative in nature. Petechiae, epistaxis, gastrointestinal bleeding, excess bleeding from superficial wounds, cuts, or tooth extraction, and easy bruisability are common manifestations of both qualitative and quantitative abnormalities. Others are listed in Table 25-1. The symptoms reflect the decreased ability of the platelets to form a primary hemostatic plug.

●
Quantitative platelet disorders

Quantitative abnormalities of platelets include those in which the platelet count is either too low or too high (Table 25-5). When the platelet count is below the lower limit of the reference range, the condition is termed *thrombocytopenia*. *Thrombocytosis* describes a platelet count above the reference range. The causes, clinical manifestations, and laboratory findings of each of these disorders will be discussed in the following section. Because platelet counts that are performed on automated instruments can be erroneously altered by several means, artifacts in platelet counting also will be discussed.

THROMBOCYTOPENIA

In most laboratories, thrombocytopenia is defined as a platelet count below 150×10^9/L. However, clinical symptoms are usually not seen unless the platelet count falls below 50×10^9/L.

When the platelet count is below 50×10^9/L, the severity of the clinical manifestations may, to some degree, parallel the platelet count. At concentrations less than 30×10^9/L, one may see menorrhagia, petechiae, or spontaneous bruising with little or no trauma. The possibility of severe and spontaneous bleeding is quite high when the platelet count is below 10×10^9/L. Fatal bleeding into the central nervous system may then occur. Also possible is spontaneous bleeding from mucous membranes, such as the gastrointestinal tract, the genitourinary tract, and

the nose. The extent of symptoms at all platelet levels vary from patient to patient and may be affected by medications, the status of the blood vessels, the activity of the platelets themselves, or concurrent disease.

In the laboratory, the platelet count obtained by either automated or chamber methods should be confirmed by estimating the concentration on a peripheral blood smear. The presence of morphologically abnormal forms, such as those larger than normal (megathrombocytes), those with decreased or absent granules (hypo- or agranular), or a combination of the two should be reported.

The bleeding time is prolonged proportionately when the platelet count is between 10 and 100×10^9/L. The linear relationship is altered if patients have abnormalities of platelet function in addition to the decreased number. Laboratory tests for coagulation factors are unaffected by thrombocytopenia.

Thrombocytopenia is the most common cause of excess or abnormal bleeding. The finding of a decreased platelet count with or without abnormalities of other hematologic parameters will alert the physician to search for a cause so that the condition can be appropriately treated.

Decreased platelets are found as a primary feature or as a secondary manifestation of several conditions. Thrombocytopenia is classified into five major categories based on pathophysiology: (1) increase in destruction or utilization; (2) decreased or ineffective production; (3) increased splenic sequestration; (4) dilution; and (5) multifactorial causes (Table 25-5).

Increased destruction The first cause of thrombocytopenia to be considered is increased destruction of platelets. The platelets in the conditions in this category have a decreased lifespan after they have been released into the peripheral blood. The function of the bone marrow is normal, and it attempts to compensate for the decreased numbers in the peripheral blood. However, the platelets are eliminated from the circulation faster than the bone marrow can produce them (Fig. 25-4). Causes of increased destruction are subdivided into two categories: immune and nonimmune (Table 25-6).

IMMUNE DESTRUCTION The immune type of platelet destruction is antibody-mediated. Immune destruction of platelets is analogous to that of erythrocytes in immune hemolytic anemias (see Chapter 12). The specificities of the antibodies, however, have not yet been determined in most instances.

The most likely mechanism of destruction is phagocytosis of antibody-sensitized platelets by splenic macrophages. These macrophages possess Fc receptors by which they recognize platelets coated with antibody (Fig. 25-5). Liver macrophages may remove platelets coated with large amounts of antibody. Antibody attachment to platelets (via the Fab fragment), in some cases, is via specific antigens on the platelet surface. Antigenic determinants related to the glycoproteins IIb/IIIa and Ib/IX complexes have been reported.[7] In other cases, nonspecific attachment of antigen-antibody complexes to platelet Fc receptors is believed to occur. The antibodies are most often of

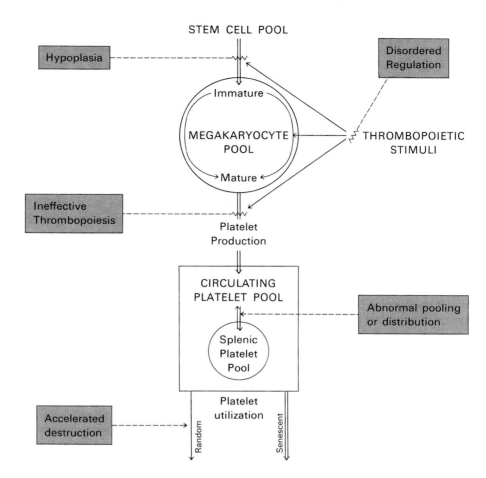

FIGURE 25-4. Schematic drawing of several mechanisms of thrombocytopenia. The solid lines indicate the normal sequence of platelet production by megakaryocytes in the bone marrow from stem cells through normal destruction by random utilization or senescence. The broken lines are sites where pathologic processes lead to thrombocytopenia. The processes are labeled in the shaded boxes. (With permission from: Bithell, T.C. Thrombocytopenia: Pathophysiology and Classification. In: Wintrobe's Clinical Hematology, 9th Ed. Edited by G.R. Lee, T.C. Bithell, J. Foerster, J.W. Athens, J.N. Lukens. Philadelphia: Lea & Febiger, 1993.)

the IgG class and can be measured as platelet associated immunoglobulin (PAIgG). IgM antibodies have been reported rarely.[8] Complement is usually not activated.

Platelet survival time is decreased as determined by ^{51}Cr tests. The lifespans may range from a few minutes to 2 or 3 days. The level to which the platelet count becomes decreased is dependent on the concentration and activity of the antibody, on the function of the macrophages Fc

TABLE 25-6   *CLASSIFICATION OF THROMBOCYTOPENIA FROM INCREASED DESTRUCTION*

IMMUNE

Idiopathic thrombocytopenia purpura

Transplacental thrombocytopenia

Alloantibodies—(transfusion or pregnancy)

Drugs

Other diseases

NONIMMUNE

Disseminated intravascular coagulation

Thrombotic thrombocytopenic purpura

Hemolytic uremic syndrome

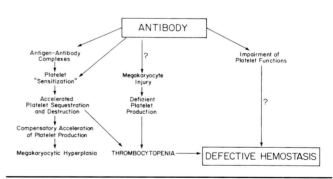

FIGURE 25-5. Immune thrombocytopenia (ITP) is caused by antibody that sensitizes platelets and leads to accelerated destruction. When bone marrow compensatory mechanisms are overwhelmed, thrombocytopenia develops. Additional proposed mechanisms are injury to the megakaryocytes and impairment of platelet function. The latter two have not yet been proven. (With permission from: Bithell, T.C.: Thrombocytopenia caused by immunologic platelet destruction: Idiopathic thrombocytopenic purpura (ITP), drug-induced thrombocytopenia, and miscellaneous forms. In: Wintrobe's Clinical Hematology. 9th Ed. Edited by G.R. Lee, T.C. Bithell, J. Foerster, J.W. Athens, J. N. Lukens. Philadelphia: Lea & Febiger, 1993.)

TABLE 25-7 *COMPARATIVE FEATURES OF ACUTE AND CHRONIC ITP*

Feature	Acute ITP	Chronic ITP
Peak age incidence	Children, 2 to 6 years	Adult, 20 to 40 years
Platelet count	$<20 \times 10^9$/L	$30-80 \times 10^9$/L
Onset of bleeding	Abrupt	Insidious
Antecedent infection	Commonly 1–3 weeks before onset	Unusual
Sex predilection	None	Females 3:1 more common than males
Eosinophilia and lymphocytosis	Common	Rare
Hemorrhagic bullae in mouth	Present in severe cases	Usually absent
Duration	2–6 weeks, rarely longer	Months or years (lifetime)
Spontaneous remissions	Occur in 80% of cases	Uncommon; course of disease fluctuates
Therapy	None, corticosteroids	Corticosteroids, splenectomy

and complement receptors, and on the ability of the bone marrow to increase platelet production to compensate for the increased loss.[8]

The mean platelet volume (MPV) as measured electronically is increased. This may be reflected on the peripheral blood smear as increased numbers of platelets that are larger than 2.5 μm in diameter.[1] An inverse relationship exists between the platelet count and the number of large platelets when the count is less than 50×10^9/L.[9]

Immune thrombocytopenia is present in several clinical situations: (1) idiopathic forms, (2) transplacental thrombocytopenia, (3) alloantibodies induced by transfusion or pregnancy, (4) drug related, or (5) conditions related to other diseases (Table 25-6).

The most common immune form of thrombocytopenia is known as *idiopathic thrombocytopenic purpura* (ITP). Two, possibly three, major forms of the disease occur based on the duration of the disease: acute, chronic, and an intermittent form. A fourth type is found in newborn infants of mothers with ITP and is called transplacental autoimmune thrombocytopenic purpura.

Acute ITP (Table 25-7) occurs most often in children 2 to 6 years of age, is not sex-dependent, and often follows a viral infection by 1 to 3 weeks. Nonspecific upper respiratory infections, chickenpox, rubella, cytomegalovirus, viral hepatitis, and so forth are some diseases that have been implicated.

Symptoms of the disease include the abrupt onset of easy bruising, petechiae on the extemities, and bleeding from mucous membranes. Spontaneous bleeding into the central nervous system, although rare, may occur. The spleen is not enlarged, and there is no fever.

The diagnosis is made by the exclusion of all other causes of thrombocytopenia. Laboratory tests should include peripheral blood counts, examination of the blood smear, and tests to rule out other diseases. A bone marrow examination may be done but is not always necessary. The platelet count is often decreased to less than 20×10^9/L. The bleeding time is usually not performed because it will be prolonged in proportion to the severity of the thrombocytopenia.

Except for thrombocytopenia, the findings on a peripheral blood smear are within normal limits for the age of the patient unless an underlying condition exists. There may be an increase in the number of lymphocytes or a mild eosinophilia in some cases.

In approximately 90% of patients with acute ITP, there is an increase in the amount of IgG immunoglobulin attached to the surface of the platelet.[7] Several laboratory procedures have been developed to identify this platelet-associated IgG. Its use, however, is limited to being positive evidence of the disease. It also may be increased in other forms of immune thrombocytopenia.

The bone marrow in ITP, if performed, is done to evaluate the megakaryocytes and rule out other causes of thrombocytopenia.[1] The granulocyte and erythrocyte precursors are normal in development, and no abnormal cells are present. Megakaryocytes, however, are increased, often markedly, reflecting stimulation by thrombopoietin to produce more platelets. In cases of severe thrombocytopenia, the marrow may increase production up to five times normal. The ploidy of megakaryocytes also is increased resulting in a larger cytoplasmic mass and eventually in increased numbers of platelets produced. A majority of the megakaryocytes may be young forms showing scant cytoplasm and lack of lobulation in the nucleus. Vacuoles in the cytoplasm have been described. These changes reflect the rapid turnover of megakaryocytes and not abnormal morphology.

Most patients (93%) with acute ITP experience a spontaneous remission within 2 to 6 weeks of the onset of the illness.[1] The disease does not recur in these patients. Some patients fail to achieve a remission by 6 months. They are then said to have the chronic form of the disease.

Treatment for patients with acute ITP primarily includes prevention of trauma to reduce the risk of bleeding. Steroids are given by some physicians in an attempt to reduce the risk of bleeding into the central nervous system.[1]

The *chronic* form of ITP (Table 25-7) is believed by some to be a different disease. This form is seen at any age but is more common in young women, 20 to 40 years of age. The female to male ratio of the disease is 3:1. In contrast to the acute form, the onset is more insidious and the platelet count higher, in the range of 30 to 80 $\times$ 10^9/L.

Serum platelet autoantibodies are found more often in the chronic form, as demonstrated by indirect tests for PAIgG. Platelet autoantibodies are believed to be directed toward the GPIIb/IIIa fibrinogen receptor on the platelet membrane in some patients, but the exact antigenic stimulation and mode of platelet destruction is unknown.[1]

The peripheral blood and bone marrow morphology are similar to that seen in the acute form of the disease.

Patients with chronic ITP are treated in an attempt to raise their platelet counts to levels of at least 40 $\times$ 10^9/L. Corticosteroids are useful in many patients. These drugs act in a variety of ways on the immune system to reduce the sequestration of the sensitized platelets by the spleen. Because the spleen is the major site of antibody production as well as platelet destruction, splenectomy is advised for all patients with chronic ITP. It is successful in a majority of patients, although relapse occurs in 10% to 12% within 1 to 5 years. In patients refractory to both corticosteroids and splenectomy, treatment with immunosuppressive drugs and high doses of gamma globulin have been attempted with limited success.

The clinical course of ITP in some patients consists of alternate periods of remissions within 6 months of the onset followed by relapse after at least 3 months. This is referred to as an *intermittent* form of the disease.

An immune form of thrombocytopenia occurs in newborn infants of mothers with ITP called *transplacental* or *neonatal thrombocytopenia*. It is estimated that ITP affects 1 to 2 of every 10,000 pregnancies.[7] Approximately 15% to 65% of infants born to mothers with ITP have thrombocytopenia. Between 6% and 70% of these will have severe thrombocytopenia with platelet counts of less than 50 $\times$ 10^9/L. The maternal platelet count does not correlate with that of the fetus. Laboratory tests for PAIgG in the mother are not useful in predicting which infants will develop severe thrombocytopenia.[7]

The condition is often self-limited. Thrombocytopenia lasts an average of 3 to 4 weeks postnatally, until the antibody is metabolized. In some cases, devastating intracranial hemorrhage occurs.[7]

Immune platelet destruction may be caused by alloantibodies that are stimulated by foreign antigens after a blood transfusion or during pregnancy. Rare patients develop thrombocytopenia 7 to 10 days after blood transfusion. Symptoms such as bleeding from mucous membranes and purpura begin abruptly and last 2 to 6 weeks. The antigenic stimulus is either the platelet specific antigen, Pl^{A1}, or Br^a in more than 95% of cases. HLA antigens also may play a role. The mechanism of platelet destruction is as yet controversial. Platelet alloantibodies are most often demonstrated circulating in the serum but do not attach to platelets in vivo, in contrast to autoantibodies.

Platelet destruction by alloantibodies is found in neonates whose mothers lack a platelet specific antigen, such as Pl^{A1}, but who have inherited the antigen from their fathers. Approximately 2% of people lack this antigen.

Transplacental passage of maternal IgG antiplatelet antibodies results in immune destruction of the infants platelets. Symptoms appear at, or shortly after birth and are self-limited. There is, however, a high mortality rate due to bleeding into the central nervous system; this may be a result of birth trauma that is complicated by low levels of coagulation proteins due to immaturity of the liver (see Chapter 26).

Another category of immune platelet destruction is that caused by drugs. Several drugs have been implicated in causing thrombocytopenia in a small percentage of patients who take them. There is, however, very little experimental evidence to establish that these drugs are the actual cause of the decreased platelet count. Many times the thrombocytopenia occurs weeks to months after the drug has first been taken. The most commonly involved drugs are quinidine, quinine, gold salts, sulfonamides and derivatives, and heparin. For these, the experimental and clinical association is more substantial. In some cases, the offending agent is a metabolite of the drug rather than the original form of the drug. Symptoms of excess bleeding appear suddenly and disappear when the suspected drug is removed. The platelet count may be very low, often less than 10 $\times$ 10^9/L.[10]

Because most drugs are too small to be immunogenic, they must attach to a larger structure to stimulate antibody formation. The structure might be a carrier protein in the plasma or it may be structural determinants on the platelets themselves, such as glycoprotein Ib/IX or IIb/IIIa. The antibodies are of the IgG type.[10]

Once the antibody is formed, there are a variety of mechanisms by which they adhere to platelets. These are analogous to the effect of drugs on erythrocytes in hemolytic anemia (see Chapter 12).[10] In one described mechanism, the drug may attach to a carrier protein in the circulation and result in antibody formation. An immune complex is formed as the antibody combines with the antigen. This complex may then adhere to the platelet, which is an "innocent bystander."[1] The process by which the immune complex attaches to the platelet is unknown. It might be by means of the Fc portion of the immunoglobulin or by adsorption of the drug on the platelet surface.[10]

Another mechanism appears to involve association of the drug or its metabolites with components of the platelet membrane. The glycoproteins Ib/IX and IIb/IIIa are typical sites of drug association. The drug may become a hapten. The resulting antibody may combine with the drug on the platelet surface by means of its Fab portions. This mechanism has been shown in quinidine sensitivity (Fig. 25-6).[10]

Alternatively, the drug may cause an alteration in the normal platelet surface, allowing the surface to become antigenic. Antibody subsequently attaches to the altered platelet surface. The level of PAIgG is increased in all cases of drug-induced thrombocytopenia, indicating attachment of the immunoglobulin to the platelet.[10]

Heparin, a drug used for prevention or treatment of thrombosis (see Chapter 26), causes thrombocytopenia in approximately 5% to 6% of patients who receive it.[10,11] In some patients, the platelet count may be below 50 $\times$

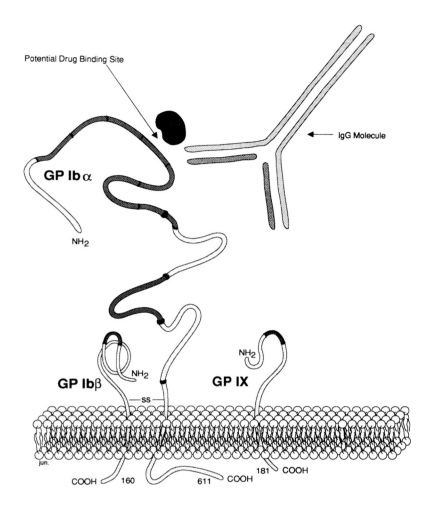

FIGURE 25-6. The proposed mechanism by which quinidine attaches to platelets and leads to drug-induced thrombocytopenia. The drug binds to a surface glycoprotein which may be glycoprotein Ib/IX, IIb/IIIa or others. Antibody attaches by the Fab portion leaving the Fc portion free. Macrophage Fc receptors may recognize the coated platelets and remove them from the circulation. (With permission from: Warkentin, T.E., Trimble, M.S., Kelton, J.G.: Thrombocytopenia due to platelet destruction and hypersplenism. In: Hematology: Basic Principles and Clinical Practice. 2nd Ed. Edited by R. Hoffman, E.J. Benz, Jr., S.J. Shattil, B. Furie, H.J. Cohen, and L.E. Silberstein. New York: Churchill Livingstone, 1995.)

10^9/L. The antiheparin IgG antibodies bind to heparin by the Fab sites possibly with the association of platelet factor 4 (Fig. 25-7). The Fc portion of the IgG then binds to the platelet Fc receptors. This leads to platelet release and activation.[10]

The thrombocytopenia induced by heparin is complicated by causing thrombosis in about 10% to 30% of patients who have antiheparin antibodies. When thrombosis occurs, the platelet count drops suddenly. For this reason, for patients receiving heparin therapy, daily platelet counts are recommended to watch for a sudden drop.

Immune thrombocytopenia occurs as a secondary feature in many diseases. While a variety of mechanisms may contribute to thrombocytopenia in many disease states, there appears to be an immune element in collagen diseases, including systemic lupus erythematosus and rheumatoid arthritis, in lymphoproliferative disorders such as Hodgkins disease and chronic lymphocytic leukemia, and in solid tumors. Additional mechanisms leading to decreased platelets in these diseases will be discussed below.

Patients with infections may develop thrombocytopenia because of immune destruction. All types of infectious agents have been implicated. The Epstein-Barr virus in infectious mononucleosis, cytomegalovirus, rubella, mumps, and nonspecific viral infections are some examples of viral agents. Thrombocytopenia occurs in more than one third of patients with bacterial septicemia. The thrombocytopenia is usually not less than 50×10^9/L and resolves when the infection is treated. The reduced platelet count is accompanied by the typical features of an immune process: shortened platelet survival, increased megakaryocytes in the bone marrow, large platelets on the blood smear, and elevated levels of PAIgG.[10] In a small number of patients with bacterial infections, a condition known as disseminated intravascular coagulation (DIC) also develops (see Chapter 26).

A thrombocytopenic disorder has been studied in homosexually active males and chronic narcotic addicts. Several patients were shown to have decreased platelet counts that were the result of platelet-adhering immune complexes and complement. Patients in this group often have AIDS, AIDS-related complex, or hepatitis.

NONIMMUNE MECHANISMS Increased destruction of platelets occurs by mechanisms other than those involving the immune system. Platelets can be destroyed by nonimmune mechanisms within the circulation in the following ways: (1) in situations when thrombin is formed intravascularly,

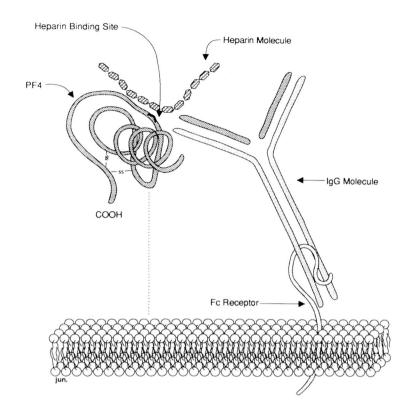

FIGURE 26-7. Proposed mechanism of binding of heparin and platelet factor 4 to the Fab binding site of an anti-heparin antibody. The Fc portion of the immunoglobulin attaches to platelet Fc receptors. The platelet becomes activated and removed from the circulation. (With permission from: Warkentin, T.E., Trimble, M.S., Kelton, J.G.: Thrombocytopenia due to platelet destruction and hypersplenism. In: Hematology: Basic Principles and Clinical Practice. 2nd Ed. Edited by R. Hoffman, E.J. Benz, Jr., S.J. Shattil, B. Furie, H.J. Cohen, L.E. Silberstein. New York: Churchill Livingstone, 1995.)

resulting in fibrin formation and platelet activation and fragmentation, (2) after damage to blood vessel endothelium so that platelets are activated by surface contact with subendothelial collagen, and (3) by mechanical destruction in patients with artificial heart valves.

Disseminated intravascular coagulation is a disorder in which fibrin formation within the blood vessels leads to platelet activation and destruction. This disease will be discussed in detail with coagulation factor deficiencies, because platelet destruction is a result of consumption combined with utilization of coagulation factors.

Diseases in which platelet utilization occurs without activation of the coagulation cascade are thrombotic thrombocytopenic purpura (TTP) and hemolytic uremic syndrome (HUS). These have been discussed with the hemolytic anemias in a previous chapter because erythrocyte destruction also is a classic feature of these disorders.

In patients with artificial heart valves or vascular grafts, platelets are used by adherence to the artificial prosthesis and also by mechanical rupture as the valves open and close.

Decreased platelet production A second category of disorders causing thrombocytopenia is characterized by failure of the bone marrow to deliver adequate numbers of platelets to the peripheral blood. The bone marrow in these disorders is abnormal, and thrombocytopenia develops secondarily. Examination of bone marrow smears and sections is required for diagnosis of the primary condition.

Decreased concentration of platelets occurs because: (1) megakaryocyte hypoplasia exists in the bone marrow,

(2) there is ineffective thrombopoiesis, or (3) the patient has a hereditary thrombocytopenic disorder (Table 25-8).

Hypoplasia of megakaryocytes (Fig. 25-4) may be the result either of decreased proliferation of megakaryocytes in the bone marrow or of replacement of the bone marrow by neoplastic, fibrous, or granulomatous tissue. Sometimes all three cell lines are affected and sometimes it is only the megakaryocytes. The most frequent cause of mar-

TABLE 25-8   *CAUSES OF DECREASED PLATELET PRODUCTION*

HYPOPLASIA OF MEGAKARYOCYTES

Decreased megakaryocyte proliferation
   Chemotherapy and radiation therapy for malignant disease
   Aplastic anemias
      Acquired
      Fanconi syndrome
      Thrombocytopenia with absent radii

Replacement of normal marrow
   Leukemias, preleukemias
   Other neoplastic disease
   Fibrous or granulomatous tissue

INEFFECTIVE THROMBOPOIESIS

Megaloblastic anemia

HEREDITARY THROMBOCYTOPENIA

Wiscott-Aldrich syndrome

Bernard-Soulier disease

May-Hegglin anomaly

row hypoplasia is drug or radiation therapy for malignant disease. Chemotherapeutic agents and radiotherapy produce generalized marrow suppression so that all three cell lines are affected. The marrow regenerates shortly after the therapy is stopped. The platelets may be the last cell line to recover.

Megakaryocytes are decreased in aplastic anemias, a bone marrow disease characterized by pancytopenia and bone marrow replacement by fat (see Chapter 9). A decreased platelet count may appear before hypoplasia of other cell lines and may be the last cell line to return to normal after recovery. Platelet size (MPV) is normal at all platelet count levels in aplastic conditions in contrast to the increased MPV seen in the thrombocytopenia of immune processes. Platelets may, however, demonstrate an increased variation in size as indicated by the platelet distribution width, PDW, on electronic instruments.

Chapter 9 discussed bone marrow aplasia and said that it is most often acquired but that it can also be inherited. Acquired aplastic anemia develops in rare individuals following infections, exposure to toxic chemicals, idiopathic disorders, and because of ingestion of certain drugs such as chloramphenicol. In constitutional aplastic anemia (Fanconi syndrome), pancytopenia is evident in childhood. It usually occurs before 10 years of age, and it may be accompanied by other anomalies. Thrombocytopenia with absent radii is another inherited condition characterized by hypoplasia of the megakaryocyte cell line but with normal erythrocyte and leukocyte precursors. Associated anomalies include absence of radii and other malformations. The syndrome is diagnosed in the newborn.

Replacement of marrow by abnormal cells results in thrombocytopenia due to decreased numbers of megakaryocytes. The diagnosis of acute leukemia is usually not considered in the absence of thrombocytopenia. Some "preleukemic" conditions or myelodysplastic syndromes have decreased platelets as part of their pathology. The bone marrow may have normal or increased numbers of megakaryocytes, many of which are micromegakaryocytes. Peripheral blood platelets also may have abnormal morphology and abnormal function, as indicated in the platelet aggregation test. Marrow replacement by solid tumors or by fibrous tissue, as in agnogenic myeloid metaplasia, may sometimes result in thrombocytopenia, although, for reasons unknown, thrombocytosis is more common. Large platelet size, independent of the platelet count, and association with hypogranular forms is reported in infiltrative marrow disease.

Megaloblastic anemias caused by a deficiency of vitamin B_{12} or folic acid are characterized by ineffective thrombopoiesis as well as ineffective erythro- and granulopoiesis (Fig. 25-4). Pancytopenia is often seen in these diseases. The bone marrow contains normal or increased numbers of megakaryocytes, but the number of platelets entering the peripheral blood is decreased. Platelets of patients with megaloblastic anemia have a decreased mean platelet volume overall, but also demonstrate greater platelet volume heterogeneity as measured by the PDW on the Coulter counter model S-plus.

Wiscott-Aldrich syndrome, Bernard-Soulier disease, and May-Hegglin anomaly are inherited disorders in which platelet production is decreased. These disorders also demonstrate other abnormalities. The Wiscott-Aldrich syndrome, an x-linked disorder, is characterized by very small platelets, thrombocytopenia, eczema, and infections. Bernard-Soulier disease is discussed later in this chapter, and May-Hegglin anomaly is discussed in Chapter 13.

Increased splenic sequestration The spleen normally stores one third of the platelets produced by the bone marrow in a pool that is in equilibrium with circulating platelets. In some conditions in which the spleen is enlarged, the number of platelets sequestered also is increased and may reach 90% of the total platelet mass.[10] Because the bone marrow production remains constant, the number of circulating platelets is decreased. The platelet count is usually above 20×10^9/L. Symptoms of excess bleeding usually are not seen.[10]

Most causes of thrombocytopenia resulting from splenomegaly are complicated by other factors that also lead to thrombocytopenia. It is rare for splenomegaly to occur as a single event. Examples of diseases in which the spleen is enlarged are hepatic cirrhosis and lymphomas. The decreased platelet count in lymphomas may be complicated by bone marrow infiltration with the malignant cells.

Some myeloproliferative disorders are characterized by splenomegaly but increased platelet counts. In these conditions, the number of platelets sequestered is increased, but the spleen also may be involved in producing platelets.

Hypersplenism is a condition in which the spleen is enlarged, but the number of macrophages also is increased. Platelets are removed by increased pooling and by increased phagocytosis. Platelet size in hypersplenism is normal. The enlarged spleen may simultaneously sequester erythrocytes and neutrophils.

Dilution Patients who experience massive hemorrhage requiring replacement of 10 to 30 units of blood may develop thrombocytopenia, if stored bank blood alone is used for transfusion. Platelets in these patients can be replaced by transfusion of platelet concentrates.[12]

Multiple factorial causes of thrombocytopenia Multiple factors contribute to thrombocytopenia in alcoholism, lymphoproliferative disease, and following cardiopulmonary bypass surgery (Table 25-9). In alcoholic patients without cirrhosis, the effect of ethanol is on the platelets alone. When cirrhosis is present, coagulation factors also are effected. Alcohol affects platelet numbers and also causes defects of aggregation, release, and procoagulant activity. Platelet production is suppressed by a direct toxic effect of alcohol on the bone marrow and also by ineffective production associated with a deficiency of folate. Patients with cirrhosis have enlarged spleens also contributing to thrombocytopenia.

In lymphoproliferative disease, when the tumor affects the bone marrow, production of platelets is impaired. Additionally, the production of autoantibodies may enhance

TABLE 25-9 *DISORDERS CHARACTERIZED BY MULTIPLE FACTORS CAUSING THROMBOCYTOPENIA*

ALCOHOLISM

Suppression of platelet production

Ineffective platelet production

Increased destruction

Splenomegaly

LYMPHOPROLIFERATIVE DISEASE

Impaired production

Immune destruction

Splenomegaly

CARDIOPULMONARY BYPASS SURGERY

Mechanical destruction

Increased utilization

TABLE 25-10 *CAUSES OF THROMBOCYTOSIS*

PRIMARY THROMBOCYTOSIS

Essential thrombocythemia

Chronic myelogenous leukemia

Polycythemia vera

Myelofibrosis with myeloid metaplasia

Idiopathic refractory sideroblastic anemia

5q-syndrome

SECONDARY THROMBOCYTOSIS

Acute hemorrhage

Surgery

Post splenectomy

Recovery from thrombocytopenia
    Alcohol-induced thrombocytopenia
    Chemotherapeutic drugs
    Therapy of vitamin B_{12} deficiency

Malignant diseases

Chronic inflammatory diseases

Iron deficiency anemia

Hemolytic anemia

Exercise

Epinephrine

platelet destruction. If splenomegaly is present, splenic sequestration may contribute to the thrombocytopenia.

During *cardiopulmonary bypass surgery*, the patient's blood circulates through a pump outside the body to be oxygenated. Several donor units of blood are used in the process. Hemostasis is altered in a variety of ways. The platelet count is decreased to approximately one half of the original level because of the dilution by donor blood. It usually remains above $100 \times 10^9/L$ during the procedure but may take several days to correct to the patient's usual concentration.[13] Additional effects of extracorporeal circulation will be discussed in later sections.

THROMBOCYTOSIS

Thrombocytosis is a general term for a condition in which the platelet count is elevated above the normal acceptable reference range. Increased numbers of platelets are the result of increased production by the bone marrow since the lifespan of the platelet is not increased.

On the peripheral smear, more than 20 platelets are seen per field, and they usually appear in large clumps on capillary or first drop smears. They may be more concentrated on the feather edge of a smear.

Megakaryocytes are increased in the bone marrow as demonstrated on histologic sections. On buffy coat smears of marrow, great numbers of megakaryocytes may be present on the feather edge.

Elevated platelet counts may result from an abnormality in the control mechanisms produced by hematopoietic growth factors, an abnormality in the megakaryocyte response to hormonal stimulation, or as a physiologic response to an appropriate stimulus. Two forms of thrombocytosis are defined on the basis of etiology of the condition as primary and secondary (Table 25-10).

Primary thrombocytosis In primary thrombocytosis, megakaryocyte proliferation and maturation bypass the normal regulatory mechanisms. Uncontrolled or autonomous production of megakaryocytes results in a marked increase in the number of circulating platelets. The platelet count is usually more than $1000 \times 10^9/L$.[14] In the bone marrow, the number of megakaryocytes as well as the volume of individual megakaryocytes is increased.

Primary thrombocytosis occurs in the chronic myeloproliferative disorders and in some forms of myelodysplasia. The myeloproliferative disorders that are associated with elevated platelet counts include essential thrombocythemia, polycythemia vera, myelofibrous with myeloid metaplasia, and chronic myelocytic leukemia. The myeloproliferative disease in which platelet proliferation predominates is known as essential thrombocythemia and has been discussed in Chapter 15. Increased platelet counts also are seen in 35% of patients with idiopathic refractory sideroblastic anemia and in the 5q-syndrome.

Patients with myeloproliferative disorders can develop symptoms of either bleeding or thrombosis. The cause of each is unknown and is probably due to multiple factors. Factors contributing to thrombotic complications are believed to be related to spontaneous platelet aggregation and release.[15] Patients with chronic myelogenous leukemia only rarely develop thrombosis.

Hemorrhagic symptoms are present in many patients despite the increased numbers of platelets. Epistaxis, bleeding from the gastrointestinal tract and from other mucous membranes can be quite profuse. Excess bruising from minor trauma also is seen. Some patients have a prolonged bleeding time, and most have abnormal in vitro platelet aggregation, most often with epinephrine, indicating some type of platelet dysfunction.[15]

Secondary thrombocytosis In secondary thrombocytosis (also called reactive thrombocytosis), the platelet count is increased because of another disease or condition. The platelet count returns to normal if the primary condition is removed.

Platelet counts are usually lower than $1000 \times 10^9/L$. The bleeding time and platelet aggregation tests are normal, and hemorrhagic and thrombotic complications are infrequent. Megakaryocytes are increased in number in the bone marrow, but the volume of individual cells is normal or may be slightly decreased. The MPV also may be decreased.[14] Conditions commonly associated with reactive thrombocytosis are: (1) After acute hemorrhage or surgery the platelet count may rise to $600 \times 10^9/L$, or greater, and will return to normal within a short period of time. (2) After splenectomy, the platelet count rises, sometimes to greater than $1000 \times 10^9/L$, and may last for several months. The count may even rise during the surgical procedure. The rise in platelet count exceeds that expected for the loss of the splenic reservoir, indicating that the spleen plays a role in regulation of platelet production. (3) Rebound thrombocytosis may follow recovery from thrombocytopenia in alcoholics, patients on chemotherapeutic drugs, or after therapy of vitamin B_{12} deficiency. (4) Thrombocytosis is common in malignant diseases, for example, carcinoma of the lung. (5) Patients with chronic inflammatory diseases, such as rheumatoid arthritis, may have thrombocytosis. (6) Platelet counts in patients with iron deficiency anemia vary from normal to over $1000 \times 10^9/L$. In those with thrombocytosis, the platelet count returns to normal after iron replacement. (7) Other miscellaneous causes include hemolytic anemia, and following exercise or epinephrine therapy.[15]

ARTIFACTS IN THE QUANTITATIVE MEASUREMENT OF PLATELETS

With increasing use of automated electronic methods for counting platelets, the laboratory must be aware of artifacts responsible for erroneously low or high platelet counts.[16] Table 25-11 is a list of the causes of pseudothrombocytopenia or pseudothrombocytosis.[16] Recognition of these artifacts may prevent misdiagnosis and inappropriate or unnecessary diagnostic procedures and therapy. In many cases, these errors can be reduced by examination of a blood smear.

The most frequent cause of spuriously low platelet counts is platelet agglutination in vitro in EDTA anticoagulated blood. This phenomenon occurs in 0.9% to 1.9% of platelet counts.[16] The aggregates that are too large to be counted as platelets by the counting device may be counted as leukocytes. This results in an erroneously high white cell count. Platelet-specific antibodies, IgM and/or IgG, which react best at room temperature and only in the presence of EDTA, are believed to cause the clumping. When EDTA platelet clumping is suspected, venous blood should be drawn using sodium citrate as the anticoagulant, or the count can be done manually using a fingerstick specimen.[16] Several additional types of platelet agglutinins have been reported.

A second cause of spuriously low platelet counts is platelet satellitism[9] (Fig. 25-8) Satellitism occurs in EDTA

TABLE 25-11 *REPORTED CAUSES OF SPURIOUS PLATELET COUNTS*

PSEUDOTHROMBOCYTOPENIA
Giant platelets
Platelet satellitism
Platelet agglutinins
Erythrocyte counts $> 6.5 \times 10^{12}/L$

PSEUDOTHROMBOCYTOSIS
Howell-Jolly bodies
Nucleated erythrocytes
Leukocyte cytoplasmic fragments
Malarial parasites
Aggregated erythrocytic stroma
Clumped Pappenheimer bodies
Heinz bodies
Microspherocytes
Severely microcytic red cells
Necrobiotic cells
Fragmented red cells
Cryoglobulin

From Evans, V.J.: Platelet morphology and the blood smear. Am. Med. Tech. *1*:689, 1984.

anticoagulated blood because platelets adhere to the surface of neutrophils and are, therefore, not counted. Both chamber and electronic counts are affected. Examination of a blood smear reveals the phenomenon.

In individuals with giant platelets, the platelets may be so large that the counter "recognizes" them as erythrocytes rather than as platelets. Review of the blood smear is helpful in this condition.

Causes of spuriously increased platelet counts include the presence of erythrocyte inclusions, erythrocyte frag-

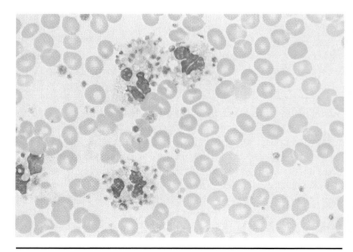

FIGURE 25-8. Platelet satellitism (PB; 250× original magnification; Wright-Giemsa stain).

ments, or otherwise small erythrocytes and malarial parasites, which are counted as platelets by the machine. The blood smear may or may not be of value in these cases.

● Qualitative (functional) platelet disorders

Abnormalities of any phase of platelet function (adhesion, aggregation, or release) may lead to the prolonged or abnormal formation of a primary hemostatic plug. Clinical symptoms vary from mild, easy bruisability to very severe, life-threatening excess bleeding, depending on the nature of the defect. The type of bleeding is similar to that seen in thrombocytopenic disorders. Common manifestations are petechiae, superficial bruises in the skin, which may appear spontaneously, bleeding from mucous membranes such as the nose or abnormal vaginal bleeding, and prolonged bleeding from cuts.

The platelet count is usually normal but could be mildly decreased in certain diseases. The bleeding time is characteristically prolonged, and in patients who also have thrombocytopenia, is increased over and above the expected range. Screening tests for coagulation factors, the prothrombin time, activated partial thromboplastin time, and tests for fibrinolysis are normal.

Platelet functional disorders are either inherited or acquired. The inheritance pattern in the hereditary types is usually autosomal recessive. Special tests for platelet function reflect the nature of the platelet defect and will be discussed with each individual defect.

HEREDITARY DISORDERS OF PLATELET FUNCTION

Hereditary platelet defects are rarely encountered clinically. However, much of the present knowledge of platelet function has been derived by the study of patients with such anomalies. Defects in each phase of platelet function have been described. Therefore, a convenient classification scheme is one that is based on the steps in platelet function. Abnormalities in function can then be related to affected portions of the platelet ultrastructure (Fig. 25-9). The most well-known disorders will be discussed in detail. Others will be mentioned briefly.

Disorders of platelet adhesion Adhesion to collagen requires the presence of both adequate amounts of functional von Willebrand factor and the presence of glycoprotein Ib on the platelet membrane (see Chapter 23). Von Willebrand factor serves as a "bridge," binding the platelet via glycoprotein Ib to collagen. Because adhesion to collagen is the major mechanism initiating platelet function, formation of the primary hemostatic plug is prolonged in patients who demonstrate abnormal platelet adhesion. Two hereditary disorders in which platelets fail to adhere to collagen are known. These are Bernard-Soulier disease and von Willebrand disease.

BERNARD-SOULIER DISEASE *Bernard-Soulier disease* is inherited as an autosomal-recessive trait. Bernard and Soulier first described the rare disorder in 1948. Patients have a lifelong bleeding tendency that may begin in infancy.

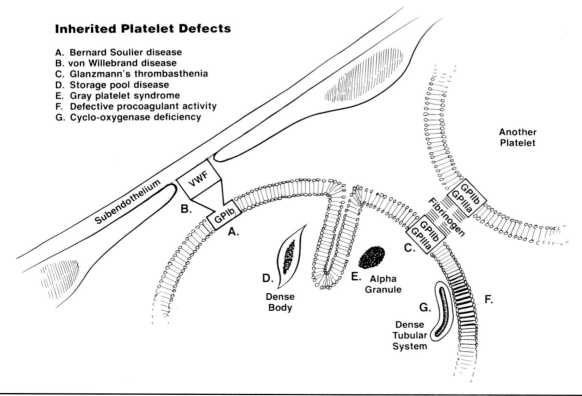

Inherited Platelet Defects

A. Bernard Soulier disease
B. von Willebrand disease
C. Glanzmann's thrombasthenia
D. Storage pool disease
E. Gray platelet syndrome
F. Defective procoagulant activity
G. Cyclo-oxygenase deficiency

FIGURE 25-9. Ultrastructural components associated with inherited disorders of platelet function.

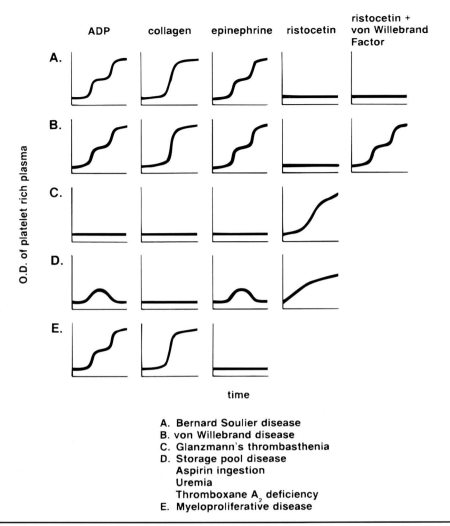

A. Bernard Soulier disease
B. von Willebrand disease
C. Glanzmann's thrombasthenia
D. Storage pool disease
   Aspirin ingestion
   Uremia
   Thromboxane A$_2$ deficiency
E. Myeloproliferative disease

FIGURE 25-10. Platelet aggregation patterns in disorders of platelet function.

Bleeding symptoms most often affect the skin and mucous membranes. Epistaxis, gastrointestinal bleeding, excessive menses, easy bruisability both ecchymotic and petechial, and excess bleeding after trauma are examples of common symptoms.

The defect in Bernard-Soulier disease is a decrease in amount or abnormal function of fractions of platelet membrane glycoprotein, including glycoprotein Ib/IX. It results from a mutation in the genes coding for glycoprotein Ibα, Ibβ, or IX. Lack of functional glycoprotein Ib/IX prevents interaction of the platelets with von Willebrand factor and prevents subsequent adhesion to collagen (Fig. 25-10A). Glycoprotein V also may be deficient, but the significance is unknown.

Laboratory tests (Table 25-12) are required to diagnose this disease and differentiate it from other platelet function disorders and from other causes of thrombocytopenia. The platelet count may be normal or slightly decreased and is variable with time in the same patient. The bleeding time is prolonged more than would be expected for the platelet count, indicating a disorder of platelet

function. Clot retraction is normal. The platelet aggregation test is normal with ADP, collagen, and epinephrine. However, aggregation with ristocetin, which requires von Willebrand factor and glycoprotein Ib/IX, is abnormal (Fig. 25-10A). Similar laboratory results are obtained in patients with von Willebrand disease (Fig. 25-10B). To differentiate these two diseases, a modification of the ristocetin aggregation test is used. The addition of some form of von Willebrand factor does not correct the ristocetin aggregation in Bernard-Soulier patients but will correct the aggregation in von Willebrand disease (Figs. 25-10A and 25-10B).

Bernard-Soulier disease is called the giant platelet syndrome because of the appearance of the platelets on a peripheral blood smear. More than 60% are increased in size with a diameter between 2.5 and 8.0 μm. The cause and significance of the large size is unknown but indicates a defect in the stem cell committed to thrombopoiesis. Platelets also have an increase in the number of dense granules.

There is no specific treatment for Bernard-Soulier dis-

TABLE 25-12 *LABORATORY TEST RESULTS IN SOME PLATELET DISORDERS*

Disorder	Abnormal Portion of Platelet	Platelet Count	Bleeding Time	Clot Retraction	Other
Bernard Soulier disease	Membrane glycoprotein Ib or IX	N or ↓	↑	N	Giant platelets
von Willebrand disease	None (plasma factor abnormality)	N	↑	N	
Glanzmann's disease	Membrane glycoproteins IIb and IIIa	N	↑	Absent	
Storage pool deficiency	Dense granule deficiency	N	↑ or N	N	
Gray platelet syndrome	Alpha granule deficiency	N	N	N	Agranular platelets

N = normal; ↓ = increased; ↑ = decreased; BT = bleeding time

ease. Supportive measures such as erythrocytes and platelet transfusions are used when needed.

VON WILLEBRAND DISEASE *von Willebrand disease* is characterized by a decreased production of von Willebrand factor, or in some variant forms, by an abnormal molecule (Fig. 25-10B). Because it is, in fact, a plasma factor disorder rather than a platelet function disorder, the disease will be discussed later in Chapter 26 as an autosomal dominant coagulation factor disorder.

Disorders of platelet aggregation

Platelet aggregation requires the presence of fibrinogen and the glycoprotein IIb/IIIa receptor on the platelet membrane. In the absence of one or more of these components, platelets will not interact with one another to produce either primary or secondary aggregation.

Congenital disorders in which there is no primary aggregation response are afibrinogenemia, the absence of fibrinogen, which will be discussed in Chapter 26, and Glanzmann thrombosthenia.

GLANZMANN THROMBASTHENIA *Glanzmann thrombasthenia* is a very rare disease that was first described in 1918. Inheritance is autosomal-recessive, and the disease is only apparent in homozygotes. Platelets of patients with Glanzmann disease are deficient in the glycoprotein IIb/IIIa complex (Fig. 25-9C).[17] Glycoproteins IIb and IIIa form the site of attachment of fibrinogen to the platelet surface. The receptor site is hidden in resting platelets and becomes "available" for binding only after stimulation by certain agonists such as ADP and thrombin.[17] When fibrinogen binds to the receptor in the presence of calcium, it becomes the connecting link between two platelets. Platelet aggregation then occurs (see Chapter 23). Other proteins such as von Willebrand factor, fibronectin, and vitronectin can bind to the glycoprotein IIb/IIIa complex, but the significance is not known.[17]

The genes for both glycoproteins are closely linked on the long arm of chromosome 17. A deficiency of the whole complex occurs when the gene for either glycoprotein IIb or IIIa are defective because production of one depends on production of the other.[17,18] The molecular defect in the gene has been studied in a few patients and varies from family to family.

Additional abnormalities of platelets occur in patients with thrombasthenia. Deficiencies of antigens such as P1^{A1} and Bak^a that are normally present on the IIb/IIIa complex are seen. Some patients have a deficiency of fibrinogen in the alpha granules the cause of which is unknown.

Patients with the disease have 5% to 20% of the complex on the platelet surface. Obligate carriers have 50% to 60% and are phenotypically normal.[17]

Because the platelets lack the site for attachment of fibrinogen, aggregation does not occur. Aspects of platelet function that are not dependent on aggregation, such as adhesion, are normal.

Bleeding symptoms may begin in infancy and involve superficial areas of the body characteristic of platelet abnormalities. Although they are usually described as moderate in severity, deaths have occurred. The symptoms do not correlate with the extent of deficiency of the proteins.

Laboratory tests are necessary to differentiate this disorder from other platelet defects. The platelet count and morphology are normal, but the bleeding time is markedly prolonged indicating platelet dysfunction. The platelet aggregation test shows no response to agonists such as ADP, epinephrine, or collagen, which depend on secretion of ADP and thromboxane A$_2$ for aggregation. Normal aggregation, however, occurs with ristocetin (Fig. 25-10C). Because the platelets lack the site for attachment of fibrinogen, aggregation cannot occur.

The clot retraction test is also abnormal (Table 25-12) although it is no longer considered a useful test in the laboratory. Retraction of the clot requires attachment of platelets to fibrin through the glycoprotein IIb/IIIa complex. On the cytoplasmic side of the platelet membrane, the complex is linked to contractile proteins of the platelet cytoskeleton. It is believed that these proteins provide the force for contraction of the fibrin clot.

No specific treatment is available for thrombasthenia patients. Supportive transfusion component therapy is used when needed, and bone marrow transplantation has been performed in rare cases.

Disorders of platelet secretion

Disorders of platelet secretion constitute a heterogenous group of defects in the mechanisms of release from platelet granules or membranes. They include defects in the content of the dense or alpha granules, defects in the mechanism of release from the granules, and defects in enzymes needed for the synthesis of thromboxane A_2 from arachidonic acid. Symptoms vary from moderate to mild bleeding tendencies depending on the abnormality. Manifestations may be easy bruising, hemorrhagia, and excess bleeding after surgery or childbirth.[17] The platelet count is normal and the bleeding time variable.

Deficiencies of dense granules occur as one of the features of several rare autosomal recessive disorders such as Chediak-Higashi syndrome, Hermansky-Pudlak syndrome and Wiscott-Aldrich syndrome. An autosomal dominant trait characterized by an isolated decrease in dense granules is called storage pool disease. The platelets in these disorders show a decrease or absence of dense bodies on electron microscopy (Fig. 25-9D), but the morphologic appearance of the platelets on stained peripheral blood smears is normal. The bleeding time is prolonged (Table 25-12), and the platelet aggregation test is abnormal with ADP, epinephrine, and with low levels of collagen (Fig. 25-10D). With ADP and epinephrine, a normal primary wave of aggregation is present, but because no ADP is released, secondary aggregation does not occur. The platelets disaggregate, and no secondary wave is seen. The platelet aggregation curve induced by collagen is normally produced by release of dense body products and is, therefore, absent. The ratio of ATP to ADP content in the dense granules, which is normally 2:3, is increased. Release of serotonin from dense bodies as well as uptake by the platelets is abnormal in these diseases.[19]

A defect in the pathway of thromboxane A_2 synthesis, particularly a deficiency of the enzyme *cyclo-oxygenase,* produces a platelet aggregation pattern that is similar to that seen in storage pool disease. This occurs because thromboxane A_2 is necessary for secretion from platelet granules (see Chapter 23) after stimulation by weak agonists such as ADP, epiniphrine, and low concentrations of collagen. Cyclo-oxygenase is localized in the dense tubular system (Figs. 25-9G and 25-10D).

Stimulation of the platelet by agonists results in enzymatic release of arachidonic acid from the second carbon of the phospholipids of membranes. Cyclo-oxygenase converts the arachidonic acid to intermediate prostaglandins (PGG_2 and PGH_2). Thromboxane A_2 is formed from the intermediates by an additional enzyme, thromboxane synthase. The thromboxane A_2 leaves the platelet and becomes an agonist by attaching to surface receptors. Secretion from the platelet granules and secondary aggregation then take place. In the absence of cyclo-oxygenase, secretion and secondary aggregation do not occur. Many other abnormalities of platelet secretion have been described. The symptoms and laboratory results are quite variable.[17]

Deficiencies of platelet alpha granules and lysosomal granules have been reported. Because alpha granules are so numerous, their absence causes the platelets to appear agranular on a peripheral blood smear. The disease is called the gray platelet syndrome. In contrast to storage pool disease, platelet aggregation studies are normal, and clinical manifestations are usually mild if present at all

(Fig. 25-9E, Table 25-12). Platelet counts often are decreased.

Disorders of platelet factor 3 release Defective procoagulant activity of platelets has been described as an additional finding in several of the above-mentioned disorders, and as a single entity in one patient (Fig. 25-9F). The clinical and diagnostic significance is as yet unknown.

ACQUIRED DISORDERS OF PLATELET FUNCTION
Platelet dysfunction is induced in a variety of conditions and with the ingestion of certain drugs. Clinical manifestations and the results of laboratory tests vary with the cause and its effect on the platelet mechanism.

Uremia A bleeding tendency in uremia, recognized for many years, was first associated with a platelet functional abnormality in 1956. The pathogenesis and severity of the platelet defect is related to the accumulation of waste products in the blood, although which of the metabolites produces harmful effects is unclear. The bleeding time is prolonged and seems to correlate with the severity of the renal failure.[20] The platelet aggregation test with collagen and secondary aggregation with ADP and epinephrine is decreased, indicating an abnormal secretory response (Fig. 25-10D). Procoagulant activity also is defective. Bleeding symptoms in uremia patients may be severe. Ecchymoses, gastrointestinal bleeding, and hemorrhages into serous cavities are some manifestations. The bleeding time shortens and symptoms lessen when the patient is receiving dialysis treatment.

Hematologic disorders The myeloproliferative disorders, chronic myelogenous leukemia, myelofibrosis with myeloid metaplasia, polycythemia vera, and essential thrombocythemia are characterized by thrombocytosis, by abnormalities of platelet morphology, and, in some instances, by abnormal megakaryocyte morphology. Despite the increased number of platelets, approximately one third of patients experience abnormal bleeding. Another third experience thrombosis. Both bleeding and thrombosis contribute to mortality in a significant number. An abnormal response to epinephrine in the platelet aggregation test is a fairly consistent abnormality. The response to ADP and collagen appears to be variable (Fig. 25-10E).

Defective platelet aggregation has been noted in patients with acute leukemia and myelodysplasia. Studies indicate abnormal storage pool of adenine nucleotides and altered release mechanism. The abnormal test results are also consistent with activation and release within the circulation. Bleeding problems in these conditions, however, are usually the result of thrombocytopenia.

Abnormal platelet function is observed in patients with dysproteinemias, multiple myeloma, and macroglobulinemia. Severe bleeding symptoms can result. Thrombocytopenia and hyperviscosity are the major causes of the bleeding tendency, but platelet function is abnormal because the paraprotein coats the platelet surface and interferes with the membrane reactions of platelet stimulation. The bleeding symptoms and the abnormal platelet function are proportional to the amount of abnormal protein in the plasma.

Abnormal tests include the bleeding time, platelet aggregation test, and platelet factor 3 availability. The results of the abnormal tests, however, do not correlate with the severity of the bleeding.

Drugs

Many drugs have been shown to contribute to platelet dysfunction. The effect of drugs on platelets of persons with normal hemostatic function is usually clinically unnoticeable. However, those with significant abnormalities in the hemostatic system are at greater risk for developing severe bleeding symptoms.

The bleeding time and platelet aggregation studies may be variably altered by drugs. The effect on these laboratory tests do not necessarily correlate with the clinical effects. The mechanisms of inhibiting platelet function also are variable and are not completely understood. Examples follow of the effects of three drugs—aspirin, alcohol, and certain antibiotic agents.

ASPIRIN Aspirin affects platelet function by irreversibly acetylating the cyclo-oxygenase enzyme, and, thereby, preventing the formation and release of thromboxane A_2. In turn, the platelet release mechanism is decreased. A single dose of 650 mg of aspirin can inhibit 95% of the function of cyclo-oxygenase in circulating platelets and also appears to affect developing megakaryocytes. The platelets affected by aspirin continue to circulate but are nonfunctional. Enzyme activity returns as new platelets are produced and may become normal after 7 days, the half-life of the affected platelets.

Laboratory tests of platelet function, therefore, may be artificially altered in patients taking aspirin. The bleeding time in normal persons may be increased by 1 to 2 minutes after taking a single dose of aspirin and may be affected for as long as 7 days. In healthy persons, though, it rarely becomes prolonged beyond the normal range. In persons with a functional abnormality of platelets (either hereditary or acquired) or von Willebrand disease, it may be prolonged far beyond that expected for the dose and may lead to serious bleeding complications. For this reason, a patient must not have ingested aspirin or any of the numerous aspirin-containing products for 7 days before performing the bleeding time.

Abnormalities in the platelet aggregation test reflect the lack of thromboxane A_2 synthesis and are similar to patients with hereditary deficiencies of enzymes in this pathway. A first wave of aggregation is seen with ADP and epinephrine, but no secondary wave is present. Aggregation does not occur with collagen and is decreased with ristocetin (Fig. 25-10D).

ALCOHOL Ingestion of large amounts of alcohol over a long period of time may lead to platelet dysfunction in some individuals. Several mechanisms have been proposed and include inhibition of prostaglandin synthesis and alterations of the storage pool of nucleotides or membrane stabilization. The platelet aggregation test may show decreased primary aggregation with ADP and may affect the release reaction.

CARBENICILLIN Antibiotics, particularly penicillins and cephalosporins, alter platelet function. Patients taking these drugs show no aggregation with ADP either in the primary or secondary wave. The bleeding time may also be prolonged. It is believed that the drug might coat the platelet membrane, block ADP and epinephrine receptors, and result in platelet inability to respond to the agonist. Serious bleeding complications can occur.

Cardiopulmonary bypass surgery

In addition to thrombocytopenia, as discussed previously, platelet function is altered during cardiopulmonary bypass surgery. The dysfunction causes the bleeding time to increase to more than 30 minutes during surgery but is corrected about 2 to 4 hours after the pump is disconnected.[13] It is believed that the platelets become activated temporarily by the abnormal surfaces to which they are exposed.

Significant bleeding develops in approximately 3% to 5% of patients after bypass surgery. Of these, approximately one half improve with additional surgery to tie the ends of severed vessels. The remaining one half may be due to a variety of defects of hemostasis. The most common of these is acquired abnormal platelet function.

SUMMARY

This chapter has described disorders associated with the primary phase of hemostasis. Patients affected by these conditions usually have an imbalance in the hemostatic system and experience hemorrhage of some form or other. Although bleeding may occur in any organ, most patients experience excess bleeding from superficial cuts, more bruising of the skin than usual, and the presence of petechiae. Occasional disorders result in excess clotting, that is, thrombosis, rather than excess bleeding.

Vascular disorders are diverse in origin and may be inherited or acquired. Diagnosis of bleeding symptoms caused by vascular disorders is usually done by excluding other causes of bleeding along with observing symptoms consistent with the underlying disorders. Laboratory tests of hemostasis, with the exception of the bleeding time, are usually normal.

Platelet disorders are broadly categorized as quantitative problems in which the platelet count is too low or too high or abnormalities in which a functional aspect of platelet function is altered. Thrombocytopenia is caused by conditions that affect the bone marrow production of megakaryocytes, by conditions that cause increased destruction of platelets after they are released into the peripheral blood, by conditions in which the spleen in increased in size, or by dilution during the need for transfusion of multiple units of banked blood within a short period of time. Thrombocytosis is seen in myeloproliferative disorders and a number of underlying problems. Functional platelet abnormalities are caused by mutations in genes that produce platelet membrane or granule constituents or may be acquired by ingestion of certain drugs such as aspirin. Laboratory tests that are helpful in establishing the cause of a platelet disorder include platelet counts, the template bleeding time, and platelet aggregation studies.

REVIEW QUESTIONS

The mother of a 4-year-old boy noticed several bruises on his arms, legs, and torso. Upon closer examination, she saw several small, pinhead-sized, brownish purple spots on the ankles. Just before leaving home for the doctor's office, the child had a moderately severe nosebleed. There had been no previous episodes of this type.

Physical examination was unremarkable except for the bruises. The child had not recently taken any medication but was recovering from the chicken pox.

Laboratory results showed:

Erythrocyte count	4.25×10^{12}/L
Hemoglobin	108 g/L
Hematocrit	0.34 L/L
MCV	80.0 fL
MCH	25.4 pg
MCHC	301 g/L
Leukocyte count	5.2×10^9/L
Platelet count	4.0×10^9/L

A bone marrow examination was scheduled but was later cancelled.

1. What disorder is most probably indicated by the patient's history?
   a. Acute leukemia
   b. Bernard-Soulier disease
   c. Immune (idiopathic) thrombocytopenic purpura
   d. Ehlers-Danlos syndrome

2. What would the bone marrow of this patient most probably show?
   a. Normal to increased numbers of megakaryocytes
   b. Large numbers of blast cells
   c. Decreased numbers of erythrocyte precursors
   d. Absence of all myeloid precursors and replacement by fat

3. What is the mechanism of platelet destruction in immune thrombocytopenia?
   a. Lysis by complement in the peripheral blood
   b. Increased sequestration of platelets by the spleen
   c. Removal of antibody-coated platelets by splenic macrophages
   d. Activation and increased utilization by forming aggregates in the blood stream

4. The small purple spots seen on this patient's ankles are most probably
   a. Petechiae
   b. Ecchymoses
   c. Allergic purpura
   d. Hematomas

5. What is the expected prognosis of this patient?
   a. Imminent death from overwhelming infection
   b. Complete spontaneous recovery within six months
   c. Similar problems for the rest of his life
   d. Recovery after a long period of steroid therapy

6. Which of the following platelet counts indicates thrombocytopenia?
   a. 200×10^9/L
   b. 2000×10^9/L
   c. 200×10^{12}/L
   d. 20.0×10^9/L

7. A patient with Bernard Soulier disease will probably have
   a. increased bleeding time
   b. increased prothrombin time
   c. increased platelet count
   d. abnormal platelet aggregation with ADP and collagen

8. A patient with Glanzmann thrombasthenia has
   a. a mutation in the gene for fibrinogen
   b. an acquired abnormality of von Willebrand factor
   c. a genetic abnormality of glycoprotein IIb or IIIa
   d. an acquired vascular disorder

9. A patient with hereditary telangiectasia has
   a. abnormal platelet adhesion to collagen
   b. thrombocytosis
   c. a deficiency of platelet dense bodies
   d. dilated capillaries on mucous membranes that are likely to cause bleeding

10. The platelet aggregation test after ingestion of aspirin will show
   a. normal pattern
   b. lack of both a primary and secondary wave of aggregation with ADP
   c. a primary wave of aggregation with ADP that returns to the baseline
   d. normal aggregation with ADP and epinephrine but not with ristocetin

11. The bleeding time is expected to be normal in
   a. vascular disorders
   b. drug-induced thrombocytopenia
   c. uremia
   d. Bernard-Soulier disease

12. Platelet adhesion is abnormal in Bernard-Soulier disease because
   a. glycoprotein Ib of the platelet membrane is defective
   b. a plasma factor needed for platelet adhesion is absent
   c. antibodies to platelet phospholipid are present
   d. abnormal proteins in the plasma coat the platelet membrane

REFERENCES

1. Bithell, T.C.: Thrombocytopenia caused by immunologic platelet destruction: Idiopathic thrombocytopenic purpura (ITP), drug-in-

duced thrombocytopenia, and miscellaneous forms. In: Wintrobe's Clinical Hematology. 9th Ed. Edited by G.R. Lee, T. C. Bithell, J. Foerster, J.W. Athens, J.N. Lukens. Philadelphia: Lea & Febiger, 1993.

2. Bithell, T.C.: Bleeding disorders caused by vascular abnormalities. In: Wintrobe's Clinical Hematology. 9th Ed. Edited by G.R. Lee, T.C. Bithell, J. Foerster, J.W. Athens, J.N. Lukens. Philadelphia: Lea & Febiger, 1993.

3. Bithell, T.C.: Qualitative disorders of platelet function. In: Wintrobe's Clinical Hematology, 9th Ed. Edited by G.R. Lee, T.C. Bithell, J. Foerster, J.W. Athens, J.N. Lukens. Philadelphia: Lea & Febiger, 1993.

4. Hanes, F.M.: Multiple hereditary telangiectasias causing hemorrhage (hereditary hemorrhagic telangiectasia). Bull. John Hopkins Hosp., 20:63, 1909.

5. Bick, R.L.: Disorders of Thrombosis & Hemostasis: Clinical and Laboratory Practice. Chicago: ASCP Press, 1992.

6. Gottlieb, A.J.: Allergic purpura. In: Hematology. 4th Ed. Edited by W.J. Williams, E. Beutler, A.J. Erslev, M.A. Lichtman. New York: McGraw-Hill, Inc., 1990.

7. McCrae, K.R., Samuels, P., Schreiber, A.D.: Pregnancy associated thrombocytopenia: Pathogenesis and management. Blood, 80:2697, 1992.

8. Bussel, J.B., Schreiber, A.D.: Immunothrombocytopenic purpura, neonatal alloimmune thrombocytopenia, and post transfusion purpura. In: Hematology: Basic Principles and Practice. Edited by R. Hoffman, E.J. Benz, Jr., S.J. Shattil, B. Furie, H.J. Cohen. New York: Churchill Livingstone, 1991.

9. Evans, V.J.: Platelet morphology and the blood smear. J. Med. Tech., 1:689, 1984.

10. Warkentin, T.E., Trimble, M.S., Kelton, J.G.: Thrombocytopenia due to platelet destruction and hypersplenism. In: Hematology: Basic Principles and Practice. 2nd Ed. Edited by R. Hoffman, E.J. Benz, Jr., S.J. Shattil, B. Furie, H.J. Cohen, L.E. Silberstein. New York: Churchill Livingstone, 1995.

11. Tollefsen, D.M. & Binder, M.A.: Heparin. In: Hematology: Basic Principles and Practice. 2nd Ed. Edited by R. Hoffman, E.J. Benz, Jr., S.J. Shattil, B. Furie, H.J. Cohen. New York: Churchill Livingstone, 1995.

12. Bithell, T. C.: Miscellaneous forms of thrombocytopenia. In: Wintrobe's Clinical Hematology. 9th Ed. Edited by G.R. Lee, T.C. Bithell, J. Foerster, J.W. Athens, J.N. Lukens. Philadelphia: Lea & Febiger, 1993.

13. Woodman, R.C., Harker, L.A.: Bleeding complications associated with cardiopulmonary bypass. Blood, 76:1680, 1990.

14. Davis, G.L., Fritsma, G.A.: Platelet disorders. In: Hemostasis and Thrombosis in the Clinical Laboratory. Edited by D.M. Corrivieau, G.A. Fritsma. Philadelphia: J.B. Lippincott Company, 1988.

15. Hoffman, R., Silverstein, M.N., Hromas, R.: Primary thrombocythemia. In: Hematology: Basic Principles and Practice. 2nd Ed. Edited by R. Hoffman, E.J. Benz, Jr., S.J. Shattil, B. Furie, H.J. Cohen, L.E. Silberstein. New York: Churchill Livingstone, 1995.

16. Payne, B.A., Pierce, R.V.: Pseudothrombocytopenia: a laboratory artifact with potentially serious consequences. Mayo Clin. Proc., 59:123, 1984.

17. Bennett, J.S.: Hereditary disorders of platelet function. In: Hematology: Basic Principles and Practice. 2nd Ed. Edited by R. Hoffman, E.J.Benz, Jr., S.J. Shattil, B. Furie, H.J. Cohen, L.E. Silberstein. New York: Churchill Livingstone, 1995.

18. Kato, A., et al: Molecular basis for Glanzmann's thrombasthenia (GT) in a compound heterozygote with glycoprotein IIb gene: A proposal for the classification of GT based on the biosynthetic pathway of glycoprotein IIb-IIIa complex. Blood, 79:3212, 1992.

19. Bennett, J.S., Shattil, S.J.: Platelet function. In: Hematology. 4th Ed. Edited by W.J. Williams, E. Beutler, A.J. Erslev, M.A. Lichtman. New York: McGraw-Hill, Inc. 1990.

20. George, J.N., Shattil, S.J.: Acquired disorders of platelet function. In: Hematology: Basic Principles and Practice. 2nd Ed. Edited by R. Hoffman, E.J. Benz, Jr., S.J. Shattil, B. Furie, H.J. Cohen, L.E. Silberstein. New York: Churchill Livingstone, 1995.

Disorders of secondary hemostasis

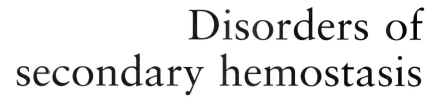

26

CHAPTER OUTLINE

KEY TERMS

chronic ITP
intermittent ITP
transplacental ITP
neonatal ITP
gray platelet syndrome
hemophilia A
hemophilia B
delayed bleeding
cryoprecipitate
factor VIII concentrate
afibrinogenemia
hypofibrinogenemia
dysfibrinogenemia
parahemophilia
hemorrhagic disease of the
  newborn
inhibitors to single factors
lupus-like anticoagulant
embolus
embolism
thromboembolism
deep vein thrombosis (DVT)
thrombophlebitis
prothrombin time ratio
streptokinase
urokinase
prourokinase
APSAC

INTRODUCTION

Chapter 24 discussed the processes of formation and lysis of fibrin after an injury has occurred. Also discussed in that chapter were the inhibitors of both processes that limit the hemostatic mechanisms to the injured area. Deficiences of any of the procoagulant or inhibitor proteins will upset the balance between clotting and lysing. Fibrin formation either will be impaired, or too much fibrin will be formed. The result will be symptoms of either excessive bleeding or inappropriate and unnecessary clotting called thrombosis.

This chapter will discuss the consequences of both situations. The disorders that result in excess bleeding will be considered first. Deficiencies of most of the fibrin-forming proteins are included in this category. For each defect, the pathophysiologic basis and the clinical manifestations will be presented. A major emphasis will be placed on the laboratory involvement in the diagnosis and treatment of the defects. Because a form of coagulation protein deficiency occurs in newborn infants, a section on newborn hemostasis also is included.

A section on thrombosis will conclude this chapter. The discussion includes the contributing factors, the mechanisms and the consequences of thrombus formation. The section concludes with a description of the laboratory methods used in evaluating effective treatment of thrombosis.

DISORDERS OF THE PROTEINS OF FIBRIN FORMATION

Disorders of the proteins (coagulation factors) of fibrin formation can arise by inheriting a defective gene that regulates the synthesis of the protein or they can be acquired secondarily to another condition during the lifetime of the individual. In the rare hereditary disorders, the genetic defect can result either in failure of synthesis of one of the proteins or in the production of a malfunctioning molecule (Fig. 26-1). In both situations, the rate of fibrin formation is slowed and ineffective.

Some clinical manifestations are listed in Chapter 25, Table 25-1. Bleeding in coagulation factor disorders tends to be into deep tissues from the rupture of arterioles as opposed to the more superficial bleeding in platelet disorders.

Clinical features found almost exclusively in coagulation factor disorders are delayed bleeding, hematomas (Chapter 25, Figure 25-1C), and bleeding into deeper muscular tissue and joints. Hematuria and retroperitoneal bleeding also are common. Bleeding may occur from several other sites.

Inherited coagulation factor disorders usually involve only one coagulation protein and, if bleeding occurs, from one site at a time. Acquired coagulation factor disorders are much more common than the inherited disorders. Bleeding in acquired disorders often occurs simultaneously from more than one site.

Early investigators of coagulation defects assumed that the factor involved was absent or decreased quantitatively. Thus, the term *deficiency* was used to describe the coagulation factor disorders. It is now known that abnormal molecules also may be synthesized. The altered molecules are nonfunctional in fibrin formation (qualitatively abnormal), both in vivo and in in vitro laboratory tests. The term deficiency, however, continues to be used and is applied to both qualitative and quantitative conditions.

To understand the concept of an abnormal molecule, consider the coagulation factors that are serine proteases. The active site of the molecule is a serine residue acting

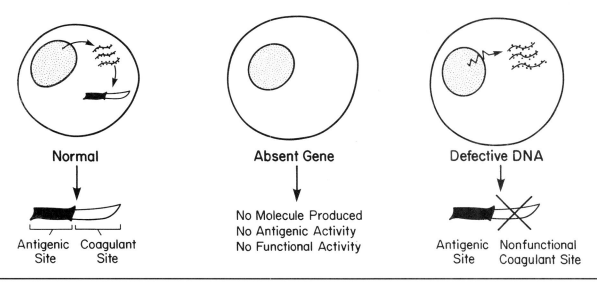

FIGURE 26-1. Diagrammatic representation of the mechanisms of unrestricted defects of hemostatic proteins. (Left) Normal synthesis with both normal function and antigenic properties, (Center) Absence of synthesis and absent antigenic properties. (Right) Production of an abnormal molecule with defective function but identifiable antigenic properties.

in conjunction with other amino acids. Certain portions of the remainder of the molecule are antigenic sites. When the protein is injected into a lower animal, it is the antigenic sites that are recognized as foreign and to which antibody specificity is directed. Antibodies produced by the animal will in turn combine with these same sites in tests designed to identify the protein immunologically. An abnormal molecule might have the antigenic sites intact but differ in amino acid sequence at the enzymatic site, causing a loss of enzymatic activity. Such a molecule could not participate in coagulation reactions in the body or in a test tube. It could, however, be identified immunologically using animal antibodies raised against it. Individuals who have a nonfunctional molecule that can be detected immunologically are said to be positive for cross-reacting material (CRM+) (Fig. 26-1). Patients in whom the clotting factor is decreased both functionally and immunologically are said to be negative for cross-reacting material (CRM−) (Fig. 26-1).

The amino acid sequence of the proteins and the nucleotide sequences of the gene structures have been determined for most of the hemostatic proteins. Molecular defects in many genes and the proteins have also been established. A variety of mutations have been characterized. Point mutations, alterations of splice junctions, deletions, and mutations resulting in stop codons are a few of the wide variety of molecular defects.

Routine laboratory tests are unable to distinguish between nonfunctional molecules and complete absence of the protein. Therefore, in quantitative and qualitative factor abnormalities, the results of screening tests, prothrombin time (PT), activated partial thromboplastin time (APTT), and thrombin time (TT) will depend on the protein that is defective (Table 26-1). The platelet count is normal with rare exceptions. The bleeding time, which is dependent on the formation of the primary hemostatic plug, is normal in most factor deficiencies. It may be abnormal if either thrombocytopenia or a decrease in fibrinogen also is present. Similar laboratory results are obtained with acquired deficiencies.

The inherited coagulation factor disorders will be classified by inheritance pattern. The autosomal dominant traits will be discussed first, followed by the sex-linked (X-linked) recessive conditions and then autosomal recessive diseases. Acquired disorders are classified under the headings of consumption disorders, liver disease, vitamin K deficiencies, and acquired pathologic inhibitors.

● Hereditary disorders

AUTOSOMAL DOMINANT INHERITANCE

Two coagulation disorders are caused by autosomal dominant inheritance of a defective protein. In these disorders, symptoms are present when just one abnormal gene is transmitted by parents to affected offspring. One of the disorders, dysfibrinogenemia, is characterized by the presence of an abnormal fibrinogen molecule, but, because other fibrinogen disorders demonstrate autosomal recessive patterns, dysfibrinogenemia is best discussed with them in a later section. The second, *von Willebrand disease*, will be considered here.

von Willebrand disease von Willebrand disease is a deficiency of von Willebrand factor. von Willebrand factor (vWF) was discussed in Chapter 23, where it was described as the bridge that, along with the glycoprotein Ib receptor, helps platelets adhere to collagen fibers after an injury. This attachment initiates the platelet response and results in the primary hemostatic plug. Disorders that cause deficiencies of either platelet glycoprotein Ib or of von Willebrand factor retard platelet adhesion and inhibit formation of the primary hemostatic plug. The deficiency of glycoprotein Ib, Bernard-Soulier disease, was discussed in the section of abnormalties of platelet adhesion. The description of von Willebrand factor deficiency is considered here with the coagulation factor deficiencies because additional aspects of the functions of von Willebrand factor affect fibrin formation as well as platelet adhesion. Consequently, laboratory tests for von Willebrand disease reflect the relationship to both platelet adhesion and fibrin formation. To understand this complex association, the molecular structure and functions of vWf will be discussed first. Clinical aspects of von Willebrand disease will follow.

NATURE OF VON WILLEBRAND FACTOR Research into the molecular biology of von Willebrand factor began in the early 1970s. At that time, there was much confusion regarding its molecular nature because of the apparent dual role in hemostasis and its affect on laboratory tests for both platelet function and fibrin formation. The fibrin formation aspect seemed to be related to a different disease called hemophilia A (discussed in the following section). von Willebrand factor was, in fact, called, or included in what was called, factor VIII, which is the hemostatic protein deficient in patients with hemophilia A. It was an elusive entity and not yet known to exist as a separate protein. Laboratory assays, such as the APTT and factor assays, were able to measure the activity of factor VIII but not of von Willebrand factor in the plasma. Using these tests, factor VIII activity was markedly decreased in patients with hemophilia A, but in patients with von Willebrand disease

TABLE 26-1 *COAGULATON SCREENING TEST RESULTS IN CONGENITAL FACTOR DEFICIENCIES*

PT	APTT	TT	Suspected Congenital Factor Deficiency
N	N	N	None
A	N	N	VII
N	A	N	XII, XI, IX, VIII, prekallikrein, HMWK, von Willebrand factor
A	A	N	X, V, II
A	A	A	Fibrinogen

N = normal; A = abnormal; PT = Prothrombin time; APTT = activated partial thromboplastin time; TT = thrombin time; HMWK = high molecular weight kininogen

the decrease was mild and the results were not always reproducible. As time went on, immunologic laboratory tests for what was called factor VIII became available. The immunologic tests further complicated matters because they showed that the factor VIII was decreased in the plasma of von Willebrand disease patients but was normal in patients with hemophilia A. The term factor VIII-related antigen was then applied to the entity measured in the immunologic tests. Questions to be answered at that time were: Why do patients with von Willebrand disease have abnormal platelet function and plasma immunologic activity of von Willebrand factor? Why do patients with hemophilia A have normal platelet function and plasma immunologic activity of von Willebrand factor? Why do both have decreased activity of plasma factor VIII? What is factor VIII and what is the factor VIII-related antigen?

These questions were answered by molecular studies. It was found that von Willebrand factor and factor VIII are two functionally and antigenically separate proteins. As they circulate in the plasma, factor VIII is noncovalently bound to some of the von Willebrand factor. The bound structure is now called the factor VIII/von Willebrand factor complex. von Willebrand factor is the protein previously identified as factor VIII-related antigen. In the complex one molecule of von Willebrand factor associates with one molecule of factor VIII. But the key to some of the confusion is that one molecule of von Willebrand factor is many times larger than one molecule of factor VIII. The factor VIII/von Willebrand factor complex defines a second role for von Willebrand factor in hemostasis. That is, it is a carrier protein for factor VIII and helps to prevent degradation of factor VIII and to localize it in the injured area. The function of factor VIII is in fibrin formation but it is not able to function, either in laboratory tests or in vivo, in the absence of von Willebrand factor. The remaining von Willebrand factor in the plasma, as well as that located in the subendothelial connective tissue matrix and the platelet alpha granules, as described in Chapter 23, functions in platelet adhesion.

von Willebrand factor, as known now, is needed for platelets to adhere to collagen and initiate the primary hemostatic plug. This function is independent of the presence or absence of factor VIII. If vWf is decreased, platelet adhesion to collagen is abnormal and the immunologic tests indicate decreased amounts circulating in the plasma. Patients with hemophilia A have decreased plasma factor VIII activity but their von Willebrand factor is normal, so they have normal platelet function and normal plasma von Willebrand factor by immunologic tests. Patients with von Willebrand disease have decreased activity of plasma factor VIII simply because factor VIII cannot function or be detected with routine laboratory tests in the absense of von Willebrand factor.

STRUCTURE AND SYNTHESIS von Willebrand factor is a glycoprotein and the larger of the two components of the factor VIII/von Willebrand factor complex. It is a group of molecules of many different sizes. Molecular weights vary from 0.5 to over 20 million Daltons. Each molecule is composed of a series of identical subunits that have a molecular

weight of 220,000 Daltons.[1] The total mass of each molecule is determined by the number of subunits it contains.

The subunits are synthesized in the endoplasmic reticulum of megakaryocytes and endothelial cells as single chain monomers, with a molecular weight of 260,000 Daltons (Fig. 26-2). Processing begins within the endoplasmic reticulum and continues in the Golgi. In the endoplasmic reticulum, simple sugars are added. Dimers are formed by attachment of two monomers at the carboxy terminal ends via disulfide bonds. The dimers are the basic building blocks of the mature multimeric molecules.

The dimers move to the Golgi region where the carbohydrates are processed to more complex forms and sulfate groups are added. In the final stages of passage through the Golgi, dimers begin to associate at the amino terminal ends with disulfide bonds to form multimers. This process continues in the cytoplasm. Finally, a sequence of 741 amino acids (22 of which are a signal peptide) is removed from the amino terminal end of each of the subunits of the multimer to form the mature protein. The molecular weight of the subunits is reduced to 220,000 and consists of 2050 amino acids.

A schematic diagram of the structure of a von Willebrand factor subunit is shown in the top part of Figure 26-3. The transcribed product (pre-pro-von Willebrand factor or pro-von Willebrand factor) is 2813 amino acids long. The first 741 amino acids consist of the signal peptide and the propeptide that are removed after polymerization. The remainder is the mature von Willebrand factor subunit. Several domains have been identified along the length of the mature von Willebrand factor corresponding to its functions. The amino end (N) contains the sites for binding to factor VIII. There are two areas for attachment to collagen and one for glycoprotein Ib. An area designated as RGD is believed to bind to glycoprotein IIb/IIIa. The lower portion of the diagram shows how a von Willebrand factor multimer might be organized. Each monomer is long and thin with a small globular region at each end. The globular C ends associate into dimers and the dimers attach to each other by the N ends.

The gene controlling the production of vWf is located on chromosome 12. It has been sequenced and cloned.[2] It has 52 exons and constitutes 178 kb of DNA, approximately 0.1% of chromosome 12.[3]

The multimers of von Willebrand factor made by the endothelial cells consist of a wide range of sizes. Smaller multimers, containing both pro-von Willebrand factor and mature von Willebrand factor, are spontaneously secreted by the endothelial cells, both into the plasma and the subendothelium. Those secreted into the plasma combine with factor VIII as they circulate. The largest multimers with mature subunits are stored in Weibel-Palade bodies of the endothelial cells. The endothelial cells secrete von Willebrand factor from the Weibel-Palade bodies after an injury has occurred and they are stimulated by thrombin, fibrin, or histamine. The von Willebrand factor from the Weibel-Palade bodies is primarily secreted into the subendothelium.[1]

The von Willebrand factor synthesized in megakaryocytes is stored in the α-granules of platelets. Approxi-

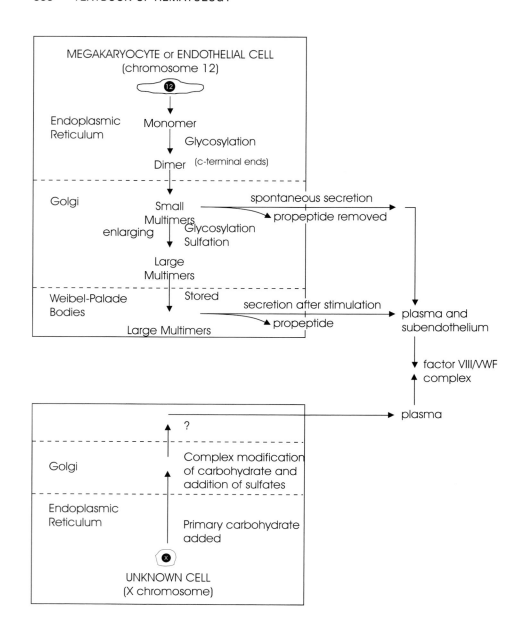

FIGURE 26-2. Synthesis and secretion of factor VIII/von Willebrand factor complex. (Top) von Willebrand factor synthesis. (Bottom) factor VIII synthesis. Both proteins are secreted into the plasma where they bind together.

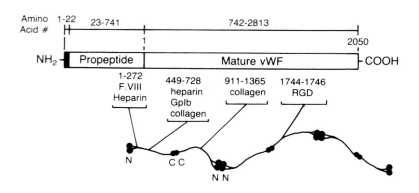

FIGURE 26-3. Organization of the von Willebrand factor molecule. Amino acids (aa) 1-22 are a signal peptide, 23-741 a propeptide that is removed after multimerization, 742-2813 the mature protein. Domains on the mature protein are aa 1-272 binding sites for factor VIII and heparin (the amino end), aa 449-728 binding sites for heparin, glycoprotein Ib and collagen, aa 911-1365 another collagen binding site, aa 1744-1746 RGD site which is a small peptide found in several adhesive proteins. Monomers of von Willebrand factor associate by the C terminal ends to form dimers. The dimers associate by the N terminal ends to form the multimers. (With permission from: Gralnick, H.R. von Willebrand disease. In Hematology. 4th Ed. Edited by W.J. Williams, E. Beutler, A.J. Erslev, M.A. Lichtman. Philadelphia, Lea & Febiger, 1990).

TABLE 26-2 *NOMENCLATURE OF THE FACTOR VIII/VON WILLEBRAND FACTOR COMPLEX*

Factor VIII—deficient in Hemophilia A
  VIII—the coagulant protein
  VIII:C—functional activity
    Functions in fibrin formation in vivo
    Functions in fibrin formation in vitro
    Function is measured by the APTT
  VIII:Ag—antigenic properties
    Antigenic determinants of VIII:C
    Measured by human homologous antibodies to factor VIII

von Willebrand Factor—deficient in von Willebrand disease
  vWf-The von Willebrand factor protein
  vWf:Ag
    Antigenic determinants of von Willebrand factor
    Measured by heterologous antisera with immunologic procedures
  Function of vWf
    Carrier of factor VIII
    Platelet adhesion—measured by bleeding time
    Ristocetin activity
      Ristocetin cofactor measured by agglutination of normal platelets
      Ristocetin induced platelet aggregation measured with autologous platelets

mately 15% of the von Willebrand factor in the plasma is in the platelets. Platelet von Willebrand factor differs from plasma von Willebrand factor in that it is not complexed with factor VIII and it contains larger multimers than are present in plasma.[1]

NOMENCLATURE In 1985, standards for nomenclature of von Willebrand factor and factor VIII were published by the International Committee on Thrombosis and Hemostasis.[4] The nomenclature defines several immunologic and functional properties based on laboratory procedures that identify them. It distinguishes between von Willebrand factor and factor VIII, which had been so muddled. The properties defined for von Willebrand factor are useful in diagnosing von Willebrand disease and in separating several variants of the disease that have since been described. The reader is cautioned to interpret older literature on this topic with caution. Indeed, even recent authors sometimes erroneously use factor VIII where von Willebrand factor is meant. Table 26-2 summarizes these properties.

CLINICAL ASPECTS von Willebrand first described the disease entity that bears his name after studying a kindred in the Aaland Islands near Sweden in 1926.[5] The laboratory tests available then were the platelet count, coagulation time, and clot retraction. All were normal. With further studies, he concluded that the disease was related to platelet dysfunction.

It was not until 1953 that the disease was found to be associated with a deficiency of factor VIII.[1] Since that time, much research has led to the conclusion that there are several types of this disease caused by a variety of abnormalities of the von Willebrand protein molecule. Inheritance of most types is autosomal dominant, although rare kindreds demonstrate an autosomal recessive trait.

In some types, synthesis of protein is decreased, in others an abnormal molecule is produced, and, in a few, there is a combination of decreased synthesis and production of abnormal molecules.

Therefore, von Willebrand disease is a group of disorders in which the von Willebrand protein is either quantitatively or qualitatively abnormal (Fig. 26-1). The factor VIII also may be affected because it depends on the presence of von Willebrand factor. The incidence of the disease is approximately 1 in 10,000 but may be higher because mild cases may be undetected.

Clinically, the disease is mild. Most individuals who have symptoms are heterozygous. Severe symptoms are present in rare patients who are homozygotes. One hallmark of the disease is its variability. The severity of the disease differs in individuals within the same kindred, among kindreds, and, occasionally, within the same individual.

Symptoms may not begin until the second decade of life in the mild forms. In the severe forms, symptoms begin early and decrease with age. There is no correlation between the clinical symptoms and the level of von Willebrand factor activity.[5]

Symptoms seen most frequently are mucosal and cutaneous hemorrhages. For example, epistaxis, gingival bleeding, easy bruising, and hypermenorrhea are common manifestations. Excessive bleeding at childbirth is comparatively rare, because in pregnancy the activity of the entire complex increases. The clinical features in mild forms resemble those seen in platelet disorders. In the severe type, the symptoms include hemarthroses and spontaneous deep bleeding, resembling coagulation factor deficiencies. Individuals with blood group O have lower levels of von Willebrand factor antigen (75%) when compared with other blood groups (125% for type AB).[3] More patients with group O have symptoms with the disease. They also are easier to diagnose with current laboratory methods.

LABORATORY ASPECTS von Willebrand factor cannot be tested for directly by the common laboratory tests for fibrin formation. The laboratory diagnosis of von Willebrand disease is based on the results of the template bleeding time, platelet aggregation test, APTT, factor VIII assay, and specially designed assays for the quantitation as well as the function of the von Willebrand factor (Table 26-3). Laboratory test results are variable, often requiring repeated testing of the same individual. DNA analysis is being used in research laboratories to explain the molecular mutations in the vWf gene that cause the disease. It is suggested that DNA screening techniques may soon be available for von Willebrand disease.[5] The disease is classified into several types according to the results of a variety of tests.

The template bleeding time, which measures platelet function, is abnormal, not because the platelets are abnormal, but because, in the absence of von Willebrand factor, the platelets are unable to adhere to collagen and initiate the series of reactions that lead to formation of the primary hemostatic plug (Chapter 25, Figure 25-8B). Following challenge with aspirin, prolongation of the bleeding

TABLE 26-3 *LABORATORY EVALUATION OF VON WILLEBRAND DISEASE AND X-LINKED RECESSIVE DISORDERS*

	von Willebrand Disease, Type I	Factor VIII Deficiency	Factor IX Deficiency
Platelet Tests			
Platelet count	N	N	N
Template bleeding	↑	N	N
Platelet aggregation			
ADP	N	N	N
Collagen	N	N	N
Epinephrine	N	N	N
Ristocetin	Absent	N	N
Coagulation factor tests			
Prothrombin time	N	N	N
Activated partial thromboplastin time	N or ↑	↑	↑
Thrombin time	N	N	N
Factor VIII assay	↓	↓	N
vWf:Ag assay	↓	N	N
Factor IX assay	N	N	↓
Fibrinolysis	N	N	N

N: normal; ↑: increased; ↓: decreased.

time is marked (aspirin tolerance test). This susceptibility to aspirin is useful in difficult diagnostic cases. It is not used as a routine test because the danger of bleeding is increased for up to a week or longer after the test.

In the platelet aggregation test, platelets respond normally to ADP, collagen, and epinephrine, but fail to aggregate with ristocetin (Chapter 25, Figure 25-9B). This pattern of aggregation is similar to that seen in Bernard-Soulier disease. However, in von Willebrand disease, the aggregation with ristocetin is normal when von Willebrand factor is added to the mixture, whereas in Bernard-Soulier disease no change is noted.

The platelet count, prothrombin time, thrombin time, and tests for fibrinolysis are normal. The APTT is used as an indirect test for von Willebrand factor because of its association with factor VIII. The APTT, a test for the intrinsic system of fibrin formation, is dependent in part on adequate amounts of functional factor VIII. If the von Willebrand factor is decreased to the level of sensitivity of the test, the coagulant factor VIII will be decreased secondarily, and the APTT will be prolonged. Some patients with mild forms of the disease may have functional factor VIII levels of 0.25 to 0.5 Um/mL (25% to 50%). In these patients, the APTT might be normal because the reagents may not be sensitive enough to detect such mild decreases. A factor assay for factor VIII may be in the range of 0.01 to 0.05 Um/mL (1% to 5%) in severe forms.

Several types of assays are available for quantitating and evaluating the functional aspects of the von Willebrand factor in the plasma. Two types of tests quantitate the level of vWf protein. One method assays the von Willebrand antigen and also correlates the amount of antigen present to the amount of protein. Several methodologies have been devised. They all use heterologous antibodies

(antibodies raised in lower animals) to identify the antigen. "Rocket" electrophoresis (Laurell) is a common technique. Measurement of von Willebrand factor antigen by the rocket technique is not believed to be reliable in all patients because the results depend greatly on the technique and are difficult to standardize.

Another method assays patient's plasma for its functional ability to support platelet aggregation in the presence of ristocetin. Patient's plasma contains the VIII/vWf complex, which is needed for platelet agglutination by ristocetin. Tests can measure the amount of ristocetin needed to agglutinate platelets, or they can quantitate the amount of aggregation induced by a fixed amount of ristocetin. If patient's platelets and patient's plasma are mixed with ristocetin, platelet aggregation can be measured on a platelet aggregometer. This test measures ristocetin-induced platelet aggregation (RIPA) in patient's platelet rich plasma. Because, as in von Willebrand disease type IIb, patient's platelets are sometimes abnormal, a better method for detection of vWf uses normal platelets with patient's plasma. This modification measures only the ristocetin cofactor, von Willebrand factor, in the patient's plasma and is not dependent on patient's platelets.

Tests for qualitative abnormalities of the molecular structure von Willebrand factor are performed by electrophoresis in gels. The molecules or multimers are separated by size corresponding to the number of subunits they contain. Two methods are common. In crossed immunoelectrophoresis, plasma containing von Willebrand factor is electrophoresed on the gel in one direction, then turned 90° and electrophoresed again with the addition of antibody. The antibody combines with and precipitates the antigen in the spot to which it has migrated. The results form an asymmetric arc of precipitate corresponding to the molecular weight distribution of the molecules.[5] In some types of von Willebrand disease, the arc is abnormal, indicating the absence of larger multimeric molecules. In the second method, the multimers are analyzed by electrophoresis of the plasma or of platelet membrane fractions in sodium dodecyl sulfate (SDS) gels, during which the various size molecules of von Willebrand factor are separated longitudinally. The gel is then incubated with radiolabeled antibody, which attaches to the antigen in the gel, and bands can be detected by photographic methods. In some forms of von Willebrand disease, the large multimeric bands of protein may be missing from plasma von Willebrand factor, platelet von Willebrand factor, or both. On SDS gel electrophoresis, normal von Willebrand factor separates in groups of three bands known as triplets. This triplet structure is abnormal in rare types of the disease.

CLASSIFICATION von Willebrand disease is the most common inherited bleeding disorder in humans. Approximately 20 clinical variants of von Willebrand disease have been described. They are classified into three major categories: types I, II, and III. There are several subtypes of types I and II. Types I and III are quantitative defects. Patients have decreased amounts of normal appearing vWf. Those with type I have a moderate decrease while those with type III have a marked decrease. The defects of the type

TABLE 26-4 *DIFFERENTIATION OF VON WILLEBRAND DISEASE*

Type	I	III	IIA	IIB	IIC†	Pseudo-vWD
Mode of inheritance	Autosomal dominant	Autosomal recessive	Autosomal dominant	Autosomal dominant	Autosomal recessive	Autosomal dominant
Template bleeding time	Normal—prolonged	Prolonged	Prolonged	Prolonged	Prolonged	Normal—prolonged
Factor VIII assay	Decreased	Severely decreased	Normal—decreased	Normal—decreased	Normal	Normal—decreased
Quantitative assays for vWf						
vWf:Ag	Decreased	Decreased—absent	Variable	Variable	Variable	Variable
Ristocetin agglutination—normal platelets	Decreased	Decreased—absent	Decreased—absent	Normal—decreased	Decreased	Decreased
RIPA‡	Decreased	Decreased—absent	Decreased—absent	Increased	Decreased	Increased
Qualitative assays for vWf						
Crossed immunoelectrophoresis	Normal	Variable	Abnormal	Abnormal	Abnormal	Abnormal
Multimeric structure in SDS gels						
Plasma	Normal	Variable	Only low-molecular-weight forms	Only low- and intermediate-molecular-weight forms present	Abnormal triplet structure	Only low- and intermediate-molecular-weight forms present
Platelet	Normal	Unknown	Only low molecular weight forms present	Normal	Abnormal triplet structure	Normal

* Based in part on Table 3 of Zimmerman, T.S., Ruggeri, Z.M., and Fulcher, C.A.: Factor III/von Willebrand factor. Prog. Hematol. *13:*279, 1983.

† Based on the study of one kindred.

‡ Ristocetin-induced platelet aggregation in patient platelet-rich plasma.

II diseases are qualitative. In type II von Willebrand disease, the largest multimers are absent.

Inheritance of most types is autosomal dominant, although some appear to be autosomal recessive traits. Classification of five forms of von Willebrand disease using results obtained with laboratory tests are shown in Table 26-4.

TYPE I Type I von Willebrand disease, known as the classic type, is seen in approximately 70% of patients and is the type originally described by von Willebrand. Inheritance is autosomal dominant with variable penetrance. The clinical course is moderate to mild. Excessive bleeding from cuts, mucosal surfaces, menses, and after surgery or trauma is the most common symptom.

In type I von Willebrand disease, there is decreased production of normal von Willebrand factor molecules. The level of von Willebrand factor is usually between 20% and 50% of normal. Both platelet and plasma von Willebrand factor are decreased, and there is a corresponding decrease in the level of factor VIII.

The template bleeding time is typically prolonged because the bleeding time is dependent on adequate platelet adhesion and requires von Willebrand factor. von Willebrand factor antigen, ristocetin cofactor activity, the RIPA, and factor VIII assay all are decreased. Crossed immunoelectrophoresis and SDS gels indicate normal multimeric structure in both the platelets and plasma. Laboratory test results vary considerably as discussed above and are helpful only 60% of the time.[6]

Several variants of type I von Willebrand disease are described. The molecular basis of type I has been studied

in a few patients but is difficult to determine because of the great size of the gene. It is believed, however, that many different mutations in the gene will be found. Rare cases appear to have homozygous autosomal recessive expression. There is almost no detectable levels of von Willebrand factor, either in plasma or platelets. These individuals have serious bleeding symptoms such as hemarthrosis and spontaneous bleeding from mucosal surfaces. It is similar to type III von Willebrand disease but distinguished by the lack of a clearly established autosomal recessive inheritance pattern.[6]

TYPE II Type II disease is characterized by decreased production of the large multimeric forms of the molecule, which are associated with adherence to platelets. Several variant types differ in the types of molecular forms that are abnormal (Table 26-4). Three of the variants will be described.

Type IIA disease is the most common type II form. Approximately 10% to 15% of all patients with von Willebrand disease have type IIA.[6] The large and intermediate multimers from both the plasma and platelets are decreased, as shown by abnormal crossed immunoelectrophoresis and multimeric analysis in SDS gels. Other parameters are decreased because of the basic deficit in protein. Point mutations in the DNA have been found in many type IIA patients using the polymerase chain reaction.[3,6] A large majority of the mutations are clustered in exon 28.[5] Bleeding in patients with type IIA von Willebrand disease is mild to moderate.

Type IIB patients have a decrease in the large multimers in the plasma only. Low and intermediate molecular weight multimers in the plasma and platelet multimers are normal. Strangely, type IIB is characterized by increased aggregation of platelets with ristocetin. This has led to the theory that the large multimers are absent from the plasma because the defect makes them more reactive with platelet or other cellular receptors. They may react with these receptors as soon as they are synthesized and are, therefore, removed from the circulation. Thrombocytopenia is also common in patients with type IIB. Several mutations in the DNA have been described.

Type IIC has been described in one family only and differs in that the structural form of the molecule is abnormal in addition to a decrease of the large multimers. This type is inherited as an autosomal recessive trait.

TYPE III Type III disease is inherited either as a homozygous or doubly heterozygous trait (i.e., a defective von Willebrand factor gene is inherited from both parents). These patients have severe disease symptoms. The von Willebrand factor is greatly decreased, factor VIII almost undetectable, and ristocetin activity markedly reduced. Some patients also have abnormal molecular structure. Type III von Willebrand disease is caused by large deletions in the DNA or by other mutations that result in total absence of functional von Willebrand factor mRNA. The first molecular abnormalities in von Willebrand disease were found in patients with type III.[5,6]

OTHER FORMS Two additional forms are an acquired type and pseudo-von Willebrand disease. The *acquired type* is found in patients with autoimmune or lymphoproliferative disease and may be immunologic in nature.

Pseudo-von Willebrand disease is also called the *platelet type* because the platelets are abnormally responsive to aggregation with ristocetin. It is similar to type IIB, but in pseudo-von Willebrand disease, the defect is in the platelet and usually results in increased binding of the larger multimers of plasma von Willebrand factor to glycoprotein Ib in vivo. This results in decreased von Willebrand factor and factor VIII in the plasma. In addition, glycoprotein IIb/IIIa receptors are exposed. Fibrinogen also binds in vivo and causes platelets to aggregate. Thrombocytopenia results.[1]

TREATMENT Treatment for von Willebrand disease is cryoprecipitate, which contains all molecular forms of von Willebrand factor. Recently, a modified antidiuretic hormone deamino-D-argenine vasopressin (DDAVP) was found to induce release of stored von Willebrand factor in endothelium. It temporarily increases the levels of von Willebrand factor; it is used in treating bleeding in patients with von Willebrand disease, and, occasionally, in patients with hemophilia A.

Therapy is given symptomatically and is monitored by the bleeding time. Aspirin and compounds containing aspirin, a host of platelet membrane activating drugs such as antihistamine, alcohol, and nonsteroid anti-inflammatory drugs should be avoided.

X-LINKED RECESSIVE DISORDERS

Two inherited coagulation factor deficiencies demonstrate X-linked inheritance. These are factors VIII and IX, which participate as a cofactor and serine protease, respectively, in the intrinsic pathway of fibrin formation (Chapter 24). The disease caused by a deficiency of these factors is known collectively as hemophilia. When factor VIII is the deficient factor, the disease is called *hemophilia A* and when factor IX is deficient, the disease is *hemophilia B.*

The disease entity has been known for several centuries. It has contributed to world history by its presence in the royal families of Europe, particularly Great Britain, Russia, and Spain.

Originally, all patients with X-linked bleeding disorders were believed to have the same disease. This idea was challenged when, in 1947, Pavlovsky observed that prolonged recalcification times on two patients with hemophilia were corrected when the test was performed on mixtures of the two plasmas.[7] In 1952, three groups of investigators reported patients who were missing a new factor that became known as factor IX. Other synonyms for factor IX are plasma thromboplastin component (PTC) and Christmas factor. Factor IX deficiency also was known as Christmas disease because Christmas was the surname of the affected family reported by one of the groups.

The overall incidence of the hemophilias is approximately 1 in 5000 males. Approximately 80% of the patients have factor VIII deficiency and the remaining 20% are deficient in factor IX. In approximately 30% of the affected individuals, there is no positive family history of the disease, indicating a high genetic mutation rate.

In hemophilia A, the coagulant portion of the factor VIII/von Willebrand factor complex is deficient, as opposed to von Willebrand disease in which the von Willebrand factor portion is decreased. Patients with hemophilia A have normal circulating levels of normal functional von Willebrand factor. Thus, their platelets adhere properly to collagen, and the formation of a normal primary hemostatic plug is not disrupted. Patients with hemophilia B have an intact VIII/von Willebrand factor complex and, likewise, have a normal primary hemostatic plug. The abnormal bleeding in both diseases is caused by delayed and inadequate fibrin formation.

Factor VIII deficiency Factor VIII is the smaller of the two components of the factor VIII/von Willebrand factor complex (see above). Plasma contains some free factor VIII but most is stabilized by vWf in a 1:1 molar ratio.

NOMENCLATURE Factor VIII is defined by the International Committee on Thrombosis and Hemostasis as the protein that circulates in the plasma and functions in the intrinsic pathway of fibrin formation. The properties of factor VIII are called VIII:C and VIII:Ag (Table 26-2). VIII:C is the activity of factor VIII in fibrin formation, also called the procoagulant or coagulant activity. The antigenic quality of factor VIII is abbreviated VIII:Ag.[4] A synonym for factor VIII is "antihemophilic factor."

STRUCTURE AND SYNTHESIS OF FACTOR VIII The molecular structure of factor VIII is shown in Figure 26-4. It is synthesized as a single chain protein with 2351 amino acids. The molecular weight is 267,039 Daltons. The molecule is organized into six domains. From the amino terminal end, the domains are called A1, A2, B, A3, C1, and C2.[8] The approximate sites of key functional components are indicated in Figure 26-4.

The cells in which factor VIII is synthesized are unknown, although the hepatocyte is strongly suggested.[8] Steps in synthesis are shown in Figure 26-2. After synthesis, the molecules are modified, first in the endoplasmic reticulum with the addition of simple carbohydrate. Further modification occurs in the Golgi with removal of a portion of the B domain between amino acids 1313 and 1648. This changes the configuration from a single to a two-chain molecule connected by a disulfide bond. The carbohydrates are modified to more complex structures. Sulfate groups are added also. Factor VIII attaches to von Willebrand factor in the plasma.[8]

The gene controlling the production of the factor VIII is located at the terminal end of the long arm of the X chromosome. It is one of the largest known genes and is composed of 26 exons and 186,000 base pairs. It constitutes 0.01% of the X chromosome. The gene has been sequenced and cloned.

MUTATIONS Genetic defects in the factor VIII gene cause hemophilia A. The mutation has been studied in hundreds of patients using restriction enzyme techniques, the polymerase chain reaction, and other methods. The molecular defect has been determined in approximately 10% of the genes studied.[9]

The genetic defects include point mutations, gross deletions, and regulatory defects.[8] The clinical severity of the disease depends on the type of mutation and the molecular functions that are disrupted. The same mutation occurs in all members of a family, resulting in a similar clinical expression of disease in affected members of the family.

The factor VIII coagulant antigen can be detected with an immunoradiometric assay. Antibodies used to detect VIII:Ag generally come from humans who have been immunized by the coagulant portion of the factor VIII/von Willebrand factor complex. Using this technique, approximately 90% of hemophilia A patients have been found to lack any detectable factor VIII antigen. These individuals are negative for factor VIII cross-reacting material (CRM−). The other 10% demonstrate normal levels of immunologically detectable factor VIII antigen. The mutation in patients who are CRM − results in lack of synthesis of detectable factor VIII. Patients who are CRM + have an abnormal nonfunctional factor VIII molecule.

Factor IX deficiency Factor IX is a vitamin K-dependent serine protease that functions in the intrinsic pathway of fibrin formation.

STRUCTURE AND SYNTHESIS OF FACTOR IX Factor IX is a glycoprotein with 415 amino acids and a molecular weight of 55,000 daltons.[10] It circulates as a single chain proenzyme and becomes a two-chain protein when activated.

Factor IX is synthesized in liver cells. The gene is located on the terminal end of the long arm of the X chromosome near the gene for factor VIII. The factor IX gene consists of 34 kb of DNA. It has 8 exons and 7 introns. The molecule includes several functional domains, each of which is coded for by a separate exon.[10]

MUTATIONS Heterogeneous mutations in the DNA of the factor IX gene or its regulatory components result in hemophilia B. As of 1992, 300 families have been studied for the defect in the DNA. Point mutations (mis-sense and

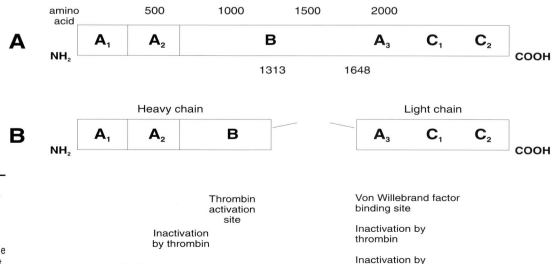

FIGURE 26-4. Organization of the factor VIII molecule. A. Sequence of the domains, A1, A2, B, A3, C1, C2. B. After activation by thrombin, a portion of the B domain is removed and two chains associate by disulfide bonds, the heavy chain and the light chain. Locations of functional sites on the active form are indicated by arrows.

nonsense) account for 95% of the abnormalities. Other rearrangements include deletions of various portions of the gene and insertions.[9,11] The clinical severity depends on the type of mutation and the part of the gene affected. Some factor IX deficient patients are CRM−, approximately one third are CRM+,[9] and some have reduced levels of antigen (CRMR) as measured by a radioimmunoassay method. The genetic defect in CRM+ hemophilia B patients is a mutation in the structural gene sequence resulting in an abnormal molecule.[9-11] Patients who are CRM− may have large deletions of the gene.

Laboratory aspects The clinical symptoms in hemophilia A and B are identical and are similar to other coagulation factor deficiencies. Therefore, the diagnosis must be made in the laboratory and the specific abnormal factor defined in order that proper therapy may be administered.

Laboratory screening tests (Tables 26-1 and 26-3) reveal a prolonged APTT, which is lengthened inversely to the level of factor present in the patient's plasma. Levels of 0.20 U/mL (20%) or less of factor IX will prolong the APTT. At levels between 0.20 and 0.50 U/mL (20% to 50%), the test will be in the upper normal range or slightly higher. The test may not be sensitive enough to detect mild deficiencies. In these cases, the physician may order a factor assay on the basis of the patient's history. The platelet count is normal, as are tests for platelet function, the bleeding time, and platelet aggregation test, including von Willebrand factor dependent ristocetin. The prothrombin time is normal since it is not dependent on either factor VIII or IX. One abnormal molecular variant, factor IXBm, causes prolongation of the prothrombin time when bovine brain thromboplastin is used as the reagent instead of rabbit thromboplastin.[12]

The thrombin time is normal because factors VIII and IX are used in the synthesis of thrombin and do not affect conversion of fibrinogen. Tests for fibrinolysis also are normal.

The definitive diagnosis is made on the basis of the results of specific factor assays. Assays determine the amount of each factor present in the patient's plasma. Factor assays were formerly reported as percentage of activity in plasma, arbitrarily assigning the value of 100% activity to normal plasma. More recently, the results are expressed in units where one unit equals the activity in 1 mL of plasma or 100 U/dL which is equal to 100% activity.

Clinical aspects Clinical manifestations of hemophilia vary with the amount of factor present (Table 26-5). Patients with less than 0.01 U/mL (1%) are considered to have severe disease, those with 0.01 to 0.05 U/mL (1% to 5%) have a moderate clinical course, and those with 0.05 to 0.25 U/mL (5% to 25%) have mild disease. Normal levels of factor VIII are 0.6 to 2 U/mL (60% to 200%)[13] and factor IX 0.5 to 1.5 U/mL (50% to 150%).

Clinical symptoms in severe disease may begin at the time of circumcision. *Hemarthrosis*, especially in the knee but in other joints as well, is the most common feature of severe hemophilia. Bleeding into a joint is accompanied by intense pain. The joint fills with blood, some of which

TABLE 26-5 *CLINICAL FINDINGS IN DEFICIENCIES OF FACTORS VIII OR IX*

Factor VII or IX Level μm/mL	Severity	Symptoms
0–1	Severe	Frequent spontaneous hemarthrosis with crippling Frequent severe, spontaneous hemorrhage (intracranial, intramuscular)
2–5	Moderate	Bleeding at circumcision Infrequent spontaneous joint and tissue bleeds Profuse bleeding after surgery or trauma Serious bleeding from minor injuries
6–20	Mild	Rare spontaneous bleeds Severe life threatening bleeding after surgery or trauma May not be discovered until bleeding episode occurs.

is not reabsorbed, causing chronic inflammation, pain, and eventual destruction of the joint and crippling. The bleeding may be preceded by trauma, which may be minor. Joint bleeds occur when the child starts to walk.

Subcutaneous hematomas may begin with slight trauma and spread to involve a large mass of tissue, causing purple discoloration of the skin. Intramuscular hemorrhages may result in contracture and deformity.

Also characteristic of coagulation factor disorders is *delayed bleeding*. Primary hemostasis is adequate to stop bleeding from a minor cut, but, because of deficient fibrin stabilization, the platelet plug is dislodged and bleeding begins a second time, and in greater proportion than would be expected for the size of the wound.

Hematomas around the tongue and throat are dangerous because blood leaking into the tissues may block the airway and lead to suffocation. Hemorrhages from the nose, mouth, gums, and other mucous membranes may potentially cause exsanguination. Other manifestations seen frequently are hematuria and excess bleeding from dental extractions. The most common cause of death is intracranial hemorrhage, which may occur after trauma or spontaneously.

Hemarthroses, and severe, spontaneous crippling bleeding into muscles are usually found only in severe disease. These symptoms are not seen in those with moderate or mild severity. More characteristic of moderate hemophilia is excessive bleeding after traumatic injury.

Mild deficiencies of the factors may be symptomless and unsuspected until a surgical procedure or major traumatic injury results in severe bleeding. While the site of bleeding varies from individual to individual, the clinical severity of deficiencies of both factors remains similar within families.

Inheritance and carrier detection X-linked disorders are inherited by sons from their mothers who have an abnormal gene on one X-chromosome and a normal gene on the other (carriers). Fifty percent of the sons will be expected to inherit the abnormal gene. Males have only one X-chromosome. If they inherit the abnormal one, they have no normal functional gene for the trait. In the case of factor VIII or IX deficiency, they are able to synthesize little or none of the factor.

Carriers of X-linked disorders are usually asymptomatic because they have one functional gene. Inactivation of one of the X-chromosomes occurs randomly in each cell of a female. Theoretically, then, in approximately 50% of the cells, the functional X-chromosome will be active. The level of factor VIII or IX is expected to be about 50% that of a noncarrier female.

Women who have hemophilic sons are obligate carriers of the disease. Daughters of obligate carriers may inherit either gene and be either carriers or normal.

Detection of carriers before they have children has become desirable for those who do not wish to have affected children. Detection of the carrier state, however, cannot be based on merely finding half of the normal activity in a factor assay. Approximately 6% to 20% of women studied may be erroneously classified either as normal or as carriers for two reasons.[14] First, random inactivation of the X-chromosomes is not always 50%. A carrier may have many more than half of her normal X chromosomes functioning, in which case her activity level may be in the normal range. Second, especially in the case of a factor VIII carrier, the protein is physiologically increased in pregnancy, exercise, fever, and several other conditions that may result in a transient rise into the normal range. Factor IX coagulant activity may rise 30% with the use of oral contraceptives. Better detection of carriers is possible by analysis of the plasma for both antigen and activity levels. In the case of factor VIII deficiency, the antigen detected is the von Willebrand factor antigen. Antigen levels in carriers should be two times the factor VIII activity levels.[13] Approximately 90% of carriers can be detected in this way. Carriers of factor IX deficiency are similarly detected by measuring the factor IX antigen by radioimmunoassay and finding it to be roughly twice the activity level as measured by a factor IX assay.[12]

Since the genes have been cloned, DNA studies have been developed to detect carriers. Restriction enzymes and PCR methods are used. Some mutations require the simultaneous use of the antigen activity method.[14]

A pregnant carrier of either disease may elect to have an aminocentesis performed for detection of sex and, if the fetus is male, blood can be obtained in utero by fetoscopy for detection of the antigen and clotting activity.[14]

Therapy Factor VIII is a labile factor and disappears on storage. Treatment for hemophilia A formerly required administration of fresh plasma. Stored plasma was used for hemophilia B. Such therapy was not satisfactory because the large volume of plasma required to reach hemostatic levels could potentially cause circulatory overload.

More recently, methods of concentrating the two factors have been developed and are more satisfactory.

Two forms of therapy are in use for factor VIII deficiency, cryoprecipitate and factor VIII concentrates.[15]

Cryoprecipitate is prepared by freezing a unit of plasma and collecting the precipitate that forms on thawing. The cryoprecipitate contains factor VIII, factor XIII, fibrinogen, and von Willebrand factor. The preparation can be centrifuged and some of the plasma removed to reduce the volume. Each unit of cryoprecipitate contains 70 to 100 units of factor VIII. It contains all molecular forms of von Willebrand factor including the large multimers, and can also be used to treat patients with von Willebrand disease.

Factor VIII concentrate is prepared by a lyophilized process. The activity of factor VIII is slightly reduced in the concentrate, and the large von Willebrand factor multimers are lost. Concentrates are used by hemophiliacs at home as prophylactic therapy to prevent extensive bleeding. Concentrates have markedly reduced crippling and enabled these individuals to lead more normal lives. To control bleeding, enough therapy is given to maintain an activity level of about 0.3 U/mL. For major surgery, 0.5 to 0.8 Um/mL (50% to 80%) activity is desired. The dose needed is calculated considering the metabolic half-life of the factor and the weight of the patient and must be continued for approximately 10 days.[13]

Major problems have been realized with the use of concentrates of factor VIII because the plasma of up to 20,000 donors is used to prepare one lot of factor VIII concentrate. Most patients who received this therapy before 1984 were exposed to hepatitis B, hepatitis C, and the HIV viruses. Since 1984, heat has been used to inactivate the HIV and hepatitis viruses, and concentrates are now considered to be safe. However, at the present time, 90% of severe factor VIII-deficient patients have HIV antibodies and antibodies to hepatitis B surface antigen.[15] To prevent this hazard, factor VIII products free of disease are being prepared by using monoclonal antibodies and recombinant factor VIII (rfactor VIII). Pure factor VIII concentrates are prepared using monoclonal antibodies raised in mice (Monoclate). A study is currently being done to evaluate the effectiveness of rfactor VIII.[16]

An alternative form of therapy in patients capable of producing some factor VIII (mildly affected hemophilia A and von Willebrand disease) is the pituitary hormone deamino-D-arginine vasopressin (DDAVP,) which stimulates storage cells to release factor VIII into the plasma.

Factor IX deficiency is treated with plasma or with concentrates that also contain factors II, VII, and X (prothrombin complex concentrates). Commercial products are Konyne (Cutter Laboratories) and Proplex (Hyland). Calculations of dosage are based on the half-life, the patient's weight, and the fact that 1 mL of plasma contains 1 unit of activity.

Factor IX concentrates are treated with heat to inactivate the hepatitis and HIV viruses as described for factor VIII. Purified factor IX concentrates called Mononine are prepared with monoclonal antibodies[17] and recombinant DNA techniques.

Complications of therapy in addition to the development of hepatitis B, hepatitis C, or AIDS, are thrombosis, with the use of factor IX concentrates, and, in some patients, formation of antibodies, also called inhibitors. In vivo antibody formation causes destruction of the factor. Inhibitors develop primarily in severely affected patients. Approximately 5% to 20% of factor VIII-deficient patients and 2% to 3% of hemophilia B patients have inhibitors. There is no way of predicting in which patients inhibitors will form.

The antibodies are of the IgG class of immunoglobulins. Attempts to prevent antibody production with immunosuppression or steroids are not effective. Treatment of patients with hemophilia A with high doses of factor (in an attempt to overwhelm the antibody) and treatment with animal factors also are used with limited success. In life-threatening hemorrhage, the patient may undergo plasma exchange to achieve hemostasis before the titer of antibody increases again.

AUTOSOMAL RECESSIVE DISORDERS

Hereditary deficiencies of the remainder of the coagulation factors are very rare. Autosomal recessive traits are expressed only in those homozygous for the defective gene, which means that the patient must inherit a rare abnormal gene from each parent. Consanguinity of the parents is frequent.

Diagnoses are suspected from the results of the PT and APTT (Table 26-1) and confirmed with subsequent specific factor assays. Tests for platelet number and function are normal, as are tests for fibrin split products and the thrombin time (Table 26-3).

Before a hereditary disease is considered, all possible causes for acquired coagulation factor deficiences must be ruled out. Clinical features of the diseases are similar to those of factor VIII and factor IX deficiencies.

Fibrinogen (factor I) deficiencies Two forms of fibrinogen deficiencies are inherited as autosomal recessive traits. *Afi-*

brinogenemia is a homozygous form in which no antigenically detectable fibrinogen is found. *Hypofibrinogenemia* is a heterozygous form in which plasma levels of fibrinogen are between 20 and 100 mg/dL. Consanguinity is found in about half of the families with afibrinogenemia.

Clinically, afibrinogenemia is the more severe disease. At birth, bleeding may occur from the umbilical cord, but, in general, patients have a milder course than severe hemophiliacs. Joint bleeds are rare, but moderate to severe bleeding from other sites, especially after trauma or surgery, has been reported. Patients with hypofibrinogenemia have few, if any, bleeding symptoms.

In afibrinogenemic patients laboratory tests based on fibrin formation (PT, APTT, and thrombin time) are abnormal because of the absence of the endpoint protein. The bleeding time is prolonged in about half of the patients, presumably because fibrinogen is required for primary aggregation in addition to fibrin formation. The platelet aggregation test is abnormal with ADP and epinephrine (Table 26-6). Diagnosis is confirmed with antigenic and functional assays for fibrinogen, which reveal almost no fibrinogen (less than 5 mg/dL). Curiously, the platelet count is decreased in 20% of patients. Erythrocytes fall precipitously in the erythrocyte sedimentation rate because of lack of fibrinogen.

In patients with hypofibrinogenemia, the PT, APTT, and thrombin times may be prolonged if the fibrinogen level is below 100 mg/dL. If the fibrinogen level is above 100 mg/dL, they will be normal. The fibrinogen functional assay is roughly equal to an antigenic assay, indicating decreased protein as opposed to abnormal protein. Platelet function tests are not affected.

Fibrinogen in the form of cryoprecipitate or fresh frozen plasma is used as therapy.

TABLE 26-6 *LABORATORY SCREENING TESTS IN AUTOSOMAL RECESSIVE COAGULATION FACTOR DISORDERS*

Disease	Platelet Tests Count/BT	Coagulation Factor Tests PT/APTT/TT/FA	Tests for Fibrin Split Products	Other
Afibrinogenemia	= N = A	A A A None	N	Abnormal platelet aggregation with ADP and epinephrine
Hypofibrinogenemia	N N	N N N A		
Dysfibrinogenemia	N N	N N A *DOT	N	
Factor II	N N	A A N N	N	
Factor V	N	A A N N	N	
Factor VII	N N	A N N N	N	
Factor X	N N	A A N N	N	Abnormal Russell viper venom test
Factor XI	N N	N A N N	N	
Factor XII	N N	N A N N	N	No bleeding tendency
Prekallikrein	N N	N A N N	N	No bleeding tendency APTT corrected with 10 minute incubation with kaolin reagents
High molecular weight kininogen	N N	N A N N	N	No bleeding tendency
Factor XIII	N N	N N N N	N	Urea solubility test

* Dependent on technique

Key to Abbreviations: BT-Bleeding Time; PT-Prothrombin Time; APTT-Activated Partial Thromboplastin Time; TT-Thrombin Time; FA-Fibrinogen assay.

A third form of fibrinogen abnormality is *dysfibrino-genemia* in which there is a structural alteration in the molecule. The structural alterations are the result of mutations in the genes controlling the synthesis of either the α, β, γ peptide of fibrogen. Over 300 abnormal fibrinogens have been identified. The molecular defect has been described in approximately 80 of them.[18] Similar to abnormal hemoglobins, the fibrinogen abnormalities are named for the city in which they were discovered.

Dysfibrinogenemia is inherited as an autosomal dominant trait. Clinically, most patients (>50%) have no bleeding symptoms or other clinical manifestations. In those who do exhibit hemorrhagic symptoms, the bleeding is mild and post-traumatic. Some of the reported patients have thrombotic disease and some have symptoms of both bleeding and thrombosis. The clinical maniferstations depend on the location and the type of gene mutation.

The functional defects in the dysfibrinogenemias vary with mutation. Defects in three phases of fibrin formation have been observed. Some patients have abnormal release of either fibrinopeptides A or B by thrombin. About half of the patients demonstrate abnormal polymerization of the fibrin monomers. The remainder have defective cross-linking of the monomers.[19]

Laboratory tests for hemostasis in patients with dysfibrinogenemia are usually normal, with the exception of the thrombin time and reptilase time, which are prolonged in most patients. Fibrinogen assays that are based on addition of thrombin and subsequent formation of a clot are incoagulable. However, determinations of fibrinogen antigenically or by a biochemical technique of precipitation and measurement of fibrinogen as protein are normal. Bleeding times and other platelet tests also are normal.

Mutations cause functional defects of the fibrinogen molecule. Functional defects of the three phases of fibrin formation have been observed. Some patients have abnormal release of either fibrinopeptides A or B by thrombin, about half demonstrate abnormal polymerization of the fibrin monomers, and the remainder have defective cross-linking of the monomers.[19]

Prothrombin (factor II) deficiency Deficiencies of prothrombin are extremely rare. Reports in the literature include 26 families diagnosed as having hypoprothrombinemia and 12 families with dysprothrombinemia. The diagnosis of hypoprothrombinemia is based on finding comparable levels of functional and antigenic activity indicative of decreased protein synthesis (Fig. 26-1). The level of prothrombin in homozygotes ranges from 0.01 to 0.25 U/mL (1% to 25%) and is usually less than 0.1 U/mL (10%). Heterozygous individuals have 0.43 to 0.75 U/mL (43% to 75%) of prothrombin protein in their plasma.

Patients with dysprothrombinemia, as with dysfibrinogenemia, have low levels of functional activity but normal immunologic activity, indicating normal amounts of a nonfunctional protein. The inheritance pattern of dysprothrombinemia is autosomal recessive.

Clinical symptoms in both dysprothrombinemia and hypoprothrombinemia are proportional to the level of functional protein and are present in both heterozygous and homozygous individuals. Homozygotes have severe bleeding after trauma or surgery, epistaxis, menorrhagia, hematuria, and easy bruising. Heterozygous patients have a milder disease, with epistaxis and bleeding after tooth extraction.[20]

Both the PT and APTT are prolonged since prothrombin is a factor in the common pathway (Tables 26-1 and 26-6). The degree to which they are prolonged varies from patient to patient. The PT time may be prolonged a few seconds in some patients and more than 60 seconds in others. Other platelet and coagulation factor tests are normal as are tests for fibrinolysis. Deficiencies of factors V and X show similar results in these screening tests. For differentiation, a specific two-stage assay[19] is suggested as the test of choice for functional prothrombin, along with immunologic tests for antigen levels.

Treatment either with fresh plasma that has been frozen or stored plasma is usually sufficient. The half-life of prothrombin is significantly longer than other factors (72 hours), which reduces the volume needed to achieve hemostasis. If needed, prothrombin complex concentrates can be used, but because of the previously mentioned risks, its use is limited. Therapy is aimed at reaching plasma levels of 0.4 to 0.5 U/mL.

Factor V deficiency The first reported case of factor V deficiency was presented by Owren in 1947. Owren, studying his patient in 1944 during the Nazi occupation of Norway, would ride his bicycle many miles at night to obtain rabbit brain for the reagent for the prothrombin time test.[21]

The incidence of factor V deficiency, also called parahemophilia, is extremely rare as fewer than 100 patients have been reported. Homozygous and heterozygous patients have been studied. The factor V level is less than 0.1 U/mL (10%) in homozygous patients and 0.3 to 0.6 U/mL (30% to 60%) in heterozygous family members. Only the homozygous individuals are symptomatic. There appears to be no correlation between the severity of symptoms and the level of factor V, and the disease has a mild course in most patients. Some patients have no abnormal bleeding. The molecular defects that cause factor V deficiency have not yet been determined. A concurrent factor VIII deficiency has been found in 30 patients.

Because factor V functions in the common pathway, the PT and APTT are both prolonged (Table 26-1). Abnormal bleeding times were reported in some, but it is unknown whether the test was influenced by ingestion of drugs, which could inhibit platelet function. Other screening tests are normal (Table 26-6). Definitive diagnosis is a factor V assay.

Treatment is with fresh or fresh frozen plasma as factor V disappears on storage. To prepare the patient for major surgery, levels of 0.25 to 0.30 U/mL are recommended.

Factor VII deficiency Factor VII deficiency is the only plasma coagulation disorder in which the prothrombin time alone is prolonged (Tables 26-1 and 26-6). The APTT, thrombin time, as well as tests for platelet numbers and function are normal. A quantitative factor VII determination provides a diagnosis. Homozygous patients usually have less than 0.1 U/mL (10%) of the factor present. Heterozygous individuals who are asymptomatic have 0.4 to 0.6 U/mL (40% to 60%) activity.

Factor VII deficiency was first described by Alexander in 1952. The condition is rare with the incidence estimated as 1 in 500,000. To date, more than 100 cases have been reported.

The genetics are heterogeneous. Factor VII abnormalities have been shown to be of the CRM + type, characterized by lack of correlation between the antigencity and functional activity, the CRM − type, with decreases in both functional and antigenic activity, and the dys-type in which the molecular structure is abnormal.

Clinical manifestations do not appear to correlate with the level of activity. Fatal intracranial hemorrhages occur frequently at an estimated rate of 16%. Homozygous patients may bleed from the umbilical cord, the nose, and the gastrointestinal tract among other sites. Hemarthroses are uncommon and, when seen, usually occur in males. Severe menstrual bleeding occurs in females. Other patients may have a mild course. Symptoms do not present until late in life in some patients.

Treatment is with fresh frozen plasma or prothrombin concentrates. Normal hemostasis is usually established when the level of factor VII is 0.2 U/mL.

Factor X deficiency   Factor X deficiency (Stuart-Prower deficiency) has been reported in 50 families. The disorder is similar to those above. Homozygous individuals have 0.1 to 0.14 U/mL (10% to 40%) of the protein in their plasma, heterozygous family members 0.4 to 0.68 U/mL (40% to 68%). Heterozygous patients are clinically asymptomatic, and homozygous patients are affected, some severely and others mildly. CRM +, CRM −, and variant molecules are described.

In the laboratory, the PT and APTT are prolonged (Tables 26-1 and 26-5). The Russell's viper venom test also is prolonged, although it may be normal in some variants.[20] Russell's viper venom reagent contains an enzyme that activates factor X. The thrombin time and platelet tests are normal. A factor X assay is the definitive test.

Treatment of homozygotes is with plasma or prothrombin complex concentrates in an attempt to raise the level to 0.4 to 0.5 U/mL, especially before surgery.

Factor XI deficiency   Factor XI deficiency (hemophilia C) is inherited as an autosomal, incompletely recessive trait. Both males and females are affected. As with the previously described autosomal recessive diseases, homozygous and heterozygous patients have been studied. Only the homozygous individuals are affected with symptoms of excess bleeding. Heterozygous patients are asymptomatic.

Factor XI deficiency has a high frequency in the Ashkenazi Jewish race. Approximately 0.2% of these individuals are homozygous, and 11% are heterozygous.[20]

The bleeding symptoms tend to be mild, occurring largely after traumatic injury, surgery, or childbirth. Often the disease is not suspected until presurgical laboratory tests are performed. Spontaneous hemorrhages have not been seen. Epistaxis, hematuria, and excess menstrual bleeding have not been reported. There is no correlation between the clinical severity and the level of factor XI activity as measured in vitro.

Laboratory screening tests reveal a prolonged APTT. Other tests are normal (Table 26-5). Factors of the intrinsic system, XII, XI, prekallikrein, and high molecular weight kininogen, VIII and IX, are considered when the APTT is the only abnormal screening test (Table 26-1). The clinical and family history is useful in arriving at a decision as to which factor assay to perform.

Specific assay for factor XI is the definitive test. Homozygous individuals have less than 0.01 to 0.1 Um/mL (1% to 10%) factor XI activity. To date, all patients studied have shown decreased antigenic activity comparable to the functional activity which is indicative of decreased production of the protein.

Laboratory testing for factor XI activity requires precautions in collection and handling of the specimen. In vitro activation of factor XI collected in glass tubes can lead to false normal results and missed diagnosis of mild deficiencies. Therefore, it is recommended that blood be drawn in plastic to minimize glass contact activation. Freezing and thawing of the specimen can also cause activation. An increase in factor XI activity may occur with storage of plasma, and as a result, cause the APTT to be in the normal range rather than low abnormal. The type of activator used by different manufacturers may affect the ability of a test system to detect a deficiency. Patients with mild factor XI deficiencies may react variably with different activators. Abnormal results may be obtained with one reagent and normal results with another. Celite was shown to detect all deficiencies, but other additives missed occasional mild deficiencies.

Treatment of factor XI deficiency is fresh frozen plasma to circulating levels of 0.35 U/mL or greater. It is better to treat the patient prophylactically than after bleeding has begun.

Factor XII deficiency   Factor XII deficiency is also called Hageman trait, named for the first patient in whom it was discovered in 1955 in Cleveland. This disease is inherited in an autosomal recessive pattern. No bleeding symptoms are associated with the disease, even after severe trauma or during surgery. Discovery of the deficiency is usually made when the APTT is done as part of a routine presurgical work-up.[20] All other hemostatic screening tests are normal (Table 26-5).

The euglobulin lysis test is prolonged, presumably because of the participation of factor XII in the activation of plasminogen.

The combination of an abnormal APTT and negative history of bleeding indicates a deficiency of either factor XII, prekallikrein, or high molecular weight kininogen. The three are differentiated by laboratory tests. A factor XII assay using specific factor XII deficient plasma will reveal less than 0.01 U/mL (1%) activity in homozygotes and 0.15 to 0.80 U/mL (15% to 80%) in heterozygotes. In heterozygotes, the APTT is normal. Antigenically, most patients show decreased production of a normal molecule (CRM−), although the CRM+ form is described.[5]

Paradoxically, patients with factor XII deficiency have increased incidence of thromboembolic disease. Mr. Hageman himself died of a pulmonary embolus. Myocardial infarction and strokes are also reported. The reason for this has been postulated to be the involvement of factor XII in activating fibrinolysis as well as complement and inflammation, but the theory has yet to be proven.

Because there is no bleeding, no treatment is needed, but treatment for thrombotic episodes is required.

Prekallikrein deficiency
A deficiency of prekallikrein was first described in 1965 in children of the Fletcher family, hence the synonym, Fletcher factor. Preoperative coagulation studies for adenoidectomy of one of the children revealed a markedly prolonged APTT. The same abnormality was found in three other siblings.

Prekallikrein deficiency is inherited in an autosomal recessive pattern. Like factor XII deficiency, no symptoms of bleeding are apparent. Patients with the disorder are likely to be discovered by chance.

The level of the APTT is sensitive to the reagent used, perhaps because of the type of activator. Reagents containing kaolin are more sensitive. A modification of the APTT is used as a screening test. Patient's plasma is incubated with a kaolin or celite-containing reagent for 10 minutes rather than the usual 2 or 3 minutes. If the prolonged APTT is corrected to normal with the longer incubation period, a prekallikrein deficiency is indicated.[20] The APTT remains prolonged in factor XII or high molecular weight kininogen deficiencies. A specific factor assay must be performed when the screening test is corrected to distinguish prekallikrein deficiency from Passovoy trait (see below).[20] The euglobulin lysis time is prolonged. Other tests are all normal.

High molecular weight kininogen deficiency
A deficiency of high molecular weight kininogen, also called Fitzgerald factor deficiency, is one of a group of disorders involving not only high molecular weight kininogen, but also variable deficiencies of low molecular weight kininogens. The low molecular weight molecules do not affect the hemostatic system so laboratory tests are not affected by their presence or absence. Concurrent absence of the low molecular weight kininogens aids in classifying the disorders, however.

In deficiency of high molecular weight kininogen, there is no bleeding tendency but the APTT is prolonged (Table 26-6) and is not corrected by longer kaolin incubation.[5] The variant molecules are known by other family names: Williams, Fleaujac, Reid, and Fujiwara. Fitzgerald and Reid traits are deficient only in high molecular weight kininogen. Both high and low are deficient in the remaining three.[20]

The euglobulin lysis time is prolonged, as in the previous two diseases. Other tests are normal. Diagnosis is made using the APTT modified by the addition of specific factor deficient plasma or an immunologic assay.[20]

Passovoy defect
Passovoy defect is a moderate bleeding disorder described in two unrelated families. Laboratory results may be confused with those seen in prekallikrein deficiency. The APTT is prolonged and corrects when the incubation period is extended to 10 minutes. The difference in the two defects is the presence of clinical bleeding in Passovoy trait and not in prekallikrein deficiency.[20]

Factor XIII deficiency
Because factor XIII functions after formation of fibrin, a deficiency does not affect the usual screening tests. In vitro clot formation, however, is abnormal. Excess red cells will be seen at the bottom of a whole blood clot tube.

A screening test for factor XIII based on dissolution of the clot in 5M urea will be positive when the factor XIII concentration is 0.005 U/mL or less. The clot will be insoluble at levels as low as 0.01 to 0.02 U/mL. Specific assays are available, some of which measure enzymatic activity and others which use immunologic techniques.

Clinically, homozygous factor XIII deficiency can be life-threatening. About 90% of patients present with umbilical cord bleeding.[20] Intracranial hemorrhage is common, and severe bleeding can develop after trauma or surgery. Abnormal scar formation has been noted in a number of patients for reasons as yet unexplained.

Factor XIII deficiency can be treated with plasma by bringing the factor XIII level to about 0.05 U/mL. The half-life of the factor is 3 to 7 days, which allows for prophylactic therapy.

α_2-antiplasmin deficiency
Four families have been described with a deficiency of α_2-antiplasmin and have severe bleeding tendencies. The function of α_2-antiplasmin is to inactivate plasmin and prevent it from circulating in the plasma. If plasmin is not inactivated because of a deficiency of its inhibitor, it will lyse protective clots that have formed and will also lyse circulating fibrinogen. An acquired deficiency of fibrinogen will develop. Both situations may result in excess bleeding. In the laboratory all screening tests are normal, but the whole blood clot lysis time and euglobulin lysis time are shortened.

Acquired disorders

Noncongenital deficiencies acquired during the lifetime of a previously normal individual are far more common than the hereditary disorders of coagulation factors. Acquired deficiencies occur in response to another disease process.

Induced deficiencies usually involve more than one coagulation factor and are produced by a variety of mechanisms. Mechanisms can involve decreased synthesis or the production of structurally altered, nonfunctional molecules which were described in the discussion of inherited diseases. In addition, mechanisms unique to the acquired disorders are either increased consumption and depletion of proteins, which are removed faster than they can be synthesized, or the presence of circulating chemical substances or antibodies that interfere with the function of normally produced factors. The conditions in which these disturbances occur are classified into the categories: disseminated intravascular coagulation, liver disease, vitamin K deficiency, and acquired pathologic inhibitors.

DISSEMINATED INTRAVASCULAR COAGULATION

Disseminated intravascular coagulation (DIC) is a condition in which the normal balance of hemostasis is altered, allowing the uncontrolled inappropriate formation of fibrin within the blood vessels. The microcirculation is primarily affected. Fibrin is deposited diffusely in the capillaries as well as arterioles and venules. As fibrin is formed, several clotting proteins, especially fibrinogen, are consumed at a faster rate than they are synthesized. The result is an acquired, multiple factor deficiency.

Platelets become caught within the fibrin mass, aggregate and are removed from the circulation. Because activation of clotting factors always results in the simultaneous activation of the fibrinolytic system, plasmin is formed. Subsequently, when fibrin degradation products are formed, they interfere with both platelet function and fibrin formation. Clinical manifestations are the result of the chain of events induced by thrombin and plasmin as they circulate within the blood stream.[20] Thus, as a result of coagulation factor and platelet consumption, and the presence of FDP, bleeding may occur at the same time that disseminated clotting occurs.

Nomenclature The term disseminated intravascular coagulation (DIC) implies systemic coagulation within the blood vessels, contrasted to normal blood coagulation that takes place extravascularly and locally. As mentioned, the clinical picture known as DIC involves not only coagulation but also fibrinolysis and is not always systemic. Consequently, several authors have advocated the use of more descriptive terms such as defibrination syndrome, consumption coagulopathy, or intravascular coagulation with fibrinolysis. Nevertheless, DIC remains the most commonly used term.

Incidence DIC occurs in approximately 1 in 1000 hospital patients. About 20% of the cases are asymptomatic and suspected only on the basis of laboratory data. It can occur at any age, although it is most often seen in the very young and in the elderly.

Etiology DIC, which is not a disease in itself, is a group of symptoms caused by a primary condition that does not normally involve coagulation. Any disease state, singly or in combination with others, may trigger the DIC syndrome.

Conditions most often associated with the development of DIC are summarized in Table 26-7. They include all types of infections, complications of pregnancy, malignant neoplasms, massive tissue injury, and vascular injury.[22] For a more complete list of causes with a literature search, the reader is referred to Bithell.[22] The effect of the conditions listed is to cause damage to either tissue, blood cells, or the endothelium. With tissue or blood cell injury, it is thought that thromboplastin-like substances enter the circulation and activate the extrinsic system. This has

TABLE 26-7 *CLINICAL CONDITIONS ASSOCIATED WITH THE DEVELOPMENT OF DIC*

Infections	Bacteria
	Virus
	Fungus
	Rickettsia
	Protozoa
Complications of pregnancy	Toxemia
	Retained placenta
	Amniotic fluid embolism
	Abrutio placentae
	Intrauterine fetal death
	Septic abortion
Neoplasms (especially malignant)	Leukemias—M3 and others
	Carcinomas
Massive tissue injury	Burns
	Traumatic injury
	Extensive surgery
	Extracorporeal circulation
Vascular injury	Shock
	Hypotension
	Hypoxia
	Acidosis
Miscellaneous	Snake bite
	Heat stroke
	Any disease

never been demonstrated, however. With endothelial rupture or damage, the intrinsic system is also activated by contact of factor XII with the exposed collagen. Figure 26-5 shows the potential portions of the hemostatic system that may become activated by triggering incidents.

Pathogenesis Activation of either the intrinsic or extrinsic pathway results in the formation of thrombin. Thrombin has many roles in hemostasis (Chapter 24). All of the roles are involved in the pathogenesis of DIC. The first function is removing fibrinopeptides A and B from fibrinogen forming fibrin monomers. Some monomers polymerize spontaneously, forming fibrin within the blood vessels. Others circulate as soluble fibrin monomers. The fibrinopeptides circulate in the blood stream, too, and are removed from the circulation by the macrophage system. Within the plasma, the fibrinogen level decreases and the level of fibrinopeptides, especially A, increases.

A second action of thrombin is activation of factors V and VIII, which are consumed as they function in the cascade of fibrin formation. In DIC, they are used at a faster rate than they can be synthesized and the plasma levels decrease. Additionally, thrombin activates factor XIII, which also is consumed. As thrombin is formed, the plasma level of prothrombin decreases. The presence of thrombin may decrease the function of liver macrophages in removing activated factors and particles, allowing them to remain for a longer time in the circulation. Finally, thrombin may contribute to thrombocytopenia by inducing platelet aggregation.

Plasmin is formed within the circulation as plasminogen is activated by tissue activators and by activated con-

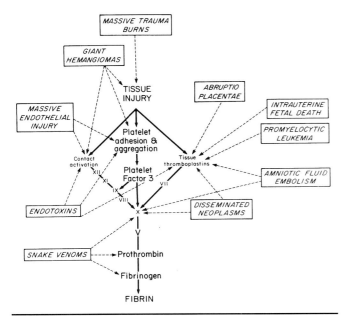

FIGURE 26-5. Conditions that initiate DIC activate the hemostatic pathways in a variety of ways. Normal hemostasis is shown by solid arrows. Processes that trigger DIC are shown in the boxes and broken arrows indicate proposed sites of activation. (With permission from: Bithell, T.C.: Acquired coagulation disorders. In Wintrobe's Clinical Hematology. 9th Ed. Edited by G.R. Lee, T.C. Bithell, J Foerster, J.W. Athens, J.N. Lukens. Philadelphia, Lea & Febiger, 1993).

tact factors (XII and prekallikrein). Consequently, plasma levels of plasminogen decrease. Plasmin digests both fibrin and fibrinogen, resulting in circulating fibrin (fibrinogen) split products (FSP). FSP act as anticoagulants forming soluble complexes with fibrin monomers, preventing them from polymerizing. They also adhere to platelet surfaces and cause decreased platelet function. Fibrinogen levels are further reduced because it is digested by plasmin. Plasmin also attacks other proteins including factors V, VIII, IX, and XI.[20] When plasmin digests crosslinked fibrin, D-D dimers are formed and circulate.

The induced deficiency of fibrinogen and factors II, V, VIII, and XIII as well as consumption of platelets leads to simultaneous bleeding and clot formation. The balance will tip in favor of bleeding or thrombosis, depending on which of the enzymes, thrombin or plasmin, predominates. Consequently, patient symptoms will be affected. If thrombin generation exceeds plasmin, more fibrin will be formed than degraded and diffuse thrombosis will result. If plasmin activity is greater, however, the fibrin will be lysed, increasing levels of circulating fibrin split products that coat platelet membranes and cause platelet dysfunction. Plasmin degradation of fibrinogen, factors V, VIII, IX and other plasma proteins, contributes to bleeding.[20]

Clinical aspects The clinical course of DIC can be either acute or chronic. The more commonly recognized acute form begins with a sudden onset of severe bleeding. The chronic form exists for a long period of time and may have either mild or no symptoms.

The acute type is seen in 80% to 90% of patients with DIC. The remaining 10% to 20% have a chronic course. Patients with acute disease tend to manifest hemorrhagic symptoms, whereas in those with chronic disease, thrombosis is more likely to occur. The mortality rate is 50% to 60%.

Thrombosis of the microvasculature and hemorrhages are responsible for the clinical manifestations. In patients with acute DIC whose disease course is hemorrhagic, bleeding begins abruptly and occurs from at least three sites at the same time.[20] Sites of bleeding tend to correspond to the tissues involved in the triggering event. Hematuria, gastrointestinal bleeding, epistaxes, oozing from needle puncture sites, ecchymoses, and petechiae are some manifestations. Bleeding may be profuse, leading to death.

Conversely, obstruction of the microvasculature by thrombi causes tissue anoxia and microinfarcts of the heart, kidney, brain, liver, and pancreas, all leading to shock. Shock is also induced because products of the complement and kinin system cause increased vascular permeability and hypotension[20] (Figure 26-6).

Laboratory aspects There is no single laboratory test that will establish a diagnosis of DIC nor any combination of tests that are specific for DIC. A battery of screening tests which include a platelet count, PT, APTT, thrombin time, and fibrinogen determination are offered by many laboratories (Table 26-8). The most useful parameters are demonstration of a progressive decrease in platelets, which may fall to 40 to 75×10^9/L and a decreased fibrinogen concentration.

The platelet count is decreased in 97% of patients, but platelet consumption may be difficult to identify in patients whose usual platelet count is in the upper normal range (300 to 440×10^9/L), unless normal base levels were previously identified. For example, a patient with a normal platelet count of 400×10^9/L may have a drop of over 50% in the circulating platelet mass before thrombocytopenia is detected. Thus, serial platelet counts may be necessary to pinpoint platelet consumption.

In severe disease, the fibrinogen may drop to 10 to 50 mg/dL. The fibrinogen level is decreased in only 23% to 71% of patients. This is probably because it is an acute phase reactant. Acute phase reactants are plasma proteins that increase in inflammatory conditions. Since many patients with DIC have underlying disease, their fibrinogen levels may have risen because of the acute phase. When DIC develops, the fibrinogen level may drop but, because it started higher than normal for the patient, may not fall below the normal range.

The PT and APTT may be prolonged because of the decrease in factors II, V, VIII, and fibrinogen. The thrombin time is increased due to the presence of fibrin split products as well as the decreased fibrinogen. Alteration of these tests is not as consistent as the platelet count. The PT is prolonged 50% to 75% of the time, APTT 50% to 60%, and the thrombin time 58%.[20] Occasionally, especially early in the disease process, these tests may be

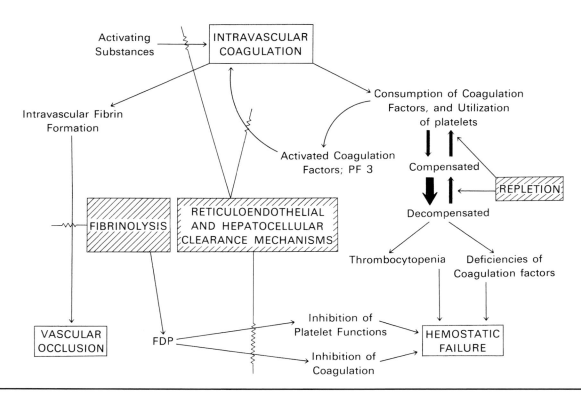

FIGURE 26-6. Pathophysiology of diffuse intravascular coagulation (DIC). Activation of the hemostatic process intravascularly by triggering processes leads to clotting and bleeding simultaneously. Intravascular fibrin formation results in occlusion of vessels. During the clotting process several coagulation factors and platelets are consumed leading to bleeding. Inhibiting processes are also activated and are shown in the hatched boxes. (With permission from: Bithell, T. C.: Acquired coagulation disorders. In Wintrobe's Clinical Hematology. 9th Ed. Edited by G.R. Lee, T.C. Bithell, J. Foerster, J.W. Athens, J.N. Lukens. Philadelphia, Lea & Febiger, 1993.)

shorter than normal, the reason for which has not been fully explained. It is believed by some to be due to the presence of factors which are already activated, and which would require less time for this phase of the test.[20,22] The presence of schistocytes on a peripheral blood smear is found in approximately half of patients with DIC. Schisto-

cytes are produced by the forcing of blood cells through the fibrin webs that clog the blood vessels.

Helpful confirmatory tests for DIC are those that demonstrate the presence of products of thrombin or plasmin cleavage, namely, the fibrin monomer, fibrinopeptides A and B, or fibrin split products. Tests evaluating the presence of fibrin monomers are the paracoagulation tests using protamine sulfate or ethanol, which detect the presence of soluble fibrin monomer complexes. These are neither specific nor sensitive. They are positive in 90% to 95% of patients with acute DIC, but are also positive in other conditions such as myocardial infarction and pulmonary embolism.[20] Proteolytic cleavage products, fibrinopeptides A and B (especially A), are potentially useful parameters, but at present, are mainly research tools. Methodology requires monoclonal antibodies and radioimmunoassay techniques, which are costly and time-consuming. Currently, the most useful procedures appear to be latex tests for the presence of fibrin split products and the D-D dimer.[20] Abnormal levels of fibrin split products have been demonstrated in 85% to 100% of patients with acute DIC, and their presence is good positive evidence in favor of the diagnosis. The D-D dimer test is elevated in 93% of patients and is also recommended.[20] The tests are performed quickly and are economical. However, FSP are also increased in several related conditions and as such

TABLE 26-8 ABNORMAL LABORATORY FINDINGS IN DIC

Test	Result
Platelet count	Decreased
Prothrombin time	Increased (sometimes decreased)
Activated partial thromboplastin time	Increased (sometimes decreased)
Thrombin time	Increased (sometimes decreased)
Fibrinogen	Decreased
Protamine sulfate test	Positive
Fibrin split products	Positive
Circulating fibrinopeptide A	Increased
Plasminogen	Decreased
Antithrombin III	Decreased
Blood smear	Schistocytes

are not specific. Values greater than 40 U/mL of FSP and greater than 200 U/dL almost always indicate DIC.[20]

A new procedure that is gaining popularity is analysis of antithrombin III, which decreases in concentration early as it combines with and inactivates thrombin and other activated serine proteases. It is decreased in 89% of patients. Analysis of this protein is possible on chemistry analyzers using chromogenic substrates.[20]

Therapy Treatment for DIC is to first eliminate the primary condition, if possible. The acute form of the disease is often self-limited and will disappear when the fibrin is completely lysed. Replacement therapy using platelets, red cells, or plasma are used when indicated.[22] The chronic form of the disease is usually secondary to disseminated carcinoma, in which elimination of the cause is difficult. Heparin therapy sometimes may be helpful if thrombosis is life-threatening because it will stop intravascular fibrin formation. It is administered with caution, however, because fatal bleeding has occurred with its use.[22]

LIVER DISEASE

Liver disease affects all hemostatic functions. Most hemostatic proteins, those which are involved in fibrin formation, fibrinolysis, and inhibitors, are synthesized in the liver (Table 26-9). The liver macrophages play a major role in removal of activated factors and products of activation, such as the fibrinopeptides, fibrin split products, and plasminogen activators. When the liver is diseased, these functions are diminished. The effects of liver disease on hemostasis are summarized in Table 26-10.

In the laboratory, liver disease may resemble DIC, and may, in fact, have an element of DIC. Differentiating the two is a difficult, sometimes impossible task for the physician. All screening coagulation tests of factors may be prolonged, including the PT, APTT, and thrombin time.[22] The fibrinogen concentration, although usually normal, is stable in the low normal range if decreased. An abnormal fibrinogen molecule is synthesized, which has an increased content of sialic acid and may cause defective clot formation.

The platelet count may be decreased for several reasons: hypersplenism from backing up of the portal blood supply when it is unable to enter the liver, alcohol toxicity of the bone marrow, or utilization if DIC is also present.

TABLE 26-9 *COMPONENTS OF HEMOSTASIS SYNTHESIZED IN THE LIVER*

Factor I (Fibrinogen)	Prekallikrein
Factor II (Prothrombin)	High molecular weight kininogen
Factor V	Antithrombin III
Factor VII:C (?)	Protein C
Factor IX	Protein S
Factor XI	α_2-macroglobulin
Factor XII	α_2-antiplasmin
Factor XIII	Plasminogen

TABLE 26-10 *THE EFFECT OF LIVER DISEASE ON HEMOSTASIS**

Decreased biosynthesis	All coagulation factors except von Willebrand factor All inhibitors of coagulation and fibrinolysis
Possible defective biosynthesis	Fibrinogen and several other factors
Decreased hepatic clearance	Activated coagulation factors Fibrin monomers and fibrinopeptides Fibrin split products Plasminogen activators
Increased destruction of coagulation factors	Lysis of fibrinogen by plasmin Possible DIC
Thrombocytopenia	Hypersplenism Folate deficiency Alcohol effect DIC
Platelet dysfunction	Fibrin split products Alcohol effect

(Modified from Wintrobe, M.M.: Clinical Hematology. 9th Ed. Philadelphia, Lea & Febiger, 1993.)

Fibrin split products are increased because of inability of the liver to remove them. Incomplete removal of plasminogen activators may result in plasmin formation systemically. Some degradation of fibrinogen may occur, resulting in a slight increase of fibrinogen degradation products. The presence of excess fibrin or fibrinogen degradation products impair blood coagulation and result in platelet dysfunction. The D-D dimer test may be normal.[20]

Clinical manifestations are minimal except in severe liver disease. Ecchymoses and epistaxis may occur. Bleeding from local lesions in the gastrointestinal tract are common. Therapy involves the use of replacement products as needed.

VITAMIN K DEFICIENCY

Vitamin K is needed by hepatic cells to complete the posttranslational alteration of factors II, VII, IX and X, protein C, and protein S. In the absence of vitamin K, the proteins are still synthesized by the hepatic cells but, because γ-carboxyglutamic acid residues are absent, calcium binding sites on the molecule are nonfunctional. Deficiency of vitamin K results in induced deficiencies of all of these factors. If the level of functional factors falls below 0.3 μm/mL, bleeding symptoms may result, and the PT and APTT will be prolonged.

Sources of vitamin K are from green, leafy vegetables in the diet and through synthesis by bacteria in the gastrointestinal tract.

Symptomatic vitamin K deficiency is most often seen in newborns in the first days of life. It is called *hemorrhagic disease of the newborn.* Because their livers are still immature, synthesis of the vitamin K-dependent factors in newborns is 30% to 50% of adult levels. Human milk contains little vitamin K and, until bacterial colonization of the intestinal tract occurs, the dependent factors are not produced. Those factors that are present at birth are metabolized so that they may become even lower during the first few days of life. In some infants, particularly those born prematurely, the levels of the proteins are low enough to cause bleeding symptoms.

Manifestations of hemorrhagic disease of the newborn are bleeding from the umbilicus or circumcision, generalized ecchymoses, large intramuscular hemorrhages, and intracranial bleeds. In the laboratory, the PT and possiby the APTT are prolonged more so than expected at this age. Specific factor assays for factors II, VII, IX, and X are markedly decreased. The bleeding time and platelet count are within normal limits.

Hemorrhagic disease of the newborn is prevented in the United States by administration of vitamin K to all newborns. In countries where this practice has recently been stopped, the disease occurs occasionally.

Other causes of vitamin K deficiency that may be seen in adults are malabsorptive syndromes such as sprue, obstruction of the biliary tract because bile salts are necessary for adsorption, and prolonged broad spectrum antibiotic therapy that abolishes normal flora of the intestine.

Vitamin K administration corrects the deficiency within 24 hours.

ACQUIRED PATHOLOGIC INHIBITORS

Acquired inhibitors, also called circulating anticoagulants, develop pathologically in patients with certain disease states, as well as in some who have no apparent underlying condition. Almost all are immunoglobulins, either IgG or IgM, with antibody specificity toward a component of fibrin formation. Some are of unknown biochemical nature. Two types of inhibitors are described: those directed toward a single factor and the lupus-like anticoagulant (LLAC).

Inhibitors of single factors

CLINICAL ASPECTS OF SINGLE FACTOR INHIBITOR Of the inhibitors to single factors, those directed against factors VIII and IX are observed most often, largely because they are associated with the hemophilias. Approximately 5% to 20% of patients with hemophilia A and 2% to 3% of patients with hemophilia B develop antibodies to the respective deficient factor.[22] Most of them have severe disease with very low coagulant levels of the affected factor. The development of antibodies is related to having received treatment with the deficient factor, but there is no correlation to the amount of exposure.[22] Some patients with mild forms of hemophilia A also develop the inhibitor.

The antibodies are of the IgG class of immunoglobulins. In hemophilia A patients, the antibody specificity is directed toward the coagulant antigen (VIII:Ag) only and not antigen associated with the von Willebrand portion of the factor VIII/von Willebrand factor complex.[22]

Clinical manifestations of patients with inhibitors resemble those of severe hemophilia. Symptoms may begin while the patient is receiving therapy, indicating a failure of treatment. In patients who have not received therapy for 1 to 2 years, the antibody level decreases, but an anamnestic response is seen within 2 to 4 days after re-exposure.

LABORATORY ASPECTS OF SINGLE FACTOR INHIBITOR Laboratory tests in patients with factor VIII or IX inhibitors resemble those found in patients with severe deficiencies. The APTT will be markedly prolonged and the other screening tests normal.

Mixing studies can be done as a screening test to distinguish between a true factor deficiency and an inhibitor. Patient's plasma is mixed in a 1:1 ratio with normal control plasma. The APTT is repeated on the mixture. If the original APTT was prolonged because of a single factor deficiency, the normal plasma will contain enough of the missing factor to correct the APTT to normal. If an inhibitor was present the test on the mixture will remain prolonged.

When an inhibitor is indicated, further tests can be done to determine the strength. The inhibitor against factor VIII depends on temperature. Its neutralization action takes place over a period of time. Assays for strength of the inhibitors have been developed in which patient plasma is incubated with normal plasma containing a known amount of factor VIII for 2 hours at 37° C.[20,23] During this time, the inhibitor, if present, will inactivate the factor VIII. After 2 hours, a factor VIII assay is performed to see how much factor VIII from the normal plasma remains. If 50% of the original factor VIII is left, the inhibitor is said to have one Bethesda unit of activity per mL. Weak factor VIII inhibitors may be detected by a sensitive procedure that uses a 4:1 mixture of patient to normal plasma. This mixture is incubated for 2 hours at 37° C. Following incubation, an APTT is performed on an aliquot of the mixture to detect loss of factor VIII activity.[23] A modification is used for factor IX inhibitors. Interpretation of the assays must be done with caution because of the variable nature of the antibodies.

THERAPY Therapy for patients with inhibitors is not always effective. For those with factor VIII inhibitors, large amounts of factor VIII may be administered in hopes of overcoming the antibody. Bovine factor VIII may be used but there is danger of anaphylactic reaction to the foreign protein. Treatment with factor IX concentrates rather than factor VIII has been attempted with limited success. Immunosuppressive therapy is used when all else fails, but also with variable results. Therapy for factor IX inhibitors is with factor IX concentrates.

Factor VIII inhibitors are found in patients other than those with hemophilia A. Some patients, otherwise healthy, develop inhibitors during or following a pregnancy. Factor VIII inhibitors are found in patients with autoimmune or lymphoproliferative diseases, or multiple myeloma. Occasionally, older patients who are otherwise healthy, develop factor VIII inhibitors. Clinical disease in these individuals is variable and the antibody may disappear spontaneously.

Inhibitors of other coagulation factors such as V, XI, XII, XIII, have been rarely described. Drugs may induce inhibitor formation at any time.

Lupus-like anticoagulant (LLAC)

The second type of inhibitor of major clinical importance is the *lupus-like anticoagu-*

lant, so called because it was first discovered in patients with systemic lupus erythematosus (SLE). Approximately 6% to 16% of patients with SLE develop the LLAC. It has subsequently been associated with a variety of other autoimmune diseases, neoplasias, the administration of drugs such as chlorpromazine or procainamide, as well as apparently normal individuals. The inhibitor is also associated with viral infections.

The lupus-like anticoagulant is a laboratory phenomenon and is not associated with clinical bleeding symptoms. Patients have undergone major surgery with no complications. Clotting factors are not inactivated by the lupus anticoagulant. Instead, the antibody, which is either IgG, IgM, or both, combines with the phospholipid surfaces of test reagents for the APTT and occasionally the PT, causing prolongation of the test(s). The lupus inhibitor is usually discovered by chance when performing routine coagulation studies.

The LLAC is difficult to identify in the laboratory. Steps in evaluating plasma for the presence of the LLAC as recommended by the Subcommittee for the Standardization of Lupus Anticoagulants are summarized in Table 26-11.[24] It must first be differentiated from other causes of a prolonged APTT such as the presence of heparin and single factor deficiencies. It must also be differentiated from a specific factor inhibitor (see above). The specimen must be collected carefully and centrifuged at high speeds for 10 to 15 minutes to remove all traces of platelets because platelets will inactivate the LLAC.[25] Heparin contamination must be ruled out first because it is the most common cause of prolonged APTTs in hospitalized patients. This can be done with a thrombin time or reptilase time.[20,26]

The next step is to perform the APTT on a 1:1 mixture of patient's plasma and normal control plasma. As de-

scribed above, the APTT will be corrected if a single factor deficiency is present. In the presence of the LLAC, no correction will be noted. It is sometimes difficult to distinguish correction, especially if the inhibitor is weak. In these cases a 4:1 ratio of patient to normal plasma may be more sensitive.[26]

Several confirmatory procedures to distinguish a specific factor inhibitor from the LLAC are described. This distinction is important because the specific inhibitors are likely to cause bleeding and needs to be identified. The test systems are based on either decreasing the phospholipid concentration by dilution to enhance the LLAC or by increasing or changing the configuration of the phospholipid in order to neutralize the LLAC.

Tests in which the phospholipid is decreased are the kaolin clotting time or the dilute Russell's viper venom time. These tests are used both to screen for and to confirm the presence of the LLAC. The tissue thromboplastin inhibition test is also used but is not recommended because it is positive in many other conditions.[26]

The platelet neutralization procedure is believed to be the most sensitive confirmatory test.[26] In this test washed, frozen and thawed platelets are added to the patient's plasma and correct the prolonged APTT. Another test in which the phospholipid is altered is the hexagonal phospholipid neutralization procedure. This test has also been shown to be very specific for LLAC.[26]

No test by itself will identify all LLACs. A combination of tests are recommended with repeated testing on different occasions.[25]

While bleeding symptoms are not seen in the presence of the LLAC, 25% of affected patients demonstrate thrombosis. Spontaneous abortions are also associated with the presence of the LLAC, presumably due to thrombosis in the blood vessels of the placenta followed by ischemia and infarction.[25] There is no test that will predict in which patients these conditions will develop.

Another group of antiphospholipid antibodies called anticardiolipin antibodies (ACLA) are associated with the presence of the LLAC. ACLAs behave in a similar manner to the LLAC. That is, they are associated with thrombosis and fetal wastage and laboratory tests are variable from time to time. They are identified by ELISA tests. Some patients who have the LLAC also have ACLA but others do not.

TABLE 26-11 *RECOMMENDED REVISED CRITERIA FOR THE IDENTIFICATION OF LUPUS-LIKE ANTICOAGULANTS**

STEP 1: Suspect from prolonged phospholipid-dependent clotting tests.
　Kaolin clotting time
　Dilute Russell's viper venom time
　Tissue thromboplastin time inhibition test
　Plasma recalcification clotting time
　APTT with reagents sensitive to LLAC

STEP 2: Differentiate inhibitor from factor deficiency by mixing studies.
　LLAC patient plasma : normal plasma mixture should be >3 SD higher than non-LLAC patient plasma : normal plasma mixture

STEP 3: Confirmation of inhibitor by correction of abnormal test.
　Platelet neutralization procedue (PNP) using lysed, washed platelets;
　Phospholipid liposome containing phosphatidyl serine or hexagonal phase phospholipids

OTHER
　Specific factor inhibitor not identified
　Rapid loss of activity in plasma diluted with saline
　Associated with positive ELISA test for antiphospholipid antibodies
　Identification as immunoglobulin

* From Exner T., Triplett, D.A., Taberner, D. and Machin, S.J.: Guidelines for testing and revised criteria for lupus anticoagulants. Thromb. Haemost. 65:320, 1991.

HEMOSTASIS IN THE NEWBORN

Blood coagulation studies in the newborn present special challenges to the laboratory. At birth, liver synthesis of several of the proteins is at a lower level than normal adults; some proteins do not reach adult levels until 9 to 12 months of age. Laboratory screening tests are prolonged and also are dependent on the age of the child and the presence of accompanying diseases. These factors influence the interpretation of the laboratory tests.

Obtaining an adequate blood specimen is of utmost importance but technically extremely difficult. A venous sample is preferred to capillary or arterial blood. Obtaining the sample from an indwelling catheter should also be avoided because of the danger of contamination of the specimen with heparin. The 3- to 5-mL sample drawn from adults is not possible in infants, especially preterm infants whose total blood mass may be only 80 to 100 mL.[27] Some suggestions for minimizing the amount of plasma needed are to eliminate duplicates when performing the PT, APTT, or TT, or to run several factor assays that use diluted plasma rather than the screening tests, thus obtaining more information from the same amount of blood.[27] Johnston and Zipursky[28] have developed micro adaptations of several routine procedures, which use 5 to 40 μL of plasma.

Adding anticoagulant to the syringe allows one to draw blood more slowly while minimizing the risk of clotting. The amount of anticoagulant must be reduced when the infant's hematocrit is above 65% because of the reduced plasma volume. Even with utmost attention to quality control, however, the possibility of spuriously altered results is always present.

●
Normal hemostasis in the newborn

Platelets and the proteins of the coagulation and fibrinolytic systems are first detected in fetuses 10 to 11 weeks of gestation. Table 26-12 shows expected values for various laboratory tests for preterm and term infants at birth.

Platelet counts reach adult levels by 27 weeks of gestation and, therefore, should be in the normal adult range at birth. As with adults, platelet counts of less than 100 × 10^9/L should be considered abnormal. Counts of 100 to 150 × 10^9/L are questionable and should be repeated. Impaired platelet aggregation with low levels of ADP, as well as to collagen, epinephrine, and thrombin are found at birth. These abnormalities disappear in infants who are several weeks old. Platelet aggregation with ristocetin, on the other hand, is increased in newborns, a fact that must be considered if the diagnosis of von Willebrand disease is attempted. The bleeding time, however, is not affected by these in vitro abnormalities and is normal in term and preterm infants. Drugs, such as aspirin, which affect platelet function when taken by the mother, will also influence hemostasis in the fetus.

Concentrations of the coagulation proteins are shown in Table 26-13. The proteins of the fibrinogen group are in the normal range at birth. These factors include fibrinogen and factors V, VIII, and XIII. Factor VIII levels are increased especially in infants delivered vaginally. The remainder of the coagulation proteins, the prothrombin group and contact factors, are decreased in amounts because of immaturity of the liver. Infants born preterm (less than 37 weeks gestation) have lower levels of these proteins than those born at term (37 to 41 weeks). The concentration of the vitamin K-dependent factors is 0.15 to 0.30 U/mL in preterm infants and increases to 0.30 to 0.50 U/mL in term babies. The contact factors are found in similar amounts. Even though the proteins are decreased in amount, hemostasis is usually not affected unless a stressful situation is present because only 20% to 30% of the proteins are necessary for normal blood clotting. They reach adult levels at varying times. Since coagulation factors do not cross the placenta, the status of the mother's proteins do not affect the infant.

Natural inhibitors that are liver dependent are decreased in newborns. These include antithrombin III which is below 0.30 U/mL in preterm infants and about 0.60 U/mL at term.[27] Adults with these levels of antithrombin III are at risk for thrombosis. Infants do not have this problem because the fibrin forming proteins that are inactivated by antithrombin III are also decreased. Levels of proteins C and S are decreased to 10% to 50% in term infants, but are not balanced by a concomitant decrease in the proteins that they inhibit.[27]

The decrease in these hemostatic factors in term and preterm infants affects coagulation tests (Table 26-12). The PT is prolonged because of the low levels of factors II, VII, and X. However, a PT of greater than 17 seconds should be considered abnormal.[29] Values in the normal adult range are usually achieved in 3 to 4 days. The APTT is also prolonged, sometimes markedly so, especially in

TABLE 26-12 *LABORATORY TESTS IN PRETERM AND TERM INFANTS AS COMPARED TO ADULTS AND OLDER CHILDREN*

Test	Preterm Infant (32–36 weeks)	Term Infant (37–41 weeks)	Adults and Older Children	Adult Level Reached
Bleeding time, (minutes)	1.5–5.5*	1.5–5.5*	2–9.3	Before birth
Platelet count, × 10^9/L	150–430	174–456	150–450	Before birth
Platelet aggregation	Abnormal	Abnormal	Normal	One month
PT (seconds)	12–21	13–20	11–13	3–4 days
APTT (seconds)	70	55	23–36	2–9 months
TT (seconds)	11–17	10–16	8–10†	Few days
Euglobulin lysis time, (minutes)	95	84	140	
Fibrin split products	Normal	Normal	Normal	Before birth

* Feusner, J.H.: Normal and abnormal bleeding times in neonates and young children utilizing a fully standardized template technic. Am. J. Clin. Pathol. 74:73, 1980.

† Oski, F.A. and Naiman, J.L.: Hematologic Problems in the Newborn. 3rd Ed. Philadelphia, W.B. Saunders, 1982.

TABLE 26-13 *LEVELS OF COAGULATION PROTEINS IN TERM AND PRETERM INFANTS AS COMPARED TO ADULTS AND OLDER CHILDREN**

Protein	Preterm Infants (27–31 weeks) (U/mL)	Term Infants (38–41 weeks) (U/mL)	Adults and Older Children (U/mL)	Age Adult Level Reached
Fibrinogen, mg/dL	256 ± 70	215 ± 35	200–400	Before birth
Factor V	0.91 ± 0.3	0.56–2.00	0.64–1.62	Before birth
Factor VIII	0.82–2.24	1.34 ± 0.54	0.50–2.00	Before birth
Factor XIII†	1.00	1.00	1.00	Before birth
Prothrombin	0.30 ± 0.08	0.54 ± 0.15	0.74–1.48	2–12 mo.
Factor VII	0.24–0.76	0.35–0.82	0.63–1.51	2–12 mo.
Factor IX	0.17–0.20	0.21–0.39	0.60–1.50	3–9 mo.
Factor X	0.14–0.70	0.33 ± 0.13	0.69–1.32	2–12 mo.
Factor XI	0.05–0.18	0.29–0.70	0.60–1.50	1–2 mo.
Factor XII	0.11–0.37	0.44 ± 0.13	0.60–1.50	9–14 days
Prekallikrein	0.13–0.38	0.36 ± 0.14	0.60–1.50	n.a.
HMWK	0.21–0.52	0.64 ± 0.10	0.60–1.50	n.a.
Plasminogen	0.24 ± 0.08	0.20–0.56	0.80–1.30	n.a.
Antithrombin III	0.29 ± 0.03	0.60 ± 0.16	0.80–1.12	n.a.
Protein C	n.a.	0.18–0.46	0.70–1.30	n.a.

Compiled from: *Montgomery, R.R., Marlar, R.A., Gill, J.C.: Newborn hemostasis. Clin. Haematol. 14:443, 1985. †Oski, F.A., Naiman, J.L.: Hematologic Problems in the Newborn. 3rd Ed. Philadelphia, W.B. Saunders, 1982. n.a. - not available

preterm infants. This test is dependent on the factors of the intrinsic system and is particularly sensitive to the contact factors. Results of this test are also highly dependent upon the reagent used.[27] Adult levels may be reached in 4 to 6 months.[29] The thrombin time is abnormal even though the fibrinogen level is normal and may be explained by the presence of an abnormal fibrinogen molecule. It becomes normal within a few days after birth. Plasminogen levels are also decreased,[27] but the fibrinolytic activity as measured by the euglobulin lysis time is increased throughout fetal life and at term. Fibrin degradation products in the fetus at any age are similar to adult values.

Common bleeding disorders in the neonate

Abnormalities of hemostasis may be present in 1% of newborns. Classification of the problems seen most often is first dependent on whether the child is considered "sick" or "well." Sick infants include those with prematurity, perinatal infection, respiratory distress syndrome, metabolic derangements, and/or birth asphyxia. Babies considered "sick" usually have either DIC isolated platelet consumption independent of a decrease in coagulation factors or liver failure. In "well" babies, the most common abnormalities of hemostasis are immune thrombocytopenia, vitamin K deficiency, hemophilia, or bleeding from a localized vascular lesion.

Bleeding manifestations in babies with DIC are similar to other patients with the syndrome and include bleeding from puncture sites and the gastrointestinal tract or from any location. The PT and APTT are markedly prolonged and thrombocytopenia is present in symptomatic babies.

Vitamin K deficiencies are characterized by bleeding 2 to 4 days after birth from the gastrointestinal tract, scalp, nose, and various other sites. Vitamin K deficiency is more common in breast fed infants because breast milk contains less vitamin K than cow's milk. Mothers taking Dilantin or other anticonvulsants may give birth to babies with vitamin K deficiency.

One of the most common causes of death in premature infants is intracranial hemorrhage. Many of these are patients who have severe respiratory distress syndrome.

Thrombosis may also occur in infants, particularly those with indwelling catheters and with diabetic mothers. The decreased level of antithrombin III may be a partial cause of thrombosis.

THROMBOSIS

A second manifestation of abnormalities of hemostasis is thrombosis, a major cause of morbidity and mortality in hospitalized patients. Thrombosis occurs when the hemostatic system is inappropriately activated to the extent that the natural anticoagulant processes are overwhelmed and a clot is allowed to form within a blood vessel. The clot consists of a mass of fibrin, platelets, and entrapped cells.

As the mass, or *thrombus,* enlarges it may occlude the blood vessel and then result in death of the tissues normally supplied by that vessel. In addition, a portion of a thrombus, called an *embolus,* may break away from the thrombus and travel to smaller vessel branches. There the embolus may become lodged in a vessel smaller than its size, obstruct the blood flow and subsequently cause tissue destruction. The obstruction is an *embolism* or *thromboembolism*.

Thrombi can develop in arteries or in veins but their composition, the factors predisposing to their formation, and their methods of treatment are different.

Thrombi also can form in capillaries where they are seen either in localized areas or diffusely throughout large areas of the body. Capillary thrombi are an expression of disseminated intravascular clotting (DIC), which has been discussed earlier in this chapter.

The diagnosis of thrombosis is often difficult and is largely a task of the radiologist and the clinician. There is no laboratory test or group of tests that can specifically identify the presence of thrombosis. However, a major portion of the workload of the coagulation laboratory is involved with the regulation of therapeutic drugs used for prevention or management of thrombosis.

The intention of this section is to briefly explain how and when thrombi are formed in arteries and veins and how the laboratory is involved in the treatment of these conditions.

Thrombus formation

ARTERIAL THROMBUS FORMATION

Arterial thrombi occur in blood vessels in which the blood flow is rapid. As the name suggests, this happens most often in arteries but also may occur in veins. These thrombi are white in color because of their composition. A white thrombus is initiated by interaction between damaged endothelium and platelets and consists primarily of layers of platelets and fibrin, among which a few leukocytes and erythrocytes have become caught.

Damage to the endothelium is associated with the presence of plaques composed of lipids, fibrous connective tissue, macrophages and excess smooth muscle cells (atherosclerosis) in the intima layer of the blood vessels (Chapter 23). When these lesions are present, the wall of a vessel becomes thicker at the expense of the lumen which, then, is narrower. Although the precise mechanisms have yet to be fully explained, it is thought that endothelial cells become injured and then detached in the areas of the plaques. This results in exposure of the platelets and the plasma to the subendothelial structures. Activation of the hemostatic elements follows. Platelets adhere to the subendothelium, aggregate and release ADP and other granule contents, as well as synthesize thromboxane A_2. Contact between the coagulation proteins and the subendothelium leads to fibrin formation. In addition, the normal anticoagulant properties of the endothelial cells, for instance, synthesis of inhibitors such as PGI_2, are diminished. The thrombus, which is the mass of platelets and fibrin, grows into the lumen of the vessel.

Factors which increase the likelihood that arterial thrombi will occur include diets rich in cholesterol, cigarette smoking, the use of oral contraceptives, and the presence of various diseases among which are arteriosclerosis, hypertension, diabetes, and nephrotic syndrome.

Symptoms develop through a number of mechanisms. An artery may become occluded by a locally developed thrombus. Or, more often, a smaller vessel in the heart, brain, or extremities is affected when an embolus from a distant site lodges in it. The products of platelet release may activate other platelets and cause small aggregates within the circulation. Released substances from platelets and similar products from leukocytes may cause damage to vessels, particularly in the heart. Clinically, the result of occlusion of vessels by thrombi and thromboemboli is slower blood flow to a particular area (ischemia) and death of the tissue (necrosis), heart attacks, and cerebral infarctions.

Laboratory tests intended to establish the presence of, or the predisposition to, the development of arterial thrombi are neither specific nor sensitive and are, therefore, of uncertain utility. Treatment includes several platelet inhibiting drugs such as aspirin, and thrombolytic agents such as streptokinase or urokinase. Laboratory involvement in these forms of treatment is minimal. Their characteristics and the ways in which laboratory tests can be used to monitor their effectiveness will be described in a later section.

VENOUS THROMBOSIS FORMATION

Venous thrombosis occurs in blood vessels in which the blood flow is slow. Slower blood flow and stagnation (stasis) occur in all veins, particularly those in the area of a valve. Damage to endothelium, which is prominent in arterial thrombosis, is not as evident in venous thrombosis. However, it is probable that because of the lower oxygen supply to the vessel's own wall, contraction of the endothelial cells produces gaps between them. Platelets could then fill the gaps by adhering to the exposed subendothelium and become activated. Activation of platelets could lead to the subsequent steps of aggregation and fibrin formation. If the natural inhibitors are overwhelmed, the thrombus will enlarge. A venous thrombus is red in color because erythrocytes are trapped among the platelet-fibrin network when the blood flow is slow. It looks similar to clotted blood in a test tube.

Most venous thrombi occur in the deep veins of the calf muscles and are lysed by natural processes without causing symptoms. Symptomatic and clinically significant venous thrombosis is called *deep vein thrombosis* (DVT). DVT may form in calf veins but usually is found in the proximal leg veins. Swelling and distension of the veins caused by the occlusion of the lumen may be accompanied by inflammation which causes pain, tenderness, redness, and warmth. The condition is then called *thrombophlebitis*.

Increased risk for developing DVT occurs with behaviors, diseases and conditions that cause stasis or that result in the entry of procoagulants into the circulation. Risk behaviors include sitting for long periods of time, sitting with crossed legs, or wearing tight garments. Diseases which require prolonged bed rest cause venostasis because of the lack of activity to aid circulation in the veins. Surgery, especially of the hips and pelvis area, congestive heart failure and cancer are examples of conditions associated with extensive tissue damage which may be accompanied by release of tissue thromboplastin into the circulation. The presence of circulating tissue thromboplastin may result in activation of the hemostatic system in the blood stream. Obesity and deficiencies of natural inhibitors of coagulation are also associated with an increased incidence of DVT. A discussion of the latter will follow in the next section. Patients who have had episodes of thrombosis are at higher risk for recurrence.

Emboli are the major complication of deep vein thrombosis. Emboli from deep veins in the legs travel through increasingly larger veins, through the right side of the heart and eventually reach the pulmonary circulation and occlude vessels in the lungs. Pulmonary emboli may be asymptomatic or they may be fatal. They cause between 50,000 and 100,000 deaths per year. Between 0.1% and 0.8% of patients who undergo general surgery and up to 5% of those who have hip surgery die of pulmonary emboli each year. Approximately 50% of patients with documented deep vein thrombosis have emboli.

It is difficult to establish a diagnosis of DVT because 70% of patients presenting with similar symptoms have some condition other than DVT. Radiologic procedures are required for demonstration of a thrombus. Laboratory tests that identify the products of fibrinolysis in the circulation are helpful as positive evidence but they are not specific for the diagnosis of DVT.

Conversely, certain laboratory tests are very important as an aid in evaluating the patient's response to some drugs used in treatment of DVT. The types of drugs and the laboratory involvement will be discussed below. Laboratory tests are not generally useful in identifying patients at risk for developing thrombosis.

● Conditions predisposing to thrombosis

Numerous conditions lead to an imbalance between clot promoting and clot inhibiting factors and might be considered to predispose the patient to thrombosis. The terms "hypercoagulable state" and "prethrombotic condition" are used to describe them. There are many discrepancies in the definitions of these terms in the literature. Some authors define "hypercoagulable state" as a condition in which there are definite measurable alterations of laboratory tests that indicate a shift of the hemostatic balance to thrombosis. The term "prethrombotic" is then used for those conditions in which there is a high likelihood that thrombosis will occur. The two terms are used interchangeably by some,[30] and others refer to the former as "primary" and the latter as "secondary" hypercoagulable states. There is overlap in any of the attempts to classify the conditions. Generally, the measurable conditions are hereditary deficiencies of one of the components of the hemostatic system. Those that cannot consistently be measured are usually secondary to another condition, that is, acquired conditions.

MEASURABLE HYPERCOAGULABLE STATES

Hypercoagulable states can be caused by deficiencies of proteins that regulate and limit fibrin formation. Hereditary deficiencies of antithrombin III, protein C, protein S,

TABLE 26-14 *HEREDITARY CONDITIONS ASSOCIATED WITH THROMBOSIS*

Antithrombin III deficiency
Protein C deficiency
Protein S deficiency
Plasminogen deficiency
Dysfibrinogenemia
Defects in fibrinolysis
Factor XII deficiency
Homocystinuria
Giant cavernous hemangioma

plasminogen, factor XII, as well as dysfibrinogenemia, have been described in families whose members have a high incidence of thrombosis (Table 26-14). Recurrent deep vein thrombosis with pulmonary emboli at a young age is the most common symptom although arterial thrombi are seen occasionally. Deficiencies of heparin cofactor II are also described but no symptoms have been associated with this condition. While this section will concentrate on the characteristics of hereditary deficiencies of the proteins listed above, conditions in which deficiencies are acquired will also be discussed.

Antithrombin III deficiency Antithrombin III functions as an inhibitor of all serine proteases including thrombin, factor Xa, and plasmin, perhaps with the exception of factor VIIa. A deficiency of antithrombin III may result in insufficient inactivation of these activated components of hemostasis and lead to the formation of fibrin within the blood vessels.

The incidence of antithrombin III deficiencies is approximately 1 in 5000. Approximately 2% to 5% of patients with DVT have this deficiency. The condition is inherited as an autosomal dominant trait, and most patients described so far have been heterozygous with plasma activity of 20% to 60% of normal.[31]

The amino acid sequence of antithrombin III and the nucleotide sequence of the antithrombin III gene have been determined. The gene for antithrombin III has seven exons and six introns and is on the long arm of chromosome 1.[31] The gene has been studied in several families with antithrombin III deficiency to determine mutations that cause the defect.

Some patients (families) have a true quantitative protein deficiency (called Type 1). Levels of both antigen and function of antithrombin III are about 50% of normal. In Type 1 deficiencies, the gene may be deleted or altered so that it cannot function and no detectable protein is produced by it. Other families appear to have immunologic activity consistent with the presence of a qualitatively abnormal molecule (types 2 and 3). These are usually point mutations in the gene. Type 2 defects affect the binding site for the serine protease and type 3 the heparin binding site (Chapter 24). A category called type 4 consists of mutations which are not included in one of these three.

Symptoms appear in the second or third decade of life. Recurrent deep vein thrombosis of the legs, pelvic and mesenteric veins, and pulmonary emboli are seen. The risk of thrombosis increases with pregnancy, injury, or surgery.

Laboratory tests for platelets, coagulation factors and fibrin split products are normal, but antithrombin III activity is decreased. Antithrombin III functional activity can be measured on automated analyzers in the presence of excess heparin using a known amount of thrombin and measuring the residual thrombin after the reaction. Immunologic methods such as radial immunodiffusion are available but these might be invalid in patients with abnormally functioning molecules (types 2 and 3). In both types of measurement, the normal range is approximately 80% to 120% of a normal control value. Testing of family members needs to be done to confirm the hereditary nature of the disorder.

The activity of antithrombin III is increased by 1000- to 10,000-fold in the presence of heparin. Heparin is often used to treat patients with thrombosis, such as deep venous thrombosis, because of its anticoagulant effect. Therefore, in patients with antithrombin III deficiency heparin therapy may be ineffective because heparin requires antithrombin III for its anticoagulant action (discussed later in this chapter). Laboratory tests for monitoring heparin dosage, such as the PTT, might not be prolonged as expected.[32] This may be the first clue to the presence of the underlying deficiency.

Patients with antithrombin III deficiency may be treated prophylactically with the warfarin type of anticoagulants, such as coumadin. These drugs lower the level of functional forms of the vitamin K-dependent coagulation proteins. Since it is primarily these proteins that are inhibited by antithrombin III the activities of coagulation proteins and AT III become more comparable and thrombosis is less likely to occur.[31,32] Coumadin compounds have been reported to increase the circulating levels of antithrombin III, presumably because less thrombin and activated serine proteases are generated. Therefore, less antithrombin III is needed to inactivate them. If thrombosis does occur, and also during times of stress such as surgery, patients may be given antithrombin III concentrate to raise the plasma level. Preparation of the concentrate destroys blood-borne pathogens and is, therefore, safe.[33]

Several conditions are associated with acquired deficiencies of antithrombin III. Normally, antithrombin III is removed from the circulation as it combines with activated serine proteases. The activity may decrease as it is utilized in DIC, and rarely during acute thrombosis. Acquired deficiencies may also occur, questionably, in patients with liver disease because of decreased synthesis, nephrotic syndrome due to protein loss, and in patients on oral contraceptive therapy. Patients on heparin therapy for more than seven days may demonstrate resistance to the heparin and the need for increased dosage.

Heparin co-factor II Heparin cofactor II (HC-II) is a protein similar to antithrombin III. As its name implies, its activity is greatly enhanced by heparin. In contrast to the action of antithrombin III, heparin cofactor II is active in inhibiting only thrombin, not other serine proteases, in in vitro tests.

Because of its similarities, HC-II can be measured and may represent a minor portion of the activity defined as antithrombin III in laboratory tests. For example, it was estimated that in the DuPont aca method for antithrombin III that HC-II might account for 5 to 10% of the activity and might lead to difficulty in recognizing some antithrombin III deficiencies.[34] Modifications in methodology are described which allow for more specific measurement of either protein.[35]

Inherited deficiencies of HC-II have been described. In two families, thrombosis was present, but more studies are needed to determine the significance.

Protein C deficiency Venous thrombosis is the clinical expression of a deficiency of Protein C. Protein C is an inhibitor of factors Va, VIIIa, and of plasminogen activator type 1 (Chapter 24). When it is deficient, the delicate balance of the hemostatic system is altered so that there is decreased control of fibrin formation and possibly less fibrinolysis.

Protein C deficiency is inherited in an autosomal dominant manner. The incidence of heterozygous individuals is thought to be quite common. In a series of healthy blood donors the frequency was 1 per 200. However, it can be difficult to identify because of the overlap between plasma levels of normal individuals in the lower range and deficient individuals in the upper abnormal range. Also, many patients in the series who were identified as deficient had no symptoms or family history of thrombosis. The fundamental genetic defect varies widely from family to family and includes deletions and point mutations in critical areas of the gene. In some, the abnormal gene produces no protein (type I) and in others a nonfunctional molecule is produced (type II).[33]

Of the patients who can be identified as heterozygous for protein C deficiency, deep vein thrombosis or pulmonary emboli develop in approximately 75% by the age of 40 years. Occasionally, heterozygotes may develop necrosis of the skin after large doses of oral anticoagulants. The necrosis is believed to occur because protein C is a vitamin K-dependent protein and, therefore, affected by the oral anticoagulants. Warfarin decreases protein C activity sooner than it affects the vitamin K-dependent factors involved in fibrin formation because protein C has a shorter half-life. This results in excess unregulated activated factors Va and VIIIa leading to thrombosis that is generalized and occludes vessels of the skin. Rarely, infants are born with a homozygous deficiency. They develop a severe type of skin necrosis called purpura fulminans, which leads quickly to death if not treated with protein C and long term anticoagulants. A protein C concentrate is being tested for use in therapy.

Two types of methods of laboratory measurement of protein C are currently available commercially. Some are immunologic assays that will detect normal as well as nonfunctional molecules and, therefore, might miss the

Type II individuals. Other assays measure the activity of the protein. The latter methodology is preferred but no method is able to detect all protein C deficiencies. By a functional assay that measures protein C activity, normal levels were found to be 4.8 to 1.0 U/mL. Newborns have 20 to 40% of normal adult levels. As with antithrombin III, plasma levels of protein C decrease with thrombosis. Therefore, the deficiency state cannot be determined during an acute thrombotic episode.

Acquired decreased levels of protein C have been reported in DIC, cirrhosis of the liver, and with warfarin anticoagulant therapy.[33]

Protein S deficiency Protein S is a vitamin K dependent protein and functions as a cofactor to increase the activity of protein C in the inactivation of factors Va and VIIIa. Protein S forms a 1:1 complex with activated protein C and enhances its binding onto the phospholipid surface. The protein is named for Seattle, the city in which it was found. A deficiency of protein S is similar to protein C deficiency in that symptoms of recurrent severe DVT or pulmonary emboli begin at 20 to 40 years of age. The deficiency is an autosomal dominant trait.

The normal level of protein S is approximately 34 U/mL or 61 to 134%. Affected persons demonstrate about half of this activity or 17 to 65%.

In the plasma, protein S circulates in two forms, bound and unbound. The unbound form or "free protein S" accounts for approximately 40% of the total and it is the only form that is functionally active. The remaining protein S in the circulation is attached to C4b binding protein.[36] Laboratory measurement of protein S is by a variety of immunologic assays that can measure total protein S or free protein S. Some assays are available commercially as kits. Methods have been proposed for functional assays but are not yet commercially available.[36] The distribution between the two forms is important in some familial abnormalities and can be differentiated by some of the methods. Some families have a decrease in both the free and bound types to about 50 % of normal total levels. Others have total level in the normal range but with most or all of the protein S bound to the C4b binding protein and therefore nonfunctional.[36]

The genetic abnormalities studied so far indicate that most families have point mutations. One family of six has been shown to have a deletion in the protein S gene.[37]

Acquired protein S deficiency occurs in pregnancy, use of oral contraceptives, DIC, nephrotic syndrome, and acute thrombosis. In conditions that manifest an increase in acute-phase proteins, of which C4b binding protein is one, the deficiency is actually a shift of the free form to the bound, nonfunctional form of protein S.[37]

Plasminogen deficiency Deficiency of plasminogen is extremely rare. It has been reported in 12 families, many of which are Japanese. All families have abnormal molecules with a variety of functional defects. Four families also have a decreased synthesis of the abnormal plasminogen. In many families, the original patient studied had symptoms of recurrent thrombosis but other family members who also had the abnormal plasminogen had no symptoms. The defect is inherited in an autosomal dominant manner.

Dysfibrinogenemia Less than 20 of the known families with dysfibrinogenemia (discussed previously) have symptoms of excess thrombosis. The molecular defect that leads to thrombosis varies. Some patients have defective release of fibrinopeptides A and B, and some have abnormal polymerization of fibrin. The reason for thrombosis has been studied in a few families, and may involve abnormal resistance of the fibrin to lysis by plasmin or decreased activation of plasminogen, both of which would lead to less fibrinolysis.

Defects in fibrinolysis Approximately 30 to 40% of patients with recurrent DVT have impaired fibrinolytic function.[39] Identification of some specific abnormalities of fibrinolysis is possible with recently developed tests.[40] The majority of patients have high levels of plasminogen activator inhibitor which inhibits plasminogen activator (tPA), and therefore decreases fibrinolysis. Increased PAI-1 activity is also associated with arterial thrombus formation. Other patients have defective release of the plasminogen activator (tPA) from the tissues. Among the laboratory tests recommended for fibrinolytic activity are the euglobulin lysis test for PAI-1 activity.

Homocystinuria Homocystinuria is a rare inborn error of amino acid metabolism. It is a deficiency of the enzyme, cystathionine beta-synthase, which is one of several enzymes in the pathway of methionine conversion to succinyl CoA. Homocystine is increased in the blood and excreted in the urine. Methionine is increased in the blood. Thrombosis occurs in arteries as well as veins.

OTHER CONDITIONS PREDISPOSING TO THROMBOSIS

Giant cavernous hemangiomas ("strawberry" hemangiomas) are congenital benign tumors of the vascular system that consist of many thin-walled vessels with abnormal endothelium (Table 26-14). They first appear about 1 month after birth and grow to a size of 0.5 to 10 cm, and then disappear. The lesions can form on the skin or internal organs. Thrombi form in the abnormal vessels, and a localized chronic type of disseminated intravascular coagulation (DIC) may develop. The DIC can occasionally become acute and cause bleeding. The association of DIC and giant cavernous hemangioma is called Kasabach-Merritt syndrome. Increased tendency to thrombosis has been associated with decreased factor XII and other deficiencies of the contact system (Table 26-14).

A higher-than-normal risk of thromboembolic disease is found as a secondary complication of a variety of clinical conditions. Many of these have been discussed previously but will be summarized here (Table 26-15). Mechanisms of inappropriate activation of the hemostatic system may involve blood vessels, platelets, or the coagulation and fibrinolytic proteins. Often more than one mechanism is proposed and most often it is difficult to identify the exact cause.

TABLE 26-15 *ACQUIRED DISORDERS ASSOCIATED WITH THROMBOSIS*

Condition	Mechanism
Malignancy	Tumor cells activate platelets Tumor cells produce procoagulant Tumor cells induce monocytes and macrophages to produce procoagulants
Venous stasis	Decreased dilution of activated factors Development of hypoxia and acidosis
Pregnancy	Increased stasis and blood viscosity Increased fibrinogen and factor VIII Decreased fibrinolysis Decreased protein S and antithrombin III
Oral contraceptives	Controversial
Estrogen therapy	Controversial
L-asparaginase therapy	Controversial
Hematologic disorders	
Polycythemia vera	Increased viscosity Platelet dysfunction
Sickle cell anemia	Increased viscosity
Hemolytic anemia	Cell breakdown
Nephrotic syndrome	Loss of antithrombin III
Diabetes mellitus	Hyperaggregability of platelets
Lupus anticoagulant	Unknown
Treatment with prothrombin complex products	Activated procoagulants

Malignancies were discussed previously as a contributing factor to the DIC syndrome. Thrombosis occurs in 5 to 15% of all patients with neoplastic disease. The incidence is higher in some types of tumors than others, with lung, pancreas, stomach, and colon cancer being most common. Several proposed mechanisms contribute to the activation of the hemostatic system. Tumor cells may interact with and activate platelets. They may produce a procoagulant tissue factor-like substance that can activate the extrinsic fibrin pathway, or they may interact with monocytes and macrophages and cause them to produce procoagulant activity.

Conditions leading to venous stasis are associated with thromboembolism. Following surgery, 70% of elderly immobilized patients develop thrombosis. Stasis interferes with the blood flow dilution of activated factors and leads to hypoxia and acidosis, which promote clotting.

Pregnancy is associated with increased risk of thrombotic disease for several reasons. Increased stasis and viscosity of the blood, an increase in the concentration of fibrinogen, an increase in factor VIII and other clotting factors, and a decrease in fibrinolysis, protein S, and antithrombin III levels are some contributing factors.

The use of oral contraceptives and estrogen therapy for arterial disease and prostate cancer is reportedly associated with a variety of thrombotic symptoms, both venous and arterial. The mechanisms involved with these condi-tions are still controversial, although protein S has been shown to be decreased in oral contraceptive therapy.

Many hematologic conditions predispose to thrombosis. Examples are the myeloproliferative disorders (MPD), sickle cell anemia, persistent thrombocytosis, following splenectomy for hemolytic anemia, paroxysmal nocturnal hemoglobinuria, and active hemolysis in immune hemolytic anemia. Patients with MPD may present with painful digital ischemia or develop characteristic thrombosis in the splenic or hepatic vessels. Neurologic symptoms caused by thrombosis of cerebral vessels are also seen. Those signs and symptoms cause the physician to suspect a myeloproliferative process. Patients with these diseases may present with either bleeding or thrombotic manifestations and during the course of their disease may change from one to another. Polycythemia vera is associated with thrombosis more often than the other MPD. The incidence is proportional to the hematocrit level, and is mainly caused by the increased viscosity of the blood because of the increased number of erythrocytes. The MPD are also associated with hyperfunction or hypofunction of platelets, which is thought to play a role in the clinical manifestations. Treatment of acute leukemia with L-asparaginase is also implicated in thrombotic disorders. Hyperviscosity may also play a role in the mechanism of thrombosis in sickle cell disease.

Other diseases associated with thrombosis are the nephrotic syndrome, thought by some to involve the loss of antithrombin III as part of the proteinuria, diabetes mellitus because of hyperaggregability of platelets, patients with the lupus anticoagulant in which the mechanism is unknown, and as previously mentioned, in patients treated with the infusion of prothrombin complex products.

● Anticoagulant therapy

Patients with thrombotic diseases are treated with drugs that either inhibit the formation of blood clots (anticoagulants) or remove clots that have formed (thrombolytic agents). The use of them is called anticoagulant therapy or thrombolytic therapy. The drugs fall into three categories: (1) drugs used to prevent initiation or extension of venous thrombosis, (2) antiplatelet drugs which prevent recurrence of arterial thromboembolic disease and (3) thrombolytic agents which cause dissolution of established clots. These are outlined in Table 26-16 and shown in Figure 26-7. The drugs interfere with normal hemostasis and can potentially cause serious hemorrhage if given in excess. If the dose isn't high enough, however, the drug will be ineffective. Because of individual response to these drugs, there is no standard dosage that is both safe and effective for all patients. The most clinically effective dose is established by trial and error, using in vitro laboratory test results as a guide. With the exception of the prothrombin time, which is used to judge the dosage in oral anticoagulant therapy, there is no reliable laboratory procedure that can be a measure of the in vivo effect of these drugs. The following discussion includes a description of the drugs used and the laboratory methods used in monitoring dosage of the anticoagulants.

TABLE 26-16 *APPROACHES TO ANTICOAGULANT THERAPY*

Prevention or extension of venous thrombosis	Heparin
	Oral anticoagulants (coumarins)
Antiplatelet drugs	Aspirin
	Dipyridamale
	Sulfinpyrazole
	Ditran
	Clofibrate
	Prostaglandins
	Phenolthiazine
	Antihistamine
Thrombolytic agents	Streptokinase
	Urokinase

DRUGS USED FOR PREVENTION OR EXTENSION OF VENOUS THROMBOSIS

Drugs used to prevent initiation or extension of venous thrombosis are heparin and the oral anticoagulants. These drugs do not dissolve clots that have already formed, but do prevent them from becoming larger while the patient's own fibrinolytic system works to remove them.

Heparin   Heparin is the anticoagulant agent used most often in medicine today. Commercial sources of heparin are porcine intestinal mucosa or bovine lung.

Heparin does not have a direct effect on blood coagulation but acts indirectly by enhancing the effect of antithrombin III. Antithrombin III, as discussed above, is a natural anticoagulant and inhibits fibrin formation by removing activated serine proteases from the circulation.

STRUCTURE   Biochemically, heparin is an acid mucopolysaccharide (glycosaminoglycan) consisting of alternating, unbranched, uronic acid (L-iduronic acid) and amino sugar residues that have undergone a series of chemical modifications. The modifications include the addition of several sulfate groups, epimerization, and deacetylation that produces a variety of components that are unevenly distributed throughout the molecule.

The primary alternating structure is synthesized attached to a core protein. Multiple copies of the heparin precursor are attached to one core protein molecule. Following synthesis, the heparin molecules are detached from the core protein by enzymatic action. The enzyme cuts are at different sites on the different heparin segments resulting in a heterogenous mixture of many different sized molecules.[41] The molecular weights range from 4,000 to 40,000 daltons. When heparin is manufactured commercially, the molecules are further degraded, which possibly adds to the heterogeniety of the preparation. Twenty-one components of heparin have been separated by molecular size. Each component has separate chemical and biologic activities and different affinities for the co-factors with which it acts.[42]

A portion of a heparin molecule that consists of five monosaccharide units is shown in Figure 26-8. This structure is the only portion of heparin that binds to antithrombin III (Chapter 24). Some sulfate groups in the pentasac-

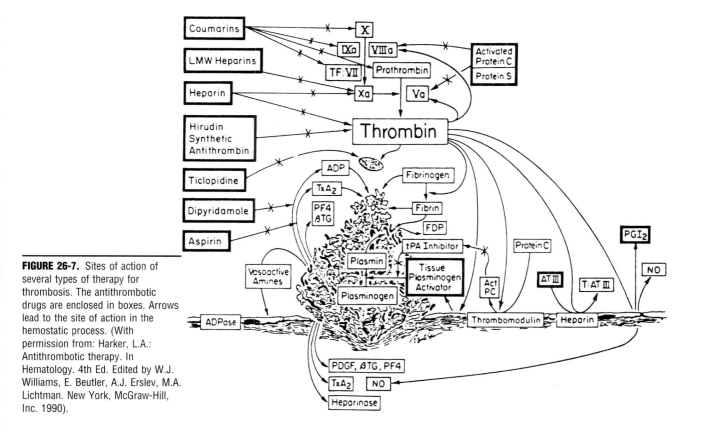

FIGURE 26-7. Sites of action of several types of therapy for thrombosis. The antithrombotic drugs are enclosed in boxes. Arrows lead to the site of action in the hemostatic process. (With permission from: Harker, L.A.: Antithrombotic therapy. In Hematology. 4th Ed. Edited by W.J. Williams, E. Beutler, A.J. Erslev, M.A. Lichtman. New York, McGraw-Hill, Inc. 1990).

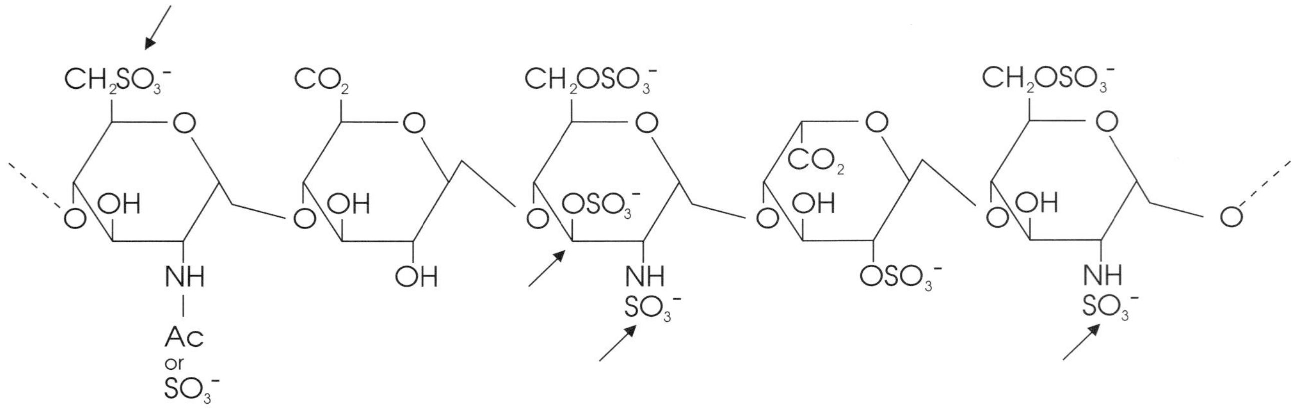

FIGURE 26-8. The pentasaccharide active component of heparin. Note the areas of sulfation. The middle residue has the highest affinity for antithrombin III binding.

charide structure, as indicated by arrows, are essential for heparin to associate with antithrombin III. The middle sulfate residue is especially important because it is found only in the five-unit antithrombin III binding site.[43] Other sulfated residues are found elsewhere in the molecule, too. Only about one-third of the heparin molecules in a commercial preparation contain the pentasccharide unit and only a few units are present on the ones that do contain it. It is distributed in the heparin molecules randomly.[43] The molecules that have the pentasaccharide unit are said to bind antithrombin III with high affinity.[44]

MECHANISMS OF ACTION Several steps in the coagulation cascade are affected by the presence of heparin. The major mechanism of the action of heparin is through its interaction with antithrombin III. Antithrombin III combines with and inactivates the serine proteases, factors XIIa, XIa, IXa, Xa, kallikrein, thrombin, and plasmin, in a 1:1 molar ratio. This process is quite slow under natural conditions but is markedly increased by the presence of heparin. Antithrombin III reacts best with thrombin, to a lesser degree with factors Xa and IXa and minimally with the others under physiologic conditions.

Interaction of the serine proteases involves reversible binding of the negatively charged sulfate groups of heparin (Figure 26-7) to a region with several positively charged lysine residues on antithrombin III. The interaction with heparin allows antithrombin III to react 1000 times faster with the serine protease, either by causing a conformational change in antithrombin III which makes the combining site more accessible to the serine protease or by acting as a template to which both molecules attach side by side.[44] After antithrombin III and the serine protease are bound together, the heparin dissociates from the complex and is free to associate with another antithrombin III molecule. The antithrombin III-serine protease complex is removed from the circulation by the monocyte-macrophage system. Each time a molecule of antithrombin III inhibits an activated serine protease, it is eliminated from the plasma. In conditions such as thrombosis, in which the number of activated serine proteases is greatly increased, an acquired defi-

ciency-like state of antithrombin III develops. The level of antithrombin III in the plasma will remain low until the liver has time to replace it.

In addition to removing activated serine proteases from the circulation, heparin also inhibits interaction between factor X and prothrombin. Platelet aggregation and function are also inhibited by heparin.

A second heparin-associated plasma protein called heparin cofactor II does not require the pentasaccharide unit to react with heparin. Combined with heparin, it is less active than antithrombin III, but will react with similar natural mucopolysaccharide substances, such as dermatan sulfate on the surface of the endothelial cells, which have no effect on antithrombin III.

CLINICAL USE Heparin is quantitated in units that are defined by international standards. One milligram of heparin contains approximately 150 units. It is commercially available as aqueous solutions of 1,000 to 40,000 units/mL.[44]

Heparin has several uses in medicine. Some of the clinical uses are:

- Treatment of thromboembolic disorders
- DVT
- Pulmonary embolism
- Prophylaxis of the above thromboembolic disorders
- Treatment of arterial thrombosis or embolism
- Treatment of DIC in some patients
- Prevention of clots in "heparin lock" arterial or venous catheters
- Prevention of clots in extracorporeal circulation and renal dialysis
- As an anticoagulant for blood sampling for selected laboratory tests

Heparin is given by injection, either intravenously or subcutaneously. Its action is immediate when it enters the bloodstream. It is not absorbed in the intestine and, therefore, cannot be given orally. The route of administration depends partially on the condition for which it is being given, and partially on the preference of the physician.

Low or "mini"-doses of standard heparin preparations are used for prophylaxis to prevent thrombosis following surgery or in patients confined to bed rest. The usual dose is 5,000 units injected subcutaneously every 8 to 12 hours. Moderate doses, 18,000 to 60,000 units, are injected either subcutaneously or intravenously. The intravenous route is by continuous drip or intermittently, every 4 to 6 hours. Higher doses are given through a continuous intravenous drip. Adjusted dose subcutaneous heparin therapy is used for pregnant women who need anticoagulant therapy but cannot use coumadin drugs. A dose is given every 12 hours and adjusted by performing laboratory tests as indicated below.

The ideal therapeutic range is between 0.2 and 0.5 units of heparin per mL of plasma. With intermittent bolus injections, the drug level is immediately very high but may fall to undetectable levels before the next injection.

A more recent variation of therapeutic heparin use is the separation by fractionation, enzymatic degradation, or chemical modification of the lower molecular weight fractions (LMW). The molecular weight of the LMW heparin ranges from 2,000 to 12,000 Daltons.[42] These preparations of heparin are also very heterogeneous in the size of the fragments and the chemical composition of the sugar residues. No two preparations are ever the same.

LMW heparin fractions differ from the standard variety in several respects. They have a greater effect on the inhibition of factor Xa than do they on thrombin.[43] The LMW heparins do not affect clot-based laboratory tests for monitoring heparin therapy. If monitoring is required, chromogenic assays using factor Xa are used. LMW heparins are more completely absorbed from the subcutaneous site of injection, so that one dose has the same effect as two doses of regular heparin preparations.[44]

The clinical usefulness of the LMW fractions is still controversial. It is hoped that fewer bleeding complications will occur but this has not been proven.

LABORATORY EVALUATION Laboratory tests are used to aid in establishing the proper heparin dosage. Because of the many sites at which heparin acts and because of each patient's individual, clinical situation, reaction to the drug varies from person to person and at different times within the same patient. There is no standard amount that provides protection from clotting while assuring that excessive bleeding will not occur. Doses are titrated by the patient's response to an in vitro laboratory test. There is, however, no laboratory test that can measure either the concentration of heparin or the effect on in vitro clot formation in whole blood or in plasma.

Whole blood tests include the obsolete Lee-White clotting time and the activated clotting time (ACT), which is designed to be performed at the patient's bedside. The prothrombin time is not useful because it is only minimally affected by the presence of heparin. The APTT, which uses plasma, has become most popular because it is already available in most laboratories as a screening test for coagulation abnormalities, and because it provides adequate information. With continuous therapy and with intermittent injections, the APTT is performed daily and the next

dose adjusted accordingly until the desired effect is achieved. With intermittent therapy, the test is usually timed 1 hour before administration of the next dose. The APTT is very sensitive to heparin. If performed too soon after an intermittent heparin dose, it will be too prolonged to measure. It is standard practice to adjust the dose of heparin so that the APTT is about 1.5 to 2 times the patient's baseline value before treatment or 1.5 to 2 times the control value. This corresponds to a heparin concentration of 0.3 to 0.5 units/mL.

Disadvantages of using the APTT for monitoring heparin therapy lie in the wide variety of instruments and reagent systems in use in clinical laboratories. Each laboratory uses its own combination of instruments and reagents, making standardization between laboratories difficult.

COMPLICATIONS Unwanted side effects of heparin therapy are possible hemorrhage or thrombocytopenia. Bleeding is a common complication of heparin therapy and may occur in 1 to 33% of patients. The patients who develop bleeding symptoms are usually those who have received high doses of heparin and/or those who have significantly prolonged monitoring tests.[44] Low dose therapy and low molecular weight heparins were developed in part to minimize the possibility of bleeding. However, clinical trials have not yet proven whether this actually happens. Patients on intermittent therapy are thought to be at greater risk than those on continuous therapy. An antidote, protamine sulfate, can be given if the bleeding becomes life-threatening.

Two types of thrombocytopenia are possible and unpredictable in patients on heparin therapy. About 25% of patients given full-dose therapy develop mild thrombocytopenia, usually unnoticed, 2 to 15 days after the first dose. The second type of heparin-associated thrombocytopenia is rare but severe. This form is related to IgG antibodies with anti-heparin properties. A platelet count should be performed before heparin therapy and 5 days into therapy to identify patients at risk for thrombocytopenia.

Oral anticoagulants Oral anticoagulants are so named because they are administered in pill form by mouth. These drugs were first discovered in 1939, when dicoumarol was found to be the cause of a hemorrhagic disease that developed in cattle after ingesting spoiled clover. Clinical trials with the drug began in 1941. Since then, oral anticoagulants have been used in the treatment of acute DVT and pulmonary embolism. Recent, well-controlled clinical trials suggest that they are also effective in preventing recurrence of disease when administered long term.

Oral anticoagulants are of three types: dicoumarols, coumarins, and indanediones. Of these, the coumarins have become the most widely used. The dicoumorals act too slowly and the indanediones have more side effects. Warfarin sodium, or coumadin sodium, is the most popular derivative of the parent compound, 4-oxycoumarin. Rat poison contains this compound.

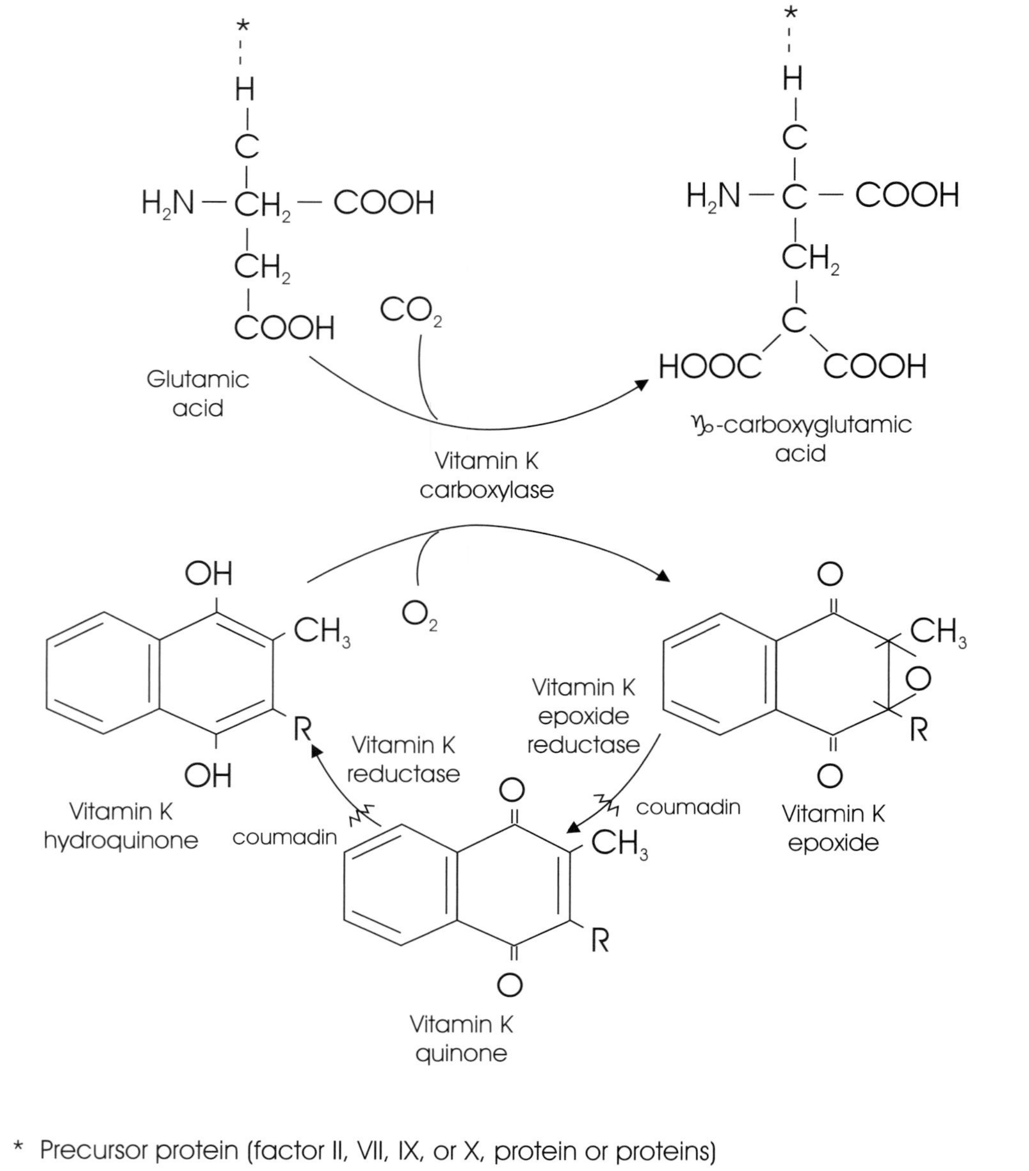

FIGURE 26-9. The vitamin K cycle in the synthesis of vitamin K dependent hemostatic proteins. Vitamin K hydroquinone form is reduced to vitamin K epoxide by vitamin K carboxylase in the presence of carbon dioxide and oxygen. During this reaction, glutamic acid residues of the vitamin K dependent proteins are carboxylated to form γ-carboxyglutamic acid residues. The vitamin K is oxidized through an intermediary step by the action of two enzymes. It is the reoxidation steps that are inhibited by coumarin drugs in oral anticoagulant therapy.

* Precursor protein (factor II, VII, IX, or X, protein or proteins)

MECHANISM OF ACTION The coumarin drugs prevent thrombin generation by inhibiting vitamin K. In the presence of coumarin, liver cells are unable to use vitamin K to carboxylate the glutamic acid residues of factors II, VII, IX and X, protein S and protein C (Chapter 24 and Figure 26-9).

This reaction normally occurs in the microsomes of liver cells by the enzyme vitamin K carboxylase. The carboxylase enzyme requires vitamin K as a cofactor. To be an active cofactor, vitamin K must be in the hydroquinone form (Figure 26-9). During the carboxylating reaction, vitamin K hydroquinone is oxidized to vitamin K epoxide. Vitamin K then must be reduced again to the hydroquinone form to participate in further reactions. This process requires two steps and two enzymes, vitamin K epoxide reductase and vitamin K reductase. Coumadin drugs block these two enzymes, preventing the reformation of the active hydroquinone form of vitamin K. Consequently, the

vitamin K-dependent hemostatic factors are not carboxylated and nonfunctional molecules of precursor protein circulate in the plasma. The result is an acquired deficiency of the prothrombin group factors and of protein C and protein S. These precursor molecules are called protein induced by vitamin K absence or PIVKA. They are detectable antigenically, but cannot bind to phospholipid micelles and participate in coagulation either in vivo or in in vitro laboratory tests.

The effect of the coumadin drugs is not present immediately as is the case with heparin. It takes a few days to metabolize the normal factors that were produced before treatment began. Metabolization is dependent on the half-life of the factors. For factor VII, this is 5 to 6 hours; factor IX, 28 to 40 hours; factor X, 40 to 50 hours; and factor II, 48 to 60 hours. The drugs begin to have an in vivo effect within 8 to 10 hours but may take 4 to 5 days to affect laboratory tests. Therapeutic anticoagulation may take 1 to 2 weeks to equilibrate and stabilize the dosage. The half life of protein C is similar to that of factor VII. Its half life becomes reduced early in therapy while there are still relatively normal levels of factors II, IX, and X. This produces a temporary imbalance between inhibition and promotion of fibrin formation and may result in thrombosis that is manifested as skin necrosis.

LABORATORY EVALUATION The dose response in different individuals is highly variable. To reach maximum effectiveness without hemorrhage, the range is from 2 mg to 18 mg. To determine the individual dosage of drug required, the prothrombin time (Chapter 24) is performed before treatment for a baseline level and then periodically, usually daily, until equilibration occurs. Most physicians adjust the dose so that the PT is 1 and $\frac{1}{2}$ to 2 times the baseline level. The prothrombin time reflects the dose given 36 to 48 hours previously.[14]

The prothrombin time is the test of choice for oral anticoagulant therapy because of the short half-life of factor VII, which is only measured by the PT and because it is dependent on two of the other affected factors. The APTT is not prolonged to a useful degree. After equilibration of the dose, the PT is checked periodically, perhaps weekly or every 2 weeks while the drug is being given.

The manner in which the results of the prothrombin time are expressed and used in conjunction with oral anticoagulant therapy is historically controversial. Laboratories that perform the prothrombin time are required to establish a normal range for the test by running the test on a sizable sample of normal individuals and then calculating the range, usually as ± 2 standard deviations (SD) from the mean. With each work shift or each time a new lot of reagent is opened, the test must also be performed on at least two plasmas for which results are known, called control plasmas. One control is expected to fall within the laboratory's normal range and the other to fall in a prolonged range corresponding to the results obtained on a patient on coumadin therapy. The results of the controls must fall within a range established by the laboratory in order for the patient's results to be considered valid. Control plasmas are available commercially from manufacturers of prothrombin time reagents.

When coumadin drugs were first monitored by the prothrombin time the scheme of fibrin formation had not yet been developed as it is today. It was thought that prothrombin alone was being measured.[45] Commercial plasmas were not then available. A standard curve was prepared by diluting normal plasma with saline and then reporting the patient's results as percent activity compared to the standard curve. This method was eventually discarded when it was shown to have a number of pitfalls. Another way of reporting the prothrombin time was to report the result of the normal control plasma with the patient value. The normal control value was used to calculate a ratio (patient value divided by control value) and to adjust the dosage of coumadin drugs in the initial stages of treatment by the result of the ratio. A more recent and valid method is to report the patient results in seconds along with the laboratory's established normal range. The

TABLE 26-17 *FACTORS CONTRIBUTING TO THE VARIABILITY OF THE PROTHROMBIN TIME TEST*

TESTING FACTORS

Source of thromboplastin reagents

Instrumentation

Source of plasma standard

PATIENT FACTORS

Patient compliance

Vitamin K intake and adsorption

Dose response

extent of alteration of the prothrombin time is related to the patient's baseline level before therapy began. Using this method, a ratio can also be calculated by dividing the patient value by the midpoint of the normal range. This is called the prothrombin time ratio.

The wide variety of commercial reagent products and instrumentation on the market today adds to the lack of standardization of the test as it is used in adjusting coumadin dosage. The reagents vary greatly from lot to lot and between manufacturers in their sensitivity to the effect of the anticoagulants. The results on an individual patient using one laboratory's protocol cannot be interchanged with those of another laboratory. Table 26-17 summarizes factors that affect the variability in the use of the prothrombin time in oral anticoagulant therapy.

The thromboplastin reagents that are commercially available are prepared in different manners from different sources. In the United States, extracts of rabbit brain, lung or placenta are most common. The reagents themselves respond differently when testing patient's plasma. For example, one specimen was tested in two different laboratories: Laboratory #1, using a thromboplastin that is quite highly responsive to the lowered levels of factors, obtained a result of 20 seconds. Laboratory #2 used a less responsive reagent and obtained results of 15 seconds. The patient would receive a much higher dose of coumadin based on the result of laboratory #2 than that of laboratory #1.

In the 1950s and 1960s, thromboplastin reagents in the United States were prepared in the laboratories using them. Subsequently, these reagents became commercially available. The commercial preparations have been shown to be less responsive than the homemade products of the past but the same criteria for dosage of patients continued to be used to adjust dosage. Therefore, patients may be unknowingly overdosed with the anticoagulant and have an increased risk of serious or even fatal bleeding. Others may not be given enough anticoagulant and have a risk of not controlling the thrombosis. Most physicians and laboratorians were unaware of the change in reagent sensitivities.[45]

To further complicate the situation, thromboplastin reagents prepared in European countries were, until recently, prepared from human brain tissue. These thromboplastins were very responsive to the coumadin effect, and the results were more reproducible than any of the animal products used in North America. They compare to or were even more responsive than earlier homemade reagents prepared in this country. The United Kingdom prepares standardized batches of their reagent that are used by almost all laboratories in that country. The results are interchangeable between different laboratories, whereas, the results between different laboratories in North America are not.

In 1977, the World Health Organization (WHO) in conjunction with other international groups, designated one of the batches of human brain thromboplastin as the First International Reference Thromboplastin (also known as the primary thromboplastin). During the next few years, they also developed a system that would relate the results of the prothrombin times performed in any laboratory to the results that would have been obtained if the primary reference reagent had been used to perform the test. The results of all prothrombin times could thus be standardized using this method, a calculation called the International Normalized Ratio (INR). The WHO have more recently begun to produce reagents from sources other than the human brain and have designated these as secondary reference thromboplastins. The secondary reagents compare to the primary reagents in sensitivity. They are the most sensitive and responsive reagents in use in the world.

Three items are needed to calculate the INR:

1. The prothrombin time of the patient
2. The midpoint of the laboratory's normal range for the prothrombin time.
3. The International Sensitivity Index (ISI) for the reagent thromboplastin. This is a figure provided by the manufacturer of the reagent and indicates the responsiveness of the particular lot of reagent compared to the international reference thromboplastin.[46]

The ISI of the primary reference is 1.0 while that of most reagents in North America is 2.0 to 2.6. The mathematical derivation of the ISI can be found in Loeliger et al.[45]

Using these items, the formula for calculating the INR is:

$$INR = \frac{\text{patient prothrombin time}^{ISI}}{\text{normal prothrombin time}}$$

The INR is the patient's prothrombin time ratio to the power equal to the ISI.

The INR is used for patients with the conditions shown in Table 26-18. A number of clinical trials have been performed on patients with each condition in an attempt to determine the optimal range of INR. Based on these studies, two categories of treatment levels are recommended. For the conditions in group A, the therapy should be less intensive with a prothrombin time ratio of 1.3 to 1.5 corresponding to an INR range of 2.0 to 3.0. The prothrombin time itself will be in the range of 14 to 17 seconds. More intensive therapy is needed for patients with the indications in group B as shown in the table.

The INR method is valid only for patients who have been stabilized on longterm oral anticoagulants for several weeks.[46] It should not be used in conjunction with the prothrombin time for evaluating the induction phase of oral anticoagulant therapy, for evaluating the hemostatic

TABLE 26-18 *RECOMMENDED THERAPEUTIC RANGE FOR PROTHROMBIN TIME IN ORAL ANTICOAGULANT THERAPY*

Clinical Condition	PT Result sec.	PT Ratio	INR
GROUP A			
Treatment of established pulmonary emboli	14–17		
		1.3–1.5	2.0–3.0
Treatment of established venous thrombosis	14–17		
		1.3–1.5	2.0–3.0
Prophylaxis of venous thrombosis			
Patients with hereditary deficiencies	14–17		
		1.3–1.5	2.0–3.0
Surgical patients	14–17	1.3–1.5	2.0–3.0
Acute myocardial infarction	14–17	1.3–1.5	2.0–3.0
Atrial fibrillation	14–17	1.3–1.5	2.0–3.0
Tissue heart valves	14–17	1.3–1.5	2.0–3.0
GROUP B			
Mechanical prosthetic heart valves	17–22	1.5–2.0	3.0–4.5
Recurrent systemic embolism	17–22	1.5–2.0	3.0–4.5

system in presurgical patients, or for evaluating hemostasis in a patient with liver disease.

The antidote for coumarin drugs is vitamin K administration. The vitamin requires 2 to 3 days to become effective, however. In an emergency situation, fresh frozen plasma that contains functional factors can be used. Prothrombin complex factors can be given, but the risk of hepatitis and HIV are greater with this therapy.

Several drugs taken concurrently can affect the response to oral anticoagulants (Table 26-19). Some potentiate the effect of the anticoagulant so that a lower dose than usual is needed. Other drugs decrease the effect of the coumarin. If the interfering drug is given steadily, the dose of the anticoagulant should be adjusted. If it is taken only periodically, the patient will be at risk of bleeding or may not be in an effective therapeutic range of the coumadin.

Combined heparin and oral anticoagulant therapy For patients with acute DVT and pulmonary emboli, the method of administering anticoagulant therapy is to first give heparin, which acts immediately. Because it is administered intravenously, however, it is inconvenient when the patient returns home. A switch is then made to oral drugs. A period of overlap of 4 to 5 days, during which both drugs are given, allows the prothrombin group factors to drop to appropriate levels.

ANTIPLATELET DRUGS

The use of platelet inhibiting drugs is gaining popularity for the prevention of arterial thromboembolic disease. Among these, aspirin is the most well known. Others are dipyridamole, ticlopidine, and sulfinpyrazone. Many clinical trials have been performed to study the effectiveness of the drugs. They are used singly or in combination with one another or with warfarin drugs.

TABLE 26-19 *EXAMPLES OF MEDICATIONS THAT INFLUENCE THE RESPONSE TO COUMARIN DRUGS*

INCREASED COUMARIN DRUG ACTION

Allopurinol	Mefanamic acid
Anabolic steroids	Methylphenidate
Antibiotics	Nalidixic acid
Chloramphenicol	Oxyphenbutazone
Chloral hydrate	Phenytoin
Cimetidine	Phenyramidol
Clofibrate	Quinidine
Diazoxide	Salicylate
Disulfiram	Sulfinpyrazone
Ethacrynic acid	Sulfonamides
Glucagon	Thyroid hormone
Indomethacin	Tolbutamide

DECREASED COUMARIN DRUG ACTION

Barbiturates	Glutethimide
Carbamazepine	Griseofulvin
Chlorthalidone	Haloperidol
Cholestyramine	Oral contraceptives
Ethchlorvynol	Phenobarbital

Laboratory monitoring of platelet-inhibiting drugs is usually not needed. The bleeding time is not always prolonged and platelet aggregation studies do not correlate with the dose of the drug.

Antiplatelet drugs may interfere with platelet function by preventing platelet adherence to subendothelial tissue, by inhibiting platelet aggregation/release, or by disaggregating platelet thrombi. Aspirin inhibits the synthesis of thromboxane A2 by the platelet, preventing platelet aggregation. It irreversibly acetylates cyclo-oxygenase, an enzyme needed for thromboxane A2 synthesis. The enzyme is inhibited for the life span of the platelet because the platelet cannot synthesize new protein. Megakaryocytes in the bone marrow may also be affected. Platelet aggregation will remain abnormal until new platelets from unaffected megakaryocytes are produced.

Dipyridamole inhibits platelet function by causing an increase in cyclic-AMP, thereby increasing intracellular calcium binding, which, in turn, leads to decreased platelet adhesiveness and aggregation. The action of sulfinpyrazole is similar to that of aspirin. It inhibits platelet cyclo-oxygenase enzyme.[20] The mechanism of action of ticlopidine is unknown.[47]

THROMBOLYTIC DRUGS

Thrombolytic drugs are enzymes which, unlike the drugs previously discussed, act on pre-existing thrombi or emboli and break them down. This type of therapy has become more popular in the last few years, particularly since DNA technology has led to the production of various types of drugs and in enough quantity to be feasible. Six drugs have been approved for use to date: Streptokinase and urokinase, which have been available for several years, plus the newer pro-urokinase, acylated plasminogen streptokinase activator complex (APSAC), and two types of tissue plasminogen activator (t-PA), a single chain type and a two-chain type. The drugs are injected intravenously and all act by activating plasminogen to plasmin which in turn lyses the fibrin. Each has different advantages and disadvantages.

Streptokinase is a bacterial enzyme derived from group C-beta hemolytic streptococci. It forms a complex with plasminogen that has been adsorbed to fibrin and activates it to plasmin. It is relatively inexpensive but is associated with allergic reactions of various types including anaphylaxis.

The remaining fibrinolytic agents are naturally occurring components of the human hemostatic system. Urokinase is produced by the kidney and is present in blood and urine. When produced commercially from cultured kidney cells or from urine, it is in a 2-chain configuration. This is the physiological form. This form of urokinase is very expensive but not as allergenic as streptokinase.

A major complication of therapy with either urokinase or streptokinase is bleeding, in part, because they both lyse circulating fibrinogen as well as the fibrin clot (see explanation below). Research is being done to find agents that will preferentially attack fibrin and leave fibrinogen intact in an attempt to diminish the bleeding complications that are inherent in the treatment. Thus far, however, success in this regard has been minimal. Four of the previously named drugs are in this category of second generation plasminogen activators. Prourokinase is a modification of urokinase and is prepared from urine or by recombinant techniques. It is an immature form of urokinase in the single-chain form. When bound to fibrin, pro-urokinase is attacked by plasmin causing formation of the two-chain active form.

APSAC is a modification of streptokinase. It is a complex of streptokinase and plasminogen which, in addition, is chemically altered. Within the complex, plasminogen is activated to plasmin followed by acylation of the plasmin. The acylated form is inactive. In the blood the plasmin is slowly deacylated to the active form. Because of this, the half life of APSAC is longer than other types of thrombolytic drugs. The same risks of allergic reactions apply to APSAC as to streptokinase.

Tissue plasminogen activator is derived from cultured melanoma cells or by recombinant DNA techniques. A single chain form is the precursor of a 2-chain form. Both are analogous to the tissue plasminogen activator produced by endothelial cells (Chapter 24). T-PA has greater specificity for fibrin than the other enzymes.

Excessive bleeding is a complication of therapy with the second generation of drugs as with the first generation. Additional preparations are being evaluated but have not as yet been approved for clinical use.

Laboratory tests are not used to monitor the dose of thrombolytic drugs as were the drugs previously described, heparin and commadins. They are given in set doses and the dose is not changed by the results of laboratory tests.

However, laboratory tests are affected by the therapy as shown in Table 26-20. The drugs injected intravenously

TABLE 26-20 *EFFECT OF THROMBOLYTIC DRUG THERAPY ON LABORATORY TESTS OF HEMOSTASIS*

Laboratory Test	Result	Biochemical Basis
Prothrombin time	Increased	Decreased fibrinogen and factor V
Activated partial thromboplastin time	Increased	Decreased fibrinogen, factors V, VIII, IX, XI, XII
Thrombin time	Increased	Decreased fibrinogen, increased fibrin split products
Fibrinogen determination	Decreased	Lysis by plasmin
Plasminogen determination	Decreased	Activation to plasmin
Fibrin/fibrinogen degradation products	Increased	From lysis of fibrin and fibrinogen by plasmin
α_2-antiplasmin	Decreased	Inhibition of increased plasmin
Plasmin	Increased	Activation of plasminogen
Euglobulin lysis time	Shortened	Circulating plasminogen activator

activate both the plasminogen adsorbed onto fibrin as the thrombus is formed and the plasminogen circulating in the plasma. Activation of the adsorbed plasminogen to plasmin is the purpose of the therapy. The plasmin formed lyses the fibrin to fibrin split products. One side effect is the activation of plasminogen in the plasma. The plasmin formed in the blood stream attacks many circulating hemostatic components: fibrinogen, factors V, VIII:C, IX, XI, and XII as well as platelet glycoprotein Ib. Platelet aggregation in vitro is affected as are other nonhemostatic functions of the platelet. The result is a decrease in circulating levels of the above factors and plasminogen and an increase in fibrin and fibrinogen split products and plasmin with blood. When the plasmin level is increased beyond the capacity of the inhibitors to inhibit the result, particularly α_2-antiplasmin, the lytic state is produced. Bleeding complications occur because of the artificial deficiency of the hemostatic elements that are affected by the circulating plasmin.

Tests for one or more of these components may be done to document that the therapy, in fact, has worked to produce the lytic state. The thrombin time is popular and would be prolonged by the fibrin split products and the decreased fibrinogen level. A fibrinogen determination may be performed but must be a method that is not affected by the increased level of fibrin split products. A determination of decreased plasminogen may also be done.

Thrombolytic drugs are used for acute myocardial infarction, DVT, pulmonary emboli, and arterial blockage. They tend to be more effective on recently formed thrombi rather than on older ones.

HIRUDIN

Hirudin is a substance first crudely extracted from medicinal leeches (Hirudo medicinalis) in Germany in 1884, and used as an anticlotting agent until the discovery of heparin. It was again studied in the 1950s when it was chemically isolated. Subsequently, its chemical structure has been sequenced and found to consist of 65 amino acids. It is now prepared by recombinant DNA techniques in enough quantity to be used clinically and is being tested for this purpose.[48]

Hirudin inhibits thrombin and can be monitored in the laboratory by the thrombin time. It has advantages over heparin in that it can be used in patients who are deficient in antithrombin III, is not as apt to cause bleeding as a side effect, and does not affect platelet function or cause thrombocytopenia.[48]

This chapter included a discussion of the conditions associated with abnormal secondary hemostasis. These conditions encompass those in which fibrin is formed too slowly or is lysed too rapidly so that excessive bleeding results, as well as conditions in which increased fibrin is formed (thrombosis). Also included is a discussion of the unique hemostatic status of newborns.

Abnormal fibrin formation occurs in patients with mutations of the genes which code for the circulating hemostatic proteins and result either in decreased synthesis or abnormal function of the protein. The most common of these disorders are X-linked deficiencies of factors VIII and IX called the hemophilias. von Willebrand disease is also discussed in this chapter because of the association of von Willebrand factor with factor VIII. Rarer deficiencies of the remaining coagulation factors and of components of fibrinolysis may result in excessive bleeding. However, in the case of factor XIII, prekallikrein and high molecular weight kininogen, no bleeding symptoms are present but rather patients have an increased risk for thrombosis. Laboratory screening tests and factor assays establish the diagnosis. Newborns are at higher risk for bleeding and may have prolonged prothrombin and activated partial thromboplastin times until vitamin K-producing intestinal bacteria and liver production of vitamin K dependent factors are established.

Thrombosis is a major cause of morbidity and mortality. Thrombi form in either arteries or veins under different conditions. Inherited deficiencies of hemostatic inhibitors result in increased risk and early onset of thrombosis. Patients with venous thrombosis are treated with anticoagulant drugs, coumarin and heparin. Laboratory tests are used to monitor the dosage of these drugs and are a major part of the workload of a coagulation laboratory.

REVIEW QUESTIONS

CASE STUDY: An 18 year-old female bled profusely following extraction of a tooth. She had a history of periodically increased menstrual bleeding and nosebleeds. She had had an appendectomy at age 10 with no unusual bleeding. A workup in the coagulation laboratory showed the following:

Laboratory test	Patient results	Laboratory normals
Platelet count	312×10^9/L	$150–400 \times 10^9$/L
Template bleeding time	9.5 minutes	2–9 minutes
Prothrombin time	12.0 seconds	10–12 seconds
Activated partial thromboplastin time	37.0 seconds	23–36 seconds
Factor VIII assay	0.2 U/mL	0.5–1.5 U/mL
Factor IX assay	1.2 U/mL	0.5–1.5 U/mL

Platelet aggregation studies showed normal aggregation with ADP, collagen, and epinephrine but no aggregation with ristocetin.

REVIEW QUESTIONS

1. Which laboratory results are outside of the normal range?
   a. all tests shown above
   b. template bleeding time, activated partial thromboplastin time, factor VIII assay
   c. platelet count, prothrombin time, factor IX assay
   d. prothrombin time, activated partial thromboplastin time, factor VIII assay

2. The results of the platelet aggregation studies indicate that the patient has a defect in
   a. factor VIII
   b. platelet adhesion
   c. fibrinolysis
   d. the intrinsic system

3. Platelet adhesion to collagen requires the presence of adequate functional
   a. thrombin and plasmin
   b. fibrinogen
   c. glycoprotein Ib and von Willebrand factor
   d. glycoprotein IIb/IIIa and ADP

4. The most probable cause of this patients bleeding is
   a. a vascular disorder
   b. hemophilia A
   c. disseminated intravascular coagulation
   d. von Willebrand disease

5. The inheritance pattern of von Willebrand disease is usually
   a. autosomal dominant
   b. autosomal recessive
   c. X-linked recessive
   d. not inherited, usually acquired

6. Type I von Willebrand disease is characterized by
   a. decreased amounts of large multimers of von Willebrand factor only
   b. increased amounts of large multimers of von Willebrand factor
   c. decreased amounts of all von Willebrand factor multimers
   d. decreased amounts of small von Willebrand factor multimers only

7. Which laboratory procedures analyze von Willebrand factor qualitatively for abnormalities of the molecular structure?
   a. ristocetin-induced platelet aggregation and template bleeding time
   b. factor VIII assay and activated partial thromboplastin time
   c. rocket electrophoresis and platelet aggregation with ristocetin
   d. crossed immunoelectrophoresis and SDS gel electrophoresis

8. von Willebrand disease is caused by
   a. genetic mutations in the factor VIII gene
   b. genetic mutations in the von Willebrand factor gene
   c. genetic mutations in the glycoprotein Ib gene
   d. exposure to dyes and chemicals

9. The structure of the von Willebrand factor molecule is
   a. two pairs of three polypeptide chains
   b. a small peptide of three amino acids
   c. a large multimer composed of several dimeric units each of varying sizes
   d. a large multimer composed of several identical dimeric subunits oriented by their N terminal ends

10. In which of the following conditions would the presence of delayed bleeding and deep muscular hematomas be most likely
    a. factor VIII deficiency
    b. antithrombin III deficiency
    c. factor XII deficiency
    d. protein C deficiency

11. Hemophilia B is a deficiency of
    a. factor XI
    b. factor VIII
    c. factor IX
    d. fibrinogen

12. In which of the following diseases would you most likely find an abnormal prothrombin time
    a. hemophilia A
    b. hemophilia B
    c. disseminated intravascular coagulation (DIC)
    d. prekallikrein deficiency

13. A deficiency of factor X would affect
    a. prothrombin time and activated partial thromboplastin time
    b. activated partial thromboplastin time and template bleeding time
    c. activated partial thromboplastin time and thrombin time
    d. thrombin time and template bleeding time

14. Acquired circulating pathologic inhibitors to single coagulation factors
    a. do not cause bleeding symptoms
    b. cause the same symptoms in the patient as an inherited deficiency of the same factor
    c. are often found in patients with Glanzmann thrombasthenia
    d. are antibodies to the phospholipid in coagulation reagents

15. In the condition known as disseminated intravascular coagulation (DIC)
  a. factors V and VIII become increased in activity
  b. fibrinolytic activity is absent
  c. the patient has a single coagulation factor deficiency
  d. fibrinogen and platelets become depleted

REFERENCES ●

1. Gralnick, H.R.: von Willebrand disease. In Hematology. 4th Ed. Edited by W.J. Williams, E. Beutler, A.J. Erslev, and M.A. Lichtman. New York, McGraw-Hill, Inc., 1990.
2. Ginsburg, D., et al.: Human von Willebrand Factor (vWf): Isolation of complementary DNA (cDNA) clones and chromosomal localization. Science 228:1401, 1985.
3. Ginsburg, D. and Bowie, E.J.W.: Molecular genetics of von Willebrand disease. Blood 79:2507, 1992.
4. Marder, V.J., et al.: Standard nomenclature for Factor VIII and von Willebrand factor: a recommendation by the International Committee on Thrombosis and Hemostasis. Thromb. Hemost. 54:871, 1985.
5. Wagner, D.D. and Ginsbsurg, D.: Structure, biology, and genetics of von Willebrand factor. In Hematology: Basic Principles and Practice. 2nd Ed. Edited by R. Hoffman, E.J. Benz, Jr., S.J. Shatill, B. Furie, H.J. Cohen, L.E. Silberstein. New York, Churchill Livingstone, 1995.
6. Ginsburg, D.: Biology of inherited coagulopathics: von Willebrand factor. Hematol./Oncol. Clin. N.A. 6:1011, 1992.
7. Pavlovsky, A.: Contribution to the pathogenesis of hemophilia. Blood 2:185, 1947.
8. Kaufman, R.J. and Antonarakis, S.E.: Structure, biology and genetics of factor VIII. In Hematology: Basic Principles and Practice. 2nd Ed. Edited by R. Hoffman, E.J. Benz, Jr., S.J. Shattil, B. Furie, H.J. Cohen, L.E. Silberstein. New York, Churchill Livingstone, 1995.
9. Furie, B. and Furie, B.C.: Molecular basis of hemophilia. Semin. Hematol. 27:270, 1990.
10. Larson, P.J. and High, K.A.: Biology of inherited coagulopathies: Factor IX. Hematol./Oncol. Clin. N.A., 6:999, 1992
11. Kurachi, K., Furukawa, M., Yao, S-N., Kurachi, S.: Biology of factor IX. Hematol./Oncol. Clin. N.A., 6:991, 1992.
12. Roberts, H.R. and Gray, T.F.: Clinical aspects of and therapy for Hemophilia B. In Hematology: Basic Principles and Practice. 2nd Ed. Edited by R. Hoffman, E.J. Benz, Jr., S.J. Shattil, B. Furie, H.J. Cohen, L.E. Silberstein. New York, Churchill Livingstone, 1995.
13. Brettler, D.B., Krause, E.M., Levine, P.H.: Clinical aspects of and therapy for Hemophilia A. In Hematology: Basic Principles and Practice. 2nd Ed. Edited by R. Hoffman, E.J. Benz, Jr., S.J. Shattil, B. Furie, H.J. Cohen, L.E. Silberstein. New York, Churchill Livingstone, 1995.
14. Sadler, J.E.: Recombinant DNA methods in hemophilia A: Carrier detection and prenatal diagnosis. Semin. Thromb. Hemost. 16:341, 1990.
15. Menitove, J.E.: Preparation and clinical use of plasma and plasma fractions. In Hematology. 4th Ed. Edited by W.J. Williams, E. Beutler, A.J. Erslev, and M.A. Lichtman. New York, McGraw-Hill, Inc., 1990.
16. Arkin, S., Rose, E., Forster, A., Aledort, L.M. for then Factor VIII Clinical Trial Group: Clinical efficacy of recombinant factor VIII. Semin. Hematol. 28:47, 1991.
17. Hrinda, M.E. et al.: Preclinical studies of a monoclonal antibody-purified factor IX, Mononine. Semin. Hematol. 28:6, 1991.
18. Galanakis, D.K.: Fibrinogen anomalies and disease. Hematol./Oncol. Clin. N.A. 6:1171, 1992.
19. Bithell, T.C.: Hereditary coagulation disorders. In Wintrobe's Clinical Hematology, 9th Ed. Edited by G.R. Lee, T.C. Bithell, J. Foerster, J.W. Athens, J.N. Lukens. Philadelphia, Lea & Febiger, 1993.
20. Bick, R.L.: Disorders of Thrombosis & Hemostasis: Clinical and Laboratory Practice. Chicago, ASCP Press, 1992.
21. Owen, C.A., Bowie, E.J.W., Thompson, J.H.: The Diagnosis of Bleeding Disorders. 2nd Ed. Boston, Little Brown & Co., 1975.
22. Bithell, T.C.: Acquired coagulation disorders. In Wintrobe's Clinical Hematology, 9th Ed. Edited by G.R. Lee, T.C. Bithell, J. Foerster, J.W. Athens, J.N. Lukens. Philadelphis, Lea & Febiger, 1993.
23. Furie, B.: Acquired anticoagulants. In Hematology. 4th Ed. Edited by W.J. Williams, E. Beutler, A.J. Erslev, and M.A. Lichtman. New York, McGraw-Hill, Inc., 1990.
24. Exner, T., Triplett, D.A., Taberner, D. and Machin, S.J.: Guidelines for testing and revised criteria for lupus anticoagulants. Thromb. Haemost. 65:320, 1991.
25. Feinstein, D.I.: Lupus anticoagulant, anticardiolipin antibodies, fetal loss, and systemic lupus erythematosus, Blood 80:859, 1992.
26. Triplett, D.A.: Laboratory diagnosis of lupus anticoagulant. Semin. Thromb. Hemost. 16:182, 1990.
27. Montgomery, R.R., Maralar, R.A., Gill J.C.: Newborn haemostasis. Clin. Haematol. 14:443, 1985.
28. Johnston, M., Zipursky, A.: Microtechnology for the study of blood coagulation system in newborn infants. Can. J. Med. Tech. 42:159, 1980.
29. Hathaway, W. and Corrigan, J. for the Subcommitee: Normal coagulation data for fetuses and newborn infants, Thromb. Haemost. 65:323, 1991.
30. Joist, J.H.: Hypercoagulability: Introduction and perspective. Semin. Thromb. Hemost. 16:1151, 1990.
31. Blajchman, M.A., Austin, R.C., Fernandez-Rachubinski, F., and Sheffield, W.P.: Molecular basis of inherited human antithrombin deficiency. Blood 80:2159, 1992.
32. Montgomery, R.R. and Scott, J.P.: Hemostasis: Diseases of the fluid phase. In Hematology of Infancy and Childhood. Edited by D.G. Nathan and F.A. Oski. Philadelphia, W.B. Saunders Company, 1993.
33. Bauer, K.A., and Rosenberg, R.D.: The hypercoagulable state. In Disorders of Hemostasis. 2nd Ed. Edited by O.D. Ratnoff and C.D. Forbes. Philadelphia, W.B. Saunders Company, 1991.
34. Hortin, G.L. Tollefson, D.L., and Santoro, S.A.: Assessment of interference by heparin cofactor II. In: the DuPont acaR antithrombin III assay. Am. J. Clin. Pathol. 89:515, 1988.
35. Tollefsen, D.M.: Laboratory diagnosis of antithrombin and heparin cofactor II deficiency. Semin. Thromb. Hemost. 16:162, 1990.
36. Comp, P.C.: Laboratory evaluation of protein S status. Semin. Thromb. Hemost. 16:177, 1990.
37. Bauer, K.A.: Hypercoaguable states. In Hematology: Basic Principles and Practice, Edited by R. Hoffman, E.J. Berry, Jr., S.J., Shattil, B. Furie, and H.J. Cohen. New York, Churchill Livinstone, 1991.
38. Robbins, K.C.: Classification of abnormal plasminogens: dysplasminogenemias. Semin. Thromb. Hemost. 16:217, 1990.
39. Wiman, B., and Hamsten, A.: The fibrinolytic enzyme system and its role in the etiology of thromboembolic disease. Semin. Thromb. Hemost. 16:207, 1990.
40. Bachman, F.: Laboratory diagnosis of impairment of fibrinolysis in patients with thromboembolic disease. Semin. Thromb. Hemost. 16:193, 1990.
41. Casu, B.: Structure of heparin and heparin fragments. Ann. N.Y. Acad. Sci. 556:1, 1989
42. Mammen, E.F.: Why low molecular weight heparin? Semin. Thromb. Hemost. 16 (suppl):1, 1990.
43. Hirsh, J. and Levine, M.N.: Low molecular weight heparin. Blood 79:1, 1992.
44. Tollefsen, D.M.: Heparin: Basic and clinical pharmacology. In Hematology: Basic Principles and Practice. 2nd Ed. Edited by R. Hoffman, E.J. Benz, Jr., S.J. Shattil, B. Furie, H.J. Cohen, L.E. Silberstein. New York, Churchill Livingstone, 1995.
45. Loeliger, E.A., et al: Questions and answers on prothrombin time standardization in oral anticoagulant control. Thromb. Haemost. 54:515, 1985.
46. Hirsh, J., et al: Optimal therapeutic range for oral anticoagulants. Chest 95 (Suppl): 55-115, 1989.
47. Harker, L.A.: Antithrombotic therapy. In Hematology. 4th Ed. Edited by W.J. Williams, E. Beutler, A.J. Erslev, and M.A. Lichtman. New York, McGraw-Hill, Inc., 1990.
48. Markwardt, F.: The comeback of hirudin as an antithrombotic agent. Semin. Thromb. Hemost. 17:79, 1991.

Laboratory methods in hematology

INTRODUCTION

This chapter is designed to introduce the clinical laboratory science student to the manual laboratory procedures performed either within the routine hematology laboratory or within a special hematology laboratory. The results obtained from these laboratory procedures are used in the definitive diagnosis of a variety of disorders including anemias, leukemias, infections, and inherited leukocyte disorders.

THE MICROSCOPE

The compound microscope[1-4] is an essential instrument in the routine hematology laboratory. The proper use of the microscope and regular preventative maintenance are critical to the reliability of the results obtained from its use. Therefore, individuals who use the microscope must understand its basic principles, its operation, and its preventative maintenance.

Principles of the compound microscope

Any discussion of the principles of the compound microscope must begin with a review of its components. The components include: eyepieces, binocular eyepiece tube, objectives located on the revolving nosepiece, microscope stage, condenser, condenser diaphragm, field diaphragm, and light source (Fig. 27-1). The condenser functions to direct the beam of light from the light source onto the specimen. As the light rays illuminate the specimen, they are altered and light is diffracted. The specimen image is produced by a combination of the diffracted light and background light from the light source.

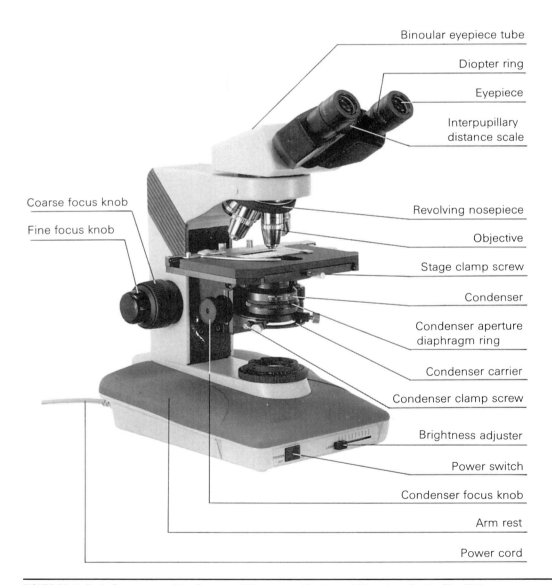

FIGURE 27-1. Basic Components of the Compound Microscope. (Courtesy of Nikon, Inc., Garden City, NY.)

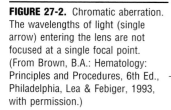
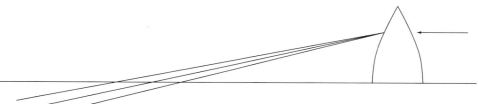

FIGURE 27-2. Chromatic aberration. The wavelengths of light (single arrow) entering the lens are not focused at a single focal point. (From Brown, B.A.: Hematology: Principles and Procedures, 6th Ed., Philadelphia, Lea & Febiger, 1993, with permission.)

The magnifying system of the compound microscope uses two sets of lenses to form an enlarged image. The first lens system is the objective. The objective projects a primary image plane. The primary image is located approximately 1 cm from the top of the body of the microscope. The distance from the back focal plane of the objective to the eyepiece is termed the optical tube length (160 mm). The second lens system is the eyepiece, which is located above the primary image plane. The total magnification is the product of the magnification of the first and second lens systems. A $10\times$ objective with a $10\times$ eyepiece produces a total magnification of $100\times$.

The resolving power (resolution) of a lens is the ability to distinguish two separate objects located close to one another and reveal the fine detail in a specimen. It is a function of the numerical aperture (NA) of the lens and the wavelength λ of the illuminating light. The numerical aperture is a designation of the amount of light entering the objective from the microscope field. The NA of the substage condenser should be equal to the NA of an objective, otherwise interference effects will occur. Since the illuminating light remains constant in light microscopy, the resolving power is determined by the numerical aperture. Thus, the higher the NA of an objective, the greater the resolving power.

Lens aberrations

An aberration is an optical defect that degrades the quality of the image. There are three important types of aberrations associated with the objectives:

(1) *Chromatic aberrations* give rise to color fringes and poor image definitions. These aberrations are due to the inability of the lens to bring the different wavelengths of light into focus at a single focal point (Fig. 27-2).

(2) *Spherical aberrations* give rise to poor image definitions and loss of contrast. In spherical aberrations, the light is refracted by the lens dependent on the area (thickness) of the lens it passes through. For example, the light passing through the periphery of the lens will be refracted more than light passing through the center. Therefore, the refracted light from the periphery will be brought to a shorter focal point than the light passing through the center (Fig. 27-3). This aberration becomes worse as the lens becomes thicker.

(3) *Field curvature aberrations* result in the periphery of the field being slightly out of focus when the center is in focus. These aberrations are the result of the image in the focal plane being slightly curved by the objective.

To compensate for these aberrations, specialized lenses are used. The achromat lens will compensate for chromatic aberrations at two colors and spherical aberrations at one color. The apochromat lens will compensate for chromatic aberrations at three colors and spherical aberrations at two colors. The field curvature aberrations may be eliminated with the use of a flat-field (plan) objective lens. A plan apochromat lens is the highest-grade, giving exceptional definition, superior color reproducibility, and prominent image flatness. This lens is most useful in the examination of morphologic detail.

Koehler illumination

Koehler illumination uses a double diaphragm illumination. The two diaphragms are the field diaphragm and the condenser diaphragm. The condenser diaphragm determines the resolution, contrast, and depth of field. As one closes the condenser diaphragm, the contrast and depth of field are increased, but the resolution is decreased. The field diaphragm determines the illuminated area on the specimen surface in relation to the field of view of the

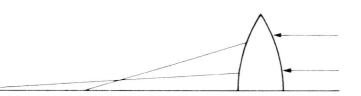

FIGURE 27-3. Spherical aberration. The wavelength of light entering the lens at its periphery is focused at a shorter focal point compared with light entering the lens at its center, which has a longer focal point. (From Brown, B.A.: Hematology: Principles and Procedures, 6th Ed., Philadelphia, Lea & Febiger, 1993, with permission.)

microscope. In Koehler illumination, the two diaphragms are adjusted so as to give uniform illumination of the field of view and optimum contrast and resolution of a specimen by focusing and centering the light path.

The procedure for Koehler illumination will vary slightly depending on the microscope manufacturer. Koehler illumination should be performed daily before using the instrument, and the procedure should be repeated for each objective. Each objective will have a different light requirement (higher NA objectives require a correspondingly higher NA setting on the condenser).

●
Preventative maintenance

A regular preventative maintenance program should be established by each laboratory. The microscope manufacturer's instruction manual will provide a preventative maintenance checklist. The following should be included in any preventative maintenance program: (1) clean the oil immersion lens daily with lens tissue and cleaner; (2) dust the optical surfaces (eyepieces, condenser, field lens, and filters) using bursts of air or a soft camel's hair brush; (3) clean external surfaces using a mild liquid soap—avoid the use of any organic solvents such as ether, alcohol, xylene; and (4) periodically inspect objectives for stubborn smudges or scratches.

●
BLOOD SMEAR EXAMINATION

●
Preparation of blood smears

The morphologic evaluation of hematopoietic cells by light microscopy requires the preparation of a well-stained blood smear.[5-8] The accuracy of the morphologic evaluation depends in part on the quality of the blood smear.

There are three types of blood smears: (1) the coverglass smear, (2) the spun smear, and (3) the wedge smear. The coverglass smear provides a smear with even distribution of the leukocytes. The disadvantages of this method are the difficulty in mastering the technique, the fragility of the coverglass, and the difficulty in staining the coverglass. The spun smear uses centrifugal force to produce a monolayer of cells with uniformly distributed leukocytes and platelets. This method requires special equipment and has the potential of creating biohazardous aerosols. The wedge smear is the method most commonly used in routine laboratory practice. Although the leukocyte distribution is poor, the technique is easily mastered, the smears are less fragile and may be stored for extended periods of time. An advantage of the leukocyte distribution in a wedge smear is that it allows for the identification of abnormal cells, which tend to locate on the edges of the smear.

In the preparation of a blood smear, a drop of EDTA-anticoagulated venous blood or capillary blood is placed on one end of a glass microscope slide. A second spreader slide, which is narrower than the glass microscope slide, is drawn into the drop of blood and the blood is allowed

TABLE 27-1 *CHARACTERISTICS OF AN OPTIMAL BLOOD SMEAR*

- minimum length of 2.5 cm
- gradual transition of smear from thick to thin
- squared or straight feather edge
- smooth, continuous margins
- margins, narrower than microscope slide
- no streaks, waves, or troughs

to spread the width of that slide. There should be a 45° angle between the spreader slide and the glass microscope slide. In one controlled movement, the blood is pulled the length of the glass microscope slide. The blood smear is dried immediately by gently waving the slide. Failure to dry the blood smear in a timely manner results in contraction artifacts of the cells, especially with increased humidity.

An optimal blood smear will have the characteristics listed in Table 27-1. Certain physiologic conditions, including anemia, polycythemia, multiple myeloma, and cold agglutinin disease may lead to less than optimal blood smears. The thickness or thinness of the blood smear may be regulated by adjusting the amount of blood used to make the drop, altering the speed with which the drop is smeared, or altering the angle at which the spreader slide is used.

●
Staining of blood smears

For more than 100 years, Romanowsky-type stains have been used in the morphologic classification of hematopoietic cells.[7-12] The Romanowsky-type stain is extremely important in the hematology laboratory because a great wealth of information may be obtained from the evaluation of a well-stained peripheral blood smear.

A Romanowsky stain is any stain consisting of methylene blue and its oxidation products and eosin Y or eosin B. The combined action of these dyes produces the Romanowsky effect, yielding purple coloration to the nuclei of leukocytes and neutrophilic granules and pinkish color to the erythrocytes. The principal components responsible for this effect are azure B (a methylene blue oxidation product) and eosin Y. The wide variation in colors and shades seen with Romanosky staining allows for subtle distinctions in cellular characteristics.

The staining properties of Romanowsky stains depend on the binding of dyes to chemical structures and the interactions between azure B and eosin Y. Acidic groupings of nucleic acids, the proteins of the cell nuclei and immature or reactive cytoplasm, will bind azure B, the basic dye. Eosin Y, the acidic dye, will bind to the basic groupings of the hemoglobin molecules and the basic proteins within certain granules.

Examples of Romanowsky stains include: Wright, Wright-Giemsa, Leishman, May-Grunwald, and Jenner stains. The most commonly used are Wright and Wright-Giemsa stains.

TABLE 27-2 *CRITERIA FOR A PROPERLY-STAINED*
  BLOOD SMEAR

Macroscopic Evaluation	Blood smear will be pinkish blue in color
Microscopic Evaluation	Blood cells will be evenly distributed
	Area between cells will be clear
	Erythrocytes will be orange-red
	Neutrophilic granules are lillac
	Eosinophilic granules are red-orange
	Basophilic granules are dark blue or purple
	Lymphocyte's cytoplasm is robin's egg blue
	Leukocyte nuclei are blue to purple
	Within nucleus, chromatin and
	parachromatin are distinct
	Precipitated stain is minimal or absent

The staining process begins with the methanol fixation step, which results in the adherence of cellular proteins to the glass microscope slide preventing the cells from being washed away during subsequent steps. Additional fixation takes place when the blood smear is flooded with Wright's stain. The actual staining begins with the addition of buffer to the Wright's stain resulting in the ionization of the dyes. After the appropriate staining time, the blood smear is thoroughly rinsed with distilled water and allowed to air dry. A properly stained blood smear will meet the criteria outlined in Table 27-2. Potential causes of an improperly stained blood smear are given in Table 27-3.

●
Peripheral blood smear examination

The examination of a well-stained peripheral blood smear is one of the most frequently requested tests in the hematology laboratory.[5,6,13–17]

The thorough examination of a peripheral blood smear may be used: (1) as a screening tool to identify illness, (2) for the definitive diagnosis of certain hematologic and nonhematologic conditions, and (3) to monitor the patient's response to therapy. The peripheral blood smear evaluation includes: a leukocyte estimate, observation for the presence of abnormal cells, abnormal erythrocyte distribution, and erythrocyte and platelet morphology, a platelet estimate, and a 100-cell leukocyte differential.

TABLE 27-3 *POTENTIAL CAUSES OF IMPROPERLY-STAINED*
  BLOOD SMEAR

If Blood Smear Is:	Potential Causes
Excessively blue or dark	prolonged staining
	inadequate washing
	too high an alkalinity of stain and/or buffer
	thick blood smear
Excessively pink or light	insufficient staining
	prolonged washing
	too high an acidity of stain and/or buffer
Presence of precipitate	unclean slides
	drying during staining process
	inadequate filtration of stain

On 100× magnification (10× objective), the peripheral blood smear is scanned to assure even distribution of leukocytes and observe for immature or abnormal cells, platelet clumps, and abnormal erythrocyte distribution patterns such as rouleaux or agglutination. The leukocyte estimate is obtained by counting the number of leukocytes in each of 5 fields of view, determining the average number of leukocytes within those 5 fields and multiplying that number by 200 (1 leukocyte = 0.2×10^9/L). The leukocyte estimate should correlate with the leukocyte count.

On 1000× magnification (100× objective), platelet morphology is observed, and a platelet estimate is obtained by counting the number of platelets in 5 to 10 fields of view, determining the average number of platelets within those fields and multiplying the number by the appropriate conversion factor (1 platelet = 20.0×10^9/L if capillary blood or 1 platelet = 15.0×10^9/L if EDTA-anticoagulated blood). The platelet estimate should correlate with the platelet count. Erythrocyte morphology is evaluated by careful observation of erythrocyte size, shape, color, and presence of inclusions. Normal erythrocytes are described as normocytic and normochromic. Any change beyond normal variation should be noted since certain variations in the erythrocytes are characteristic of specific hematologic disorders. A detailed discussion of possible morphologic changes can be found in Chapter 5.

The leukocyte differential is performed by counting 100 cells per slide using the "battlement" track method for examination (Fig. 27-4). Each leukocyte encountered must be identified and placed in the appropriate category; distorted cells should be included only if they are clearly identifiable. Nucleated erythrocytes are not included within the differential but are tabulated separately. The results of the differential are reported as a percentage of all leukocytes counted. The nucleated erythrocytes are expressed per 100 leukocytes. Finally, leukocytes are observed for changes in morphology (i.e., Dohle bodies, hypersegmented neutrophils, etc.). Morphologic changes may be the result of an underlying hematologic disorder, presence of excess anticoagulant, or failure to prepare the blood smears within four hours of collection. Typical anticoagulant changes include: cytoplasmic vacuolization, degranulation, karyorrhexis, karyolysis, and changes in nuclear shape.

The leukocyte differential reference values for adult males and females can be found in Table B on the inside

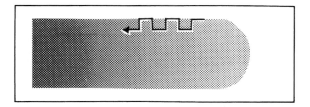

FIGURE 27-4. Pathway for the differential cell count. (From Brown, B.A.: Hematology: Principles and Procedures, 6th Ed., Philadelphia, Lea & Febiger, 1993, with permission.)

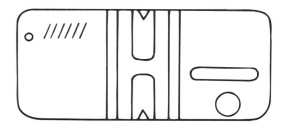

FIGURE 27-5. Neubauer hemacytometer. (From Brown, B.A.: Hematology: Principles and Procedures, 6th Ed., Philadelphia, Lea & Febiger, 1993, with permission.)

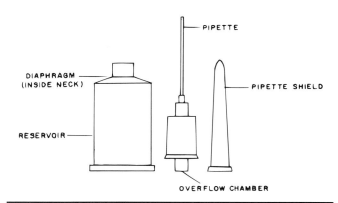

FIGURE 27-7. Unopette System. (From Brown, B.A.: Hematology: Principles and Procedures, 6th Ed., Philadelphia, Lea & Febiger, 1993, with permission.)

cover. The reference values will vary in children as shown in Table E in the Appendix.

CELL ENUMERATION BY HEMACYTOMETER

The hemacytometer consists of two identically ruled glass platforms mounted in a glass holder (Fig. 27-5).[7,18] Each platform contains a ruled square measuring 3 × 3 mm (9 mm²), and is subdivided according to the "improved Neubauer ruling" (Fig. 27-6). This ruling subdivides the ruled square into 9 large squares, each measuring 1 × 1 mm (1 mm²). The four corner squares labeled "W" are used for leukocyte counts, and each is further divided into 16 smaller squares.

The center large square (1 mm²) is used for platelet and

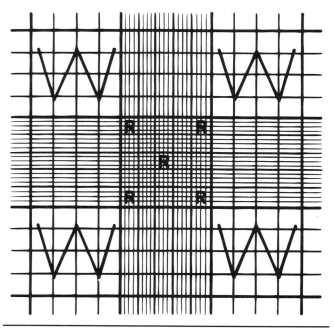

FIGURE 27-6. Neubauer hemacytometer, counting area. "W" indicates the squares used for leukocyte counts, while "R" indicates the squares used for erythrocyte counts. The entire center square is used for platelet counts. (From Brown, B.A.: Hematology: Principles and Procedures, 6th Ed., Philadelphia, Lea & Febiger, 1993, with permission.)

erythrocyte counts. This square is divided into 25 smaller squares, each with an area of 0.04 mm². Each of the 25 squares is further divided into 16 smaller squares. The five squares labeled "R" are used in performing the erythrocyte count, whereas the entire center square is used in performing the platelet count.

On either side of the two ruled glass platforms of the hemacytometer is a raised ridge on top of which is placed a coverglass. The distance between the coverglass and the surface of the ruled area (depth) is exactly 0.1 mm.

The Unopette system is a fast and accurate method for collecting and diluting blood for cell counts.[19-22] For each laboratory determination performed, the Unopette consists of the following elements: the reservoir, the pipet, and the pipet shield (Fig. 27-7). The reservoir contains a premeasured volume of diluting fluid, which is specific for the cell count to be performed.

Manual leukocyte (white blood cell) count

Whole blood is diluted with a 3% acetic acid solution, which hemolyzes mature erythrocytes and facilitates leukocyte counting. The standard dilution for leukocyte counts is 1:20. This dilution may be prepared using the leukocyte Unopette system[19] or leukocyte diluting pipets. The dilution is mixed well and mounted on a hemacytometer. The cells are allowed to settle, and then are counted in four corner squares of the hemacytometer chamber using the low power (10×) objective. With proper light adjustment, the leukocytes should appear as dark dots.

The number of leukocytes are calculated per μL (× 10⁹/L) of blood. To make this determination, the total number of cells counted must be corrected for the initial dilution of blood and the volume of blood used (Fig. 27-8). The typical dilution of blood for leukocyte counts is 1:20; therefore the dilution factor is 20. The volume of blood used is based on the area and depth of the counting area. The area counted is 4 mm² and the depth is 0.1 mm; therefore, the volume factor (area × depth) is 0.4 mm³.

Reference intervals for leukocyte counts in adult males and females can be found in Table A on the inside cover.

Total number of cells counted • dilution factor • 1/volume factor = cells/mm³

Example:	Total number of cells (one side of hemacytometer)	200 cells
	Dilution	1:20
	Area counted	4 mm²
	Depth	0.1 mm
	Volume factor (area × depth)	0.4 mm³

$200 \cdot 20 \cdot 1/0.4 \text{ mm}^3 = 10,000/\text{mm}^3 \ (\mu L) \text{ or } 10.0 \times 10^9/L$

FIGURE 27-8. Calculation formula for hemacytometer cell counts.

The reference values will vary in children as shown in Table E in the Appendix. Conditions commonly associated with increased or decreased leukocyte counts are shown in Table 27-4.

Manual erythrocyte (red blood cell) count

Whole blood is diluted with a 0.85% saline solution, which prevents erythrocyte lysis and facilitates erythrocyte counting. The standard dilution for erythrocyte counts is 1:200. This dilution may be prepared using the erythrocyte Unopette system[20] or erythrocyte diluting pipets. The dilution is mixed well and mounted on a hemacytometer. The cells are allowed to settle and then are counted in five of the smaller squares within the large center square (labeled "R" in Fig. 27-6) using the high dry objective (40×).

The number of erythrocytes are calculated per μL ($\times 10^{12}$/L) of blood using the calculation formula for hemacytometer cell counts (Fig. 27-8). The variations will be in the dilution factor and the volume factor. For erythrocyte counts, the dilution factor is 200 and the volume factor is 0.02 mm³ (area = 0.2 mm²; depth = 0.1 mm).

The reference intervals for erythrocyte counts in adult males and adult females can be found in Table A on the inside cover. The reference values will vary with age as shown in Table D in the Appendix. Conditions commonly associated with increased or decreased erythrocyte counts are shown in Table 27-4.

Manual platelet count

Whole blood is diluted with a 1% ammonium oxalate solution. The isotonic balance of the diluent is such that all erythrocytes are lysed while the leukocytes, platelets, and reticulocytes remain intact. The standard dilution for platelet counts is 1:100. This dilution may be prepared using the leukocyte/platelet Unopette system[21] or erythrocyte diluting pipets. The dilution is mixed well and mounted on both sides of the hemacytometer. The cells are allowed to settle. Using the high dry objective (40×), the platelets are counted in the large center square (1 mm²) of both counting chambers (total area counted is 2 mm²). With phase microscopy, the platelets appear as round or oval bodies.

A second method for manual platelet counts is the Rees-Ecker method. Using the erythrocyte diluting pipet, a 1:100 dilution of whole blood is prepared with the Rees-Ecker solution containing brilliant cresyl blue. The brilliant cresyl blue stains the platelets a light bluish color. The platelets are then counted using a standard hemacytometer and bright field microscopy.

The number of platelets are calculated per μL ($\times 10^9$/L) of blood using the calculation formula for hemacytometer cell counts (Fig. 27-8). The variations will be in the dilution factor and the volume factor. For platelet counts, the dilution factor is 100 and the volume factor is 0.2 mm³ (area = 2 mm²; depth = 0.1 mm).

The reference interval for platelet counts is 150 to 440 $\times 10^9$/L. Conditions commonly associated with increased or decreased platelet counts are shown in Table 27-4.

Eosinophil count (Unopette method)

The eosinophil count is performed by diluting whole blood with a staining solution. The staining solution contains phyloxine B which stains the eosinophils red; all other leukocytes are preserved but not stained.[22,24] The diluted specimen is mixed well and mounted on both sides of the hemacytometer. The cells are allowed to settle. Using the low power objective (10×), the eosinophils are counted in the entire ruled area (9 mm²) of both counting chambers. Eosinophils appear bright orange-red and are clearly distinguishable from other leukocytes. The direct

TABLE 27-4 *CONDITIONS COMMONLY ASSOCIATED WITH CHANGES IN ERYTHROCYTE, LEUKOCYTE, AND PLATELET CONCENTRATIONS*

	Increased Concentration	Decreased Concentration
Erythrocyte	Polycythemia Myeloproliferative disorders Dehydration	Anemia Acute leukemia Myelodysplastic syndromes Hemorrhage Hemolysis
Leukocyte	Bacterial infections Inflammation Metabolic intoxication Hemolysis Hemorrhage Tissue necrosis After strenuous exercise Anxiety or stress Acute leukemia Myeloproliferative disorders	Viral infections Aplastic anemia Megaloblastic anemia Drug-induced leukopenia Myelodysplastic syndromes
Platelet	Following splenectomy Hemorrhage Iron deficiency anemia Myeloproliferative disorders	Immune thrombocytopenic purpura Aplastic anemia Megaloblastic anemia Myelodysplastic syndromes Acute leukemia

eosinophil count is inherently inaccurate due to the low number of eosinophils. In order to improve the accuracy of the eosinophil count, at least 100 eosinophils should be counted.[25] This involves the repeated charging of the hemacytometer and counting eosinophils until this number is met. The final calculation is based on the total volume counted.

The number of eosinophils are calculated per μL ($\times 10^9/L$) of blood using the calculation formula for hemacytometer cell counts (Fig. 27-8). The variations will be in the dilution factor and the volume factor. For eosinophil counts, the dilution factor for the Unopette system is 32. The volume factor will vary depending on the total area needed to count 100 eosinophils and the depth of the hemacytometer (e.g., Fuchs-Rosenthal hemacytometer = 0.2 mm depth).

The reference interval for adults is 0 to $0.45 \times 10^9/L$. However, reference values will vary with age as shown in Table E in the Appendix.

● ROUTINE HEMATOLOGY PROCEDURES

● Hemoglobin concentration

Whole blood is diluted in cyanmethemoglobin reagent. The diluting fluid hemolyzes the erythrocytes releasing hemoglobin into the solution. The ferrous ions (Fe^{2+}) of the hemoglobin molecules are oxidized by potassium ferricyanide to ferric ions (Fe^{3+}). This oxidation results in the formation of methemoglobin. Methemoglobin combines with the cyanide ions (CN^-) to form cyanmethemoglobin, a stable compound that can be quantitated using spectrophotometry.[26,27] All hemoglobin derivatives except sulfhemoglobin are converted to cyanmethemoglobin.

When measured spectrophotometrically at 540 nm, the absorbance of cyanmethemoglobin follows Lambert-Beer's law and is directly proportional to the concentration of hemoglobin in the blood. A reference (standard) curve is prepared using cyanmethemoglobin standard solutions of known hemoglobin concentrations (Fig. 27-9). An unknown hemoglobin concentration may be calculated from the measured absorbance, read from a standard calibration curve, or read directly from the instrument scale of specialized instruments. The reference values for hemoglobin will vary with age and sex as shown in Table D in the Appendix.

There are several physiologic conditions, which lead to turbidity in the cyanmethemoglobin reagent-patient specimen mixture (Table 27-5). Any turbidity in the mixture will result in falsely elevated values. It is important to recognize the falsely elevated result and take the appropriate corrective action to obtain the true hemoglobin value.

● Hematocrit

The hematocrit of a blood specimen is the packed cell volume (PCV), denoting the percentage of erythrocytes in a known volume of whole blood.[28,29,30] It is one of the simplest and most reproducible of any laboratory test. The

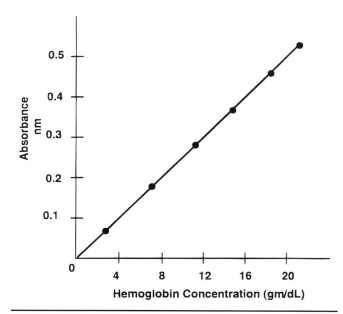

FIGURE 27-9. Hemoglobin standard calibration curve. Absorbance in nm is on the y-axis and hemoglobin concentration in gm/dL is on the x-axis.

hematocrit is useful in the detection of anemia and polycythemia. Together with the total number of erythrocytes and hemoglobin determination, it is used to calculate the erythrocyte indices, mean cell volume (MCV) and mean cell hemoglobin concentration (MCHC).

In the microhematocrit method, a capillary tube is filled with anticoagulated whole blood and centrifuged in a microhematocrit centrifuge at 10,000 to 15,000 g for 5 minutes. The volume occupied by the erythrocytes is expressed as a percentage of the total volume (packed cell volume). This method has a number of advantages including small

TABLE 27-5 *PHYSIOLOGIC SOURCES OF ERROR IN HEMOGLOBIN DETERMINATION AND CORRECTIVE ACTIONS*

Physiologic Condition	Corrective Action
Extremely high leukocyte count ($>30.0 \times 10^9/L$)	Centrifuge hemoglobin mixture and use supernatant to determine hemoglobin concentration
Presence of hemoglobin S or hemoglobin C	Use a 1:2 dilution of the hemoglobin mixture with distilled water to determine hemoglobin concentration (multiply hemoglobin by 2)
Presence of lipemia	Use a patient blank or replace patient's plasma with isotonic saline to determine hemoglobin concentration
Presence of abnormal globulins (e.g. those found in Multiple myeloma or Waldenstrom's macroglobulinemia)	Increase the alkalinity of the cyanmethemoglobin reagent by adding potassium carbonate, then repeat hemoglobin determination

TABLE 27-6 *ERYTHROCYTE INDICES*

Calculation	Example	Reference Interval
*MCV = $\dfrac{\text{Hct (\%)}}{\text{RBC } (\times 10^{12}/\text{L})} \cdot 10$	$\dfrac{42.6}{4.88} \cdot 10 = 87$ fL	80–100 fL
MCH = $\dfrac{\text{Hb (g/dL)}}{\text{RBC } (\times 10^{12}/\text{L})} \cdot 10$	$\dfrac{14.2}{4.88} \cdot 10 = 29$ pg	26–34 pg
**MCHC = $\dfrac{\text{Hb (g/dL)}}{\text{Hct (\%)}} \cdot 100$	$\dfrac{14.2}{42.6} \cdot 100 = 33$ g/dL	32–36 g/dL

* If hct is expressed in L/L multiply by 1000 instead of 10.
** If hct is expressed in L/L do not multiply by 100.

sample size, high centrifuge speed resulting in less trapped plasma, and shorter centrifugation time.

The reference values will vary with age and sex as shown in Table D in the Appendix.

Erythrocyte indices

In 1929, Wintrobe introduced the erythrocyte indices, MCV, mean cell hemoglobin (MCH), and MCHC.[12,18,31] These indices are calculated from the erythrocyte count, hemoglobin concentration, and hematocrit (Table 27-6). With the advent of automation in hematology, the erythrocyte indices are measured and/or calculated from data collected by erythrocyte analysis. The electrical impedance analyzers measure the MCV by averaging the heights of the voltage pulses. The MCH, MCHC, and Hct are calculated from the measured values. The automated MCV eliminates the problem of a falsely elevated MCV due to trapped plasma which may occur in the centrifuged hematocrit specimen. Likewise, the MCHC also may be affected in cases of increased trapped plasma (e.g., sickle cell anemia). The MCHC calculated from centrifuged hematocrits will be lower than that obtained from the automated instrument. When the hematocrit is corrected for trapped plasma, the erythrocyte indices calculated from the centrifuged hematocrit agree with those obtained from automated instruments. The erythrocyte indices are used in the morphologic classification of anemias, defining normocytic, microcytic, and macrocytic anemias with the MCV.

Erythrocyte sedimentation rate

The erythrocyte sedimentation rate (ESR) is a measurement of the rate at which the erythrocytes settle from the plasma.[32–35] The rate of erythrocyte settling is dependent on: (1) the protein composition of the plasma, (2) the size and shape of the erythrocytes, and (3) the erythrocyte concentration.

Increasing levels of plasma proteins (primarily fibrinogen, alpha globulins, or gamma globulins) result in a decrease of the zeta potential surrounding the erythrocytes. With a lower zeta potential, the erythrocytes are able to join together in rouleaux formation and settle from the plasma at a faster rate.

Likewise, the size and shape of the erythrocytes affect the rate of fall. Macrocytes will settle faster than normal erythrocytes and microcytes will settle slower. Due to their irregular shape, poikilocytes are unable to form rouleaux and settle at a slower rate.

The erythrocyte concentration directly affects the ESR. The higher the erythrocyte concentration, the lower the ESR. An anemic individual will appear to have an increased ESR. Therefore, it is important to follow NCCLS' recommendations to eliminate the effect of erythrocyte concentration on the ESR.[32]

The ESR is used to demonstrate the presence of inflammation and/or tissue destruction. It is a "nonspecific" test indicating tissue destruction but not specifying the cause (i.e., disease state responsible). Table 27-7 lists a number of conditions associated with an elevated ESR.

Two principal methods have been used to measure the ESR: the Westergren method and the Wintrobe method. The Wintrobe method utilizes undiluted whole blood and the Wintrobe tube. The Wintrobe tube is filled to the "0" mark and allowed to sit in a vertical position for 60 minutes. The ESR is read as the distance (mm) between the meniscus of the plasma and the top of the erythrocytes. The resulting distance is the erythrocyte sedimentation rate in mm/hr. The disadvantages of this method include: too short free fall time as a result of the short tube and problems arising due to the narrow bore of the tube and the use of undiluted blood. The NCCLS' recommended method is the Westergren method.[32] In the modified Westergren method, EDTA-anticoagulated whole blood is diluted with 0.85% NaCl. The diluted blood is aspirated into a calibrated Westergren pipet and the cells are allowed to settle for a period of exactly one hour. Like the Wintrobe method, the distance in millimeters between the meniscus of the plasma and the top of the sedimented erythrocyte column is read.

The reference interval for ESR varies with age and sex. For adult males and children, the reference interval is 0

TABLE 27-7 *CONDITIONS ASSOCIATED WITH AN ELEVATED ESR*

Inflammatory conditions with increased acute phase reactants
Systemic lupus erythematosus
Rheumatoid arthritis
Acute and chronic infections
Pulmonary tuberculosis
Subacute bacterial endocarditis
Rheumatic fever
Hepatitis
Myocardial infarctions
Multiple myeloma
Waldenstrom's macroglobulinemia
Pregnancy
Menstruation
Oral contraceptives

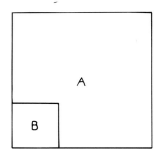

FIGURE 27-10. Miller disk. Reticulocyte counting area = A; Erythrocyte counting area = B. (From Brown, B.A.: Hematology: Principles and Procedures. 6th Ed., Philadelphia, Lea & Febiger, 1993, with permission.)

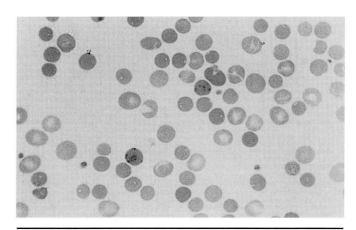

FIGURE 27-11. Reticulocytes identified by new methylene blue stain. The reticulocytes are the cells containing particulate inclusions. (250× original magnification.)

to 10 mm/hr. The reference interval for adult females is 0 to 20 mm/hr.

DIAGNOSTIC PROCEDURES FOR ANEMIA

Reticulocyte count

Reticulocytes are immature non-nucleated erythrocytes containing residual RNA. In the erythrocyte maturation sequence, the reticulocyte spends 2 days in the bone marrow and 1 day in the peripheral blood. As the reticulocyte matures, the amount of RNA decreases. The quantitation of reticulocytes present in the peripheral blood provides a method of evaluating the bone marrow's erythropoietic activity. This evaluation is used in the differential diagnosis of anemias and in monitoring a patient's erythropoietic response to therapy.[36,37]

Using a supravital stain (new methylene blue), residual ribosomal RNA is precipitated within the reticulocytes.[38] A blood smear is prepared from the mixture of anticoagulated whole blood and supravital stain. The smear is examined microscopically using the oil immersion lens fitted with a field restricted ocular (Fig. 27-10). An erythrocyte containing two or more particles of blue-stained material is a reticulocyte (Fig. 27-11). The number of reticulocytes is expressed as a percentage of the total number of erythrocytes counted.

Other erythrocyte inclusions (Pappenheimer bodies, Howell-Jolly bodies, and Heinz bodies) also will be stained with new methylene blue and must be distinguished from reticulocytes. Howell-Jolly bodies and Heinz bodies may be distinguished from precipitated reticulum by their shape and staining characteristics. Heinz bodies appear as light blue green inclusions located at the periphery of the erythrocyte. Howell Jolly bodies are usually one or two round, deep purple staining inclusions and are also visible on Romanowsky stains. Pappenheimer bodies are indistinguishable from reticulum of reticulocytes. If Pappenheimer bodies are suspected, a Prussian blue iron stain should be performed to verify their presence. Reticulum will not stain with the Prussian blue iron stain.

Misinterpretations may result when reporting only the percentage of reticulocytes present in the peripheral blood because the reticulocyte result is dependent on the total number of erythrocytes present in the peripheral blood.[31,40–42] If the total erythrocyte count is decreased, the reticulocyte percentage does not accurately reflect the bone marrow's production of new erythrocytes. The corrected reticulocyte count and the reticulocyte production index may be used to avoid interpretation errors due to the total erythrocyte count and increased bone marrow stimulation. These calculations are discussed in Chapter 5.

With the advent of flow cytometry and its expanding role in the laboratory, automated reticulocyte counts can now be performed. A discussion of the application of flow cytometry to automated reticulocyte enumeration is found in Chapter 29.

Sodium metabisulfite test

The sodium metabisulfite procedure is a screening test for the presence of hemoglobin S (Hb S).[43] Sodium metabisulfite ($Na_2S_2O_5$) is a strong reducing agent that deoxygenates hemoglobins. When erythrocytes containing Hb S are exposed to sodium metabisulfite, the deoxygenated Hb S crystallizes and the erythrocytes become sickle shaped. In this procedure, whole blood is mixed with a 2% sodium metabisulfite solution, a portion of the suspension is placed on a glass microscope slide and covered with a coverslip. Thus, the erythrocyte suspension is incubated within an oxygen-free environment. The erythrocyte suspension is observed microscopically for the presence of sickled or "holly-leaf" cells (Fig. 27-12). The appearance of either shape indicates a positive test result. This procedure does not distinguish hemoglobin S disease from hemoglobin S trait. A hemoglobin electrophoresis procedure should be performed to differentiate between the two states.

Solubility test for hemoglobin S

The solubility test is the more commonly used screening test for the presence of Hb S. It is based on the relative

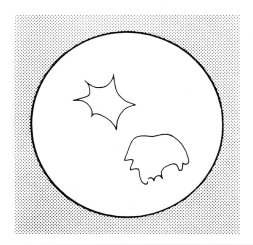

FIGURE 27-12. Holly leaf-shaped red blood cells. (From Brown, B.A.: Hematology: Principles and Procedures. 6th Ed., Philadelphia, Lea & Febiger, 1993, with permission.)

insolubility of hemoglobin S when combined with a reducing agent (sodium dithionite).[44-47] When anticoagulated whole blood is mixed with the reducing agent, erythrocytes will lyse due to the presence of saponin and hemoglobin will be released. If hemoglobin S is present, it will form liquid crystals and give a turbid appearance to the solution (Fig. 27-13). A transparent solution is seen with other hemoglobins that are more soluble in the reducing agent.

Like the sodium metabisulfite test, the solubility test will not differentiate hemoglobin S disease from hemoglobin S trait and a hemoglobin electrophoresis procedure should be performed to differentiate the two states. In addition, there are several abnormal hemoglobin variants that cause sickling and will give a positive solubility test.

These variants include Hb C Harlem, Hb S Travis, and Hb C Ziguinchor. The hemoglobin electrophoresis procedure is used to differentiate these variants from Hb S.

● Hemoglobin electrophoresis using cellulose acetate

Electrophoresis is the movement of charged molecules in an electric field. In hemoglobin electrophoresis, hemoglobin A (adult hemoglobin) takes on a negative charge at an alkaline pH and moves toward the anode (positive electrode). Abnormal hemoglobin variants will have altered charges due to single amino acid substitutions on their globin chains. This change in electrical charge allows for the separation of the majority of abnormal hemoglobin variants from hemoglobin A at an alkaline pH.[48-50]

In the hemoglobin electrophoresis procedure, the electrophoretic patterns and hemoglobin percentages of the unknown specimens are compared to those of the control sample containing Hb A, F, S, and C and a known adult sample. The detection and preliminary identification of hemoglobinopathies and thalassemias may be obtained using hemoglobin electrophoresis with cellulose acetate at an alkaline pH. Cellulose acetate electrophoresis allows for the separation of Hb A, F, S, and C into distinct bands (Fig. 27-14). However, there are other abnormal hemoglobin variants that have the same electrophoretic mobility as Hb S and Hb C. Hb D and Hb G have the same mobility as Hb S whereas, Hb E and Hb O$_{Arab}$ have the same mobility as Hb C. Additional tests must be used to confirm the presence of abnormal hemoglobin variants. The solubility test may be used to confirm Hb S and citrate agar electrophoresis may be used to confirm the presence of Hb A, F, S, and C.

Citrate agar electrophoresis separates Hb F, A, S, and

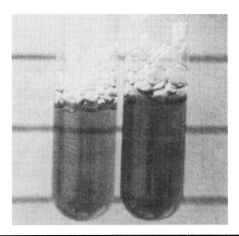

FIGURE 27-13. Sodium dithionite tube test. Negative results are indicated by the clear solution, where the black lines on the reader scale are visible through the test solution. Positive results are shown as a turbid solution, where the reader scale is not visible through the test solution. (From Brown, B.A.: Hematology: Principles and Procedures. 6th Ed., Philadelphia, Lea & Febiger, 1993, with permission.)

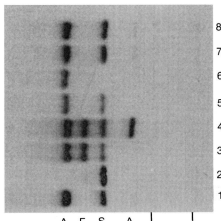

8. AA$_2$S, D or G

7. AA$_2$S, D or G

6. AA$_2$

5. AS, D or G

4. AFSC Control

3. AFSA$_2$ Control

2. Homozygous S, D or G

1. AA$_2$S, D or G

A   F   S   A$_2$ Application Point
          D   C
          G   E   Carbonic Anhydrase

FIGURE 27-14. Electrophoretic mobilities of hemoglobins on cellulose acetate at pH 8.6. (Courtesy of Helena Laboratories, Beaumont, TX.)

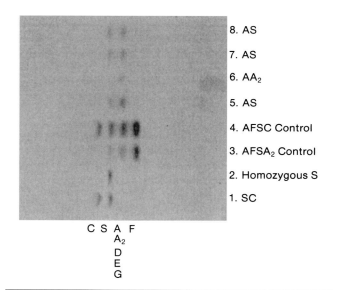

8. AS

7. AS

6. AA₂

5. AS

4. AFSC Control

3. AFSA₂ Control

2. Homozygous S

1. SC

C S A F
A₂
D
E
G

FIGURE 27-15. Electrophoretic mobilities of hemoglobins on citrate agar at pH 6.2, showing separation of hemoglobins 5 and C from other hemoglobins. (Courtesy of Helena Laboratories, Beaumont, TX.)

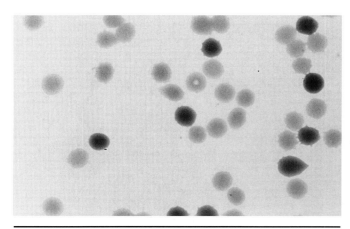

FIGURE 27-16. Acid elution test for determination of hemoglobin F. Erythrocytes containing hemoglobin F appear as dark-staining cells. The light staining cells are erythrocytes which contain adult hemoglobins.

C into distinct bands (Fig. 27-15). Because no other hemoglobin variants travel with Hb S and Hb C on citrate agar, it is used to confirm the presence of Hb S and Hb C. It also is useful in differentiating other hemoglobin variants, which travel together with Hb S and Hb C on cellulose acetate electrophoresis; these hemoglobin variants (Hb D, Hb G, Hb E, and Hb O_Arab) have the same mobility as Hb A on citrate agar.[51,52] Rare abnormal hemoglobin variants may be positively identified with globin chain analysis and structural studies.

Due to the small amount of sample used, the presence of low concentrations of hemoglobin variants may be undetectable and increases in Hb A₂ concentration may not be detected. Anion exchange column chromatography is a more accurate method to detect increases in Hb A₂.

Acid elution for hemoglobin F

The acid elution test for fetal hemoglobin (HbF) may be used in the differentiation of hereditary persistence of fetal hemoglobin (HPFH) from other conditions associated with high levels of HbF. HPFH is characterized by an even or uniform distribution of HbF within the erythrocytes whereas, other conditions with high levels of Hb F are characterized by an uneven or non-uniform distribution of Hb F within the erythrocytes. Conditions such as beta-thalassemia minor, beta-thalassemia major, sickle cell anemia, hereditary spherocytosis, and aplastic anemia are associated with high levels of Hb F. This stain also may be used to detect the presence of fetal cells in the maternal circulation (fetal-maternal bleed) during problematic pregnancies.

In an acid solution, all hemoglobins are eluted from the erythrocytes except hemoglobin F (fetal hemoglobin).[53–55] Blood smears are fixed in 80% ethanol and then incubated in a citrate-phosphate buffer (pH 3.3). The slide is stained with acid hematoxylin and counterstained with eosin. The slide is observed microscopically using the oil immersion lens to determine the distribution of Hb F within the erythrocytes and the percentage of Hb F-containing erythrocytes. Erythrocytes containing fetal hemoglobin stain bright pink or red with the eosin B stain (Fig. 27-16). The rest of the erythrocytes appear as pale ghosts. Intermediate erythrocytes (pink colored, but not intense) are sometimes seen. The acid hematoxylin stains the leukocyte's nuclei a faint gray-purple color.

Quantitation of hb F by alkali denaturation

Fetal hemoglobin (Hb F) is resistant to denaturation by strong alkali solutions while other hemoglobins are not resistant.[56–59] The addition of a strong alkali solution (1.27 M NaOH) to a hemolysate containing a known concentration of hemoglobin results in hemoglobin denaturation. The denaturation process is stopped by adding a saturated solution of ammonium sulfate. Ammonium sulfate lowers the pH of the reaction mixture and precipitates all denatured hemoglobins. After filtration, the concentration of the remaining alkali-resistant hemoglobin is determined. The alkali-resistant hemoglobin is expressed as a percentage of the total hemoglobin concentration. The hemoglobin concentrations (alkali-resistant and total) are determined by the cyanmethemoglobin method. Each laboratory should establish its own reference interval. In general, adult levels of Hb F are less than 2%.

Hb F levels also may be determined by column chromatography or radial immunodiffusion techniques. Column chromatography is more accurate at HbF levels greater than 40% and radial immunodiffusion is more accurate at HbF levels less than 2%.

Hemoglobin A₂ by column

HbA₂ is a normal adult hemoglobin present in small amounts (up to 3.5%). Increased amounts of HbA₂ are characteristic of beta-thalassemia minor. Therefore, the quantitation of HbA$_2$ is useful in its presumptive diagnosis. Slight increases in HbA$_2$ concentration have been noted in persons with Hb S trait, Hb S disease, unstable hemoglobin variants, or megaloblastic anemia. Decreased HbA$_2$ concentrations may be seen in iron deficiency anemia or alpha-thalassemia.

Hemoglobin A$_2$ may be quantitated with anion exchange chromatography.[60–62] The anion exchange resin is a preparation of cellulose covalently coupled to small positively charged molecules. Thus, the anion exchange resin will attract negatively charged molecules. Hemoglobins, like other proteins, contain positive and negative charges due to the ionizing properties of the component amino acids. In the anion exchange chromatography of hemoglobin A$_2$, the ionic strength of the buffer and pH levels are controlled to cause different hemoglobins to possess different net negative charges. These negatively charged proteins are attracted to the positively charged cellulose and bind accordingly. Following binding, the hemoglobins are removed selectively from the resin by altering the pH or ionic strength of the elution buffer. Due to the solubility of hemoglobin A$_2$ in the elution buffer, hemoglobin A$_2$ is eluted from the resin as the elution buffer moves through the column. The other normal, and most abnormal, hemoglobins are retained by the resin. The percentage of hemoglobin A$_2$ is determined by comparing the absorbance of the hemoglobin A$_2$ fraction to the absorbance of the total hemoglobin fraction at 415 nm using a spectrophotometer. Each laboratory must establish its own reference interval for HbA$_2$ levels. The CDC National Hemoglobinopathy Laboratory reference interval for HbA$_2$ is 1.8% to 3.5%.

Values between 3.5% and 8% are considered indicative of beta-thalassemia trait. Values greater than 8% indicate the presence of additional hemoglobin variants such as S, C, E, O, D, S-G hybrid, and HPFH, which elute with HbA$_2$. HbA$_2$ cannot be differentiated from several abnormal hemoglobin variants such as hemoglobins C, E, and O, which have a net electrical charge similar to HbA$_2$. If abnormal hemoglobin variants are suspected, hemoglobin electrophoretic techniques should be performed to confirm their presence. HbA$_2$ levels may be normal when iron deficiency anemia coexists with beta-thalassemia minor. In this situation, HbA$_2$ levels must be considered together with family history, laboratory data including serum iron, total iron-binding capacity, erythrocyte morphology, Hb, Hct, and MCV. HbA$_2$ also may be quantitated using cellulose acetate electrophoresis followed by elution or densitometry. However, these methods are less accurate than HbA$_2$ measurement by anion exchange chromatography.

● Heat stability test for unstable hemoglobin

Unstable hemoglobins are hemoglobin variants, which result from a variety of amino acid substitutions or deletions that affect the intramolecular interactions of the hemoglobin molecule. These hemoglobin variants are susceptible to spontaneous denaturation resulting in Heinz body formation and erythrocyte hemolysis. Unstable hemoglobins become insoluble at higher temperatures (50° C), whereas normal hemoglobin remains soluble.[7,42,63–65] The hemoglobin concentrations for heated and unheated fractions are determined by the cyanmethemoglobin method. The concentration of unstable hemoglobin is expressed as a percentage of the total hemoglobin concentration (unheated fraction).

Unstable hemoglobins are a cause of congenital nonspherocytic hemolytic anemias. Examples of unstable hemoglobins are: hemoglobin Koln, hemoglobin Hammersmith, hemoglobin Zurich, hemoglobin Seattle, and hemoglobin Bristol. A positive heat instability test should be confirmed by other test methods that identify unstable hemoglobins such as tests for erythrocyte inclusions and the isopropanol precipitation test. Low concentrations of unstable hemoglobin result in false-negative results.

● Heinz body stain

Heinz bodies represent denatured hemoglobin inclusions. These inclusions are usually round or oval in shape and appear refractile. They tend to locate adjacent to the erythrocyte membrane. Heinz bodies are only visible on supravital stained smears and are not visible on Wright's stained smears. Heinz bodies may be present in glucose-6-phosphate dehydrogenase deficiency and related enzyme disorders when the individual is exposed to oxidizing agents such as primaquine or sulfanilamide. In addition, they may be found in individuals with unstable hemoglobins or thalassemias. They are occasionally found in senescent erythrocytes of normal individuals.

A specific dye for Heinz bodies is brilliant green.[66] Using this method, EDTA-anticoagulated whole blood is first mixed with 0.5% neutral red. The mixture is counterstained with 0.5% brilliant green. Several thick smears are prepared from the final mixture. The smears are observed microscopically for the presence of Heinz bodies. Heinz bodies stain green, while reticulocytes and Howell-Jolly bodies stain a deep red. The erythrocytes will stain light red. The percentage of erythrocytes containing Heinz bodies may be determined by counting the number of erythrocytes containing Heinz bodies within 500 erythrocytes.

The specificity of the brilliant green dye for Heinz bodies eliminates problems that arise with the use of other supravital stains such as methyl violet or crystal violet. With these supravital stains, Howell-Jolly bodies, basophilic stippling, and reticulum stain the same as Heinz bodies. This often leads to difficulties in the interpretation of the stain.

● Fluorescent spot test for glucose-6-phosphate dehydrogenase

The fluorescent spot test for glucose-6-phosphate dehydrogenase (G-6-PD) is a screening test to detect G-6-PD deficiency.[67–69] In this procedure, whole blood is added

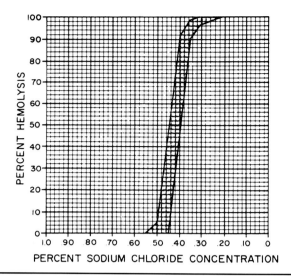

FIGURE 27-17. Normal osmotic fragility curve. The osmotic fragility curve of a normal individual would fall within the area defined by the two sigmoid curves. A curve to the left of normal indicates decreased fragility and a curve to the right increased fragility. (From Brown, B.A.: Hematology: Principles and Procedures. 6th Ed., Philadelphia, Lea & Febiger, 1993, with permission.)

to a mixture of glucose-6-phosphate, NADP, and saponin. Saponin hemolyzes the erythrocytes releasing their contents into solution. If the erythrocytes contain G-6-PD, NADP will be converted to NADPH. Using ultraviolet light, the presence of NADPH is detected by its fluorescence. Lack of G-6-PD is identified by no fluorescence, since NADP will not fluoresce under ultraviolet light. The fluorescent spot test should not be used to assess the degree of G-6-PD deficiency. A quantitative measurement of G-6-PD activity should be performed.

Osmotic fragility test

In this procedure, whole blood is added to increasingly hypotonic solutions of buffered sodium chloride (0.85% to 0.00%) and the solutions are incubated 20 minutes at room temperature.[70] The amount of hemolysis at each concentration is determined by measuring the absorbance of the supernatants spectrophotometrically. An osmotic fragility graph is prepared by plotting the percent of hemolysis of each solution against its concentration, and the results are compared with a normal control. In normal individuals, an almost symmetrical sigmoid shaped curve is obtained (Fig. 27-17). Normal erythrocytes will begin to hemolyze at approximately 0.50% NaCl concentration and hemolysis will be complete at 0.30% NaCl. The normal values for osmotic fragility with each sodium chloride concentration are given in Table K in the Appendix.

In the osmotic fragility test, spherocytes with a decreased surface area-to-volume ratio have a limited ability to expand in hypotonic solutions. They will lyse at higher concentrations of saline than normal biconcave erythrocytes and are said to have an increased osmotic fragil-

ity.[7,70–72] Target cells or sickle cells have a large surface area-to-volume ratio. This increased surface area-to-volume ratio translates into a greater ability to expand in hypotonic solutions. These cells will lyse at lower concentrations of sodium chloride than normal cells, and are said to have a decreased osmotic fragility.

An increased osmotic fragility is associated with hemolytic anemias in which spherocytes are present, in particular, hereditary spherocytosis. Conditions associated with a decreased osmotic fragility include thalassemia, sickle cell anemia, and those conditions in which target cells are observed. Figure 27-18 depicts the increased osmotic lysis of spherocytes in a hypotonic medium.

An incubated osmotic fragility test is performed to identify patients with mild hereditary spherocytosis in which the standard osmotic fragility test is normal. In the incubated osmotic fragility test, patient's blood and control blood are incubated for 24 hours at 37° C under sterile conditions. A significantly increased osmotic fragility after incubation is characteristic of hereditary spherocytosis.

Sugar-water screening test

A "sugar-water" solution (10%) provides a low ionic strength solution, which promotes the attachment of complement to susceptible paroxysmal nocturnal hemoglobinuria erythrocytes.[73] Upon attachment of complement, the erythrocytes hemolyze. Normal erythrocytes do not hemolyze under these conditions. A positive "sugar-water" test is presumptive evidence for paroxysmal nocturnal hemoglobinuria (PNH). The acidified serum test should be used to confirm PNH, since the "sugar-water" test is not specific. If the "sugar-water" test is negative, no further testing is required because the test is sensitive for PNH.

Acidified serum test (Ham test)

The erythrocytes of paroxysmal nocturnal hemoglobinuria (PNH) are unusually sensitive to hemolysis by complement.[7,74,75] In the acidified serum test, complement attaches to the erythrocytes at a slightly acidic pH (6.5 to 7.0) and is activated by an alternate pathway, not involving the presence of antibodies. The activation of complement results in the hemolysis of the erythrocytes. Table 27-8 outlines the procedural set-up for the acidified serum test and the expected results in PNH. A diagnosis of paroxysmal nocturnal hemoglobinuria is suggested if hemolysis occurs in tubes 2 and 5. No hemolysis should be seen in tube 3 because PNH red blood cells require complement for hemolysis.

A false-positive test may be seen in hereditary spherocytosis. Spherocytes may undergo hemolysis in test tubes 2, 3, and 5. If hemolysis occurs in test tube 2 and 7, but not in test tube 5, a warm hemolysin antibody may be present in the patient's serum. The acidified serum test also may be positive in hereditary erythroblastic multinuclearity with positive acidified serum test (HEMPAS). Two differentiating features of this disorder are (1) the patient's (HEMPAS) erythrocytes are not lysed

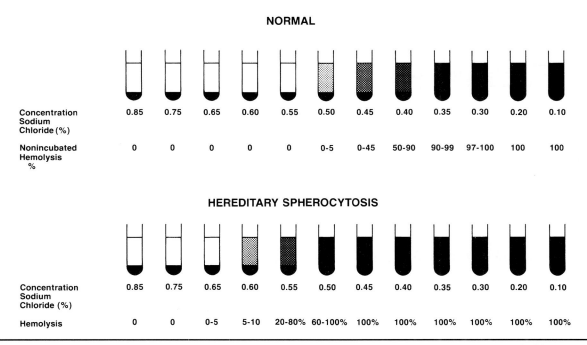

NORMAL

Concentration Sodium Chloride (%)	0.85	0.75	0.65	0.60	0.55	0.50	0.45	0.40	0.35	0.30	0.20	0.10
Nonincubated Hemolysis %	0	0	0	0	0	0-5	0-45	50-90	90-99	97-100	100	100

HEREDITARY SPHEROCYTOSIS

Concentration Sodium Chloride (%)	0.85	0.75	0.65	0.60	0.55	0.50	0.45	0.40	0.35	0.30	0.20	0.10
Hemolysis	0	0	0-5	5-10	20-80%	60-100%	100%	100%	100%	100%	100%	100%

FIGURE 27-18. The osmotic fragility test demonstrates the increased osmotic lysis of spherocytes in a hypotonic medium compared with normal red cells.

by the patient's own acidified serum and (2) the sucrose hemolysis test is negative.

CYTOCHEMICAL STAINS

Leukocyte alkaline phosphatase

The leukocyte alkaline phosphatase (LAP) score is useful in differentiating chronic myelogenous leukemia from a leukemoid reaction.[76-79] Chronic myelogenous leukemia, paroxysmal nocturnal hemoglobinuria, and hereditary hypophosphatasia are associated with abnormally low or absent staining. Conversely, leukemoid reactions, physiologic leukocytosis, polycythemia vera, and myelofibrosis

are associated with markedly elevated LAP scores. Blood or other tissues are fixed to a slide. The sites of alkaline phosphatase activity are identified by incubating the specimen in naphthol AS-BI phosphate at an alkaline pH. As a result of the phosphatase activity, naphthol-AS is liberated. The liberated naphthol immediately couples with a diazonium salt (e.g., fast red violet) forming an insoluble, visible pigment. The sites of alkaline phosphatase activity will appear as red granules. The leukocyte alkaline phosphatase activity (LAP) score is obtained by rating 100 consecutive segmented and band neutrophils using a scale of 0 to 4 + according to the appearance and intensity of the precipitated dye (Table 27-9). The number of cells counted in each cell rating is multiplied by the cell rating value, and a total LAP score is obtained (Table 27-10). Normal healthy individuals exhibit minimal alkaline

TABLE 27-8 *ACIDIFIED SERUM PROCEDURAL OUTLINE WITH EXPECTED RESULTS IN PNH*

TUBE	1	2	3	4	5	6	7
Patient Serum (mL)	0.5	0.5				0.5	0.5
Control Serum (mL)			0.5*	0.5	0.5		
0.2 N HCl (mL)		0.05	0.05		0.05		0.05
Patient RBC (mL)	0.05	0.05	0.05	0.05	0.05		
Control RBC (mL)						0.05	0.05
Results observed in PNH	0	+	0	0	+	0	0

* Serum was heat inactivated

0 = No hemolysis

+ = Hemolysis

TABLE 27-9 *LEUKOCYTE ALKALINE PHOSPHATASE: CELL RATING AND STAINING CHARACTERISTICS*

Cell Rating	Amount (%)*	Size of Precipitated Dye Granule	Intensity of Staining
0	None		None
1+	<50	Small	Faint
2+	50–80	Small to medium	Moderate
3+	80–100	Medium to large	Strong
4+	100	Medium and large	Brilliant

* Percentage of volume of cytoplasm occupied by diazonium dye precipitate.

phosphatase activity within neutrophils. An elevated alkaline phosphatase score may be associated with the use of oral contraceptives or cortisol and stress.

Leukocyte peroxidase (myeloperoxidase)

Myeloperoxidase is an enzyme capable of catalyzing the oxidation of substances by hydrogen peroxide. Myeloperoxidase activity is detected by incubating the fixed specimen in a solution of hydrogen peroxide, p-phenylenediamine, and catechol.[80,81] The sites of myeloperoxidase activity will be identified by an insoluble brown-black reaction product. This enzyme is present in neutrophils, eosinophils, and monocytes.

Neutrophils and their precursors exhibit brown-black intracellular granulation. Monocytes stain less intensely than neutrophils. Lymphocytes do not exhibit myeloperoxidase activity. The myeloperoxidase stain is useful in the differentiation of acute myeloid leukemias from acute lymphocytic leukemias (Table 27-11).

Sudan black B stain

Sudan black B is a diazo dye that stains phospholipids, neutral fats, and sterols. Staining occurs because the Sudan black B dye is more soluble in intracellular lipids than in the alcohol solvent of the stain.[82,83] Cellular components containing lipids will stain brown-black with the

TABLE 27-10 *CALCULATION OF LAP SCORE*

Cell Rating	Number of Cells Counted	LAP Score
0	45	0
1+	30	30
2+	15	30
3+	5	15
4+	5	20
Total LAP Score		95

Sudan black B stain. Sudan black B will stain primary and secondary granules of the granulocytic cell line. Auer rods have a rich phospholipid membrane that is demonstrated by the Sudan black B stain. Neutrophils, neutrophil precursors, and eosinophils show blue-black intracellular granulation. Monocytes will stain less intensely than neutrophils. Lymphocytes do not stain with Sudan black B. The Sudan black B stain results parallel those results seen with the myeloperoxidase stain. Therefore, it is useful in the differentiation of acute myeloid leukemias from acute lymphocytic leukemias (Table 27-11).

Chloroacetate esterase stain

Chloroacetate esterase activity is detected by incubating the specimen in naphthol AS-D chloroacetate at an acid pH.[84–86] As a result of the esterase activity, there is enzymatic hydrolysis of ester linkages and free naphthol compounds are liberated. The liberated naphthol immediately couples with a diazonium salt (e.g., fast red violet), forming an insoluble, visible pigment at the site of enzyme activity. Naphthol AS-D chloroacetate esterase is considered specific for the granulocytic cell line. The sites of enzyme activity show bright red granulation. Enzyme activity is weak or absent in monocytes and lymphocytes. Similar to the myeloperoxidase stain and Sudan black B stain, the chloroacetate esterase stain is useful in differentiating acute myeloid leukemias from acute lymphocytic leukemias (Table 27-11)

α-naphthyl esterase stain

α-naphthyl esterase activity is detected by incubating the specimen in α-naphthyl acetate at an alkaline pH.[84–86] As a result of the esterase activity, there is enzymatic hydrolysis of ester linkages and free naphthol compounds are liberated. The liberated naphthol immediately couples with a diazonium salt (e.g., fast blue BB), forming an insoluble, visible pigment at the site of enzyme activity. α-naphthyl acetate esterase is detected primarily in monocytes. The sites of enzyme activity show black granulation. Enzyme activity may be detected in megakaryocytes, macrophages, and histiocytes and is virtually absent in granulocytes. Lymphocytes and mature granulocytes will occasionally exhibit enzyme activity. In addition, enzyme activity may be detected in the erythroblasts of erythroleukemia and focal enzyme activity may be observed in lymphoblasts of acute lymphocytic leukemia.

α-naphthyl butyrate also may be used as a substrate. α-naphthyl butyrate exhibits strong activity in the monocytic cell line but very weak or absent activity in neutrophils, megakaryocytes, and lymphocytes. The α-naphthyl acetate esterase stain is useful in the diagnosis of acute monocytic leukemias and acute myelomonocytic leukemias (Table 27-11).

To differentiate monocytes from those cells that occasionally show positivity, sodium fluoride may be added

TABLE 27-11 *CYTOCHEMICAL STAINS USEFUL IN THE DIAGNOSIS OF LEUKEMIAS*

Stain	Specimen Type	Stained Cellular Components	Cell Specificity	Interpretation
Myeloperoxidase	Smears, imprints, or frozen sections	Primary granules; Auer rods	Neutrophils & precursors—strong positivity Monocytes—weak positivity	Differentiates acute myelogenous leukemia from acute lymphocytic leukemia
Sudan Black B	Smears, imprints, or frozen sections	Primary & secondary granules; Auer rods	Neutrophils & precursors—strong positivity Monocytes—weak positivity	Parallels the myeloperoxidase stain
Chloracetate Esterase	Smears, imprints, frozen sections, or paraffin-embedded sections	Cytoplasm	Neutrophils & precursors—strong positivity	Similar to the myeloperoxidase stain and Sudan black B stain
α-Naphthyl Esterase (acetate & butyrate)	Smears, imprints, or frozen sections	Cytoplasm	Monocytes & precursors—strong positivity Neutrophils & precursors—weak positivity or negative T lymphocytes—focal positivity Megakaryocytes & platelets—positive with acetate only	Useful in the diagnosis of acute monocyte leukemia (M5) and acute myelomonocyte leukemia (M4); erythroblasts of erythroleukemia may exhibit enzyme activity
Periodic acid-Schiff	Smears, imprints, frozen sections, or paraffin-embedded sections	Glycogen	Neutrophils, monocytes, megakaryocytes—degree of positivity varies	Useful in diagnosis of erythroleukemia; erythroblasts exhibit strong PAS positivity
Acid Phosphatase	Smears, imprints, or frozen sections	Cytoplasm	Without tartaric acid, most hematopoietic cells will exhibit acid phosphatase activity including hairy cells; with tartaric acid, only hairy cells will exhibit acid phosphatase activity	Useful in the diagnosis of hairy cell leukemia

to the incubation mixture. Sodium fluoride inactivates the monocytic enzyme. This is referred to as the fluoride inhibition test. In the inhibition test, two incubation mixtures are prepared, one without fluoride and the other with fluoride. Slides are incubated in the incubation mixtures and the two slides are compared with their staining results. Observation of the slide stained in the incubation mixture containing fluoride will show an inhibition of staining in monocytes but not in other cell lines.

Periodic acid–Schiff reaction

Periodic acid oxidizes 1,2 glycol groups to dialdehydes. These aldehyde groups combine with Schiff's reagent to produce a red-colored product. Cellular components containing polysaccharides, mucopolysaccharides and glycoproteins possess the 1,2 glycol groups and will be stained.[87–89] Periodic acid–Schiff (PAS) staining is seen in almost all normal hematopoietic cells. In the granulocytic cell line, the intensity of the staining increases with maturity. Monocytes exhibit a diffuse staining pattern while lymphocytes may be negative or show a few PAS positive granules. Megakaryocytes and platelets stain intensely. Normal erythroblasts do not stain with PAS. However, PAS activity is strongly positive in erythroleukemia (AML-M6). In this disease early erythroblasts will exhibit coarse,

granular positivity but later stages of erythroblasts exhibit a fine, diffuse positivity. Lymphoblasts in acute lymphoblastic leukemia (L1 and L2) may exhibit PAS positivity, either coarse granular or block-like positivity. The use of this stain in the diagnosis of acute leukemia is summarized in Table 27-11.

Acid phosphatase stain

Acid phosphatase activity is detected by incubating the specimen in naphthol AS-BI phosphoric acid.[90–93] As a result of the enzyme activity, naphthol AS-BI is liberated. The liberated naphthol immediately couples with a diazonium salt (e.g., fast garnet) forming an insoluble, visible pigment at the site of enzyme activity. Acid phosphatase activity is present in most normal leukocytes appearing as purplish-dark red intracellular granules. The hairy cells of hairy cell leukemia also will exhibit acid phosphatase activity. Hairy cells may be differentiated from like-appearing leukocytes using tartrate inhibition. The acid phosphatase activity within normal leukocytes will be inhibited by tartrate, while enzyme activity within hairy cells is resistant to tartrate inhibition. The acid phosphatase stain is useful in the diagnosis of hairy cell leukemia (Table 27-11). The acid phosphatase activity within T lymphocytes is characteristic; T lymphocytes exhibit focal acid phosphatase activity.

Terminal deoxynucleotidyl transferase

This is an example of an indirect immunofluorescence technique. Rabbit anti-calf TdT is applied to the specimen slide. If the nuclei of the cells contain terminal deoxynucleotidyl transferase (TdT), anti-calf TdT will bind to it.[94] Excess anti-calf TdT is washed away. Fluorescein isothiocyanate-conjugated F(ab')$_2$ goat anti-rabbit IgG antiserum is used to identify the rabbit anti-calf TdT-TdT complex. The nucleus of the cells containing TdT will fluoresce.

Terminal deoxynucleotidyl transferase is a nuclear enzyme that polymerizes a single stranded deoxynucleotidyl sequence onto a primer without the need of a template. TdT may be found in thymocytes, prethymic cells and pre-B cells. It is not normally present in peripheral lymphocytes or lymph node lymphocytes. Increased levels of TdT are associated with T-cell acute lymphocytic leukemia, Pre-B cell acute lymphocytic leukemia and acute undifferentiated leukemia.[95,96] TdT is not elevated in B-cell acute lymphocytic leukemia. TdT is a primitive cell marker and may be valuable in differentiating acute lymphocytic leukemias from acute myeloid leukemias. However, it also is seen in up to 5% of acute myeloid leukemias.

Prussian blue iron stain

The Prussian blue iron stain is designed to demonstrate the presence of hemosiderin (storage iron) in the bone marrow and stainable iron in erythroblasts (sideroblasts) and/or erythrocytes (siderocytes).[42] In this stain, a weak acid solution is needed to free the iron from the loose protein bonds present in the hemosiderin molecule. The freed iron combines with potassium ferrocyanide to produce ferric ferrocyanide, a blue-green insoluble compound. Freed iron will appear as greenish-blue diffuse material and nuclei will appear red. Hemosiderin (storage iron) may be reported as normal, increased, or decreased amounts based on low power (100×) examination of bone marrow specimens. The Prussian-blue reaction may be performed on Wright-stained smears that are several years old with successful results. Deparaffinization may lead to leaching of the iron; therefore, the interpretation of storage iron from paraffin sections should be done with caution.

The determination of bone marrow storage iron is useful in the classification of anemias associated with defective hemoglobin synthesis. Storage iron is markedly decreased or absent in iron deficiency anemia; normal or increased in anemia of chronic disease and thalassemia trait; and increased in sideroblastic anemia. The presence of ringed sideroblasts (siderotic granules arranged in ring around cell nucleus) is diagnostic for sideroblastic anemia. However, ringed sideroblasts may be observed in a number of conditions: other myelodysplastic syndromes, hematologic malignancies, following chemotherapy, and megaloblastic anemia.

The presence of Pappenheimer bodies may be confirmed with the Prussian-blue reaction. Pappenheimer bodies are iron deposits usually found at the periphery of the cell. Since they will stain with Wright's stain, they may be confused with other erythrocyte inclusions.

BONE MARROW EXAMINATION

A thorough examination of a well-stained peripheral blood smear provides a wealth of information concerning an individual's hematopoietic status. However, there are instances when the peripheral blood picture does not adequately reflect the activity or alterations taking place in the hematopoietic bone marrow. The bone marrow examination is important in the diagnosis and monitoring of a wide variety of hematologic disorders including megaloblastic anemia, acute leukemia, myelodysplastic syndromes, thrombotic thrombocytopenic purpura, myeloproliferative disorders, Hodgkin's disease and non-Hodgkin's lymphomas.

Specimen collection and processing

A bone marrow aspirate and trephine biopsy are obtained using a Jamshidi needle and/or Illinois needle.[19,31,97] In the adult and the majority of children, the bone marrow aspirate and biopsy can be easily obtained through the iliac crest at the posterior superior iliac spine using a Jamshidi needle. The trephine biopsy is obtained first, followed by relocation of the needle and aspiration of the bone marrow. Alternatively, in the adult, a bone marrow aspirate can be obtained from the sternum using an Illinois needle. A bone marrow biopsy cannot be obtained from this site. There are two additional aspiration sites in children. A bone marrow aspirate can be obtained from the tibia in children younger than 2 years of age or the spines of the most prominent vertebral segments (L1 and L2) in older children. A bone marrow biopsy is not obtained from either site.

From the bone marrow aspirate, direct smears of bone marrow fluid are prepared immediately following collection. A portion of the bone marrow aspirate is anticoagulated with EDTA. This EDTA-anticoagulated bone marrow is further processed in the laboratory. EDTA-anticoagulated bone marrow is placed in a Wintrobe tube and centrifuged. After centrifugation, four layers are present: fat and perivascular; plasma; buffy coat (all nucleated cells and platelets); and erythrocytes. One or two smears of the fat and perivascular layer are prepared and stained with the Prussian blue reaction. Concentrate smears are prepared from the buffy coat which is resuspended in a portion of the plasma. The bone marrow particle crush preparations are prepared by placing a drop of bone marrow aspirate containing a bone marrow particle on a glass microscope slide or coverslip. Another coverslip is placed diagonally across the coverslip containing the marrow particles. The top coverslip is gently dragged across the bottom coverslip to spread the marrow particles evenly.

The remaining bone marrow particles are aggregated with 2 drops of 0.015 M $CaCl_2$. The aggregated particles are fixed, embedded in paraffin, sectioned and stained in a manner similar to the trephine biopsy. The direct smears, concentrate smears, and particle crush smears are stained with Wright's stain.

Immediately after obtaining the specimen, the bone marrow trephine is imprinted two to four times on several glass microscope slides. These touch preparations are stained with Wright's stain. The bone marrow trephine is placed in a fixative solution. After fixation, the trephine is processed by embedding in paraffin, sectioning the paraffin-embedded trephine, and staining the sectioned material with hematoxylin and eosin.

●
Microscopic examination

Well-stained bone marrow aspirate smears and trephine biopsy sections are examined microscopically. The bone marrow aspirate smear evaluation includes: performing a 500-cell differential, evaluating cellular morphology, observing for the presence of abnormal cells, estimating overall cellularity, and determining the myeloid:erythroid ratio (M:E).[19,31,97–99] The identification of dysplastic changes within hematopoietic cells is useful in the diagnosis of a number of hematologic disorders. Dysplasia includes: megaloblastic changes, multinucleation, karyorrhexis, karyolysis, pseudo-Pelger Huet changes, hypogranulation, giant agranular platelets, abnormal megakaryocytes.

The bone marrow trephine biopsy evaluation includes: identifying abnormal cells and observing bone marrow architecture and cellularity. The bone marrow cellularity refers to the percentage of hematopoietic tissue (red marrow) as compared to adipose tissue (yellow marrow). Normal bone marrow cellularity in the adult is approximately 50%. A hypercellular marrow contains a cellularity of 75% or greater, while a hypocellular marrow contains a cellularity of 30% or less.

Each type of slide preparation from the bone marrow aspirate and trephine biopsy should be evaluated in the total assessment of an individual's hematopoietic status. The evaluation of the direct bone marrow smear provides morphologic detail of the cells within the bone marrow. A bone marrow differential may be performed on a direct bone marrow smear. The concentrate bone marrow smear permits the observer to examine a large number of randomly distributed marrow cells. There may be some anticoagulant associated changes; however, morphologic detail is acceptable. This smear is especially useful for performing a bone marrow differential on a hypoplastic or aplastic marrow. In addition, the concentrate smear may be used for estimation of megakaryocyte numbers. The particle crush preparation allows the demonstration of the spatial relationship of cells within the bone marrow particle and cellularity, while the particle clot section reveals both architecture and cellularity of the marrow. Identification of focal marrow involvement with Hodgkin's disease, granulomatuous disease, or non-Hodgkin's lymphoma may be observed in the particle clot section.

The evaluation of trephine biopsy touch preparations permits the evaluation of cellular morphology and the detection of tumor clusters. Tumor clusters are less likely to be disrupted in a touch preparation than a direct smear; therefore, these preparations permit good morphologic detail of tumor cells. The trephine biopsy sections provide an estimation of overall cellularity of the bone marrow and adequacy of megakaryocytes, observation of fibrosis, granulomas, necrosis or serous atrophy, and examination of individual cellular morphology.

The perivascular-fat smear provides a good estimation of storage iron. Further evaluation of iron status can be obtained by performing an iron stain on a bone marrow trephine section or bone marrow aspirate smear. This will allow determination of the percentage of sideroblasts and observation of ringed sideroblasts.

The reference values for bone marrow differentials in adults can be found in Table F in the Appendix.

●
SUMMARY

This chapter reviewed the manual laboratory procedures performed in the hematology laboratory including their applications and potential sources of error. The results of these procedures are utilized in the diagnosis, prognosis, and therapeutic monitoring of a variety of disorders. The accuracy and reliability of the results depend on the clinical laboratory scientist's knowledge of the test procedure and its application, as well as the possible problems that may arise in the performance of the test. For example, a Wright-stained peripheral blood smear may be used as a screening tool to identify illness or monitor patient's response to therapy, but its usefulness will be limited if the smear is improperly prepared or improperly stained.

●
REVIEW QUESTIONS

1. In the microscopic examination of a Wright-stained peripheral blood smear, the erythrocytes appeared bright red and the nuclei of the leukocytes were pale. What is the best explanation for this occurrence?
   a. The blood smear was too thick.
   b. The buffer was too acidic.
   c. The staining process was prolonged.
   d. The Wright stain was too alkaline.

2. A manual leukocyte count was performed on an EDTA-anticoagulated specimen. The specimen was diluted 1:20 and a total of 165 leukocytes were counted in the four corner squares of the hemacytometer. What is the leukocyte count?
   a. 1.3×10^9/L
   b. 3.3×10^9/L
   c. 4.1×10^9/L
   d. 8.3×10^9/L

3. An elevated platelet count is associated with:
   a. hemorrhage
   b. megaloblastic anemia

   c. myelodysplastic syndromes

   d. immune thrombocytopenic purpura

4. Any turbidity in a peripheral blood specimen will result in a falsely elevated hemoglobin determination. Which of the following is NOT a potential source of turbidity?

   a. lipemia

   b. increased leukocyte count (60×10^9/L)

   c. increased levels of carboxyhemoglobin

   d. presence of hemoglobin S

5. The following erythrocyte data were obtained from an EDTA-anticoagulated specimen: erythrocyte count = 2.84×10^{12}/L, hemoglobin = 7.2 g/dL, hematocrit = 26% (.26 L/L), calculate the MCV.

   a. 25.3 fL

   b. 27.7 fL

   c. 65.9 fL

   d. 91.5 fL

6. Which of the following is not a condition associated with an elevated ESR?

   a. rheumatoid arthritis

   b. polycythemia vera

   c. multiple myeloma

   d. chronic infection

7. Which stain is commonly used to perform a reticulocyte count?

   a. Wright stain

   b. crystal violet

   c. new methylene blue

   d. neutral red

8. Which of the following is an appropriate screening test for the presence of hemoglobin S?

   a. diothionate solubility test

   b. hemoglobin electrophoresis

   c. heat instability test

   d. acid elution test

9. Which of the following stains is not useful in the differentiation of acute myelogenous leukemia from acute lymphocytic leukemia?

   a. chloroacetate esterase stain

   b. Sudan black B stain

   c. myeloperoxidase stain

   d. periodic acid–Schiff stain

10. Based on the results obtained from the evaluation of a leukocyte alkaline phosphatase (LAP) stain, what is the total LAP score?

Cell Rating	Number of Cells Counted
0	35
1+	40
2+	20
3+	5
4+	0

   a. 65

   b. 75

   c. 95

   d. 130

REFERENCES

1. Nikon: Instructions for the Labophot-2. Garden City, NY: Nikon Inc.
2. Nikon: Introduction to the Microscope: Operation and Preventive Maintenance Using the Nikon Labophot. Garden City, NY: Nikon, Inc.
3. Locquin, M., Langeron, M.: Handbook of Microscopy. Boston: Butterworths, 1983.
4. Koenig, A.S., Day, J.C., Sodeman, T.M., Alpert, N.L.: Laboratory Instrument Verification & Verification Maintenance Manual. 3rd Ed. Skokie, IL: College of American Pathologists, 1982.
5. National Committee for Clinical Laboratory Standards: Reference Leukocyte Differential Count (Proportional) and Evaluation of Instrumental Methods. vol 12 no 1. Villanova, PA: NCCLS, 1992.
6. Koepke, J.A.: Differential white cell counting and the NCCLS method. In Advances in Hematologic Methods: The Blood Count. Edited by O.W. van Assendelft and J.M. England. Boca Raton, FL: CRC Press, 1982.
7. Dacie, J.V., Lewis, S.M.: Practical Hematology. 6th Ed. New York: Churchill Livingstone, 1984.
8. Steine-Martin, E.A.: Causes of poor leukocyte distribution in manual spreader slide blood films. Am. J. Med. Tech., 46:624, 1980.
9. National Committee for Clinical Laboratory Standards: Romanowsky Blood Stains. vol 6 no 2. Villanova, PA: NCCLS, 1986.
10. Marshall, P.N.: Romanowsky Staining: State of the Art and Ideal Techniques. In Differential Leukocyte Counting. Edited by J.A. Koepke. Skokie, IL: The College of American Pathologists, 1979.
11. Marshall, P.N.: Romanowsky and Reticulocyte Stains. In CRC Handbook Series in Clin. Lab. Sci. Section I. Hematology, Vol. II. Edited by R.M. Schmidt. Bocan Raton, FL: CRC Press, 1980.
12. Henry, J.B. (ed): Clinical Diagnosis and Management by Laboratory Methods. 18th Ed. Philadelphia: W.B. Saunders, 1991.
13. Koepke, J.A.: Standardization of the manual differential leukocyte count. Lab. Med., 11:371, 1980.
14. vanAssendelft, O.W., McGrath, C., Murphy, R.S., Schmidt, R.M.: The Differential Distribution of Leukocytes. In Differential Leukocyte Counting. Edited by J.A. Koepke. Skokie, IL: The College of American Pathologists, 1977.
15. Koepke, J.A., Dotson, M.A., Shifman, M.A.: A critical evaluation of manual/visual differential leukocyte counting method. Blood Cells, 11:173, 1985.
16. Koepke, J.A.: Practical Laboratory Hematology. New York: Churchill Livingstone, 1991.
17. vanAssendelft, O.W.: Reference values for the total and differential leukocyte count. Blood Cells, 11:77, 1985.
18. Wintrobe, M.M.: Clinical Hematology, 8th Ed. Philadelphia, Lea & Febiger, 1981.
19. Becton-Dickinson: Unopette WBC Determination for Manual Methods. Rutherford, NJ: Becton, Dickinson, and Company, 1974.
20. Becton-Dickinson: Unopette Erythrocyte Determination for Manual Methods. Rutherford, NJ: Becton, Dickinson, and Company.
21. Becton-Dickinson: Unopette WBC/Platelet Determination for Manual Methods. Rutherford, NJ: Becton, Dickinson, and Company, 1984.
22. Becton-Dickinson: Unopette Eosinophil Determination for Manual Methods. Rutherford, NJ: Becton, Dickinson, and Company, 1974.
23. Brecher, G., Cronkite, E.P.: Morphology and enumeration of human blood platelets. J. Appl. Physiol., 3:365, 1950.
24. Costello, R.T.: A unopette for eosinophil counts. Am. J. Clin. Pathol., 54:249, 1970.
25. MacFarlane, J.C.W., Cecil, G.W.: Eosinophil counting: A modification of Pilot's method. Br. Med. J., 2:1187, 1951.
26. National Committee for Clinical Standards: Reference Procedure for the Quantitative Determination of Hemoglobin in Blood. vol. 4, no. 3. Villanova, PA: NCCLS, 1984.
27. International Committee for Standardization in Hematology: Recommendations for reference method for hemoglobinometry in human blood and specifications for international hemiglobincyanide reference preparation. J. Clin. Pathol., 31:139, 1978.
28. National Committee for Clinical Laboratory Standards: Procedure

for Determining Packed Cell Volume by the Microhematocrit Method, vol. 5, no. 5. Villanova, PA: NCCLS, 1985.

29. International Committee for Standardization in Hematology: Selected Methods for the determination of packed cell volume. In Advances in Hematologic Methods: The Blood Count. Edited by O. W. van Assendelft and J. M. England. Bocan Raton, FL: CRC Press, 1982.

30. International Committee for Standardization in Hematology Expert Panel on Blood Cell Sizing: Recommendation for reference method for determination by centrifugation of packed cell volume of blood. J. Clin. Pathol., 33:3, 1980.

31. Williams, W.J., Nelson, D.A., Morris, M.W.: Examination of the blood. In Hematology, 4th Ed. Edited by W.J. Williams. New York: McGraw-Hill, 1989.

32. National Committee for Clinical Standards: Reference Procedure for Erythrocyte Sedimentation Rate (ESR) Test. vol. 8, no. 3. Villanova, PA: NCCLS, 1988.

33. International Committee for Standardization in Hematology: Recommendation for measurement of erythrocyte sedimentation rate of human blood. Am. J. Clin. Pathol., 68:505, 1977.

34. Gambino, S.R., Dire, J.J., Monteleone, M., Budd, D.C.: The Westergren sedimentation rate, using K₃EDTA. Am. J. Clin. Pathol., 43:173, 1965.

35. International Committee for Standardization in Hematology: Reference method for the erythrocyte sedimentation rate (ESR) test on human blood. J. Clin. Pathol., 27:310, 1973.

36. Davis, B.H., Bigelow, N.C.: Flow cytometric reticulocyte quantification using thiazole orange provides clinically useful reticulocyte maturity index. Arch. Pathol. Lab. Med., 113:684, 1989.

37. Hackney, J.R., Cembrowski, G.S. Prystowsky, M.B., Kant, J.A.: Automated reticulocyte counting by image analysis and flow cytometry. Lab. Med., 20:551, 1989.

38. National Committee for Clinical Laboratory Standards: Method for Reticulocyte Counting. vol 5 no 10. Villanova, PA: NCCLS, 1985.

39. Gilmer, P.R., Koepke, J.A.: The reticulocyte: an approach to definition. Am. J. Clin. Pathol., 66:272, 1976.

40. Peebles, D.A., Hochberg, A., Clark, T.D.: Analysis of manual reticulocyte counting. Am. J. Clin. Pathol., 76:713, 1981.

41. Savage, R.A., Skoog, D.P., Rabinovitch, A.: Analytical inaccuracy and imprecision of reticulocyte counting: a preliminary report from the College of American Pathologists Reticulocyte Project. Blood Cells, 11:97, 1985.

42. Brown, B.A.: Hematology: Principles and Procedures. 6th Ed. Philadelphia: Lea & Febiger, 1993.

43. Daland, G.A., Castle, W.B.: A simple and rapid method for demonstrating sickling of the red cells: The use of reducing agents. J. Lab. Clin. Med., 33:1082, 1948.

44. National Committee for Clinical Laboratory Standards: Solubility Test for Confirming the Presence of Sickling Hemoglobins; Approved Standard. vol. 6, no. 10. Villanova, PA: NCCLS, 1986.

45. Itano, H.A.: Solubilities of naturally occurring mixtures of human hemoglobin. Arch. Biochem. Biophys., 47:148, 1953.

46. Nalbandian, R.M., et al.: Dithionite tube test—a rapid, inexpensive technique for the detection of hemoglobin S and non-S sickling hemoglobin. Clin. Chem., 17:1028, 1971.

47. Diggs, L.W., Walker, R.: Technical points in the detection of sickle cell hemoglobin by the tube test. Am. J. Med. Tech., 37:33, 1971.

48. National Committee for Clinical Laboratory Standards: Detection of abnormal hemoglobin using cellulose acetate electrophoresis. vol. 6, no. 9. Villanova, PA: NCCLS, 1985.

49. Schneider, R.G.: Methods for detection of hemoglobin variants and hemoglobinopathies in the routine clinical laboratory. CRC Crit. Rev. Clin. Lab. Sci., 9:243, 1978.

50. Helena Laboratories: Hemoglobin Electrophoresis Procedure, Beaumont, TX: Helena Laboratories, 1985.

51. National Committee for Clinical Laboratory Standards: Citrate Agar Electrophoresis for Confirming the Identification of Variant Hemoglobins. vol. 8, no. 6. Villanova, PA: NCCLS, 1988.

52. Schneider, R.G., Hosty, T.S., Tomlin, G., Atkins, R.: Identification of hemoglobins and hemoglobinopathies by electrophoresis on cellulose acetate plates impregnated with citrate agar. Clin. Chem., 20:74, 1974.

53. Sigma Diagnostics: Fetal Hemoglobin-Acid Elution, Semi-quantitative Procedure for Blood Smears. St. Louis: Sigma Diagnostics, 1990.

54. Oski, F.A., Naiman, J.L.: Hematologic Problems in the Newborn. 3rd Ed. Philadelphia: W.B. Saunders, 1982.

55. Clayton, E.M., Feldhaus, W.D., Phythyon, J.M.: The demonstration of fetal erythrocytes in the presence of adult red blood cells. Am. J. Clin. Pathol., 40:487, 1963.

56. National Committee for Clinical Laboratory Standards: Quantitative Measurement of Fetal Hemoglobin Using the Alkali Denaturation Method. vol. 9, no. 18. Villanova, PA: NCCLS, 1989.

57. Betke, K., Marti, H.R., Schlicht, I.: Estimation of small percentages of foetal haemoglobin. Nature, 184:1877, 1959.

58. Pembury, M.E., McWade, P., Weatherall, J.: Reliable routine estimation of small amounts of foetal hemoglobin by alkali denaturation. J. Clin. Pathol., 25:738, 1972.

59. International Committee for Standardization in Haematology: Recommendations for fetal hemoglobin reference preparations and fetal hemoglobin determination by the alkali denaturation method. Br. J. Haematol., 42:133, 1979.

60. National Committee for Clinical Laboratory Standards: Chromatographic (Microcolumn) Determination of Hemoglobin A₂. vol. 9, no. 17. Villanova, PA: NCCLS, 1989.

61. Centers for Disease Control: Laboratory Methods for Detecting Hemoglobinopathies. Division Host Factors, Center for Infectious Diseases, Center for Disease Control, Atlanta, GA, 1984.

62. Helena Laboratories: Sickle-Thal Quik Column Procedure. Beaumont, TX: Helena Laboratories, 1988.

63. Huisman, T.H.J., Jonxis, J.H.P.: The Hemoglobinopathies: Techniques of Identification. New York: Marcel Decker, 1977.

64. Huehns, E.R.: Diseases due to abnormalities of hemoglobin structure. Ann. Rev. Med., 21:157, 1970.

65. Lehmann, H., Huntsman, R.G.: Man's Hemoglobins. Philadelphia: J. B. Lippincott, 1974.

66. Schwab, M.L., Lewis, A.E.: An improved stain for Heinz bodies. Am. J. Clin. Pathol., 39:673, 1969.

67. Sigma Diagnostics: Glucose-6-Phosphate Dehydrogenase Deficiency: Qualitative, Visual Fluorescence Screening Procedure. St. Louis: Sigma Diagnostics, 1989.

68. Beutler, E.: A series of new screening procedures for pyruvate kinase deficiency, glucose-6-phosphate dehydrogenase deficiency, and glutathione reductase deficiency. Blood, 28: 553, 1966.

69. Beutler, E, et al.: International Committee for Standardization in Hematology: Recommended methods for red-cell enzyme analysis. Br. J. Hem., 35:331, 1977.

70. Becton-Dickinson: UNOPETTE RBC Osmotic Fragility Determination for Manual Methods Procedure. Rutherford, NJ: Becton, Dickinson and Company.

71. Dacie, J.V., Vaughan, J.M.: The fragility of the red blood cells: Its measurement and significance. J. Path. Bact., 46:341, 1938.

72. Parpart, A.K., et al.: The osmotic resistance (fragility) of human red cells. J. Clin. Invest., 27:636, 1947.

73. Hartmann R.C., Jenkins, D.E.: The "sugar-water" test for paroxysmal nocturnal hemoglobinuria. N. Engl. J. Med., 275:155, 1966.

74. Wolf, P.: Practical Clinical Hematology Interpretations and Techniques. New York: John Wiley and Sons, 1973.

75. Ham, T.H.: Studies on destruction of erythrocytes. Arch. Int. Med., 66:1271, 1939.

76. National Committee for Clinical Laboratory Standards: Proposed Standard: Histochemical Method for Leukocyte Alkaline Phosphatase. vol. 4, no. 14. Villanova, PA: NCCLS, 1984.

77. Kaplow, L.S.: Cytochemistry of leukocyte alkaline phosphatase. Am. J. Clin. Pathol., 39:439, 1963.

78. Kaplow, L.S.: A histochemical procedure for localizing and evaluating levels of leukocyte alkaline phosphatase activity in smears of blood and marrow. Blood, 10:1023, 1955.

79. Sigma Diagnostics: Alkaline phosphatase, leukocyte: Histochemical semiquantitative demonstration in leukocytes. St. Louis: Sigma Diagnostics, 1990.

80. Sigma Diagnostics: Leukocyte Peroxidase (Myeloperoxidase) Procedure No. 390. St. Louis: Sigma Diagnostics, 1988.

81. Hanker, J.S., Yates, P.E., Metz, C.B., Rustioni, A.: A new specific, sensitive and non-carcinogenic reagent for the demonstration of horseradish peroxidase. Histochem. J., 9:789, 1977.

82. Sheehan, H.L., Storey, G.W.: An improved method of staining leukocyte granules with Sudan black B. J. Pathol. Bacteriol., 59:336, 1947.

83. Sigma Diagnostics: Sudan Black B Staining System, Procedure No. 380. St. Louis: Sigma Diagnostics, 1989.

84. Sigma Diagnostics: Naphthol AS-D Chloroacetate Esterase and alpha-naphthyl acetate esterase, Procedure No. 91. St. Louis: Sigma Diagnostics, 1990.

85. Li, C.Y., Lam, K.W., Yam, L.T.: Esterases in human leukocytes. J. Histol. Cytol., 21:1, 1973.

86. Yam, L.T., Li, C.Y., Crosby, W.H.: Cytochemical identification of monocytes and granulocytes. Am. J. Clin. Pathol., 55:283, 1971.

87. Sigma Diagnostics: Periodic Acid-Schiff Staining System, Histochemical Demonstration of Glycol-containing Cellular Components in Blood or Bone Marrow Films, Procedure No. 395. St. Louis: Sigma Diagnostics, 1986.

88. Wislocki, G.B., Rheingold, J.J., Dempsey, E.: The occurrence of the periodic acid–Schiff reaction in various normal cells of blood and connective tissue. Blood, 4:562, 1948.

89. Hotchiss, R.D.: A microchemical reaction resulting in the staining of polysaccharide structures in fixed tissue preparations. Arch. Biochem., 16:131, 1949.

90. Sigma Diagnostics: Acid Phosphatase, Leukocyte, Procedure No. 387. St. Louis: Sigma Diagnostics, 1988.

91. Yam, L.T., Li, C.Y., Lam, K.W.: Tartrate-resistant acid phosphatase isoenzyme in the reticulum cells of leukemic reticuloendotheliosis. N. Engl. J. Med., 284:357, 1971.

92. Li, C.Y., Yam, L.T., Lam, K.W.: Acid phosphatase isoenzyme in human leukocytes in normal and pathologic conditions. J. Histochem. Cytochem., 18:473, 1970.

93. Catvosky, D., et al.: Acid-phosphatase reaction in acute lymphoblastic leukemia. Lancet, 1:749, 1978.

94. Sun, T, Li, C.Y., Yam, L.T.: Altas of Cytochemistry and Immunochemistry of Hematologic Neoplasms. Chicago: American Society of Clinical Pathologists Press, 1985.

95. Bollum, F.J.: Terminal deoxynucleotidyl transferase as a hematopoietic cell marker. Blood, 54:1203, 1979.

96. Kung, P.C., et al.: Terminal deoxynucleotidyl transferase in the diagnosis of leukemia and malignant lymphoma. Am. J. Med., 64:788, 1978.

97. Brynes, R.K., McKenna, R.W., Sundberg, R.D.: Bone marrow aspiration and trephine biopsy: an approach to a thorough study. Am. J. Clin. Pathol., 70:753, 1978.

98. Trubowitz, S., Davis, S.: The Human Bone Marrow: Anatomy, Physiology, and Pathophysiology. Boca Raton, FL: CRC Press, 1982.

99. Kass, L.: Bone Marrow Interpretation. Philadelphia: J.B. Lippincott, 1979.

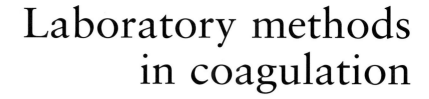

Laboratory methods in coagulation

28

KEY TERMS

hypercoagulable state
platelet-poor plasma
platelet-rich plasma
reference interval
von Willebrand disease
aggregating reagent
petechiometer
INR
ISI
platelet factor 4
paraprotein
fibrin degradation product
circulating inhibitor
normal pooled plasma
adsorbed plasma
aged serum
von Willebrand factor
factor VIII inhibitor
D dimer
chromogenic assay

INTRODUCTION

This chapter is designed to introduce the clinical laboratory science student to laboratory tests performed in the coagulation laboratory. The results obtained from these tests are used to assess an individual's coagulation status. Tests are grouped according to the part of the coagulation system that they assess: primary hemostasis, secondary hemostasis, and fibrinolysis. The last section of this chapter deals with laboratory tests used to assess hypercoagulable states.

SPECIMEN COLLECTION AND PROCESSING

Specimen collection

Whole blood should be collected aseptically by venipuncture using an evacuated tube system or a syringe. When using the evacuated tube system, the second or third tube collected should be the coagulation specimen. When using the two-syringe technique, part of the blood from the second syringe should be used for the coagulation specimen. The possibility of heparin contamination must be considered when blood is collected from an indwelling catheter. The line should be flushed with saline and the first 5 mL of blood discarded.[1]

The anticoagulant of choice for coagulation studies is 3.2% sodium citrate. The proper ratio of anticoagulant to whole blood is 1:9. If the patient's hematocrit is greater than 55%, the use of a collection tube containing the standard amount of anticoagulant will result in an over-anticoagulated sample. In this situation, there must be an adjustment to the amount of anticoagulant used (Fig. 28-1).

Specimen processing

Citrate anticoagulated whole blood is separated by centrifugation to obtain plasma for coagulation testing. Depending on the test, either platelet-poor or platelet-rich plasma may be required.

$$X = \frac{100 - Hct}{(595 - Hct)} \cdot Vol$$

Where,   X = volume of anticoagulant required for proper anticoagulation of volume of blood (vol)
Hct = patient's hematocrit
Vol = volume of blood to be anticoagulated

Example: Patient's Hct = 62%
Volume of blood = 5 mL

$$X = \frac{100 - 62}{(595 - 62)} \times 5 \, ml = 0.36 \, mL$$

FIGURE 28-1. Correction formula for proper volume of anticoagulant. This correction formula is used when the patient's hematocrit exceeds 55%. The final concentration of sodium citrate in the final blood mixture should be 10.9–12.9 mmol/L.

PLATELET-POOR PLASMA

Proper processing of the specimen is required to obtain reliable results. To obtain platelet-poor plasma, the specimen is centrifuged for 10 minutes at a minimum RCF of $1000 \times$ g as soon as possible after collection. Platelet-poor plasma should be separated from the packed cells using a nonwettable pipet and placed in a covered nonwettable container. If testing can not be performed immediately, platelet-poor plasma may be stored at room temperature (22° C to 24° C) for 2 hours; at 2° C to 4° C for 4 hours; at −20° C for 2 weeks; at −70° C for 6 months (must be rapidly frozen). Frozen samples are to be thawed rapidly at 37° C and should be tested immediately.[1]

PLATELET-RICH PLASMA

Several coagulation procedures require the use of platelet-rich plasma, rather than platelet-poor plasma (e.g., platelet aggregation studies). To obtain platelet-rich plasma, the specimen is centrifuged for 10 minutes at 200 g as soon as possible after collection. Platelet-rich plasma should be separated from the packed cells using a nonwettable pipet and placed in a covered nonwettable container. If testing is not to be performed immediately, platelet-rich plasma may be stored at room temperature (22° C to 24° C) for 3 hours.

LABORATORY INVESTIGATION OF PRIMARY HEMOSTASIS

Bleeding time

Primary hemostasis is best evaluated by the bleeding time. It is an "in vivo" measurement of platelet function. Several factors affect the bleeding time including platelet numbers, platelet function, and vascular integrity.[2]

Several methods have been used to perform the bleeding time. The oldest method, "Duke bleeding time," used a lancet to make a puncture in the ear lobe. In 1941, Ivy improved the bleeding time technique by creating a constant venous pressure with a blood pressure cuff (40 mmHg) and performing the test on the forearm with a lancet. The "template" bleeding time used today is a modification of the Ivy bleeding time. The incision is a consistent length and depth. Disposable bleeding time devices are currently available to perform the template bleeding time.

In the template bleeding time, a blood pressure cuff is placed on the patient's arm above the elbow and inflated to 40 mmHg to create venostasis. A standardized horizontal incision is made on the volar surface of the forearm using a disposable bleeding time device. A stopwatch is started and at 30-second intervals the blood is blotted away using filter paper. The bleeding time is the length of time required for bleeding to cease. Each laboratory should establish its own reference interval. The general reference interval is 1 to 9 minutes.

To be a true reflection of in vivo platelet function, the patient should avoid the use of aspirin or aspirin-like drugs for 7 days before the bleeding time since the ingestion of aspirin and many aspirin-like drugs will result in a prolonged bleeding time. Likewise, a platelet count should be performed before the bleeding time since a platelet count less than $100.0 \times 10^9/L$ will result in a prolonged bleeding time. If the above conditions are met, a prolonged bleeding time will indicate platelet dysfunction. Possible causes of platelet dysfunction include: hereditary and acquired platelet dysfunctions, von Willebrand disease, afibrinogenemia, severe hypofibrinogenemia, and some vascular bleeding disorders.

Platelet aggregometry

The addition of an aggregating reagent to a stirred suspension of platelet-rich plasma results in platelet shape change and aggregation. These changes can be monitored as an increasing percent transmittance by an aggregometer. The aggregometer records the changes in percent transmittance in the form of a graph (curve). A battery of aggregating reagents is used in the performance of platelet aggregation studies. Commonly used aggregating reagents include ADP, epinephrine, collagen, ristocetin, and arachidonic acid. The resultant platelet aggregation curves are interpreted by the clinical laboratory scientist to identify qualitative platelet disorders.[3,4] Platelet aggregation studies should not be performed on any patient who has ingested aspirin 7 days before the test. Aspirin inhibits platelet aggregation and will mask the presence of any qualitative platelet abnormality.

Depending on the aggregating reagent used, aggregation occurs in one or two waves. The primary wave represents the direct response of the platelets to the aggregating reagent. It represents platelet shape change and the formation of small aggregates. The secondary wave represents complete aggregation, which occurs as a result of endogenous ADP release from cytoplasmic organelles. An aggregating reagent, which results in both a primary and secondary wave, is said to produce a biphasic curve, whereas an aggregating reagent, which results in only one wave, is said to produce a monophasic curve. Aggregating reagents have typical aggregation patterns (Fig. 23-17).

ADP

When used in optimal concentration ($2 \times 10^{-5}M$), ADP results in a biphasic curve. ADP-induced platelet aggregation abnormalities such as aspirin-like release disorders or storage pool disorder are characterized by a primary wave only. However, Glanzmann's thrombasthenia is characterized by no response to ADP.

EPINEPHRINE

Epinephrine results in a biphasic curve. Aggregation curve abnormalities are similar to those seen with ADP. Epinephrine may be used to confirm the responses seen with ADP.

COLLAGEN

The aggregation curve associated with collagen lacks a primary wave. It is a monophasic curve characterized by

a secondary wave only. The single wave represents secondary wave platelet aggregation resulting from the release of cytoplasmic organelle contents, primarily endogenous ADP. No response to collagen is associated with Glanzmann's thrombasthenia, aspirin-like release disorders, storage pool disorder, and uremia.

RISTOCETIN

Ristocetin may result in a monophasic or biphasic curve. Ristocetin induces immediate platelet agglutination, which produces a primary wave. The release reaction follows agglutination, which produces secondary aggregation. The action is dependent on the presence of von Willebrand factor and the platelet membrane receptor, glycoprotein Ib (GP Ib). Abnormal ristocetin aggregation curves are associated with von Willebrand disease and Bernard-Soulier syndrome. In von Willebrand disease, the abnormal aggregation curve may be corrected by the addition of von Willebrand factor.

ARACHIDONIC ACID

Arachidonic acid results in a monophasic curve. An abnormal arachidonic acid curve is associated with abnormalities in the thromboxane pathway of platelets. If the patient has ingested aspirin, the curve will be suppressed.

Capillary fragility test

The capillary fragility test is used in the investigation of blood vessel disorders.[4–6] A petechiometer creates negative pressure through a suction cup. The suction cup is placed on the volar surface of the forearm. The negative pressure is maintained for 1 to 2 minutes, then released. After several minutes, the area under the suction cup is examined for petechiae. A capillary fragility test is considered positive if one or more petechiae are present. The presence of petechiae indicates increased permeability of the blood vessels. An advantage of the capillary fragility test is the ability to perform the test several times to increase the accuracy of the results. The capillary fragility test will be positive in vascular disorders, thrombocytopenia, and decreased fibrinogen levels.

An alternative method to measure capillary fragility is the tourniquet test. A blood pressure cuff is placed on the upper arm and inflated to a pressure half way between the individual's diastolic and systolic pressure. Pressure is maintained for 5 minutes, then released. Several minutes later, the arm is observed for the presence of petechiae distal to where the cuff had been placed. If more than five petechiae are observed in a 3-cm diameter, the test is considered positive.

LABORATORY INVESTIGATION OF SECONDARY HEMOSTASIS

Screening tests

PROTHROMBIN TIME

The prothrombin time (PT) is an important screening test for the laboratory evaluation of patients with inherited or

$$INR = R^{ISI}$$

Where, R = PT ratio obtained with the working thromboplastin

PT ratio = patient's PT/mean normal PT

ISI = International sensitivity index (provided by manufacturer)

Example: Patient's PT = 21.5 seconds

Mean normal PT = 12.0 seconds

ISI = 1.35

$$INR = (21.5/12.0)^{1.35} = 2.2$$

FIGURE 28-2. International Normalized Ratio (INR) calculation formula.

acquired deficiencies in the extrinsic or common pathway of the coagulation cascade and for monitoring the effectiveness of oral anticoagulant therapy.[7-10] The addition of prewarmed, (37° C) platelet-poor plasma to prewarmed thromboplastin-calcium reagent activates the coagulation cascade via formation of the thromboplastin (TF)/factor VII complex. The time required for clot formation is recorded. Clot formation may be detected by optical or electromechanical methods using manual, semiautomated, or automated devices. PT results are recorded to the nearest half second. Reported results should include the patient's result, the reference interval, and the median of the reference interval. Each laboratory should establish its own reference interval.

The World Health Organization (WHO) and the International Committee on Thrombosis and Haemostasis recommend using the International Normalized Ratio (INR) for reporting PT results when monitoring long-term oral anticoagulant therapy. Because the INR results are independent of the reagents and methods used to determine PT, these results allow for better assessment of long-term oral anticoagulant therapy. The INR is the PT ratio obtained by using the WHO International Reference Preparation as the source of thromboplastin in the performance of a PT. The PT ratio determined by the use of another thromboplastin may be converted to the INR by using the equation: $INR = R^{ISI}$ (Fig. 28-2). The international sensitivity index (ISI) is determined for each thromboplastin reagent; it is specific for manufacturer and lot number. An individual receiving oral anticoagulants for a hypercoagulable state should have an INR between 2.0 and 2.5; occasionally the ratio must be higher.

ACTIVATED PARTIAL THROMBOPLASTIN TIME

The activated partial thromboplastin time (APTT) is an important screening test for the laboratory evaluation of patients with inherited or acquired deficiencies in the intrinsic pathway of the coagulation cascade, for monitoring the effectiveness of heparin anticoagulant therapy, and for detecting inhibitors of blood coagulation (lupus-like anticoagulants).[11] Deficiencies in the common pathway also will affect the APTT. Platelet-poor plasma is added to an equal volume of activated partial thromboplastin reagent and warmed to 37° C for an exact incubation time. Prewarmed (37° C) calcium chloride reagent (0.025 M) is

added to this mixture to activate the coagulation cascade at factor XII. The time required for clot formation is recorded. Clot formation may be detected by optical or electromechanical methods using manual, semiautomated, or automated devices. APTT results are recorded to the nearest second. Reported results should include the patient's result, the reference interval, and the median of the reference interval. Each laboratory should establish its own reference interval.

If the APTT is used in monitoring heparin therapy, there are four influencing factors that should be considered. (1) The time of collection is important since heparin has an immediate anticoagulant effect and this effect decreases rapidly. The in vivo half-life of heparin is approximately 1.5 hours. The term "half-life" refers to the time required for one half the amount of a given substance to be metabolized by the body. In other words, if a patient receives 500 units of heparin at 1:30 pm, only 250 units would remain at 3:00 pm. (2) The specimen should be collected with a minimum of trauma, and care should be taken to centrifuge the sample adequately to remove all platelets. Platelets are a source of platelet factor 4, a heparin-neutralizing factor. (3) When using the APTT to monitor heparin therapy, the testing procedure should not be delayed. A delay in testing will result in prolonged APTT results. (4) There is no standardization ratio for APTT results. Therefore, care should be exercised in using APTT for heparin monitoring, and one should avoid interchange of test methodologies as well as reagents.

THROMBIN TIME

The thrombin time measures the conversion of fibrinogen to an insoluble fibrin clot. This conversion is initiated by the addition of thrombin to platelet-poor plasma.[12] Clot formation may be detected by optical or electromechanical methods using manual, semiautomated, or automated devices. The results are reported to the nearest second. Each laboratory should establish its own reference interval. The normal thrombin time is between 10 and 16 seconds.

Prolonged thrombin times are associated with hypofibrinogenemia, dysfibrinogenemia, presence of paraproteins, and the presence of circulating anticoagulants including heparin, fibrin degradation products FDP, and plasmin.

If a prolonged TT is the result of heparin contamination or other antithrombin activity, protamine sulfate can be added to the specimen. Protamine sulfate will neutralize the heparin and correct the thrombin time.

QUANTITATIVE FIBRINOGEN

Several methods can be used to determine the fibrinogen concentration, including precipitation or denaturation methods, turbidimetric method, immunologic assays, ultraviolet measurement of fibrin clot, and the clot-based Clauss assay. The reference method for quantitative determination of fibrinogen is the clot-based Clauss assay.[13,14] In this assay, an excess of thrombin is added to the appropriate dilution (1:10) of either patient's platelet-poor plasma or a control plasma. The time required for clot

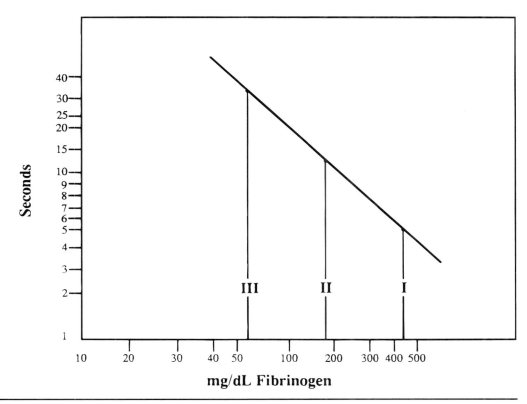

FIGURE 28-3. Fibrinogen standard curve. I, II, and III represent reference plasmas of known fibrinogen concentrations. The thrombin time in seconds is on the y-axis and the fibrinogen concentration in mg/dL is on the x-axis.

formation is recorded. Clot formation may be detected by optical or electromechanical methods using manual, semiautomated, or automated devices.

The fibrinogen concentration is inversely proportional to the thrombin time of diluted plasma. Therefore, a reference (standard) curve must be prepared using known fibrinogen concentrations vs. the respective thrombin times (Fig. 28-3). The fibrinogen results for patients and controls are read from this curve using their respective clotting times. Each laboratory should establish its own reference interval. In general, the reference interval for fibrinogen is 150 to 350 mg/dL.

● Tests to evaluate factor deficiency

MIXING STUDIES
When the PT and/or APTT are abnormal, further testing may be done to identify the specific abnormality. Mixing studies are performed to differentiate a factor deficiency from a circulating inhibitor.[3,6] The coagulation test with abnormal results is repeated using several different dilutions of the patient's plasma and normal pooled plasma (Table 28-1). The testing is performed immediately and after incubation at 37° C. Clot formation may be detected by optical or electromechanical methods using manual, semiautomated, or automated devices. The clotting times for the various dilutions and time intervals are compared

to determine if the patient's clotting time has been corrected. Clotting times will tend to increase with time due to the loss of labile factors; therefore, it is important to compare the patient's diluted sample results with the result obtained from the normal pooled plasma (Tube 1). A clotting time is considered prolonged if it is longer than the normal pooled plasma's clotting time (Tube 1). The presence of a factor deficiency is indicated by the correction of the prolonged test result by the normal pooled plasma. The normal pooled plasma supplies the deficient factor. A circulating inhibitor is indicated by no correction of the prolonged test by normal pooled plasma. The patient's circulating inhibitor also will inhibit the normal plasma's coagulation factors. The detection of a circulating inhibitor should be followed by a specific test to identify and

TABLE 28-1 *DILUTIONS FOR MIXING STUDIES*

Tube	Patient's Plasma	Normal Pooled Plasma	0.85% NaCl
1	—	0.5 mL	0.5 mL
2	0.1 mL	0.9 mL	—
3	0.2 mL	0.8 mL	—
4	0.5 mL	0.5 mL	—
5	1.0 mL	—	—

TABLE 28-2 *DILUTIONS FOR SUBSTITUTION STUDIES*

Tube	1	2	3	4
Patient Plasma	0.1 mL	0.1 mL	0.1 mL	0.1 mL
Normal Plasma	0.1 mL			
Adsorbed Plasma		0.1 mL		
Aged Serum			0.1 mL	
0.85% NaCl				0.1 mL

quantitate the inhibitor. If a factor deficiency is detected, substitution studies and factor assays should be performed to identify and quantitate the activity of the specific factor.

In the case of a circulating inhibitor, the performance of the test after incubation reveals the time and temperature dependency of the inhibitor. Factor VIII inhibitors are time- and temperature-dependent. Patient plasma that contains inhibitors which are time- and temperature-dependent will exhibit correction immediately after mixing with normal pooled plasma. However, on incubation, the result will become prolonged. Lupus-like anticoagulants tend to act immediately; however, they may exhibit time dependency.

SUBSTITUTION TEST

The substitution test is performed to identify a specific factor deficiency or to narrow the possibilities when the APTT or PT is prolonged.[3] The prolonged coagulation test (PT or APTT) is repeated using dilutions of patient's plasma and substitution reagents (Table 28-2). The substitution reagents are adsorbed plasma, aged serum, and normal plasma. The substitution reagents contain different combinations of coagulation factors (Table 28-3). If the substitution reagent contains the deficient factor in the patient's plasma, the coagulation time will normalize. The clot formation may be detected by optical or electromechanical methods using manual, semiautomated, or automated devices.

The clotting times for adsorbed plasma and aged serum are compared with the clotting time of the original (undiluted) patient plasma. The adsorbed plasma or aged serum

TABLE 28-3 *COAGULATION FACTORS PRESENT AND ABSENT IN SUBSTITUTION REAGENTS*

Reagent	Factors Present	Factors Absent
Adsorbed Plasma	I V VIII XI XII	II VII IX X
Aged Serum	VII IX X XI XII	I II V VIII

TABLE 28-4 *PROBABLE COAGULATION DEFICIENCIES BASED ON THE APTT AND PT SUBSTITUTION TEST RESULTS*

APTT	PT	Adsorbed Plasma		Aged Serum		Probable Deficiency
		APTT	PT	APTT	PT	
N	N	—	—	—	—	No deficiency
A	N	C	—	C	—	XI or XII
A	N	NC	—	C	—	IX
A	A	NC	NC	C	C	X
A	A	C	C	NC	NC	V
N	A	—	NC	—	C	VII
A	N	C	—	NC	—	VIII
A	A	NC	NC	NC	NC	II

N = Normal result. A = Abnormal (prolonged result). C = Corrected result. NC = Not corrected.
(From Brown, BA: Hematology: Principles & Procedures 6th Ed., Lea & Febiger, Philadelphia, 1993, with permission.)

result is considered corrected if the difference between the original result and adsorbed plasma or aged serum result is 90% or greater than the difference between the original result and the established upper limit of normal for the APTT or PT. Tube 4 (patient plasma and 0.85% NaCl) represents the uncorrected patient result. Table 28-4 can be used to interpret the substitution test results and determine the factor deficiency. The identification of a specific factor deficiency should be followed by the performance of a specific factor assay to determine the activity of the factor. Substitution studies using adsorbed plasma and aged serum are qualitative tests designed to identify single factor deficiencies. If multiple factor deficiencies are suspected, 1:1 dilutions of patient's plasma and a battery of specific factor deficient plasmas should be tested.

REPTILASE TIME

Reptilase is a serine protease found in the venom of Bothrops atrox snake. This thrombin-like enzyme cleaves fibrinopeptide A from the fibrinogen molecule, whereas, thrombin cleaves both fibrinopeptide A and B.[15,16] The addition of reptilase to platelet-poor plasma initiates clot formation. The clot formation may be detected by optical or electromechanical methods using manual, semiautomated, or automated devices. Each laboratory should establish its own reference interval. The normal reptilase time for this procedure is between 18 and 22 seconds.

The reptilase time (RT) will be prolonged in hypofibrinogenemia, dysfibrinogenemia, presence of fibrin degradation products, and other circulating inhibitors. The reptilase time is useful in the detection of heparin contamination and the differentiation of dysfibrinogenemia from presence of fibrin degradation products when compared with the thrombin time. In the case of heparin contamination, the reptilase time is not prolonged, but the thrombin time (TT) is prolonged. In dysfibrinogenemia,

TABLE 28-5 *DILUTIONS FOR FACTOR ASSAYS*

Tube (#)	Buffer (mL)	Plasma (mL)	Activity (%)	Dilution
1	0.9	0.1	100	1:10
2	1.9	0.1	50	1:20
3	0.5	0.5 mL from tube #2	25	1:40
4	0.5	0.5 mL from tube #3	12.5	1:80
5	0.5	0.5 mL from tube #4	6.3	1:160
6	0.5	0.5 mL from tube #5	3.2	1:320

(From Brown, BA: Hematology: Principles & Procedures 6th Ed., Lea & Febiger, Philadelphia, 1993, with permission.)

the RT will be more affected than the TT, but in the presence of FDPs, the TT is more affected than the RT.

FACTOR ASSAYS, PROTHROMBIN TIME

Factor assays are performed to confirm a specific factor deficiency and determine the actual activity of that factor within the plasma.[3] The prothrombin procedure provides a mechanism of determining the factor activity of the coagulation proteins within the extrinsic (VII) and common (X, V, and II) pathways of the coagulation cascade. The basis of a factor assay is the ability of the patient's plasma to correct a prolonged PT of a known factor deficient substrate. The PT is performed on specific factor deficient substrate containing varying dilutions of patient plasma (1:10 and 1:20). In addition, the PT is performed on spe-

cific factor deficient substrate containing dilutions of a reference plasma (Table 28-5). A factor activity curve is prepared by plotting the PT clotting times for the reference plasma dilutions against the percent factor activity of each respective dilution (Fig. 28-4). The factor activity for the patient is determined by comparing the patient's results with those results obtained using reference plasma. Each laboratory should establish its own reference interval based on the reagents used and the methodology. Generally, the normal factor activity range is 50% to 150%.

FACTOR ASSAYS, PARTIAL THROMBOPLASTIN TIME

Factor assays are performed to confirm a specific factor deficiency and determine the actual concentration of that factor within the patient's plasma.[3,17] The APTT procedure provides a mechanism of determining the factor activity of the coagulation proteins within the intrinsic (XII, XI, IX, VIII) and common (X, V, and II) pathways of the coagulation cascade. The basis of a factor assay is the ability of the patient plasma to correct a prolonged APTT of a known factor deficient substrate. The APTT is performed on specific factor deficient substrate containing varying dilutions of patient plasma (1:10 and 1:20). In addition, the APTT is performed on specific factor deficient substrate containing dilutions of a reference plasma (Table 28-5). A factor activity curve is prepared by plotting the APTT clotting times for the reference plasma dilutions against the percent factor activity of each respective dilution (Fig. 28-4). The factor activity for the patient is

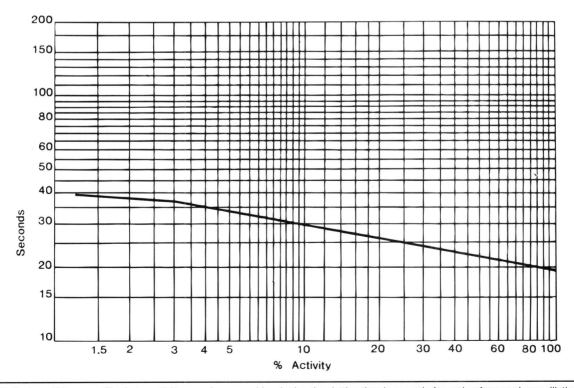

FIGURE 28-4. Factor activity curve. The factor activity curve is prepared by plotting the clotting time in seconds for each reference plasma dilution on the y-axis and the percent factor activity of each dilution on the x-axis. (From Brown, B.A.: Hematology: Principles and Procedures, 6th Ed., Philadelphia: Lea & Febiger, 1993, with permission.)

determined by comparing the patient's results with those results obtained using reference plasma. Each laboratory should establish its own reference interval based on the reagents used and the methodology. Generally, the normal factor activity range is 50% to 150%.

PREKALLIKREIN SCREENING TEST
Individuals with a prekallikrein (Fletcher factor) deficiency will have a prolonged APTT. The prolonged APTT result will be shortened by increasing the incubation period of patient's plasma with partial activated thromboplastin reagent to 10 minutes before the addition of calcium chloride (0.025 M).[3] Kaolin is the recommended activator for the detection of prekallikrein deficiency. The longer incubation period increases contact activation. Therefore, the correction of the patient's APTT result following the extended incubation period is indicative of prekallikrein deficiency. The normal control plasma's APTT result should remain within or near the normal range after the extended incubation period. Confirmation of a prekallikrein deficiency is accomplished by performing a factor assay using prekallikrein deficient substrate.

FACTOR XIII SCREENING TEST
Factor XIII activity is necessary for the formation of a stable fibrin clot. Factor XIII is a transamidase that is responsible for forming covalent bonds between the fibrin monomers. The covalent linkage of fibrin monomers results in a stabilized fibrin polymer. If Factor XIII is present, the fibrin clot formed is insoluble in 5 M urea when left at room temperature for 24 hours.[3] The patient's platelet-poor plasma is clotted with 0.025 M calcium chloride, and 5 M urea is added to this clot. If the patient's clot dissolves within the 24-hour period, the result is indicative of a Factor XIII deficiency of less than 1% to 2%. The normal control plasma's clot should be insoluble in 5 M urea after 24 hours.

VON WILLEBRAND FACTOR ASSAY
von Willebrand factor (vWF) is responsible for the in vitro platelet aggregation in the presence of ristocetin; therefore, the biologic activity of vWF can be measured in a modified ristocetin platelet aggregation study.[3,18] Patient's platelet-poor plasma is added to a standard mixture of ristocetin and platelets. The resultant platelet aggregation is measured using a platelet aggregometer. The reference (standard) curve is prepared by plotting the slope values for the reference plasma dilutions against the percent activity (100%, 75%, 50%, 25%, 12.5%) of each dilution. The patient results are compared with this curve. The percent activity of vWF is determined by the comparison. The reference interval is 60% to 180%. Each laboratory should establish its own reference interval.

LAURELL ROCKET IMMUNOELECTROPHORESIS (VON WILLEBRAND FACTOR ANTIGEN)
Laurell rocket electrophoresis is used to measure von Willebrand factor antigen (vWF:Ag). vWF:Ag is electrophoresed in an agar gel containing antibodies directed against vWF:Ag. A rocket-like immunoprecipite is formed. The rocket height is directly proportional to the concentration of vWF:Ag expressed as a percentage of vWF activity.[19] A reference (standard) curve is prepared using the results obtained from the dilutions of normal pooled plasma representing 100%, 50%, 25%, and 12.5% vWF activity. The height of the rocket is plotted against the concentration of vWF:Ag expressed in percent of normal. A best-fit line is drawn through the four points. The percent of vWF:Ag in the patient's sample is determined from the reference curve. The reference interval is 43% to 150%. Each laboratory should establish its own reference interval.

This procedure measures antigen activity, not biologic activity. Measurement of vWF:Ag is useful in the diagnosis of von Willebrand's disease, hemophilia A, and the detection of carriers of hemophilia A. vWF:Ag also can be measured by enzyme-linked immunosorbent assay (ELISA) or immunoradiometric assay (IRMA).

● Tests to evaluate circulating inhibitors

The two most common circulating inhibitors are lupus-like anticoagulant and factor VIII inhibitor. The following three procedures can be used to determine the specificity of the circulating inhibitor. The platelet neutralization procedure and the lupus-like anticoagulant procedure are used in the diagnosis of lupus-like anticoagulants, and the factor VIII inhibitor assay is used in the evaluation of factor VIII inhibitor.

PLATELET NEUTRALIZATION PROCEDURE
Lupus-like anticoagulants have anti-phospholipid activity and can be inactivated in a suspension of phospholipids.[20-22] Ruptured platelets serve as a source of phospholipid. The patient's platelet-poor plasma is mixed with a suspension of ruptured platelets and APTT reagent. The addition of 0.025 M calcium chloride activates the coagulation system. The clotting time is determined and compared with the APTT clotting times of the patient's platelet-poor plasma and the saline control (1:2 dilution of saline and patient's platelet-poor plasma). If lupus-like anticoagulants are present, the clotting time will be significantly shorter than the original APTT and the saline control APTT. False-positive results are seen with patients receiving heparin or other anticoagulant therapies.

LUPUS ANTICOAGULANTS
Molecules of purified phosphatidylethanolamine undergo structural rearrangement into hexagonal H_{II} phase at 37° C in aqueous solution. Hexagonal phase phosphatidylethanolamine consists of hexagonally packed cylinders of lipid surrounding central aqueous channels toward which the polar head groups are orientated. Lupus-like antiphospholipid antibodies specifically recognize these structures.[23] The addition of H_{II} phase phosphatidylethanolamine to a plasma containing lupus-like anticoagulants will correct the prolonged APTT. An advantage of this procedure over the platelet neutralization procedure is the elimination of false-positive results seen in patients receiving

$$= \frac{\text{Residual factor activity (\%)}}{\frac{\text{Factor activity for the patient dilution}}{\text{Factor activity for normal pooled plasma}}} \cdot 100$$

Example: Factor activity for patient dilution = 50%
Factor activity for normal pooled plasma = 100%

50/100 · 100% = 50% Residual factor activity

FIGURE 28-5. Residual factor VIII activity calculation for factor VIII inhibitor assay.

Dilution factor · Bethesda units (Table 28-6)
= Bethesda units of factor VIII inhibitor per milliliter (mL) of plasma.

Example: Patient dilution = 1 : 5
Residual factor VIII activity = 50%
Bethesda unit factor = 1.00

5 × 1.00
= 5 Bethesda units of Factor VIII inhibitor per mL of plasma

FIGURE 28-6. Calculation of Bethesda units for factor VIII inhibitor assay.

heparin or other anticoagulant therapy with the PNP procedure.

In addition to the platelet neutralization procedure and the lupus-like anticoagulant procedure, the Kaolin clotting time (KCT) and the dilute Russell's Viper venom test (DRVVT) can be used to confirm the presence of lupus-like anticoagulant.

FACTOR VIII INHIBITOR ASSAY

Factor VIII inhibitor can be quantitated by preparing several dilutions of the patient's plasma with a normal pooled plasma containing a known amount of Factor VIII activity.[3] After incubation, the "residual" factor VIII activity is measured by the factor VIII assay. The residual factor VIII activity is calculated from the comparison of factor VIII activity in the patient plasma dilution with the activity in the normal pooled plasma (Fig. 28-5). The residual factor VIII activity is converted to a Bethesda unit using Table 28-6 and the calculation formula (Fig. 28-6). One Bethesda unit of inhibitor is defined as the amount of inhibitor that will inactivate 50% of the factor VIII activity present.

The Bethesda titer assay was originally developed to measure factor VIII inhibitors. The assay can be modified to assay factor V and factor IX inhibitors. A weak factor VIII inhibitor may not be detected by this procedure. To detect weaker inhibitors, the incubation temperature and length should be altered. The dilutions should be incubated at 37° C for an increased period of time. The inhibitor titer does not correlate with or predict bleeding. The characteristics of an inhibitor vary from patient to patient.

LABORATORY INVESTIGATION OF FIBRINOLYTIC SYSTEM

Fibrin degradation products

The detection of fibrin and/or fibrinogen degradation products (FDP) in patient's plasma indicates increased fibrinolytic activity. Conditions associated with increased FDPs are disseminated intravascular coagulation (DIC), liver disease, alcoholic cirrhosis, kidney disease, cardiac disease, postsurgical complications, carcinoma, myocardial infarction, pulmonary embolism, deep vein thrombosis, and conditions of eclampsia. The FDP assay represents one of the screening tests used in the diagnosis of DIC. The FDP assay does not distinguish between fibrin degradation products and fibrinogen degradation products.

Fibrin and/or fibrinogen degradation products (FDPs) are identified through a specific antigen-antibody reaction.[24] Latex particles coated with monoclonal antihuman FDP antibodies are mixed with patient sample. The sensitivity of the test system and the choice of specimen will vary depending on the manufacturer. Most procedures require the preparation of two dilutions for each sample (i.e., 1 : 2 and 1 : 8), which allows a gradation of results. Macroscopic agglutination in both dilutions corresponds to a FDP level greater than 20 μg/mL. If macroscopic agglutination is observed in the 1 : 2 dilution but not the 1 : 8 dilution, the results correspond to an FDP level greater than 5 μg/mL but less than 20 μg/mL FDP. No macroscopic agglutination with either dilution indicates a FDP level less than 5 μg/mL. Normally, individuals have FDP levels less than 5 μg/mL.

D-dimer test

The D-dimer is a specific marker for fibrinolysis involving plasmin's degradation of fibrin. The D-dimer is a fibrin degradation product that contains the factor XIIIa crosslinked fibrin portion (see Fig. 24-24). The presence of D-dimers indicates plasmin degradation of crosslinked fibrin and is an excellent marker for DIC with secondary fibrinolysis.[25] D-dimers also are found in pulmonary embolism, deep vein thrombosis, arterial thromboembolism, and sickle cell disease.

Latex particles coated with monoclonal antibodies directed against D-dimer are mixed with a dilution of the patient's plasma. If D-dimers are present, agglutination of

TABLE 28-6 *BETHESDA UNIT FACTOR CHART*

Residual Factor %	Bethesda Units Factor	Residual Factor %	Bethesda Units Factor	Residual Factor %	Bethesda Units Factor
93	0.10	61	0.70	38	1.40
87	0.20	57	0.80	35	1.50
81	0.30	53	0.90	33	1.60
75	0.40	50	1.00	30	1.70
70	0.50	46	1.10	28	1.80
66	0.60	43	1.20	26	1.90
		41	1.30	25	2.00

the latex particles will occur. Most procedures test undiluted and diluted sample (1:2), which allows a gradation of results. Macroscopic agglutination in neither dilution corresponds to a D-dimer level of less than 0.5 μg/mL. If macroscopic agglutination is in the undiluted plasma but not the 1:2 dilution, the results correspond to a D-dimer level of 0.5 to 1.0 μg/mL. The observation of macroscopic agglutination in both dilutions corresponds to a D-dimer level of greater than 1.0 μg/mL. Normal individuals will have less than 0.5 μg/mL.

Euglobulin clot lysis

The euglobulin clot lysis is useful in the detection of increased fibrinolytic activity.[3,6] Conditions associated with increased fibrinolytic activity are DIC, liver disease, surgery, certain malignancies, and women receiving oral contraceptives, or during menstruation. The euglobulin fraction of plasma consists of fibrinogen, plasminogen, and the activators of plasminogen. This fraction is isolated from plasma by precipitation with 1% acetic acid. The precipitated euglobulin fraction is dissolved in buffered saline and thrombin is added to clot the euglobulins. The resulting clot serves as substrate for plasmin, which is generated from plasminogen by the plasminogen activators. The resulting clot is incubated at 37° C for 2 hours. At 30-minute intervals, the clot is observed for evidence of lysis. The euglobulin lysis of the clot is the time required for complete degradation of the clot. In normal individuals, the time required for complete euglobulin clot lysis is longer than 2 hours. Increased fibrinolytic activity is indicated by lysis in less than 2 hours.

LABORATORY EVALUATION OF HYPERCOAGULABLE STATES

Antithrombin III

Antithrombin III (AT-III) activity can be measured by a chromogenic assay. The powerful AT-III action in the presence of heparin is determined in a coupled reaction.[26] The first reaction involves the incubation of plasma with a known excess of thrombin in the presence of heparin. The second reaction determines the residual thrombin activity by its enzymatic activity on a chromogenic substrate. Thrombin activity results in the release of p-nitroaniline (pNA) from the chromogenic substrate. The released pNA is measured spectrophotometrically at 405 nm. The residual thrombin activity is inversely proportional to the AT-III level in the plasma. A reference (standard) curve is prepared by plotting the AT-III activity (%) for each reference plasma dilution against its corresponding absorbance. The results for patients and controls are read from this curve using their respective absorbance readings. Each laboratory should establish its own reference interval following a recommended procedure. However, the normal AT-III level for this procedure is between 85% and 122%.

Inherited deficiencies of AT-III may involve a decrease in the protein or a dysfunctional protein. Acquired deficiencies of AT-III are associated with DIC, liver disease (cirrhosis), in women taking oral contraceptives or receiving estrogen therapy, and malignancy. Antigenic levels of AT-III are determined by immunologic techniques such as ELISA or radial immunodiffusion (RID).

Protein C

Protein C activity can be measured by a chromogenic assay. Protein C is activated by a specific activator derived from the venom of Agkistrodon c. contortrix.[27] Plasma is incubated with this activator. The quantity of activated protein C is measured by its enzymatic activity on a chromogenic substrate. The enzymatic activity results in the release of pNA from the chromogenic substrate. The released pNA is measured spectrophotometrically at 405 nm. The absorbance of pNA is directly proportional to the quantity of activated protein C. A reference (standard) curve is prepared by plotting the protein C activity (%) for each reference plasma dilution against its corresponding absorbance. The results for patients and controls are read from this curve using their respective absorbance readings. Each laboratory should establish its own reference interval. The normal protein C level for this procedure is between 60% and 150%.

Inherited deficiencies of protein C include the quantitative type, which is characterized by decreased antigenic and functional levels, and the qualitative type, which is characterized by dysfunctional protein C. A chromogenic assay will detect quantitative and qualitative deficiencies. Acquired deficiencies of protein C are associated with DIC, Vitamin K deficiency, liver disease, oral anticoagulant therapy, and after surgery. Antigenic levels of protein C are determined by immunologic techniques such as ELISA or RID.

Protein S

Protein S exists in two forms: free and bound. Sixty percent of protein S is bound to C4b binding protein. In this form, protein S is nonfunctional. The remaining 40% of protein S is free. Free protein S serves as a cofactor for protein C enhancing its activity. The cofactor activity of protein S is measured by a clotting system using human plasma which is protein S-free, a reagent containing activated protein C and a reagent that is rich in factor Va, the principal substrate of activated protein C.[28] The clotting time will be prolonged in the presence of protein S.

A reference (standard) curve is prepared using dilutions of pooled normal plasma representing 100%, 75%, 50%, and 25% protein S activity. The protein S activity for each plasma and control is read from this curve. Each laboratory should establish its own reference interval. The normal protein S level for this procedure is between 66% and 122%.

Inherited deficiencies of protein S may involve a decrease in the protein or a dysfunctional protein. This procedure will detect both quantitative and qualitative deficiencies. Acquired deficiencies of protein S are associated with liver disease, pregnancy, DIC, Type I diabetes mellitus, and oral anticoagulant therapy. Total protein S is determined by immunologic techniques such as ELISA.

Plasminogen

Plasminogen is analyzed in a coupled enzymatic procedure.[29] The first reaction involves the incubation of plasma with a known excess of streptokinase. A plasminogen-streptokinase complex is formed that possesses plasmin-like activity. The second reaction determines the quantity of plasminogen-streptokinase complex by its enzymatic activity on a chromogenic substrate. The enzymatic activity results in the release of pNA from the chromogenic substrate. The released pNA is measured spectrophotometrically at 405 nm. The absorbance of pNA is directly proportional to the quantity of plasminogen. A reference (standard) curve is prepared by plotting the plasminogen activity (%) for each reference plasma dilution against its corresponding absorbance. The results for patients and controls are read from this curve using their respective absorbance readings. Each laboratory should establish its own reference interval. The normal plasminogen level for this procedure is between 74% and 124%.

Measurement of circulating plasminogen levels is useful in monitoring hepatic regeneration of plasminogen during discontinuous treatment with streptokinase and to control and adjust the rate of infusion if plasminogen is being given to the patient.

Inherited deficiencies of plasminogen include the quantitative type, which is characterized by decreased antigenic and functional levels, and the qualitative type, which is characterized by dysfunctional protein. Acquired deficiencies of plasminogen are associated with DIC, liver disease, and leukemias. Antigenic levels of plasminogen are determined by immunologic techniques such as ELISA or RID.

Antiplasmin

The primary biochemical inhibitor of plasmin is α2-antiplasmin. This inhibitor is analyzed by a coupled reaction.[30] The first reaction involves the incubation of plasma with a known excess of plasmin. The second reaction determines the residual plasmin activity by its enzymatic activity on a chromogenic substrate. Plasmin activity results in the release of pNA from the chromogenic substrate. The released pNA is measured spectrophotometrically at 405 nm. The residual plasmin activity is inversely proportional to the α2-antiplasmin level in the plasma. A reference (standard) curve is prepared by plotting the α-2-antiplasmin activity (%) for each reference plasma dilution against its corresponding absorbance. The results for patients and controls are read from this curve using their respective absorbance readings. Each laboratory should establish its own reference interval. The normal antiplasmin level for this procedure is between 80% and 120%.

Measurement of circulating α2-antiplasmin levels is useful in monitoring fibrinolytic therapy. A decrease in α-2-antiplasmin levels reflects the efficacy of the therapy.

Acquired deficiencies of α2-antiplasmin are associated with severe liver disease, DIC, and septicemia.

SUMMARY

This chapter reviewed the laboratory tests performed in the coagulation laboratory. The tests are grouped according to the part of the coagulation system that they assess, primary hemostasis or secondary hemostasis. A combination of tests from these groups can be selected to screen for a disorder of the coagulation system. For instance, a bleeding time, prothrombin time, and activated partial thromboplastin time can be used to identify a defect in primary hemostasis or secondary hemostasis. Once this defect is identified, specific laboratory tests can be selected for a definitive diagnosis of the coagulation disorder. If labortory tests for the investigation of fibrinolysis are included in the selected screening tests, fibrinolytic disorders such as primary fibrinolysis may be diagnosed. The last section of this chapter reviewed laboratory tests which are used in the evaluation of hypercoagulable states. Laboratory investigation of hypercoagulable states represents the newest area of the coagulation laboratory.

REVIEW QUESTIONS

1. The hematology laboratory informs you that the hematocrit on patient Z is 57% (.57 L/L). For the proper anticoagulation of a 5.0 mL sample of patient Z's blood, how much 3.2% sodium citrate should be used?
   a. 0.22 mL
   b. 0.40 mL
   c. 0.57 mL
   d. 0.96 mL

2. The laboratory test used to monitor oral anticoagulant therapy is:
   a. reptilase time
   b. bleeding time
   c. prothrombin time
   d. activated partial thromboplastin time

3. Platelet aggregation studies revealed normal aggregation curves with collagen, epinephrine, and ADP, but an abnormal aggregation curve with ristocetin. Based on these findings, what is the differential diagnosis?
   a. von Willebrand disease and Bernard-Soulier syndrome
   b. Glanzmann's thrombasthenia and von Willebrand disease
   c. Storage pool disease and Glanzmann's thrombasthenia
   d. Bernard-Soulier syndrome and storage pool disease

4. The activated partial thromboplastin time (APTT) is used as a screen for the laboratory evaluation of inherited or acquired deficiencies in the:
   a. extrinsic pathway of the coagulation cascade
   b. intrinsic pathway of the coagulation cascade

c. platelets

d. vascular system

5. The combination of a prolonged APTT and a prolonged test with the mixing study procedure indicates the presence of:

a. circulating inhibitor

b. factor VIII deficiency

c. anti-platelet antibodies

d. excessive vitamin K

6. Which coagulation factor is NOT present in adsorbed plasma?

a. factor V

b. factor VIII

c. factor X

d. factor XII

7. Based on the following data, what is the most likely factor deficiency?

PT	normal
APTT	prolonged
APTT + normal plasma	correction
APTT + adsorbed plasma	no correction
APTT + aged serum	correction

a. factor V

b. factor VIII

c. factor IX

d. factor XI

8. The observation of a normal reptilase time and a prolonged thrombin time is indicative of:

a. presence of fibrin degradation products

b. dysfibrinogenemia

c. hypoplasminogenemia

d. presence of heparin

9. Which laboratory test is specific for fibrinolysis?

a. D-dimer test

b. fibrin degradation products

c. euglobulin clot lysis

d. antithrombin III

10. Which laboratory test is NOT used to investigate the hypercoagulable states?

a. antithrombin III

b. protein S

c. plasminogen

d. activated partial thromboplastin time

●
REFERENCES

1. National Committee for Clinical Laboratory Standards: Collection, Transport, and Processing of Blood Specimens for Coagulation Testing and Performance of Coagulation Assays, 2nd Ed., vo. 11, no. 23, Villanova, PA: NCCLS, 1991.

2. Mielke, C.H.: International Committee Communications: Measurement of the bleeding time. Thromb. Haemost., 52:210, 1984.

3. Brown, B.A.: Hematology: Principles and Procedures, 6th Ed., Philadelphia: Lea & Febiger, 1993.

4. Corriveau, D.M., Fritsma, G.A.: Hemostasis and Thrombosis in the Clinical Laboratory. Philadelphia: J.B. Lippincott Company, 1988.

5. Ens, G.E.: Hemostasis: part III. Platelet function testing and hereditary and acquired disorders of platelet function. Am. J. Med. Tech., 48:119, 1982.

6. Sirridge, M.S., Shannon, R.: Laboratory Evaluation of Hemostasis and Thrombosis, 3rd Ed. Philadelphia: Lea & Febiger, 1983.

7. National Committee for Clinical Laboratory Standards: One-Stage Prothrombin Time Test (PT), vol. 12, no. 22. Villanova, PA: NCCLS, 1992.

8. Poller, L.: A simple nomogram for the derivation of international normalised ratios for the standardization of prothrombin times. Thromb. Haemost., 60:18, 1988.

9. International Committee for Standardization in Hematology, International Committee on Thrombosis and Hemostasis: ICSH/ICTH recommendations for reporting prothrombin time in oral anticoagulant control. Thromb. Haemost., 53:155, 1985.

10. Biggs, R., Denson, K.W.E.: Standardization of the one-stage prothrombin time for the control of anticoagulant therapy. Br. Med. J., 1:84, 1967.

11. National Committee for Clinical Laboratory Standards: Activated Partial Thromboplastin Time Test (APTT), vol. 12, no. 23. Villanova, PA: NCCLS, 1992.

12. American Bioproducts Company: Thrombin Prest: Calcium Thrombin for the Determination of the Thrombin Time, Parsipany, NJ: American Bioproducts Company, 1991.

13. Ortho Diagnostic Systems, Inc.: ORTHO Quantitative Fibrinogen Assay, Raritan, NJ: Ortho Diagnostic Systems, Inc., 1990.

14. National Committee for Clinical Laboratory Standards: Standardized Procedure for the Determination of Fibrinogen in Biological Samples, vol. 2, no. 13, Villanova, PA: NCCLS, 1982.

15. Abbott Diagnostic Systems: Reptilase-R, Abbott Laboratories, Diagnostics Division, North Chicago, IL, 1978.

16. Funk, C., Gumer, J., Herold, R., Straub, P.W.: Reptilase-R-A: A new reagent in blood coagulation. Br. J. Hematol., 21: 43, 1971.

17. National Committee for Clinical Laboratory Standards: Determination of Factor VIII Coagulant Activity (VIII:C), vol. 6, no. 6, Villanova, PA: NCCLS, 1986.

18. Weiss, H.J., et al.: Quantitative assay of a plasma factor deficient in von Willebrand's disease that is necessary for platelet aggregation. J. Clin. Invest., 52:2808, 1973.

19. Laurell, C.B.: Quantitative estimation of proteins by electrophoresis in agarose gel containing antibodies. Anal. Biochem., 13: 45, 1966.

20. Triplett, D.A., Brandt, J.T., Kaczor, D, Schaeffer, J.: Laboratory diagnosis of lupus inhibitors: A comparison of the tissue thromboplastin inhibition procedure with a new platelet neutralization procedure. Am. J. Clin. Pathol., 79:678, 1983.

21. Lupus Anticoagulant Working Party, BCSH Hemostasis and Thrombosis Task Force: Guidelines on testing for the lupus anticoagulant. Am. J. Clin. Pathol., 44:885, 1991.

22. Jensen, R., Ens, G.E.: Advances in the diagnosis of lupus anticoagulant. Clin. Hemostasis. Rev., 7:1, 1993.

23. American Bioproducts Company: LA: Detection of Lupus Anticoagulants. Parsipany, NJ: American Bioproducts Company, 1992.

24. American Bioproducts Company: FDP Plasma: Determination of FDP in Plasma by Latex Agglutination. Parsippany, NJ: American Bioproducts Company, 1992.

25. American Bioproducts Company: D-Di TEST: Latex Agglutination Slide Test for the Qualitative and Semi-quantitative Determination of D-Dimer. Parsippany, NJ: American Bioproducts Company, 1990.

26. American Bioproducts Company: ATIII: Colorimetric Assay of Antithrombin III. Parsipany, NJ: American Bioproducts Company, 1990.

27. American Bioproducts Company: Protein C: Colorimetric Assay of Protein C. Parsipany, NJ: American Bioproducts Company, 1989.

28. American Bioproducts Company: Protein S: Clotting Assay of Protein S. Parsipany, NJ: American Bioproducts Company, 1992.

29. American Bioproducts Company: Plasminogen: Rapid photometric analysis of Plasminogen. Parsipany, NJ: American Bioproducts Company, 1991.

30. American Bioproducts Company: Antiplasmin: Colorimetric Assay of Fast-Acting Antiplasmin. Parsipany, NJ: American Bioproducts Company, 1991.

Automation in hematology

CHAPTER OUTLINE

KEY TERMS

threshold limit
histogram
red cell distribution width
  (RDW)
mean platelet volume (MPV)
platelet distribution width
  (PDW)
hydrodynamic focusing
scattergram
continuous flow analysis
isovolumetric focusing
cell hemoglobin
  concentration mean
  (CHCM)
hemoglobin distribution width
  (HDW)
cytogram
viscosity
PT clotting curve

INTRODUCTION

Automation is firmly established within the hematology/coagulation laboratory. This chapter reviews examples of instrumentation that are currently used. The basic principles of operation are discussed for each instrument. Using examples of erythrocyte, leukocyte, or platelet abnormalities, histograms and scattergrams are compared for their ability to detect these abnormalities. Finally, clinical applications are discussed for the flow cytometry, the newest addition to the clinical hematology laboratory.

AUTOMATED BLOOD CELL COUNTING INSTRUMENTS

Introduction

The evolution of instrumentation in hematology began in the mid-1950s. Clinical laboratory scientists at that time were performing manual hemacytometer blood cell counts, spun hematocrits, spectrophotometrically determined hemoglobins, and microscopic blood smear evaluations. With the advent of the first single automated blood cell counter, manual hemacytometer blood cell counts for erythrocyte enumeration and leukocyte enumeration were replaced. In general, automated blood cell counters provide data with increased reliability, precision, and accuracy.

With the many advances in hematology instrumentation, automation currently encompasses the primary testing in the hematology laboratory. A complete blood cell count including the platelet count and the five-part differential can be performed using instrumentation. A number of principles for cell counting and differential analysis have been used in the past. The two principles of blood cell counting currently used by the hematology instruments are impedance and optical light scattering.

The impedance principle of blood cell counting is based on the increased resistance that occurs when a blood cell with poor conductivity passes through an electrical field. The number of pulses indicate the blood cell count, and the amplitude of each pulse is proportional to the volume of the cell. Examples of instruments using this principle are the Coulter Counter instruments, the TOA Sysmex instruments, and the Abbott Cell-Dyn instruments.

The optical light scattering principle of blood cell counting is based on light scattering measurements obtained as a single blood cell passes through a beam of light (optical or laser). Blood cells create forward scatter and side scatter, which are detected by photodetectors. The degree of forward scatter is a measurement of cell size, while the degree of side scatter is a measurement of cell complexity or granularity. This principle is used by the Technicon H System instruments.

This section will review the basic operating principles of several hematology instruments seen in the field. Other instruments use a combination of these principles.

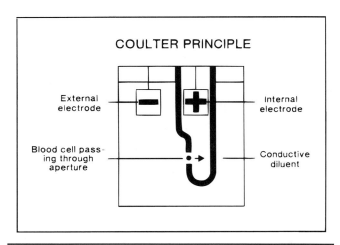

FIGURE 29-1. Coulter principle. (From Pierre, R.: Seminar & Case Studies: The Automated Differential, Hialeah, FL: Coulter Electronics, Inc., 1985, with permission.)

Impedance instruments

COULTER COUNTER S-PLUS SERIES

In 1983, Coulter Corporation introduced the Coulter Counter S-Plus IV, a multiparameter, automated analyzer. Blood cell counting was based on the Coulter principle of impedance. Blood cells were diluted in an electrically conductive diluent, and two electrodes separated by an aperature were suspended in this dilution (Fig. 29-1). As individual blood cells pass through the aperture, there is an increase in resistance between the two electrodes proportional to the volume of the cell. Threshold limits were established for the enumeration of each cell population based on cell volume. Like previous Coulter instruments, there were two counting chambers that operated simultaneously (one counting chamber for erythrocyte and platelet enumeration and another for leukocyte enumeration). Each counting chamber has three separate apertures for triplicate analysis and internal comparison of results to identify errors.

Histograms (size distribution curves) are created for erythrocyte (RBC), leukocyte (WBC), and platelet (PLT) populations based on cell volume (fL) and relative cell number (Fig. 29-2). These histograms allow the visualization of subpopulations of cells, their average size in relation to the rest of the population, and their relative number.[1,2]

The data obtained from the erythrocyte/platelet dilution include the RBC count by direct measurement (particles greater than 36 fL), mean cell volume (MCV), and red cell distribution width (RDW), which are derived from the RBC histogram (Fig. 29-3). The hematocrit is calculated from the MCV and the RBC count. The mean cell hemoglobin (MCH) and the mean cell hemoglobin concentration (MCHC) are calculated from the RBC count, the MCV, and the hemoglobin concentration, which is obtained from the leukocyte counting chamber.

Histogram

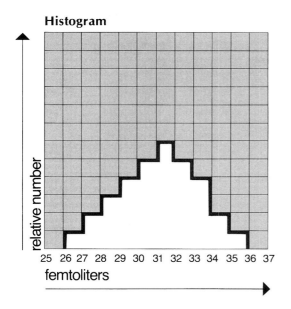

FIGURE 29-2. Histogram or size distribution curve. (From Significant Advances in Hematology, Coulter Electronics, Inc., Hialeah, FL, 1983, with permission.)

The platelet count also is obtained from this dilution. Particles between 2 and 20 fL are counted as platelets, and a raw platelet histogram is obtained (Fig. 29-4). The raw platelet histogram is evaluated to determine if it is a log normal curve. The raw platelet histogram is electronically smoothed and extrapolated over 0 to 70 fL. The platelet count is derived from the extrapolated histogram. Two additional parameters are obtained from the platelet histogram, mean platelet volume (MPV), which is analogous to the MCV, and platelet distribution width (PDW), which is analogous to the RDW.

The leukocyte count is directly measured from the leukocyte dilution after a lytic agent has been added. The lytic agent serves to lyse the erythrocytes, convert free hemoglobin to cyanmethemoglobin, and shrink the leuko-

cyte cell membrane and cytoplasm. Therefore, the leukocyte count represents a measure of the cell volume rather than native cell size as it passes through the aperture. Particles greater than 35 fL are counted as leukocytes. A WBC histogram is created from the data obtained as the cells pass through the aperture. A three-part differential is obtained based on the relative sizes of the leukocytes evaluated. Lymphocytes are found between 35 and 90 fL; mononuclear cells are found between 90 and 160 fL; granulocytes are found between 160 and 450 fL (Fig. 29-5).

The concentration of cyanmethemoglobin is determined by photometry at 525 nm. Through the application of Beer's law, the concentration of cyanmethemoglobin is proportional to the concentration of free hemoglobin. This instrument uses a reagent blank at the beginning of each operating cycle.

The instrument's computer analyzes the data obtained from the erythrocyte/platelet dilution and the leukocyte dilution. The instrument's computer corrects the counts for coincidence (two or more cells pass through the aperture simultaneously) and evaluates the triplicate results from each dilution for replication. If two or three results do not agree, the result is not reported but recorded as "vote-out." The accepted results are averaged and displayed on a computer screen or printed to hard copy for the clinical laboratory scientist's review. If abnormalities are detected by the instrument, the abnormal results are either backlighted or flagged. Backlighting is primarily used for out-of-range results or vote-out situations. Region flags are used for the WBC histogram and differential. These flags alert the clinical laboratory scientist to the presence of interferences within one or more of the WBC histogram regions.[2-6] For example, the presence of nucleated erythrocytes or clumped platelets is indicated if the Region 1 flag is reported.[3]

COULTER COUNTER STKS

The Coulter STKS uses a combination of technologies to enumerate erythrocytes, platelets, and leukocytes and to determine a five-part differential.[7] The basic counting principle of impedance is used to enumerate the cell counts and derive the erythrocyte and platelet histograms. The

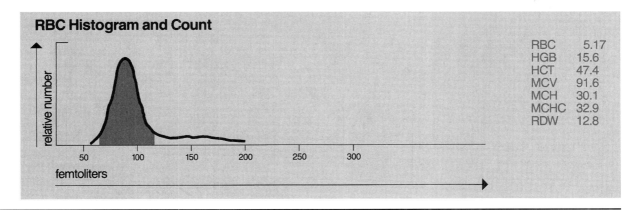

			RBC	5.17
			HGB	15.6
			HCT	47.4
			MCV	91.6
			MCH	30.1
			MCHC	32.9
			RDW	12.8

FIGURE 29-3. RBC histogram and count. The shaded area represents those cells used in the RDW calculation. The excluded cells may represent large platelets, platelet clumps, or electrical interference on the left and RBC doublets, RBC triplets, RBC agglutinates, or aperature artifacts on right. (From Significant Advances in Hematology, Coulter Electronics, Inc., Hialeah, FL, 1983, with permission.)

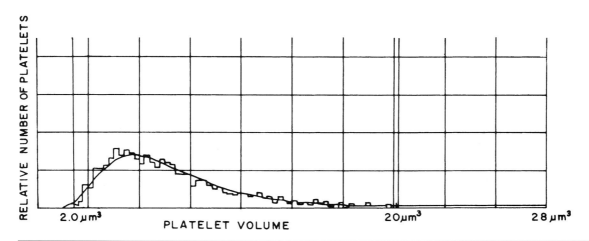

RELATIVE NUMBER OF PLATELETS

PLATELET VOLUME

2.0 μm³   20μm³   28 μm³

FIGURE 29-4. Normal platelet histogram, Coulter Counter S Plus. The jagged line represents the raw data collected from 2-20 fL. The smooth line represents the extrapolated histogram from 0-70 fL. (From Brown, B.A.: Hematology: Principles and Procedures, 6th Ed., Philadelphia, Lea & Febiger, 1993).

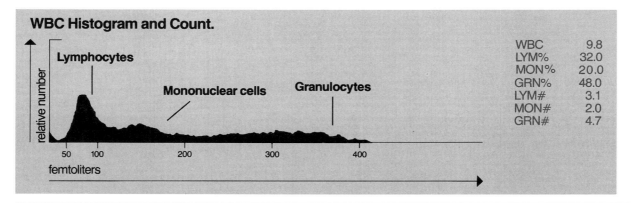

WBC Histogram and Count.

relative number

Lymphocytes

Mononuclear cells   Granulocytes

50 100   200   300   400

femtoliters

WBC	9.8
LYM%	32.0
MON%	20.0
GRN%	48.0
LYM#	3.1
MON#	2.0
GRN#	4.7

FIGURE 29-5. WBC histogram and count. In a normal patient, the lymphocyte region represents lymphocytes, the mononuclear region represents monocytes, and the granulocyte region represents neutrophils, eosinophils, and basophils. (From Significant Advances in Hematology, Coulter Electronics, Inc., Hialeah, FL, 1983, with permission.)

five-part differential is determined by VCS (volume·conductivity·scatter) technology.

The instrument aspirates a sample of EDTA anticoagulated blood and divides this sample three ways. As with previous Coulter instruments, erythrocyte and platelet counts are determined within one aperture bath, and leukocyte counts and hemoglobin determinations are obtained from a second aperture bath. The data from each bath are accumulated and reviewed by the instrument's computer. The cell counts, histograms, and other erythrocyte and platelet parameters are sent to the data management system.

The third portion of the blood sample is sent to a mixing chamber where a dilution is prepared using a lytic agent that removes erythrocytes but maintains leukocytes in their near-native state. A stabilizer also is added to preserve the integrity of the leukocytes. This dilution is analyzed within the flow cell of the triple transducer to obtain the five-part differential. The cells pass through the flow cell singly by hydrodynamic focusing. As each cell passes

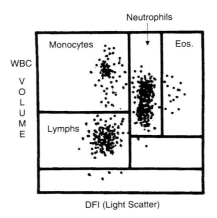

Neutrophils

WBC
VOLUME

Monocytes   Eos.

Lymphs

DFI (Light Scatter)

FIGURE 29-6. DF1 scatterplot, Coulter STKS. DF1 scatterplot graphs volume vs light scatter and reveals the locations of four leukocyte populations. The basophil population is located behind the lymphocytes. (From Brown, BA: Hematology: Principles and Procedures, 6th Ed., Philadelphia, Lea & Febiger, 1993).

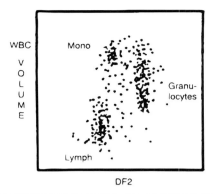

FIGURE 29-7. DF2 scatterplot, Coulter STKS. DF2 scatterplot graphs volume vs conductivity and reveals the locations of three leukocyte populations. The granulocyte population represents neutrophils, eosinophils, and basophils. (From Brown, B.A.: Hematology: Principles and Procedures, 6th Ed., Philadelphia, Lea & Febiger, 1993).

through the flow cell, three separate measurements are taken simultaneously. These measurements include cell volume, cell conductivity, and the cell's light scatter characteristics. Cell volume is determined by impedance, cell conductivity is determined by a high-frequency electromagnetic probe, and light scatter characteristics are determined by helium–neon laser.[6–11] The instrument system analyzes these measurements and classifies the cell into one of five normal populations. From these measurements, the percentage value of each cell type is obtained, and the absolute number is calculated. The two-dimensional scatterplots are created and displayed by the data management system. The DF1 (discriminant function 1) scatterplot is the two-dimensional scatterplot most commonly included in the STKS report form and shows data derived from volume and light scatter (Fig. 29-6). The DF2 scatterplot shows data derived from volume and conductivity analysis (Fig. 29-7). The basophil population, which is hidden by the lymphocyte population on the DFI

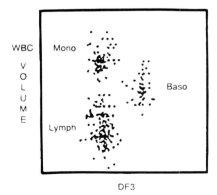

FIGURE 29-8. DF3 scatterplot, Coulter STKS. This scatterplot also graphs volume vs conductivity, but the neutrophil and eosinophil populations are gated out of the granulocyte population to reveal the basophils. (From Brown, B.A.: Hematology: Principles and Procedures, 6th Ed., Philadelphia, Lea & Febiger, 1993).

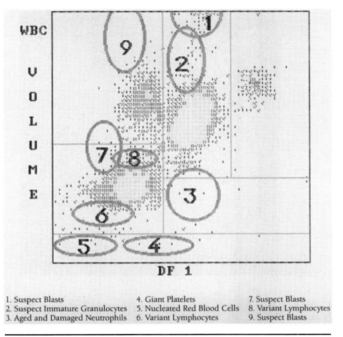

1. Suspect Blasts	4. Giant Platelets	7. Suspect Blasts
2. Suspect Immature Granulocytes	5. Nucleated Red Blood Cells	8. Variant Lymphocytes
3. Aged and Damaged Neutrophils	6. Variant Lymphocytes	9. Suspect Blasts

FIGURE 29-9. Location of abnormal cell types on the scatterplot, Coulter STKS. (From Brown, B.A.: Hematology: Principles and Procedures, 6th Ed., Philadelphia, Lea & Febiger, 1993).

scatterplot, is observed on the DF3 scatterplot (Fig. 29-8). Scatterplots and histograms also may be used to detect abnormalities or subpopulations of cells (Fig. 29-9).[6–11]

The microcomputer system analyzes and compiles all data obtained from the instrument. The results are displayed on a computer screen or printed to hard copy for clinical laboratory scientist's review (Fig. 29-10). Abnormalities in the results are identified by a cell classification system. This system consists of software-generated flags (suspect flags) or user-defined flags (definitive flags). The clinical laboratory scientist uses this information to correlate complete blood count (CBC) data with peripheral blood morphology to improve the identification and confirmation of abnormalities.

The newest methodology added to the Coulter STKS instrument is reticulocyte analysis. Reticulocyte analysis uses the supravital stain, new methylene blue, to stain residual RNA. The stained sample is analyzed by VCS technology to determine the reticulocyte count. With this additional methodology, the Coulter STKS is capable of performing a CBC with differential and a reticulocyte count.

SYSMEX NE-8000

The Sysmex NE-8000 is a fully-automated hematology instrument manufactured by TOA Medical Electronics Company. This instrument is capable of performing blood cell counts, hemoglobin determinations, and five-part differentials. Blood cell counting is based on the impedance principle with both cell counts and histograms obtained through the analysis of a blood cell dilution. The five-part differential is obtained through a combination of technol-

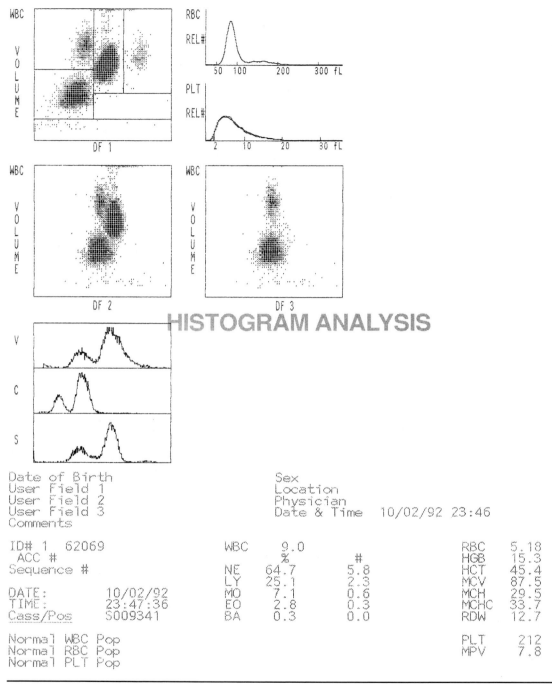

FIGURE 29-10. Coulter STKS report from a normal individual. (Courtesy of Linda Nash, MT(ASCP), Southwest Texas Methodist Hospital, San Antonio, TX.)

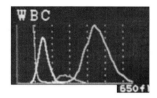

FIGURE 29-11. Tri-modal histogram revealing the lymphocyte, monocyte, and granulocyte regions, Sysmex NE-8000. (From Brown, B.A.: Hematology: Principles and Procedures, 6th Ed., Philadelphia, Lea & Febiger, 1993, with permission.)

ogies: impedance, radio frequency, and differential cell lysis.[12]

Erythrocytes and platelets are counted from one dilution, and the leukocyte count and hemoglobin determination are obtained from a second dilution that contains a mild lytic agent. The lytic agent lyses the erythrocytes and converts the free hemoglobin to cyanmethemoglobin but maintains leukocytes in their native state. The use of hydrodynamic focusing in the cell counting process minimizes the problems due to coincidence, erythrocyte deformability, and the recirculation of counted cells. Instead of using established threshold limits for the differentiation of cell populations, the NE-8000 uses automatic discrimination. Automatic discriminators (floating threshold limits) allow for patient to patient variation by adjusting with each sample, therefore more clearly defining each cell population.[9,12] In addition to the cell counts, histograms also are generated for the erythrocyte and platelet counts. Like other impedance counters, the instrument's computer reviews the data obtained from each dilution and derives or calculates additional erythrocyte and platelet parameters. The erythrocyte parameters include the RDW-CV, the coefficiant of variation of the erythrocyte distribution width, and the RDW-SD, the distribution width of the

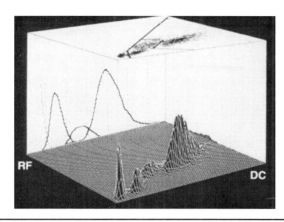

FIGURE 29-13. Isometric histogram from normal individual, Sysmex NE-8000. RF refers to radio frequency and reflects the complexity of the cell. DC refers to direct current (impedance) and reflects the volume of the cell. (From Brown, BA: Hematology: Principles and Procedures, 6th Ed., Philadelphia, Lea & Febiger, 1993).

erythrocyte population. Together, these parameters are used to identify erythrocyte abnormalities.

Information obtained from three separate detection blocks is compiled to give the five-part differential. The first detection block uses a combination of impedance and radio frequency to generate a trimodal histogram (Fig. 29-11) and two-dimensional scattergram (Fig. 29-12) representing the lymphocyte, monocyte, and granulocyte populations. Radio frequency provides information on nuclear size and cellular density, and impedance reflects the cell size. Automatic discriminators allow clearer delineation of the three cell populations. By combining this information with particle numbers, a three-dimensional histogram is created (Fig. 29-13). Eosinophils and basophils are enumerated in separate detection blocks using specific cell lytic agents and impedance. Histograms are generated for these two cell populations. Figure 29-14 is an example of an eosinophil histogram. The neutrophil count is obtained by subtracting the eosinophil and basophil counts from the granulocyte population.

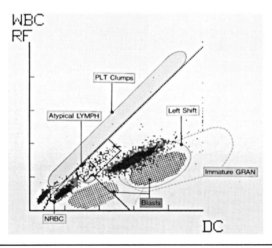

FIGURE 29-12. WBC scattergram shows normal WBC scatter and location of abnormal WBC and platelets, Sysmex NE-8000. (From Brown, BA: Hematology: Principles and Procedures, 6th Ed., Philadelphia, Lea & Febiger, 1993).

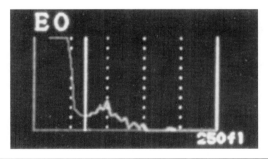

FIGURE 29-14. Eosinophil histogram, Sysmex NE-8000. This histogram represents the eosinophil population following differential lysis of the leukocytes. (From Garrity, P., Walters, J.: Concepts in New Age Hematology: A Hematology Monograph. McGaw Park, IL, Baxter Healthcare Corp., Scientific Products Division, 1990, with permission.)

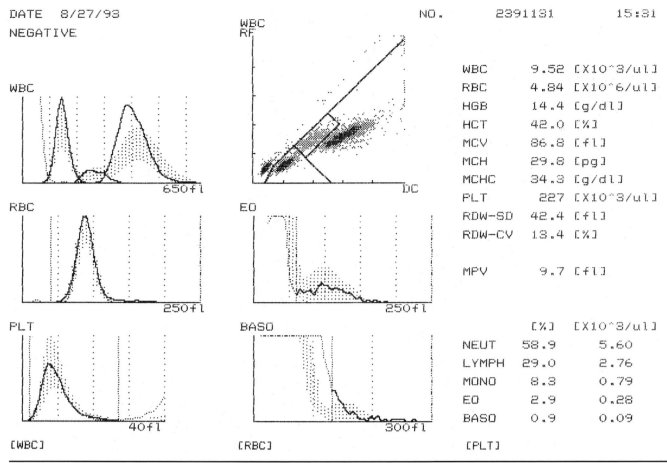

FIGURE 29-15. Sysmex NE-8000 report from a normal individual. (Courtesy of Dora Mae Parker, MS, MT(ASCP), Baylor University Medical Center, Dallas, TX.)

All data, including cell counts, histograms, and scattergrams, are analyzed by the computer system. The results are displayed on the computer screen or printed to hard copy (Fig. 29-15). An extensive flagging program with interpretive comments alerts the clinical laboratory scientist to abnormal results. Use of the flagging system and observation of the scattergrams and histograms allows the clinical laboratory scientist to focus on specific abnormalities when performing a peripheral blood smear evaluation. [6,9,10,13]

The NE-Alpha is an integrated system consisting of the SP-1 slide preparation unit, the NE-8000 hematology analyzer, and a control unit. The Sysmex R-3000, an automated reticulocyte analyzer, also can be added to this system. This integrated system of instruments introduces complete automation to the hematology laboratory.

The newest edition to the Sysmex instruments is the SE-9000, a discrete analyzer. The instrument performs discrete testing of specific components of the CBC (i.e., Hb, Hct, PLT only) through user-defined menus or preset menus. The basis of cell counting and the determination of the five-part differential are the same as the NE-8000.

In addition, the SE-9000 has an immature cell channel, which provides a clearer delineation of immature neutrophils and blasts. [14] Together, the five-part differential and the data from the immature cell channel may be used by the clinical laboratory scientist for the interpretation of specific abnormalities.

In addition, the data analysis component creates a radar chart (Fig. 29-16) from the patient's results for the eight CBC parameters. The comparison of the patient's radar chart to a normal radar chart may be used by the clinical laboratory scientist as another tool in the investigation of hematologic abnormalities (Fig. 29-16). [14]

● Light-scattering instruments

TECHNICON H*1 SYSTEM

Technicon Instruments Corporation has been involved in hematology instrumentation since the early 1970s. The first instruments were based on continous flow analysis similar to their chemistry instruments. The Hemolog D performed leukocyte differentials based on continuous

RADAR CHART

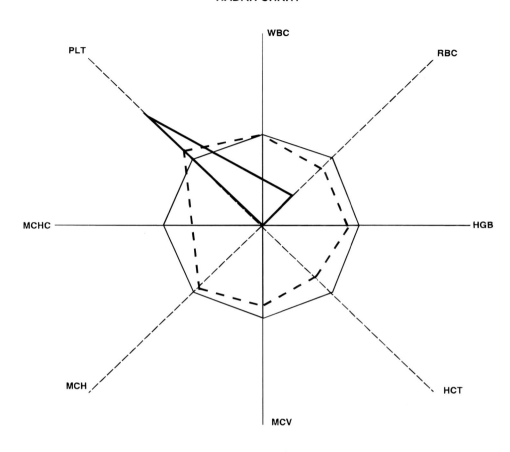

FIGURE 29-16. A radar chart showing a comparison of the pattern seen in iron deficiency (bold line) to the pattern of a normal patient (dotted line). The single line represents normal reference points.

——————	**Defines normal limits**
— — — —	**Normal patient**
————————	**Iron Deficiency Anemia**

flow analysis and peroxidase cytochemical staining. The Technicon H-6000 was capable of performing a complete blood cell count and five-part differential using continuous flow analysis and an improved cytochemical staining method. The Technicon H*1 was the first of a series of instruments to combine these principles of cell detection and identification with flow cytometry.[15]

The Technicon H*1 aspirates a sample of EDTA anticoagulated blood and processes portions of that sample through four separate channels. The erythrocyte/platelet channel determines erythrocyte and platelet counts by the analysis of light scattering measurements obtained as the diluted cells pass singly through a helium–neon laser beam. The diluent used for erythrocyte and platelet counts causes isovolumetric sphering of the erythrocytes. Isovolumetric sphering of erythrocytes eliminates cell volume errors due to variations in erythrocyte shape.[16,17] The erythrocytes are counted and sized by both high-angle and low-angle light scattering measurements (Fig. 29-17).

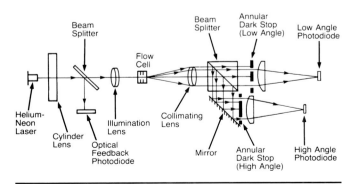

FIGURE 29-17. Cytometer measuring differential light scattering. (From Proceedings of Technicon H*1 Hematology Symposium, Tarrytown, NY, Technicon Instruments Corp., October 11, 1985, with permission.)

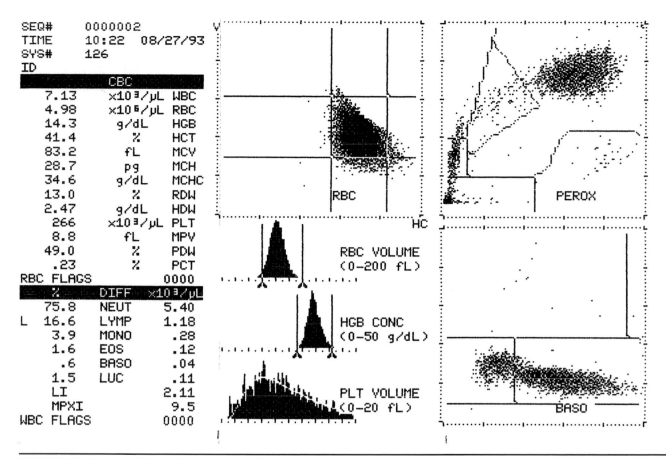

SEQ#	0000002	
TIME	10:22	08/27/93
SYS#	126	
ID		

CBC		
7.13	x10³/µL	WBC
4.98	x10⁶/µL	RBC
14.3	g/dL	HGB
41.4	%	HCT
83.2	fL	MCV
28.7	pg	MCH
34.6	g/dL	MCHC
13.0	%	RDW
2.47	g/dL	HDW
266	x10³/µL	PLT
8.8	fL	MPV
49.0	%	PDW
.23	%	PCT
RBC FLAGS		0000

%	DIFF	x10³/µL
75.8	NEUT	5.40
L 16.6	LYMP	1.18
3.9	MONO	.28
1.6	EOS	.12
.6	BASO	.04
1.5	LUC	.11
	LI	2.11
	MPXI	9.5
WBC FLAGS		0000

RBC VOLUME (0-200 fL)

HGB CONC (0-50 g/dL)

PLT VOLUME (0-20 fL)

PEROX

BASO

FIGURE 29-18. Technicon H*1 report from a normal individual depicting the erythrocyte cytogram, erythrocyte and platelet histogram, a hemoglobin concentration histogram, a WBC peroxidase cytogram and basophil/lobularity cytogram.

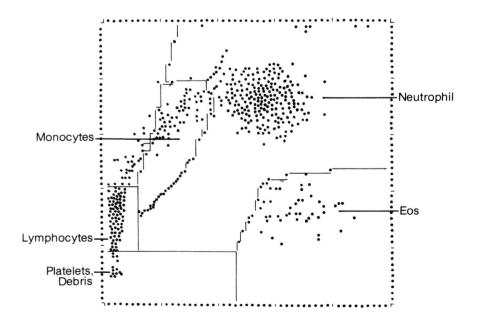

FIGURE 29-19. WBC/peroxidase cytogram, Technicon H*1. (From Brown, BA: Hematology: Principles and Procedures, 6th Ed., Philadelphia, Lea & Febiger, 1993).

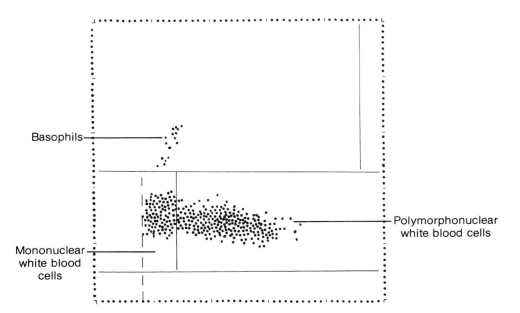

FIGURE 29-20. Basophil/lobularity cytogram, Technicon H*1. (From Brown, BA: Hematology: Principles and Procedures, 6th Ed., Philadelphia, Lea & Febiger, 1993(.

Individual erythrocyte hemoglobin concentration and cell volume can be determined from these measurements; thus, the mean cell volume (MCV) and cellular hemoglobin concentration mean (CHCM) are obtained.[17–19] The red cell distribution width (RDW) and the hemoglobin distribution width (HDW) are derived from these measurements. Platelet enumeration and sizing are accomplished using one detector that is set at an increased gain. Together, these measurements allow for the generation of an erythrocyte cytogram and erythrocyte, hemoglobin concentration, and platelet histograms (Fig. 29-18).

Within the hemoglobin channel, a portion of EDTA-anticoagulated blood is mixed with the hemoglobin diluent. The erythrocytes are lysed and free hemoglobin is converted to cyanmethemoglobin. The concentration of cyanmethemoglobin is determined photometrically at 546 nm.

The leukocyte count and five-part differential are obtained using two different methods and two separate channels, the peroxidase channel and the basophil/lobularity channel. In the peroxidase channel, neutrophils, monocytes, and eosinophils are identified by the degree of peroxidase positivity and the amount of forward light scatter. Lymphocytes and large unstained cells (LUCs) are identified by the amount of forward light scatter and the fact that they remain unstained by this peroxidase cytochemical staining method. Erythrocytes are removed before peroxidase staining by lytic action. The amount of forward scatter and degree of positivity are detected as the cells pass through a tungsten-based flow cell. Within the basophil/lobularity channel, a fourth portion of EDTA-anticoagulated blood is mixed with basophil diluent. The basophil diluent lyses erythrocytes and platelets and strips all leukocytes except basophils of their cytoplasm. This dilution is measured by the helium–neon laser flow cell. Basophils will have large, low angle scattered signatures, and the remaining cell nuclei will be classified as mononuclear or polymorphonuclear based on their high angle scatter signatures.

The normal cell pattern as depicted on the basophil/lobularity cytogram is referred to as the "worm," with the head region representing the mononuclear cells and the body region representing the polymorphonuclear cells. The WBC peroxidase cytogram represents measurements obtained by the peroxidase channel (Fig. 29-19), while the basophil/lobularity cytogram represents the measurements obtained by the basophil/lobularity channel (Fig. 29-20).

The absolute count for each leukocyte population is obtained from both channels. The computer compares the corresponding cell counts and generates flags if the results do not compare. The percentage values are calculated from the absolute cell counts. In the peroxidase channel,

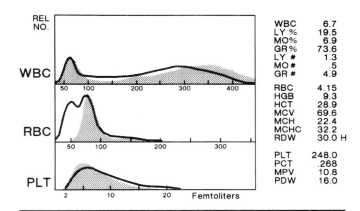

FIGURE 29-21. Coulter S-Plus report illustrating changes associated with iron deficiency anemia. Observe the bimodal RBC population. The left peak represents the microcytic erythrocytes and the right peak represents a combination of normal transfused erythrocytes and the reticulocyte response associated with iron therapy. The solid lines represent patient data. The shaded area is a reference range (normal) for comparison. (From Pierre, R.: Seminar & Case Studies: The Automated Differential, Hialeah, FL, Coulter Electronics, Inc., 1985, with permission.)

basophils and lymphocytes fall in the same region; therefore, the total lymphocyte count is determined by subtracting the basophil count obtained from the basophil/lobularity channel. An advantage of this method of determining cell counts is the capability of performing WBC counts and differentials on specimens with very low counts (WBC less than 0.1×10^9/L).

The Technicon H*1 evaluates the information from the two flow cells and displays the information on the computer screen. The results can be printed to hard copy for record-keeping (Fig. 29-18). If abnormalites are detected in cell counts, histograms, or cytograms, the instrument flags the appropriate result or results. The flagging critieria assist the clinical laboratory scientist in defining the abnormalities to be reviewed by peripheral blood smear examination.[6,9–11,18–22]

The Technicon H*3 is the newest version of the Tech-

nicon H* System instruments. This instrument is capable of performing a complete blood cell analysis, five-part differential, and a reticulocyte analysis. The reticulocytes are stained with oxazine 750 and evaluated by the helium–neon laser beam of the erythrocyte/platelet channel.[23] The reticulocyte analysis provides additional measurements, including a measure of the reticulocyte mean cell volume and the reticulocyte cellular hemoglobin concentration mean. In combination with the reticulocyte count, these two results may be used to provide information related to the bone marrow's responsiveness to therapy.

Comparison of histograms, scattergrams, and cytograms in selected disorders

This section is designed to provide a broad comparison of abnormalities that can be detected by automated hema-

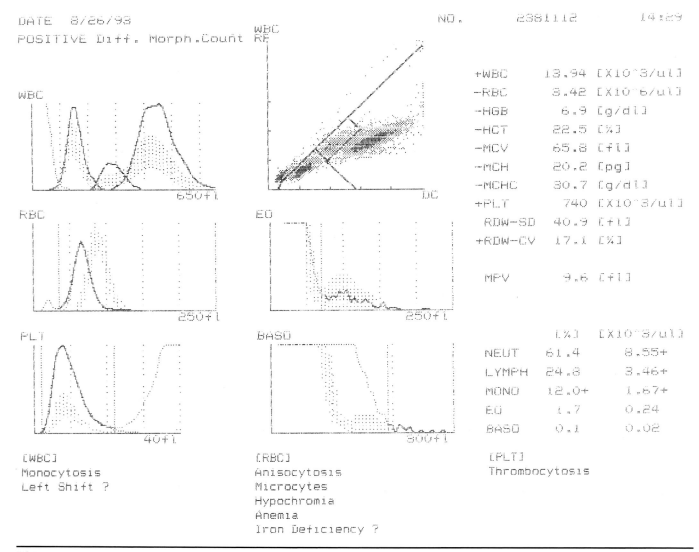

FIGURE 29-22. Sysmex NE-8000 report illustrating changes associated with iron deficiency anemia. Observe the shift to the left of the RBC population indicating microcytosis. The lines represent patient data and the shaded area is the reference range (normal) for comparison. (Courtesy of Dora Mae Parker, MS, MT(ASCP), Baylor University Medical Center, Dallas, TX.)

tology instruments. Selected disorders have been chosen to compare the histograms, scattergrams, cytograms, and other significant data. Histogram, scattergram, or cytogram analysis may be the first clue as to the presence of a RBC or WBC abnormality. However, further laboratory studies often are required to confirm the diagnosis.

IRON DEFICIENCY ANEMIA

Iron deficiency is the most common cause of a hypochromic microcytic anemia. The detection of microcytic erythrocytes is made from the observation of the RBC histogram using the Coulter S Plus, Coulter STKS, or Sysmex NE-8000 and from the observation of the RBC histogram and RBC cytogram using the Technicon H*1. The Coulter Counters RBC histogram (Fig. 29-21) and the Sysmex NE-8000 RBC histogram (Fig. 29-22) will show a shift to the left in the RBC population. The RBC cytogram will show a wide distribution of cells extending to the left and lower regions of cytogram (Fig. 29-23). Hypochromasia is detected by a shift to the left in the hemoglobin concentration histogram using the Technicon H*1 (Fig. 29-23). For all instruments, significant data will include decreased hemoglobin concentration, decreased MCV, decreased MCHC, and increased RDW. With each instrument, suspect flags will alert the clinical laboratory scientist as to the possible abnormalities.

The differential diagnosis of hypochromic microcytic anemia often includes thalassemia, in addition to iron deficiency anemia. The Sysmex NE-8000 reviews the MCV,

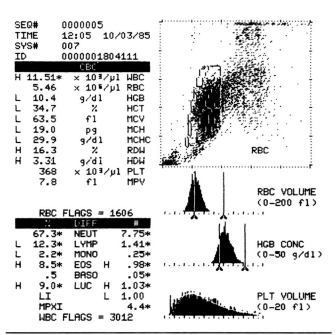

FIGURE 29-24. Technicon H*1 report illustrating changes associated with beta thalassemia minor. Observe the shift to the left of the RBC population and the tighter cluster of erythrocytes compared to the RBC cytogram associated with iron deficiency (Fig. 29-23). (Proceedings of Technicon H*1 Hematology Symposium. Tarrytown, NY, Technicon Instruments Corp., October 11, 1985, with permission.)

RDW-SD, and RDW-CV results to differentiate the two anemias. In iron deficiency anemia, the RDW-SD and RDW-CV are increased compared with the computer established value; however, thalassemia is characterized by RDW values equal to or below the computer established value. In thalassemia, the RBC cytogram of the Technicon H*1 shows a tighter cluster of cells that is shifted to the left (Fig. 29-24).

MEGALOBLASTIC ANEMIA

The observations made from the RBC histogram (Coulter S Plus, Coulter STKS, Sysmex NE-8000, and Technicon H*1) and the RBC cytogram (Technicon H*1) are useful in the detection of macrocytic anemias. The RBC histograms will show a shift to the right indicating the presence of macrocytic erythrocytes (Figs. 29-25 and 29-26). The RBC cytogram will show a movement in the erythrocyte population to the upper right quadrant and a very wide distribution of erythrocytes (Fig. 29-27). For all instruments, significant data will include increased MCV and increased RDW. Suspect flags will alert the clinical laboratory scientist to the possibility of a macrocytic anemia.

COLD AGGLUTININS

Cold agglutinins are autoantibodies that react at room temperature or below and are associated with a variety of disorders. The presence of cold agglutinins can be detected by careful review of the RBC values, RBC histograms, and RBC cytograms. The Sysmex RBC histogram

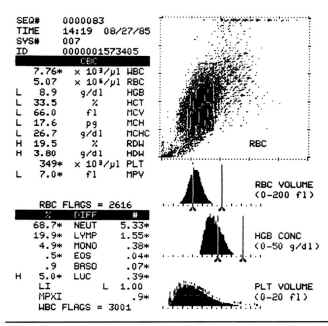

FIGURE 29-23. Technicon H*1 report illustrating changes associated with iron deficiency anemia. The RBC cytogram reveals a wide distribution of erythrocytes and a shift to the lower left region which is typical of microcytosis. The hemoglobin histogram reveals a shift to the left indicating hypochromasia. (Proceedings of Technicon H*1 Hematology Symposium. Tarrytown, NY, Technicon Instruments Corp., October 11, 1985, with permission.)

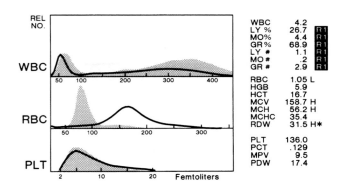

WBC	4.2
LY %	26.7 R1
MO%	4.4 R1
GR%	68.9 R1
LY #	1.1 R1
MO #	.2 R1
GR #	2.9 R1
RBC	1.05 L
HGB	5.9
HCT	16.7
MCV	158.7 H
MCH	56.2 H
MCHC	35.4
RDW	31.5 H*
PLT	136.0
PCT	.129
MPV	9.5
PDW	17.4

FIGURE 29-25. Coulter S-Plus report illustrating changes associated with severe folate deficiency (macrocytic anemia). Observe the shift to the right of the RBC population indicating macrocytosis. (From Pierre, R.: Seminar & Case Studies: The Automated Differential, Hialeah, FL, Coulter Electronics, Inc., 1985, with permission.)

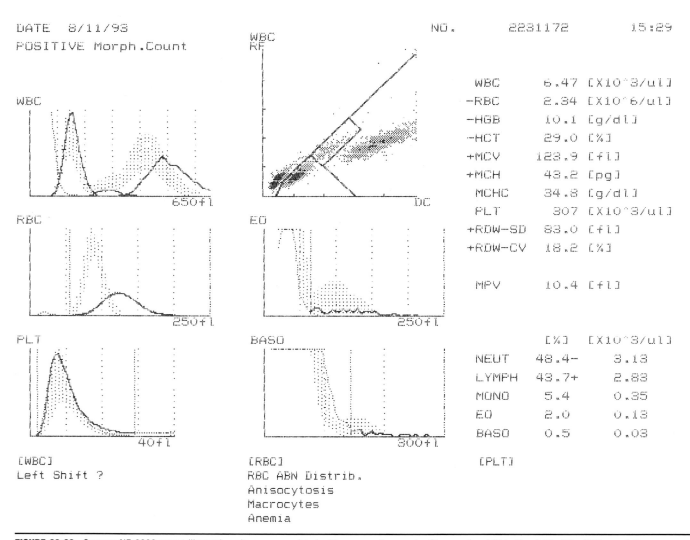

FIGURE 29-26. Sysmex NE-8000 report illustrating changes associated with macrocytic anemia. Observe the shift to the right of the RBC population indicating macrocytosis. (Courtesy of Dora Mae Parker, MS, MT(ASCP), Baylor University Medical Center, Dallas, TX.)

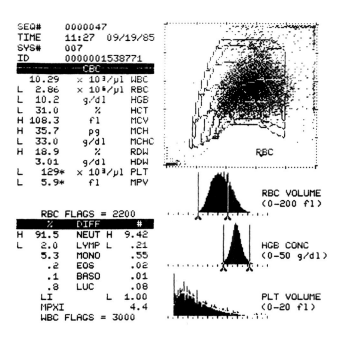

```
SEQ#      0000047
TIME      11:27  09/19/85
SYS#      007
ID        0000001538771
          CBC
    10.29   x 10 3/µl  WBC
L    2.86   x 10 6/µl  RBC
L   10.2    g/dl       HGB
L   31.0    %          HCT
H  108.3    fl         MCV
H   35.7    pg         MCH
L   33.0    g/dl       MCHC
H   18.9    %          RDW
     3.01   g/dl       HDW
L   129*    x 10 3/µl  PLT
L    5.9*   fl         MPV

    RBC FLAGS = 2200
       %    DIFF       #
H   91.5    NEUT H   9.42
L    2.0    LYMP L    .21
     5.3    MONO      .55
      .2    EOS       .02
      .1    BASO      .01
      .8    LUC       .08
    LI          L    1.00
    MPXI             4.4
    WBC FLAGS = 3000
```

RBC

RBC VOLUME
(0-200 fl)

HGB CONC
(0-50 g/dl)

PLT VOLUME
(0-20 fl)

FIGURE 29-27. Technicon H*1 report illustrating changes associated with macrocytic anemia. The RBC cytogram reveals a very wide distribution of erythrocytes and a shift to the upper right region, which is typical of macrocytosis. (From Proceedings of Technicon H*1 Hematology Symposium. Tarrytown, NY, Technicon Instruments Corp., October 11, 1985, with permission.)

will show a broad peak with a slight shift to the right representing the agglutinated erythrocytes (Fig. 29-28). The Technicon H*1 RBC cytogram reveals a cluster of cells within the macrocytic normochromic region above the normal erythrocyte population, which represents the agglutinated erythrocytes (Fig. 29-29). The NE-8000 will flag for RBC agglutination, whereas the Technicon H*1 will flag for anisocytosis and macrocytosis. An advantage of the MCHC/CHCM comparison with the Technicon H*1 is the increased sensitivity of the instrument to the presence of cold agglutinins. The presence of a CE flag indicates a RBC/MCV/Hgb problem, which is resolved by performing a spun hematocrit.

NUCLEATED ERYTHROCYTES

The presence of nucleated erythrocytes in the peripheral blood is an indication of increased erythropoietic activity within the bone marrow or infiltration of the bone marrow. Careful observation of the WBC scatterplot (Coulter STKS), WBC scattergram (Sysmex NE-8000), and WBC cytograms (Technicon H*1) will indicate their presence. In the WBC scattergram, the nucleated erythrocytes will obscure the discriminator line and appear below the lymphocyte region and to the right of the erythrocyte population (Fig. 29-30). The WBC peroxidase cytogram shows the population of nucleated erythrocytes in a parallel line of cells from the debri region into the lymphocyte region (Fig. 29-31). The basophil/lobularity cytogram shows the nucleated erythrocytes falling below the normal cell population or belly of the worm (Fig. 29-31). With both instruments, a suspect flag for the presence of nucleated erythrocytes will alert the clinical laboratory scientist to review the peripheral blood smear.

INFECTIOUS MONONUCLEOSIS

Infectious mononucleosis is characterized by the presence of atypical lymphocytes. The WBC scatterplot (Coulter STKS), WBC scattergram (Sysmex NE-8000), peroxidase cytogram (Technicon H*1), and basophil/lobularity cytogram (Technicon H*1) will detect the presence of these abnormal cells. The WBC scatterplot will show an increased number of cells within the lymphocyte region as well as a wide distribution of cells within that region (Fig. 29-32). Suspect flags will be generated alerting the clinical laboratory scientist to the possibility of atypical lymphocytes or blasts. In the WBC scattergram, the atypical lymphocytes will be located within the lymphocyte region, not the monocyte region, due to automatic discrimination (Fig. 29-33). The peroxidase cytogram will show an increased number of large unstained cells (LUCs), which are flagged as atypical lymphocytes (Fig. 29-34). Some atypical lymphocytes are in active mitosis and have swollen or enlarged nuclei. In the basophil/lobularity cytogram, these cycling cells are observed as a stream of dots extending from the mononuclear cell cluster and vertically above the basophil threshold (Fig. 29-34). This phenomenon results in a falsely increased basophil count. Atypical lymphocytes are distinguished from blasts based on their location within the basophil/lobularity cytogram. Blasts fall in a lower channel (channel 8) than atypical lymphocytes (Fig. 29-36).

ACUTE LYMPHOBLASTIC LEUKEMIA

Acute lymphoblastic leukemia may be detected in the peripheral blood by the presence of lymphoblasts. In the Coulter WBC scatterplot, lymphoblasts are indicated by an increased number of cells within the lymphocyte region and a wider distribution of cells within the region (Fig. 29-35). In the Technicon H*1 peroxidase cytogram, this will be evident by the presence of increased cells within the LUC population and a cluster of blasts within the lymphocyte "box" (Fig. 29-36). The abnormal cell population will be in a parallel line to the y-axis of the cytogram since

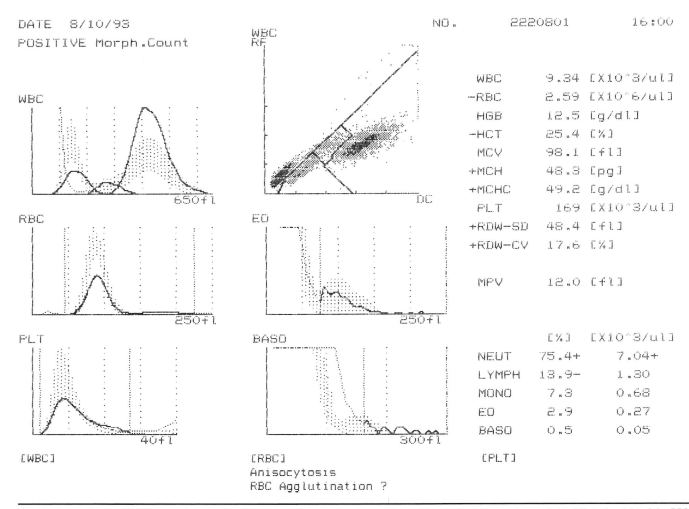

FIGURE 29-28. Sysmex NE-8000 report illustrating changes associated with cold agglutinins. Observe the broad peak and slight shift to the right of the RBC population representing the agglutinated erythrocytes. (Courtesy of Dora Mae Parker, MS, MT(ASCP), Baylor University Medical Center, Dallas, TX.)

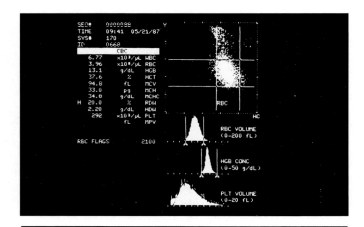

FIGURE 29-29. Technicon H*1 report illustrating changes associated with cold agglutinins. The agglutinated erythrocytes are located within the macrocytic normochromic region above the normal erythrocyte population. (From Simson, E., Ross, D.W., Kocher, W.D.: Atlas of Automated Cytochemical Hematology. Tarrytown, NY, Technicon Instruments Corp., 1988, with permission.)

lymphoblasts do not contain peroxidase. The basophil/lobularity cytogram also will provide evidence of the presence of blasts. The presence of blasts is indicated by a cluster of cells extending as a vertical band from the mononuclear cell cluster into the basophil region (Fig. 29-36). Suspect flags are generated indicating the presence of blasts or atypical lymphocytes.

ACUTE MYELOMONOCYTIC LEUKEMIA

Acute myelomonocytic leukemia is characterized by the involvement of the myeloid cell line and monocytic cell line. Myeloblasts, monoblasts, and various myeloid and monocytic precursors may be detected in the peripheral blood. The WBC scatterplot (Coulter STKS), WBC scattergram (Sysmex NE-8000), and WBC cytograms (Technicon H*1) will reflect this diversity. The Coulter STKS WBC scatterplot would show the majority of cells within the monocyte region. There would be an extension of cells from the lymphocyte region into the monocyte region representing the blasts, monocytic cells, and immature myelocytes. In the Technicon H*1 WBC peroxidase cytogram, the abnormal cell population appears almost parallel to

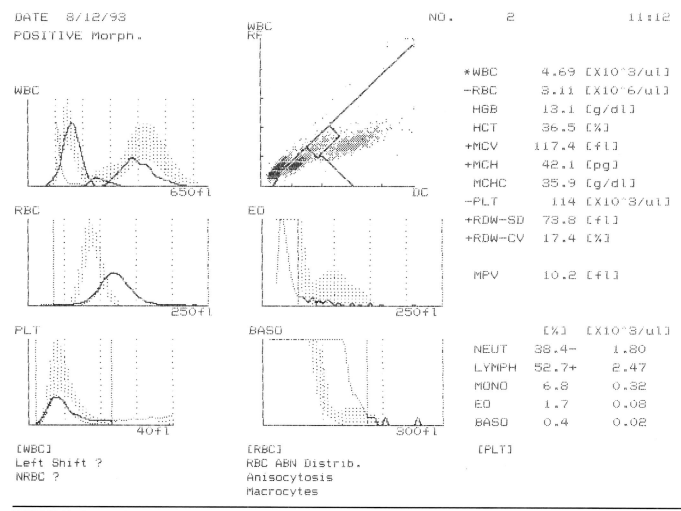

DATE 8/12/93   NO.   2   11:12
POSITIVE Morph.

*WBC	4.69	[X10^3/ul]
—RBC	3.11	[X10^6/ul]
HGB	13.1	[g/dl]
HCT	36.5	[%]
+MCV	117.4	[fl]
+MCH	42.1	[pg]
MCHC	35.9	[g/dl]
—PLT	114	[X10^3/ul]
+RDW-SD	73.8	[fl]
+RDW-CV	17.4	[%]
MPV	10.2	[fl]

	[%]	[X10^3/ul]
NEUT	38.4—	1.80
LYMPH	52.7+	2.47
MONO	6.8	0.32
EO	1.7	0.08
BASO	0.4	0.02

[WBC]
Left Shift ?
NRBC ?

[RBC]
RBC ABN Distrib.
Anisocytosis
Macrocytes

[PLT]

FIGURE 29-30. Sysmex NE-8000 report illustrating changes associated with the presence of nucleated erythrocytes. The nucleated erythrocytes are located below the lymphocyte population and to the right of the RBC population obscuring the discriminator line. (Courtesy of Dora Mae Parker, MS, MT(ASCP), Baylor University Medical Center, Dallas, TX.)

the x-axis beginning in the lymphocyte region and spreading into the LUC, monocyte, and neutrophil regions (Fig. 29-37). This pattern reflects the peroxidase positivity of the myeloblasts and monoblasts. In the basophil/lobularity cytogram, the malignant cell population reshapes the worm (Fig. 29-37). The head region becomes less compact, and there is a wide distribution of cells within the tail region extending into the basophil region (butterfly pattern).

CHRONIC MYELOCYTIC LEUKEMIA

Leukocytosis with immature myeloid cells and an absolute basophilia is observed in chronic myelocytic leukemia (CML). The WBC scatterplots (Coulter STKS), scattergrams (Sysmex NE-8000), and cytograms (Technicon H*1) will reflect this change in cell populations. In the WBC scatterplot, the majority of cells will be in the neutrophil region. The presence of the immature myeloid cells will be observed in the upper area of the neutrophil region

(Fig. 29-38). Observation of the DF3 scatterplot would reveal the increased number of basophils (Fig. 29-8). The peroxidase cytogram shows the cells spreading in a broad band diagonally across the cytogram (Fig. 29-39). The basophil/lobularity cytogram is classic for CML with a spray of cells extending from the head and body of the worm into the basophil region (Fig. 29-39). This represents the actively mitotic cells of CML.

CHRONIC LYMPHOCYTIC LEUKEMIA

In chronic lymphocytic leukemia, there is an absolute lymphocytosis. This absolute lymphocytosis will be observed in the WBC scatterplot (Coulter STKS), WBC scattergram (Sysmex NE-8000), and WBC cytograms (Technicon H*1). The WBC scatterplot shows the malignant population as a cluster of cells within the lymphocyte region (Fig. 29-40). In the WBC scattergram, the malignant cell population will be observed in the lymphocyte region, but falling below the normal lymphocyte population area (Fig. 29-41). This would indicate a smaller cell with a mature

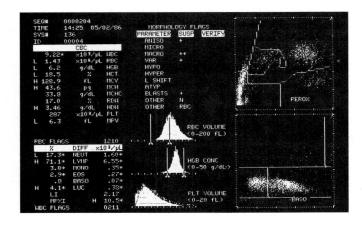

FIGURE 29-31. Technicon H*1 report illustrating the changes associated with the presence of nucleated erythrocytes in a case of hemolytic disease of the newborn. In the WBC peroxidase cytogram, the nucleated erythrocytes are located in a parallel line of cells from the debri region into the lymphocyte region. In the basophil/lobularity cytogram, the nucleated erythrocytes fall in the belly of the worm below the normal cell population. (From Simson, E., Ross, D.W., Kocher, W.D.: Atlas of Automated Cytochemical Hematology. Tarrytown, NY: Technicon Instruments Corp., 1988, with permission.)

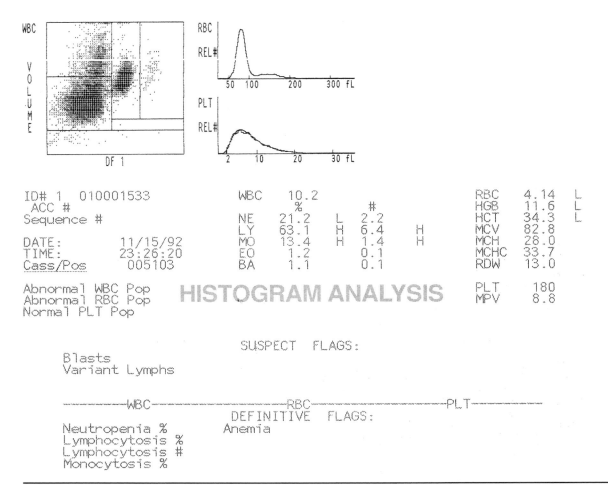

FIGURE 29-32. Coulter STKS report illustrating changes associated with infectious mononucleosis. The presence of atypical lymphocytes is indicated by the wide distribution of cells within the lymphocyte region. (Courtesy of Linda Nash, MT(ASCP), Southwest Texas Methodist Hospital, San Antonio, TX.)

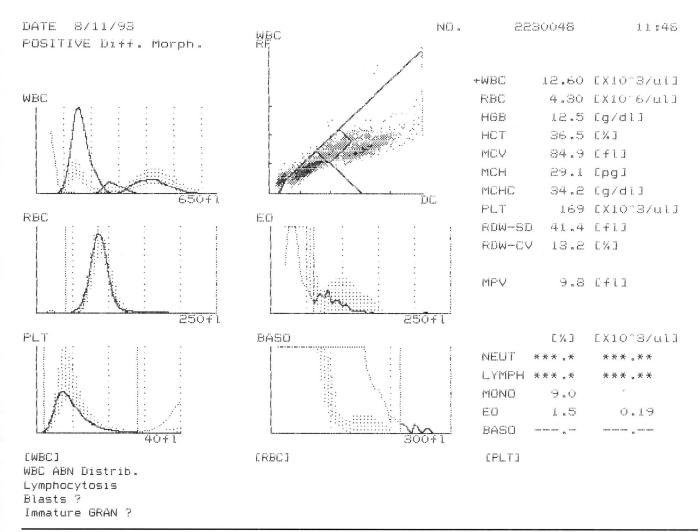

FIGURE 29-33. Sysmex NE-8000 report illustrating changes associated with Infectious mononucleosis. Note the expansion of the lymphocyte population. The atypical lymphocytes are located within the upper portion of the lymphocyte region. (Courtesy of Dora Mae Parker, MS, MT(ASCP), Baylor University Medical Center, Dallas, TX.)

condensed nucleus. The WBC peroxidase cytogram will have a similar pattern (Fig. 29-42). The basophil/lobularity cytogram will show the majority of cells within the head region of the worm with some cells spraying into the basophil region reflecting malignant cells in active mitosis (Fig. 29-42).

MYELOPEROXIDASE DEFICIENCY

Since the Technicon H*1 uses peroxidase activity in its differentiation of white blood cell types, the presence of neutrophil myeloperoxidase deficiency can be detected by this instrument. The cytogram patterns for this deficiency are distinctive. The peroxidase cytogram shows no neutrophil cluster; however, the basophil/lobularity cytogram shows the normal pattern of lymphocyte and neutrophil clusters (Fig. 29-43).

PLATELET CLUMPING

Observation of the WBC scatterplot (Coulter STKS), WBC scattergram (Sysmex NE-8000), and WBC cytograms (Technicon H*1) will indicate the presence of platelet clumps. The platelet clumps will appear in the debri region of DF1 scatterplot (Fig. 29-6). With the Sysmex NE-8000, the platelet clumps will appear above the discriminator line in the WBC scattergram (Fig. 29-44). Therefore, there is little interference with the WBC count. In the WBC peroxidase cytogram, the platelet clumps will be represented by interference, which rises from the debri region into the lymphocyte and monocyte region (Fig. 29-45). The basophil/lobularity cytogram will be unaffected. For each instrument, a suspect flag indicating the presence of platelet clumps will be generated.

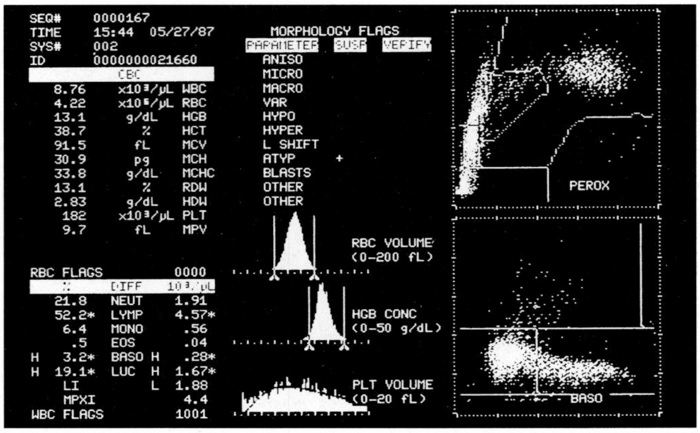

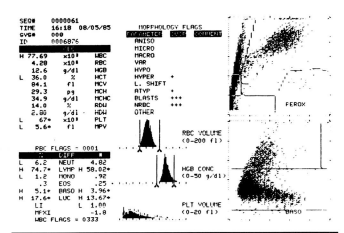

FIGURE 29-34. Technicon H*1 report illustrating changes associated with infectious mononucleosis. In the WBC peroxidase cytogram, atypical lymphocytes are located in the large unstained cell region. Atypical lymphocytes are also detected in the basophil/lobularity cytogram. Observe the stream of cells extending above the head of the "worm." (From Simson, E., Ross, D.W., Kocher, W.D.: Atlas of Automated Cytochemical Hematology. Tarrytown, NY, Technicon Instruments Corp., 1988, with permission.)

FIGURE 29-36. Technicon H*1 report illustrating changes associated with L1 acute lymphoblastic leukemia. In the WBC peroxidase cytogram, lymphoblasts extend in a parallel line of cells extending from the lymphocyte region into the large unstained cell (LUC) region. In the basophil/lobularity cytogram, a cluster of lymphoblasts extends above the mononuclear region into the basophil region. (From Proceedings of Technicon H*1 Hematology Symposium. Tarrytown, NY, Technicon Instruments Corp., October 11, 1985, with permission.)

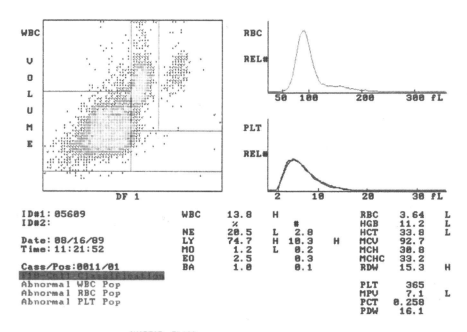

FIGURE 29-35. Coulter STKS report illustrating changes associated with L1 acute lymphoblastic leukemia. The presence of lymphoblasts is indicated by the increased number of cells within the lymphocyte region and their wide distribution. Note the cluster is shifted to the right. (Courtesy of Coulter Electronics, Inc., Hialeah, FL.)

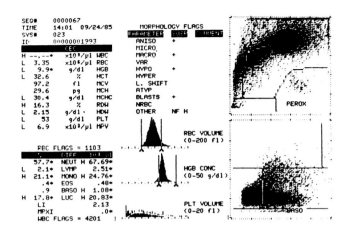

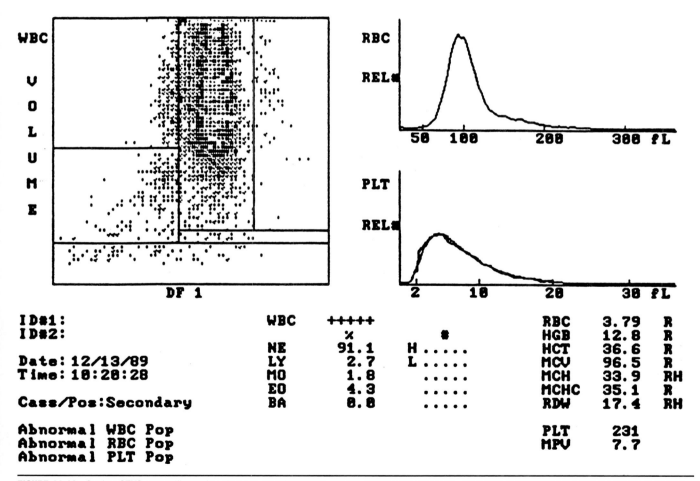

FIGURE 29-37. Technicon H*1 report illustrating changes associated with acute myelomonocytic (M4) leukemia. In the WBC peroxidase cytogram, the presence of myeloblasts and monoblasts is indicated by the abnormal cell population which extends from the upper lymphocyte region into the large unstained cell region, monocyte region, and neutrophil region. In the basophil/lobularity cytogram, the presence of myeloblasts and monoblasts is indicated by a "butterfly" pattern extending from the tail region into the basophil region. (From Proceedings of Technicon H*1 Hematology Symposium. Tarrytown, NY, Technicon Instruments Corp., October 11, 1985, with permission.)

FIGURE 29-38. Coulter STKS report illustrating changes associated with chronic granulocytic leukemia. Immature neutrophils are indicated by the extension of the cells into the upper neutrophil region. (From Rappaport, E.S., Helbert, B.J.: Three Dimensional Leukocyte Imaging. Scott & White Clinic and Texas A&M University College of Medicine, Temple, TX, with permission.)

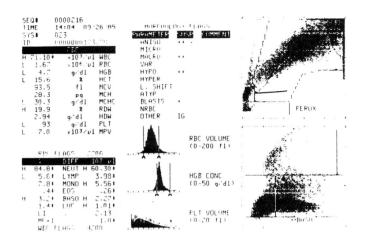

FIGURE 29-39. Technicon H*1 report illustrating changes associated with chronic myelocytic leukemia. The presence of all stages of neutrophil maturation is indicated by the broad band of cells which extends diagonally across cytogram. In the basophil/lobularity cytogram there is a spray of cells extending from the head and body of the worm into the basophil region. (From Proceedings of Technicon H*1 Hematology Symposium. Tarrytown, NY, Technicon Instruments Corp., October 11, 1985, with permission.

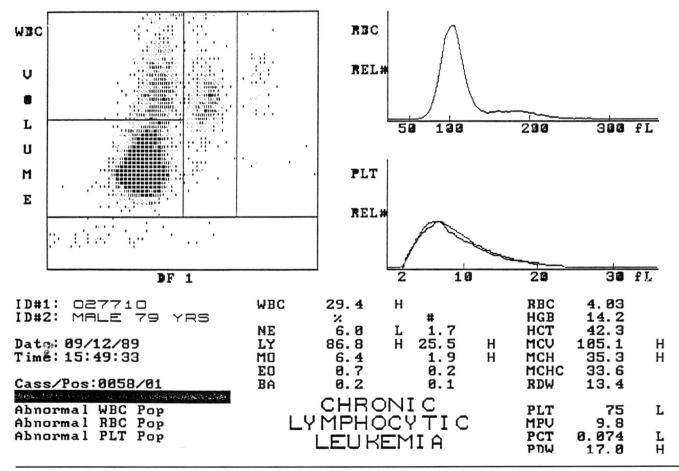

FIGURE 29-40. Coulter STKS report illustrating the changes associated with chronic lymphocytic leukemia. Malignant lymphocytes are located in a tight cluster within the lymphocyte region. (Courtesy of Coulter Electronics, Inc., Hialeah, FL.)

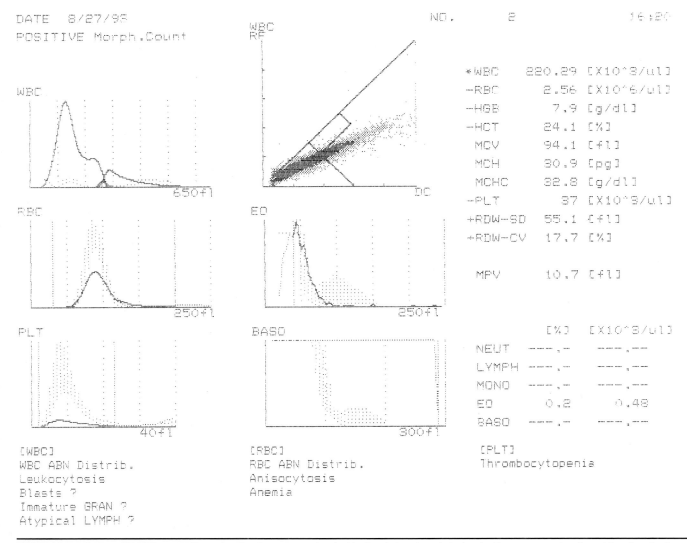

FIGURE 29-41. Sysmex NE-8000 report illustrating the changes associated with chronic lymphocytic leukemia. The presence of malignant lymphocytes is indicated by a downward shift in the lymphocyte cluster. This extended band of cells is typical of CLL. (Courtesy of Dora Mae Parker, MS, MT(ASCP), Baylor University Medical Center, Dallas, TX.)

AUTOMATED COAGULATION INSTRUMENTS

Introduction

Instrumentation was actually introduced into coagulation testing in the early 20th century. These first instruments, like the majority of instruments used today, analyzed the coagulation system through the detection of clot formation. The coaguloviscometer developed by Kottman in 1910 determined clotting times by measuring the change in blood viscosity as it clotted. The change in viscosity was determined by plotting the voltage against time. A second method of clot detection was introduced by Kugelmass in 1922. He adapted the nephelometer to coagulation testing. In nephelometry, the clotting time was determined by measuring variations in transillumination as registered by a galvanometer. The photoelectric technique

for the determination of clotting times was introduced by Baldes and Nygaard in 1936. With their instrument, clotting times were determined by the measurement of increasing optical density as the plasma clotted. Coagulation instrumentation continued to improve and by the 1960s semiautomated coagulation instruments began to replace manual coagulation techniques in the clinical laboratory. These first instruments were based on electromechanical methods or optical density methods of clot detection. The 1970s saw an evolvement in coagulation testing with the introduction of fully-automated instruments capable of performing multiple coagulation assays.

With the new directions in coagulation testing including chromogenic and immunologic methods, newer coagulation instruments are capable of performing these test methods and the clot-based tests. The introduction of instrumentation into coagulation testing has led to increased

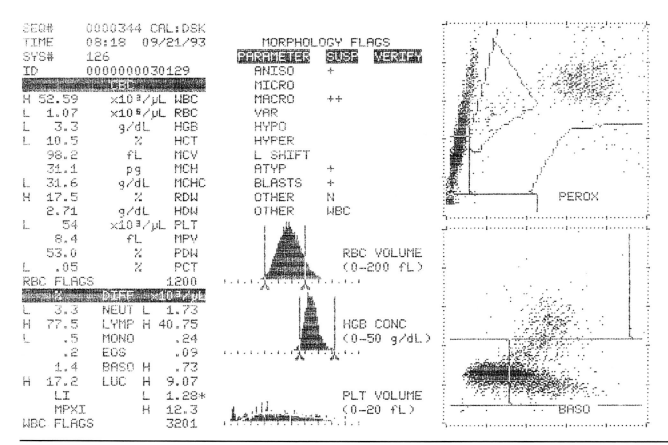

FIGURE 29-42. Technicon H*1 report illustrating the changes associated with chronic lymphocytic leukemia. In the WBC peroxidase cytogram, the malignant lymphocytes are located in a cluster within the lymphocyte region and extending into the LUC region. In the basophil/lobularity cytogram, malignant lymphocytes are located in the head of the "worm" with some cells spraying into the basophil region.

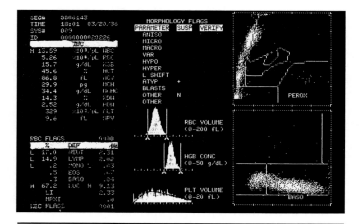

FIGURE 29-43. Technicon H*1 report illustrating the changes associated with myeloperoxidase deficiency. Observe the absence of a neutrophil cluster in the WBC peroxidase cytogram, but the presence of a normal pattern of neutrophil and lymphocyte clusters in the basophil/lobularity cytogram. (From Simson, E., Ross, D.W., Kocher, W.D.: Atlas of Automated Cytochemical Hematology. Tarrytown, NY, Technicon Instruments Corp., 1988, with permission.)

precision and accuracy and, therefore, improved diagnostic testing and monitoring of therapeutic interventions.

The two principles of clot-based detection currently used by coagulation instruments are electromechanical and optical density. This section will review these principles and how they have been adapted to several coagulation instruments, which may be seen in the clinical laboratory. Other available instruments use a combination of these principles.

Electromechanical instruments

BBL FIBROSYSTEM

The FibroSystem, a semiautomated coagulation instrument, was introduced in the 1960s. This system is composed of a Fibrometer coagulation timer (Fig. 29-46), thermal prep block to prewarm reagents and samples to 37° C, and an automatic pipet to deliver the appropriate amount of sample or reagent to the test cuvet. The Fibrometer probe, which is an integral part of the Fibrometer coagulation timer, serves as the clot detector. The probe consists of two sensory electrodes (stationary and moving) and a probe foot, which is an extension of the moving electrode extending beyond the base of the probe assembly

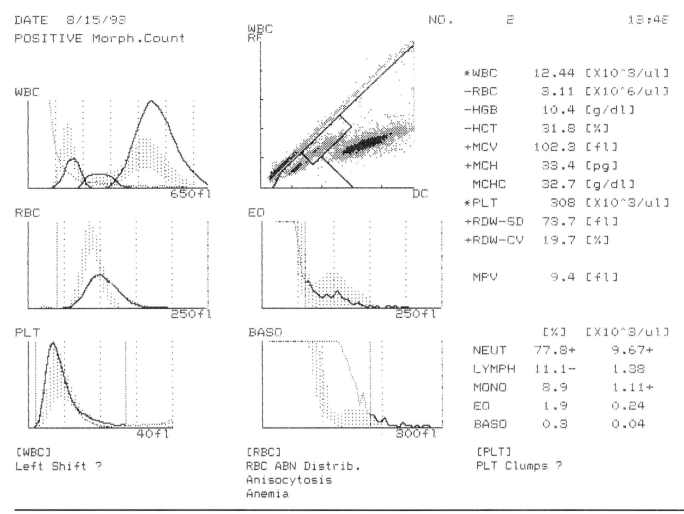

DATE 8/15/93
POSITIVE Morph.Count

NO.   2   13:46

*WBC	12.44	[X10^3/ul]
-RBC	3.11	[X10^6/ul]
-HGB	10.4	[g/dl]
-HCT	31.8	[%]
+MCV	102.3	[fl]
+MCH	33.4	[pg]
MCHC	32.7	[g/dl]
*PLT	308	[X10^3/ul]
+RDW-SD	73.7	[fl]
+RDW-CV	19.7	[%]
MPV	9.4	[fl]

	[%]	[X10^3/ul]
NEUT	77.8+	9.67+
LYMPH	11.1-	1.38
MONO	8.9	1.11+
EO	1.9	0.24
BASO	0.3	0.04

[WBC]
Left Shift ?

[RBC]
RBC ABN Distrib.
Anisocytosis
Anemia

[PLT]
PLT Clumps ?

FIGURE 29-44. Sysmex NE-8000 report illustrating the changes associated with platelet clumping. Observe the stream of platelet clumps along the discriminator line. (Courtesy of Dora Mae Parker, MS, MT(ASCP), Baylor University Medical Center, Dallas, TX.)

(Fig. 29-47). In the timing sequence, the moving electrode cycles through the reaction mixture in an elliptical pattern created by the raising and lowering of the probe foot. The stationary electrode remains in the reaction mixture and is responsible for establishing the electric potential between the two electrodes. The moving electrode becomes electrically active when it is above the reaction mixture. As the fibrin clot is formed, it is picked up by the small hook on the tip of the moving electrode. The electric circuit is completed when the moving electrode becomes activated as it moves out of the reaction mixture; current flows from the stationary electrode through the reaction mixture and fibrin clot to the moving electrode. The creation of this electric circuit causes the timing device to stop and the clotting time in seconds is recorded. Thus, the principle of clot detection is the electromechanical principle.[24–27] An advantage of the FibroSystem is that it can be adapted to any coagulation assay that is clot-based.

AMERICAN BIOPRODUCTS ST-4 CLOT DETECTION INSTRUMENT

The ST-4 Clot Detection instrument is a semiautomated instrument for coagulation testing that is based on the electromechanical clot detection principle. This is a stand-alone instrument consisting of a 16-position incubator with four separate incubation channels and timers, a dispensing pipet, room temperature and 37° C-thermostated reagent storage wells, four separate sample analysis wells, and a microprocessor system. This variation of the electromechanical clot detection principle is based on the increasing viscosity of plasma as clot formation occurs.[28,29] The increasing viscosity is detected by the movement of an iron ball located at the bottom of the reaction cuvet. A constant pendular swing of the ball is created by alternating an electromagnetic field on opposite sides of the cuvet using two independent driving coils. As clot formation begins, the plasma viscosity increases and there is a corresponding decrease in ball movement. The clotting time is determined from an algorithm of the variations in oscillation ampli-

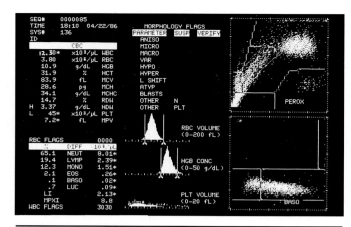

```
SEQ#    0000085
TIME   18:10  04/22/86          MORPHOLOGY FLAGS
SYS#   136                    PARAMETER  SUSP  VERIFY
ID                             ANISO
          CBC                  MICRO
   12.30*  x10³/µL  WBC        MACRO
    3.80   x10⁶/µL  RBC        VAR
   10.9    g/dL     HGB        HYPO
   31.9    %        HCT        HYPER
   83.9    fL       MCV        L SHIFT
   28.6    pg       MCH        ATYP
   34.1    g/dL     MCHC       BLASTS
   14.7    %        RDW        OTHER    N
 H  3.37   g/dL     HDW        OTHER    PLT
 L    45*  x10³/µL  PLT
    7.2*   fL       MPV
                                        RBC VOLUME
                                        (0-200 fL)
 RBC FLAGS          0000
        .   DIFF    10³/µL
   65.1   NEUT    8.01*
   19.4   LYMP    2.39*                 HGB CONC
   12.3   MONO    1.51*                 (0-50 g/dL)
    2.1   EOS      .26*
     .1   BASO     .02*
     .7   LUC      .09*
        LI        2.13*
        MPXI      8.8                    PLT VOLUME
 WBC FLAGS         3030                  (0-20 fL)
```
PEROX
BASO

FIGURE 29-45. Technicon H*1 report illustrating the changes associated with platelet clumping. The platelet clumps are indicated by interference extending from the debri region into the lymphocyte and monocyte regions. (From Simson, E., Ross, D.W., Kocher, W.D.: Atlas of Automated Cytochemical Hematology. Tarrytown, NY, Technicon Instruments Corp., 1988, with permission.)

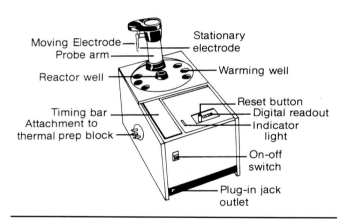

FIGURE 29-46. Fibrometer. (From Brown, B.A.: Hematology: Principles and Procedures, 6th Ed. Philadelphia, Lea & Febiger, 1993, with permission.)

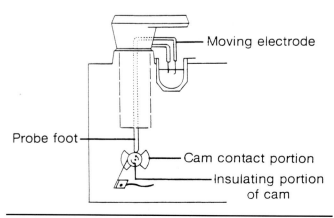

FIGURE 29-47. Fibrometer Probe. (From Brown, B.A.: Hematology: Principles and Procedures, 6th Ed. Philadelphia, Lea & Febiger, 1993).

tude. Clotting time results are displayed on the liquid crystal display screen and printed results are obtained from the thermal printer. This instrument can be adapted to any coagulation assay, which is clot-based.

Optical density instruments

MLA ELECTRA 900

The MLA Electra 900 is an automated coagulation instrument capable of performing multiple test assays by random access. It is a stand-alone instrument consisting of a cuvet transport system, computer system with display monitor and keypad, reagent storage system, and reagent heater system. This instrument relies on manual sampling of the patient specimen but automatic sampling of the reagents. The test procedure to be performed is programmed by the specific colored reaction cuvet (e.g., pink cuvets for PT and blue cuvets for APTT). The movement of a reagent from its refrigerated storage reservoir, through a heating trough, and into the reaction cuvet is accomplished by the action of a peristaltic pump. The cuvet transport system moves the reaction cuvet into position for monitoring by a photodetector. The addition of the final prewarmed reagent initiates the timer. As fibrin clot formation begins, the amount of light detected by the photodetector decreases, causing a change in the electrical signal output from the detector. The electrical signal is analyzed by the computer to determine the clotting time.[30] Four optical channels are present, allowing for simultaneous analysis of as many as four reaction cuvets. Test assays that can be performed on this instrument include PT, APTT, TT, fibrinogen, and factor assays, as well as user-defined clotting assays. In addition, an estimate of the fibrinogen concentration can be derived from the PT clotting curve. The fibrinogen concentration is calculated from the change in optical density (Δ OD) over a period of 100 seconds.[30] A hardcopy printout of the results, temperature status, error messages, and standard curves is obtained from the thermal printer.

ORGANON TEKNIKA COAG-A-MATE X2

The Coag-A-Mate X2 is an automated instrument using the change in optical density that occurs with clot formation as its principle of clot detection.[26,31] The instrument consists of a refrigerated reagent storage system, reagent heater system, incubation test plate, photodetection system, and microprocessing system. The clinical laboratory scientist manually places the specimens for APTT testing into the outer channel cuvets of the testing tray and specimens for PT testing into the inner channel cuvets. The test procedures are programmed using the touch entry keypad. The test tray is placed on the incubation test plate to maintain the samples at a cool temperature before testing. To assure correct test procedures are performed, the station number displayed by the station number indicator must correspond to the cuvet number of the first sample to be tested. Reagents are prewarmed as they pass through the reagent incubator arm and are dispensed into the appropriate test cuvet. Four test cuvets enter the heating zone at one time. The reaction mixture is warmed to 37° C. The addition of the final reagent to the test cuvet initiates the timer. The photoelectric cell detects the sudden change in optical density occurring with fibrin formation, and the timer is stopped.[31]

The results are printed on printer tape. This instrument is capable of performing two tests simultaneously: two different tests or two like tests in duplicate or four like tests performed singularly. This instrument is capable of performing the majority of clot-based coagulation assays.

ORTHO DIAGNOSTIC SYSTEMS KOAGULAB 60-S

The KoaguLab 60-S and KoaguLab 60-S Autoloader combine to produce a fully-automated coagulation system. The Koagulab 60-S is composed of a message display panel, membrane keypanel, four reagent wells, four peristaltic reagent pumps, a reagent arm, sample carousel with four photodetectors, and a thermal printer. The centrifuged patient samples are placed into the autoloader's sample carousel, and the test procedures to be performed on each sample are programmed into the autoloader via the autoloader keypad or the barcode reader. Optionally, the test information can be directed from the Koagulab 60-S computer. The patient samples are then pipeted into a disposable cuvet tray. The autoloader is capable of performing sample dilutions for fibrinogen assays or factor assays. The sample probe is rinsed with distilled water between each specimen. When the sample pipeting is complete, the disposable cuvet tray is placed within the sample carousel of the Koagulab 60-S. The testing cycle is initiated by pressing RUN. After the appropriate incubation period, the first four test cuvets will reach the test area. The refrigerated reagents are prewarmed to 37.5° C as they pass through the reagent arm before being dispensed into the test cuvets. With the addition of the final reagent into the test cuvet, the timing mechanism is initiated. A photodetector cell detects the change in optical density as clot formation occurs and the timer is stopped. Four test cuvets can be measured simultaneously. Clot formation is monitored during the entire reaction providing a graphic representation of the reaction's turbidity versus the reaction time for any assay being performed.[26,32] This graphic representation is referred to as the clot signature or clotting curve. The clot signature of the prothrombin time can be used to give a qualitative fibrinogen measurement. Clot signatures may become a valuable visual tool allowing for the identification of patients with abnormally low fibrinogen values and alerting the laboratory that a quantitative fibrinogen determination may be appropriate.[33] The majority of clot-based coagulation assays can be performed on this instrument.

●
Chromogenic/clot detection instruments

Several coagulation instrument manufacturers currently market coagulation instruments that combine the traditional clot-based detection principle with chromogenic analysis.

Since the coagulation cascade is a series of enzymatic reactions catalyzed by serine proteases, the activity of these enzymes can be measured by conventional clinical chemistry methods. Chromogenic analysis is an example of a clinical chemistry methodology that has been adapted to coagulation testing. In a chromogenic analysis, the enzyme of interest (activated coagulation factor) cleaves the chromogenic substrate at a specific site releasing the chromophore tag. The color intensity is measured spectrophotometrically and is proportional to the concentration of the enzyme. Through the choice of substrates used in a specific assay, chromogenic assays can be used for the testing of individual coagulation proteins, biochemical inhibitors, and fibrinolytic proteins. In addition to coagulation instruments, chromogenic assays have been adapted for use on a number of spectrophotometric chemistry analyzers.

MLA ELECTRA 1000C

The MLA Electra 1000C is a fully-automated coagulation instrument consisting of two units, an MLA Electra 900C and an automatic primary tube sampler. The instrument is capable of performing clot-based assays and chromogenic assays.[26,34] The clot-based assays are performed in the same manner as the MLA Electra 900 with the addition of automatic patient sampling. To perform chromogenic assays, the reagents and reagent tubing must be changed. The instrument is programmed to perform the specific chromogenic assay using the test selection mode. The automatic primary tube sampler dispenses the appropriate amount of patient sample into the reaction cuvet and places the cuvet on the cuvet transport belt. When the reaction cuvet reaches the test station, reagent is added through the action of the peristaltic pump. A photodetector monitors the rate of change in optical density as the colored product is formed. The reaction between the reagent substrate and the analyte releases the chromophore paranitroaniline, which is measured at 405 nm. The instrument takes a series of OD readings and determines the linearity of the data and the change in absorbance per minute. This absorbance change is compared with the reference calibration curve programmed into the instrument by the laboratory. The final result is determined from this curve and is reported in the appropriate units. A hard copy printout of the results, temperature status, error messages, and standard curve is obtained from the thermal printer.

INSTRUMENTATION LABORATORY ACL 3000

The ACL 3000 is a fully-automated, centrifugal coagulation instrument capable of performing clot-based assays and chromogenic assays.[26,35] The instrument is programmed to perform the specific test assays on each patient specimen through the test selection mode. The patient specimens are loaded into the sample tray. The pipeting of samples and reagents is performed by the arm assembly. Samples and reagents are pipeted into the reaction cuvets of a disposable rotor. Initially, the sample and reagents are separated by a dividing ridge. When all reagents and samples are pipeted into the rotor, the rotor spins at a speed of 1200 rpm, and the reaction temperature is stabilized at 38.5° C. The centrifugal movement forces

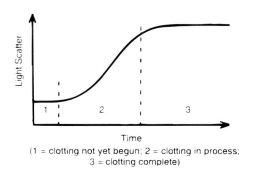

FIGURE 29-48. Normal clotting curve, ACL 3000. (From Brown, B.A.: Hematology: Principles and Procedures, 6th Ed. Philadelphia, Lea & Febiger, 1993).

the samples and reagents together in the outer well of the reaction cuvet. The centrifuge stops abruptly, resulting in a homogeneous reaction mixture. The rotor spins again for a specified time period, and the monitoring of the assay's reaction occurs.

The measuring system for the clot-based assays is nephelometry.[26,35] In nephelometry, the photodetector measures light scattered at right-angles (90°) to the light path. Before fibrin clot formation, the amount of light scatter will be low because of the presence of finely dispersed particles. With fibrin clot formation, larger particles will be seen, and the amount of light scatter will increase. The clotting time is determined from the clotting curve (Fig. 29-48). In addition, the fibrinogen concentration can be determined from the prothrombin time clotting curve, and the observation of all clotting curves can be used for the detection of problems.[26,36]

The measuring system for chromogenic assays is photometry. The final enzymatic reaction in the chromogenic assays yields paranitroaniline. The photodetector cell monitors the change in optical density over the reaction period. A clotting curve created by plotting the change in optical density against time is compared with the appropriate calibration curve. The patient results are calculated from this comparison and are reported in the appropriate units.

FLOW CYTOMETRY

Introduction

Flow cytometry was introduced to the clinical laboratory in the 1980s. The evolution of flow cytometry occurred as a result of the development of monoclonal antibodies in the 1970s. Flow cytometric instruments were available before that time but had limited application in the clinical laboratory. Monoclonal antibodies conjugated with a fluorescent tag allow for the study of a cell's physical and biological properties. The information obtained through flow cytometric analysis has improved the ability to diagnose certain disease states, stage these disease states, and monitor their therapeutic interventions.[37–39]

This section will review the basic principles of flow cytometry and its clinical applications.

Basic principles of flow cytometry

Flow cytometry is the analysis of cellular characteristics as the cells pass singly in a fluid suspension through a beam of light.[40–43] The scattered light and fluorescence intensity is measured by a set of photodiodes. The data collected by these photodiodes are transmitted to the computer for further processing and data output. The basic components of a flow cytometer are the fluid system, the optical system, the signal detector system, and the data management system.

The fluid system is responsible for the movement of the sample through the flow chamber from sample aspiration to sample waste disposal. Through hydrodynamic focusing, a single cell suspension is created within the sheath fluid. As the sample is aspirated, a pressure differential between the sample flow and sheath fluid flow creates a central sample stream surrounded by sheath fluid (laminar flow) and prevents the mixing of sample with sheath fluid (Fig. 29-49). The cells pass through the laser beam single file at a rate of approximately 5000 cells per second.

In the clinical laboratory, the most commonly used light source for flow cytometry is the argon-ion laser. The important characteristics of laser light are high radiance, stability, and spectral purity. The advantage of laser light is the ability to focus the monochromatic light beam to an area equal to the dimensions of the cell.[41–43] The focusing of the laser is accomplished by a series of beam-shaping lenses (Fig. 29-50).

As the cell passes through the laser beam, the cell scatters light and fluorochromes absorb light and re-emit it at a different wavelength (fluoresence). The light is scattered at different angles. Forward (low angle) scatter defines the cell size, and side (90° angle) scatter defines cell granularity or nuclear structure. Fluorescence intensity is proportional to the amount of fluorochrome present on or in the cell.

The collection of the scattered light and fluorescent emission is accomplished through a set of interference filters and/or dichroic mirrors, which direct the light to photodiodes and photomultiplier tubes (Fig. 29-50). Photodiodes change light photons into electronic signals, which are proportional to the amount of light photons detected. Photomultiplier tubes (PMT) are useful in the collection and amplification of the weaker side scatter light and fluorescent emissions.[40,41] The flow cytometer will have a forward scatter detector, side scatter detector, and fluorescence detector. The number of fluorescence detectors will depend on the number of different wavelengths to be detected. The majority of flow cytometers used in the clinical laboratory are capable of either two-color or three-color analysis. A list of common fluorochromes used in clinical flow cytometry are found in Table 29-1.

The signal processing electronic component converts the electronic signals into voltage pulses and processes the pulses to eliminate background and/or stray noise. The peak voltages for each analyzed cell are sent to the data

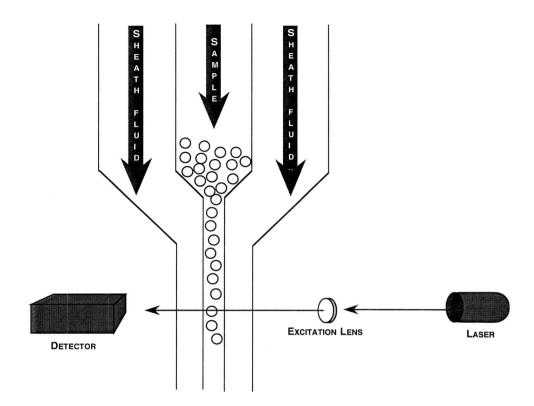

FIGURE 29-49. Flow chamber illustrating hydrodynamic focusing.

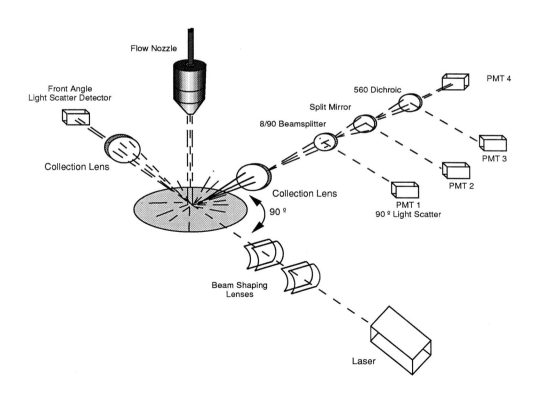

FIGURE 29-50. Schematic drawing of flow cytometer.

TABLE 29-1 *COMMON FLUOROCHROMES UTILIZED IN CLINICAL FLOW CYTOMETRY*

Fluorochrome	Absorbance (nm)	Emission (nm)
Fluorescein isothiocynate (FITC)	488	530
Phycoerythrin (PE)	492	580
Phycoerythrin-Texas Red (PE:TR)	488	620
Peridinin Chlorophyll Protein (PerCP)	488	680
Thiazole orange	488	530
Auramine O	432	533
Propidium iodide (PI)	488	620

management system. The data can be stored by the computer or analyzed through the use of histograms. Specific information about a cell population can be obtained through the use of a two-variable histogram or dot-plot (Fig. 29-51). The cell population can be isolated for analysis by operator-generated electronic gates (Fig. 29-52). Subsequent dot-plots can be built on data within the electronic gates (Fig. 29-53). Through this technique, specific information can be obtained concerning a defined cell population.[40-43]

The flow cytometric instruments used in the clinical laboratory have these basic principles of operation in common. The Becton-Dickinson FACScan instruments and Coulter EPICS instruments are examples of flow cytometers that can be adapted to any number of clinical applications, whereas the TOA Sysmex R-3000, Technicon H*3, and Coulter instruments have limited application. The TOA Sysmex R-1000 and Coulter instruments perform only automated reticulocyte counts. In addition to automated reticulocyte analysis, the Technicon instruments can be adapted to perform lymphocyte immunophenotyping (i.e., T-helper and T-suppressor ratios).

● Clinical applications

LYMPHOCYTE IMMUNOPHENOTYPING
Lymphocyte immunophenotyping was the clinical application that led to flow cytometry's entry into the clinical laboratory. The development of monoclonal antibodies that not only differentiate B-lymphocytes from T-lymphocytes but subclassify T-lymphocytes into their respective effector category (e.g., CD4-helper T-lymphocyte and CD8-suppressor T-lymphocyte) allowed for further investigation and diagnosis of immunodeficiency disorders. Currently, lymphocyte immunophenotyping is used in the diagnosis, staging, and therapeutic intervention of HIV-infected individuals.[37-39]

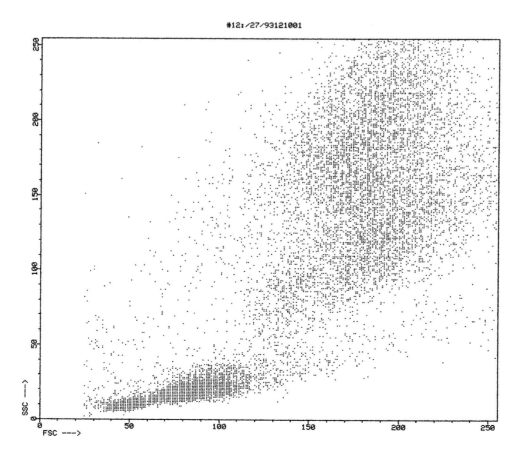

#12:/27/93121001

FIGURE 29-51. Dot-plot histogram of leukocytes (forward scatter vs side scatter). (Courtesy of Linda Nash, MT(ASCP), Southwest Texas Methodist Hospital, San Antonio, TX.)

#12:/27/93121001

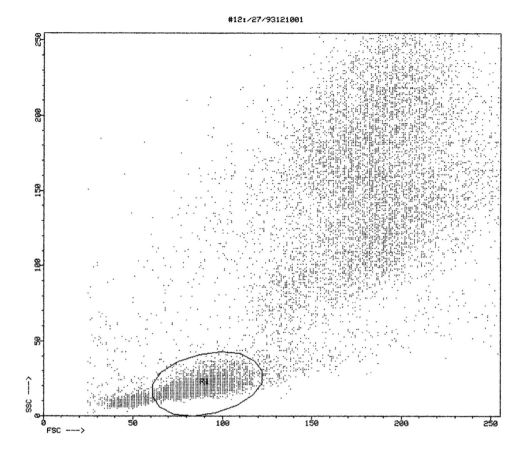

FIGURE 29-52. Dot-plot histogram (Fig. 29-51) with electronic gating of the lymphocyte population (within circle). (Courtesy of Linda Nash, MT(ASCP), Southwest Texas Methodist Hospital, San Antonio, TX.)

LEUKEMIA/LYMPHOMA IMMUNOPHENOTYPING

Lymphocytic leukemias and malignant lymphomas are classified as B, T, or pre-B cell processes using immunophenotyping. Also, immunophenotyping aids in the diagnosis of certain myeloid leukemias, in particular, acute myeloid leukemia with minimal differentiation (AML-MO), acute erythroblastic leukemia (AML-M6), and acute megakaryoblastic leukemia (AML-M7). By immunophenotyping a patient after bone marrow transplantation, one can verify the lack of the malignant process or identify an early relapse of malignancy. The immunophenotyping of malignancy has led to earlier diagnosis, better therapeutic interventions, and improved prognosis.[38]

DNA PLOIDY ANALYSIS

DNA ploidy analysis is useful in the identification of tumor cells. Normal cells are diploid (2N), whereas tumor cells tend to be aneuploid. To determine the DNA content of the cell, the cell nuclei is stained with a fluorescent stain (i.e., propidium iodide). The flow cytometer quantitates the amount of DNA present in each cell and displays it as a histogram. From the histogram, one can determine the ploidy of the tumor cells and if the tumor cells differ from normal cells. The presence of aneuploidy is a reliable indicator of neoplasia. DNA ploidy analysis is useful in

determining the prognosis of the malignancy and monitoring the effectiveness of treatment.[37-39]

RETICULOCYTE ENUMERATION

The enumeration of reticulocytes is used to evaluate the bone marrow's erythropoietic activity. Evaluation of the erythropoietic activity is useful in the differentiation of anemias, the monitoring of a patient's response to therapy, and the assessment of erythropoietic activity after a bone marrow transplant.[37-39] Traditionally, the reticulocyte count has been performed manually using a supravital stain (e.g., new methylene blue). In the reticulocyte enumeration by flow cytometry, a fluorescent dye (e.g., thiazole orange) is used to stain the residual RNA. The flow cytometer analyzes approximately 10,000 cells to determine the reticulocyte percentage as well as the absolute reticulocyte count. Newer instrumentation for flow cytometric analysis of reticulocytes allows the determination of reticulocyte maturity. Reticulocytes with a high fluorescence ratio represent the earliest cells with the most RNA content, and those with a low fluorescence ratio represent the most mature reticulocytes. Reticulocytes with a middle fluorescence ratio are the intermediate reticulocytes. The ability to distinguish the maturity of the reticulocytes will increase the usefulness of flow cytometric reticulocyte analysis in the evaluation

#12:/27/93121004

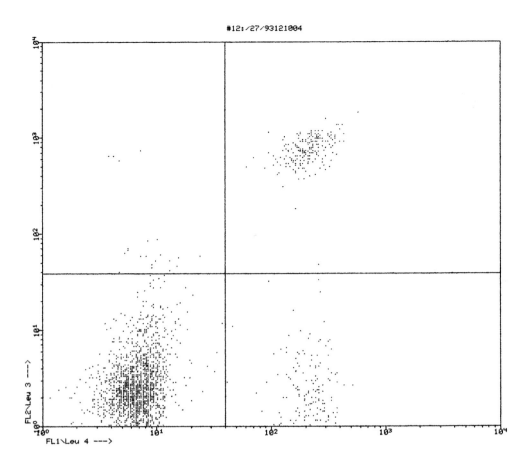

FIGURE 29-53. Dot-plot histogram of gated lymphocyte population (Fig. 29-52) identifying helper T-lymphocytes with Leu4(CD3) and Leu3(CD4) in quadrant 2 in upper right. (Courtesy of Linda Nash, MT(ASCP), Southwest Texas Methodist Hospital, San Antonio, TX.)

of erythropoietic activity. The TOA Sysmex R-3000 is an example of a fully-automated flow cytometer for reticulocyte analysis.

FUTURE APPLICATIONS

With the continuing improvement in flow cytometry instrumentation, the development of new fluorochromes and the increasing number of monoclonal antibodies, additional applications of flow cytometry in the clinical laboratory will be discovered. Already, there is research investigation into the use of flow cytometry in chromosome analysis, platelet assays, cell function assays, and immune complex quantitation.[38,39] Clearly, the future of flow cytometry in the clinical laboratory is bright.

SUMMARY

This chapter has briefly reviewed the ever increasing technology within the automated hematology laboratory. To operate these instruments to their fullest potential, it is important that qualified individuals evaluate the data created by the instrument's analysis of individual cell's characteristics or clotting characteristics. Through careful review of these data, new applications of these instruments may arise that will aid in the early detection of abnormalities. For example, careful review of numerous Technicon

WBC cytograms revealed a new method of detecting myeloperoxidase deficiency, as discussed earlier in this chapter. Automation has increased precision and accuracy within the hematology laboratory and shortened the amount of time needed for analysis, but it has increased the need for the individual's interpretative skills.

REVIEW QUESTIONS

1. Blood cell counting in this instrument is based on optical light scattering:
   a. Coulter S-Plus instrument
   b. Sysmex NE-8000 instrument
   c. Cell-Dyn 3000 instrument
   d. Technicon H*1 instrument

2. What information is needed to create a histogram?
   a. cell volume and relative cell number
   b. cell size and cell complexity
   c. nuclear size and cellular density
   d. cell forward scatter and cell side scatter

3. For the Sysmex NE-8000, which of the following technologies is NOT used in the categorization of leukocyte cell types?
   a. impedence
   b. radio frequency

c. optical light scatter

d. differential cell lysis

4. Using the Technicon H*1 instrument, what leukocyte cell type is located in the body of the worm of the basophil/lobularity cytogram?

a. basophils

b. mononuclear leukocytes

c. polymorphonuclear leukocytes

d. eosinophils

5. If the erythrocyte histogram shows a shift to the right, which of the following erythrocyte abnormalities would be indicated?

a. iron deficiency anemia

b. beta thalassemia minor

c. aplastic anemia

d. megaloblastic anemia

6. In the Technicon H*1 peroxidase cytogram, the presence of cells extending in a parallel line to the y-axis from the lymphocyte region into the LUC region indicates:

a. presence of monocytosis

b. presence of lymphoblasts

c. presence of immature granulocytes

d. presence of agglutinated erythrocytes

7. In the Sysmex NE-8000, the presence of a stream of cells located above the discriminator line indicates:

a. presence of clumped platelets

b. presence of nucleated erythrocytes

c. presence of erythrocyte fragments

d. presence of atypical lymphocytes

8. Which of the following coagulation instruments uses electromechanical detection of clots?

a. MLA Electra 900 instrument

b. ST-4 clot detection instrument

c. Coag-A-Mate X2 instrument

d. ACL 3000 instrument

9. Which of the following fluorochromes is used for DNA ploidy analysis?

a. fluorescein isothiocynate

b. thiazole orange

c. propidium iodide

d. phycoerythrin

10. Which of the following statements concerning flow cytometry is INCORRECT?

a. Fluorescence intensity is proportional to the number of antigenic sites.

b. Side scatter of the laser beam defines the cell's granularity.

c. The data are analyzed through the use of dot-plots.

d. Polyclonal antibodies provide increased specificity for the detection of antigens.

● REFERENCES

1. Mattern, C.F.T., Brackett, F.S., Olson, B.: Determination of number and size of particles by electrical gating: Blood cells. J. Appl. Physiol., 10:56, 1957.

2. Cox, C.J., et al.: Evaluation of the Coulter Counter Model S-Plus IV. Am. J. Clin. Pathol., 84:297, 1985.

3. Griswold, D.J., Champagne, V.D.: Evaluation of the Coulter S-Plus IV three-part differential in an acute care hospital. Am. J. Clin. Pathol., 82:49, 1985.

4. Allen, J.K., Batjer, J.D.: Evaluation of an automated method for leukocyte differential counts based on electronic volume analysis. Arch. Path. Lab. Med., 109:534, 1985.

5. Barnard, D.F., et al.: Detection of important abnormalities of the differential count using the Coulter STKR blood counter. J. Clin. Path., 42:772, 1989.

6. Krause, J.R.: Automated differentials in the hematology laboratory. Am. J. Clin. Pathol., 93:S11, 1990.

7. Coulter Corporation: Coulter STKS Operator's Guide, Hialeah, FL, Coulter Corporation, 1991.

8. Warner, B.A., Reardon, D.M.: A field evaluation of the Coulter STKS. Am. J. Clin. Pathol., 95:207, 1991.

9. Poulsen, K.B., Bell, C.A.: Automated hematology: Comparing and contrasting three systems. Clin. Lab. Sci., 4:16, 1991.

10. Warner, B.A., Reardon, D.M., Marshall, D.P.: Automated hematology analysers: a four-way comparison. Med. Lab. Sci., 47:295, 1990.

11. Swaim, W.R.: Laboratory and clinical evaluation of white blood cell differential counts. Comparison of the Coulter VCS, Technicon H.1, and 800-cell manual method. Am. J. Clin. Pathol., 95:381, 1991.

12. TOA Medical Electronics (USA) Inc.: NE-8000 Operator's Manual, McGaw, IL, Baxter Scientific Products Division, 1988.

13. Corberand, J.X.: Discovery of unsuspected pathological states using a new hematology analyser. Med. Lab. Sci., 48:80, 1991.

14. Houwen, B., et al.: Performance evaluation of the Sysmex SE-9000 Hematology Workstation.

15. Technicon Instruments Corp.: Technicon H*1 System Operator's Guide, Tarrytown, NY, Technicon Instruments Corp., 1985.

16. Kim, Y.R., Ornstein, L.: Isovolumetric sphering of erythrocytes for more accurate and precise cell volume measurement by flow cytometry. Cytometry, 3:419, 1983.

17. Mohandas, N., et al.: Accurate and independent measurement of volume and hemoglobin concentration of individual red cells by laser light scattering. Blood, 68:506, 1986.

18. Watson, J.S., Davis, R.A.: Evaluation of the Technicon H*1 Hematology System. Lab. Med., 18:316, 1987.

19. Bollinger, P.B., et al.: The Technicon H*1—an automated hematology analyzer for today and tomorrow. Am. J. Clin. Pathol., 87:71, 1987.

20. Nelson, L., Charache, S., Wingfield, S., Keyser, E.: Laboratory evaluation of differential white blood cell count information from the Coulter S-Plus IV and Technicon H*1 in patient populations requiring rapid "turnaround" time. Am. J. Clin. Pathol., 91:563, 1989.

21. Jovin, T.M., et al.: Automatic sizing and separation of particles by ratios of light scattering intensities. J. Histochem. Cytochem., 24:269, 1976.

22. Ross, D.W., Bardwell, A.: Automated cytochemistry and the white cell differential in leukemia. Blood Cells, 6:455, 1980.

23. Brugnara, C., Goldberg, M.A.: Recent insights into red cell and reticulocyte characteristics during accelerated erythropoiesis. In: The Emerging Importance of Accurate Reticulocyte Counting. Miles Diagnostics Division, Tarrytown, NY, Technicon Instruments Corp., 1993.

24. Ens, G.E., Jensen, R.: Coagulation instrumentation review. Clin. Hemostasis Rev., 7:1, 1993.

25. Sabo, M.G.: Coagulation instrumentation and reagent systems. In: Laboratory Evaluation of Coagulation. Edited by D.A. Triplett. Chicago, ASCP Press, 1982.

26. Brown, B.: Hematology: Principles and Procedures. 6th Ed. Philadelphia, Lea & Febiger, 1993.

27. BBL: The FibroSystem Manual, Cockeysville, MD, Division of Becton Dickinson and Company, June 1976.

28. American Bioproducts Company: ST-4 Operator's Manual, Parsippany, NJ, American Bioproducts Company.

29. Ledford, M.R., Kaczor, D.A.: Evaluation of the ST4 Clot Detection Instrument. Lab. Med., 23:172, 1992.

30. Medical Laboratory Automation, Inc.: Electra 900C Operator's Manual, Pleasantville, NY, 1990.
31. Organon Teknika Corp.: Coag-A-Mate X2 Operations Manual, Durham, NC, Organon Teknika Corp, 1981.
32. Ortho Diagnostic Systems, Inc.: KoaguLab 60-S Operator's Manual, Raritan, NJ, Ortho Diagnostic Systems, Inc, 1990.
33. Carroll, J.J., et al.: The clot signature and new aspects in coagulation testing. Raritan, NJ: Ortho Diagnostic Systems, Inc, 1989.
34. Medical Laboratory Automation, Inc.: Electra 1000C Operator's Manual, Pleasantville, NY, 1992.
35. Instrumentation Laboratory: ACL 3000 Coagulation System Operator's Manual, Milan, Italy, 1991.
36. Chantarangkul, V., Tripodi, A., Mannucci, P.M.: Evaluation of a fully automated centrifugal analyzer for performance of hemostasis tests. Clin. Chem., 33:1888, 1987.
37. Byers, C.D.: Clinical applications of flow cytometry. Clin. Lab. Sci., 6:174, 1993.
38. Goetzman, E.A.: Flow cytometry: Basic concepts and clinical applications in immunodiagnostics. Clin. Lab. Sci., 6:177, 1993.
39. Keren D.F., ed.: Flow Cytometry In Clinical Diagnosis. Chicago, ASCP Press, 1989.
40. Johnson, K.L.: Basics of flow cytometry. Clin. Lab. Sci., 5:22, 1992.
41. Bogh, L.D., Duling, T.A.: Flow cytometry instrumentation in research and clinical laboratories. Clin. Lab. Sci., 6:167, 1993.
42. Melamed, M.R., Lindmo, T., Mendelsohn, M.L., eds.: Flow cytometry and sorting. 2nd Ed. New York, Wiley-Liss, 1990.
43. Shapiro, H.M.: Practical Flow Cytometry. 2nd Ed. New York, Alan R. Liss, Inc., 1988.

ANSWERS TO REVIEW QUESTIONS

ANSWERS TO REVIEW QUESTIONS

Chapter 1
1. A
2. D
3. B
4. C
5. A
6. B
7. C
8. D

Chapter 2
1. B
2. D
3. A
4. B
5. C
6. C
7. D
8. A
9. D
10. B

Chapter 3
1. A
2. C
3. D
4. C
5. D
6. D
7. B
8. A
9. B
10. A
11. B
12. C

Chapter 4
1. C
2. B
3. C
4. C
5. D
6. D
7. B
8. A
9. C
10. C

Chapter 5
1. A
2. C
3. D
4. A
5. D
6. C
7. D
8. C
9. D
10. A

Chapter 6
1. C
2. D
3. A
4. B
5. B
6. A
7. C
8. A
9. B
10. D

Chapter 7
1. C
2. D
3. B
4. D
5. C
6. B
7. C
8. D
9. A
10. A

Chapter 8
1. C
2. B
3. B
4. A
5. D
6. B
7. C
8. A
9. C
10. A

Chapter 9
1. B
2. C
3. A
4. C
5. D
6. A
7. B
8. D
9. C
10. A

Chapter 10
1. D
2. B
3. C
4. C
5. A

Chapter 11
1. A
2. B
3. B
4. A
5. C*
6. D
7. D
8. B
9. C
10. C

Chapter 12
1. D
2. D
3. A
4. C
5. B
6. C
7. A
8. C
9. B
10. A

Chapter 13
1. C
2. C

* The MCHC is just over 36g/dL, the upper limit of normal, so technically you may describe the cells as normocytic, hyperchromic. The reticulocyte count is very high, and the MCHC is an average of all cells. Therefore, the MCHC of the reticulocytes may be keeping the MCHC lower than expected. The peripheral blood smear may help you decide the terminology. If many densely stained spherocytes without a central area of pallor were present, you would be correct in stating that the cells were normocytic, hyperchromic.

3. A
4. B
5. D
6. C
7. A
8. D
9. A
10. D

Chapter 14
1. A
2. B
3. B
4. A
5. C
6. A
7. C
8. D
9. A
10. C

Chapter 15
1. B
2. A
3. C
4. B
5. C
6. D
7. A
8. D
9. D
10. B

Chapter 16
1. B
2. C
3. A
4. D
5. C
6. D
7. A
8. B
9. D
10. A

Chapter 17
1. C
2. A
3. C
4. A
5. D
6. A
7. B
8. C
9. A
10. C
11. C
12. C
13. D
14. B

15. B
16. C

Chapter 18
1. B
2. D
3. A
4. C
5. D
6. A
7. C
8. B
9. C
10. D

Chapter 19
1. C
2. A
3. D

Chapter 20
1. B
2. D
3. C

Chapter 21
1. C
2. C
3. D
4. B
5. A
6. C
7. B
8. D
9. D
10. D

Chapter 22
1. C
2. C

Chapter 23
1. B
2. C
3. A
4. D
5. A
6. C
7. B
8. D
9. A
10. B

Chapter 24
1. A
2. C
3. D
4. B
5. A
6. C
7. B
8. D
9. B

10. A
11. C
12. A
13. C
14. D
15. B
16. D
17. A
18. B
19. D
20. B

Chapter 25
1. C
2. A
3. C
4. A
5. B
6. D
7. A
8. C
9. D
10. C
11. A
12. A

Chapter 26
1. B
2. B
3. C
4. D
5. A
6. C
7. D
8. B
9. D
10. A
11. C
12. C
13. A
14. B
15. D

Chapter 27
1. B
2. D
3. A
4. C
5. D
6. B
7. C
8. A
9. D
10. C

Chapter 28
1. B
2. C
3. A
4. B
5. A
6. C

7. C
8. D
9. A
10. D

Chapter 29
1. D
2. A

3. C
4. C
5. D
6. B
7. A
8. B
9. C
10. D

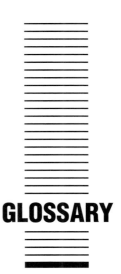

Acanthocyte: an abnormally shaped erythrocyte with spicules of varying length irregularly distributed over the cell membrane's outer surface; also known as a spur cell.

Acquired aberration: chromosome aberration (either numerical or structural) that occurs at some time after birth and involves only one cell line that is neoplastic.

Acrocentric: chromosome that has the centromere close to the terminal end so that the short arm is much shorter than the long arm. The short arm in an acrocentric chromosome consists only of a stalk and a small amount of DNA called a satellite.

Acrocyanosis: a condition precipitated by cold or stress in which arterial spasms cause cyanotic discoloration, coldness, and sweating of the extremities, especially the hands. Warming produces vasodilation and the blue becomes mottled with red. This is also known as Raynaud's phenomenon.

Activated lymphocyte: see reactive lymphocyte.

Activation: the changes that take place in platelets and other cells after stimulation.

Actomyosin: a contractile protein of the platelet similar to that found in smooth muscle and composed of actin and myosin.

Acute idiopathic thrombocytopenic purpura (ITP): a common, immune form of thrombocytopenia that occurs in children; occurs abruptly, often following a viral infection and ends with spontaneous recovery.

Acute leukemia: a stem cell disorder characterized by a neoplastic proliferation and accumulation of immature hematopoietic cells in the bone marrow. The cells are unable to differentiate into normal functional blood cells. Blasts are typically present in the peripheral blood.

Adenyl cyclase: a cellular membrane enzyme that synthesizes cyclic AMP from ATP. Cyclic AMP is an important regulator of cellular processes.

Afibrinogenemia: a condition in which there is absence of fibrinogen in the peripheral blood. It may be caused by a mutation in the gene controlling the production of fibrinogen or by an acquired condition in which fibrinogen is pathologically converted to fibrin.

Agglutinate: clumping together of erythrocytes as a result of interactions between membrane antigens and specific antibodies.

Agranulocytosis: an absence of granulocytes.

AIDS: Acquired Immunodeficiency Syndrome; a disease caused by infection with human immunodeficiency virus type I (HIV-I). The virus selectively infects helper T-lymphocytes causing rapid depletion of these cells. This causes a deficiency in cell-mediated immunity. The patients have repeated infections with multiple opportunistic organisms and an increase in malignancies.

Alder-Reilly anomaly: a benign condition characterized by the presence of leukocytes with large purplish granules in their cytoplasm when stained with a Romanowsky stain. The cells are functionally normal.

Allele: one of several alternate forms of a gene. In a particular person's genome, there are usually two different alleles of each gene, one inherited from mother and the other from father. For example, one allele of the β-globin gene lies on the chromosome 11 inherited from mother, and the other allele of the β-globin gene lies on chromosome 11 inherited from father. Differences between the two alleles may be referred to as polymorphisms.

Alloantibodies: antibodies produced in one individual in response to the antigens of another individual of the same species.

Allogeneic: pertains to an allograft in which donor and host belong to the same species but are not genetically identical.

Alloimmune hemolytic anemia: a hemolytic anemia generated when blood cells from one person are infused into a genetically unrelated person. Antigens on the infused donor cells are recognized as foreign by the recipient's lymphocytes stimulating the production of antibodies. The antibodies react with the donor cells and cause hemolysis.

Alloimmune: immune to an alternate form of an antigen within a species. This usually occurs as a result of transfusion or pregnancy in which one who lacks the alternate form is exposed to it. Blood group antigens are an example of antigens that provoke an alloimmune response.

Alpha granules: platelet storage granules containing a variety of proteins that are released into an injured area after an injury.

Anaphylaxis: an allergic reaction to foreign protein to which the immune system has been previously sensitized.

Anemia: a condition that occurs when the body's hemoglobin content is less than that required to fulfill the oxygen demands of the body. This results from a disequilibrium between erythrocyte loss and erythrocyte production. Increased erythrocyte loss may be caused by hemorrhage, chronic bleeding or hemolysis. Decreased production may be the result of deficiency of a vital nutrient such as iron, intrinsic abnormalities of hematopoietic cells or deficiency of hematopoietic growth factors.

Aneuploid: number of chromosomes per cell that does not equal a multiple of the haploid number, n. For example, in human cells a chromosome count of 45, 47, 48, etc.

Anisocytosis: a term used to describe a general variation in erythrocyte size.

Antibody: an immunoglobulin produced in response to an antigenic substance.

Antigen-dependent lymphopoiesis: development of immunocompetent lymphocytes into effector T- and B-lymphocytes that mediate the immune response through production of lymphokines and antibodies. The process is initiated when mature lymphocytes come into contact with an antigen. This process occurs in secondary lymphoid tissue.

Antigen-independent lymphopoiesis: development of lymphoid stem cells into immunocompetent T and B lymphocytes (virgin lymphocytes). This process occurs in the primary lymphoid tissue under the regulation of hematopoietic growth factors.

Antigen: any foreign substance that evokes antibody production (an immune response) and reacts specifically with that antibody.

Antihuman globulin (AHG) test: laboratory procedure used to detect the presence of antibodies that are directed against erythrocyte antigens on the erythrocyte membrane.

Anti-oncogene: see tumor suppressor gene.

Aplasia: the failure of tissue or organs to develop; in hematology aplasia refers to the failure of hematopoietic cells to generate and develop in the bone marrow.

Aplastic anemia: an anemia characterized by peripheral blood pancytopenia and hypoplastic bone marrow. It is considered a pluripotential stem cell disorder.

Apoferritin: a cellular protein that combines with iron to form ferritin. It is only found attached to iron, not in free form.

APSAC: Acylated Plasminogen Streptokinase Activator Complex; a modification of the enzyme, streptokinase, that is a chemically altered complex of streptokinase and plasminogen and is used as a thrombolytic agent in the treatment of thrombosis.

Arachidonic acid: an unsaturated essential fatty acid, usually attached to the second carbon of the glycerol backbone of phospholipids, released by phospholipase A_2 and a precursor of prostaglandins and thromboxanes.

Arachnoid mater: delicate membrane that covers the central nervous system; middle layer of the meninges.

Arterioles: arterial blood vessels that are less than 200 μm in diameter. Their function is regulation of blood pressure and hemostasis.

Ascitic fluid: fluid that has abnormally collected in the peritoneal cavity of the abdomen.

Ataxia: an abnormal condition in which the ability to coordinate movement is impaired.

Atypical lymphocyte: see reactive lymphocyte.

Auer rods: reddish-blue staining needle-like inclusions within the cytoplasm of leukemic myeloblasts that occur as a result of abnormal cytoplasmic granule formation. Their presence on a Romanowsky stained smear is helpful in differentiating acute myeloid leukemia from acute lymphoblastic leukemia.

Autoantibodies: antibodies in the blood that are capable of reacting with the subject's own antigens.

Autohemolysis: lysis of subject's own erythrocytes by hemolytic agents in the subject's serum.

Autoimmune hemolytic anemia (AIHA): anemia that results when individuals produce antibodies against their own erythrocytes. The antibodies are usually against high incidence antigens.

Autoimmunization: an immune response (antibody production) to the subject's own tissue.

Autosome: chromosomes that do not contain genes for sex differentiation; in humans, chromosome pairs 1–22.

Autosplenectomy: extensive splenic damage secondary to infarction. This is often seen in older children and adults with sickle cell anemia.

Azurophilic: refers to the predilection of some granules (primary granules) within myelocytic leukocytes for the aniline component of a Romanowsky type stain. These granules appear bluish-purple or bluish-black when observed microscopically on a stained blood smear. They first appear in the promyelocyte. In leukemia, these granules may appear in blasts (type II and type III blasts).

Band granulocyte: the immediate precursor cell of the mature granulocyte. This cell can be found in either the bone marrow or peripheral blood. The nucleus is elongated and nuclear chromatin condensed. The cytoplasm stains pink and there are many specific granules. The cell is 9–15 μm in diameter. Also called a stab, unsegmented neutrophil, or band.

Base pair: a nucleotide pair of A with T, or G with C, in double-stranded DNA. The length of a DNA sequence is measured in base pairs (bp), or in thousands of base pairs = kilobases (kb).

Basophilia: an increase in the concentration of circulating basophils.

Basophilic normoblast: a nucleated precursor of the erythrocyte that is derived from a pronormoblast. The cell is 10–16 μm in diameter. The nuclear chromatin is coarser than the pronormoblast and nucleoli are usually absent. Cytoplasm is more abundant and it stains deeply basophilic. The cell matures to a polychromatophilic normoblast. Also called a prorubricyte.

Basophilic stippling: erythrocyte inclusions composed of precipitated ribonucleoprotein and mitochondrial remnant. Observed on Romanowsky stained blood smears as diffuse or punctate bluish-black granules in toxic states such as drug (lead) exposure. The diffuse, fine basophilic stippling may occur as an artifact.

Basophil: a mature granulocytic cell characterized by the presence of large basophilic granules. These granules are purple-blue or purple-black with Romanowsky stain. The cell is 10–14 μm in diameter and the nucleus is segmented. Granules are cytochemically positive with periodic-acid-schiff (PAS) and peroxidase. The granules contain histamine and heparin peroxidase. The granules containing histamine and heparin have been called "suicide bags" because the release of large numbers of granules in anaphylactic shock may cause death. Basophils constitute < 0.2 × 10^9/L or 0–1% of peripheral blood leukocytes. The basophil functions as a mediator of inflammatory responses. The cell has receptors for IgE.

Bernard-Soulier disease: a rare hereditary platelet disorder characterized by a genetic mutation in the gene coding for platelet glycoprotein Ib resulting in inability of the platelets to adhere to collagen.

Bilineage acute leukemia: an acute leukemia that has two separate populations of leukemic cells. One that phenotypes as lymphoid and the other as myeloid.

Bilirubin: a breakdown product of the heme portion of the hemoglobin molecule. Initial steps in the degradation of hemoglobin result in a water insoluble form (unconjugated or direct bilirubin) that travels in the blood stream to the liver where it is converted to a water soluble form (conjugated or indirect bilirubin) that can be excreted into the bile.

Biphenotypic acute leukemia: an acute leukemia that has myeloid and lymphoid markers on the same population of neoplastic cells.

Birefringence: physical property such that light is transmitted unequally in different directions. Also referred to as double refraction. This indicates a bonding of molecules or ions such as is seen in crystals.

2,3-bisphosphoglycerate (2,3-BPG): see 2,3-diphosphoglycerate.

Blackwater fever: a condition that results as a complication of chronic infection with the parasite *Plasmodium falciparum*. There is sudden onset of fever; tender, enlarged liver and spleen; hemoglobinuria; epigastric pain; vomiting; jaundice; and shock.

Blood cell differential: microscopic evaluation of a Romanowsky stained blood smear that includes enumeration of the relative number (percentage) of each leukocyte type present. Usually a total of 100 leukocytes are counted. This evaluation also includes performing an evaluation of the morphology of all cell types, and an estimate of the absolute number of leukocytes and platelets present.

Blood clot: a mass of aggregated platelets, fibrin and entrapped cells that forms after activation of the hemostatic system, either in vivo or in vitro.

Blood coagulation: formation of a blood clot or thrombus, usually considered a normal process.

Bohr effect: the effects of pH on hemoglobin-oxygen affinity. This is one of the most important buffer systems in the body. As the H$^+$ concentration in tissues increases, the affinity of hemoglobin for oxygen is decreased permitting unloading of oxygen.

***Bordetella pertussis*:** a gram-negative aerobic coccobacilli that is the cause of whooping cough. The hematologic picture in whooping cough is leukocytosis with lymphocytosis. The lymphocytes are small cells with folded nuclei.

Buffy coat: the layer of white blood cells and platelets that lies between the plasma and erythrocytes in a centrifuged blood sample.

Cabot ring: reddish-violet erythrocyte inclusion resembling the figure 8 on Romanowsky stained blood smears that can be found in some cases of severe anemia.

Capillaries: the smallest blood vessels which are the site of exchange of gases, nutrients and waste products between the blood and the tissues.

Carboxyhemoglobin: a compound that results when hemoglobin is exposed to carbon monoxide. This form of hemoglobin is incapable of oxygen transport.

Cardiac tamponade: accumulation of fluid in the pericardial sac which is either sudden and/or large in amount causing restriction of the normal heart beat.

cDNA (complementary DNA): synthetic DNA transcribed from an RNA template by the enzyme reverse transcriptase.

Cell-mediated immunity: an event in the immune response mediated by T-lymphocytes. The event requires interaction between histocompatible T-lymphocytes and macrophages with antigen. There are at least three important T-lymphocyte subsets involved: helper, suppressor and cytotoxic. When activated, these cells proliferate and produce lymphokines.

Central nervous system: anatomically defined by the brain and spinal cord.

Centriole: cytoplasmic organelle that is the point of origin for the contractile protein known as the spindle fiber.

Centromere: primary constriction that attaches sister chromatids in a chromosome, dividing the chromatids into long and short arms.

Cerebriform: having the appearance of a brain.

Cerebrospinal fluid: fluid that is normally produced to protect the brain and spinal cord. It is produced by the choroid plexus cells, absorbed by the arachnoid pia and circulates in the subarachnoid space.

Chediak-Higashi anomaly: a multi-system disorder inherited in an autosomal recessive fashion and characterized by recurrent infections, hepatosplenomegaly, partial albinism, CNS abnormalities; neutrophil chemotaxis and killing of organisms is impaired. There are giant cytoplasmic granular inclusions in leukocytes and platelets.

Chiasmata: crossing of non-sister chromatids during formation of the synaptonemal complex. This may result in a physical exchange between the chromatids.

Chimerism: cells from two different zygotes expressed in one individual.

Chloroma: extramyeloid tissue (mass) that appears green. The green color is probably due to myeloperoxidase. The color fades to dirty yellow upon exposure to air.

Chlorosis: a term used to describe iron-deficiency anemia between 1870–1920. Refers to the greenish-hue of the skin in iron deficient subjects.

Chromatid: structure of DNA during G_0 and G_1 of the cell cycle. After S-phase, DNA has replicated and the chromosome consists of two parallel, identical chromatids held together at the centromere.

Chromosome: nuclear structure seen during mitosis and meiosis consisting of supercoiled DNA with histone and non-histone proteins. Consists of two identical (sister) chromatids attached at the centromere.

Chronic idiopathic thrombocytopenic purpura (ITP): an immune form of thrombocytopenia that occurs most often in young adults and lasts longer than six months.

Chronic myelocytic leukemia (CML): a myeloproliferative disorder characterized by a neoplastic growth of primarily myeloid cells in the bone marrow and an extreme elevation of these cells in the peripheral blood. There are two phases to the disease: chronic and blast crisis. Also referred to as chronic granulocytic leukemia.

Chronic myelomonocytic leukemia (CMML): a subgroup of the myelodysplastic syndromes. There is anemia and a variable total leukocyte count. An absolute monocytosis ($>1 \times 10^9$/L) is present and immature erythrocytes and granulocytes may also be present. There are less than 5% blasts in the peripheral blood. The bone marrow is hypercellular with proliferation of abnormal myelocytes, promonocytes and monoblasts and there are <20% blasts.

Chronic nonspherocytic hemolytic anemia: a group of chronic anemias characterized by premature erythrocyte destruction. Spherocytes are not readily found differentiating these anemias from hereditary spherocytosis.

Chylous: term used to describe fluid that is thick and milky in appearance due to the presence of lymph fluid and chylomicrons.

Circulating leukocyte pool: the population of neutrophils actively circulating within the peripheral blood stream.

Clot retraction: the cohesion of a fibrin clot that requires adequate, functionally normal platelets. Retraction of the clot occurs over a period of time and results in the expression of serum and a firmer mass of cells and fibrin. The clot retraction test was formerly used to determine whether platelets were functionally normal.

Coagulation factors: soluble inert plasma proteins that interact to form fibrin after an injury.

Codocyte: an abnormally shaped erythrocyte. The cell appears as a target with a bull's eye center mass of hemoglobin, surrounded by an achromic ring and an outer ring of hemoglobin. The osmotic fragility of this cell is decreased. Also called a target cell or Mexican hat cell.

Cold autoimmune hemolytic anemia: anemia resulting from the action of IgM autoantibodies that react at room temperature with one's own erythrocyte antigens mediating destruction of the cell via complement.

Common pathway: one of three interacting pathways in the coagulation cascade. The common pathway includes three rate-limiting steps 1) activation of factor X by the intrinsic and extrinsic pathways. 2) Conversion of prothrombin to thrombin by activated factor X and, 3) cleavage of fibrinogen to fibrin.

Compensated hemolytic disease: a disorder in which the erythrocyte life span is decreased but the bone marrow is able to increase erythropoiesis enough to compensate for the decreased erythrocyte life span. Anemia does not develop.

Complement: any of the eleven serum proteins that when sequentially activated, causes lysis of the cell membrane.

Complete antibody: antibody capable of agglutinating saline-suspended erythrocytes. These are usually IgM antibodies.

Congenital aberration: chromosome aberration (either numerical or structural) that is present at the time of birth in all cell lines, or in several cell lines in the case of mosaicism.

Congenital Heinz body hemolytic anemia: a clinical term used to describe congenital hemolytic anemias that are caused by the presence of unstable hemoglobin variants. The instability results from amino acid substitutions in the internal residues that prevent the hemoglobin molecule from folding into its normal conformation, alter the α-helix structure or subunit interaction sites, or impair the binding of heme to globin. The unstable hemoglobin denatures in the form of Heinz bodies which attach to the cell membrane causing membrane injury and premature cell destruction.

Contact group: a group of coagulation factors in the intrinsic pathway that are involved with the initial activation of the coagulation system and require contact with a negatively charged surface for activity. These factors include factors XII, XI, prekallikrein and high molecular weight kininogen.

Cryoprecipitate: a preparation of proteins containing fibrinogen, von Willebrand factor and factor VIII, and used for replacement therapy in patients with hemophilia A and von Willebrand disease. It is prepared by freezing and thawing plasma.

Culling: selection or filtering; in hematology, the selection and phagocytosis of damaged or senescent erythrocytes by the spleen or liver.

Cyanosis: a bluish discoloration of the skin and mucous membranes caused by an excess of deoxygenated hemoglobin in the blood.

Cyclooxygenase: a cellular membrane enzyme that synthesizes the precursor of prostaglandins and in the platelet is essential for the production of thromboxane A_2.

Cytocentrifuge: instrument that is used to prepare slides of cells contained in fluid other than peripheral blood. The specimen is directly centrifuged onto a glass slide.

Cytochemistry: chemical staining procedures used to identify various constituents (enzymes and proteins) within white blood cells. Useful in differentiating blasts in acute leukemia, especially when morphologic differentiation on Romanowsky stained smears is impossible.

Cytogenetics: the study of chromosome morphology particularly as it relates to a normal or abnormal state.

Cytoplasm: the protoplasm of a cell outside the nucleus.

Dacryocyte: an abnormally shaped erythrocyte with a single elongated or pointed extremity. Also known as a tear-drop cell or tennis racquet cell.

Decay accelerating factor (DAF): a regulating protein found on cell membranes that accelerates decay (dissociation) of membrane bound complement (C3bBb). An absence of this factor leads to excessive sensitivity of these cells to complement lysis.

Deep vein thrombosis (DVT): formation of a thrombus, or blood clot, in the deep veins (usually a leg vein).

Delayed bleeding: a symptom of severe coagulation factor disorders in which a wound bleeds a second time after initial stoppage of bleeding because the primary hemostatic plug is not adequately stabilized by the formation of fibrin.

Dense bodies: platelet storage granules containing nonmetabolic ADP, calcium and serotonin along with other compounds that are released into an injured area.

Diapedesis: the passage of blood cells through the unruptured capillary wall. For leukocytes, this involves active locomotion.

2,3-diphosphoglycerate (2,3-DPG): a product of the glycolytic pathway that affects the oxygen affinity of hemoglobin. It serves in the biochemical feedback system that regulates the amount of oxygen released to the tissues. As the concentration of 2,3-DPG increases, hemoglobin's affinity for oxygen decreases and more oxygen is released to the tissue. Also referrred to as 2,3-bisphosphoglycerate (2,3-BPG).

Diploid: number of chromosomes in somatic cells that is 2n. For human cells 2n = 46.

Direct antihuman globulin test (DAT): a laboratory test used to detect the presence of antibody and/or complement that is attached to the erythrocyte. The test uses antibody directed against human immunoglobulin and/or complement.

DNA (deoxyribonucleic acid): the blueprint that cells use to catalog, express, and propagate information. DNA is the fundamental substance of heredity that is carried from one generation to the next. DNA is a double-stranded molecule composed of complementary nucleotide sequences. The two strands of DNA are held together by hydrogen bonds formed according to the following rules of complementary nucleotide pairing: G bonds with C, A bonds with T, while other combinations cannot bond.

Döhle body: an oval aggregate of rough endoplasmic reticulum that stains light grey-blue (with Romanowsky stain) found within the cytoplasm of neutrophils and eosinophils. It is associated with severe bacterial infection, pregnancy, burns, cancer, aplastic anemia and toxic states.

Donath-Landsteiner antibody: a biphasic IgG antibody associated with paroxysmal cold hemoglobinuria. The antibody reacts with erythrocytes in capillaries at temperatures below 15°C and fixes complement to the cell membrane. Upon warming, the terminal complement components on erythrocytes are activated causing cell hemolysis.

Downey Cell: an outdated term used to describe morphologic variations of the reactive lymphocyte.

Drepanocyte: an abnormally shaped erythrocyte; the cell usually has a sickle, crescent or boat shape. These cells contain polymerized hemoglobin S; also called a sickle cell.

Drug-induced hemolytic anemia: hemolytic anemia precipitated by ingestion of certain drugs. The process may be immune mediated or non-immune mediated. In the immune mediated type four mechanisms have been identified: drug adsorption; immune complex mediated; autoantibody induction; nonspecific adherence. Nonimmune mediated hemolysis usually occurs secondary to a erythrocyte metabolic defect such as glucose 6-phosphate dehydrogenase (G6PD) deficiency.

Dura mater: dense membrane covering the central nervous system. Outer most layer of the meninges.

Dutcher body: intranuclear membrane bound inclusions found in plasma cells from patients with dysproteinemias and in neoplastic plasma cells. The body stains with periodic-acid-Schiff (PAS) indicating it contains glycogen or glycoprotein.

Dysfibrinogenemia: a hereditary condition in which there is a structural alteration in the fibrinogen molecule.

Dyshematopoiesis: abnormal formation and/or development of blood cells within the bone marrow.

Dysplasia: abnormal cell development.

Dyspoiesis: in hematology, abnormal development of blood cells frequently characterized by asynchrony in nuclear to cytoplasmic maturation and /or abnormal granule development.

Easy bruisability: a condition in which there are a greater than normal number of bruises that occur with less trauma than usual.

Ecchymosis (pl. ecchymoses): bruise (bluish-black discoloration of the skin) which is greater than 3 mm in diameter caused by bleeding from arterioles into subcutaneous tissues without disruption of intact skin.

Echinocyte: a spiculated erythrocyte with short, equally spaced projections over the entire outer surface of the cell.

Effector lymphocytes: antigen stimulated lymphocytes that mediate the efferent arm of the immune response.

Effusion: abnormal accumulation of fluid.

Elliptocyte: an abnormally shaped erythrocyte. The cell is an oval to elongated ellipsoid with a central area of pallor and hemoglobin at both ends; also known as ovalocyte, pencil cell or cigar cell.

Embolism: the blockage of an artery by an embolus, usually by a portion of a blood clot but can be other foreign matter, resulting in obstruction of blood flow to the tissues.

Embolus: a piece of blood clot or other foreign matter that circulates in the blood stream and usually becomes lodged in a small vessel obstructing the blood flow.

Endomitosis: a nuclear DNA synthesis without cytoplasmic division.

Endoplasmic reticulum (ER): a cytoplasmic organelle in eukaryocytic cells that consists of a network of interconnected tubes and flattened membranous sacs. If the ER has ribosomes attached, it is known as granular or rough endoplasmic reticulum (RER) and if ribosomes are not attached it is known as smooth endoplasmic reticulum (SER). The amount of RER and SER in a cell is determined by its function. Those cells that secrete proteins are rich in RER. The protein is synthesized on the attached ribosomes and then transported through the RER to the Golgi apparatus for packaging.

Endothelial cells: flat cells that line the cavities of the blood and lymphatic vessels, heart and other related body cavities.

Eosinophil: a mature granulocytic cell characterized by the presence of large acidophilic granules. These granules are pink to orange-pink with Romanowsky stains. The cell is 12–17 μm in diameter and the nucleus has 2–3 lobes. Granules contain acid phosphatase, glycuronidase cathepsins, ribonuclease, arylsulfatase, peroxidase, phospholipids and basic proteins. Eosinophils have a concentration of less than 0.45×10^9/L in peripheral blood. The cell membrane has receptors for IgE and histamine.

Eosinophilia: an increase in the concentration of eosinophils in the peripheral blood ($>0.45 \times 10^9$/L). Associated with parasitic infection, allergic conditions, hypersensitivity reactions, cancer and chronic inflammatory states.

Epitope: a structural portion of an antigen that reacts with a specific antibody. Also called the antigenic determinant.

Erythroblast: see normoblast.

Erythroblastic island: a composite of erythroid cells in the bone marrow that surrounds a central macrophage. These groups of cells are usually disrupted when the bone marrow smears are made but may be found in erythroid hyperplasia. The central macrophage is thought to transfer iron to the developing cells. The least mature cells are closest to the center of the island and the more mature cells on the periphery.

Erythroblastosis fetalis: hemolytic anemia occurring in newborns as a result of fetal-maternal blood group incompatibility involving the Rh factor or ABO blood groups. It is caused by an antigen-antibody reaction in the newborn when maternal antibodies traverse the placenta and attach to antigens on the fetal cells. Rh hemolytic reactions are usually more severe than ABO reactions.

Erythrocyte: a mature red blood cell (RBC). The cell is anuclear and about 7 μm in diameter. It contains the respiratory pigment hemoglobin, which readily combines with oxygen to form oxyhemoglobin. The cell develops from the pluripotential stem cell in the bone marrow under the influence of the hematopoietic growth factor, erythropoietin, and is released to the peripheral blood as a reticulocyte. The average life span is about 120 days after which the cell is removed by cells in the mononuclear-phagocyte system. The average concentration is about 5×10^{12}/L for males and 4.5×10^{12}/L for females.

Erythrocytosis: an abnormal increase in the number of circulating erythrocytes as measured by the erythrocyte count, hemoglobin or hematocrit. This may be due to an absolute increase in the erythrocyte concentration or a relative increase in the erythrocyte concentration due to a decrease in plasma volume.

Erythrophagocytosis: phagocytosis of an erythrocyte by a histiocyte; the erythrocyte can be seen within the cytoplasm of the histiocyte as a pink globule or, if digested, as a clear vacuole on stained bone marrow or peripheral blood smears.

Erythropoiesis: production and maturation of erythrocytes. This normally occurs in the bone marrow under the influence of the hematopoietic growth factor, erythropoietin.

Erythropoietin: a hormone, secreted by the kidney, that regulates erythrocyte production by stimulating the stem cells of the bone marrow to mature into erythrocytes. Its primary effect is on the committed stem cell, CFU-E.

Essential thrombocythemia: a myeloproliferative disorder affecting primarily the megakaryocytic element in the bone marrow. There is extreme thrombocytosis in the blood (usually $>1,000 \times 10^9$/L). Also called primary thrombocythemia, hemorrhagic thrombocythemia and megakaryocytic leukemia.

Euchromatin: region of the chromosome that contains genetically active DNA, is lighter staining and replicates early in S phase of the cell cycle. (See heterochromatin)

Evan's syndrome: a condition characterized by a warm autoimmune hemolytic anemia and concurrent severe thrombocytopenia.

Excess bleeding: bleeding from a wound that is more profuse than normal.

Extracorpuscular: occurring outside the blood corpuscle.

Extramedullary hematopoiesis: the formation and development of blood cells in tissue outside the bone marrow. (See medullary hematopoiesis).

Extravascular: occurring outside of the blood vessels.

Extrinsic Pathway: one of three interacting pathways in the coagulation cascade. The extrinsic pathway is initiated when tissue factor comes into contact with blood and forms a complex with factor VII. This complex activates factor X. The term "extrinsic" is used because the pathway requires a factor extrinsic to blood, tissue factor.

Exudate: effusion that is formed by increased vascular permeability and/or decreased lymphatic resorption. This indicates a true pathologic state in the anatomic region, usually either infection or tumor.

Factor VIII concentrate: a lyophilized preparation of concentrated factor VIII used for replacement therapy of Factor VIII in patients with hemophilia A.

Fagot cells: promyelocytes containing bundles of Auer rods. Found in the hypergranular variant of acute promyelocytic leukemia (FAB subgroup M3).

Familial aplastic anemia: a subset of Fanconi's anemia but with no congenital abnormalities. Pancytopenia and bone marrow hypoplasia are present.

Fanconi's anemia: an autosomal recessive disorder associated with a variety of congenital anomalies, progressive bone marrow hypoplasia and peripheral blood pancytopenia.

Favism: sensitivity to a species of bean, *Vicia faba*. It is commonly found in Sicily and Sardinia in individuals who have inherited glucose-6-phosphate dehydrogenase deficiency. It is characterized by fever, acute hemolytic anemia, vomiting and diarrhea after ingestion of the bean or inhalation of the plant pollen.

Ferritin: an iron-phosphorus-protein compound formed when iron complexes with the protein apoferritin; it is a short term storage form of iron found primarily in the bone marrow, spleen, and liver. This readily available iron store can be incorporated into hemoglobin molecules.

Fibrin Monomer: the structure resulting when thrombin cleaves the A and B fibrinopeptides from the α and β chains of fibrinogen.

Fibrin Polymer: a complex of covalently bonded fibrin monomers. The bonds between glutamine and lysine residues are formed between terminal domains of γ-chains and polar appendages of α-chains of neighboring residues.

Fibrinogen Group: a group of coagulation factors that are consumed during the formation of fibrin and therefore absent from serum. Includes factors I, V, VIII, XIII. Also called the consumable group.

Fibrinolysis: breakdown of fibrin.

Fibrosis: abnormal formation of fibrous tissue.

Flame cell: a plasma cell with reddish-purple cytoplasm. The red tinge is caused by the presence of a glycoprotein and the purple by ribosomes.

Forssman antibody: a heterophil antibody produced by a variety of infectious agents and occurring in almost all human sera. This antibody reacts with sheep erythrocytes and is not associated with infectious mononucleosis.

Fragment D: see fragment E.

Fragment E: a product formed from plasmin digestion of fibrinogen. This fragment is produced when fragment Y is cleaved between the E and D domains. This cleavage produces fragment E and fragment D.

Fragment X: a product formed from plasmin digestion of fibrinogen. This fragment is produced when a few small peptides from the exposed polar appendages in the C-terminal region of the Aα-chains of fibrinogen are cleaved.

Fragment Y: a product formed from plasmin digestion of fibrinogen. This fragment is produced when fragment X is cleaved by plasmin in the coiled region, midway between the D-terminal domain and the E-central domain. This produces the uninodular fragment D and a binodular fragment E,D. The binodular fragment is called fragment Y.

Free erythrocyte protoporphyrin (FEP): protoporphyrin within the erythrocyte that is not complexed with iron. The concentration of FEP increases in iron deficient states. It is now known that in the absence of iron, erythrocyte protoporphyrin combines with zinc to form zinc protoporphyrin (ZPP).

G-band: differential pattern of light and dark chromosome bands using Giemsa stain with various types of pre-treatment.

Gammopathy: an abnormal condition in which there is an increase in serum immunoglobulins.

Gene: a functional segment of DNA that serves as a template for RNA transcription and protein translation. Regulatory sequences control gene expression, so that only a small fraction of the estimated 100,000 genes are ever transcribed by a given cell.

Gene rearrangement: a process in which segments of DNA are cut and spliced to produce new DNA sequences. During normal lymphocyte development, rearrangement of the immunoglobulin genes and the T cell receptor genes results in new gene sequences that encode the antibody and surface antigen receptor proteins necessary for immune function.

Genome: the total aggregate of inherited genetic material. In humans, the genome consists of 3 billion base pairs of DNA divided among 46 chromosomes, including 22 pairs of autosomes numbered 1–22 and the two sex chromosomes.

Genotype: the genetic constitution of a particular person.

Glanzmann's thrombasthenia: a rare hereditary platelet disorder characterized by a genetic mutation in one of the genes coding for the glycoproteins IIb or IIIa and resulting in the inability of platelets to aggregate.

Globin: the protein portion of the hemoglobin molecule. There are four globin chains that occur in pairs in each hemoglobin molecule: α_2, β_2, δ_2, and γ_2. The combination of the pairs determines the type of hemoglobin. There are three types of hemoglobin normally found in the adult: A (α_2, β_2), A$_2$ (α_2, δ_2), F (α_2, γ_2).

Glucose-6-phosphate-dehydrogenase: an enzyme within erythrocytes that is important in carbohydrate metabolism. It dehydrogenates glucose-6-phosphate to form 6-phosphogluconate in the hexose monophosphate shunt. This reaction produces NADPH from NADP. This provides the erythrocyte with reducing power protecting the cell from oxidant injury.

Glutathione: a tripeptide that takes up and gives off hydrogen and prevents oxidant damage to the hemoglobin molecule. Deficiency of this enzyme is associated with hemolytic anemia.

Glycocalicin: a portion of glycoprotein Ib of the platelet membrane that is external to the platelet surface and contains binding sites for von Willebrand factor and thrombin.

Glycocalyx: an amorphous coat of glycoproteins and mucopolysaccharides covering the surface of cells, particularly the platelets and endothelial cells.

Glycolysis: a metabolic process that involves the anaerobic conversion of glucose to lactate and pyruvate resulting in the production of energy through a series of metabolic pathways.

Glycoprotein Ib: a glycoprotein of the platelet surface that contains the receptor for von Willebrand factor and is critical for initial adhesion of platelets to collagen after an injury.

Glycoprotein IIb/IIIa complex: a complex of membrane proteins on the platelet surface that is functional only after activation by agonists and then becomes a receptor for fibrinogen and von Willebrand factor. It is essential for platelet aggregation.

Glycosylated hemoglobin: hemoglobin that has glucose attached to the terminal amino acid of the beta chains. Also called hemoglobin A_{1c}.

Golgi apparatus: a cytoplasmic organelle composed of flattened sacs or cisternae arranged in stacks. In secretory cells it functions in concentrating and packaging secretory products. The size of the Golgi depends upon the cell type and function. The Golgi apparatus in blood cells does not stain with Romanowsky stains and appears as a clear area usually adjacent to the nucleus.

Gower hemoglobin: an embryonic hemoglobin detectable in the yolk sac for up to eight weeks gestation. Gower I hemoglobin is composed of two zeta (ζ) chains and two epsilon (ϵ) chains. Gower II hemoglobin is formed from two alpha (α) and two ϵ chains.

Granulocytopenia: a decrease in granulocytes below 2 $\times$ 10^9/L.

Granulocytosis: an increase in granulocytes. Usually seen in bacterial infections, inflammation, metabolic intoxication, drug intoxication and tissue necrosis.

Gray platelet syndrome: a rare hereditary platelet disorder characterized by the lack of alpha granules.

Ham test: a specific laboratory test for paroxysmal nocturnal hemoglobinuria (PNH). When erythrocytes from a patient with PNH are incubated in acidified serum the cells lyse due to complement activation. Also called the acid-serum lysis test.

Haploid: number of chromosomes in a gamete that is n; consists of one of each of the autosomes and one of the sex chromosomes. For human cells n = 23.

Haptoglobin: a plasma glycoprotein whose function is to transport hemoglobin that has been released into the blood to the liver.

Heinz body: an erythrocyte inclusion composed of denatured or precipitated hemoglobin. Appears as purple staining body on supravitally (crystal violet) stained smears.

Hematocrit: the packed volume of erythrocytes in a given volume of blood following centrifugation of the blood sample. Expressed as a percentage of total blood volume or liter of erythrocytes per liter of blood (L/L). Also referred to as packed cell volume (PCV).

Hematology: the study of blood and blood-forming tissue.

Hematoma: a localized collection of blood under the skin or in other organs caused by a break in the wall of a blood vessel.

Hematopoiesis: the production and development of blood cells normally occurring in the bone marrow under the influence of hematopoietic growth factors.

Hematopoietic growth factors: cytokines secreted by a variety of different cells that influence the production and differentiation of hematopoietic cells. Hematopoietic cells have specific receptors for different growth factors.

Hematopoietic inductive microenvironment (HIM): the local environment of developing hematopoietic cells in the bone marrow that has a modifying influence on stem cells and their path of differentiation.

Hematopoietic system: the blood-forming tissue and organs, including the bone marrow, lymph nodes, spleen, liver, thymus.

Hematuria: refers to the presence of intact erythrocytes in the urine.

Heme: the nonprotein portion of hemoglobin and myoglobin that contains iron nestled in a hydrophobic pocket of a porphyrin ring (ferroprotoporphyrin). It is responsible for the characteristic color of hemoglobin.

Hemochromatosis: a clinical condition resulting from abnormal iron metabolism. Characterized by accumulation of iron deposits in body tissues.

Hemodialysis: a mechanical means of removing impurities and waste from the blood providing the function of the kidneys in cases of renal failure.

Hemoglobin: a protein-iron compound composed of a heme group and four globin chains found within erythrocytes. It is responsible for carrying oxygen and carbon dioxide between the lungs and the tissues.

Hemoglobinemia: the presence of excessive hemoglobin in the plasma.

Hemoglobinopathies: a group of genetically determined diseases caused by abnormalities in the structure or synthesis of the globin portion of the hemoglobin molecule. Those that are caused by abnormal synthesis are known specifically as thalassemia.

Hemoglobinuria: the presence of hemoglobin in the urine.

Hemolysis: destruction of erythrocytes resulting in the release of hemoglobin. In hemolytic anemia this term refers to the premature destruction of erythrocytes.

Hemolytic anemia: a disorder characterized by a decreased erythrocyte concentration due to premature destruction of the erythrocyte.

Hemolytic Disease of the Newborn (HDN): an alloimmune disease characterized by fetal red blood cell destruction as a result of incompatibility between maternal and fetal-blood groups.

Hemolytic uremic syndrome (HUS): a disorder characterized by a combination of microangiopathic hemolytic anemia, acute renal failure and thrombocytopenia.

It occurs most often in children. The etiology is unknown.

Hemopexin: a plasma glycoprotein (β-globulin) that binds the heme molecule in the absence of haptoglobin.

Hemophilia A: a sex-linked (x-linked) hereditary hemorrhagic disorder caused by a genetic mutation of the gene coding for coagulation factor VIII.

Hemophilia B: a sex-linked (x-linked) hereditary hemorrhagic disorder caused by a genetic mutation of the gene coding for coagulation factor IX.

Hemorrhagic disease of the newborn: a severe bleeding disorder in the first week of life caused by deficiencies of the vitamin K dependent clotting factors due to vitamin K deficiency.

Hemosiderin: a water insoluble, heterogeneous iron-protein complex found primarily in the cytoplasm of cells (normoblasts and histiocyte) in the bone marrow, liver, and spleen; the major long-term storage form of iron. Readily visible microscopically in unstained tissue specimens as irregular aggregates of golden brown granules. It may be visualized with Prussian blue stain as blue granules. The granules are normally distributed randomly or diffuse.

Hemosiderosis: a relative or absolute increase in the amount of storage iron in the body.

Hemosidinuria: the presence of hemosiderin in the urine. Occurs as a result of intravascular hemolysis and disintegration of renal tubular cells.

Hemostasis: the localized, controlled process that results in arrest of bleeding after an injury.

Hemostatic plug: the mass of platelets and fibrin that forms in a blood vessel after an injury and results in the arrest of bleeding.

Heparin: a polysaccharide that inhibits coagulation of blood by preventing thrombin from cleaving fibrinogen to form fibrin. Commercially available in the form of a sodium salt for therapeutic use as an anticoagulant.

Hereditary elliptocytosis: an autosomal dominant condition characterized by the presence of increased numbers of elongated and oval erythrocytes. The abnormal shape is due to a defect in the erythrocyte cytoskeleton. Overt hemolysis is present in only 10% of individuals with this disorder.

Hereditary pyropoikilocytosis (HPP): a rare but severe hemolytic anemia inherited as an autosomal recessive disorder. Characterized by marked erythrocyte fragmentation. The defect is most likely a spectrin abnormality in the erythrocyte cytoskeleton. These cells are thermally unstable, fragmenting when heated to 45°C. Normal erythrocytes will fragment at 49°C.

Hereditary spherocytosis: a chronic hemolytic anemia caused by an inherited erythrocyte membrane disorder. The underlying defect is an abnormality in spectrin or its association with other cytoskeletal proteins. The defect causes membrane instability and progressive membrane loss. Secondary to membrane loss, the cells become spherocytes and are prematurely destroyed in the spleen. The condition is usually inherited as an autosomal dominant trait.

Hereditary stomatocytosis: a rare hemolytic anemia inherited in an autosomal dominant fashion. The erythrocyte membrane is abnormally permeable to sodium and potassium. The cell becomes overhydrated resulting in the appearance of stomatocytes. The specific membrane abnormality has not been identified.

Hereditary xerocytosis: a hereditary disorder in which the erythrocyte membrane is abnormally permeable. The erythrocyte becomes dehydrated and appears as either targeted, or contracted and spiculated. The cells are rigid and are trapped in the spleen.

Heterochromatin: region of the chromosome that contains genetically inactive DNA, is dark staining, and replicates late in S phase of the cell cycle.

Heterophil antibodies: antibodies that can react against a heterologous antigen that did not stimulate the antibody's production. In infectious mononucleosis, heterophil antibodies are produced in response to infection with Epstein-Barr virus, and react with sheep, horse and beef erythrocytes.

Heterozygous: in genetics, used to describe the condition of possessing two different alleles at a given locus on homologous chromosomes. A person who is heterozygous for a particular characteristic has inherited a gene for that characteristic from one parent and an alternate gene from the other parent.

Hexose-monophosphate shunt: a metabolic pathway that converts glucose 6-phosphate to pentose phosphate. This pathway couples oxidative metabolism with the reduction of nicotinamide adenine dinucleotide-phosphate (NADPH) and glutathione. This provides the cell with reducing power and prevents injury by oxidants.

HIV-I (human immunodeficiency virus type-I): a virus that causes acquired immunodeficiency syndrome (AIDS).

Hodgkin's disease: malignancy that most often arises in lymph nodes and is characterized by the presence of Reed-Sternberg cells and variants with a background of varying numbers of benign lymphocytes, plasma cells, histiocytes and eosinophils. The origin of the malignant cell is still controversial.

Homozygous: in genetics, used to describe the condition of possessing identical alleles at a given locus on homologous chromosomes. A person who is homozygous for a particular characteristic has inherited two identical genes for that characteristic, one from each parent.

Howell-Jolly body: an erythrocyte inclusion composed of nuclear remnants (DNA). On Romanowsky stained blood smears, it appears as a dark purple spherical granule usually near the periphery of the cell. Commonly associated with megaloblastic anemia and splenectomy.

Humoral immunity: immunity imparted as a result of B-lymphocyte activation. The B-lymphocyte differentiates to a plasma cell which produces antibodies specific to the antigen that stimulated the response.

Humoral: pertaining to any fluid in the body.

Hybridization: the process in which one nucleotide strand binds to another strand by formation of hydrogen bonds between complementary nucleotides.

Hydrops fetalis: a genetically determined hemolytic disease resulting in production of an abnormal hemoglobin (hemoglobin Bart's, γ_4) that is unable to carry oxygen. There is a macrocytic hypochromic anemia, enlargement of the spleen and liver and generalized edema. Infants are stillborn or die shortly after birth.

Hyperdiploid: number of chromosomes per cell that is greater than 2n. For human cells, this would be >46.

Hyperplasia: an increase in the number of cells per unit volume of tissue. This can be brought about by an increase in the number of cells replicating, by an increase in the rate of replication or by prolonged survival of cells. The cells usually maintain normal size, shape and function. The stimulus for the proliferation may be acute injury, chronic irritation or prolonged, increased hormonal stimulation: in hematology, a hyperplastic bone marrow is one in which the proportion of hematopoietic cells to fat cells is increased.

Hyperplastic: pertaining to hyperplasia.

Hypersplenism: a disorder characterized by enlargement of the spleen and pancytopenia in the presence of a hyperactive bone marrow.

Hypochromic: a lack of color; used to describe erythrocytes with an enlarged area of pallor due to a decrease in the cell's hemoglobin content. The mean corpuscular hemoglobin concentration (MCHC) and mean corpuscular hemoglobin (MCH) are decreased.

Hypodiploid: number of chromosomes per cell that is less than 2n. For human cells, this would be <46.

Hypofibrinogenemia: a condition in which there is an abnormally low fibrinogen level in the peripheral blood. It may be caused by a mutation in the gene controlling the production of fibrinogen or by an acquired condition in which fibrinogen is pathologically converted to fibrin.

Hypogammaglobulinemia: a condition associated with a decrease in resistance to infection as a result of decreased γ-globulins (immunoglobulins) in the blood.

Hypoplasia: a condition of underdeveloped tissue or organ usually caused by a decrease in the number of cells; in hematology a hypoplastic bone marrow is one in which the proportion of hematopoietic cells to fat cells is decreased.

Hypoproliferative: decreased production of any cell type(s).

Hypovolemia: diminished volume of circulating blood.

Hypoxia: a deficiency of oxygen to the cells.

Idiopathic thrombocytopenic purpura (ITP): an acquired condition in which the platelets are destroyed by immune mechanisms faster than the bone marrow is able to compensate. Platelets are decreased.

Idiopathic: pertains to disorders or diseases in which the pathogenesis is unknown.

Immune hemolytic anemia: an anemia that is caused by premature, immune mediated, destruction of erythrocytes. Diagnosis is confirmed by the demonstration of immunoglobulin (antibodies) and/or complement on the erythrocytes.

Immune response (IR): the response of a host to foreign antigens. The response results in the production of antibodies by B-lymphocytes and/or cell-mediated immunity by T-lymphocytes. Initial exposure to the antigen results in a primary immune response with the production of IgM and then IgG antibodies. Memory T- and B-lymphocytes are produced. These memory cells are sensitized and primed to react to that antigen immediately upon re-exposure. The secondary immune response is more rapid and occurs when an individual is re-exposed to the same antigen. The memory cells proliferate and produce antibodies or mediate cellular immunity.

Immune tolerance: T-suppressor lymphocyte inhibition of the antibody producing activity of B-lymphocytes against self-antigens. Loss of immune tolerance results in antibody production against self-antigens (autoimmune disorder).

Immunoblast: a T- or B-lymphocyte that is mitotically active as a result of stimulation by an antigen. The cell is morphologically characterized by a large nucleus with prominent nucleoli, a fine chromatin pattern, and abundant, deeply basophilic, cytoplasm.

Immunocompetent: the ability to respond to stimulation by an antigen.

Immunoglobulin: protein synthesized by B-lymphocytes and plasma cells that is capable of acting as an antibody. There are five antigenically distinct types of immunoglobulin: IgG, IgA, IgD, IgE and IgM.

Immunophenotyping: the process of identifying cellular membrane markers (receptors/antigens) using monoclonal antibodies.

In situ hybridization: detection of DNA or RNA by hybridization of a probe directly to a cell or tissue on a glass slide. In a variation of this procedure called fluorescence in situ hybridization (FISH), the target is a karyotypic preparation of chromosomes.

Incomplete antibodies: a term used to describe antibodies that fail to agglutinate erythrocytes in saline solution. These antibodies are usually of the IgG subclass. If incomplete antibodies are attached to patient's erythrocytes they can be detected by the antihuman globulin (AHG) test.

Indirect antihuman globulin (AHG) test: laboratory test used to detect the presence of serum antibodies against specific erythrocyte antigens.

Infectious lymphocytosis: an infectious, contagious disease of young children that may occur in epidemic form. The most striking hematologic finding is a leukocytosis of 40–50 $\times$ 10^9/L with 60–97% small normal appearing lymphocytes.

Infectious Mononucleosis: a self-limiting lymphoproliferative disease caused by infection with Epstein-Barr virus (EBV). The leukocyte count is usually increased which is related to an absolute lymphocytosis. Various forms of reactive lymphocytes are present. Serologic tests to detect the presence of heterophil antibodies are helpful in differentiating this disease from more serious diseases.

Inhibitors to single factors: pathologic antibodies directed against single clotting factors that circulate in the peripheral blood. They may arise spontaneously or, in patients with severe clotting factor deficiencies, following treatment with commercial blood products.

Integral proteins: proteins embedded between phospholipids within a cell membrane.

Intermittent idiopathic thrombocytopenic purpura (immune ITP): a form of ITP in which the platelet count is decreased at separated intervals.

Intravascular: occurring within the blood vessels.

Intrinsic factor: substance found in gastric juice secreted by parietal cells that is necessary for the absorption of cobalamin.

Intrinsic Pathway: one of three interacting pathways in the coagulation cascade. The intrinsic pathway is initiated by exposure of the contact coagulation factors (Factors XII, XI, prekallikrein and high molecular weight kininogen) with vessel subendothelial tissue. The intrinsic pathway activates factor X. The term "intrinsic" is used because all intrinsic factors are contained within the blood.

Ischemia: deficiency of blood supply to a tissue, caused by constriction of the vessel or blockage of the blood flow through the vessel.

Jaundice: yellowing of the skin, mucous membranes, and the whites of the eye caused by accumulation of bilirubin.

Karyorrhexis: disintegration of the nucleus resulting in the irregular distribution of chromatin fragments within the cytoplasm

Karyotype: a systematic display of a cell's chromosomes that determines the number of chromosomes present and their morphology.

Keratocytes: abnormally shaped erythrocytes with one or several notches and projections on either end that look like horns. Also called helmet cells and horn-shaped cells. The shape is caused by trauma to the erythrocyte.

Knizocyte: an abnormally shaped erythrocyte that appears on stained smears as a cell with a dark stick-shaped portion of hemoglobin in the center and a pale area on either end. The cell has more than two concavities.

Lecithin-cholesterol acyl transferase (LCAT): the enzyme responsible for catalyzing the reaction that results in the formation of cholesterol esters from cholesterol.

Leptocyte: an abnormally shaped erythrocyte that is thin and flat with hemoglobin at the periphery. It is usually cup-shaped.

Leukemia: a progressive, malignant disease of the hematopoietic system characterized by unregulated, clonal proliferation of the hematopoietic stem cells. The malignant cells eventually replace normal cells. It is generally classified into chronic or acute and lymphocytic or myelocytic.

Leukemic hiatus: a phase in leukemia in which there is a gap in the maturation sequence of leukocytes characterized by the presence of many blasts and some mature cells but few intermediate stages. Often seen in acute leukemias.

Leukemoid reaction: a transient, reactive condition resulting from certain types of infections or tumors char-

acterized by an increase in the total leukocyte count to greater than 30×10^9/L with many circulating immature leukocyte precursors.

Leukoerythroblastic reaction: a condition characterized by the presence of nucleated erythrocytes and a shift-to-the-left in neutrophils in the peripheral blood. Often associated with myelophthisis.

Leukocyte alkaline phosphatase (LAP): an enzyme in the cytoplasm and secondary granules of neutrophils. Semiquantitation of this enzyme through the use of special staining techniques is useful in differentiating certain disease states (i.e. CML from a leukemoid reaction and polycythemia vera from secondary erythrocytosis).

Leukocyte: white blood cell (WBC). There are five types of leukocytes: neutrophils, eosinophils, basophils, lymphocytes, monocytes. The leukocyte develops from the pluripotential stem cell in the bone marrow. Differentiation into the various types of leukocytes is influenced by hematopoietic growth factors. The function of these cells is defense against infection and tissue damage. The normal reference range for total leukocytes in peripheral blood is $3.5–11.0 \times 10^9$/L. A differential is often performed with the total leukocyte count to determine the concentrations of various leukocyte types. This can be done by automated instruments or by microscopic examination of a Romanowsky stained blood smear.

Leukocytoid lymphocyte: see reactive lymphocyte.

Leukocytosis: an increase in leukocytes greater than 11.0×10^9/L.

Leukopenia: a decrease in leukocytes below 3.5×10^9/L.

Leukophoresis: a procedure in which leukocytes are removed from the circulation.

Linkage analysis: the process of following the inheritance pattern of a particular gene in a family based on its tendency to be inherited together with another locus on the same chromosome.

Locus: a specific position on a chromosome.

Loffler's syndrome: a benign, self-limited pulmonary form of hypereosinophilic syndrome (HES) which subsides in a few weeks. Clinical findings include malaise, fever and cough.

Lupus-like anticoagulant: a circulating anticoagulant that arises spontaneously in patients with a variety of conditions (originally found in patients with lupus erythematosus) and directed against phospholipid components of the reagents used in laboratory tests for clotting factors.

Lymphadenopathy: abnormal enlargement of lymph nodes.

Lymphoblast: a lymphocytic precursor cell found in the bone marrow. The cell is 10–20 μm in diameter and has a high nuclear/cytoplasmic ratio. The nucleus has a fine (lacy) chromatin pattern with one or two nucleoli. The cytoplasm is agranular and scant. It stains deep blue with Romanowsky stain. The cell contains terminal deoxynucleotidyltransferase (TdT) but no peroxidase, lipid, or esterase.

Lymphocyte: a mature leukocyte with variable size depending on the state of cellular activity and amount of cytoplasm. The nucleus is usually round with condensed chromatin and stains deep, dark purple with Romanowsky stains. The cytoplasm stains a light blue. Nucleoli are usually not visible. A few azurophilic granules may be present. These cells interact in a series of events that allow the body to attack and eliminate foreign antigen. Lymphocytes have a peripheral blood concentration in adults from $1.5-4.0 \times 10^9$/L (20–40% of leukocytes). The concentration in children less than 10 years old is higher.

Lymphocytopenia: a decrease in the concentration of lymphocytes in the peripheral blood ($<1.5 \times 10^9$/L). Also called lymphopenia.

Lymphocytosis: an increase in peripheral blood lymphocyte concentration ($>4 \times 10^9$/L in adults or $>9 \times 10^9$/L in children).

Lymphokines: substances released by sensitized lymphocytes and responsible for activation of macrophages and other lymphocytes. Lymphocytes can affect the function of a variety of cells.

Lymphoma: malignant proliferation of lymphocytes. Most cases arise in lymph nodes, but it can begin at many extranodal sites. The lymphomas are classified as to B- or T-cell, and low, intermediate or high grade.

Lymphoproliferative disorders: broad term that refers to any abnormal proliferation of lymphocytes in peripheral blood, bone marrow, or tissue.

Lymphosarcoma: old term used for tissue based malignancy of lymphocytes (lymphoma).

Lysosomal granules: granules containing lysosomal enzymes.

Lysosome: membrane bound sacs in the cytoplasm that contain various hydrolytic enzymes. These enzymes are important in breaking down proteins and certain carbohydrates. Lysosomes combine with phagosomes after phagocytosis releasing enzymes that help destroy and digest the phagocytosed particle.

Macrocyte: an abnormally large erythrocyte. The mean corpuscular volume (MCV) is typically >100 fL and its diameter greater than 7.5 μm on a stained smear.

Macro-ovalocyte: an abnormally large erythrocyte with an oval shape. This cell is characteristically seen in megaloblastic anemia.

Macrophage: a large tissue cell (10–20 μm) derived from monocytes. The cell secretes a variety of products which influence the function of other cells. It plays a major role in both nonspecific and specific immune responses.

Marginal pool: refers to the population of neutrophils that are attached to or marginated along the vessel walls and not actively circulating. This is about one-half the total pool of neutrophils in the vessels.

Mean cell volume (MCV): an indicator of the average volume of individual erythrocytes reported in femtoliters. This measurement may be determined by use of an automated instrument or calculated manually from the hematocrit and erythrocyte count:

$$\text{MCV (fL)} = \frac{\text{Hematocrit (L/L)}}{\text{Erythrocyte count } (\times 10^{12}/\text{L})} \times 1000$$

This parameter is useful when evaluating erythrocyte morphology on a stained blood smear. The MCV will correlate with the diameter of the erythrocytes observed microscopically. The reference interval for MCV is 80–100 fL.

Mean Corpuscular Hemoglobin (MCH): an indicator of the average weight of hemoglobin in individual erythrocytes reported in picograms. This parameter is calculated manually from the hemoglobin and erythrocyte count:

$$\text{MCH (pg)} = \frac{\text{Hemoglobin (g/dL)}}{\text{Erythrocyte count } (\times 10^{12}/\text{L})} \times 10$$

The reference interval for MCH is 26–34 pg.

Mean Corpuscular Hemoglobin Concentration (MCHC): a measure of the average concentration of hemoglobin in grams per deciliter of erythrocytes. The MCHC is useful when evaluating erythrocyte hemoglobin content on a stained smear. This parameter will correlate with the extent of chromasia exhibited by the stained cells and is calculated from the hemoglobin and hematocrit as follows:

$$\text{MCHC (g/dL)} = \frac{\text{Hemoglobin (g/dL)}}{\text{Hematocrit (L/L)}}$$

The reference interval for MCHC is 32–36 g/dL

Medullary hematopoiesis: the production and development of hematopoietic cells in the bone marrow. (see extramedullary hematopoiesis).

Megakaryocytes: a large cell found within the bone marrow characterized by the presence of a large or multiple nuclei and abundant cytoplasm. Gives rise to the blood platelets.

Megakaryopoiesis: the production and development of megakaryocytes from which platelets are formed. This development is under the control of hematopoietic growth factors.

Megaloblastic: asynchronous maturation of any nucleated cell type characterized by delayed nuclear development in comparison to the cytoplasmic development. The abnormal cells are large. They are characteristically found in pernicious anemia or other megaloblastic anemia.

Meninges: membranes that cover and protect the central nervous system: dura mater, arachnoid mater, and pia mater.

Metacentric: chromosome that has the centromere near center so that the short arm and long arms are of equal length.

Metamyelocyte: a granulocytic precursor cell normally found in the bone marrow. The cell is 10–15 μm in diameter. The cytoplasm stains pink and there is a predominance of specific granules. The nucleus is indented with a kidney-bean shape. The nuclear chromatin is condensed and stains dark purple.

Metaplasia: conversion of normal cells into abnormal cells.

Methemoglobin reductase pathway: a metabolic pathway that uses methemoglobin reductase and NADH to maintain heme iron in the reduced state (Fe^{++}).

Methemoglobin: hemoglobin in which the iron has been oxidized to the ferric state (Fe^{+++}). This form of hemoglobin is incapable of combining with oxygen.

Mexican hat cell: see codocyte.

Microangiopathic hemolytic anemia: term used to describe any hemolytic process that is caused by prosthetic devices or lesions of the small blood vessels.

Microcyte: an abnormally small erythrocyte. The MCV is typically less than 80 fL and its diameter less than 7.0 μm on a stained smear.

Microfilament: a contractile filament composed of actin and found in most cells. The filament supports and moves cell membranes; together, the microfilaments form the contractile ring during mitosis.

Microtubule: a cylindric structure (20–27 μm in diameter) composed of protein subunits. It is a part of the cytoskeleton, helping some cells maintain shape. The microtubules increase during mitosis and form the mitotic spindle fibers. They also assist in transporting substances in different directions. In the platelet, a band of tubules located on the circumference is thought to be essential for maintaining the disc shape in the resting state.

Mitochondrium (pl. mitochondria): a microscopic rod (0.5μm) within the cytoplasm of a cell that is the principal site of energy production for the cell through oxidative phosphorylation and adenosine triphosphate (ATP) synthesis. It is also involved in protein synthesis and lipid metabolism. This organelle is sometimes referred to as the cell's "power plant."

Mitotic pool: the population of cells within the bone marrow that is capable of DNA synthesis. Also called the proliferating pool.

Mixed lineage acute leukemia: an acute leukemia that has both myeloid and lymphoid populations present or blasts that possess myeloid and lymphoid markers on the same cell.

Monoblast: the monocytic precursor cell found in bone marrow. It is about 14–18 μm in diameter with abundant agranular, blue-grey cytoplasm. The nucleus may be folded or indented. The chromatin is finely dispersed and several nucleoli are visible. The monoblast has nonspecific esterase activity that is inhibited by sodium fluoride.

Monoclonal gammopathy: an alteration in immunoglobulin production that is characterized by an increase in one specific class of immunoglobulin.

Monoclonal: arising from a single cell.

Monocyte: a mature leukocyte found in bone marrow or peripheral blood. Its morphology depends upon its activity. The cell ranges in size from 12–30 μm with an average of 18 μm. The blue-grey cytoplasm is evenly dispersed with fine dust-like granules. There are two types of granules. One contains peroxidase, acid phosphatase and arylsulfatase. Less is known about the content of the other granule. The nuclear chromatin is loose and linear forming a lacy pattern. The nucleus is often irregular in shape.

Monocytopenia: a decrease in the concentration of circulating monocytes ($<0.2 \times 10^9$/L).

Monocytosis: an increase in the concentration of circulating monocytes ($>0.8 \times 10^9$/L).

Mononuclear-phagocyte system: a collection of monocytes and macrophages, found both intravascularly and extravascularly. The primary functions of this system are phagocytic and immunologic. It was formerly known as the reticulo-endothelial system.

Morulae: basophilic, irregularly shaped granular, cytoplasmic inclusions found in leukocytes in an infectious disease called ehrlichiosis.

Mott cell: a pathologic plasma cell whose cytoplasm is filled with colorless globules. These globules most often contain immunoglobulin (Russell bodies). The globules form as a result of accumulation of material in the RER, SER or Golgi complex due to an obstruction of secretion. The cell is associated with chronic plasmocyte hyperplasia, parasitic infection and malignant tumors. Also called a grape cell.

Mutation: any change in the nucleotide sequence of DNA. In instances where large sequences of nucleotides are missing, the alteration is referred to as a deletion.

Myeloblast: the first microscopically identifiable granulocyte precursor. It is normally found in the bone marrow. The cell is large (15–20 μm) with a high nuclear/cytoplasmic ratio. The nucleus has a fine chromatin pattern with nucleoli. There is a moderate amount of blue, agranular cytoplasm.

Myelocyte: a granulocytic precursor cell normally found in the bone marrow. The cell is 12–18 μm in diameter with a pinkish, granular cytoplasm. There are both primary and secondary granules present.

Myelodysplastic syndromes: a group of primary, neoplastic pluripotential stem cell disorders characterized by one or more cytopenias in the peripheral blood together with prominent maturation abnormalities in the bone marrow. The FAB classification includes five subgroups: refractory anemia, refractory anemia with ringed sideroblasts, refractory anemia with excess blasts, refractory anemia with excess blasts in transformation and chronic myelomonocytic leukemia.

Myelodysplastic: in hematology, pertaining to abnormal development of blood cells.

Myelofibrosis with myeloid metaplasia: a myeloproliferative disorder characterized by excessive proliferation of all cell lines as well as progressive bone marrow fibrosis and blood cell production at sites other than the bone marrow such as the liver and spleen. Also called agnogenic myeloid metaplasia and primary myelofibrosis.

Myeloid to erythroid ratio (M:E ratio): the ratio of granulocytes and their precursors to nucleated erythroid precursors derived from performing a differential count on bone marrow nucleated hematopoietic cells. Monocytes and lymphocytes are not included. The normal ratio is usually between 1.5 to 1 and 3.5 to 1 reflecting a predominance of myeloid elements.

Myeloperoxidase stain: a cytochemical stain used to identify the enzyme myeloperoxidase within primary granules of myelocytic and monocytic cells.

Myeloperoxidase: an enzyme present in the primary granules of myeloid cells including neutrophils, eosinophils and monocytes.

Myelophthisic anemia: an anemia resulting from replacement of normal bone marrow tissue with a tumor or other tissue. The erythrocytes in the peripheral blood are usually misshapen (poikilocytes) often in the form of teardrops (dacryocytes).

Myeloproliferative: term used to describe a group of neoplastic, clonal disorders characterized by excess proliferation of one or more cell types in the bone marrow.

Necrosis: morphological changes that indicate death of tissue.

Neonatal idiopathic thrombocytopenic purpura (neonatal ITP): a form of ITP that occurs in newborns because of the transfer of maternal alloantibodies.

Neoplasm: abnormal formation of new tissue (such as a tumor) that serves no useful purpose.

Neoplastic: pertaining to the formation of new, abnormal tissue such as a tumor.

Neutropenia: a decrease in neutrophils below 2×10^9/L.

Neutrophilia: an increase in neutrophils over 7×10^9/L. Seen in bacterial infections, inflammation, metabolic intoxication, drug intoxication and tissue necrosis.

Nondisjunction: an error in segregation that occurs in mitosis or meiosis so that sister chromatids do not disjoin. A spindle fiber malfunction results in one daughter cell with an extra chromosome (trisomy) and one daughter cell with a missing chromosome (monosomy).

Nonspecific granules: large blue-black granules found in promyelocytes. The granules have a phospholipid membrane that stains with Sudan black B and contain acid phosphatase, myeloperoxidase, acid hydrolases, lysozyme, sulfated mucopolysaccharide and other basic proteins. Also called azurophilic or primary granules.

Normoblast: nucleated erythrocyte precursor cell found in the bone marrow. Also called an erythroblast.

Nuclear cytoplasmic asynchrony: a term used to describe a cell when the nuclear and cytoplasmic development do not occur together. The nuclear development lags behind cytoplasmic development. Thus, the nucleus takes on the appearance of a nucleus associated with a younger cell than its cytoplasmic development indicates. This is a characteristic of megaloblastic anemias.

Nuclear to cytoplasmic ratio (N:C ratio): the ratio of the volume of the cell nucleus to the volume of the cell's cytoplasm. This is usually estimated as the ratio of the diameter of the nucleus to the diameter of the cytoplasm. In immature hematopoietic cells the N:C ratio is usually greater than in more mature cells. As the cell matures, the nucleus condenses and the cytoplasm expands.

Nucleolus (pl: nucleoli): a spherical body within the nucleus in which ribosomes are produced. It is not present in cells that are not synthesizing proteins or that are not in mitosis or meiosis. It stains a lighter blue than the nucleus with Romanowsky stains.

Nucleotide: the basic building block of DNA, composed of a nitrogen base (A = adenine, T = thymine, G = guanine, or C = cytosine) attached to a sugar (deoxyribose) and a phosphate molecule.

Nucleus (pl: nuclei): the characteristic structure in the eukaryocytic cell that contains chromosomes and nucleoli. It is separated from the cytoplasm by a nuclear envelope. It is the site of DNA replication and transcription. The structure stains deep bluish-purple with Romanowsky stains. In young, immature, hematopoietic cells, the nuclear material is open and dispersed in a lacy pattern. As the cell becomes mature, the nuclear material condenses and appears structureless.

Oncogene: a gene that contributes to the development of cancer. Most oncogenes are altered forms of normal genes that function to regulate cell growth and differentiation.

Opsonin: an antibody or complement that coats microorganisms or other particulate matter found within the blood stream so that the foreign material may be more readily recognized and phagocytized by leukocytes.

Orthochromatic normoblast: a nucleated precursor of the erythrocyte that develops from the polychromatophilic normoblast. The cell is found in the bone marrow but may also be found in the peripheral blood in hematologic disorders and in the newborn. As the cell matures, it loses its nucleus and becomes a reticulocyte. The cell is 8–10 μm in diameter. The nuclear chromatin is structureless, and the nucleus may be fragmented. The cytoplasm is pink or orange-pink with only a tinge of blue. Also called a metarubricyte.

Osmotic fragility: a laboratory procedure employed to evaluate the ability of erythrocytes to withstand different salt concentrations; this is dependent upon the erythrocyte's membrane, volume, surface area, and functional state.

Oxidant: an oxidizing agent.

Oxygen-affinity: the ease with which hemoglobin binds and releases oxygen. This affinity is physiologically adjustable. An increase in CO_2, acid and heat decrease oxygen affinity while an increase in pO_2 increases oxygen affinity.

Oxyhemoglobin: the compound formed when hemoglobin combines with oxygen.

Pancytopenia: marked decrease of all blood cells in the peripheral blood.

Panhypercellular: an increase in all blood cells in the peripheral blood.

Panhyperplasia: an abnormal increase in all cell types.

Pappenheimer body: a blue staining erythrocyte inclusion composed of iron containing granules; visible near the periphery of the cell in Romanowsky stained smears and often occurs in clusters. Also stains with Prussian blue stain.

Parahemophilia: an alternate name, no longer used, for a deficiency of coagulation factor V.

Paroxysmal cold hemoglobinuria: an autoimmune hemolytic anemia characterized by hemolysis and hematuria upon exposure to cold.

Paroxysmal nocturnal hemoglobinuria (PNH): a stem cell disease in which the erythrocyte membrane is abnormal making the cell more susceptible to hemolysis by complement. There is a lack of decay accelerating factor (DAF) and C8 binding protein (C8bp) on the membrane which normally is responsible for preventing amplification of complement activation. The deficiency of DAF and C8bp is due to the lack of glycosyl phosphatidyl inositol (GPI) a membrane glycolipid that serves to attach (anchor) proteins to the cell membrane. Intravascular hemolysis is intermittent. Often the first sign of the disease is passage of bloody urine upon awakening.

Pelger-Huet anomaly: an inherited benign condition characterized by the presence of functionally normal neutrophils with a bi-lobed nucleus. Cells with this appearance are called "pince-nez" cells.

Pericardial cavity: anatomic region between the outermost portion of the heart and innermost portion of the pericardial sac.

Pericardium: thin membrane that lines the outermost portion of the heart (visceral pericardium) and is continuous with the innermost portion of the pericardial sac (parietal pericardium).

Peripheral protein: protein that is attached to the cell membrane by ionic or hydrogen bonds but is outside the lipid framework of the membrane.

Peritoneal cavity: anatomic region between the outermost portion of the intestine, liver, and pelvic dome, and the innermost portion of the abdominal wall.

Peritoneum: thin membrane that lines the outermost portion of the intestine, liver, and pelvic dome (visceral peritoneum) and is continuous with the innermost portion of the abdominal wall (parietal peritoneum).

Pernicious anemia: megaloblastic anemia resulting from a lack of intrinsic factor. The intrinsic factor is needed to absorb cobalamin (vitamin B12) from the gut.

Petechiae: small, pinhead-sized purple spots caused by blood escaping from capillaries into intact skin. These are associated with platelet and vascular disorders.

Phagocytosis: the process by which certain types of cells destroy micro-organisms and cellular debris by means of ingestion and digestion of the particulate matter.

Phagolysosome: a digestive vacuole (secondary lysosome) formed by the fusion of lysosomes and a phagosome. The hydrolytic enzymes of the lysosome digest the phagocytosed material.

Phospholipase A$_2$: a cell membrane enzyme that hydrolyzes the fatty acid from the R$_2$ position of a phospholipid. This is usually arachidonic acid and in the platelet leads to the production of thromboxane A$_2$.

Phospholipase C: a cell membrane enzyme that hydrolyzes phosphatidylinositol on cell membranes and begins a series of reactions that transfers messages from the external environment to the inside.

Pia mater: thin membrane directly covering the central nervous system; middle layer of the meninges.

Pica: a perversion of appetite that leads to bizarre eating practices; a clinical finding in some individuals with iron deficiency anemia.

Pitting: a function of the spleen in which abnormal inclusions are removed from erythrocytes and the intact cells released into the circulation.

PIVKA (protein-induced by vitamin-K absence or antagonist): these factors are the nonfunctional forms of the prothrombin group coagulation factors. They are synthesized in the liver in the absence of vitamin-K and lack the carboxyl (COOH) group necessary for binding the factor to a phospholipid surface.

Plasma cell: a transformed, fully differentiated B-lymphocyte normally found in the bone marrow and medullary cords of lymph nodes. May be seen in the circulation in certain infections and disorders associated with increased serum γ-globulins. The cell is characterized by the presence of an eccentric nucleus containing condensed, deeply staining chromatin and deep basophilic cytoplasm. The large Golgi apparatus next to the nucleus does not stain leaving an obvious clear paranuclear area. The cell has the PC-1 membrane antigen and cytoplasmic immunoglobulin.

Plasmacytoid Lymphocyte: a term used to describe an intermediate stage in the transformation of an antigen stimulated B-lymphocyte to a plasma cell. The cell ranges in size from 15–20 μm. The chromatin is less clumped than that of a plasma cell and a nucleolus may be visible. The cytoplasm is deeply basophilic. The membrane antigens include CD19, CD20, and PC-1.

Plasmacytosis: the presence of plasma cells in the peripheral blood or an excess of plasma cells in the bone marrow.

Plasmin: a proteolytic enzyme with trypsin-like specificity that digests fibrin or fibrinogen as well as other coagulation factors. Plasmin is formed from plasminogen.

Plasminogen activator inhibitor-1 (PAI-1): the primary inhibitor of tissue plasminogen activator (t-PA) and urokinase-like plasminogen activator (tcu-PA) released from platelet α-granules during platelet activation.

Plasminogen activator inhibitor-2 (PAI-2): an inhibitor of tissue plasminogen activator and urokinase-like plasminogen activator. Secretion of PAI-2 is stimulated by endotoxin and phorbol esters. Increased levels impair fibrinolysis and are associated with thrombosis.

Plasminogen: a β-globulin, single chain glycoprotein that circulates in the blood as a zymogen. Large amounts of plasminogen are absorbed with the fibrin mass during clot formation. Plasminogen is activated by intrinsic and extrinsic activators to form plasmin.

Platelet adhesion: platelet attachment to collagen fibers.

Platelet aggregation: platelet to platelet interaction that results in a clumped mass; may occur in vitro or in vivo.

Platelet factor 3: the procoagulant property of platelet phospholipids that enables activated coagulation factors and cofactors to adhere to the platelet surface during fibrin formation.

Platelet procoagulant activity: the properties of platelets that enables activated coagulation factors and cofactors to adhere to the platelet surface during the formation of fibrin.

Plateletpheresis: a procedure in which platelets are removed from the circulation.

Platelet: a round or oval structure in the peripheral blood formed from the cytoplasm of megakaryocytes in the bone marrow. Platelets play an important role in primary hemostasis adhering to the ruptured blood vessel wall and aggregating to form a platelet plug over the injured area. Platelets are also important in secondary hemostasis by providing platelet factor 3 (PF3) important for the activation of coagulation proteins. The normal reference range for platelets is $150-440 \times 10^9$/L.

Pleomorphism: having varied morphology within a single cell population. Commonly used in reference to white blood cells.

Pleura: thin membrane that lines the outermost portion of both lungs (visceral pleura) and is continuous with the innermost portion of the chest wall (parietal pleura).

Pleural Cavity: anatomic region between the outermost portion of the lungs and the innermost portion of the chest wall.

Plumbism: lead poisoning.

Pluripotential stem cell: a hematopoietic stem cell that has the potential to self-renew, proliferate and differentiate into erythrocytic, myelocytic, monocytic, lymphocytic and megakaryocytic blood cell lineages.

Poikilocytosis: a term used to describe the presence of variations in the shape of erythrocytes.

Polychromatophilia: the quality of being stainable with more than one stain; the term is commonly used to describe erythrocytes that stain with a greyish or bluish tinge with Romanowsky stains. These cells are young erythrocytes with residual RNA which takes up the blue portion of the dye. When stained supravitally, these cells are identified as reticulocytes.

Polychromatophilic erythrocyte: a red blood cell that stains a bluish-grey with Romanowsky stains due to the presence of residual RNA. These are young cells that have been released from the bone marrow in the last 24 to 48 hours. They are usually larger than more mature red blood cells. If stained with new methylene blue, these cells would show reticulum and would be identified as reticulocytes.

Polychromatophilic normoblast: a nucleated precursor of the erythrocyte that is derived from the basophilic normoblast. The cell is found in the bone marrow and matures to the orthochromatic normoblast. The cell is $10-12$ μm in diameter. The nuclear chromatin is irregular and coarsely clumped. There is abundant cytoplasm that stains bluish-grey. Also called a rubricyte.

Polyclonal gammopathy: an alteration in immunoglobulin production that is characterized by an increase in immunoglobulins of more than one class.

Polyclonal: arising from different cell clones.

Polycythemia: an increase in cellular blood elements; most commonly used to describe an increase in total erythrocyte mass.

Polymerase chain reaction: a procedure for copying a specific DNA sequence many-fold.

Polymorphonuclear neutrophil (PMN): a mature granulocyte found in bone marrow and peripheral blood.

The nucleus is segmented into 2 or more lobes. The cytoplasm stains pinkish and there is abundant specific granules. The cell is $9-15$ μm in diameter. This is the most numerous leukocyte in the peripheral blood ($2-7 \times 10^9$/L). Its primary function is defense against foreign antigens. It is active in phagocytosis and killing of microorganisms. Also called a segmented neutrophil or seg.

Polyploid: number of chromosomes per cell that is a multiple of n other than one or two. e.g., 3n(69), 4n(92), etc.

Pores: small openings in the cytoplasm of endothelial cells that allow for the movement of cells or substances.

Porphyrins: a highly unsaturated tetrapyrrole ring bonded by four methene ($-CH=$) bridges. Substituents occupy each of the eight peripheral positions on the four pyrrole rings. The kind and order of these substituents determine the type of porphyrin. Porphyrins are only metabolically active when they are chelated. When iron is chelated to porphyrin, it is known as heme, a constituent of hemoglobin and myoglobin.

Portland hemoglobin: an embryonic hemoglobin found in the yolk sac and detectable up to eight weeks gestation. It is composed of two zeta (ζ) chains and two gamma (γ) chains.

Post-mitotic pool: also called the maturation-storage pool; the neutrophils in the bone marrow that are not capable of mitosis. These cells include metamyelocytes, bands and segmented neutrophils. Cells spend about 5-7 days in this compartment before being released to the peripheral blood.

Primary aggregation: the earliest association of platelets in an aggregate that is reversible.

Primary fibrinolysis: a clinical situation that occurs when there is a release of excessive quantities of plasminogen activators into the blood in the absence of fibrin clot formation. Excess plasmin degrades fibrinogen and the clotting factors leading to a potentially dangerous hemorrhagic condition.

Primary hemostasis: the initial arrest of bleeding that occurs with blood vessel/platelet interaction.

Primary hemostatic plug: an aggregate of platelets that initially halts blood flow from an injury.

Primitive erythropoiesis: the production and development of primitive erythroblasts in the yolk sac of the embryo.

Probe: a tool for identifying a particular nucleotide sequence of interest. A probe is composed of a nucleotide sequence that is complementary to the sequence of interest and is therefore capable of hybridizing to that sequence. Probes are labeled in a way that is detectable, such as by radioactivity.

Procoagulant: an inert precursor of a natural substance that is necessary for blood clotting or a property of anything that favors formation of a blood clot.

Prolymphocyte: the immediate precursor cell of the lymphocyte; normally found in bone marrow. It is slightly smaller than the lymphoblast and has a lower nuclear to cytoplasmic ratio. The nuclear chromatin is somewhat clumped and nucleoli are usually present. The cytoplasm stains light blue and is agranular. The cell matures to a lymphocyte.

Promonocyte: a monocytic precursor cell found in the bone marrow. The cell is 14–18 μm in diameter with abundant blue-grey cytoplasm. Fine azurophilic granules may be present. The nucleus is often irregular and deeply indented. The chromatin is finely dispersed and stains a light purple-blue. Nucleoli may be present. Cytochemically the cells stain-positive for nonspecific esterase, peroxidase, acid phosphatase and arylsulfatase. The cell matures to a monocyte.

Promyelocyte: a granulocytic precursor cell normally found in the bone marrow. The cell is 15–21 μm in diameter. The cytoplasm is basophilic and the nucleus is quite large. The nuclear chromatin is lacy, staining a light purple-blue. Several nucleoli are visible. The distinguishing feature is the presence of large blue-black primary (azurophilic) granules. The granules have a phospholipid membrane that stains with Sudan black B. The granules contain acid phosphatase, myeloperoxidase, acid hydrolases, lysozyme, sulfated mucopolysaccharides and other basic proteins. The promyelocyte matures to a myelocyte. Also called a progranulocyte.

Pronormoblast: a precursor cell of the erythrocyte. The cell is derived from the pluripotential stem cell and is found in the bone marrow. The cell is 12–20 μm in the diameter and has a high nuclear/cytoplasmic ratio. The cytoplasm is deeply basophilic with Romanowsky stains. The nuclear chromatin is fine and there is one or more nucleoli. Also called a rubriblast. The cell matures to a basophilic normoblast.

Prothrombin group: the group of coagulation factors that are vitamin-K dependent for synthesis of their functional forms and that require calcium for binding to a phospholipid surface. Includes factors II, VII, IX, X. Also known as vitamin-K dependent factors.

Prothrombin time ratio: a calculation derived by dividing the patient's prothrombin time result by the midpoint of the laboratory's normal range and used to calculate the international normalized ratio (INR).

Prothrombinase complex: a complex formed by coagulation factors Xa, and V, calcium and phospholipid. This complex activates prothrombin to thrombin.

Proto-oncogene: a gene that when activated or altered forms an oncogene. Oncogenes can cause cancer/tumors.

Prourokinase: an immature, single-chained form of urokinase that is prepared from urine and by recombinant DNA techniques and can be activated to an active two-chain form by plasmin.

Pseudochylous: Fluid that appears chylous due to the presence of many inflammatory cells; does not contain lymph fluid or chylomicrons.

Pseudodiploid: a cell that has a chromosome count of 2n, however, with a combination of numerical and/or structural aberrations. e.g., 46,XY, -5, -7, 2D8, 2D21.

Pseudoneutropenia: a decrease in the concentration of neutrophils in the circulation ($<2.0 \times 10^9$/L) due to a temporary shift of cells from the circulating pool to the marginal pool. This occurs in some infections and hypersensitivity.

Pseudoneutrophilia: an increase in the concentration of neutrophils in the peripheral blood ($>7.0 \times 10^9$/L) occurring as a result of cells from the marginating pool entering the circulating pool. The response is immediate but transient. This redistribution of cells accompanies vigorous exercise, epinephrine administration, anesthesia, convulsions and anxiety states. Also called immediate or shift neutrophilia.

Pseudopods: spiny projections from the surface of activated platelets.

Pure red cell aplasia (PRCA): a disease characterized by a selective decrease in erythroid precursor cells in the marrow accompanied by peripheral blood anemia.

Purpura: (1) Purple discoloration of the skin caused by petechiae and/or ecchymoses; (2) a diverse group of disorders that are characterized by the presence of petechiae and ecchymoses.

Pyknotic: pertaining to degeneration of the nucleus of the cell in which the chromatin condenses to a solid, structureless mass and shrinks in size.

Pyrogen: a fever-producing substance.

Q-band: differential pattern of bright and dull fluorescent bands following quinacrine (fluorescent) staining.

Rapoport-Leubering shunt: a metabolic pathway in which 2,3-diphosphoglycerate (DPG) is synthesized from 1,3-diphosphoglycerate]. 2,3-DPG facilitates the release of oxygen from hemoglobin in the erythrocyte. 2,3-DPG is also refferred to as 2,3-BPG (bisphosphoglycerate).

Raynaud's phenomenon: secondary disorder resulting from vaso-arterial spasms in the extremities of the body when exposed to the cold. Characterized by blanching of the skin, followed by cyanosis and finally redness when the affected area is warmed; also referred to as acrocyanosis.

Reactive lymphocyte: an antigen stimulated lymphocyte that exhibits a variety of morphologic features. The cell is usually larger than resting lymphocytes and has an irregular shape. The cytoplasm is more basophilic. The nucleus is often elongated and irregular with a finer chromatin pattern than that of the resting lymphocyte. Often this cell is increased in viral infections; also called a virocyte, or stimulated, transformed, atypical, activated or leukocytoid lymphocyte.

Reactive neutrophilia: an increase in the concentration of peripheral blood neutrophils ($>7.0 \times 10^9$/L) as a result of reaction to a physiologic or pathologic process.

Refractory anemia with excess blasts (RAEB): a subgroup of the FAB classification of the myelodysplastic syndromes. There are usually cytopenias and signs of dyspoiesis in the peripheral blood with <5% blasts. The bone marrow is usually hypercellular with dyspoiesis in all hematopoietic cell lineages. Bone marrow blasts vary from 5%-20%.

Refractory anemia with excess blasts in transformation (RAEB-T): a subgroup of the FAB classification of the myelodysplastic syndromes. There is/are cytopenia(s) in the peripheral blood with more than 5% blasts. The bone marrow is usually hypercellular with dyspoiesis and 20%-30% blasts.

Refractory anemia with ringed sideroblasts (RARS): a subgroup of the FAB classification of the myelodysplastic syndromes characterized by <1% blasts in the peripheral blood, anemia and/or thrombocytopenia and/or leukopenia. There are more than 15% ringed sideroblasts and <5% blasts in the bone marrow.

Refractory anemia: a subgroup of the FAB classification of the myelodysplastic syndromes. Anemia refractory to all conventional therapy is the primary clinical finding. Blasts constitute <1% of nucleated peripheral blood cells. The bone marrow shows signs of dyserythropoiesis.

Refractory: pertains to disorders or diseases that do not respond readily to therapy.

Release: energy dependent discharge or secretion of the contents of platelet granules that occurs after stimulation of the platelets by agonists.

Replication: the process by which DNA is copied during cell division. Replication is carried out by the enzyme DNA polymerase that recognizes single stranded DNA and fills in the appropriate complementary nucleotides to produce double stranded DNA. Synthesis is initiated at a free 5′ end where double stranded DNA lies adjacent to single stranded DNA, and replication proceeds in the 5′ direction. In the laboratory, DNA replication can be induced as a means of copying DNA sequences, as exploited in the polymerase chain reaction.

Restriction endonuclease: an enzyme that cleaves double-stranded DNA at specific nucleotide sequences. For example, HindIII cleaves DNA only where the sequence 5′-AAGCTT-3′ is present. A variety of other enzymes are known to cut various specific target sequences.

Reticulocytosis: the presence of excess reticulocytes in the peripheral blood.

Reticulocyte production index (RPI): an indicator of the bone marrow response in anemia. This calculation corrects the reticulocyte count for the presence of marrow reticulocytes in the peripheral blood. It is calculated using the following formula:

$$\frac{\text{Patient hematocrit (L/L)}}{0.45\ (\text{L/L})} \times \text{reticulocyte count (\%)}$$

$$\times \frac{1}{\substack{\text{maturation time of shift} \\ \text{reticulocytes}}} = \text{RPI}$$

Reticulocyte: a young erythrocyte that contains residual RNA but no nucleus. The RNA is visualized as granules or filaments within the cell when stained supravitally with new methylene blue. Normally reticulocytes constitute approximately 1% of the circulating erythrocyte population.

Rh system: a blood group that may be present on erythrocytes. When present, the blood type is Rh positive and when absent the blood type is Rh negative. An Rh negative mother may become sensitized by an Rh positive fetus. In future pregnancies, if the fetus is Rh positive, the mother may produce antibodies against the Rh antigen on fetal cells. These antibodies can cross the placenta and destroy fetal erythrocytes. This condition is known as erythroblastosis fetalis or hemolytic disease of the newborn.

Ribosomes: a cellular particle composed of ribonucleic acid (RNA) and protein whose function is to synthesize polypeptide chains from amino acids. The sequence of amino acids in the chains is specified by the genetic code of messenger RNA. Ribosomes appear singly or in reversibly dissociable units and may be free in the cytoplasm or attached to endoplasmic reticulum. The cytoplasm of blood cells that contain a high concentration of ribosomes stains bluish-purple with Romanowsky stains.

RNA (ribonucleic acid): a single stranded molecule composed of ribonucleotides (A,C,G and U = uracil). RNA is produced by transcription of genes on a DNA template, and RNA in turn serves as a template for protein translation.

Rhopheocytosis: an energy and temperature dependent process by which iron enters cells.

Rough endoplasmic reticulum: see endoplasmic reticulum.

Rouleau (plural rouleaux): erythrocyte distribution characterized by stacking of the erythrocytes like a roll of coins. This is due to abnormal coating of the cell's surface with increased plasma proteins which decreases the zeta potential between cells.

Russell body: globule filled with immunoglobulin found in pathologic plasma cells called Mott cells. (See Mott cell).

Satellite: DNA containing many tandem repeats. Morphologically, it appears as a small ball-like structure making up the short arm of acrocentric chromosomes. This is the locus of the nucleolar organizing region.

Schistocyte: fragment of an erythrocyte; a schistocyte may have a variety of shapes including triangles, helmets, commas.

SCID (severe combined immunodeficiency disease): an inherited condition in which there are deficient T- and B-lymphocytes resulting in severe immune deficiency. Lymphopenia is usually due to a deficiency of both T- and B-lymphocytes but occasionally only T-lymphocytes. Immunoglobulins are decreased. Clinically, there is recurrent opportunistic infections. The disease is usually fatal within the first two years of life.

Secondary aggregation: irreversible aggregation of platelets that occurs over a period of time.

Secondary fibrinolysis: a clinical condition characterized by excessive fibrinolytic activity in response to disseminated intravascular clotting.

Secondary hemostasis: the formation of fibrin which stabilizes a primary platelet aggregate.

Secondary hemostatic plug: a primary platelet aggregate that has been stabilized by fibrin formation during secondary hemostasis.

Secretion: energy dependent discharge or release of products usually from glands in the body but also pertaining to the contents of platelet granules that are released after stimulation of the platelets by agonists; also, the product that is discharged or released.

Sensitize: development of specific antibodies in response to an antigen.

Septicemia: the presence of micro-organisms in the blood stream resulting in a systemic infection.

Shape change: transformation of platelets from discs to spiny spheres that occurs after stimulation by agonists.

Shift neutrophilia: see pseudoneutrophilia.

Shift-to-the-left: term used to describe the appearance of increased numbers of immature leukocytes in the peripheral blood.

Sickle-cell anemia: a genetically determined disorder in which hemoglobin S is inherited in the homozygous state. No hemoglobin A is present. Hemoglobins S, F, A_2 are present.

Sickle-cell trait: a genetically determined disorder in which hemoglobin S is inherited in the heterozygous state. The patient has one normal β-globin gene and one β^s-globin gene. Both hemoglobin A and hemoglobin S are present.

Sideroachrestic: pertaining to a defect in iron utilization.

Sideroblast: normoblast within the bone marrow that contains stainable iron granules.

Siderocyte: an erythrocyte that contains stainable iron granules.

Sideropenia: a condition of a deficiency in iron.

Sideropenic: pertaining to iron deficiency

Smooth endoplasmic reticulum (SER): see endoplasmic reticulum.

Somatic: pertaining to the body.

Southern blot: a procedure first described by Ed Southern for determining DNA structure. In this procedure, DNA is cleaved with restriction endonucleases that cut DNA at specific nucleotide sequences. The resulting DNA fragments are electrophoresed in an agarose gel to separate them by size, and then treated with a solution of high pH that separates double-stranded DNA into two single-stranded parts. The single-stranded fragments are then transferred to a membrane where they can be hybridized to a complementary labeled probe. Probe hybridization permits identification of the DNA fragments containing the sequence of interest. The size and number of those fragments reflects the structure of the DNA. (See Figure 3 in Chapter 21)

Specific granules: granules that appear at the myelocyte stage of neutrophil development. Also called secondary granules. They contain alkaline phosphatase, lysozyme, amino peptidase, collagenase and basic proteins.

Spherocyte: an abnormally round-shaped erythrocyte with dense hemoglobin content (increased MCHC). The cell has no central area of pallor as it has lost its biconcave shape.

Splenectomy: removal of the spleen.

Splenomegaly: abnormal enlargement of the spleen.

Stab: see band.

Steatorrhea: increased amounts of fat in the stool.

Stimulated lymphocyte: a lymphocyte that has encountered an antigen. This cell may differentiate into an effector cell that mediates the immune response or a memory cell.

Stomatocytes: an abnormal erythrocyte shape characterized by a slit-like area of central pallor. This cell has a uniconcave, cup-shape.

Streptokinase: a bacterial enzyme derived from group C-beta hemolytic streptococci that activates plasminogen to plasmin and is used as a thrombolytic agent in the treatment of thrombosis.

Subendothelium: tissue of the wall of blood vessels beneath the endothelial cell monolayer.

Submetacentric: chromosome that has the centromere positioned off-center so that the short arm is shorter in length than the long arm.

Sucrose hemolysis test: a screening test to identify erythrocytes that are abnormally sensitive to complement lysis. In this test, erythrocytes, serum and sucrose are incubated together. Cells abnormally sensitive to complement will lyse. The test is used to screen for paroxysmal nocturnal hemoglobinuria. Also called the sugar-water test.

Sudan black B: a lipophilic dye that stains intracellular lipid. Granular cells (i.e., myeloid cells) develop increasing amounts of cytoplasmic lipids as they mature. Therefore myeloid cells stain positive with this dye. Lymphoid cells are negative.

Sulfhemoglobin: hemoglobin that results when sulfur combines with the heme portion of the hemoglobin molecule. This is a very stable compound that is incapable of carrying oxygen.

Synaptonemal complex: close, gene-for-gene association of homologous pairs of chromosomes during stage I of meiosis.

Synovium: continuous membrane that lines the bony, cartilaginous, and connective tissue surfaces of a joint.

Telangiectasis: persistent dilation of superficially located veins.

Thalassemia: a group of genetically determined microcytic, hypochromic anemias resulting from a decrease in synthesis of one or more globin chains in the hemoglobin molecule. The disorder may occur in the homozygous or heterozygous state. Heterozygotes may be asymptomatic but homozygotes typically have a severe, often fatal, disease. Thalassemia occurs most frequently in populations from the Mediterranean area and Southeast Asia.

Thrombocytopathy: abnormal platelet function.

Thrombocytopenia: a decrease in the number of platelets in the peripheral blood below the normal range for an individual laboratory (usually below 150×10^9/L).

Thrombocytosis: an increase in the number of platelets in the peripheral blood above the normal range for an individual laboratory (usually over 440×10^9/L).

Thromboembolism: dislodgment of a blood clot that was formed in the heart, arteries or veins and movement through blood vessels until reaching a smaller vessel and blocking further blood flow.

Thrombomodulin: an intrinsic membrane glycoprotein present on endothelial cells that serves as a cofactor with thrombin to activate protein C. It forms a 1:1 complex with thrombin inhibiting thrombin's ability to cleave fibrinogen to fibrin but enhances thrombin's ability to activate protein C.

Thrombophlebitis: thrombosis within a vein that is accompanied by an inflammatory response, pain and redness of the area.

Thrombopoietin: a humoral factor that regulates the maturation of megakaryocytes and the production of platelets.

Thrombosis: Formation of a blood clot or thrombus, usually considered to be under abnormal conditions within a blood vessel.

Thrombosthenin: an out-dated term for properties of the platelet now known to be related to the contractile proteins actin and myosin.

Thrombotic thrombocytopenic purpura: acute disorder of unknown etiology that affects young adults. Characterized by microangiopathic anemia, decreased number of platelets, renal failure as well as neurological symptoms.

Thrombus: a blood clot within the vascular system.

Tissue factor: a coagulation factor present on subvascular cells that forms a complex with factor VII when the vessel is ruptured. This complex activates factor X. Tissue factor is an integral protein of the cell membrane.

Tissue plasminogen activator (tPA): a serine protease that activates plasminogen to plasmin. It forms a bimolecular complex with fibrin increasing the catalytic efficiency of t-PA for plasminogen activation.

Total iron binding capacity (TIBC): the capacity of the plasma proteins, primarily transferrin, to bind iron.

Toxic granules: large dark blue-black primary granules in the cytoplasm of neutrophils that are present in certain infectious states. Usually seen in conjunction with Döhle bodies.

Toxoplasmosis: a condition that results from infection with *Toxoplasma gondii*. Acquired infection may be asymptomatic or symptoms may resemble infectious mononucleosis. There is a leukocytosis with relative lymphocytosis or rarely an absolute lymphocytosis and the presence of reactive lymphocytes.

Transcription: synthesis of RNA from a DNA template.

Transferrin: a plasma β_1-globulin responsible for the binding of iron and its transport from the intestine into the bloodstream. Each gram of transferrin can bind 1.25 mg of iron. The capacity of transferrin to bind iron is functionally measured as the total iron binding capacity (TIBC).

Transformed lymphocyte: see reactive lymphocyte

Transfusion reaction: any adverse response as a result of the transfusion of blood or blood component. The reaction can vary from a relatively benign allergic reaction to a severe acute hemolytic reaction.

Transfusion: infusion of whole blood or blood components into the blood stream.

Transient erythroblastemia of childhood (TEC): a temporary suppression of erythropoiesis that frequently occurs after a viral infection in infants and children. Therapy is supportive and patients usually recover within two months.

Translation: synthesis of protein from an RNA template.

Translocation: an abnormal chromosomal rearrangement whereby part of one chromosome breaks off and becomes attached to another chromosome. The site of juxtaposition between the two chromosomes is referred to as the breakpoint.

Transplacental idiopathic thrombocytopenic purpura (ITP): a form of ITP that is present in newborns because of maternal transfer of platelet-destroying antibodies.

Transudate: effusion that is formed due to increased hydrostatic pressure or decreased osmotic pressure; does not indicate a true pathologic state in the anatomic region.

Tumor suppressor gene: a gene that codes for a normal substance that suppresses tumor formation. Maturation and/or absence of both alleles allows tumor growth.

Tunica adventitia: the outermost layer of the wall of a blood vessel consisting of connective tissue with embedded fibroblasts.

Tunica intima: the innermost layer of the wall of blood vessels consisting of the endothelial cells and basement membrane.

Tunica media: the middle layer of the wall of arteries and veins consisting of connective tissue and varying numbers of smooth muscle cells.

Unilineage stem cell: a cell in which it is restricted to develop into only one blood cell lineage, i.e., erythrocytes.

Urokinase-like tissue plasminogen activators (u-PA): a secreted, extrinsic plasminogen activator. It exists in two forms: single-chain type glycoprotein (scu-PA) and two-chain type glycoprotein (tcu-PA). The scu-PA has significant fibrin specificity but it is not effective in activating plasminogen. scu-PA is converted to tcu-PA by plasmin. tcu-Pa has no specific affinity for fibrin but is more effective than scu-PA in activation of plasminogen.

Urokinase: an enzyme found in urine that activates plasminogen to plasmin and is used as a thrombolytic agent in the treatment of thrombosis.

Vascular permeability: the property of endothelial cells of blood vessels which selectively allows for exchange of gasses, nutrients and waste products.

Vasculitis: inflammation of a blood vessel.

Vaso-occlusive crisis: a condition caused by blockage of the microvasculature by sickled cells occurring spontaneously in sickle cell anemia. The crises may be triggered by infection, dehydration, decreased oxygen pressure or slow blood flow. Often the crisis occurs without a known cause. There is pain, fever, organ dysfunction and tissue necrosis in the blockaded area. The crisis lasts for one to two weeks and subsides spontaneously.

Vasoconstriction: narrowing of the lumen of blood vessels that occurs immediately following an injury.

Venules: venous blood vessels that are less than 200 μm in diameter and are the major site of hemostasis.

Vesicles: small sacs in the cytoplasm of cells used to transfer nutrients or waste products.

Virocyte: see reactive lymphocyte.

Vitamin-K dependent factors: see prothrombin group.

Warm autoimmune hemolytic anemia: anemia resulting from the presence of IgG autoantibodies that are reactive at 37° C with antigens on subject's erythrocytes. The antibody/antigen complex on the cell membrane sensitizes the erythrocyte which is removed in the spleen or liver.

Zeta potential: an electrostatic potential created by a difference in charge density of the inner and outer layers of the ionic cloud of erythrocytes suspended in saline. This force tends to keep the erythrocytes about 25 nm apart.

Zymogen: an inactive precursor that can be converted to the active form by an enzyme, alkali or acid. The inert coagulation factors are zymogens. Also called a proenzyme.

GLOSSARY FOR HEMATOLOGY/COAGULATION PROCEDURES

Adsorbed plasma: platelet-poor plasma that is adsorbed with either barium sulfate or aluminum hydroxide to remove the coagulation factors II, VII, IX, X (the prothrombin group). Factors V, VIII, XI, XII, and fibrinogen (I) are present in adsorbed plasma. This plasma is one of the reagents used in the substitution studies to determine a specific factor deficiency.

Aged serum: serum that lacks the coagulation factors fibrinogen (I), prothrombin (II), V, and VIII. Aged serum is prepared by incubating normal serum for 24 hours at 37°C. Factors VII, IX, X, XI, and XII are present in aged serum. This serum is one of the reagents used in the substitution studies to determine a specific factor deficiency.

Aggregating reagent: a chemical substance (agonist) that promotes platelet activation and aggregation by attaching to a receptor on the platelet's surface. Common platelet aggregating reagents include ADP, epinephrine, collagen, ristocetin, and arachidonic acid.

Alpha globulins: a group of serum proteins identified by similar electrical net charge (pI 4.0–5.4) and molecular size (40,000–400,000 D). These proteins travel in the alpha regions (α1 and α2) on protein electrophoresis using cellulose acetate at pH 8.6. Haptoglobin, ceruloplasmin, and α1-antitrypsin are examples of alpha globulins.

Anticoagulant: a chemical substance added to whole blood to prevent blood from coagulating. Depending on the type of anticoagulant, in vitro coagulation is prevented by the removal of calcium (EDTA) or the inhibition of the serine proteases such as thrombin (heparin).

Beta globulins: a group of serum proteins identified by similar electrical net charge (pI 5.8–6.0) and molecular size (60,000–400,000 D). These proteins travel in the beta region on protein electrophoresis using cellulose acetate at pH 8.6. Fibrinogen, transferrin, and hemopexin are examples of beta globulins.

Bone marrow aspirate: fluid withdrawn from the bone marrow by aspiration using a special needle (e.g., Jamshidi needle) and syringe. It represents the specialized soft tissue that fills the medullary cavities between the bone trabeculae. Examination of the bone marrow aspirate is useful in evaluating cellular morphology, distribution and development, observing for presence of abnormal cells, and estimating cellularity.

Bone marrow trephine biopsy: removal of a small piece of the bone marrow core that contains marrow, fat, and trabecula. Examination of the trephine biopsy is useful in observing the bone marrow architecture and cellularity and allows interpretation of the spatial relationships of bone, fat, and marrow cellularity.

Cell hemoglobin concentration mean (CHCM): an erythrocyte index that represents the average hemoglobin concentration of the individual cells analyzed. CHCM is derived from the hemoglobin histogram (individual cell's hemoglobin concentration and relative cell number). CHCM is compared with the MCHC to help determine if there is interference with the hemoglobin measurement, such as turbidity or lipemia. CHCM is a parameter provided by the Technicon instruments.

Chromogenic assay: a spectrophotometric measurement of an enzyme's activity based on the release of a colored pigment following enzymatic cleavage of the pigment-producing substrate (chromogen). In the majority of chromogenic assays, increasing concentration of colored pigment corresponds to increased enzyme activity. This technique is used to measure coagulation factor activity.

Circulating inhibitors: acquired pathologic proteins, primarily immunoglobulins (IgG or IgM), with antibody specificity toward a factor involved in fibrin formation. Circulating inhibitors interfere with the activity of the factor. The inhibitors are associated with a number of conditions, such as hemophilia, autoimmune diseases, malignancies, certain drugs, and viral infections.

Column chromatography: a separation method based on the differential distribution of a liquid or gaseous sample (mobile phase) that flows through a column of specific substance (stationary phase). Depending on the chemical characteristics of the stationary phase, the substance of interest may bind to the stationary phase and remain in the column or directly pass through the column and remain in the mobile phase. If the substance of interest remains in the column, a second mobile phase is used to release the substance from the stationary phase and allow it to pass through the column. This released substance can then be measured.

Continuous flow analysis: an automated method of analyzing blood cells that allows measurement of cellular characteristics as the individual cells flow singly through a laser beam.

Cyanmethemoglobin: a hemoglobin derivative that is produced when whole blood is added to a solution of potassium cyanide and potassium ferricyanide. This is a two-step process: (1) the ferrous ion is oxidized to the ferric ion creating methemoglobin and (2) the resulting methemoglobin combines with cyanide ions to form cyanmethemoglobin. The conversion of hemoglobin to cyanmethemoglobin results in a stable compound which is measured spectrophotometrically in the determination of hemoglobin concentration.

Cytogram: a dot-plot histogram of two cellular characteristics that allows definition of the cell population. For example, the peroxidase cytogram differentiates the leukocyte population based on each cell's size and its peroxidase activity. Lymphocytes are small in size and lack peroxidase activity, whereas neutrophils are large in size and have increased peroxidase activity. Cytograms are generated by the Technicon instruments.

D dimer: a cross-linked fibrin degradation product that is the result of plasmin's proteolytic activity on a fibrin clot. The presence of D dimers is specific for fibrinolysis.

Densitometry: a method that determines the pattern and concentration of protein fractions separated by electrophoresis. It measures the amount of light absorbed by each dye-bound protein fraction as the fraction passes a slit through which light is transmitted. The amount of light absorbed (optical density) is directly proportional to the protein's concentration.

Factor VIII inhibitor: an IgG immunoglobulin with antibody specificity to Factor VIII. The inhibitor inactivates the factor. The antibodies are time and temperature dependent. Factor VIII inhibitors are associated with hemophilia.

Fibrin degradation product: the breakdown products of fibrin or fibrinogen that are produced when plasmin's proteolytic action cleaves these molecules. The four main products are fragments X, Y, D and E. The presence of fibrin degradation products is indicative of either fibrinolysis or fibrinogenolysis.

Hemoglobin distribution width: a measure of the distribution of hemoglobin within an erythrocyte population. It is derived from the hemoglobin histogram generated by the Technicon instruments.

Hereditary erythroblastic multinuclearity with positive acidified serum test (HEMPAS): Type II congenital dyserythropoietic anemia (CDA). CDA is characterized by both abnormal and ineffective erythropoiesis. Type II is distinguished by a positive acidified serum test (Ham test) but a negative sucrose hemolysis test.

Histogram: a plot of the number of cells within a defined parameter. For example, an erythrocyte histogram plots the number of erythrocytes within specific size ranges. Histograms are generated by cell analyzers.

Hydrodynamic focusing: a technique used in optical flow cytometer designs in which a sample fluid containing cells is injected into the central portion of a flowing stream of cell-free fluid (sheath fluid). This process is used to transport the cells to and through the path of the laser beam.

Hypercoagulable state: a condition associated with an imbalance between clot promoting and clot inhibiting factors. This leads to an increased risk of developing thrombosis.

INR (international normalized ratio): a method of reporting prothrombin time results when monitoring long-term oral anticoagulant therapy. Results are independent of the reagents and methods used. It is the ratio obtained by dividing the patient prothrombin time by the laboratory's mean prothrombin time raised to the power of the international sensitivity index for the thromboplastin reagent used.

ISI (international sensitivity index): This figure is provided by the manufacturer of thromboplastin reagents. It indicates the responsiveness of the particular lot of reagent compared to the international reference thromboplastin. It is used to calculate the INR.

Isovolumetric focusing: a method employed by the Technicon H*1 hematology analyzer system in which a specific buffered diluent is used to isovolumetrically sphere and fix erythrocytes. The cells resemble homogeneous dielectric spheres. As a result, erythrocyte membrane effects are ignored and errors in determining erythrocyte volume are eliminated.

Karyolysis: destruction of the nucleus.

Lambert-Beer's law: The law forming the mathematical basis for colorimetry; the absorbance (A) of a colored solution is equal to the product of the concentration of the substance being measured (C), times the depth of solution through which the light travels (L) times a constant (K). ($A = C \times L \times K$) Also referred to as Beer's law.

Mean platelet volume (MPV): the mean volume of a platelet population; analogous to the MCV of erythrocytes.

Normal pooled plasma: platelet-poor plasma collected from at least 20 normal individuals; normal is defined by the PT and APTT. The plasma should give PT and APTT results within the laboratory's reference range. The plasma is pooled and used in mixing studies to differentiate a circulating inhibitor from a factor deficiency.

Paraprotein: abnormal serum globulins.

Petechiometer: an instrument that provides negative pressure using a suction cup. A petechiometer is used to determine capillary fragility. The device is placed on the forearm for 1 to 2 minutes. The area under the cup is then examined for the presence of petechiae.

Phase microscopy: a type of light microscopy in which an annular diaphragm is placed below or in the substage condenser and a phase shifting element is placed in the rear focal plane of the objective. This causes alterations in the phases of light rays and increases the contrast between the cell and its surroundings. This methodology is used to count platelets.

Platelet distribution width (PDW): coefficient of variation of platelet volume distribution; analogous to RDW.

Platelet factor 4: a protein present in platelet's alpha granules that is capable of neutralizing heparin.

Platelet-poor plasma (PPP): citrated plasma containing less than 15×10^9/L platelets. It is prepared by centrifugation of citrated whole blood at a minimum RCF of $1000 \times$ g for 15 minutes. PPP is used for the majority of coagulation tests.

Platelet-rich plasma (PRP): citrated plasma containing approximately $200-300 \times 10^9$/L platelets. It is prepared by centrifugation of citrated whole blood at an RCF of $150 \times$ g for 5-10 minutes. PRP is used in platelet aggregation studies.

PT clotting curve: represents a graph of the changing optical density or light scatter versus time as a fibrin clot is formed in the prothrombin time test procedure. The results of the PT clotting curve can alert the clinical laboratory scientist to low fibrinogen levels.

Red cell distribution width (RDW): the coefficient of variation of red cell volume distribution.

Reference (standard) curve: a curve made by measuring the optical density (or other property) of solutions of known concentration of a substance and plotting concentration versus optical density or percent transmittance of light (or other property).

Reference interval: the test value range which is considered normal. It is used to evaluate test values of patients. Generally the range is determined to include 95% of the reference population.

Scattergram: a dot-plot histogram of two cellular characterics, (1) radio frequency which provides information on nuclear size and celluar density and (2) direct current (impedance) which provides information on overall cell size. Together, these two characteristics allow the definition of the leukocyte population. Lymphocytes are small mononuclear cells with no granules, whereas neutrophils are large polymorphonuclear cells with granulation. Scattergrams are generated by Sysmex instruments.

Sensitivity: the ability to detect small quantities of a component.

Specificity: the ability to determine only the component meant to be detected or measured.

Supernatant: clear liquid remaining on top of a solution after centrifugation of the particulate matter.

Supravital stain: a stain used to stain cells or tissues while they are still living.

Threshold limit: in automated cell analyzers, the level above which pulses of particles will be counted. In the Coulter analyzers, a voltage pulse will be produced as a particle passes through an aperature through which a current flows. The amplitude of the pulse is directly proportional to the volume of the cell. Adjusting the threshold allows different types of cells to be counted.

Turbidity: a physical property of a solution or suspension that refers to its cloudiness.

Viscosity: resistance to flow; this physical property is dependent on the friction of component molecules in a substance as they pass one another.

von Willebrand disease: an autosomal dominant hereditary bleeding disorder in which there is a lack of von Willebrand factor (vWf). This factor is needed for platelets to adhere to collagen. Platelet aggregation is abnormal with ristocetin. The bleeding time is also abnormal. The APTT may be prolonged due to a decrease in the factor VIII molecule secondary to a decrease in vWf.

von Willebrand factor (vWf): a plasma factor needed for platelets to adhere to collagen. It binds to the platelet glycoprotein Ib. It is synthesized in megakaryocytes and endothelial cells. The vWf is a molecule of multimers. It is noncovalently linked to factor VIII in plasma.

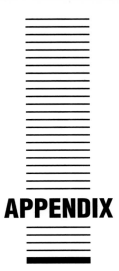

APPENDIX

TABLE I *MEASURES OF HEMOGLOBIN (Hb) DESTRUCTION*

Measurement	95% Limits
Icterus index (units)	5–7.5
Bilirubin, total (mg/dl)	0.5–1.0 (high critical limit 15 [SD 5])
Bilirubin, direct (mg/dl)	0.01–0.10
Urobilinogen, urine[8] (Ehrlich units/2 hr)	0.1–1.5
Urobilinogen, fecal	
Ehrlich units/100 g	50–300
mg/day	40–280
mg/100 g Hb/day	11–21
Bilirubin production (mg/kg/day)	2.6–5.0
Endogenous carbon monoxide production (μmol/hr)	12.3–25.1
Serum hemoglobin (mg/dl)	<1.0
Serum haptoglobin (g Hb/dl)	
type 1—1	1.0–1.73
type 2—1	0.71–1.45
Type 2—2	0.48–1.16
All types	0.40–2.08
Urine iron (mg/day)	<0.1

(With permission: Lee, GR, Bithell, TC, Foerster, J., Athens, JW, Lukens, JN. Wintrobe's Clinical Hematology. 9th Edition. Philadelphia: Lea & Febiger, 1993.)

TABLE J *PORPHYRINS AND PORPHYRIN PRECURSORS IN FECES, URINE, AND ERYTHROCYTES*

Porphyrin or Precursor	Feces	Urine	Erythrocytes
Aminolevulinic acid	—	3.0 (0.4–5.6) mg/L* 2.3 (1.3–5.4) mg/day	—
Porphobilinogen	—	1.5 (0.5–2.5) mg/L 1.4 (0.4–2.4) mg/day	—
Uroporphyrin	0–0.06 mg/day	8 (0–40) μg/day	0
Coproporphyrin	8 (0–27) μg/g†	50 (1–180) μg/day	1.3 (0.7–2.3) μg/dl
Protoporphyrin	22 (0–75) μg/g†	None	39 (16–67) μg/dl
Total porphyrin	(0–95) μg/g† 4 mg/day	<0.2 mg/day	—

* 95% limits given in parentheses.
† Dry weight.

(With permission: Lee, GR, Bithell, TC, Foerster, J., Athens, JW, Lukens, JN. Wintrobe's Clinical Hematology. 9th Edition. Philadelphia: Lea & Febiger, 1993.)

TABLE K *NORMAL VALUES FOR OSMOTIC FRAGILITY*

Sodium Chloride (Conc. in g/dl)	% Hemolysis	
	Before Incubation	After Incubation
0.85	0	0
0.75	0	0–2
0.65	0	0–19
0.60	0	0–40
0.55	0	5–70
0.50	0–5	36–88
0.45	0–45	54–96
0.40	50–90	65–100
0.35	90–99	72–100
0.30	97–100	80–100
0.20	100	91–100
0.10	100	100

(By permission of Grune & Stratton from Cartwright G.E.: *Diagnostic Laboratory Hematology*, 4th Ed. New York: Grune & Statton, 1968.)

(With permission: Lee, GR, Bithell, TC, Foerster, J., Athens, JW, Lukens, JN. Wintrobe's Clinical Hematology. 9th Edition. Philadelphia: Lea & Febiger, 1993.)

TABLE L   *LEUKOCYTE ALKALINE PHOSPHATASE SCORES IN NORMAL SUBJECTS*

Group	Number	Mean	95% Limits
Male	51	73	22–124
Female	50	91	33–149
Total	101	82	25–139

(By permission of Grune & Stratton from Cartwright G.E.: *Diagnostic Laboratory Hematology,* 4th Ed. New York: Grune & Stratton, 1968.)

(With permission: Lee, GR, Bithell, TC, Foerster, J., Athens, JW, Lukens, JN. Wintrobe's Clinical Hematology. 9th Edition. Philadelphia: Lea & Febiger, 1993.)

TABLE M   *COMMONLY USED LEUKOCYTE DIFFERENTIATION ANTIGENS*

CD Notation	Other Names	Molecular Weight (kd)	Function
T cell lineage			
CD1a, 1b, 1c	T6, Leu6	49,45,43	
CD2	T11, Leu5	50	Sheep erythrocyte receptor
			Interacts with adhesion molecule LFA-3
			Alternate T cell activation
CD3	T3, Leu4	5 proteins:	Complex with T cell receptor
		$\gamma, \delta, \epsilon, \zeta, \eta$	Signal transduction
CD4	T4, Leu3	60	T helper cell marker
			Interacts with class II MHC
			HIV receptor
CD5	T1, Leu1	67	Present on CLL cells
CD6	—	120	
CD7	Leu9	40	FcR for IgM
			Precursor cells
CD8	T8, Leu2	32	T cytotoxic cells
			Interacts with class I MHC
CD27	—	107	Activation antigen
B cell lineage			
CD10	J5, Calla, BA-3	100	Pre-B cells
			Neutral endopeptidase (NEP)
CD19	B4, Leu12	95	
CD20	B1, Leu16	35	
CD21	B2	140	Receptor for C3d (CR2)
			Receptor for Epstein-Barr virus
CD22	Leu14	135	
CD23	Blast-2	45	Low affinity receptor for IgE (FcϵR II)
CD24	BA-1	45–55	
CD40	p50, Bp50	50	Growth factor receptor
			Growth regulation of human carcinomas
			Similar to nerve growth factor receptor
Myeloid-monocytic lineage			
CD13	My7	150	
CD14	My4, MO2, UCHM1	55	
CD15	My1, LeuM1	50–180	
CD16	Leu11, HNK-1, NKH-1	50–60	Fc receptor for IgG (FyγRIII)
			Present on NK cells, neutrophils, but absent in patients with paroxysmal nocturnal hemoglobinuria
CD17			
CDw32			Fc receptor for IgG (FcγRII)
CD33	My9	67	Myeloid precursors
CD34	My10	115	Stem cell marker
Others			
CD11a		175	α-chain of LFA-1 (adhesion molecule)
CD11b	Mac1	165	α-chain of complement receptor CR3
CD11c		150	α-chain of complement receptor CR4
CD18		95	β-chain for CD11a, b, c
CD25	Tac	55	Low affinity receptor for interleukin 2 (β-chain)
CD35		220	Receptor for C3b (CR1)
CD38	T10	45	Activation marker T cells, plasma cells
CR45	2H4, OX22, UCHL1	180–220	Leukocyte common antigen
			Cell interactions
CD52	LFA-3		Adhesion molecule, interacts with CD2
CD54	I-CAM	90–115	Adhesion molecule, interacts with LFA-1
CD71	VIP-1		Transferrin receptor

(With permission: Lee, GR, Bithell, TC, Foerster, J., Athens, JW, Lukens, JN. Wintrobe's Clinical Hematology. 9th Edition. Philadelphia: Lea & Febiger, 1993.)

TABLE N *WORKSHOP-DEFINED CLUSTER GROUPS FOR MONOCLONAL ANTIBODIES TO HUMAN LEUKOCYTES*

Cluster	Specificity Group	MW of Antigen	Periph. Blood Normal Range (% of Lymphs)	Monoclonal Antibodies
CD1a 1b 1c	(Langerhans' cells) Common thymocyte	49/12K 45K 43K	0%	Leu6, T6, OKT6, BL6, NA1/34, VIT6 4A76, NUT2, WM-25 L161, M241, 7C6, PHM3
CD2	E-rosette receptor LFA-3 (CD58) receptor T, NK-cells	45–50K	83 ± 5%	Leu5, T11, 35.1, 6F10-3, 9.6, OKT11, 9-2, MT910
CD2R	Activated T-cells			D66, T11.3, VIT13
CD3	T-cell Ag receptor associated	22–28K	75 ± 7%	Leu4, 41F, UCHT1, X35, OKT3, T3, CRIS-7
CD4	T-helper/inducer cells, monocytes	59K	45 ± 10%	Leu3a, T4, 91.D6, BL4, OKT4(4A)
CD5	Mature thymocytes, T-cells, some sIg$^+$ CLL, some T-ALL	67K	72 ± 7%	Leu1, OKT1, HH9, BL1a, L17F12, T101, T1, DK23 6-2, 10.2, UCHT2
CD6	Thymocytes, mature T-cells, some B-cells	100K	0%	T12, 12.1, T411
CD7	T-cells, NK cells, most T-ALL (Fc$_u$R?)	40K	75%	Leu-9, CL1.3, G3-7 4H9, 3A1, T55, DK24
CD8	T cytotoxic/suppressor cells Class I MHC receptor α chain β chain	32K	28 ± 9%	 OKT8, T-8, Leu2a, UCHT4, M236, T811, B9-11, OKT5 T8/2T8, 5H7
CD9	Lymphopoietic bone marrow progenitor cells	24K	0%	BA2, ALB6, FMC56
CD10	Common acute lymphoblastic leukemia Ag (CALLA)	100K	0%	anti-CALLA, ALB1, J5, BA-3, VILA1
CD11a 11b 11c	Leukocytes α-chain LFA-1 (β2 family) NK subset, monocytes (C3bi recept) α-chain Leu CAMb (β2 family) NK subset, monocytes, granulocytes α-chain MAC 1 (β2 family)	180K 150K 170K	30 ± 5	2F12, CRIS-3, 25.3.1, VEP13 OKM1, Leu15, Mo1, MAC1, 5A4.C5 KiM1, L29, BL-4H4
CDw12	Monocytes, PMN, platelets	90–120K	0%	M67
CD13	Monocytes, granulocytes some CFU-C (marrow) (Aminopeptidase N)	150K	0%	MY7, 44H, TUK1, MOU28, MCS-2
CD14	Monocytes (>90%), some granulocytes (Folicular dendritic reticular cells)	55K	0%	LeuM3, MY4, Mo2, VIM13, MoP15, UCHM1, Bear-2
CD15	Monocytes (80–100%) (gpLNPIII) mature granulocytes (>95%) (Reed-Sternberg cells)		0%	LeuM1, VIM-D5, 80H5, My1, MCS1
CD16	IgG Fc receptor on NK cells and neutrophils Fc$_{gamma}$ receptor (FcRIII)	50–60K	15 ± 7%	Leu11, L23, HUNK2, VEP13, 3G8, BW209, 80H3
CDw17	PMN, monocytes, platelets (Lactosylceramide)		0%	T5A7, 6035, GO35, Huly-m13
CD18	Leukocytes (integrin β2 chain LEU CAM complexes w LFA α-chain: CD11a,b,c)	95K	(100%)	BL5, M232, 11H6, CLB54, MHM23
CD19	B-cells	95K	10 ± 5%	Leu12, B4, HD37, AB-1
CD20	B-cells (ion channel?)	32–37K	10 ± 5%	Leu16, B1, IF5
CD21	mature B-cells (CR$_2$)/ (C3dR) EBV receptor	140K	5–15%	LeuCR$_2$, HB5, BL13, B2, CRII, BL-10
CD22	B-cells (95% blood B-cells, mantle & germinal center B-cells in nodes)	135K	10 ± 5%	Leu14, B3, HD39, To15, S-HCL1, BL-9

(continued)

TABLE N *(continued)*

Cluster	Specificity Group	MW of Antigen	Periph. Blood Normal Range (% of Lymphs)	Monoclonal Antibodies
CD23	Fc$_E$ (low-affinity) recept. (FceRII) B-cell subset, activated eosinophils	45–50K		BLAST-2, B6, MHM
CD24	Immature leukocytes, some B-cells, granulocytes	45, 55, 65K		BA-1, VIBE3, ALB9
CD25	Interleukin-2 recept. β chain (activated T-cells and B-cells) (Hairy cell Leukemias)	55–60K	0%	anti-IL 2 recept. TAC, 7G7/B6, B1.49.9, IL-2R1, 2A3 ACT1, 33.B3.1
CD26	activated T-cells (Dipeptidylpeptidase IV)	120K	0%	134-2C2, Tal, TS145
CD27	T-cell subset, plasma cells	55K		OKT18a, VIT14, S152
CD28	T-cell subset	44K		9.3, Kolt-2
CD29	Regulatory subpopulations of CD4 and CD8 cells, platelets gpIIa (integrin β1-chain; VLA1-6)	135K		4B4, K20, A-1A5
CD30	Activated T- and B-cells (Reed-Sternberg cells)	120K		Ki-1, BerH4, HSR4
CD31	PMN, monocytes, platelets (gpIIa)	130–140K	0%	SG134, TM3, HEC-75, ES12F11
CDw32	Fc$_{gamma}$ RII (PMN, monocytes, platelets, B-cells)	40K	0%	2E1, C1KM5, IV3, 41H16, IV.3, KB61
CD33	Early myeloid progenitors (myelogenous leukemia)	67K	0%	MY9, LeuM6, L4F3, H153
CD34	Early myeloid progenitors (myeloid and lymphoblastic leukemia)	105–120K	0%	12-8, B1-3C5, HPCA-1, My10, ICH-3
CD35	B-cells, PMN, monocytes (CR$_1$) C3b receptor	220K		TO5, CBO4, J3D3
CD36	Monocytes, plts (gpIV)	90K	0%	5F1, C1Meg1, ESIVC7
CD37	B-cells	40–45K		G28-1, HD28, HH1, G28-1, BL14
CD38	Plasma cells, activated T-cells, Lymphocyte progenitors	45K	0%	OKT10, Leu-17, T16, HB7
CD39	B-cells, macrophages	70–100K		G28-2, AC2
CD40	B-cell subset (some carcinomas) (homology to NGF receptor)	50K		G28-5, MA6
CD41a	Platelets gpIIb/IIIa (integrin β3 family) (Fibrinogen receptor)		0%	J15, PL273, PBM 6.4
CD41b	Platelets gpIIb (integrin β3 family)	125 + 25K		PLT-1
CD42a	Platelets (gpIX) (von Willebrand's factor receptor)	23K	0%	FMC25, BL-H6, GR-P
CD42b	Platelets (gpIb) Platelet CD42a/42b (gpIbIX complex)	25/135K	0%	PHN89, AN51, GN287 HLe-1
CD43	T-cells, granulocytes, monocytes, brain (leukosialin)	95K		G10-2, OTH 71C5, G19-1, MEM-59
CD44	T-cells, pre-B, brain, granulocytes, RBC	80–95K		1-173, GRHL1, BRIC35, F10-44-2, 33-3B3
CD45	Pan-leukocyte (leukocyte common antigen)	200K	(100%)	T29/33, T-200/LCA, 2311, ROS 220, KC56
CD45RA	T-subsets, B-cells, granulocytes, monocytes (restricted T200)	220K		73.5, G1-15, F8-11-13
CD45RB	T-subsets, B-cells, granulocytes, monocytes (restricted T200)	220K		PTD/26
CD45RO	T-subsets (some CD4 and CD8 cells), NK cells, and some B-cells	220K	77 ± 15%	Leu-18, 2H4, 3AC5, HB10, HB11, UCHL1

(continued)

TABLE N *(continued)*

Cluster	Specificity Group	MW of Antigen	Periph. Blood Normal Range (% of Lymphs)	Monoclonal Antibodies
CD46	Leukocytes (membrane cofactor protein)	56/66K		HULYM5, 122-2, J48
CD47	Broad pan-leukocyte (N-linked glycan)	47–52K		BRIC 126, CIKM1, BRIC 125
CD48	Leukocytes (Platelet-linked)	41K		WM68, J4-57, LO-MN25
CDw49a	Platelets (α1-chain VLA-1)	200K		
CDw49b	Platelets gpla, cultured T-cells (α2-chain VLA-2)	165K		Gi14, CLB-thromb/4
CDw49c	Platelets (α3-chain VLA-3)	135 + 25K		
CDw49d	Thymocytes, T-cells, B-cells, monocytes, Langerhans' cells (epidermis) (α4-chain VLA-4)	150K		
CDw49e	Platelets gplc (α5-chain VLA-5)	140K		
CDw49f	Platelets gplc, (T-cells) (α6-chain VLA-6)	140K		GoH3
CDw50	Leukocytes	108/148K		101-1D2, 140-1
CD51	Platelets (α-chain Vitronectin receptor) (integrin β3 and β4 family)			MKI-M7, NKI-M9, 13C2, 23C6
CDw52	Leukocytes	21–28K		097, YTH66.9, YTH34.5
CD53	Leukocytes	32–40K		HI29, HI36, MEM-53, HD77
CD54	Broad specificity (ICAM-1)			7F7, WEHI-CAMI, RR1/1
CD55	Broad specif. (Decay Accelerating Factor, DAF)			BRIC 110, BRIC 128, 143-30, F2B-7.2
CD56	NK (pan-NK Ag), T-subset	135/220K		Leu 19, NKH-1, FP2-11.14, L185
CD57	NK, T-cell subsets B-cell subsets, (brain)	110K	$20 \pm 7\%$	Leu 7, L183, L186
CD58	Leukocytes, epithelium (LFA-3)	40–65K		G26, BRIC 5, TS2/9
CD59	Broad specificity	18–20K		YTH53.1, MEM-43
CDw60	T-cell subset (NeuAc-NeuAc-Gal-)			M-T32, M-T21, M-T41, UM4D4
CD61	Platelets gpIIIa (integrin β3 chain) (Vitronectin Receptors)	105K		Y2/51, VL-PL2, BL-E6, CLB-thromb/1
CD62	Platelet activation (GMP-140) (PADEGM LEC-CAM)	140K		CLB-thromb/6, RUU-SP1.18.1
CD63	Platelets activation, monocytes, some T-, B-cells, granulocytes. (α-granules)	53K		RUU-SP2.28, CLB-gran/12
CD64	Monocytes (FcRI)	75K		MAb32.2, MAb22
CDw65	Granulocytes, monocytes (Ceramide-dodecasaccharide 4c)			VIM2, VIM8, HE10, CF4
CD66	Granulocytes	180–200K		CLB-gran/10, YTH71.3
CD67	Granulocytes	100K		B13.9, G10F5, JML-H16
CD68	Macrophages	110K		Ki-M6, Ki-M7, EBM11, Y2/131, Y-1/82A
CD69	Activated B- and T-cells	28/32K		MLR3, L78, FN50, BL-Ac/p26
CDw70	Activated B- and T-cells (Reed-Sternberg cells)			Ki-24, HNE 51, HNC 142
CD71	Proliferating cells, macrophages (Transferrin receptor)			OKT-9, 138-18, 120-2A3, MEM-75, VIP-1, Nu-TfR2, BK19.9, B3/25
CD72	Pan B-cell (B-cell activation marker?)	39/43K	$10 \pm 5\%$	BU-40, BU-41, S-HCL2, J3-109
CD73	B-cell subset (70% CD19+) T-cell subset (20% CD3+) (ecto-5'-nucleotidase)	69K	20%	1E9.28.1, AD2, 7G2.2.11

(continued)

TABLE N *(continued)*

Cluster	Specificity Group	MW of Antigen	Periph. Blood Normal Range (% of Lymphs)	Monoclonal Antibodies
CD74	B-cells, monocytes (HLA II assoc. invar. chain)	33/35/41K		LN2, BU-43, BU-45
CDw75	mature B-cells (germinal center) T-cell subset	53K		LN1, HH2, EBU-141
CD76	mature B-cells T-cell subset	67/85K		HD66, CRIS-4
CD77	B-cells (Gb3) (Globotriaosylceramide)			38.13(BLA), 424/4A11, 424/3D9
CDw78	B-cells, monocytes			Anti Ba, 1588, LO-panB-a
Other Specificities, not clustered				
Regulatory subpopulations of CD4$^+$ and CD8$^+$ cells; some B-cells, neutrophils, and monocytes		80K	68 ± 7%	Leu-8, TQ1
HLA Antigens (class II):				
HLA-DR: B-cells, monocytes, activated T-cells		28–34K	11 ± 4%	anti-HLA-DR, I2, ILR2
HLA-DQ: B-cells, monocytes		27, 32K	10 ± 5%	Leu-10
HLA-DP: B-cells, monocytes		25, 35K	10 ± 5%	anti-HLA-DP
Platelet and Endothelial Cell Receptor Complexes				
CD 36 (gpIIIboulV)		Thrombosponden Receptor		
CD61 + CD 41b (gpIIIa + gpIIb/IIb)		Vitronectin (Fibrinogin) Receptor		
CD49f (gpIc)		Fibronectin Receptor		
CD31 + CD49f (gpIIa + gpIc)		Laminin Receptor		
CD49b (gpIIa + gpIa)		Collagen Receptor		
CD42a + CD42b (gpIX + gpIb/gpIb)		Von Willebrand's Factor Receptor		
CD54 (I-CAM)		Receptor for LFA-1 (CD11a)		

List compiled by: T. Vincent Shankey and Thomas M. Ellis. Loyola Univ. Med. Cntr. 1/91. With permission from: Bauer KD, Duque RE, Shankey TV.: Clinical Flow Cytometry. Baltimore: Williams & Wilkins, 1993.

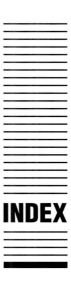

INDEX

Page numbers followed by "t" indicate tables. Page numbers italicized are figures.

A

Aberration
chromosomal, 422; *see also*
Chromosome; Molecular genetics
microscope lens, 603
Abetalipoproteinemia, 249–250
ABO blood group incompatibility, 270t, 272
Absolute hemoglobin concentration, 93
Absorption
of cobalamin, 189–190
of iron, 124t, 124–125
Acanthocyte, *105*, 106
Acanthocytosis, 230–231, 249–250
Achlorhydria, iron deficiency and, 131
Achromat lens, 603
Acid
amino
hemoglobinopathy and, 152
hemostatic proteins and, 564
arachidonic; *see* Arachidonic acid
hydrochloric, 191
methylmalonic, 193
nucleic, 420
Acid elution test of hemoglobin, 150
Acid phosphatase, leukemia and, 366
Acid phosphatase stain, 617–618
Acidified serum test (Ham test), 232, 614–615, 615t
Aciduria, orotic, 194t
ACL 3000 instrument, 661–662
Acquired immunodeficiency syndrome, 303–304, 304t, 307
hemophilia treatment and, 573–574
Acrocentric chromosome, 420

Acrocyanosis, 264
Actin, platelets and, 487, 492
Activated partial thromboplastin time, 529–531, 531t
disseminated intravascular coagulation and, 579–580
factor assays and, 629–630
factor VIII and, 572
factor XI deficiency and, 576
factor XII deficiency and, 576–577
heparin therapy and, 593
high molecular weight kininogen deficiency and, 577
in newborn, 584–585
oral anticoagulant and, 595
platelet neutralization and, 630
prekallikrein and, 577
procedure for, 626
prothrombin deficiency and, 575
von Willebrand factor and, 567, 568
Activation, platelet, 490–493, *491–494*
Actomyosin, platelet and, 492
Acute idiopathic thrombocytopenic purpura, 546
Acute leukemia; *see* Leukemia
Addison, William, *57*
Adenocarcinoma, 464, *466*
cerebrospinal fluid and, *471*
morphology of, 465t
Adenosine diphosphate, platelets and, 495–496, 556
aggregometry and, 625
Adenosine triphosphate
in blood cells, 6

Embden-Myerhoff pathway and, 233
erythrocytes and, 39
membrane permeability of, 225
spleen and, 13
Adenyl cyclase, 492
Adenylcobalamin, 189
Adhesion, platelet, 489–490
Adhesion deficiency, leukocyte, 289
Adhesion molecule
of immune response, 86, 87t
neutrophils and, 63–64, 64t
Adipocyte, 16
Adsorbed plasma, 628
Adult T-cell leukemia/lymphoma, 412
Adventitial cell, 17
Afibrinogenemia, 574–575
Agammaglobulinemia
leukemia and, 362
X-linked, 306–307
Age
erythrocyte concentration and, 40
globin chain synthesis in, 45
Aged serum, 628
Agenesis, red cell, 208–209
Agglutination, 111, 111t, *112*
granulocyte, 284
hemolytic anemia and, 258
infectious mononucleosis and, 300
Agglutinin
cold, 647–648
hemolytic anemia and, 255t
cold autoimmune, 264t, 264–265, 265t
Aggregating reagent, 626

TABLE E   LEUKOCYTE COUNTS AND DIFFERENTIAL COUNTS REFERENCE VALUES IN CHILDREN

Age	Total Leukocytes Mean	(Range)	Neutrophils Mean	(Range)	%	Lymphocytes Mean	(Range)	%	Monocytes Mean	%	Eosinophils Mean	%
Birth	18.1	(9.0–30.0)	11.0	(6.0–26.0)	61	5.5	(2.0–11.0)	31	1.1	6	0.4	2
12 hours	22.8	(13.0–38.0)	15.5	(6.0–28.0)	68	5.5	(2.0–11.0)	24	1.2	5	0.5	2
24 hours	18.9	(9.4–34.0)	11.5	(5.0–21.0)	61	5.8	(2.0–11.5)	31	1.1	6	0.5	2
1 week	12.2	(5.0–21.0)	5.5	(1.5–10.0)	45	5.0	(2.0–17.0)	41	1.1	9	0.5	4
2 weeks	11.4	(5.0–20.0)	4.5	(1.0–9.5)	40	5.5	(2.0–17.0)	48	1.0	9	0.4	3
1 month	10.8	(5.0–19.5)	3.8	(1.0–9.0)	35	6.0	(2.5–16.5)	56	0.7	7	0.3	3
6 months	11.9	(6.0–17.5)	3.8	(1.0–8.5)	32	7.3	(4.0–13.5)	61	0.6	5	0.3	3
1 year	11.4	(6.0–17.5)	3.5	(1.5–8.5)	31	7.0	(4.0–10.5)	61	0.6	5	0.3	3
2 years	10.6	(6.0–17.0)	3.5	(1.5–8.5)	33	6.3	(3.0–9.5)	59	0.5	5	0.3	3
4 years	9.1	(5.5–15.5)	3.8	(1.5–8.5)	42	4.5	(2.0–8.0)	50	0.5	5	0.3	3
6 years	8.5	(5.0–14.5)	4.3	(1.5–8.0)	51	3.5	(1.5–7.0)	42	0.4	5	0.2	3
8 years	8.3	(4.5–13.5)	4.4	(1.5–8.0)	53	3.3	(1.5–6.8)	39	0.4	4	0.2	2
10 years	8.1	(4.5–13.5)	4.4	(1.8–8.0)	54	3.1	(1.5–6.5)	38	0.4	4	0.2	2
16 years	7.8	(4.5–13.0)	4.4	(1.8–8.0)	57	2.8	(1.2–5.2)	35	0.4	5	0.2	3
21 years	7.4	(4.5–11.0)	4.4	(1.8–7.7)	59	2.5	(1.0–4.8)	34	0.3	4	0.2	3

* Numbers of leukocytes are in thousands per mm^3, ranges are estimates of 95% confidence limits, and percentages refer to differential counts. Neutrophils include band cells at all ages and a small number of metamyelocytes and myelocytes in the first few days of life.
(From: Dallman P.R.: in *Pediatrics,* 16th Ed. ed A.M. Rudolph. New York: Appleton-Century-Crofts, 1977; Lubin B.H.: Reference values in infancy and childhood. In *Hematology of Infancy and Childhood,* 3rd Ed, eds D. G. Nathan, F.A. Oski, Philadelphia: W.B. Saunders, 1987.)
(With permission: Lee, GR, Bithell, TC, Foerster, J., Athens, JW, Lukens, JN. Wintrobe's Clinical Hematology. 9th Edition. Philadelphia: Lea & Febiger, 1993.)

TABLE F   DIFFERENTIAL COUNTS OF BONE MARROW ASPIRATES FROM 12 HEALTHY MEN

	Mean (%)	Observed Range (%)	95% Confidence Limits (%)
Neutrophilic series (total)	53.6	49.2–65.0	33.6–73.6
Myeloblasts	0.9	0.2–1.5	0.1–1.7
Promyelocytes	3.3	2.1–4.1	1.9–4.7
Myelocytes	12.7	8.2–15.7	8.5–16.9
Metamyelocytes	15.9	9.6–24.6	7.1–24.7
Band	12.4	9.5–15.3	9.4–15.4
Segmented	7.4	6.0–12.0	3.8–11.0
Eosinophilic series (total)	3.1	1.2–5.3	1.1–5.2
Myelocytes	0.8	0.2–1.3	0.2–1.4
Metamyelocytes	1.2	0.4–2.2	0.2–2.2
Band	0.9	0.2–2.4	0–2.7
Segmented	0.5	0–1.3	0–1.1
Basophilic and mast cells	0.1	0–0.2	
Erythrocytic series (total)	25.6	18.4–33.8	15.0–36.2
Pronormoblasts	0.6	0.2–1.3	0.1–1.1
Basophilic	1.4	0.5–2.4	0.4–2.4
Polychromatophilic	21.6	17.9–29.2	13.1–30.1
Orthochromatic	2.0	0.4–4.6	0.3–3.7
Lymphocytes	16.2	11.1–23.2	8.6–23.8
Plasma cells	1.3	0.4–3.9	0–3.5
Monocytes	0.3	0–0.8	0–0.6
Megakaryocytes	0.1	0–0.4	
Reticulum cells	0.3	0–0.9	0–0.8
M : E ratio	2.3	1.5–3.3	1.1–3.5

(With permission: Lee, GR, Bithell, TC, Foerster, J., Athens, JW, Lukens, JN. Wintrobe's Clinical Hematology. 9th Edition. Philadelphia: Lea & Febiger, 1993.)